EMERGENCY TOXICOLOGY
Second Edition

Emergency Toxicology
Second Edition

Edited by

Peter Viccellio, M.D., F.A.C.E.P.
Vice Chairman
Department of Emergency Medicine
State University of New York at Stony Brook
School of Medicine
Stony Brook, New York

Tod Bania, M.D.
New York, New York

Jeffrey Brent, M.D., Ph.D., F.A.C.E.P.,
F.A.C.M.T., F.A.A.C.T.
Associate Clinical Professor
Department of Medicine, Surgery, and Pediatrics
University of Colorado Health Sciences Center,
  Toxicology Associates
Denver, Colorado

Robert S. Hoffman, M.D.
Assistant Professor
Department of Surgery and Emergency Medicine
New York University School of Medicine
New York, New York

Ken W. Kulig, M.D.
Associate Clinical Professor
Department of Surgery
Division of Emergency Medicine and Trauma
University of Colorado
Denver, Colorado

Howard C. Mofenson, M.D., F.A.A.P.,
F.A.A.C.T., F.A.B.M.T.
Professor of Pediatrics and Emergency Medicine
State University of New York at Stony Brook
Long Island Regional Poison Control Center
Winthrop University Hospital
Mineola, New York

Harold H. Osborn, M.D.
Professor and Chairman
Department of Emergency Medicine
New York Medical College, Lincoln Hospital
Bronx, New York

Richard Y. Wang, D.O.
Assistant Professor of Medicine
Department of Emergency Medicine
Brown University/Rhode Island Hospital
Providence, Rhode Island

Paul M. Wax, M.D., F.A.C.M.T., F.A.C.E.P.
Associate Professor
Department of Emergency Medicine
University of Rochester Medical Center
Rochester, New York

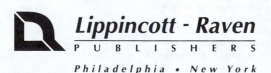
Lippincott - Raven
P U B L I S H E R S
Philadelphia • New York

Acquisitions Editor: Elizabeth Greenspan
Developmental Editors: Susan Rhyner/Rebecca Irwin Diehl
Manufacturing Manager: Dennis Teston
Production Manager: Kathleen Bubbeo
Production Editor: Mary Ann McLaughlin
Cover Designer: Karen Quigley
Indexer: Mary Kidd
Compositor: Circle Graphics
Printer: Donnelley/Crawfordsville

Printed in the United States of America

9 8 7 6 5 4 3 2 1

Library of Congress Cataloging-in-Publication Data

Emergency toxicology / edited by Peter Viccellio. — 2nd ed.
    p.   cm.
    Rev. ed. of: Handbook of medical toxicology. 1st ed. c1993.
    Includes bibliographical references and index.
    ISBN 0-316-90237-3 (soft cover)
    1. Toxicological emergencies—Handbooks, manuals, etc.
  2. Poisoning—Handbooks, manuals, etc. I. Viccellio, Peter.
  II. Handbook of medical toxicology.
    [DNLM: 1. Poisoning—diagnosis handbooks. 2. Poisoning—therapy
handbooks. 3. Poisons—adverse effects handbooks. QV 39 E53 1998]
RA1224.5.E485 1998
615.9—dc21
DNLM/DLC
for Library of Congress   98-15949
                                                  CIP

In memorium

David Kreis
Nina Mazur
Tom Coffee

Contents

Contributing Authors

Gregory L. Almond, M.D. *Associate Clinical Professor of Emergency Medicine, Department of Emergency Medicine, New York Medical College, Metropolitan Hospital Center, 1901 First Avenue, New York, New York 10029*

Angela C. Anderson, M.D., A.B.MT. *Assistant Professor, Department of Pediatrics, Brown University School of Medicine, Rhode Island and Hasbro Children's Hospitals, 593 Eddy Street, Providence, Rhode Island 02903*

Tod Bania, M.D. *New York, New York 10024*

Paula Jane Barclay, M.D. *Outpatient Family Medicine & Internal Medicine, Allergy & Immunology, Minor Emergencies, X-Ray, & Lab, 150 Midland Avenue, P.O. Box 1369, Basalt, Colorado 81621*

David Barlas, M.D. *Clinical Instructor and Attending Physician, Department of Emergency Medicine, New York University School of Medicine; North Shore University Hospital, 300 Community Drive, Manhasset, New York 11030*

Carol Barsky, M.D. *New York, New York 10014*

Amy S. Baruch, M.D. *Attending Physician, Department of Emergency Medicine, St. Lukes Regional Hospital, 190 East Bannock, Boise, Idaho 83712*

William David Binder, M.D. *Assistant in Emergency Medicine, Department of Emergency Medicine, Massachusetts General Hospital, Harvard University, 55 Fruit Street, Boston, Massachusetts 02114*

Jay L. Bock, M.D., Ph.D. *Department of Pathology, State University of New York at Stony Brook, HSC L3-532 Niccolls Road, Stony Brook, New York 11794-7300*

Jonathan Borak, M.D. *Associate Clinical Professor, Department of Internal Medicine, Yale Medical School, 234 Church Street, New Haven, Connecticut 06510*

Jeffrey Brent, M.D., Ph.D., F.A.C.E.P., F.A.C.M.T., F.A.A.C.T. *Associate Clinical Professor, Department of Medicine, Surgery, and Pediatrics, University of Colorado Health Sciences Center, Toxicology Associates, 2555 South Downing Street, Suite 260, Denver, Colorado 80210*

Gerald M. Brody, M.D.   *Clinical Assistant Professor, Department of Emergency Medicine, State University of New York at Stony Brook; Adjunct Associate Professor of Pharmacy, St. John's University; Department of Emergency Medicine, Winthrop University Hospital, 259 First Street, Mineola, New York 11501*

Gerard X. Brogan, M.D.   *Associate Professor, Department of Emergency Medicine, State University of New York at Stony Brook, Stony Brook, New York 11794-7400*

Jeffrey R. Brubacher, M.D., F.R.C.P.C. (EM.), A.B.E.M., A.B.M.T.   *Clinical Instructor, University of British Columbia, Department of Emergency Medicine, Vancouver General Hospital, 855 West 12th Avenue, Vancouver, British Columbia, Canada V6N 2G7*

G. Richard Bruno, M.D.   *Assistant Residency Director, Department of Emergency Medicine, SUNY-HSCB, Attending Physician, Kings County Hospital, 45 Clarkson Avenue, Brooklyn, New York 11203*

Jonathan L. Burstein, M.D.   *Instructor in Medicine, Division of Emergency Medicine, Harvard Medical School; Department of Emergency Medicine, Beth Israel Deaconess Medical Center, UL 202, 330 Brookline Avenue, Boston, Massachusetts 02215*

Francine D. Cantor, M.D.   *Department of Emergency Medicine, State University of New York at Stony Brook, Stony Brook, New York 11794-7400*

Kimberle F. Capes, Pharm.D.   *Lifespan Poison Center, Rhode Island Hospital, 593 Eddy Street, Samuel Building, Second Floor, Providence, Rhode Island 02903*

Thomas R. Caraccio, Pharm.D., R.P.H.   *Assistant Professor of Emergency Medicine, State University of New York at Stony Brook, Long Island Regional Poison Control Center, Winthrop University Hospital, 259 First Street, Mineola, New York 11501*

Rosemarie Carnevale, B.S.   *Pharmacist and Poison Information Specialist, Pharmacy, Rhode Island Hospital, 593 Eddy Street, Providence, Rhode Island 02920*

Stuart N. Chale, M.D.   *Department of Emergency Medicine, State University of New York at Stony Brook, University Hospital, Stony Brook, New York 11794-7400*

Adam L. Church, M.D.   *Department of Emergency Medicine, North Shore University Hospital, 300 Community Drive, Manhasset, New York 11030*

Cathleen Clancy, M.D.   *Medical Director, Maryland Poison Center; Clinical Assistant Professor, University of Maryland, Baltimore, School of Pharmacy, 20 North Pine Street, Baltimore, Maryland 21201-1180; Attending Physician and Clinical Instructor, Department of Emergency Medicine, Georgetown University Medical Center, 3800 Reservoir Road, Washington, D.C. 20007; Medical Toxicologist, National Capital Poison Center; Adjunct Assistant Professor, Department of Emergency Medicine, George Washington University Medical Center, 3201 New Mexico Avenue, Suite 310, Washington, D.C. 20016*

Daniel J. Cobaugh, Pharm.D.   *Director, Finger Lakes Regional Poison and Drug Information Center, Assistant Professor of Emergency Medicine, Department of Emergency Medicine, University of Rochester Medical Center, 601 Elmwood Avenue, Box 321, Rochester, New York 14608*

Jeffrey M. Cox, M.D. *Associate Clinical Instructor, Department of Surgery, Brown University, Rhode Island Hospital, 593 Eddy Street, Providence, Rhode Island 02903*

Sandra A. Craig, M.D. *Associate Residency Director, Department of Emergency Medicine, Carolinas Medical Center, 1000 Blythe Boulevard, P.O. Box 32861, Charlotte, North Carolina 28232-2861*

Cameron Cushing, M.D. *Resident Physician, Department of Emergency Medicine, Brown University, Rhode Island Hospital, 593 Eddy Street, Providence, Rhode Island 02906*

Mark S. DeManuelle, M.D. *Metairie, Louisiana 70005-3342*

Francis J. DeRoos, M.D. *Assistant Professor, Department of Emergency Medicine, University of Pennsylvania, 3400 Spruce Street, Philadelphia, Pennsylvania 19104*

Scott T. Elberger, M.D. *New York Medical College, 38 Sheppard Street, Rockville Center, New York 11570*

Jeffrey S. Fine, M.D. *Assistant Professor, Department of Pediatrics, Pediatric Emergency Medicine, New York University School of Medicine/Bellevue Hospital, 462 First Avenue, Room 1, South 6, New York, New York 10016*

Warren L. Fisher, M.D. *Seattle, Washington 98103*

Laura J. Fochtmann, M.D. *Department of Psychiatry, State University of New York at Stony Brook, HSC T10-020, Stony Brook, New York 11794-8101*

Marsha Ford, M.D. *Department of Emergency Medicine, Charlotte Memorial Hospital, P.O. Box 32861, Charlotte, North Carolina 28232-2861*

P. N. Galaska, M.D. *Assistant Professor, Department of Emergency Medicine, Virginia Commonwealth University, Medical College of Virginia, 11928 Blandfield Street, Richmond, Virginia 23233*

Victor M. Garcia-Prats, M.D. *Department of Emergency Medicine, Alton Ochsner Medical Foundation, 1516 Jefferson Highway, New Orleans, Louisiana 70121*

Raquel L. Gibly, M.D. *Instructor of Clinical Surgery and Fellow of Medical Toxicology, Division of Emergency Medicine, University Medical Center, 1501 North Campbell, P.O. Box 245057, Tucson, Arizona 85724*

William L. Haith, M.D. *Department of Emergency Medicine, Rhode Island Hospital, 593 Eddy Street, Providence, Rhode Island 02903*

Richard J. Hamilton, M.D. *Assistant Professor of Emergency Medicine, Department of Emergency Medicine, Allegheny University Hospital, 3300 Henry Ave., Philadelphia, Pennsylvania 19129-1121*

Michael T. Handrigan, M.D. *San Antonio, Texas 78247-5902*

Stephen R. Hayden, M.D.   *Department of Emergency Medicine, University of San Diego Medical Center, 200 West Arbor Drive, San Diego, California 92103*

William Heino, D.O.   *Long Island Regional Poison Control Center, Winthrop University Hospital, 259 First Street, Mineola, New York 11501*

Mark C. Henry, M.D.   *Professor and Chairman, Department of Emergency Medicine, School of Medicine, State University of New York at Stony Brook, Stony Brook, New York 11794-7400*

Kenneth A. Hirsch, M.D.   *Emergency Department Attending Physician and Hyperbaric Physician, Department of Emergency Medicine, J. T. Mather Memorial Hospital, Port Jefferson, New York 11777; Clinical Associate Professor, State University of New York at Stony Brook, University Hospital, Stony Brook, New York 11794-7400*

Robert S. Hoffman, M.D.   *Assistant Professor, Department of Surgery and Emergency Medicine, New York University School of Medicine, 455 First Avenue, Room 123, New York, New York 10016*

Judd E. Hollander, M.D.   *Villanova, Pennsylvania 19085*

King F. Hom, M.D., F.A.A.P.   *Pediatric Practice, Intermountain Health Care, 3905 Harrison Boulevard, Suite W-609, Ogden, Utah 84403*

Clark S. Homan, M.D.   *Department of Emergency Medicine, State University of New York at Stony Brook, University Hospital, Level 4-515, Stony Brook, New York 11794-7400*

Rivka S. Horowitz, M.D., Ph.D.   *Clinical Assistant Professor of Medicine, Division of Biology and Medicine, Brown University, 593 Eddy Street, Providence, Rhode Island 02903*

Philip I. Hubel, M.D.   *Department of Emergency Medicine, North Shore Long Island Jewish Health System, 200 Community Drive, Great Neck, New York 11021*

Oliver L. Hung, M.D.   *Fellow, Medical Toxicology, New York City Poison Control Center; Department of Emergency Medicine, Bellevue Hospital Center, New York University Medical Center, 462 First Avenue, New York, New York 10016*

Matthew Jenkins, M.D.   *Department of Emergency Medicine, Carolinas Medical Center, P.O. Box 32861, Charlotte, North Carolina 28232-2861*

Lester Kallus, M.D.   *Setauket, New York 11733*

Paul Krochmal, M.D.   *Guilford, Connecticut 06437*

Ken W. Kulig, M.D.   *Associate Clinical Professor, Department of Surgery, Division of Emergency Medicine and Trauma, University of Colorado, 2555 South Downing, Suite 260, Denver, Colorado 80210*

Fred Landes, M.D.   *Attending Physician, Department of Emergency Medicine, Berkshire Medical Center, 725 North Street, Pittsfield, Massachusetts 01201*

Thomas G. Lemke, M.D. *Assistant Professor of Medicine, Department of Emergency Medicine, Brown University, Rhode Island Hospital, 593 Eddy Street, Providence, Rhode Island 02903*

Kathleen A. Leonard, M.D. *Blood Bank and Transfusion Service, F-540, The New York Hospital, 525 East 68th Street, New York, New York 10021*

William J. Lewander, M.D. *Associate Professor, Department of Pediatrics and Emergency Medicine, Brown University Medical School, Hasbro Children's Hospital, 593 Eddy Street, Providence, Rhode Island 02903*

Jeffrey L. Margulies, M.D. *Stony Brook, New York 11790*

John D. Markman, M.D. *Clinical Fellow, Department of Neurology, Harvard University Medical School, 330 Mount Auburn Street, Cambridge, Massachusetts 02238*

Nina Mazur, M.D. *Deceased*

Charles F. McCuskey, M.D. *New York, New York 10029*

Maria Micalone, M.D. *Emergency Medicine Resident, Department of Emergency Medicine, Rhode Island Hospital, Brown University, 593 Eddy Street, Providence, Rhode Island 02903*

Howard C. Mofenson, M.D., F.A.A.P., F.A.A.C.T., F.A.B.M.T. *Professor of Pediatrics and Emergency Medicine, State University of New York at Stony Brook, Long Island Regional Poison Control Center, Winthrop University Hospital, 259 First Street, Mineola, New York 11501*

James P. Morgan, M.D. *Assistant Professor of Medicine, Department of Internal Medicine, Loyola University—Chicago, 2160 South First Avenue, Maywood, Illinois 60153*

Lewis S. Nelson, M.D. *Assistant Professor of Clinical Surgery/Emergency Medicine, Department of Emergency Services, New York University, Bellevue Hospital, 455 First Avenue, Room 123, New York, New York 10016*

R. Scott Orava, M.D. *Department of Emergency Medicine, Valley Lutheran Hospital, 6644 East Baywood Avenue, Mesa, Arizona 85206*

Harold H. Osborn, M.D. *Professor and Chairman, Department of Emergency Medicine, New York Medical College, Lincoln Hospital, 234 East 149th Street, Bronx, New York 10451*

Michael Osmundson, M.D. *Department of Emergency Medicine, Swedish Hospital, 700 Minor Avenue, Seattle, Washington 98104*

Monica Parraga, M.D. *Assistant Professor and Assistant Director, Residency Program, Department of Emergency Medicine, Metropolitan Hospital, 1901 First Avenue, New York, New York 10028*

William S. Pearl, M.D. *Assistant Professor, Department of Emergency Medicine, Emory University School of Medicine, 69 Butler Street SE, Atlanta, Georgia 30303*

Jeanmarie Perrone, M.D. *Assistant Professor, Department of Emergency Medicine, University of Pennsylvania, 3400 Spruce Street, Philadelphia, Pennsylvania 19104*

Rama B. Rao, M.D.   *Fellow in Medical Toxicology, New York City Poison Control Center, Clinical Instructor, Department of Surgery/Emergency Medicine, New York University Medical Center, 455 First Avenue, New York, New York 10016*

Sean M. Rees, M.D.   *Senior Resident, Department of Emergency Medicine, Bellevue Hospital Medical Center, 27th Street and First Avenue, New York, New York 10016*

Philip L. Rice, M.D.   *Brooklyn, New York 11215*

David S. Rosen, M.D.   *Department of Emergency Medicine, Medical College of Pennsylvania, 3300 Henry Avenue, Philadelphia, Pennsylvania 19129*

Jonathan Rudolph, M.D.   *Staff Physician, Department of Emergency Medicine, Shore Memorial Hospital, Somers Point, New Jersey 08244*

James G. Ryan, M.D.   *Assistant Professor, Department of Emergency Medicine, North Shore University Hospital, 300 Community Drive, Manhasset, New York 11030*

Joseph J. Sachter, M.D.   *Bronx, New York 10471-1804*

Bruce Sanderov, M.D.   *Attending Physician, Department of Emergency Medicine, Winthrop University Hospital, 259 First Street, Mineola, New York 11501*

Scott M. Sasser, M.D.   *Emergency Medical Services Fellow, Department of Emergency Medicine, Carolinas Medical Center, 1000 Blythe Boulevard, Charlotte, North Carolina 28232-2861*

Diane Sauter, M.D.   *Metropolitan Hospital, 1901 First Avenue, New York, New York 10029*

Daniel L. Savitt, M.D.   *Director, Emergency Medicine Residency Training Program, Rhode Island Hospital and Brown University, 593 Eddy Street, Samuels Building, Floor 2, Providence, Rhode Island 02903*

Frederick M. Schiavone, M.D.   *Department of Emergency Medicine, State University of New York at Stony Brook, University Hospital, Stony Brook, New York 11794-7400*

Richard D. Shih, M.D.   *Department of Emergency Medicine, Morristown Memorial Hospital, 100 Madison Avenue, Morristown, New Jersey 07962*

Frederick R. Sidell, M.D.   *Bel Air, Maryland 21014*

Bonnie Simmons, M.D., F.A.C.E.P.   *Director, Department of Emergency Medicine, North General Hospital, Mt. Sinai Affiliate, 1879 Madison Avenue, New York, New York 10035*

Adam J. Singer, M.D.   *Assistant Professor, Department of Emergency Medicine, State University of New York at Stony Brook, University Hospital and Medical Center, Stony Brook, New York 11794-7400*

Karl A. Sporer, M.D.   *Associate Clinical Professor, Department of Surgery, University of California at San Francisco, Emergency Services, San Francisco General Hospital, 1001 Potrero Avenue, San Francisco, California 94110*

Mara J. Stankovich, M.D. *Resident Physician, Department of Emergency Medicine, Brown University, Rhode Island Hospital, 593 Eddy Street, Samuels Building, Second Floor, Providence, Rhode Island 02903*

Lisa Torraca, M.D. *Department of Emergency Medicine, Central Maine Medical Center, 300 Main Street, Lewiston, Maine 04240*

Patricia L. VanDevander, M.D. *Department of Emergency Medicine, Lutheran Medical Center, 8300 West 38th Avenue, Wheat Ridge, Colorado 80033*

Susi U. Vassallo, M.D. *Clinical Assistant Professor of Surgery/Emergency Medicine, and Assistant Director, Medical Toxicology Fellowship Program, Department of Emergency Medicine, New York University Medical School, Bellevue Hospital Center, 26th Street and First Avenue, New York, New York 10016*

Peter Viccellio, M.D. *Vice Chairman, Department of Emergency Medicine, State University of New York at Stony Brook School of Medicine, Stony Brook, New York 11794-7400*

Richard Y. Wang, D.O. *Assistant Professor of Medicine, Department of Emergency Medicine, Brown University, Rhode Island Hospital, 593 Eddy Street, Providence, Rhode Island 02903*

Paul M. Wax, M.D., F.A.C.M.T., F.A.C.E.P. *Associate Professor, Department of Emergency Medicine, University of Rochester Medical Center, 601 Elmwood Avenue, Box 4-9200 Rochester, New York 14642*

James M. West, M.D. *Santa Fe, New Mexico 87501*

Richard E. Westfal, M.D. *Associate Professor of Clinical Emergency Medicine, New York Medical College; Associate Director, Department of Emergency Medicine, Saint Vincents Hospital, 153 West 11th Street, New York, New York 10011*

James V. Writer, M.P.H. *Walter Reed Army Institute of Research, Building 40, Washington, D.C. 20307-5100*

Jason Yuan, M.D. *West Orange, New Jersey 07052*

John S. Yuthas, M.D. *Noble, Oklahoma 73068*

Preface

This book is for physicians, residents, medical students, nurses, physicians' assistants, and pharmacists who participate in the care of poisoned patients. Toxicology can be a frustratingly descriptive, empiric discipline. Diagnosis is often difficult, proper management can be controversial, and end points are unknown. There are few prospective randomized trials to justify the paths we choose in therapy. The physician responsible for the care of a patient with a potentially lethal exposure often has a superficial knowledge at best of the complexities at hand. Many lethal exposures must be diagnosed and treated long before the physician has any confirmatory evidence that he or she made the correct assessment. More than in other areas of medicine, a good understanding of biochemistry and physiology, quick thinking, and careful detective work constitute the delightful challenge of toxicology.

The purpose of this book is to give physicians and other health care providers an easily accessible, but in-depth, resource on toxicology. The outline format of the handbook allows for particularly rapid review of essential information. However, this is not accomplished at the expense of inadequate detail. It is critical to the lives of the patients whom we treat that we manage, not by recipe, but by an understanding of what is unfolding in front of us and how our interventions affect the patients.

The first two sections cover the general aspects of toxicology. Many of these chapters are rich in detail and deserve careful study by the health care provider not intimately familiar with the subjects. Also, the second section contains a number of tables that provide invaluable clues to proper diagnosis and therapy. Any health care provider who treats the poisoned patient should have mastery over the material in these two sections.

The remaining sections cover particular toxicologic entities. Peculiar presentations, co-ingestions, and complicating factors restrict the efficacy of empiric, "recipe" approaches to toxicology. The authors of these chapters have, therefore, provided, where possible, a pathophysiologic description of the relevant toxin to enhance the physician's understanding. Many of our therapeutic interventions are ill-founded or, at best, controversial. We have tried to highlight these controversies and discuss alternatives in a way that allows the physician to adopt the best therapy for his or her patient. As always, consultation with the local poison center will minimize the possibility of therapeutic misadventure, and ensure that your treatment is current with what is the best understanding from the medical literature.

Peter Viccellio
State University of New York at Stony Brook
aviccellio@epo.hsc.sunysb.edu

Acknowledgments

My many thanks to all the people who participated in the writing of this book. Their extraordinary efforts are evident. My particular thanks go to the section editors—Dr. Howard Mofenson, Dr. Tod Bania, Dr. Richard Wang, Dr. Paul Wax, Dr. Robert Hoffman, Dr. Jeffrey Brent, Dr. Kenneth Kulig, and Dr. Harold Osborn; the folks at Lippincott–Raven—Elizabeth Greenspan and Susan Rhyner; and most of all to Connie Meade, for her tireless efforts and her ability to deal with my tiresome ways.

PART I

Introduction

Emergency Toxicology, Second Edition,
edited by Peter Viccellio.
Published by Lippincott–Raven Publishers, Philadelphia.

1

Epidemiology and Prevention

James V. Writer

Walter Reed Army Institute of Research, Washington, D.C. 20307-5100

Who is poisoned, how they are exposed, to what they are exposed, and where they are exposed varies greatly with age, psychological and social influences, environment, and occupation. Young children, for example, who overall are at the greatest risk of becoming poisoning victims, are most likely to be unintentionally exposed to drugs or household chemicals in the home. The Consumer Product Safety Commission estimates that 110,000 children under age 5 were treated for accidental poisoning in hospital emergency departments (EDs) in 1983 (1). During adolescence and young adulthood, the exposures are more likely to be intentional, either through suicide attempts or experimentation with drugs or alcohol. Adult men have been reported to be more at risk of occupational exposures than adult women (2). Among the elderly, unintentional exposures become important again.

Nearly everyone is at risk of acute and chronic toxic exposures to hazardous substances in the ambient environment. Unintentional acute exposures due to transport accidents, such as the release of white phosphorus from a derailed train in Miamisburg, Ohio, in 1986, may send hundreds of exposed people to EDs for treatment and reassurance (3). Intentional exposures to toxins through terrorist acts like the release of military nerve agent in the Tokyo subway in 1995 are rare but possible.

This short chapter presents an overview of the broad topic of the epidemiology of poisoning and makes some recommendations for preventing unintentional exposures. The epidemiology described is based on readily available data from the Vital Statistics of the United States and the annual report of the American Association of Poison Control Centers. Therefore, it is mostly a description of the epidemiology of unintentional poisonings.

I. What is a poison?

Before discussing epidemiology of poisonings it is important to define poison. Paracelsus, a 16th century physician, wrote that all substances known to humans are poisons, and only the dose determines the effect. This axiom continues to be the basis for determining the dose of therapeutics with the lowest risk/benefit ratio, acceptable levels of chemicals in the environment, and when or how to treat people exposed to potentially toxic substances.

II. History

The history of poisoning is as old as human history itself. Since the earliest times, humans have been updating and refining their knowledge of toxins. Early humans probably learned

---

The views of the author do not purport to reflect the position of the Department of the Army or the Department of Defense.

quickly that the domestication of fire required ventilation of areas where fires were burning to avoid smoke inhalation and carbon monoxide exposure. Attempts to identify and use safe forage, naturally occurring pharmaceuticals, and toxins, one can postulate, took a great deal of experimentation. As the toxic properties of plants and animal venom were identified, however, they found uses as medicines, agents of warfare, and to remove undesirable individuals from society.

Hemlock, for example, was the state poison of ancient Greece. During the 4th century B.C., poisoning was reported to be epidemic in Rome. However, it was not until 82 B.C. that the Romans issued the *Lex Cornelia,* the first law against poisoning. During the Middle Ages, the art of poisoning matured, and its use for political, personal, or financial gain became relatively common. During this period and into the Renaissance, poisoning was considered a normal hazard of living. As the Dark Ages ended and the Renaissance began, the science of poisons and their antidotes advanced. By the mid-1800s the science of toxicology was founded by Spanish physician Mattieu Joseph Bonaventura Orfila (1787–1853).

III. Epidemiology

An understanding of the following basic statistical measures of the distribution and occurrence of poisoning in a population are required to interpret epidemiologic data.

  A. The mortality rate is the number of deaths occurring per unit of population over a given defined unit of time, e.g., 230 deaths per 10,000 persons per year.

  B. A similar measure of new cases of a disease or other adverse health event occurrence (rather than deaths) per unit of population per defined period of time is the attack rate or morbidity rate.

  C. The incidence rate is the number of new cases of a poisoning per unit of population over a given period of time, e.g., 300 poisonings per 100,000 persons per year. This is an excellent measure of acute events like most poisoning events.

  D. The prevalence rate is a measure of new and existing cases of a disease or adverse health event per unit of population per unit of time. This measure is less applicable to poisonings but is a better measure of the burden or impact of longer lasting conditions. It could be applied to the sequelae of poisonings, e.g., 50 cases of lead associated peripheral neuropathy per 10,000 bridge painter union members per year. Point prevalence is the prevalence of a condition at given point in time such as on a single day rather than over a period of time.

  E. The case fatality rate is the number of deaths per unit of persons afflicted with a given condition per unit time, e.g., 56 deaths per 10,000 person exposed per year. However, a more common use of this statistic, especially during an acute outbreak such a release of a toxic substance into the ambient environment, may simply be the number of deaths divided by the number ill. Because the unit time component is removed in this usage this measure is not truly a rate but is a proportion or ratio.

Today, poisonings, both accidental and intentional, are a significant contributor to mortality and morbidity in the United States. It has been estimated that 7% of all emergency room (ER) visits are the result of toxic exposures (4). Household cleaners, over-the-counter and prescription drugs, cosmetics, and solvents comprise the most frequent human toxic exposures (7). Table 1-1 compares the 10 most common causes of injury and death attributed to poisons in the United States during 1987.

TABLE 1-1. *Most common human poison exposures and most common causes of death due to poison exposure*

Most common poison exposures	Most common poison exposures resulting in death
Cleaning substances	Analgesics
Analgesics	Antidepressants
Cosmetics/personal care products	Sedatives and hypnotics
Plants	Stimulants and street drugs
Cough/cold preparations	Cardiovascular drugs
Food products/food poisoning	Alcohols
Bites and envenomations	Gases and fumes
Pesticides and rodenticides	Asthma therapies
Topicals	Automotive products
Foreign bodies	Chemicals

Data from ref. 7.

1. **Mortality**
   a. In 1990, there were 5,803 people who died because of **accidental poisonings** (5). Another 5,424 died of self-inflicted poisonings. While media attention and volumes of mystery literature devoted to assaults by poison suggest they are more common, there were only 445 homicides by poisoning in 1990. However, among 1,223 deaths involving poison, the intent was undetermined.
   b. Although accidental poisonings account for 3.9% of all accidental injury deaths, they were the **fifth leading cause** of such deaths.
   c. A larger percentage of **suicides** result from poisonings; 17.5% of all suicides in 1990 were attributed to poison, in contrast to about 0.2% of homicides.
   d. **Trends.** U.S. deaths due to poisoning increased from 10,112 deaths in 1968 to 12,381 deaths in 1990 (5,6). Most of this increase has been due to accidental poisoning by illicit drugs, medications, and biologicals, e.g., venoms or plant poisons. The 1968 and 1990 data are summarized in Table 1-2. A breakdown of poisoning by age and substance for the two time periods is presented in Table 1-3. Note that for total salicylates, total solid and liquids, cleaning and polishing products, petroleum products, pesticides, and caustics there is a reduction in deaths of those under 5 years of age. The reduction may

TABLE 1-2. *Poisoning deaths in the United States, 1968 and 1990*

Toxin	Accidental		Suicide		Unknown cause		Total	
	1968	1990	1968	1990	1968	1990	1968	1990
Drugs	1,692	4,506	[a]	2,920	[a]	749	1,692	8,175
Solids/liquids	89	549	3,276	223	911	257	4,276	1,029
Gases/vapors	1,526	784	2,408	2,281	182	112	4,116	3,177
Total	3,307	5,839	5,684	5,424	1,093	1,118	10,084	12,381

[a] Drug data are included in Solids/liquids.
In 1968 there were 28 homicides by poisoning. In 1990 there were 45 homicides by poisoning.
Data from refs. 5 and 6.

TABLE 1-3. *Accidental U.S. poisoning deaths by age groups, 1968 and 1990*

Toxin	1968		1990	
	<5 yr	≥5 yr	<5 yr	≥5 yr
Drugs/medications	150	1,542	38	4,468
Barbiturates	11	310	0	22
Salicylates	61	59	1	43
Sedatives/hypnotics	2	504	0	26
Solids/liquids	134	757	31	12
Alcohols	2	180	2	367
Cleaning/polishing products	13	10	1	14
Petroleum products	70	37	4	76
Pesticides and fertilizers	31	41	2	8
Caustics	6	22	0	12
Gases and vapors	48	1,478	10	574
Utility gases and carbon monoxide	22	1,024	8	123
Total	332	3,777	79	5,054

Data from refs. 5 and 6.

be attributable to a decrease in aspirin use, poison prevention education, poison control centers, or the Poison Prevention Packaging Act of 1970, which mandated child-resistant caps on some hazardous products.

2. **Poison control center data**
   a. Although more than 12,000 deaths in 1990 could be attributed to poisonings, this number represents a relatively small percentage of people who are poisoned each year. The American Association of Poison Control Centers estimates that more than 2.3 million human poison exposures occurred in 1994 (7). Based on these estimates, fewer than 1.0% of exposed individuals die.
   b. **Mortality data** are relatively complete and an accurate source of data for poisoning deaths, but they are a poor indicator of incidence. Poison control center statistics are a better indicator of accidental poison exposures than local, state, or national mortality figures. In addition to the fact that fewer than 1% of the exposed population dies, intentional poisonings are possibly given more weight in the mortality data, and certain poisons may be overrepresented because they are fast-acting, are difficult to treat, or occur with minimal participation of the host, e.g., accidental intoxication by carbon monoxide.
   c. **Poison control center data,** however, are not without limitations. In 1994, the national reporting system covered 83% of the U.S. population (7). Not all poisonings occurring in a region may be reported to the local poison center, especially industrial poisonings, suicide attempts, and common or easily treated poisonings. For example, nationwide poison control centers reported 38 deaths due to carbon monoxide exposure in 1994, whereas the Vital Statistics of the United States reported 582 deaths in 1990, which represents significant underreporting even when taking into account the fact that only about 83% of the U.S. population were served by a poison control center in 1994.

d. **Suicide attempts and drug abuse** are most likely underrepresented in poison control data. People making a real attempt at suicide rather than a suicidal gesture probably do not contact a poison control center. These people may become medical examiners' cases, with no intervening treatment. Likewise, a drug abuser is less likely to consult a poison control center than someone who is accidentally exposed to a toxin.

e. **Accidental poisonings in children** may be overrepresented in poison center data. Children under 5 years of age account for 1% to 2% of poisoning mortalities but more than 50% of poison control center calls for assistance. Parents and caregivers may be more likely to contact a poison control center for a child than for themselves or other adults. Additionally, parents of young children are the target of poison control center marketing campaigns and may be more inclined to contract a center before seeking other medical advice. Given these caveats, the data are still an important source of epidemiologic data on the incidence of poisonings.

f. **Number of exposures.** More than 1.9 million poison exposures in humans were reported to the 65 poison control centers participating in the American Association of Poison Control Centers in the United States in 1994. These centers serve approximately 215.9 million people. An estimated 83% of all human toxic exposures occurring in the United States occur in poison control center catchment areas.

g. **Age.** Of the more than 1.9 million reported exposures, 40.2% were in children younger than 3 years of age and 54.1% in children younger than 6 years of age. More than 67.6% of all poison exposures occur in children and adolescents younger than 20 years of age (Fig. 1-1). Exposures are equally reported in males and females: 48.7% and 50.5%, respectively.

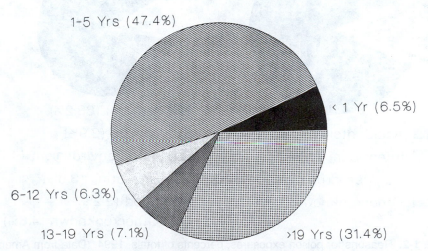

FIG. 1-1. Age distribution of poison exposure cases, 1994. (Data from American Association of Poison Control Centers, 1995.)

h. The **exposure** was reported as accidental in 86.4% of all cases; intentional in 11.1% cases; and the result of an adverse drug reaction in 1.8% of all cases (Fig. 1-2).

In **children** younger than 6 years of age, 99.5% of the incidents were due to accidental exposures. Accidental exposure accounted for 91.2% of exposures in 6- to 12-year-olds, 50.8% in 13- to 19-year-olds, and 70.2% in those older than 19-years of age.

i. **The most common route of entry** of toxins reported to poison control centers was ingestion, 74.3%; 7.9% of exposures were transdermal; 6.2% were ophthalmic; and 6.7% were by inhalation. The remainder of exposures were divided between bites and stings, parenteral exposure, and other (or unknown) routes. Only one toxin was involved in more than 93.2% of the cases.

j. **Site of exposure** was a residence in 90.4% of all calls to poison control centers, followed by the workplace (2.9%), schools (1.2%), and health facilities (0.4%). Most calls to poison control centers came from residences (80.4%), followed by health care facilities (12.7%), workplaces (1.8%), and schools (0.6%).

k. **Most poison exposures do not result in clinical toxicity** (Fig. 1-3). Forty-two percent of reported exposures had no effect on the subject or were reported as nontoxic. Another 43.5% resulted in a minor effect or were minimally toxic exposures. Children under 6 years of age were most likely to be reported as exposed with no ensuing or minimal toxicity; 59.2% of these exposures were nontoxic or resulted in no adverse effect. A similar pattern

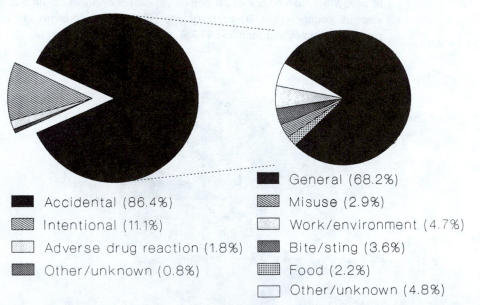

General (68.2%)

Accidental (86.4%)   Misuse (2.9%)

Intentional (11.1%)   Work/environment (4.7%)

Adverse drug reaction (1.8%)   Bite/sting (3.6%)

Other/unknown (0.8%)   Food (2.2%)

Other/unknown (4.8%)

FIG. 1-2. Reasons for poison exposures, percents of totals, 1994. (Data from American Association of Poison Control Centers, 1995.)

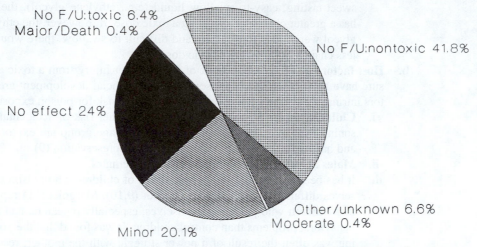

No F/U:toxic 6.4%
Major/Death 0.4%
No F/U:nontoxic 41.8%
No effect 24%
Other/unknown 6.6%
Moderate 0.4%
Minor 20.1%

FIG. 1-3. Medical effects on poison exposure victims, 1994. (Data from American Association of Poison Control Centers, 1995.)

has been reported in England (8), where 65% to 78% of childhood exposures did not result in toxicity. Among the poison control center data, 18.6% of exposures in people older than 19 years of age did not result in toxicity. The age-dependent differences in outcomes are due in part to intent; adult exposures are more likely to be intentional exposures, and many adults seek treatment or consultation for exposures in children that they would not follow up on in themselves or other adults.

3. **Epidemiologic model**

   a. Poisonings can be explained using the **classic epidemiologic model** of host-agent/vehicle-environment interaction. In the epidemiologic model, enabling factors in each of these three areas must be present for a poisoning to occur. Change any of the enabling factors, and the poisoning may not occur. Unfortunately, many factors are not changeable.

      i. The **host** is the person exposed to the poison. Factors particular to the host put the host at risk of being poisoned: his or her age, gender, physical or mental maturity, and personality.

      ii. **Environment** greatly contributes to the probability of a toxic exposure. Environmental factors include supervision of children by parents, how and where potential toxins are stored, the socioeconomic level of the family, and the level of stress in the family.

      iii. The **agent** is the energy, usually chemical, that causes injury, e.g., acetylsalicylic acid. The agent is carried by a vehicle (e.g., for salicylic acid the **vehicle** is the aspirin tablet). Although the term agent is often used when discussing the vehicle, it is important to remember the difference between the two because alterations to the vehicle can lessen the likelihood of injury from the agent. For example, if the vehicle is a sweet-tasting, easy-to-swallow liquid (e.g., ethylene glycol), the host has a greater chance of ingesting a toxic dose. If, however, the ethylene glycol were made foul-tasting and difficult to swallow, there would be less chance of ingesting a toxic dose.

   b. **Host factors** that increase the risk of poisoning or injury from a toxic exposure have been described. Age, sex, and psychosocial development are factors intrinsic to the host that may lead to a higher risk for poison exposure.

      i. **Children under 5 years of age** are at a higher risk of accidental poisoning than older children. Children in this age group are exploratory and have a limited sense of danger and self-preservation (9).

      ii. **Males are at a slightly higher risk** than females.

      iii. It has been shown that the **personalities** of children who poison themselves differ from children who do not (9,10). Margolis (11) reported that children who poisoned themselves, especially repeaters, had more behavioral problems than control children. It was found that the poisoning was often the result of a power struggle with the mother, resulting from an abnormal parent-child relationship (characterized by hyperactivity, destructiveness, uncooperativeness, negativism, and attention demands by the child). These young patients were reported to be more deviant by their mothers and teachers than were the control children.

   c. **Intentional exposures.** Accidental poisonings are rare in older children. The provider must be alert to patients whose exposure may have been self-inflicted. Appropriate psychiatric care is indicated following these events.

   d. The patient's **environment** contributes greatly to the risk of poisoning.

      i. Common sense tells us that accessibility of poisons should be an important factor, but it does not appear to be a major factor (12).

      ii. For children it appears that **family stress** and the quality and quantity of **parental supervision** may be the leading environmental contributors to accidental poisoning incidents (9,10,13).

      iii. Siebert (14) reports significantly more **stress** in families with a poisoning than in control families. Serious family illness during the month before the interview, pregnancy, a recent family move, one parent away from home, and anxiety or depression in parents were reported more often in case families than in control families.

      iv. Sobel (13) studied 347 families in rural New Hampshire and Vermont and indicated that accidental poisoning is primarily a function of **parental psychopathology** and **family disturbance.** The most significant associations were those between accidental poisonings and the mother's psychopathology.

IV. Prevention

  A. The **Poison Prevention Packaging Act of 1970** has led to a decline in the number of poisoning incidents due to regulated items (15). However, there has been an increase among unregulated substances.

  B. One study reported increased risk of accidental poisonings from indoor pesticide residues (16). **Education** must therefore continue to be a major component of any poison prevention program. It is important for the health care worker to remember that preventing future poisoning should be an important part of treating a poisoned patient, especially a child.

C. A key risk factor in **childhood poisoning** is a **previous exposure.** In a study of 1943 potentially toxic ingestions Litovitz et al. (12) showed that 30.1% of the children under age 6 had a previous exposure.

   1. The physician and other health professionals should discuss with parents or other caregivers ways to separate the child from the poison and other steps to prevent future episodes.

   2. Discussion of quality of supervision, family stress, and the child's behavior should be undertaken to identify host or environment factors that may have contributed to the incident.

D. Prevention of poisoning in **older age groups** is more complex than in children.

   1. **Young and middle-aged adults** are more likely to intentionally expose themselves to poisons or may be exposed at their workplace through the accidental release of toxins or because of poor industrial hygiene.

   2. **Older adults** are special cases in terms of poison prevention (17). The elderly are prone to senility and confusion, which may contribute to accidental poisoning in the 64+ age group. These adults must be particularly vigilant, especially as they may be exposed to a wide range of potentially toxic pharmaceuticals. The elderly are also less able to recover from poisoning incidents than more resilient, younger persons. Many of the prevention tips outlined below apply to them. In general, older adults must exercise care when taking medications to make sure they are taking the correct dose at the right time and in the right combination with other drugs. It is largely the physician's responsibility to be aware of potentially toxic drug interactions and to make sure their patients understand and are able to execute the medication instructions.

E. Preventing accidental poisoning requires **interrupting the host-agent/vehicle-environment interaction.** The easiest of the three to modify may be the environment, where the goal is to separate potential victims from potential poisons. Modification of host factors may not be feasible, particularly age, sex, behavioral problems, and psychosocial maturation. Likewise, altering the agent/vehicle may not be possible for the individual consumer. However, if constructing physical barriers between the child and the toxin is likely to be ineffective, it may be possible to store some poisons in quantities that would be nontoxic or would produce a low level toxicity after exposure.

F. **Pharmaceuticals** are the leading cause of accidental poisoning.

   1. **Agent or vehicle factors** that may contribute to a poisoning include the packaging of the product, labeling, form of the vehicle, flavor, fragrance, color route of exposure, and how the agent is used (18).

   2. **To produce injury**, the agent's energy must reach the host at levels above the host injury threshold.

   3. **Preventive measures.** By reducing the amount of available toxin through using smaller containers, making substances less easily accessible, and giving them a less palatable taste, an exposure may take place without injury. In home situations

where children are at a high risk of being poisoned, parents may want to consider buying smaller quantities of pharmaceuticals or buying household chemicals in aerosol or powder form, when possible, rather than liquid.

G. **Poison prevention strategies**

1. Keep all household poisons separate from food.
2. Keep all products in their original containers.
3. Always read all labels carefully *before* using the product.
4. Never give or take any medication in the dark.
5. Dispose of all products in a safe and proper manner.
6. Encourage periodic home hunts and dispose of old medicines.
7. Never refer to medicine or vitamins as candy.
8. Teach children never to take medication unless given by an adult they know and trust.
9. Buy only those drugs supplied in childproof packaging.
10. Once a child has been poisoned, be on the alert for repeat episodes.
11. Teach children not to eat plants or berries.
12. Store all drugs or potentially toxic substances out of sight and out of reach; use cabinet locks.
13. Encourage parents to purchase and have ready a 1-oz bottle of syrup of ipecac. It should be made clear that it is not to be administered except at the direction of a physician or the local poison control center.
14. Keep the telephone number for the local poison control center at each telephone. Do not be afraid to call if an incident should occur.

References

1. Leads from *MMWR*. Update: childhood poisonings—United States. *JAMA* 1985;253:1857.
2. Bresnitz EA. Poison control center follow-up of occupational disease. *Am J Public Health* 1990;80:711–712.
3. Ohio Department of Health. Unpublished data, 1987.
4. Guzzardi LJ. Role of the emergency physician in the treatment of the poisoned patient. *Emerg Med Clin North Am* 1984;2:3–13.
5. National Center for Health Statistics. *Vital statistics of the United States, 1990. Vol. II. Mortality, part A*. DHHS Publ. No. (PHS)95-1101, Public Health Service, Washington, DC: U.S. Government Printing Office, 1995.
6. National Center for Health Statistics. *Vital statistics of the United States, 1968. Vol. II. Mortality, part A*. DHEW Publ. No. (HSM)72-1101. Public Health Service. Rockville, MD: U.S. Government Printing Office, 1972.
7. Litovitz TL, et al. 1994 annual report of the American Association of Poison Control Centers national data collection system. *Am J Emerg Med* 1995;13:551–597.
8. Calnan MW, Dale JW, de Fonseka CP. Suspected poisoning in children, study of the incidence of true poisoning and poisoning scare in a defined population in North East Bristol. *Arch Dis Child* 1976;51:180–185.
9. Katz J. Psychiatric aspects of accidental poisoning in childhood. *Med J Aust* 1976;2:59–62.
10. Steward MA, Bradley TT, Freidin MR. Accidental poisoning and the hyperactive child syndrome. *Dis Nerv Syst* 1970; 31:403–407.
11. Margolis JA. Psychosocial study of childhood poisoning: a 5-year follow-up. *Pediatrics* 1971;47:439–444.
12. Litovitz TL, et al. Recurrent poisoning among paediatric poisoning victims. *Med Toxiol Adverse Drug Exp* 1989; 4:381–386.
13. Sobel R. The psychiatric implications of accidental poisoning in children. *Pediatr Clin North Am* 1970;17:653–685.
14. Siebert R. Stress in families of children who have ingested poisons. *Br Med J* 1975;3:87–89.
15. Done AK. The toxic emergency. *Emerg Med* 1982;11:39–54.
16. Fenske RA, et al. Potential exposure and health risks of infants following indoor residential pesticide applications. *Am J Public Health* 1990;80:689–693.
17. Klein-Schwartz W, Oderda GM, Booze L. Poisoning in the elderly. *J Am Geriatr Soc* 1983;31:195–199.
18. Olson DK, et al. An epidemiological view of poisoning. *Vet Hum Toxicol* 1985;27:402–408.

Emergency Toxicology, Second Edition,
edited by Peter Viccellio.
Lippincott–Raven Publishers, Philadelphia © 1998.

2

Pharmacokinetics

Thomas R. Caraccio and Howard C. Mofenson

Department of Emergency Medicine, Long Island Regional Poison Control Center, Winthrop
University Hospital, Mineola, New York 11501

I. Definitions

A. ***Pharmacokinetics*** is a study of the changes in body drug concentration with respect to absorption, distribution, metabolism (biotransformation), and excretion. Pharmacokinetics is important in establishing a safe dosage of anticonvulsants, antidysrhythmics agents, digitalis preparations, and theophylline (1,2).

B. ***Pharmacodynamics*** is the interaction of the drug with biologic receptors and mechanisms of action. It is the basis for the therapeutic or toxic effects produced. Pharmacodynamics is important in understanding the effects of antihypertensive agents, sedative-hypnotics, antidysrhythmics agents, and hormones (Fig. 2-1) (2).

C. ***Pharmacogenetics.*** This branch of pharmacology concerns genetically determined factors that alter drug responses. Knowledge of the existence of a pharmacogenetic trait within a family is important in the provision of care to members of that family. Whenever an unusual drug reaction is observed in a patient, the possibility that pharmacogenetic factors underlie such a reaction should be considered. Some conditions with a pharmacogenetic basis are listed below.

1. **Glucose-6-phosphate dehydrogenase (G6PD) deficiency.** The G6PD enzyme is responsible for making nicotine adenosine phosphate (NADPH) to prevent hemolysis caused by oxidative stress. G6PD deficiency incidence is about 100 million worldwide. About 13% black American males are deficient. It is an X-linked recessive deficiency. In G6PD deficiency, the patients have resistance conferred to malaria due to *Plasmodium falciparum*. However, oxidative stress in these patients causes hemolysis. **Some causes of oxidative stress** include antimalarials, dimercaprol, fava beans, methylene blue, nalidixic acid, naphthalene, nitrofurans, probenecid, salicylate (controversial), sulfonamides, and vitamin K analogs.

2. **Pseudocholinesterase deficiency. Congenital deficiency of plasma cholinesterase** exists in 1:50,000, and it is decreased in fetuses, in infants, in the elderly, usually in pregnancy, and in liver disease. These individuals, when exposed to cocaine, may be at increased risk for life-threatening toxicity (3). In a study of 191 patients with a plasma cholinesterase deficiency, the plasma cholinesterase was lowest in patients with life-threatening toxicity. The study was limited by no follow-up plasma cholinesterase levels (4). The cocaine lethality in mice, when adminis-

```
Dose------------Blood Level-----------Effect
    Pharmacokinetics              Pharmacodynamics
    (What body does to drug)   (What drug does to body)
```

FIG. 2-1. Pharmacokinetics and pharmacodynamic actions of drugs.

tered tetraisopryl pyrophosphoramide (parathion), supported this observation (5). Infusion of human purified plasma cholinesterase in mice was found to decrease the lethality of cocaine intoxication (5,6). One in 3,000 persons who are homozygous for one of the genetic defects exposed to succinylcholine will degrade it very slowly or not at all, and endotracheal intubation and assisted ventilation will be required for hours. This period can be shortened by transfusion of normal plasma. It is autosomal recessive. It is evaluated by dibucaine, a choline ester, for sensitivity. This is manifested by succinylcholine and depolarizing neuromuscular blockers sensitivity and may play a role in the severity of cocaine intoxication and its complications and possibly organophosphate insecticides toxicity.

3. **Debrisoquine polymorphism.** This is an autosomal recessive deficiency in the cytochrome P-450 isoenzyme that have slow and fast metabolism. Approximately 5% to 10% of caucasians are slow metabolizers. Slow metabolizers accumulate the parent drug of Class Ib and 1c antidysrhythmic agents mexiletine, encainide, flecainide, and propafenone (which metabolizes to active 5-hydroxypropafenone). Both phenotypes of propafenone respond to the drug with suppression of the dysrhythmia, but the slow metabolizers have more neurological side effects, which are due to the parent drug. Other agents with slow metabolism in this type of deficiency are dextromethorphan and codeine.

4. **Hepatic porphyria inducers stimulate delta aminolevulinic acid** which can produce the signs of porphyria, including paralysis. The neuropsychiatric symptoms are precipitated by anticonvulsants, barbiturates, griseofulvin, and corticosteroids.

5. **Acetylation.** Slow acetylation is inherited by autosomal recessive patients and involves hydralazine, isoniazid, and procainamide. The enzyme *N*-acetyltransferase-2 is deficient. This occurs in 50% of blacks and whites, 15% of Japanese, and 5% of Eskimos. Isoniazid slow acetylators are more prone to peripheral neuropathy, and the fast acetylators are more likely to develop hepatitis. Hydralazine rapid acetylators are more likely to develop the drug-induced lupus syndrome. Slow acetylators are more likely to develop bladder cancer from carcinogenic amines, which are substrates of naphthalene amines.

6. Methemoglobin reductase deficiency (see Methemoglobinemia)

D. *Adverse drug reactions* are either dose-dependent (toxicity), dose-independent, immunologic (allergic), or nonimmunologic (isoniazid hepatitis).

E. *Toxicokinetics* is a mathematical conceptualization of clinical pharmacology in an overdose patient. Basic principles of kinetics will allow one to determine when peak blood concentrations and therapeutic effects will occur as well as when manifestations will occur or resolve. The duration of action, half-life, and mode of excretion may explain why some compounds are more easily removed from the body by extracorporeal methods.

F. Knowledge of pharmacokinetics and toxicokinetic principles of a specific toxin will allow the physician to plan a rational approach to the definitive management of the intoxicated patient after the vital functions have been stabilized.

G. *Miscellaneous terms*

1. **LD$_{50}$.** Lethal does for 50% of experimental animals.

2. **MLD.** Minimum lethal dose. (Both these terms, LD$_{50}$ and MLD, are seldom relevant in human intoxications, but indicate potential toxicity of substance.)

3. **Bioavailability** refers to the efficiency of absorption of oral route versus intravenous route. The liver biotransforms some drugs during the initial pass from the portal circulation after oral administration. Therefore, a large portion of the drug fails to reach the systemic circulation in the original form.

4. **Volume of distribution** (V_d) is a hypothetical volume of body fluid that would be necessary if the total amount of drug were distributed at the same concentration as plasma. It can be calculated by the following equation: $V_d = $ dose$/C_p$, where the V_d is expressed in L/kg or mL/kg; dose = mg or g of drug administered per kg; and C_p = peak concentration in mg/L, g/L, or µg/mL. **Example 1:** A 50-kg patient ingests 500 mg of a drug; what is volume distribution if the peak blood concentration is 20 µg/mL?

$$V_d = \text{dose mg/kg} = 500 \text{ mg/50 kg/plasma peak level } (C_p)$$
$$(20 \text{ µg/mL or mg/L}) = 0.5 \text{ L/kg}$$

5. **Half-life** ($t_{1/2}$) is the time required to reduce the blood concentration in half. It is calculated by the following equation: $t_{1/2} = 0.693/K_e$. The $t_{1/2}$ is expressed in time units such as minutes, hours, or days. K_e is the elimination rate constant in reciprocal units such as min^{-1}, h^{-1}, or days^{-1}. It is the fraction or percentage of the total amount of drug in the body removed per unit of time and is a function of clearance and volume of distribution. It is also expressed by the following equation when the clearance is considered:

$$0.693 \times V_d/\text{clearance} = \text{half-life}$$

6. **pK$_a$** is the pH at which a substance exists half in the ionized and half in the non-ionized form. This helps predict which substances may benefit from manipulation of urinary pH in order to enhance ion trapping and increase excretion.

7. **Therapeutic blood range** is the concentration of any drug at which the majority of the treated population can be expected to receive therapeutic benefit.

8. **Toxic blood range** is the concentration at which the majority would be expected to have toxic manifestations.

9. **Blood concentrations** (C) may be a quantitative aid in determining whether more specific measures are needed to be instituted in the therapy of a poisoning. In some cases, they may correlate with the clinical manifestations. **Peak blood concentrations**. The peak blood concentration is expressed in mg/L, g/L, or µg/mL. The height of the peak is the function of the dose. The slope of decay after the peak can reflect the rate of elimination or the rate of absorption whichever is much *slower*. The height of the peak is the function of the volume of distribution. Peak levels

occur when the rate of absorption equals the rate of clearance not when the absorption is complete. It can be calculated by the following equation: C_p = dose/V_d, where total amount is in mg and V_d = the volume of distribution in L/kg or mL/kg. **Example 2:** A 10-kg child ingests 10 mL of 100% methanol (V_d 0.6 L/kg); the peak blood level of methanol can be predicted as follows: dose = 10 mL of 100% = 10 g;

$$C_p = 10,000 \text{ mg } (10 \text{ kg} \times 0.6) = 10,000/6 = 1,666 \text{ mg/L or } 166 \text{ mg/dL}$$

Example 3: A 37-year-old 60-kg woman ingested 30 tablets of 200 mg of aminophylline. Predict the peak plasma concentration of theophylline.

$$6,000 \text{ mg } (60 \text{ kg} \times 0.45 \text{ L/kg}) = 222 \text{ mg/L}$$

Aminophylline is a salt that contains 80% of theophylline, so this must be taken into account to avoid overestimating the theophylline level above.

$$6,000 \text{ mg} \times 0.80 \times \text{bioavailability } (100\%)/60 \text{ kg} \times 0.45 = 178 \text{ mg/L}$$

However, it is unlikely to reach this peak concentration because the elimination is occuring continuously, so that the level has begun to decline when it is measured.

10. **Clearance** is the amount of body fluid sufficient to account for all the drug removed per unit time.

Clearance = F (fraction of the drug absorbed) $\times$ dose/dosing interval $\times$ clearance
$Cl = K_e \times V_d$
$K_e = \text{Ln}(C_1 - C_2)/\text{time}$

11. **Pharmacokinetic principles**
A. Initial loading dose = peak blood concentration $\times V_d$
B. Steady state maintained = fraction absorbed $\times$ maintenance dose/Dosing interval $\times$ clearance
C. *Ethanol loading dose*
   1. **Intravenous** 10 mL/kg 10% ethanol (1.0 mL/kg 95% absolute ethanol) The i.v. absolute ethanol is diluted to 10%.
   2. **Oral** 1 mL/kg 95% of ethanol should be diluted in twice its volume of fruit juice to give approximately a 30% solution in order to avoid gastritis.
D. *Ethanol maintenance dose.* The average maintenance is 0.1 g/kg/h or 0.15 mL/kg/h of 95% or 1.4 mL/kg/h 10% in D5W. **Example 4:** Calculate the loading dose of ethanol needed to produce a blood ethanol concentration of 100 mg/dL using a 10% solution for a 28-year-old 70-kg man with serum methanol concentration of 60 mg/dL. The loading dose is 10 mL/kg of 10% ethanol. 10 mL/kg $\times$ 70 kg = 700 mL of 10% ethanol is needed. **Example 5:** Using the same parameters as in Example 4, determine what amount or volume of a bottle of 100 proof vodka would be needed to give as a loading dose. Answer: One-hundred proof vodka is 50%. The loading dose is 700 mL of 10% needed. What you have is what you want. 70 mL $\times$ 100% available = volume desired $\times$ desired percentage (50%). 700 mL $\times$ 10% = X mL $\times$ 50%. 700 mL = 0.5X. X = 140 mL of 50% is needed.

E. *Summary ETOH dose in treatment of methanol intoxication*

Dose	Intravenous	Oral
Loading[a]	20 mL/kg 5% solution 10 mL/kg 10% solution	2.0 mL/kg 50% solution
Maintenance solution[a]	2.80 mL/kg/h 5% solution 1.40 mL/kg/h 10% solution	0.28 mL/kg 50% solution
Maintenance during dialysis	3 to 5 mL/kg/h 5% solution 1.5 to 2.5 mL/kg/h 10% solution up to 91 mL/h	0.3 to 0.5 mL/kg/h solution

[a]Maintenance and loading dose should be given concomitantly.

II. **Body compartment models.** Body compartments, blood plasma, or serum may be a reflection of the amount and concentration of the drug in the blood or various tissues of the body. The possible movements of a drug from its sites of administration to the sites of elimination are depicted schematically in Fig. 2-2 (7).

    A. *Single compartment model.* In this situation, the drug rapidly equilibrates with all tissues of the body. The rate at which the drug is eliminated (metabolized or excreted) depends on the amount present at a specific time. Figure 2-3 illustrates blood concentrations when the drug follows first-order kinetics or when concentration is the major factor influencing drug movement (8).

    B. *Multicompartment model.* In a two-compartment model, there is a central compartment composed of the plasma volume and highly perfused tissues such as the brain, heart,

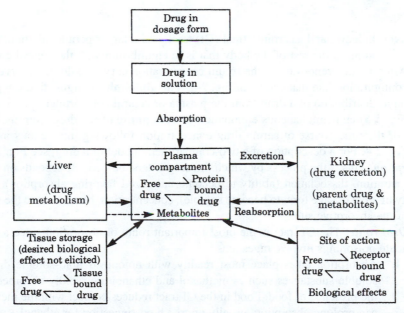

FIG. 2-2. Possible movements of a drug from site(s) of administration to site(s) of elimination, showing the factors that affect drug concentration at the site of action.
(From ref. 7, with permission.)

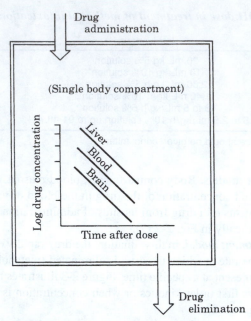

FIG. 2-3. Illustrates blood concentration when the drug follows first-order kinetics or when concentration is the major factor influencing drug movement.

liver, kidneys, and gastrointestinal (GI) tract, and a larger peripheral compartment corresponding to the rest of the body that is in equilibrium with the central compartment. After an intravenous dose, the serum concentration curve would be observed to have a configuration like that shown in Fig. 2-4. **The alpha phase** in this figure represents the rapid distribution of a drug from the plasma or central compartment into tissues (k1 in Fig. 2-5) and simultaneous elimination or **beta phase** of the drug from the body (kel). For the time course of serum drug concentration following intravenous injection, see Fig. 2-4. For a description of a two-compartment model of a drug, see Fig. 2-5.

III. *Absorption.* This is the process by which the drug enters the body. It depends on the route of administration, dissociation (ability to become unionized favoring absorption), dissolution (ability of solid dosage form to become soluble), concentration, blood flow to the site, and the area of the absorptive site.

   A. *Oral route.* The GI tract is the most important route of absorption since a majority of acute poisonings involve ingestions.

   1. Absorption takes place most readily with unionized lipid-soluble drugs. Lipid-soluble substances such as methanol and ethanol are rapidly absorbed, except in the presence of food. Food in the GI tract reduces contact with the membrane and can prolong absorption, usually up to 3 h postingestion for ethanol.

   2. The small intestine absorbs most drugs, and malabsorption or decreased gastric emptying can delay absorption and toxicity (Table 2-1).

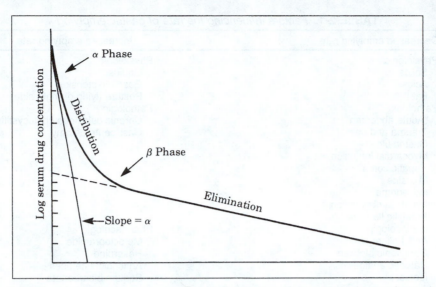

FIG. 2-4. The alpha phase represents rapid distribution of drug from plasma; beta phase represents the slower elimination phase of drug.

3. **Reduction of gastric cell function and consequent decreases in the acidity** can lead to increased levels of acid-labile medications such as levodopa, penicillins, and erythromycin. Substances such as ketoconazole and iron are decreased since they are better absorbed in an acid media.

4. Reduced **motility and decreased gastric emptying time** may decrease the absorption but not to any significant extent. In the small intestine, the decreased motility may decrease absorption and transport.

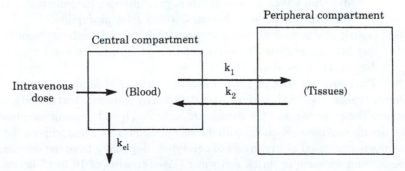

FIG. 2-5. Two-compartment model.

TABLE 2-1. *Factors influencing the rate of gastric emptying*

Decreased emptying rate	Increased emptying rate
Physiologic	Physiologic
Solids	Liquids
Acids	Gastric distension
Fat	Posture (lying on right side)
Pathologic	Pathologic
"Acute abdomen"	Chronic calculous cholecystitis
Trauma and pain	Gastroenterostomy
Gastric ulcer	
Myocardial infarction	
Hepatic coma	
Migraine	
Myxedema	
Intestinal obstruction	
Paralytic ileus	
Pharmacologic	Pharmacologic
Anticholinergics	Metoclopramide
Ganglionic blockers	Reserpine
Narcotic analgesics	Anticholinesterases
Isoniazid	Sodium bicarbonate
Aluminum hydroxide	
Drugs with anticholinergic side effects	

Adapted from ref. 23.

5. **A reduction in the active transport** may impair the absorption of nutrients, calcium, thiamine, vitamins, and iron which occurs with advancing age. Most medications are absorbed by passive transport. Drugs that have a **high extraction ratio** such as **lidocaine, pentazocine, propranolol,** and **tocainide** may have increased bioavailability, due to decreased hepatic blood flow.

6. Pathologic factors and concurrent medications are important factors in the absorption of medication. Antacids can decrease absorption of cimetidine, digitalis, tetracycline, phenytoin, iron, quinolones, and ketoconazole.

7. **Common drugs that decrease gastric emptying** include aspirin, anticholinergics, alcohol, barbiturates, iron, and opiates. Sustained release formulations of drugs such as theophylline, aspirin, and lithium cause marked delays in absorption and toxicity. Drugs such as aspirin, iron, glutethimide, meprobamate, and ethchlorvynol form **concretions or bezoars,** which delay absorption.

8. Gastric acids can limit the absorption of drugs such as benzylpenicillin, whereas metabolizing enzymes in the brush border of the intestine can impair absorption of drugs such as levodopa.

9. The **comatose state** can also decrease motility and delay absorption.

B. *Dermal route.* The skin is composed of the epidermis, dermis, and underlying subdermal tissue. The epidermis and the dermis are separated by a basement membrane, whereas the dermis remains continuous with the subcutaneous tissue and adipose tissue. The epidermis is composed of five layers of cell types. Beginning from the outside of the skin, the stratum corneum or "brick and water" layer consists of 10 to 15 layers of flattened cornified cells, which are the bricks, and the lipid-rich intracellular matrix consisting of the mortar, the stratum lucidum, stratum granulosum, stratum spinosum, and stratum basale. In the dermis lie hair folicles, sebaceous glands, apocrine glands, and exocrine sweat glands—all supported by a rich vascular network. The cornified layer of the stratum corneum is the rate-limiting step to drug penetration. Lipid solubility of a substance is an important factor affecting the degree of absorption through the skin. The currently available medications for transcutaneous delivery include clonidine, scopolamine, estradiol, fentanyl citrate, nitroglycerin, and nicotine.

1. **Organophosphate insecticides** are lipid-soluble and readily absorbed from the skin and can present a hazard to medical personnel who handle the patient.

2. **Organic solvents** such as carbon tetrachloride, methanol, and others that are present as vehicles for some chemicals, which may enhance skin absorption.

3. **Dimethyl sulfoxide (DMSO),** a common solvent used commercially, is very efficient as a carrier or transporter for carrying other substances into the skin to be absorbed.

4. **Inflammation, rubbing,** and other causes of increased skin flow may increase absorption.

5. **Application of ice or tourniquets** for envenomations may retard absorption.

6. **The mucosal surfaces** may allow significant absorption of such drugs such as viscous lidocaine. Lidocaine has almost an immediate onset of action from mucosal surfaces and open wounds, and has resulted in seizures in infants when applied topically for teething pain (9).

C. *Inhalation route.* Toxic fumes, particulates, and noxious gases may be absorbed through the lungs.

1. **Irritant gases** can be subdivided by their degree of water solubility.

   a. **Water-soluble gases** such as ammonia and chlorine produce immediate symptoms and primarily irritate the upper respiratory tract.

   b. **Less water-soluble** gases such as nitrogen dioxide or phosgene produce little upper respiratory tract irritation and a delayed onset of symptoms, and affect primarily the lower respiratory tract and parenchyma.

2. **Particle size** is another important factor influencing lung retention of a particular substance. Only particles less than 1 μm in diameter can penetrate the lower airways. Generally, the only means of reducing absorption through the lungs is by removing the patient from the toxic atmosphere.

D. *Intramuscular route.* This route is unreliable and varies from patient to patient. Phenytoin is slowly absorbed from this route and has precipitated crystals at the injection site. Poor perfusion during shock will leave medication at the site to be absorbed when circulation is re-established (6).

E. *Intravenous route.* The intravenous route is the most reliable and provides the most rapid clinical response.

1. **"Layering out"** of drugs in the intravenous tubing may alter the intended drug concentration at the point of entry into the body.

2. Extraction of drugs by **in-line filters** may interfere with this supposedly direct route, so that the medication does not enter the body in the expected dosage or composition (10).

3. **Other factors.** Intravenous drug abusers, malfunctioning infusion devices, incorrect dosage calculations, "Munchausen's" syndrome, and "Munchausen by proxy" syndrome (administration of drugs to children to produce factitious disease by caretakers) (10) are all responsible for patients developing toxicity from this route of administration.

F. **Other routes.** In cases where the intravenous route is not feasible or in emergencies, the endotracheal route may be used for epinephrine, atropine, lidocaine, or naloxone. A second emergency route of administration is by intraosseous infusion. Almost any emergency drug, as well as resuscitation fluids like saline and blood, may be administered by this route. Drugs and solutions instilled into the bone marrow are absorbed as rapidly as when administered intravenously. In contrast to peripheral veins, the intramedullary vessels will not collapse in shock (11).

G. **Rectal route.** The rectal route is generally considered to produce erratic absorption and may lead to toxicity with drugs such as theophylline. Rectally administered drugs, like those absorbed from the oral mucosa, do not pass through the liver before entering the general circulation.

IV. **Volume of distribution.** The apparent volume of distribution is a useful pharmacokinetic parameter that relates the plasma or serum concentration of a drug to the total amount of drug in the body (1,2). The volume of fluid within the body into which the drug appears to distribute with the concentration equal to plasma is defined as "volume of distribution"; this term is simplistic because it assumes the body acts as a single compartment.

A. **In reality, this value does not refer to any actual physiologic space.** The real distribution volume of a drug is related to body water and cannot exceed total body water, which is about 60% body weight in an adult. This corresponds to approximately 40 L in an average 70-kg adult.

B. **Total body water is divided into three separate compartments:** plasma water, interstitial water, and intracellular water. Extracellular water is a combination of plasma water and interstitial water. Intracellular fluid also includes the fluids in the erythrocytes and other formed elements.

C. **When the volume of distribution is large,** the tissue concentration is large and the plasma concentration is small. When the volume of distribution is small, most of the drug remains in the plasma.

D. **The volume of distribution may be affected by a number of different factors:** proportion of body fat, increased fat increases V_d; muscle lean mass, increased lean muscle mass decreases V_d; protein binding of the drug decreases V_d, acidic agents bind to albumin and basic agents bind to alpha-1 glycoprotein; tissue binding of drugs; and physiologic and pathologic conditions.

E. **Duration of action** of a drug depends on volume distribution (V_d), metabolism (mostly by the liver), clearance of the drug (mostly by the kidneys) or a combination of these factors. As the body size decreases a decrease in the dose may be required to avoid reaching a toxic blood concentration.

F. **The proportion of adipose tissue** increases with aging. The body **fat** is 18% to 33% in young adults (18% in males and 36% in females) and **increases** to 36% to 45% in the elderly (36% in males and 48% in females). Therefore, there is an increased volume distribution of lipid-soluble drugs causing a prolonged half-life in the elderly. This is important for medications that affect the central nervous system such as barbiturates and benzodiazepines. Drugs that are **fat-soluble (lipophilic)** theoretically have an increased **volume of distribution** (V_d) and **prolonged effect,** but **lower peak concentrations** than expected. Examples are benzodiazepines diazepam, digoxin, pentobarbital, and ethchlorvynol.

G. There is a **decrease in the total body water** by as much as 15% (both extracellular and intracellular) between the ages from 20 to 80 years, therefore, there is a decreased volume distribution of water-soluble drugs. The V_d of water-soluble substances such as lithium, cimetidine and ethanol is decreased and can result in increased serum concentrations. Diuretics reduce the extracellular fluid volume further.

H. There is a **decrease in muscle mass and plasma proteins, particularly the albumin,** which results in more free fraction of the drug. The increased body fat combined with decreased total body water leads to **decreased lean body mass.** Digoxin binds to muscle Na–K-adenosine triphosphate which decreases because of the reduced muscle mass with aging. The concentration of digoxin may increase as a result of decreased V_d. Digoxin toxicity may occur at doses of the drug that are therapeutic for the younger patients. If the elderly are **dosed according to ideal body weight** this leads to smaller volume distribution and a higher plasma concentration for water-soluble drugs. **Hydrophilic medications,** such as acetaminophen and many antibiotics, may have a **decreased** V_d, resulting in **higher than expected peak concentrations** which may lead to toxicity.

I. **In toxicology the volume of distribution can be useful in several ways:**

1. **In calculating the amount of substance** in the body to help verify the history of the quantity ingested,

2. In **predicting the peak blood concentration** of drug taken

3. In deciding whether to attempt to **apply extracorporeal elimination** of the toxic substance. **Examples** illustrating the usefulness of volume distribution will be given for each of these three indications. **Case 6:** A 70-kg patient states she ingested approximately thirty 100 mg phenobarbital tablets. Volume of distribution (V_d) listed is 0.75 L/kg. Peak blood concentration measured by laboratory was 60 mg/L. The history can be verified as follows: Dose = $V_d \times$ conc = (0.75 L/kg $\times$ 70 kg) $\times$ 60 mg/L = 3150 mg. This represents approximately 31 tablets of 100 mg phenobarbital. **Case 7:** A 60-kg patient presents with history of ingesting 20 phenytoin capsules, 100 mg each, 15 min ago. How can you predict what the peak concentration is to determine if this patient will develop any manifestations of phenytoin toxicity?

$$\text{Answer: Conc} = \text{dose}/V_d = 20 \times 100 \text{ mg}/0.75 \text{ L/kg} \times 60 \text{ kg}$$
$$= 2{,}000 \text{ mg}/45 \text{ L} = 44.4 \text{ mg/L}$$

You would expect phenytoin toxicity since this is above the normal therapeutic range of 10 to 20 mg/L. **Case 8:** A patient ingests an unknown amount of lithium capsules and has a peak concentration of 5 mEq/L. The patient is very agitated. Is this drug dialyzable? Answer: Since the V_d is 0.7 L/kg, the drug is dialyzable. Drugs with small volumes of distribution (less than 1 L/kg) are present in substantial amounts in the circulation. Both low volume of distribution and low protein binding (less than 50%), are important variables in determining if a drug can be removed by extracorporeal measures. Other factors may be important as well, but they will be discussed in the section on Principles of Elimination of Toxin: Enhancing Elimination.

V. **Protein binding**

   A. **Drugs are transported in the blood stream either attached to carrier proteins or unbound in solution.**

   1. **Bound drugs** are unable to cross cell membranes and consequently are unable to exert biological effects.

   2. **Only unbound or free drugs** are able to cross lipoprotein membranes and are able to exert pharmacologic effects. This principle is routinely used in the management of patients with cyclic antidepressant overdose.

   3. **Alkalinization** of the blood by sodium bicarbonate to keep the pH at 7.5 has been shown to increase the protein binding of these agents and decrease the amount of free drug that can produce toxicity.

   B. **Drugs that are highly bound to protein** have small volumes of distribution. A drug with a greater affinity for plasma proteins can displace weakly bound drugs from their plasma protein binding sites and under certain circumstances elevate free drug concentrations at tissue receptor sites with resultant clinical toxicity. Such examples include phenytoin and anticoagulants (1,2).

   C. The concentration of plasma protein and protein binding tends to decrease in the elderly. The albumin concentration is often decreased 15% to 25% in the elderly (due to decreased production in liver, chronic illness, and hospitalized or institutionalized patients), compared with young adults. This results in increased free pharmacologically active fractions of medication, which are usually extensively bound to albumin and inactive. Consequently, this may produce an **enhanced response to a particular drug,** due to the higher free fraction. This is important for **highly protein bound (more than 90%) acidic medications** such as phenylbutazone, phenytoin, salicylates, theophylline, tolbutamide, and warfarin.

   D. **Alpha-1 acid glycoprotein** is an acute-phase reactant that can increase with advancing age in the presence of inflammation. The **basic medications** have an affinity for alpha acid glycoproteins which are increased and decrease the amount of unbound drug. The drugs may require higher doses. Examples are lidocaine, meperidine, propranolol. Drugs also **compete for drug binding sites.** A recently added medication can displace a drug on a binding site that has been in therapeutic range and lead to potential toxicity. **Free drug concentrations** rather than protein bound are often desirable in the elderly, although they are not always clinically available. **Most drug concentration determinations** measure the total drug (protein-bound and free levels), and this may not accurately reflect the drug activity when the plasma protein is decreased. Whenever possible, measure the free drug (12).

VI. **Metabolism**

   A. Metabolism is the biochemical transformation of a drug. It is the process by which the body transforms a drug and makes it more water-soluble so that the drug may be eliminated more rapidly via the kidney into the urine.

B. Biotransformation can produce metabolites that are pharmacologically active and toxic.
C. For example, parathion is metabolized into paraoxon, its toxic metabolite. Drugs with active metabolites are listed in Table 2-2 and chemicals with active metabolites are listed in Table 2-3. The rate of drug metabolism by the liver is determined by the hepatic blood flow and hepatic function. The **hepatic blood flow** is decreased by 0.3% to 1.5% per year due to decreased cardiac output and the liver size by 37% in the elderly as compared with younger adults, resulting in a higher bioavailability due to reduction in first-pass metabolism (9). The elderly are more susceptible to toxic effects of **rapidly hepatic metabolized drugs** such as calcium channel blockers, diazepam, lidocaine, morphine, propranolol and tricyclic antidepressants because their rate of metabolism is dependent on hepatic blood flow or **"perfusion-dependent"** (1). Drugs that have a limited capacity

TABLE 2-2A. *Active metabolites of drugs*

Drug	Active metabolite(s)
Sulfate conjugation	
Acetaminophen O → P450	Acetaminophen sulfate
	N-Acetyl-p-benzoquinoneimine
Acetohexamide	Hydroxyhexamide
Acetylsalicylic acid	Salicylic acid
Allopurinol	Alloxanthine
Deamination	
Amphetamines O →	Phenylacetone
Amitriptyline	Nortriptyline
Antidepressants	Various
Benzodiazepines	Various
Amitriptyline	Nortriptyline
Alcohol dehydrogenase	
Chloral hydrate O →	Trichloroethanol
Nitroreduction	
Chloramphenicol O →	"Arylamine" glycolic acid metabolite
Sulfoxidation	
Chlorpromazine O →	Chlorpromazine sulfoxide
Codeine	Morphine
Cortisone	Cortisol
Diazepam	Desmethyldiazepam, oxazepam
Digitoxin	Digoxin
Digoxin	Digoxigenin derivatives
O-Dealkylation	
Encainide O →	O-Demethylencainide
Glutethimide	4-OH-glutethimide
N-Dealkylation	
Imipramine O →	Desipramine
Acetylation	
Isoniazide	Acetylated isoniazid
Lidocaine	Desethyllidocaine
N-Oxidation	
Meperidine O →	Meperidine N-oxide → normeperidine
Glucuronide	
Morphine	Morphine-3-glucuronide

O →, biotransformed by oxidation.

TABLE 2-2B. *Active metabolites of drugs*

Drug	Active metabolite(s)
Methylation	
Norepinephrine	Normetanephrine
Hydroxylation of aromatic rings	
Phenobarbital O →	p-Hydroxyphenobarbital
Phenylbutazone	Oxyphenylbutazone
Hydroxylation of aromatic rings	
Phenytoin O →	P-Hydroxyphenytoin
Prednisone	Prednisolone
Azoreduction	
Prontosil O →	Sulfanilamide
Primidone	Phenobarbital
Procainamide	N-Acetylprocainamide
Propranolol	4-Hydroxypropranolol
Quinidine	3-Hydroxyquinidine
Glycine conjugation	
Salicylates	Salicl-CoA → salicylic acid
Theophylline	Caffeine
Side chain oxidation (aliphatic hydroxylation)	
Tolbutamide O →	Hydroxytolbutamide
Verapamil	Norverapamil

O →, biotransformed by oxidation.
Modified from ref. 8.

TABLE 2-3. *Active metabolites of chemicals*

Drug	Active metabolite(s)
Acetonitrile	Cyanide
Aflatoxins	Aflatoxin M1
Aromatic hydrocarbons (polyclic)	Epoxides
(e.g., anthracene)	
Benzene	Epoxides
Benzyl alcohol	Benzoic acid, hippuric acid
Nonmicrosomal oxidation	
Ethanol O →	Acetaldehyde
Ethylene glycol	Oxalic acid, glycolaldehyde, glycolate, glyoxylate
Isopropyl alcohol	Acetone
Malathion	Maloxone
Methylene chloride	Carbon monoxide
Methanol	Formic acid
Naphthalene	Epoxides
Desulfonation	
Parathion O →	Paraoxon
Paraquat	Superoxide radical
Trichloroethylene	Trichloroethanol

O →, biotransformed by oxidation.

to be metabolized by the liver, including barbiturates, phenytoin, theophylline, and warfarin, have a rate that is determined by enzymes activity and are **"perfusion-independent."** When two perfusion-independent drugs are administered concurrently, the body has a limited capacity to metabolize them and metabolism of both occurs at a slower rate.

D. **First-pass effect.** The liver biotransforms some drugs during the initial first pass from the portal circulation after oral administration. Therefore, a large portion of the drug fails to reach the systemic circulation in the original form. The first-pass effect accounts for the difference in peak plasma levels between the oral and intravenous doses.

1. **Common examples** of drugs that have rapid hepatic clearance due to this are: guanethidine, hydralazine, lidocaine, isoproterenol, propranolol and testosterone.

2. Variations in **hepatic blood flow** in diseases such as congestive heart failure can delay the metabolism and cause toxicity at usual pharmacologic doses of some drugs, such as theophylline.

E. *Biotransformation.* Biotransformation reactions convert drugs from less polar, more lipophilic-soluble compounds to more polar, hydrophilic compounds that are more readily excreted predominantly via the kidney. Biotransformation in humans is grouped into **Phase I reactions,** which includes oxidation (hydroxylation), reduction, hydrolysis and carboxylation reactions, and **Phase II reactions** involving synthesis processes such as conjugations (Fig. 2-6). Some drugs require only Phase I reactions for inactivation; others must pass through both phases for complete inactivation; and some drugs undergo Phase II reactions immediately. **Phase II synthetic reactions** involves glucuronidation, sulfation, or acetylation of the molecule. The result is usually a pharmacologic inactive metabolite. Phase II metabolism remains relatively unchanged with aging. Therefore, it is more desirable to use medications that undergo phase II metabolism, such as the benzodiazepines lorazepam, oxazepam, procainamide (slow and fast acetylation), temazepam or lorazepam. **Medications** reach a steady state in four to five times the half-life. Alprazolam and diazepam undergo oxidative (phase I) metabolism which produces active metabolites, contributing to a prolonged duration of action in the elderly. In contrast lorazepam, oxazepam and triazolam undergo conjugation (phase II) metabolism which is unaffected by normal aging and does not result in prolonged action.

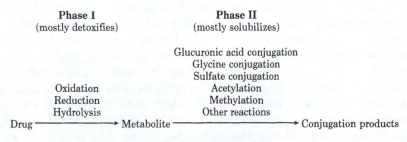

FIG. 2-6. Biotransformation.

1. **Phase I reactions** is the addition of reactive groups by microsomal oxidations, non-microsomal oxidations, reductions, and hydrolysis. **Phase I oxidative metabolism** is performed by the microsomal enzyme mixed function oxidase system (chromosome P-450) and produces metabolites that may be pharmacologically active. Phase I metabolism decreases with aging. The medications metabolized via the **hepatic oxidative pathways** such as barbiturates, clorazepate (Tranxene), diazepam, flurazepam, lidocaine, propranolol, quinidine and theophylline, triazolam have significantly longer half-lives, resulting in accumulation and enhanced effects. Examples include the **oxidation** of aromatic substance such as naphthalene or bromobenzene; highly reactive epoxides may spontaneously rearrange to form hydroxylated metabolites. Examples of **reduction** if the transfer of electrons from NADPH to $R-NO_2$ (a nitrite) forming $R-NH_2$ (an amine). The most clinically important oxidative reaction is hydroxylation of lipid-soluble aromatic substances such as benzene (including bromobenzene) and naphthalene. The **cytochrome P-450** mono-oxygenase or P450 mixed function oxidase gets it name from the fact when reduced (Fe+2) binds to carbon monoxide and its maximum absorption spectrum occurs at P450. **Oxidative-reduction** reactions may change the polarity of substrates and are usually mediated through the iron/porphyrin-containing cytochrome oxidases NAD or NADP. The electrons extracted are transferred to molecular oxygen through the mitochondrial oxygen through the electron transport system and the hexose-monophosphate shunt which serves as a major source of NADPH.

2. **Phase II reactions** link foreign compounds to an endogenous conjugate such as glucuronic acid and sulfate to make the conjugate more polar and hydrophilic. The elimination of the glucuronide complexes is facilitated by the biliary and active renal transport. An example of this type of reaction is the conjugation of acetaminophen with glutathione. **Glutathione conjugations** catalyze many toxic compounds. Following complexation, the glycine and glutamate residues are cleaved and the molecule acetylated resulting in mercapturic acid metabolite. Bromobenzene is metabolized by glutathione transferase. The rate-limiting process is the availability of reduced glutathione. Examples of these reactions include the addition of hydroxy group (-OH), sulfhydryl (-SH), amino ($-NH_2$), carboxyl (-COOH) to foreign molecules.

E. *Enzyme induction and inhibition.* Induction of enzyme activity will increase the rate of clearance of a drug by enhancement of its metabolism. Conversely, inhibition will decrease the rate of clearance by reduction of the drug's metabolism. **Enzyme induction** is associated with the growth of smooth endoplasmic reticulum (microsomal drug-metabolizing system) in the liver cells, which enlarge as a result. Enzyme induction is associated with increased synthesis of the cytochrome oxidase P-450, NADPH-cytochrome C reductase, and other enzymes involved in drug metabolism. Induction usually requires repetitive administration of the inducing agent over a period of several days and, once started, may continue for 2 to 3 weeks. It is variable and unpredictable. Drug metabolism may increase two- to fourfold during induction (Table 2-4): *inducers,* (*poppers*)—**p**henobarbital, **o**rganochlorine insecticides, **p**henytoin, **p**hencycidine, **e**thanol (chronic), **r**ifampin; *inhibitors* (*Kidde soap*)—**k**etoconazole, **i**soniazid, **d**icu-

TABLE 2-4. *Common enzyme inducers and inhibitors*

Inducers	Inhibitors
Antipyrine	Allopurinol
Carbamazepine	Chlordiazepoxide
Cigarette smoking[a]	Chloramphenicol[a]
DDT, lindane[a]	Chlorpromazine
Ethanol (chronic use)[a]	Cimetidine[a] (warfarin, theophylline)
Glutethimide	Dextropropoxyphene[a]
Phenobarbital[a]	Dicumarol[a]
Phenylbutazone[a]	Disulfiram[a]
Phenytoin (methadone)[a]	Erythromycin (CBZ, cimetidine)[a]
Primidone	Ethanol (acute use)[a]
Rifampin (CBZ, OC)[a]	Imipramine
Metronidazole[a]	Isoniazid[a]
	Ketoconizole and fluconazole[a]
	Oral contraceptives[a]
	Phenylbutazone
	Prochlorperazine
	Sulfonamides
	Warfarin

[a]CBZ, carbamazepam (increase risk of seizures); OC, oral contraceptive (failure contraception); INH, isoniazid (failure TB therapy and danger of toxic hepatitis).

marol, **d**isulfiram, **e**rythromycin, **s**ulfonamides, **o**ral contraceptives, **a**llopurinol, **p**henothiazines; *drugs that inhibit astemizole*—macrolids (erythromycin, azithromycin, clarithromycin), ketoconazole and fluconazole; *multifactoral*—quinidine and cyclosporine elevate digitalis level by decreasing digitalis clearance and decreasing the V_d of digitalis; additive effects—loop diuretics and aminoglycosides increase ototoxicity. Verapamil and digoxin have additive inhibitory effects on cardiac conduction and heart rate.

G. *Interactions*

1. Direct chemical. Interactions of cations in antacids or iron with tetracycline to decrease tetracycline absorption.

2. Effects on absorption. Tetracycline reduces metabolism of digoxin by intestinal flora resulting in increased digitalis levels.

3. Alterations in protein binding

a. **Drugs bound to albumin** ("A" drugs) are acidic, anticonvulsants, aspirin-like and anticoagulants. The drugs have a small volume distribution and are expressed in mg/dL. Most interactions occur with "A" drugs. Acidic drugs have two sites: site 1, warfarin and bilirubin; site 2, diazepam.

b. **Drugs bound to alpha-2 glycoprotein** are basic drugs like tricyclic antidepressants. These drugs have a larger volume distribution and are expressed in concentrations of µg/mL. Basic drugs bind to alpha-glycoprotein, a phase reactant which increases with some illness less free drug.

H. *Drugs that influence the absorption of other medications.* Antacids decrease absorption of the following: chlorpromazine, digitoxin, isoniazid, penicillinamine, phenytoin, propranolol, ranitidine, tetracyclines, theophylline. Metoclopramide increases the absorption of the following: acetaminophen, chlorthiazide, cimetidine, digoxin, ethanol, lithium.

I. *Significant food-drug interaction*
1. Anticoagulants. Limit foods high in vitamin K. Limit citrus fruits, egg yolks, fish, potato chips, leafy green vegetables.
2. Cardiac glycosides. Limit foods high in calcium. Withhold milk, give after meals. No kaopectate or antacids.
3. Erythromycin. Limit acidic food, carbonated beverages. Give before or 3 h after meals.
4. MAO inhibitors. Limit foods high in pressor amines. Limit cheese, wine, beer, chocolate, yeast, liver, herring.
5. Penicillin. Limit acid fruit or fruit juices. Give on empty stomach with water.
6. Tetracycline. Limit foods high in calcium. Give before or 2 h after meals.
7. Thiazides. Imported licorice (cause hypokalemia).
8. Grapefruit juice interactions by inhibition of presystemic (first-pass) metabolism of some drugs metabolized by the cytochrome P-450 isoenzymes (CYP3A4, CYP1A2, CP2A6) has been reported (13,14), CY3A4 metabolizes calcium channel blockers (15), cyclosporine (16) and terfenidine (17) and inhibition of metabolism may increase serum concentrations. Inhibition of CYP1A2 metabolism may influence the serum concentration of caffeine (18), theophylline (19) and tarcine (14). The clinical effect has yet to be determined.

J. **Drugs that displace other medication from binding sites:**

Drug displaced	Causative medication
Warfarin	Chloral hydrate, clofibrate, diazoxide, ethacrynic acid, mefenamic acid, nalidixic acid, phenylbutazone, phenytoin, salicylates
Diazepam	Heparin, valproate
Phenytoin	Phenylbutazone, salicylates, tolbutamide
Tolbutamide	Phenylbutazone, salicylates, dicumarol

K. **Other examples.** Bilirubin displacement, sulfonamides, ceftriaxone. Phenylbutazone decreases the binding of tolbutamide and warfarin to albumin increasing the anti-coagulant effect.

L. **Renal elimination or excretion.** Excretion is the final means of drug elimination, either as metabolites or unchanged parent drug. Excretion through the lungs is the major route for gaseous substances. In the case of nonvolatile water-soluble drugs, the kidneys are the most important route of excretion. Additional routes include: sweat, saliva, tears, nasal secretions, milk, bile, and feces. **Altered renal clearance** by diuretics and non-steroidal anti-inflammatory drugs (NSAID) decreases lithium clearance. NSAIDs, probenecid and salicylate decrease methotrexate clearance by decreased renal tubular excretion. **Glomerular filtration rate and renal plasma blood flow** decreases by 1% per year; decreases by 40% from 30 to 80 years. These parameters are reduced by 50% at 90 years of age. **Active secretion** decreases with aging, leading to an increase in the half-life (prolonged effect) of medications eliminated primarily by the kidneys. Examples of such medications are antibiotics (aminoglycosides, imipenem, pyrazinamide, vancomycin), benzodiazepines, digoxin, lithium, meperidine (normeperidine), procainamide (*N*-acetylprocainamide), sulfonylurea (chlorpropamide, acetohexamide) and vancomycin. These medications may accumulate with increased toxicity. In assessing renal function it is important to **look not only at the creatinine,** (since the lean muscle mass decreases with aging, therefore the daily endogenous creatinine production decreases and the serum creatinine decreases) but at the **creatinine clearance,** whereby creatinine clearance is estimated based on the sex, age, weight, and serum creatinine. The serum creatinine may be "normal" in the elderly while the renal function may be considerably reduced. This finding can seriously mislead the physician when confronted with an overdose of aminoglycosides, digoxin or sulfonylurea in the elderly. The serum creatinine is not a reliable accurate measure of renal function in the elderly. Aminoglycosides, atenolol, digoxin and lithium accumulations can result when there is a decreased renal function. The **Cockroft-Gault equation for the creatinine clearance** (CrCl):

CrCl (mL/min) = (140 – age [years]) weight ($\times$ 0.85 for females)/serum creatinine $\times$ 72

It is estimated that the creatinine clearance decreases 35% between the ages of 20 and 90 without evidence of renal disease. When creatinine clearance is less than 30 mL/min, this is significant. **Example 9:** A 35-year-old 50-kg woman with a creatinine of 1.0 mg/dL has a CrCl 62 mL/min. An 85-year-old 50-kg woman with a creatinine of 1.0 mg/dL has a CrCl 32 mL/min. Drugs prescribed with low renal clearance and low therapeutic index including aminoglycosides, digoxin, lithium, procainamide, vancomycin require close monitoring of the plasma drug level. Renal function in elderly patients, especially those with decreased circulating blood volume, is strongly dependent on prostaglandin-mediated blood flow, which is inhibited by nonsteroidal antiinflammatory drugs (NSAIDs).

1. ***Lungs.*** The body excretes volatile anesthetics primarily by the lungs. Toxic gases such as hydrogen sulfide, carbon monoxide, and cyanide are excreted by the lungs. Factors affecting rate of excretion include tidal volume, minute ventilation, solubility, and ventilation/perfusion ratio.

2. ***Bile.*** Drugs and chemicals excreted into the bile enter the intestine and are subsequently either reabsorbed into the blood or eliminated in the feces. Some drugs are excreted as water-soluble glucuronide conjugates which are hydrolyzed by intestinal bacteria resulting in reformation of the parent drug or metabolite and are readily reabsorbed into the blood. This process of excretion into bile and reabsorption into the intestine is known as ***Enterohepatic circulation.*** A list of substances reported to undergo enterohepatic circulation is found in Table 2-5. Repeated doses of activated charcoal have been shown to be very effective in some of these cases by preventing reabsorption. Continuous gastric suctioning has also been shown to be useful for removing substances which undergo enterohepatic recirculation.

3. ***Kidneys.*** Particular attention must be given to those drugs with a narrow therapeutic range that are eliminated principally through the kidneys. Drugs with a narrow therapeutic range, where kidney function is important, are amphotericin B, chloramphenicol, lithium, warfarin, digoxin, phenytoin, aminoglycoside, isoniazid,

TABLE 2-5. *Substances with enterohepatic circulation*

Chloral hydrate
Colchicine
Digitalis preparations (digoxin, digitoxin)
Glutethimide
Halogenated hydrocarbons (DDT derivatives)
Isoniazid
Methaqualone
Nonsteroidal anti-inflammatory agents
Phencyclidine
Phenothiazines
Phenytoin
Salicylates
Tricyclic antidepressants

and procainamide. The **fraction of a drug that is excreted unchanged** may vary from below 0.1 for lipid-soluble drugs to above 0.9 for water-soluble drugs. The more polar (highly ionized) compounds that are water-soluble are excreted relatively unchanged by the kidney (penicillins and aminoglycosides). Renal impairment can prolong the half-life of these agents and require dosage adjustments to avoid toxicity, especially with the aminoglycosides. Drugs primarily excreted by the renal route include the agents mentioned previously plus: acetohexamide, allopurinol, cephalexin, chlorpropamide, chlorothiazide, methenamine salts, nitrofurantoin, phenobarbital, and warfarin. Table 2-6 contains a list of substances that produce acute renal and hepatic failure.

VII. **Ion trapping.** Drugs can be weak acids or bases. They become ionized in solution when they lose or gain a hydrogen ion. Ionized (polar) compounds do not easily cross cell membranes and become trapped in the compartment in which they are more ionized. If the urine pH favors the ionized form of the drug, trapping will occur in the renal tubular space, resulting in increased excretion. Weak acids (e.g., aspirin and phenobarbital) are better reabsorbed in acid media and better excreted in alkaline media. Weak bases (e.g.,

TABLE 2-6. *Substances that produce acute renal and hepatic failure*

Renal	Hepatic
Aminoglycoside	Acetaminophen
Arsenic	Arsenic
Amphotericin B	Carbon tetrachloride
Chromium	Cyclopeptides (mushroom)
Cisplatin	Iron
Cyclosporine	Methotrexate
Cyclopeptides (mushroom)	Phosphorous (yellow)
Halogenated hydrocarbons	Phosphine
Mercury	
Ethylene glycol	
Orellanine (mushroom)	

quinidine, phencyclidine, and amphetamines) are better reabsorbed in alkaline environments and better excreted in acid urine. In toxicology these principles can be applied to these agents by manipulating the urine pH. Alkalinization with sodium bicarbonate can be used to hasten the excretion of salicylates and phenobarbital. Acidification of the urine, although previously used for phencyclidine and amphetamines, is no longer recommended to hasten elimination because of the possible precipitation of myoglobin in the renal tubules in a patient with rhabdomyolysis.

VIII. *Clearance (CL).* The elimination of drugs from the body can also be described by the term "clearance." This is a quantitative measure of the volume of blood cleared of drug per unit of time usually expressed in mL/min: $CL = 0.693 \, (V_d)/(t_{1/2}) = $ mL/min; $V_d = $ mL/kg; $t_{1/2} = $ half-life in minutes or hours.

IX. *First-order, zero-order, and Michaelis-Menten elimination.* Drugs are eliminated in one of three ways: first-order elimination, zero-order elimination, or a combination of the two.

    A. Drugs that are charged or highly polar are excreted directly by the kidneys, which represents first-order elimination.

    B. Drugs that are highly lipid-soluble are first metabolized by the liver and made highly polar to be excreted.

    C. Liver enzymes responsible for metabolism can become saturated and cause zero-order elimination.

    D. "Michaelis-Menten kinetics" is a term that refers to a drug elimination pattern whereby the drug exhibits a combination of both zero-order and first-order kinetics.

        1. First-order kinetics. Concentration is the major factor influencing the drug movement in first-order kinetics. The rate at which the drug is eliminated (metabolized or excreted) depends on the amount present at a specific time. As the concentration falls, the process proceeds at a slower rate.

        2. First-order kinetics is a decline in the drug level to a constant **percentage** of the remaining amount in the plasma per unit of time. The drug concentration versus time profile will be **curvilinear on linear coordinate plot ("sunken belly") and linear when the logarithmic concentration is plotted** against time at lower concentrations (dose-dependent). For practical purposes, most drugs follow first-order kinetics within the therapeutic range. As an example: if the initial concentration of a particular drug was determined to be 20 μg/mL and the half-life was 6 h, then the concentration would fall to 10 μg/mL in 6 h, 5 μg/mL in 12 h, and 2.5 μg/mL in18 h. The reduction in the concentration is less during successive half-lives, although the fraction remains constant.

        3. The half-life for first-order elimination is a constant. It can be a useful kinetic parameter as long as renal function is normal. For example, in the drug excreted by first-order elimination, a plasma concentration of 200 μg/mL will fall to 100 μg/mL after one half-life, to 50 μg/mL after two half-lives, and so on. **A rule of thumb** is that after five to six half-lives, there will be no significant amount of drug effect. Table 2-7 shows the number of half-lives it would take to reach steady state. At least five half-lives are required for a drug to reach 97% of steady state.

TABLE 2-7. *Half-life versus steady state*

No. of half-lives	Percentage of steady-state concentration
1	50
2	75
3	88
4	94
5	97
6	98
7	99

From ref. 7.

4. The half-life of a drug has **practical implications.** Drugs with short half-lives accumulate in the body minimally and require multiple doses to reach steady-state concentrations shortly after initiation of therapy. They also leave the body rapidly once therapy has been discontinued. For drugs with long half-lives the converse is true; that is, they accumulate extensively in the body with multiple doses, reach steady-state concentration slowly, and leave the body slowly on termination of therapy.

F. *Zero-order kinetics* (dose-dependent, capacity limited). When the rate of a process is independent of concentration it is said to follow zero-order kinetics.

1. A fixed amount of drug is eliminated over a period of time. **This is a linear process on linear graph paper (nonlinear on semi-log paper)** which is limited by the capacity of the enzymes involved which become saturated near the upper limits of the therapeutic range.

2. **Zero-order kinetics** (when a constant **quantity** of drug is eliminated from the body per unit of time and the drug concentration versus time profile is **linear on linear coordinates plot and curvilinear on logarithmic plot ("pot belly")** of concentration versus time (or saturation, dose-independent) at the higher therapeutic plasma concentrations. Acetylsalicylic acid, phenytoin, and ethanol are common examples of drugs that follow zero-order kinetics.

3. The significance of zero-order kinetics is that small increments in the dose may produce large increases in plasma concentration.

4. **The proportion of drug elimination** falls as the drug concentration rises, resulting in longer elimination half-life. As an example an overdose of phenytoin may change the drug's usual elimination half-life from 22 h to 4 days because first-order elimination is changed to zero-order when the enzyme system is saturated. A 50% increase in the maintenance dose of aspirin has resulted in a 300% increase in steady-state salicylate concentrations in the plasma. Therefore, the half-life for drugs such as phenytoin, salicylates, and theophylline may not be constant, even in therapeutic doses, but can change as a result of the amount of drug in the body. (Table 2-8 provides a comparison of first-order kinetics versus "zero"-order kinetics.)

X. *Blood concentrations in toxicology*

A. **The time of exposure** is important in estimating when the onset of the symptoms would be expected, when the peak action would be reached and how long it might last. It is important in determining when to obtain a blood sample for quantitative analysis and interpreting the plasma concentrations.

TABLE 2-8. *Michaelis-Menten kinetics*

Zero order	First order
Synonyms—saturation, capacity limited, dose dependent, nonlinear on semilog paper	Synonyms—linear (on semilog paper)
Independent of concentration	Dependent on concentration
No predictable half-life ($t_{1/2}$) decline	Half-life decline
Constant amount eliminated	Fixed fraction eliminated
Rate remains constant	Rate slows as concentration falls
Limited by enzyme capacity	Not limited by enzyme capacity
Example: initial concentration 24 µg/mL, in 6 h falls 4 to 20 µg/mL, in 12 h 16 µg/mL, in 18 h 12 µg/mL, etc.	Example: initial concentration 24 µg/mL and half-life ($t_{1/2}$) 6 h, in 6 h falls to 12 µg/mL, in 12 h to 6 µg/mL, in 18 h to 3 µg/mL, etc.
Drugs: probenecid, acetylsalicylic cyclic acid, phenytoin, ethanol, warfarin	Drug: most drugs in their therapeutic range

B. Table 2-9 contains a list of substances that require quantitative analysis to evaluate toxicity and determine appropriate managements including antidotal therapy in poisoned patients.

C. Drugs such as acetaminophen, aspirin and digoxin have delayed peak blood levels especially in an overdose. As a result one must obtain a careful history in order to determine when the peak levels will occur in an acute overdose to determine a specific course of management to administer.

XI. *Age-dependent factors in pharmacokinetics*

A. *Pediatrics*

1. In the first few weeks of life, achlorhydria, delayed gastric emptying and irregular intestinal motility result in decreased absorption of agents such as acidic drugs (penicillin, sulfonamide, barbiturates, and acetaminophen.) Erratic absorption occurs with phenytoin. Topical application has produced systemic toxicity in newborns and young infants because of increased skin permeability due to an immature striatum corneum (Table 2-10).

2. *Distribution.* Throughout childhood there is a relative change in the amount of tissue mass, especially lymphatic and neural tissues, which may alter distribution. The total body water may account for as much as 85% of the premature infant's body weight. This decreases as the child matures. Extracellular water decreases after birth and intracellular water increases. As a result of these changes, the volume of distribution of water-soluble drugs would be greater in the neonate than in the adult. Conversely, because the fraction of body weight present as fat increases with increasing age, the volume of distribution of a fat-soluble drug would be larger in a neonate than in an adult (11).

3. *Metabolism*

a. At birth, the neonate has immature enzyme systems and a reduced capacity to metabolize drugs, especially drugs that are **hydroxylated or conjugated with glucuronic acid.** Drugs that are eliminated chiefly by these paths will tend to persist in the body in active form for longer periods.

b. Although the rate of oxidation and glucuronidation is often reduced in the newborn, the demethylation and sulfate conjugation seem to proceed at adult levels of activity. **Decreased oxidation** has been demonstrated in newborns

TABLE 2-9. *Substances where quantitative blood values are necessary*

Substance	Specimen	Time postingestion to obtain specimen	Toxic concentration
Acetaminophen	Serum	After 4 h	>150 µg/mL @ 4 h
Amikacin	Serum	1 h; predose	>30; >8 µg/mL
Carboxyhemoglobin	Blood	Stat	Extrapolate
Carbamazepine	Serum	Stat/steady-state (e.g., 2–5 d)	>12 µg/mL
Chloramphenicol	Serum	Predose	>25 µg/mL
Digoxin	Serum	6 to 8 h	>2 ng/mL adult, > 4 ng/mL child
Ethanol	Serum	1/2 to 1 h	>80 mg/dL (800 µg/mL)
Ethylene glycol	Serum	1/2 to 1 h	>20 mg/dL (200 µg/mL)
Euthosuximide	Serum	Predose	>100 µg/mL
Gentamicin	Serum	1 h; predose	>6; >2 µg/mL
Imipramine	Serum	Steady-state (e.g., 3d)	>500 ng/mL
Lead	Blood	Any time	>25 µg/dL (may be >10)
Iron			
Liquid	Serum	2 h	>350 µg/dL (3.5 µg/mL)
Tablet	Serum	4 h	>350 µg/dL (3.5 µg/mL)
Isopropanol	Serum	1/2 to 1 h	>50 mg/dL (500 µg/mL)
Lithium	Serum	6 to 8 h	>2.0 mEq/L
Kanamycin	Serum	1 h; predose	>30; >6 µg/mL
Lidocaine	Serum	Steady-state (e.g., 7.5 h)	>6.0 µg/mL
Methanol	Serum	1/2 to 1 h	>20 mg/dL (200 µg/mL)
Methemoglobin	Blood	Stat	>30%
Nitroprusside	Serum	On infusion for 72 h >2 µg/kg/min	120 µg/mL thiocyanate
Paraquat	Plasma	8 h	>1 µg/mL within 24 h
Pentobarbital	Serum	Steady-state (e.g., 3–10 d)	>6 µg/mL
Phenobarbital	Serum	Stat/steady-state (e.g., 10–25 d)	>40 µg/mL
Phenytoin	Serum	1–2 h steady-state (e.g., 5–7 d)	>20 µg/mL
Primidone	Serum	Stat	>12 µg/mL as primidone
Procainamide	Serum	Steady-state (e.g., 24 h)	>10 µg/mL
Salicylate	Serum	After 6 h	>300 µg/mL (30 mg/dL)
Theophylline	Serum		
Liquid		1 h	>20 µg/mL
Regular tablet		1–3 h	>20 µg/mL
Slow release		3–10 h	>20 µg/mL
Tobramycin	Serum	1 h; predose	>10; >2 µg/mL
Vancomycin	Serum	1 h	>40 µg/mL

Ethylene glycol, red blood cell cholinesterase, serum cyanide are difficult to obtain. In an acute overdose situation of these agents, the aim should be to draw levels during their peak times and follow serial levels for a trend.

Stat, draw level immediately on admission; steady-state, draw the level when at least five to six $t_{1/2}$ have passed from the last dose change for it to be most useful for therapeutic purposes; ( ), examples of when drug is expected to be at steady-state.

for acetaminophen, phenytoin, phenobarbital, diazepam, lidocaine, and nortriptyline (Aventyl). **Decreased glucuronidation** has been demonstrated for chloramphenicol, salicylate, and nalidixic acid.

  c. After the first month's dramatic increase in enzyme efficiency, there is a slow increase in maturity of the enzymes approaching adult levels at one year.

  d. If a neonate is exposed to a liver enzyme-inducing agent (e.g., phenytoin or phenobarbital) during intrauterine life, however, the enzyme systems of the neonate may be near the adult level at birth.

TABLE 2-10. *Topical agents producing toxicity in neonates or small infants*

Agent	Effect
Hexachlorophene	Brain vacuolization
Iodides	Hyperthyroidism
Aniline dye	Methemoglobinemia
Naphthalene	Hemolysis in G6PD-deficient patients
Boric acid	Red lobster syndrome
Glucocorticosteroids	Adrenal suppression
Diphenhydramine	Toxic encephalopathy
Phenylmercuric diaper rinse	Mercury poisoning and acrodynia
Salicylate	Salicylate poisoning

4. ***Excretion***
   a. Renal function is incompletely developed at birth. The newborn's glomerular filtration rate is **35% to 50% that of older children and adults** (in the newborn it is 10 mL/min/m^2; in the adult it is 70 mL/min/m^2 or about 100 L/m^2/day) (11).
   b. The tubular function (both secretory and absorptive capacities) of the newborn's kidney is decreased by adult standards. Some of the drugs that would be affected by this immaturity are salicylic acid, penicillins, and phenylbutazone.
   c. The pH of the newborn's urine is acidic, which allows reabsorption of the slightly acidic drugs, such as penicillins, furosemide, ethacrynic acid, phenytoin, phenobarbital, indomethacin, and chlorates.
   d. The newborn's renal plasma flow is only 20% to 40% that of an adult. Renal function quickly improves by four weeks of age. Full adult capacity may not be reached until the first year of life.

B. **Elderly.** Elderly patients are likely to develop toxicity from medications because of the following factors: altered pharmacokinetics (Table 2-11); greater use of multiple medications because of chronic disease states; greater potential for drug interactions because of increased drugs; and poor compliance or chronic confused states.
   1. ***Absorption.*** There is evidence to suggest that substances such as calcium, iron, and thiamine are absorbed less with increasing age. Physiologic changes such as an increase in gastric pH can lead to delayed gastric emptying. Clinically, these changes may have an effect in patients receiving anticholinergics and cyclic anti-

TABLE 2-11. *Age-related changes and effects on drug distribution*

Age-related change	Effect on drug distribution
Body water decrease	Drug concentration per unit volume increase
Change in lean body weight/fat ratio	
Lean body weight decrease	V_D for water-soluble drugs decreases
Fat increases	V_D for lipid-soluble drugs increases
Protein binding	
Albumin levels decrease	If highly bound (mostly lipophilic), free fraction increased

depressants due to delayed gastric emptying (9). Bioavailability has been shown to decrease with digoxin.

2. ***Distribution.*** Lean muscle mass decreases in the elderly, whereas fat increases by 20% compared to their original amount during their second decade of life (8,9). Total body water decreases 17%, extracellular water 40% and plasma volume 8%.

    a. Drugs or chemicals mainly distributed in muscle will result in higher blood levels if the dose is based on total body weight.

    b. Conversely for lipophilic drugs, the volume of distribution increases and there may be prolonged drug action.

    c. Plasma protein concentration, especially of serum albumin, also decreases. Clinically, this has resulted in the elderly being at increased risk of toxicity due to more free drug being present.

    d. Organ blood flow decreases, as does cardiac index. This may contribute to decreased absorption of high lipid-soluble agents or for agents that show high first-pass effects such as lidocaine. For a summary of age related changes in drug distribution (12,20), see Table 2-11.

3. ***Elimination***

    a. Hepatic blood flow decreases and thereby reduces the first-pass effect for drugs such as propranolol and lidocaine.

    b. Mixed function oxidase activity (cytochrome p450 pathway) decreases with age leading to reduced enzyme induction.

    c. Alcohol, barbiturates, corticosteroids, haloperidol, phenacetin, estrogens, testosterone, and chlordiazepoxide cause some limited enzyme induction in the elderly leading to a net decrease in metabolism.

    d. Renal plasma flow and glomerular filtration decrease up to 50% between 40 and 90 years of age. Effect is not predicted by creatinine alone because both production and clearance are reduced.

XII. Summary. Lipid-solubility increases the volume of distribution of diazepam, lidocaine, and amitriptyline. **Intracellular water** decreases the V_d and the protein binding, which increases the free drug in those drugs over 90% protein bound. Liver extraction decreases phase I reaction oxidation (diazepam and phenytoin accumulate). A decrease in the glomerular filtration rate (GFR) increases lithium, aminoglycosides, and *N*-acetylprocainamide (NAPA) metabolite of procainamide. **In overdose and poisoning,** the pharmacokinetics are disturbed. The absorption may be delayed and prolonged, the half-life lengthened, the liver enzymes saturated (thus slowing elimination), the volume of distribution altered, and the body clearance lengthened. These kinetic effects may be even further distorted by poor perfusion of liver and kidneys. Multiple drug overdoses introduce the possibilities of dangerous interactions. Nevertheless, the pharmacokinetics serve as a focus of determining vital toxicologic information such as time of onset, duration of action, and peak action. The bioavailability may influence the degree of toxicity of the ingested dose, food may delay absorption, metabolites produced by the liver may prolong toxicity, and renal dysfunction may prolong excretion of substances excreted primarily by the kidneys. Treatment modalities, such as repeated doses of activated charcoal, changing the pH of the blood for protein binding, or the pH in the urine, are beneficial techniques commonly used in toxicology. Pharmacokinetic parameters such as volume of distribution and protein binding can also influence the susceptibility of extra-corporeal measures to remove various toxins from the blood stream.

References

1. Gibaldi M, Levy G. Pharmacokinetics in clinical practice. *JAMA* 1976;235:1864–1867.
2. Gibaldi M, Levy G. Pharmacokinetics in clinical practice. *JAMA* 1976;235:1987–1992.
3. Stewart DJ, Inaba T, Lucassen M, et al. Cocaine metabolism: cocaine and norcocaine hydrolysis by the liver and serum esterases. *Clin Pharm Ther* 1979;25:464.
4. Hoffman RS, Henry G, Howland MA. Association between life-threatening cocaine toxicity and plasma cholinesterase activity. *Ann Emerg Med* 1992;21:247–253.
5. Hoffman RS, Henry GC, Wax PM, et al. Decreased plasma cholinesterase activity enhances cocaine toxicity in mice. *J Pharmacol Exp Ther* 1992;263:698–702.
6. Hoffman RS, Morasco R, Goldfrank LR. Human plasma cholinesterase protects against cocaine toxicity in mice [Abstract]. *Vet Hum Toxicol* 1993;35:349.
7. Pippenger C. Rationale and clinical application of therapeutic drug monitoring. *Pediatr Clin North Am* 1980;27:891–925.
8. Roberts RS. *Drug therapy in infants: pharmacologic principles and clinical experience*. Philadelphia: WB Saunders, 1984.
9. Mofenson HC, Caraccio TR. Lidocaine toxicity from topical mucosal application. *Clin Pediatr* 1983;22:190–193.
10. Shnaps Y, Frand M, Rotem Y, et al. The chemically abused child. *Pediatrics* 1981;68:119.
11. Mofenson HC, Caraccio TR. General principles of pediatric pharmacology and pharmacokinetics. *Drug Protocol* 1987;2:9–25.
12. Lamy PP. Comparative pharmacokinetic changes and drug therapy in an older population. *J Am Geriatr Soc* 1982;30:511–519.
13. Merkel U, Sigusch H, Hoffmann A, et al. Grapefruit juice inhibits 7-hydroxyylation of coumarin in healthy volunteers. *Eur J Clin Pharmacol* 1994;46:175.
14. Anom. Grapefruit juice interactions with drugs. *Med Lett* 1995;37:73–74.
15. Soons PA, Vogels BA, Roosemalen MC, et al. Grapefruit juice and cimetidine inhibits steroselective metabolism of nitrendipine in humans. *Clin Pharmacol Ther* 1991;50:394–403.
16. Bailey DG, Arnold JM, Spence JD. Grapefruit juice and drugs. How significant is this interaction? *Clin Pharmacol Ther* 1994;26:91–98.
17. Ducharme MP, Warbasse LH, Edwards DJ. Disposition of intravenous and oral cyclosporine after administration with grapefruit juice. *Clin Pharmacol Ther* 1995;57:485–491.
18. Honig P, Wortham MD, Lazarev LR, et al. Pharmacokinetic and cardiac effects of terfenadine in poor metabolizers receiving concomitant grapefruit juice. *Clin Pharmacol Ther* 1995;57:185–187.
19. Fuhr U, Doehmer J, Battula N, et al. Biotransformation of caffeine and theophylline in mamalian cell line genetically engineered for expression of single cytochrome p450 isoforms. *Biochem Pharmacol* 1992;43:225–235.
20. Schmucker D. Drug desposition in the elderly: a review of the critical factors. *J Am Geriatr Soc* 1982;30:511–519.
21. Weisman RS, Howland MA, Reynolds JR, Smith C. Pharmacokinetics and toxicokinetics principles. In: Goldfrank LR, et al., eds. *Goldfrank's toxicologic emergencies*. 5th ed. Norwalk, CT: Appleton & Lange, 1994:85–98.
22. Abdel-Magid EHM, Ahmed FREA. Salicylate intoxication in an infant with ichthyosis transmitted through skin ointment: case report. *Pediatrics* 1994;94:939–940.
23. Nimmo WS. Drugs, diseases and altered gastric emptying. *Clin Pharmacokinet* 1976;1:194–195.

Emergency Toxicology, Second Edition,
edited by Peter Viccellio.
Lippincott–Raven Publishers, Philadelphia © 1998.

3

Psychiatric Assessment and Management

Laura J. Fochtmann

Department of Psychiatry, State University of New York at Stony Brook, Stony Brook,
New York 11794-8101

I. During the toxicologic emergency, psychiatric aspects are integral to the patient's care. Many psychiatric symptoms and syndromes may be produced by toxic ingestions (1–3). Conversely, underlying psychiatric disorders may result in toxic ingestions. For example, depressed patients often attempt suicide via medication overdose. Thus, when dealing with toxicologic emergencies, it is important to understand the relevant aspects of psychiatric emergency assessment and management.

II. **Priorities during the initial psychiatric approach** to the patient (4–11).

    A. **Psychiatric assessment** should never preempt medical evaluation or treatment of the medical aspects of the toxicologic emergency.

    B. Whenever possible, obtain a **brief description of the case** before encountering the patient. This will allow adequate security and backup personnel to be summoned if indicated.

    C. **Search the patient and remove all potential weapons.** Also remove additional toxic substances that the patient may try to ingest even after entering the emergency department (ED).

    D. **Maximize patient comfort and dignity** while simultaneously maintaining safety for other patients and staff. Interview the patient in as private an area as possible, away from excessive stimuli, potentially dangerous objects, and family or friends. Always explain the rationale behind interventions even if the patient does not seem receptive or able to understand.

    E. **Professionals should be respectful and empathic,** not judgmental or punitive. Do not provoke the patient by arguing, challenging, or being sarcastic. Rather, use a soft and calm but firm tone of voice. Demonstrate your wish to be of help to the patient by words and actions. For example, to a patient who is beginning to pace about the area, one might say "You seem really upset right now, Mr. Jones. We want to help with what's bothering you. Would you like to sit down so we can talk?" An offer of food or drink is often useful for forging an alliance with the patient.

    F. Always **exercise caution and be alert for signs of potential violence** (threats or boasts of violence, tense body posture, loud speech, suspiciousness, hostility, or delusional beliefs, particularly about staff). Patients at particular risk for violence in the ED include those with a recent history of violence and those intoxicated with alcohol, cocaine, amphetamines, or hallucinogens.

    G. **Do not turn your back on the patient.** When not actively engaged in medical interventions, maintain at least an arm's length distance from the patient.

    H. **Convey the expectation that the patient will behave in an appropriate manner and that violence will not be tolerated.** For example, if a patient is beginning to become threatening, one might say "We can't allow people to get hurt here so we need you to get yourself back under control. Is there some way you'd like us to help you with that?" One can also emphasize to the patient that it takes strength to stay in control and thereby appeal to the patient's desire to show how powerful they are. If the patient does not respond to such verbal interventions and becomes violent, staff must be prepared to immediately restrain them (see **III.B.**).

    I. **Documentation** at all stages of the evaluation is crucial.

III.   **Ensure the safety of the patient and staff** while the medical evaluation proceeds.

    A. **Assess the need for one-to-one observation** while the medical evaluation is in progress.

        1. Patients who present to the ED after a suicide attempt should be observed carefully throughout their stay. A number of factors will determine whether additional staff should be assigned to stay directly beside the patient on a continuous basis. These include the layout of the area (open versus closed rooms), the patient's proximity to potentially dangerous objects, the density of staff, and the presence of at least one staff person in the area at all times. If the physician has any doubts about the ability of staff to observe the patient closely and prevent further attempts at self-harm, the patient should be placed on one-to-one observation until a thorough assessment of suicide risk can be completed. Any patient reporting continued thoughts of self-harm while in the ED should also be placed on one-to-one observation.

        2. On the basis of available history or observed behavior, patients believed to be at risk to themselves or others should be prevented from eloping from the ED until the medical and psychiatric evaluations can be completed. This may require stationing medical staff or hospital security staff outside the patient's room.

    B. **Assess the need for physical or pharmacologic restraint** while the medical evaluation is in progress.

        1. Unless there is an immediate danger of patient self-injury or harm to others, alternative approaches should be used before relying on physical or pharmacologic restraints. These measures typically include verbal intervention or one-on-one supervision by staff (11–14).

        2. **Clinical indications** exist for pharmacologic or physical restraint or seclusion in the emergency setting.

            a. To prevent clear, imminent harm either to the patient or to others when control by other means is ineffective or inappropriate

            b. To prevent significant disruption of the treatment program or damage to the physical surroundings (11–14).

        3. **Legal aspects of restraint**

            a. The Supreme Court decision, Youngberg v. Romeo serves as a constitutional basis for the use of seclusion or restraint prior to a violent act if a clinician concludes in good faith that an emergency intervention is required (13,15).

The Court stated "the decision {for seclusion or restraint}, if made by a professional, is presumptively valid . . . liability may be imposed only when the decision by the professional is such a substantial departure from accepted professional judgment, practice or standard that the person responsible actually did not base the decision on such a judgment" (16). In other emergency situations, courts consistently hold in favor of physicians who have treated when immediate care was needed to eliminate an imminent threat of death or harm to the patient or others (5).

    b. Each physician is also required to meet standards set by state statutes, institutional policy, and regulations of administrative bodies such as the Joint Commission on the Accreditation of Hospitals (JCAH) (17).

    c. Although much has been made of the concept of the "least restrictive intervention," there is no clinical consensus as to which method of restraint is actually "least restrictive" (18–20). Such determinations typically depend more on the staff member's subjective perceptions than on the patient's clinical needs (13). No specific legal precedent governs, but in *Youngberg* v. *Romeo* the court stated "it is not appropriate for the courts to specify which of several professionally acceptable choices should have been made . . . in determining what is reasonable, . . . courts must show deference to the judgment exercised by a qualified professional" (16). Thus, the physician's best judgment should determine which form of restraint to use with a particular patient (13).

    d. Regardless of which method of restraint is chosen, close **monitoring** by the physician and full documentation of the rationale for restraint are essential (11,14,21).

    e. **Documentation** should include a discussion of the emergent nature of the patient's condition and the risks and benefits of intervening (13,14).

C. Clinical guidelines for choosing a mode of restraint

    1. As a general rule, physical restraint should be utilized initially. This is particularly true with unknown or mixed toxic ingestions since use of additional pharmacologic agents may complicate the toxicologic picture.

    2. In some cases, restraint alone may sufficiently calm the patient so that further assessment can proceed.

    3. If the toxicologic ingestion has been identified and if the patient's behavior is escalating gradually, it is sometimes possible to convince them to voluntarily accept oral medications.

    4. Since medications require time to take effect, most individuals who are agitated enough to need some form of restraint will require physical restraint at least briefly. With extremely agitated individuals, pharmacologic and physical restraint may need to be applied simultaneously.

    5. The use of seclusion alone does not permit adequate ongoing monitoring of the medical aspects of the toxicologic emergency and therefore should not be used (5,13,14).

    6. Pharmacologic interventions are also indicated for extremely or persistently agitated patients since prolonged combativeness while in restraints may result in rhabdomyolysis (22), sprains, or fractures (5).

D. Procedure for pharmacologic restraint

    (1) As shown in Table 3-1, **a number of agents** are available that safely and effectively provide pharmacologic restraint of agitated patients (4,5,10,12,23–26). The selection of a particular drug should be individualized based upon patient characteristics and on the therapeutic and adverse effects of each drug class. For example, for a patient with psychotic symptoms or existing respiratory depression, a neuroleptic would be a more reasonable choice than a benzodiazepine. Drug selection also depends on the nature of the toxicologic emergency. One would not want to exacerbate a toxic ingestion by administering a medication of the same class. The advantages and disadvantages of the various approaches are discussed below.

2. Neuroleptics

  a. Choice of neuroleptic

    (1) In the toxicologic emergency patient, no indications exist for the use of low-potency neuroleptics such as chlorpromazine (Thorazine) or thioridazine (Mellaril) (37,47).

    (2) In comparison with high-potency neuroleptics, low-potency agents are associated with much higher rates of hypotension, greater decreases in seizure threshold and more anticholinergic properties (making them more likely to induce or exacerbate delirium) (29,48–50).

    (3) Although high-potency agents do have higher rates of extrapyramidal side effects (EPSEs) than low-potency agents, these can be treated with anticholinergic drugs such as benztropine (Cogentin) or diphenhydramine (Benadryl) (29,48). To prevent EPSEs, medically stable psychiatric patients are often treated simultaneously with an anticholinergic drug. This is not indicated in the toxicologic emergency patient because of possibly exacerbating an unknown anticholinergic ingestion. Also, patients who already have an anticholinergic loading from an ingestion would be unlikely to exhibit EPSEs and require additional doses of anticholinergic agents.

    (4) If added sedation is desired in the toxicologic emergency patient, benzodiazepines or droperidol are better choices than low-potency neuroleptics.

  b. Among the high-potency agents (haloperidol, fluphenazine, thiothixene), neuroleptic choice is largely a matter of physician preference, although **haloperidol** is most commonly used (25,29,51). The only high-potency neuroleptic with unique properties is droperidol (Inapsine). Although it is only approved by the U.S. Food and Drug Administration (FDA) as a preanesthetic sedative medication, droperidol has also been used to treat acute agitation (27,40,52–55). Its advantages over conventional high-potency neuroleptics are its somewhat more rapid onset of action, its shorter half-life and its sedative properties.

  c. Guidelines for neuroleptic administration in agitated patients

    (1) For treating agitation, the high-potency neuroleptics are generally given intramuscularly (24,25,29–31).

TABLE 3-1. *Comparison of pharmacologic treatments for agitation*

Generic (and trade) name/route	Usual dose (mg)	Time to peak level (min)	Elimination half-life (h)	Comments	Refs.
Haloperidol (Haldol)					
p.o.	5–15	150	15–37	Oral concentrate has better absorption than tablets and achieves peak concentrations almost as rapidly as IM injection.	27–38
i.m.	5–10	20	21	Administer every 30–60 min until sedated (maximum daily dose 100 mg).	
i.v.	2.5–10	<10	14.5		
Droperidol (Inapsine)					27,30,39,40
i.m./i.v.	2.5–7.5	<10	2.2	Administer every 30–60 min until sedated (maximum daily dose 40 mg).	
Lorazepam (Ativan)					27,41–46
p.o.	2–4	60–120	14.1	Administer every 2–4 h until calm.	
i.m.	1–2	45–75	15	Monitor respiratory function carefully during administration.	
i.v.	1–2	5–10	12.2		

Note: In elderly patients, begin at about half the noted dosages. Lower dosages should also be used in patients with hepatic dysfunction.

    (2)   Usual doses of **haloperidol, fluphenazine,** and **thiothixene** are 5 to 10 mg i.m. with dosages varying with patient age and size (5,25,29,31,56).

    (3)   The usual dosage of **droperidol** is 2.5–7.5 mg i.m. Doses may be given every 30 to 60 min with good control of agitation generally occurring after one to three doses. The usual maximum amount given in a 24-h period is six doses (25,27,40,52,54).

    (4)   Haloperidol and droperidol can also be administered intravenously, although the risk of hypotension is somewhat greater by this route. Here the usual dose is 5 to 20 mg/h via i.v. drip or 2.5–10.0 mg i.v. bo-luses (with a maximal administration rate of 10 mg/min) repeated every 30 to 60 min (35,37,53,57,58).

    (5)   With cooperative patients, oral concentrate allows more rapid and complete absorption than tablets (38). When given orally the usual dosage is 5 to 15 mg p.o. (29,38).

3. Benzodiazepines

    a.   Comparisons with neuroleptics for treating agitation

        (1)   In comparison to parental high-potency neuroleptics, benzodiazepines have a number of **advantages** (30,45,59). They lack extrapyramidal side effects, they increase (rather than decrease) seizure threshold, and they have a greater sedative effect.

        (2)   Their **disadvantages** are higher rates of associated cognitive changes, increased risks of respiratory depression, and slower onsets of action when given intramuscularly or by mouth (27,60–64). In addition, some studies suggest that parenteral benzodiazepines are associated with increased rates of nausea and vomiting (30,44), whereas neuroleptics have antiemetic properties (27,48,65). In some patients treated with benzodiazepines, paradoxical behavioral disinhibition may occur (27,51,66,67).

        (3)   In patients who are **acutely intoxicated with alcohol or sedative-hypnotics,** the cognitive and sedative effects of benzodiazepines are potentiated (68,69) and the duration of intoxication may be prolonged as well. **Chronic alcoholics and substance abusers** may be relatively resistant to the benzodiazepine's effects and require much larger doses of drug (70). Thus, in treating agitation in the intoxicated patient, benzodiazepines should be used with caution and high-potency neuroleptics may be a better choice. Concerns about lowering seizure threshold in alcoholics given neuroleptics seem to be theoretical rather than observed (56,71–73).

    b.   Choice of benzodiazepine

        (1)   Of the benzodiazepines, **lorazepam** (Ativan) has the best intramuscular absorption and is therefore, most appropriate for use with agitated patients (30,74,75). It also has a relatively short half-life and no active metabolites.

        (2)   In contrast, **diazepam** (Valium) has erratic i.m. absorption and multiple active metabolites some of which have long half-lives (74–76). The

resulting accumulation of psychotropic drug levels increases the risk of delirium in the toxicologic emergency patient. Thus, lorazepam is preferable to diazepam even when administered intravenously to circumvent problems with absorption.

(3) **Midazolam** has been suggested by some for treating agitation because of its ultrashort half-life (77,78). Because it has been associated with relatively high rates of respiratory arrest and confusion, midazolam use is not recommended (79–81).

c. **Guidelines for benzodiazepine administration in agitated patients**

(1) For treating agitation, lorazepam is usually given in a dose of 1 to 2 mg i.m. or 2 to 4 mg p.o. every 2 to 4 h. Although most patients are well controlled after two to four doses, psychotic patients may require a two- to threefold increase in dosage for eventual behavior control (30,44,45,70).

(2) Benzodiazepines can also be administered intravenously, although this method further increases the rate of respiratory depression. Usual dosages of lorazepam are 1 to 2 mg i.v. every 4 h until sedation is achieved (27).

4. **Other approaches to pharmacologic restraint**

a. **Barbiturates,** such as sodium amytal, have been used in the past with agitated psychiatric patients. Sodium amytal has a somewhat faster onset of action but no other advantages over lorazepam. Its narrow therapeutic index and tendency to cause respiratory depression are clear disadvantages. Thus, sodium amytal is not recommended for use.

b. **Combined neuroleptic/benzodiazepine treatment** (10,82)

(1) Combinations of haloperidol and lorazepam have been used successfully in agitated psychotic patients and in delirious cancer patients. The usual i.m. or i.v. dosages are 5 mg of haloperidol and 1 to 4 mg of lorazepam (46,58,83).

(2) Combination treatment seems to control agitation with significantly lower doses of neuroleptic and fewer apparent side effects.

(3) Given the need to minimize confounding effects of multiple drugs, this approach should be used cautiously in the toxicologic emergency patient if at all.

E. **Procedure for physical restraint** (4,8,11,14,82,84,85).

1. Before beginning the restraint process, the area should be cleared of all uninvolved people and sufficient staff should be gathered. Generally five individuals are required (one to restrain each limb and one to stabilize the head and prevent biting). Such a "show of force" is often helpful in and of itself in enlisting the patient's cooperation. All staff involved in a restraint should remove neckties, earrings, or other objects the patient could grab and use as a weapon.

2. Avoid physical pain or injury to the patient during the restraint process.

3. Do not continue to bargain with the patient once the decision to restrain has been made.

4. At a signal from the team leader, each team member grasps the assigned body part. Control of the patient is most easily achieved by immobilizing the knee or elbow joint of the respective limb. The patient is then carried to the bed or stretcher.

5. Restraints are now applied. Two major types of restraint can be used. Standard four-point restraints, made of leather or heavy vinyl, are used to immobilize the patient's extremities. The net or sheet restraint is a nylon net with padding at the neck and arms. Extremely agitated patients may require both net and the four-point restraints. Handcuffs are not appropriate restraints for prolonged periods. If continued restraint is indicated in handcuffed patients, standard restraints should be exchanged for handcuffs once adequate staff are available.

6. Once restraints are in place, blood can be obtained for laboratory studies and medications can be administered.

7. With any restrained patient, special care must be taken to avoid restricting the circulation to the extremities. Circulation checks should be performed every 15 min. In addition, care should be taken to preserve access to an intravenous site and maintain a patent airway. When sheet restraints are used they must not be so tight as to compromise movement of respiratory cage muscles.

8. The risk of aspiration is always of concern in the restrained patient. The best preventive measure is to avoid oversedation. With all restrained patients, continuous visual observation must be maintained. If vomiting or choking occurs, staff must be prepared to immediately loosen restraints and assist the patient. In avoiding aspiration, it is best to have patients lie on their sides. Unfortunately, it is difficult to keep a seriously agitated individual restrained in this position. Prone restraint is also possible, but respiration can be compromised in this position particularly with obese patients. In most psychiatric settings, patients are restrained in a face-up position, which is generally the most secure and comfortable for the patient (15).

9. Nursing care of the restrained patient should ensure proper hygiene, administration of fluids, and regular toileting (at least every 4 h).

10. Physician documentation of the restraint should include a description of the patient's condition, the need for restraint, special precautions, and plans for further monitoring.

IV. **Once the patient is medically stable,** the psychiatric evaluation can begin.

  A. The focus of the evaluation varies with the consultative question being asked. Psychiatric aspects of toxicologic emergencies generally fall into one of several categories:

    1. Assessing and treating **psychiatric symptoms secondary to toxic ingestions.**

    2. Assessing suicide risk in patients with toxic ingestions resulting from an **apparent suicide attempt.** Since it is not always clear whether overdoses are accidental or intentional, all overdoses should be considered suicide attempts until proven otherwise.

    3. Assessing the "competence" of patients who present with toxicologic emergencies and who **attempt to sign out against medical advice.** Although competence is a legal determination, the psychiatric evaluation *can* document the presence (or absence) of psychiatric disorders, psychosis, or cognitive impairments that would influence an individual's ability to understand the risks of leaving the emergency room and refusing treatment (15).

B. **If the patient is intoxicated,** serial mental status examinations are indicated. Any final decisions about psychiatric disposition can be made only after the acute intoxication resolves.

C. **Collecting relevant history**

   1. **Identifying information** should include the patient's name, age, race, and gender as well as the source of referral, if any.

   2. The **chief complaint** should be recorded in the patient's own words.

   3. The **history of the present illness** should be obtained and recorded in as much detail as possible.

      a. It should include information about the onset and duration of symptoms, as well as recent stressors or precipitants.

      b. In all patients, changes in vegetative functions (sleep, appetite, weight, libido, diurnal variation), activity, concentration, personality, or social or occupational function should be noted.

      c. Family members, friends, and other sources can provide important historical information, particularly when patients are uncooperative or have altered levels of consciousness. When consulting other informants, remember to protect the patient's confidentiality insofar as possible. In an emergency situation, informants can be consulted even without a formal release. If the patient's cooperation can be enlisted before contacting such sources, however, it often benefits the physician–patient alliance.

   4. **Psychiatric history**

      a. Age of initial psychiatric presentation

      b. Psychiatric hospitalizations

         (1) When

         (2) Where

         (3) Duration of hospitalization

         (4) Treatment received and response to treatment

      c. Previous outpatient treatment

      d. Current outpatient treatment, if any

         (1) Treating therapist (obtain therapist's phone number when possible)

         (2) Dates of most recent and next scheduled appointments

         (3) Current psychiatric medications and recent medication changes. It is also helpful to know the name of the prescribing physician if it is other than the patient's primary therapist.

         (4) Degree of compliance with medications and outpatient follow-up.

   5. Alcohol and substance use history

      a. Types of substance used

      b. For each substance used note the frequency of use, time of last use, route of administration, usual symptoms associated with use, and relation of use to current presentation

      c. History of treatment for alcohol or substance abuse or dependence

      d. History of legal or social problems associated with use

      e. History of past or current withdrawal symptoms

6. **Medical history**
   a. Although usually obtained during the medical evaluation of these patients, this should include significant medical or surgical illnesses, allergies, current medications (including over-the-counter preparations) and use of tobacco and caffeine.
   b. Pay particular attention to historical evidence that suggests medical conditions often resulting in psychiatric syndromes (i.e., thyroid abnormalities or neurologic disorders) or medications that may precipitate psychiatric symptoms (1–3).
7. **Family history**
   a. Suicide or suicide attempts
   b. Psychiatric treatment or hospitalization
   c. Depression
   d. Alcohol or substance abuse
8. **Relevant personal history**
   a. Living situation
   b. Marital/relationship status
   c. Children
   d. Educational level
   e. Employment status
   f. Legal problems, including current charges or court dates
   g. Baseline level of function and premorbid personality
   h. Insurance status
   i. The **possibility of abuse or neglect** should always be considered in children and adolescents.

D. **Mental status examination**
   1. The patient's **appearance and behavior** should be noted including the state of dress, grooming, and hygiene; degree of distress; attitude toward the examiner; level and stability of consciousness; level of psychomotor activity (normal versus agitated versus slowed); and the presence of hallucinatory behaviors, posturing, or abnormal movements.
   2. A description of the patient's **speech** should include its rate, rhythm, volume, amount, and articulation as well as an assessment of the flow of thought.
   3. Both the patient's subjective description of their **mood** and the examiner's assessment of the apparent mood should be noted.
   4. The range, stability, and appropriateness of the patient's **affect** should be described.
   5. The presence or absence of auditory, visual, or tactile **hallucinations** should be documented.
   6. A description of the patient's **thought content** should address the presence or absence of:
      a. **Delusions**
         (1) These may be delusions of grandeur, persecution, reference (believing that other people, objects, or events refer specifically to them), or passivity (believing that the mind or body is being controlled by some external force).

       (2)   Other delusional beliefs most commonly seen with depressive disorders include delusions of poverty, somatic delusions, or delusional guilt or self-blame.

       (3)   Thought insertion, thought withdrawal, and thought broadcasting are more commonly seen with schizophrenic patients. These terms refer to the patient's perceptions that thoughts which are not their own are being put into their minds, taken from their minds, or broadcast over the television, radio, or loudspeakers.

  b.   **Suicidal ideation.**

       (1)   Suicidal ideation may fall anywhere on a continuum ranging from no thoughts of self-harm, to nonspecific thoughts of death, to thoughts of self-harm without suicidal intentions, to vague thoughts of suicide without a clear plan, to clear-cut suicidal ideation with both a plan and an intention to carry it out.

       (2)   With patients who have made **suicide attempts** or have **current suicidal thoughts,** determine whether a current plan for suicide is present and whether the patient intends to act on it. If the patient does have a suicide plan, its availability and degree of lethality should be assessed.

       (3)   Also important are the patient's degree of hopelessness about the future and whether he or she has begun to make preparations for death, such as writing a suicide note or putting affairs in order.

       (4)   The examiner should also identify whether the suicidal impulses are related to hallucinatory experiences or delusional beliefs.

  c.   **Homicidal ideation.** As with suicidal ideation, the examiner should establish the specificity of any plan, the degree of intention to carry out the plan, the availability and relative lethality of the plan and the relation between the homicidal ideas and any psychotic symptoms the patient is experiencing.

  d.   Assessing the patient for **obsessions, compulsions, or phobias** is part of the formal evaluation of mental state but is rarely relevant to patients presenting with toxicologic emergencies.

7. **Cognitive examination** should at least include an assessment of **orientation, memory function, and attention and concentration.**

  a.   Memory may be assessed by formal testing of registration, recent recall, and remote memory. In less cooperative patients, a general sense of memory function is provided by their ability to recall relevant historical details.

  b.   Concentration and attention can be assessed through simple calculations, serial 3's or 7's or spelling words forward and then backward. A more gross assessment of concentration can be obtained by noting whether the patient requires frequent repetitions of questions.

  c.   In cases where serial examinations of cognitive function are indicated, formal tests are useful (86). Examples of brief tests with quantifiable results are the Mini-Mental Status Examination (87) and the Cognitive Capacity Screening Examination (88). Both tests include assessments of orientation, cognitive processing, immediate recall, recent memory, and language. In addition, the

Mini-Mental Status Examination assesses attention and registration, visuo-motor function, and praxis (87).

8. The patient's **insight and judgment** should be described particularly as it relates to the appropriateness of recent behavior, the presence of illness, the need for treatment, and the potential for dangerousness to self or others.

V. **Recommendations** made on the basis of the psychiatric evaluation depend on whether the patient requires medical inpatient treatment.

A. **If the patient is being medically admitted,** the key question to be addressed is whether the patient requires one-to-one observation on the medical service. This determination depends on the degree of suicidal risk (see **V. B. 1. a**), the level of agitation, and the environment and staffing intensity on the unit where the patient is admitted. For example, patients admitted to an intensive care unit rarely need an additional order for one-to-one observation. However, as a general rule, a patient with a suicidal ingestion serious enough to require inpatient medical treatment should be placed under continuous observation.

B. **If the patient is medically ready for discharge,** the key issue is whether the patient requires psychiatric admission. Crucial determinants in making such a decision include:

1. **Is the patient at significant risk for suicide?**

   a. **Risk factors for suicide** (89–93)

      (1) Patients with a **psychiatric diagnosis** of major affective disorder comprise about 65% of completed suicides (89,91,94–97), with suicide generally occurring during the depressive phase of the illness. Patients with alcoholism or substance abuse comprise 25% of completed suicides (91,96,98). In suicide completers under the age of 30, the incidence of substance abuse is even higher (53% in one study) (99,100). In alcohol or substance abusers, completed suicides are frequently precipitated by recent losses (98,101). Schizophrenic patients are also at increased risk (91,102,103). Those who commit suicide are typically young, single, white men who use highly lethal methods and fail to communicate their suicidal intent.

      (2) The presence of **psychotic symptoms** increases risk, particularly in patients with a diagnosis of psychotic depression or in those with command hallucinations instructing them to harm or kill themselves.

      (3) In general, suicide risk increases with increasing **age** (89–92). Recently, increases in suicide rates have been seen among adolescents and young adults. Young adult suicide completers are increasingly using firearms in their attempts (104). Rates of alcohol and substance abuse are also increased in this population (99).

      (4) **Marital status** influences suicide risk with greater suicide rates in single patients than in married individuals.

      (5) **Gender** is an additional determinant. Females attempt suicide three times more frequently than men, but males complete suicide three times more often than females (91,92,105,106). Males tend to use more lethal methods of suicide (hanging, jumping, firearms) than females (107).

    (6) **Race** is a factor, with suicide rates being greater among whites (91,92,106).

    (7) **Concurrent medical illnesses** are associated with increased rates of suicide (108). This is particularly true of illnesses that are terminal or associated with chronic, unrelenting pain or disfigurement.

    (8) In both inpatient and outpatient populations, **hopelessness** about the future has been shown to be a long-term predictor of eventual suicide (109).

    (9) A **recent interpersonal loss,** a personal history of **previous suicide attempts,** and a **family history of suicide** increase risk (89–91,93, 98,101,110,111).

b. With patients who have made **actual suicide attempts,** assessment of their current risk depends on a number of additional factors.

    (1) What was the actual and intended lethality of the attempt? Highly lethal methods or intent place the patient at higher risk (93).

    (2) What was the patient's chance for rescue? This factor depends on whether others were present at the time of the attempt and if the patient was discovered purposely or accidentally. Weisman and Worden (112) have developed a quantitative suicide risk assessment scale which combines the probability of rescue and the risk of lethality.

    (3) Was the attempt impulsive or planned, with preparations made for death? Suicide attempts that are planned over extensive periods imply greater suicidal intent and are more worrisome in terms of future risk than those arising out of fleeting impulses.

    (4) Were drugs or alcohol used at the time of the attempt? This information alerts the physician to strongly consider an alcohol or drug abuse diagnosis, which increases risk. In addition, a true assessment of current suicidality cannot be completed until the acute intoxication has resolved.

    (5) Was the patient disappointed or relieved at the lack of success of the suicide attempt? Patients who are disappointed at still being alive are at persistent risk of further attempts even if they do not report active ideation.

    (6) Were suicidal threats or statements made before the attempt? What were the circumstances and manner in which these statements were made? Statements made in a dramatic fashion in the heat of an argument immediately followed by a dramatic but low lethality attempt generally connote low risk.

    (7) Have the precipitants to the suicide attempt changed as a result of the attempt? If so, the risk of further attempts is decreased. This is frequently the case after dramatic and impulsive suicide attempts.

c. **Guidelines for hospitalization decisions in suicidal patients**

    (1) Our current abilities to predict suicide are poor (113,114). Studies to assess suicidal risk factors are difficult because low base rates of suicide in the population yield high false-positive prediction rates. Thus, there are no clear-cut rules for psychiatric hospitalization of patients with suicidal features.

(2) Because the ability to assess suicide risk improves with experience (115), psychiatric consultants should be utilized whenever they are available. Psychiatric hospitalization (which has disadvantages as well as advantages) can often be avoided in cases with intermediate risk.

(3) If no psychiatric consultant is available, the emergency physician should err on the side of admitting patients with intermediate risk for suicide.

(4) As a general rule, patients who have current suicidal ideation with a highly lethal and available method or a high degree of intent should be admitted to the hospital.

(5) Likewise, patients should be also admitted who have made a suicide attempt with high lethality or intent, low probability of rescue, and high degree of planning before the attempt. Expressing disappointment about being alive after an attempt is also reason for hospitalization.

(6) Patients with psychotic symptoms (hallucinations or delusions) should be admitted even if they only display modest degrees of suicidal ideation. More moderate suicidal ideation is also an indication for admission of patients with an escalating pattern of suicidal behaviors or numerous other suicide risk factors. This is particularly true if the patient has a diagnosis of major depression or diagnoses of both substance abuse and another psychiatric disorder.

2. **Is the patient a significant risk to others?**
   a. **Risk factors for dangerousness** (5,12,14,116)
      (1) For psychiatric inpatients, an increased risk of violence is associated with a **psychiatric diagnosis** of mania, schizophrenia, mental retardation, or other organic disorder. In the outpatient setting, the largest number of violent individuals carry diagnoses of substance abuse or personality disorder. Many crimes are committed by criminally violent patients whose only psychiatric diagnosis is antisocial personality disorder. Nonetheless, violent behavior is seen in a minority of individuals with serious mental illness, generally in the setting of medication noncompliance or concurrent substance abuse (116).

      (2) The presence of **psychotic symptoms,** particularly persecutory delusions or command hallucinations, is associated with increased risk (117).

      (3) Risk is also increased by a history of **previous violence,** particularly if violence or impulsivity have recently escalated or if severe injury has been inflicted on others.

      (4) Other factors associated with increased risk include male **sex, age** in late adolescence or early adulthood, low **educational level, history of family violence** or marital or family disruption, income at or below the poverty level, and physically crowded or hot **environment.**

   b. As with suicidal patients, when **assessing the risk of violence,** it is crucial to consider the specificity of the violent plan, the availability of a method, the lethality of the method, and the lethality of violent intent as ascertained during the mental status examination.

   c. **Guidelines for hospitalization decisions in violent patients**
- **(1)** Like suicide risk, risk of violence is difficult to predict accurately. As with suicidal patients, however, general guidelines can be formulated regarding need for hospitalization because of dangerousness to others.
- **(2)** Individuals with a specific plan or available method and lethal intent are at high risk for violence and should be hospitalized.
- **(3)** Individuals with thoughts or threats of violence in the setting of psychosis or thought disorder generally require admission.
- **(4)** In studies of patient characteristics in those hospitalized for dangerousness, high impulsivity was highly associated with the need for hospitalization (118,119).
- **(5)** Specification of a particular victim by an individual with violent method or intent is a situation requiring additional action on the part of the physician. In the landmark *Tarasoff* v. *Regents of the University of California* decision, psychotherapists were stated to have a "duty to warn" a specific intended victim (120). At the rehearing of the Tarasoff case, this "duty to warn" was amended to a "duty to protect" others against foreseeable harm from dangerous patients (121). Part of this "duty to protect" includes some intervention on the therapist's part to decrease the risk of dangerousness by the patient. It may include hospitalization, medications, or more intensive outpatient treatment (122). The "duty to warn" is another component of this "duty to protect" and may involve giving specific warnings to the intended victim or to law enforcement personnel. In some cases, subsequent to the Tarasoff decision, this "duty to protect" has been upheld even without a specific intended victim named by the patient (123). In most jurisdictions, the Tarasoff decision does not constitute law and there are no clear legal precedents involving nonpsychiatrists. Nevertheless, the "duty to protect" has become a national standard of practice suggesting that this responsibility would extend to all physicians (13,82,124).

3. **Does the patient have significant psychosis,** indicating a need for admission?
- **a.** A high degree of disorganization may place the patient at an indirect risk of self-harm or make the patient unable to provide adequately for himself or herself.
- **b.** The magnitude of the psychotic symptoms or a lack of insight into the presence of psychotic symptoms may make it difficult for the patient to be maintained in the community or to pursue outpatient treatment.

4. **Factors that influence the need for admission**
- **a.** Strength and availability of social supports
- **b.** Presence of an established ongoing therapeutic alliance with an outpatient herapist
- **c.** Immediate availability of outpatient follow-up
- **d.** History of compliance with outpatient treatment
- **e.** Positive response to outpatient intervention in the past
- **f.** Presence of internal controls on behavior

C. If the patient requires admission, physician must determine whether the patient should be admitted **under a voluntary or an involuntary status.** This decision varies with the degree of risk as determined above and with specific state mental health statutes. Patients referred elsewhere for psychiatric admission should be medically stable and transported via ambulance. The name of the physician at the receiving hospital who accepts the patient must be clearly documented.

D. If the patient does not require psychiatric admission, he or she should be:

   1. Discharged with phone numbers for the ED and for local hotlines as well as appropriate outpatient referrals.

   2. Discharged with supportive friends or family members whenever possible and family members instructed to remove all potential weapons from the home.

   3. Discharged with prescriptions only under rare circumstances. If prescriptions are written, they should be in small quantities which would not be harmful in an overdose.

References

1. Anonymous. Drugs that cause psychiatric symptoms. *Med Lett Drugs Ther* 1993;35:65–70.
2. Frame DS, Kercher EE. Acute psychosis. Functional versus organic. *Emerg Med Clin North Am* 1991;9:123–136.
3. Popkin MK, Tucker GJ. "Secondary" and drug-induced mood, anxiety, psychotic, catatonic, and personality disorders: a review of the literature. *J Neuropsychiatry Clin Neurosci* 1992;4:369–385.
4. Tardiff K. Management of the violent patient in an emergency situation. *Psychiatr Clin North Am* 1988;11:539–549.
5. Rice MM, Moore GP. Management of the violent patient. Therapeutic and legal considerations. *Emerg Med Clin North Am* 1991;9:13–30.
6. Reid WH. Clinical evaluation of the violent patient. *Psychiatr Clin North Am* 1988;11:527–537.
7. Lane FE. Utilizing physician empathy with violent patients. *Am J Psychother* 1986;40:448–456.
8. Weissberg M. Safe strategies for recognizing and managing violent patients. *Emerg Med Rep* 1987;8:169–175.
9. Hughes DH. Assessment of the potential for violence. *Psychiatr Ann* 1994;24:579–583.
10. Tupin JP. The violent patient: a strategy for management and diagnosis. *Hosp Comm Psychiatry* 1983; 34:37–40.
11. Tardiff K. *Concise guide to assessment and management of violent patients*. Washington, DC: Amercan Psychiatric Press, 1989.
12. Tardiff K. The current state of psychiatry in the treatment of violent patients. *Arch Gen Psychiatry* 1992;49:493–499.
13. Simon RI. *Clinical psychiatry and the law*. 2nd ed. Washington, DC: American Psychiatric Press, 1992.
14. Fisher WA. Restraint and seclusion: a review of the literature. *Am J Psychiatry* 1994;151:1584–1591.
15. Lavoie FW. Consent, involuntary treatment, and the use of force in an urban emergency department. *Ann Emerg Med* 1992;21:25–32.
16. *Youngberg v. Romeo.* 457 US 307, 1982.
17. Joint Commission on Accreditation of Healthcare Organizations. *Consolidated standards manual*. Chicago: Joint Commission on Accreditation of Healthcare Organizations, 1991.
18. Gutheil TG, Appelbaum PS, Wexler DB. The inappropriateness of "least restrictive alternative" analysis for involuntary procedures with the institutionalized mentally ill. *J Psychiatr Law* 1983;11:7–17.
19. Perr IN. The most beneficial alternative: a counterpoint to the least restrictive alternative. *Bull Am Acad Psychiatry Law* 1978;6:4–8.
20. Wexler DB. Seclusion and restraint: lessons from law, psychiatry, and psychology. *Int J Law Psychiatry* 1982;5:285–294.
21. American Psychiatric Association Task Force. *Seclusion and restraint: the psychiatric uses*. Washington, DC: American Psychiatric Association, 1985.
22. Jermain DM, Crismon ML. Psychotropic drug-related rhabdomyolysis. *Ann Pharmacother* 1992;26:948–954.
23. Tesar GE. The agitated patient. Part II: pharmacologic treatment. *Hosp Comm Psychiatry* 1993;44:627–629.
24. Jacobs D. Psychopharmacologic management of the psychiatric emergency patient. *Gen Hosp Psychiatry* 1984;6:203–210.
25. Dubin WR, Feld JA. Rapid tranquilization of the violent patient. *Am J Emerg Med* 1989;7:313–320.

26. Dubin WR, Weiss KJ, Dorn JM. Pharmacotherapy of psychiatric emergencies. *J Clin Psychopharmacol* 1986;6:210–222.
27. Crippen DW. The role of sedation in the ICU patient with pain and agitation. *Crit Care Clin* 1990;6:369–392.
28. Fernandez F, et al. Treatment of severe, refractory agitation with a haloperidol drip. *J Clin Psychiatry* 1988;49:239–241.
29. Milton GV, Jann MW. Emergency treatment of psychotic symptoms. Pharmacokinetic considerations for antipsychotic drugs. *Clin Pharmacokinet* 1995;28:494–504.
30. Dubin WR. Rapid tranquilization: antipsychotics or benzodiazepines? *J Clin Psychiatry* 1988;49:5–12.
31. Donlon PT, Hopkin J, Tupin J.P. Overview: efficacy and safety of the rapid neuroleptization method with injectable haloperidol. *Am J Psychiatry* 1979;136:273–278.
32. Forsman A, Ohman R. Pharmacokinetic studies on haloperidol in man. *Curr Ther Res* 1976;20:319–336.
33. Froemming JS, et al. Pharmacokinetics of haloperidol. *Clin Pharmacokinet* 1989;17:396–423.
34. Holley FO, et al. Haloperidol kinetics after oral and intravenous doses. *Clin Pharmacol Ther* 1983;33:477–484.
35. Dudley DL, Rowlett DB, Loebel PJ. Emergency use of intravenous haloperidol. *Gen Hosp Psychiatry* 1979;1:240–246.
36. Cressman WA, et al. Plasma level profile of haloperidol in man following intramuscular administration. *Eur J Clin Pharmacol* 1974;7:99–103.
37. Moulaert P. Treatment of acute nonspecific delirium with i.v. haloperidol in surgical intensive care patients. *Acta Anaesthesiol Belg* 1989;40:183–186.
38. Dubin WR, et al. Rapid tranquilization: the efficacy of oral concentrate. *J Clin Psychiatry* 1985;46:475–478.
39. Cressman WA, Plostnieks J, Johnson PC. Absorption, metabolism and excretion of droperidol by human subjects following intramuscular and intravenous administration. *Anesthesiology* 1973;38:363–369.
40. Resnick M, Burton BT. Droperidol vs. haloperidol in the initial management of acutely agitated patients. *J Clin Psychiatry* 1984;45:298–299.
41. Greenblatt DJ. Clinical pharmacokinetics of oxazepam and lorazepam. *Clin Pharmacokinet* 1981;6:89–105.
42. Greenblatt DJ, et al. Pharmacokinetics and bioavailability of intravenous, intramuscular, and oral lorazepam in humans. *J Pharm Sci* 1979;68:57–63.
43. Greenblatt DJ, et al. Clinical pharmacokinetics of lorazepam. II. Intramuscular injection. *Clin Pharmacol Ther* 1977;21:222–230.
44. Modell JG. Further experience and observations with lorazepam in the management of behavioral agitation. *J Clin Psychopharmacol* 1986;6:385–387.
45. Salzman C, et al. Parenteral lorazepam versus parenteral haloperidol for the control of psychotic disruptive behavior. *J Clin Psychiatry* 1991;52:177–180.
46. Salzman C, et al. Benzodiazepines combined with neuroleptics for management of severe disruptive behavior. *Psychosomatics* 1986;27:17–22.
47. Shy KE, Rund DA. Psychotropic medications. In: Tintinalli JE, Ruiz E, Krome RL, eds. *Emergency medicine: a comprehensive study guide.* McGraw-Hill: New York, 1996 pp. 1340–1344.
48. Schwartz JT, Brotman AW. A clinical guide to antipsychotic drugs. *Drugs* 1992;44:981–992.
49. Oliver AP, Luchins DJ, Wyatt RJ. Neuroleptic induced seizures. *Arch Gen Psychiatry* 1982;39:206–209.
50. Man P, Chen C. Rapid tranquilization of acutely psychotic patients with intramuscular haloperidol and chlorpromazine. *Psychosomatics* 1973;14:59–63.
51. Durbin C. Sedation of the agitated, critically ill patient without an artificial airway. *Crit Care Clin* 1995;11:913–936.
52. Szuba MP, et al. Safety and efficacy of high-dose droperidol in agitated patients. *J Clin Psychopharmacol* 1992;12:144–146.
53. Frye MA, et al. Continuous droperidol infusion for management of agitated delirium in an intensive care unit. *Psychosomatics* 1995;36:301–305.
54. Ayd FJ. Parenteral droperidol for acutely disturbed behavior in psychotic and non-psychotic individuals. *Int Drug Ther Newsletter* 1980;15:13–16.
55. Granacher R, Douglas D. Droperidol in acute agitation. *Curr Ther Res* 1979;25:361–365.
56. Clinton JE, et al. Haloperidol for sedation of disruptive emergency patients. *Ann Emerg Med* 1987;16:319–322.
57. Seneff MG, Mathews RA. Use of haloperidol infusions to control delirium in critically ill adults. *Ann Pharmacother* 1995;29:690–693.
58. Menza MA, et al. Controlled study of extrapyramidal reactions in the management of delirious, medically ill patients: intravenous haloperidol versus intravenous haloperidol plus benzodiazepines. *Heart Lung* 1988;17:238–241.
59. Lenox RH, et al. Adjunctive treatment of manic agitation with lorazepam versus haloperidol: a double-blind study. *J Clin Psychiatry* 1992;53:47–52.
60. Scharf MB, et al. Differential amnestic properties of short- and long-acting benzodiazepines. *J Clin Psychiatry* 1984;45:51–53.

61. King DJ. Psychomotor impairment and cognitive disturbances induced by neuroleptics. *Acta Psychiatr Scand Suppl* 1994;380:53–58.
62. Gudex C. Adverse effects of benzodiazepines. *Soc Sci Med* 1991;33:587–596.
63. Lister RG, et al. Clinical relevance of effects of benzodiazepines on learning and memory. *Psychopharmacol Ser* 1988;6:117–127.
64. Plasky P, Marcus L, Salzman C. Effects of psychotropic drugs on memory: part 2. *Hosp Comm Psychiatry* 1988;39:501–502.
65. Roberts CJ, Millar JM, Goat VA. The antiemetic effectiveness of droperidol during morphine patient-controlled analgesia. *Anaesthesia* 1995;50:559–562.
66. Gardos G. Disinhibition of behavior by antianxiety drugs. *Psychosomatics* 1980;21:1025–1026.
67. Little JD, Taghavi EH. Disinhibition after lorazepam augmentation of antipsychotic medication. *Am J Psychiatry* 1991;148:1099–1100.
68. Hollister LE. Interactions between alcohol and benzodiazepines. *Recent Dev Alcohol* 1990;8:233–239.
69. Mattila MJ, Aranko K, Seppala T. Acute effects of buspirone and alcohol on psychomotor skills. *J Clin Psychiatry* 1982;43:56–61.
70. Modell JG, Lenox RH, Weiner S. Inpatient clinical trial of lorazepam for the management of manic agitation. *J Clin Psychopharmacol* 1985;5:109–113.
71. Benforado JM, Houden D. The use of haloperidol to control agitation/violence during admission to an alcohol detoxification center. *Curr Alcoholism* 1979;7:331–338.
72. Palestine ML, Alatorre E. Control of acute alcoholic withdrawal symptoms: a comparative study of haloperidol and chlordiazepoxide. *Curr Ther Res* 1976;20:289–299.
73. Lenehan GP, Gastfriend DR, Stetler C. Use of haloperidol in the management of agitated or violent, alcohol-intoxicated patients in the emergency department: a pilot study. *J Emerg Nurs* 1985;11:72–79.
74. Greenblatt DJ, et al. Kinetic and dynamic study of intravenous lorazepam: comparison with intravenous diazepam. *J Pharmacol Exp Ther* 1989;250:134–140.
75. Peppers MP. Benzodiazepines for alcohol withdrawal in the elderly and in patients with liver disease. *Pharmacotherapy* 1996;16:49–58.
76. Divoll M, et al. Absolute bioavailability of oral and intramuscular diazepam: effects of age and sex. *Anesth Analg* 1983;62:1–8.
77. Mendoza R, et al. Midazolam in acute psychotic patients with hyperarousal. *J Clin Psychiatry* 1987;48:291–292.
78. Wyant M, et al. The use of midazolam in acutely agitated psychiatric patients. *Psychopharmacol Bull* 1990;26:126–129.
79. Graham MA. Misuse of midazolam. *J Clin Psychiatry* 1988;49:244.
80. Taylor JW, Simon KB. Possible intramuscular midazolam-associated cardiorespiratory arrest and death. *DICP* 1990;24:695–697.
81. Boxed warning added to midazolam labeling. *FDA Bull* 1988;18:15–16.
82. Dwyer B. Safe strategies for recognizing and managing violent patients. *Emerg Med Rep* 1987;8:169.
83. Garza-Trevino ES, et al. Efficacy of combinations of intramuscular antipsychotics and sedative-hypnotics for control of psychotic agitation. *Am J Psychiatry* 1989;146:1598–1601.
84. American Psychiatric Association. *The psychiatric uses of seclusion and restraint.* Washington, DC: American Psychiatric Association, 1984.
85. Soloff PH, Gutheil TG, Wexler DB. Seclusion and restraint in 1985: a review and update. *Hosp Comm Psychiatry* 1985;36:652–657.
86. Baker FM. Screening tests for cognitive impairment. *Hosp Comm Psychiatry* 1989;40:339–340.
87. Folstein MF, Folstein SE, McHugh PR. "Mini-mental state." A practical method for grading the cognitive state of patients for the clinician. *J Psychiatr Res* 1975;12:189–198.
88. Jacobs JW, et al. Screening for organic mental syndromes in the medically ill. *Ann Intern Med* 1977;86:40–46.
89. Buzan RD, Weissberg MP. Suicide: risk factors and therapeutic considerations in the emergency department. *J Emerg Med* 1992;10:335–343.
90. Forster P. Accurate assessment of short-term suicide risk in a crisis. *Psychiatr Ann* 1994;24:571.
91. Hirschfeld R, Davidson L. Clinical risk factors for suicide. *Psychiatr Ann* 1988;18:628.
92. Moscicki EK. Epidemiology of suicidal behavior. *Suicide Life Threat Behav* 1995;25:22–35.
93. Hofmann DP, Dubovsky SL. Depression and suicide assessment. *Emerg Med Clin North Am* 1991;9:107–121.
94. Fawcett J, et al. Clinical predictors of suicide in patients with major affective disorders: a controlled prospective study. *Am J Psychiatry* 1987;144:35–40.
95. Goldstein RB, et al. The prediction of suicide. Sensitivity, specificity, and predictive value of a multivariate model applied to suicide among 1906 patients with affective disorders. *Arch Gen Psychiatry* 1991;48:418–422.
96. Hillard JR, et al. Suicide in a psychiatric emergency room population. *Am J Psychiatry* 1983;140:459–462.

97. Carlson GA, et al. Secular trends in psychiatric diagnoses of suicide victims. *J Affect Disord* 1991;21:127–132.
98. Murphy GE, et al. Multiple risk factors predict suicide in alcoholism. *Arch Gen Psychiatry* 1992;49:459–463.
99. Fowler RC, Rich CL, Young D. San Diego Suicide Study. II. Substance abuse in young cases. *Arch Gen Psychiatry* 1986;43:962–965.
100. Rosenberg ML, et al. The emergence of youth suicide: an epidemiologic analysis and public health perspective. *Annu Rev Public Health* 1987;8:417–440.
101. Rich CL, et al. San Diego Suicide Study. III. Relationships between diagnoses and stressors. *Arch Gen Psychiatry* 1988;45:589–592.
102. Breier A, Astrachan BM. Characterization of schizophrenic patients who commit suicide. *Am J Psychiatry* 1984;141:206–209.
103. Caldwell CB, Gottesman II. Schizophrenia—a high-risk factor for suicide: clues to risk reduction. *Suicide Life Threat Behav* 1992; 22:479–493.
104. Boyd JH, Moscicki EK. Firearms and youth suicide. *Am J Public Health* 1986;76:1240–1242.
105. Canetto SS, Lester D. Gender and the primary prevention of suicide mortality. *Suicide Life Threat Behav* 1995;25:58–69.
106. Diekstra RF. The epidemiology of suicide and parasuicide. *Acta Psychiatry Scand Suppl* 1993;371:9–20.
107. Rich CL, et al. Some differences between men and women who commit suicide. *Am J Psychiatry* 1988;145:718–722.
108. Mackenzie T, Popkin M. Suicide in the medical patient. *Int J Psychiatry Med* 1987;17:3–20.
109. Beck AT. Hopelessness as a predictor of eventual suicide. *Ann NY Acad Sci* 1986;487:90–96.
110. Heikkinen M, Aro H, Lonnqvist J. Recent life events, social support and suicide. *Acta Psychiatry Scand Suppl* 1994;377:65–72.
111. Murphy GE, Wetzel RD. Family history of suicidal behavior among suicide attempters. *J Nerv Ment Dis* 1982; 170:86–90.
112. Weisman AD, Worden JW. Risk-rescue rating in suicide assessment. *Arch Gen Psychiatry* 1972;26:553–560.
113. Murphy GE. The prediction of suicide: why is it so difficult? *Am J Psychother* 1984;38:341–349.
114. Pokorny AD. Prediction of suicide in psychiatric patients. Report of a prospective study. *Arch Gen Psychiatry* 1983;40:249–257.
115. Meyerson AT, et al. Influence of experience on major clinical decisions. Training implications. *Arch Gen Psychiatry* 1979;36:423–427.
116. Torrey EF. Violent behavior by individuals with serious mental illness. *Hosp Comm Psychiatry* 1994;45:653–662.
117. Junginger J. Command hallucinations and the prediction of dangerousness. *Psychiatr Serv* 1995;46:911–914.
118. Segal SP, et al. Civil commitment in the psychiatric emergency room. III. Disposition as a function of mental disorder and dangerousness indicators. *Arch Gen Psychiatry* 1988;45:759–763.
119. Mezzich JE, et al. Symptoms and hospitalization decisions. *Am J Psychiatry* 1984;141:764–769.
120. *Tarasoff v. Regents of the University of California.* 17 Cal 3d 425, 131 Cal Rptr 14, 551 P 2d 334, 1976.
121. *Tarasoff v. Regents of the University of California.* 17 Cal 3d at 440–41, 551 P 2d at 347, 167 Cal Rptr at 30, 1976.
122. Appelbaum PS. Tarasoff and the clinician: problems in fulfilling the duty to protect. *Am J Psychiatry* 1985;142:425–429.
123. Mills MJ, Sullivan G, Eth S. Protecting third parties: a decade after Tarasoff. *Am J Psychiatry* 1987;144:68–74.
124. Pointer JE, Small LB. Emergency physicians' duty to warn and protect: a critique and guidelines. *J Emerg Med* 1986;4:75–78.

Selected Readings

Hillard JR ed. *Manual of clinical emergency psychiatry.* Washington, DC: American Psychiatric Press, 1990.
Hyman SE, Tesar GE, ed. *Manual of psychiatric emergencies.* 3rd ed. Boston: Little, Brown, 1994.
Kaplan HI, Sadock BJ. Pocket handbook of emergency psychiatric medicine. Baltimore: Williams & Wilkins, 1993.
Simon RI. *Concise guide to psychiatry and law for clinicians.* Washington, DC: American Psychiatric Press, 1992.
Slaby AE. *Handbook of psychiatric emergencies.* 4th ed. Norwalk, CT: Appleton & Lange, 1994.

PART II

General Approach to the Poisoned Patient

Emergency Toxicology, Second Edition,
edited by Peter Viccellio.
Lippincott–Raven Publishers, Philadelphia © 1998.

4

Initial Evaluation and Management of the Poisoned Patient

Howard C. Mofenson, Thomas R. Caraccio, and Gerald M. Brody

*Department of Emergency Medicine, Long Island Regional Poison Control Center, Winthrop
University Hospital, Mineola, New York 11501*

All substances are poisons. There is none, which is not. The right dose differentiates a poison and a remedy.
—Paracelsus (1495–1541)

I. **Introduction**. The purpose of this chapter is to provide guidelines for the evaluation of the severity of an exposure to a potentially toxic substance, clues to the identity of the offending substance by its clinical effects on the vital functions, its odor and its effect on the skin, and, most importantly, how to initially manage the severely intoxicated patient. To accomplish these aims, the evaluation and identification have been presented separately from the management; however, these procedures obviously are often performed concomitantly.

   A. Any substance that can injure or kill a living organism is a poison. Exposure to a poison means to endanger by contact but does not necessarily indicate contamination. **Contamination** usually indicates the poison has entered the body and may interfere with biologic functions. **Overdose** means exposure to an excess amount, which may be accidental, intentional, recreational substance abuse, child abuse, or homicidal. The field of **medical toxicology** is concerned with the chemical and physical properties of poisons, the pharmacokinetics of toxic agents, the physiologic and behavioral effects of these poisons on humans, and the effective prevention and management of those effects. The **routes of exposure of poisons** include ingestion, which is the commonest route (79%), dermal (7%), ophthalmologic (6%), inhalation (5%), insect bites and stings (3%), and parenteral injections (0.3%).

   B. It is estimated that **4 million potentially toxic exposures** occur each year in the United States. According to the Office of Public Affairs, Centers for Disease Control, poisoning accounted for 11,894 deaths (including carbon monoxide) and 218,000 hospitalizations in 1988 (latest year available) (1). Poisoning accounts for 3% of total injuries but ranks fourth in the cost of injuries (1).

   C. **Hospital visits and admissions.** Poisoning makes up 2% to 5% of pediatric admissions, 10% of adult admissions, and 5% of ambulance calls. About 5% of hospital admissions of the elderly (over 65 years) are for drug-related disorders. In one urban hospital, overdoses and other drug-related emergencies account for 38% of the emergency department (ED) visits (2). Toxicologic emergencies admissions to the **medical intensive care unit**

(ICU) and a step-down medical ICU over a 3-month period of a urban hospital were 47 of 239 admissions (19.7%) (3).

D. Pharmaceutical preparations are involved in 40% of poisonings. The 1994 American Association of Poison Control Centers National Data Collection System Report on over 1.9 million exposures revealed that the number one pharmaceutical exposure is acetaminophen (4). **The leading pharmaceuticals** causing **fatalities** in 1994 were the **analgesics** with 205 (0.113%) deaths. Other leading causes of death are **tricyclic antidepressants** 175 (0.355%), sedative/hypnotics/psychotics 99 (0.166%), stimulant and street drugs 91 (0.312%), other cardiovascular drugs 90 (0.307%), and alcohols 76 (0.15%) (4).

E. Other fatalities in 1994 were due to gases and fumes 56 (0.154%), asthma therapies 36 (0.204%), automotive products 33 (0.25%), chemicals 26 (0.055%), hydrocarbons 26 (0.04%), antihistamines 23 (0.06%), and cleaning substances 22 (0.011%) (4). The number one poisonous killer is carbon monoxide which is not reflected in poison control statistics because it is not routinely reported to poison control centers (PCCs) (1).

F. Fewer than 1% of overdose cases reaching the hospitals result in fatality; however, some of these poisonings result in permanent disability. Patients presenting in **deep coma** to medical care facility, however, have a fatality rate of 13% to 35% (5). According to a study of 500 patients, the largest single cause of coma of unapparent etiology was drug poisonings (5). **About 25% of suicide** are attempted with drugs. Suicides represent about 10% of exposures but 60% to 90% of the fatalities.

II. Evaluation of the patient (Fig. 4-1)

A. Criteria for appropriate ED visit. PCCs avoid many unnecessary visits to EDs; however, it is important that medical insurance companies acknowledge PCC ED referrals without prior physician approval. The American College of Emergency Physicians has appropriate categories for these referrals under "threat of vital signs and mental status changes" and the "referral is from another source" (6-9). Tables 4-1a and 4-1b indicate the small amounts of medication that may be fatal in a 10-kg toddler (10). The **evaluation** of any toxicologic emergency begins with the initial rapid assessment and resuscitation if necessary; a secondary survey for infection, trauma, metabolic derangements or other problems; definitive care with continuous reassessment, monitoring, measures to identify the toxic agent, to prevent further absorption, to administer effective antidotal therapy (if available), and to enhance the elimination of the toxic substance; and to maintain vital functions; and the disposition of the patient. The evaluation starts with assessment of the patient's vital functions.

B. The initial assessment of all medical emergencies follows the principles of advanced cardiac life support. Determine the adequacy of the patient's airway, degree of ventilation, and circulatory status. Establish and maintain the vital functions. Vital signs should be measured accurately and frequently and should include body core temperature (Table 4-2).

    1. Airway—Ensure the airway and protect the cervical spine.

    2. Breathing—Assess ventilation and if necessary assist with bag-valve-mask and/or intubation. Administer supplemental 100% oxygen. Any unknown unconscious patient who requires assistance with a bag-valve-mask or a patient in shock should be intubated. All unconscious or shock patients benefit from intubation.

Exposure to Potential Toxin

Primary survey Identify life threatening problems and resuscitate

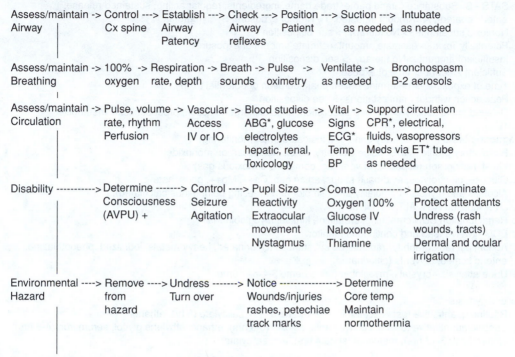

Assess/maintain -> Control ---> Establish ---> Check ---> Position ---> Suction ---> Intubate
Airway .... Cx spine ..... Airway .... Airway ... Patient ...... as needed ... as needed
.... Patency ...... reflexes

Assess/maintain -> 100% -> Respiration -> Breath -> Pulse -> Ventilate -> Bronchospasm
Breathing .... oxygen ... rate, depth ... sounds ... oximetry ... as needed ... B-2 aerosols

Assess/maintain -> Pulse, volume -> Vascular -> Blood studies -> Vital -> Support circulation
Circulation ...... rate, rhythm ... Access ...... ABG*, glucose ... Signs ... CPR*, electrical,
.... Perfusion .... IV or IO ..... electrolytes ...... ECG* ... fluids, vasopressors
.... hepatic, renal, ... Temp ... Meds via ET* tube
.... Toxicology .... BP ..... as needed

Disability ----------> Determine -------> Control ----> Pupil Size -----> Coma -------------> Decontaminate
.... Consciousness ... Seizure ...... Reactivity ...... Oxygen 100% ... Protect attendants
.... (AVPU) + ... Agitation ..... Extraocular ..... Glucose IV ..... Undress (rash
.... movement .... Naloxone .... wounds, tracts)
.... Nystagmus .... Thiamine .... Dermal and ocular
.... irrigation

Environmental ----> Remove ----> Undress -------> Notice ---------------> Determine
Hazard .... from .... Turn over ...... Wounds/injuries ...... Core temp
.... hazard .... rashes, petechiae ..... Maintain
.... track marks .... normothermia

Secondary Survey - History, complete physical, diagnostic tests

History -> "Ps" from Paramedics, Parents, Pals, Physician, Pharmacists, PMH, Allergies

Physical -> Examine wallet, clothes, shoes, hat, look for MediAlert bracelet necklace
1. Vital signs, general appearance, weight, temperature
2. Toxidromes recognized (depressant, stimulant, hallucination, anticholinergic cholinergic
3. Neurological -> level of consciousness (LOC), motor function/tone, focal sign cranial nerves,
   pupils (size, reactivity), EOM, nystagmus, dysconjugate gaze, fundi, corneal.
4. Cardiovascular -> pulses rate rhythm, volume; heart sounds, ECG monitor, perfusion (LOC, skin)
5. Respiratory -> rate, depth; breath sounds, chest expansion, air entry, odor on breath
6. Gastrointestinal -> oral mucosal burns, bowel sounds, tenderness, blood in stools
7. Skin -> tract marks, tatoos, bulla, moisture, color, warmth, burns, wounds, bleeding, rash, pressure sores.
   Mark on diagram of body.
8. Genitourinary -> bladder distention, rectal ot vaginal drugs, blood in urine monitor urinary output.
9. Potential toxicity -> time of exposure, estimate amount.
10. Need to know, toxcity, toxic amount, symptoms, onset of action, peak action delayed toxicity,
    duration of action, and management?

Call Poision Control Center

(continued)

FIG. 4-1. Exposure to potential toxin.

|

Evaluate Toxicity

Toxicity

1. SATS - **S**=Substance (brand name, trade name, ingredients, regular acting, sustained release, enteric coated), **A**=Amount ingested, **T**=Time of exposure, **S**=Symptoms
2. Nontoxic substance -> No therapy -> see disposition
3. Potentially Toxic -> estimate amount, estimate amount of exposure
   Insufficient amount ->No therapy -> see disposition
   Sufficient amount -> time of exposure
4. Time of exposure -> determine onset, peak, duration of potential toxin
   Peak action without manifestations -> see disposition
   Delayed onset toxicity -> delayed absorption, anticholinergeric action, produces toxic metabolite

|

Diagnostic tests (if not already done/or if indicated or for monitoring)

1. Respiratory profile - ABG, pulse oximetry, co-oximeter (carbon monoxide) chest radiograph (especially if vomiting, comatose or noxious gas)
2. Glucose, electrolytes, acid-base status, anion gap, Ca++. Mg++, phosphate
3. Alcohols and glycols - osmolality and osmolor gap (freezing point minus calculated).
4. Liver function AST, ALT, PT, bilirubin
5. Renal function BUN/creatinine, creatinine kinase, myoglobinuria
6. ECG - twelve-lead and continuous monitor.
7. Abdominal radiograph for radiopague substances (chlorinated, heavy metals, iodinized, phenothiazine, enteric coated, solvents (chlorinated)
8. Urine analysis - crystals, myoglobin (urine heme 3-4+, <10rbc

|

Toxicology tests

1. Routine quantitative tests : acetaminopen (4 and 6 hrs), salicylate (6 hr), ethanol
2. Specific quantitative tests anticonvulsants, digoxin (6-8 hrs), ethanol ethylene glycol, serum iron (4-6 hrs), lithium (stat, 6-12 hrs), methanol (state 4 hrs), and salicylates

|

Defensive Care

|

Frequent assessment - LOC, vital signs, temperature, ECG, urine output.

|

Administration of effective antidote

|

Decontamination

Syrup Ipecac - children > 1 year at home immediate, less than $\frac{1}{2}$ hour
Gastric Lavage - adults, less 1 hour with airway protection if necessary
Activated charcoal/cathartic - less then 2 hours
Whole bowel irrigation - sustained release, "body packers" and "stuffers"

|

Enhancement of Elimination

1. Multiple dose Activated charcoal initially with cathartic - (Phenobarbital, dapsone, salicylates, quinine, theophylline)
2. Alkaline diuresis (Salicylate, phenobarbital)
   Hemodialysis
3. Charcoal hemoperfusion

|

Observe for sequela

Stimulants, sympathomimetics, convulsive Substances - convulsion precautions
Intention - suicide precautions, cannot sign out

FIG. 4-1. *Continued*

Dispositions and Consultation

Holding area - Observe several hours past known onset and peak action

Admission - to floor, to telemetry, to intensive care, to psychiatry (stable and medically cleared)

Discharge procedures
1. Accidental -> preventive education
2. Substance abuse -> Treatment alternatives
3. Child chemical abuse -> Child Protective Services
4. Occupational -> Office Occupation Safety and Health
5. Food Poisoning - Local Health Department, Food and Drug Administration
6. Environmental Hazard - Hazmat unit, Health Department, Environmental protection Agency
   Intentional - Psychosocial evaluation

Key: *ABE = Arterial blood gases. CPR = Cardiorespiratory resuscitation. **ECG = Electrocardiogram, LOC level of consciousness, ET = endotracheal tube, AVPU = **A**lert-responds to **V**erbal stimuli, responds to **P**ainful stimuli, **U**nconscious

FIG. 4-1. *Continued*

3. **Circulation**—Take pulse and assess volume, rate and rhythm. Assess perfusion of the skin. Place on ECG monitor. Establish vascular access, and obtain blood specimens.
4. **Disability** (neurological status)—Assess level of consciousness by immediate AVPU scale (see **14.a**) and or later by Glasgow (Table 4-3) or Reed (Table 4-4) Coma scale or Severity of Stimulants (Table 4-5). Determine pupil size and reactivity, extraocular movements, oculovestibular response (assuming the C-spine is normal), motor response and focality, and pattern of breathing. Administer 100% oxygen, thiamine, glucose, naloxone.
5. **Exposure**—Complete exposure by removing clothes and other items that interfere with a full evaluation.

TABLE 4-1A. *Medications potentially fatal to 10-kg toddler if one tablet, capsule, or teaspoonful ingested*

Medication	Minimal fatal dose	Maximum unit dose available	Amount to produce potential fatality
Camphor	100 mg/kg	60 mg/5 mL	<1 tsp
Chloroquine	20 mg/kg	500 mg	1 tablet (500 mg)
Clonidine	0.1 mg	0.2 mg	1 tablet
Cyanide	—	—	—
Hydroxychloroquine	20 mg/kg	200 mg	1 tablet
Imipramine	20 mg/kg	150 mg	1 tablet (150 mg)
Quinine	80 mg/kg	650 mg	1 tablet (650 mg?)
Methylsalicylate	200 mg/kg	1,400/mg/ml	<1 tsp (7,400 mg)
Podophyllin	—	25%	—
Theophylline	8.4 mg/kg	300 mg	1 tablet/capsule (300 mg)
Thioridazine	15 mg/kg	200 mg	1 tablet (200 mg)

TABLE 4-1B. *Selected medications and their potential fatal amount in 10-kg toddler*

Medication	Minimum potentially fatal dose	Maximum unit available	Amount to produce potential fatality
MAOI	25 mg/kg	15 mg	15 tablets
Diphenoxylate (Lomotil)	30 mg/kg	2.5 mg	15 (120) tsp or (120) tablets
Codeine	15 mg/kg	60 mg	3 tablets
Pentazocine (Talwin)	45 mg/kg	50 mg	9 tablets
Dimenhydrinate (Dramamine)	25 mg/kg	10 mg	3 (25) tablets
Diphenhydramine (Benadryl)	25 mg/kg	50 mg	5 tablets
Elemental iron	60 mg/kg	60 mg	10 tablets
Orphenadrine (Dispal)	25 mg/kg	50 mg	5 tablets

Modified from Koren G. Medications which can kill a toddler with one tablet or one teaspoonful. *Clin Toxicol* 1993;31:407–413.

TABLE 4-2. *Important measurements and vital signs*

Age	BSA (m²)	Wt[a] (kg)	Ht (cm)	Pulse[b] (bpm resting)	BP[c] (hypertension) Significant	BP[c] (hypertension) Severe	RR[d] (rpm)
Newborn	0.19	3.5	50	70–190	96	106	30–60
1–6 mo	0.30	4–7	50–65	80–160	104	110	30–50
6 mo to 1 yr	0.38	7–10	65–75	80–160	104	110	20–40
1–2 yr	0.50–0.55	10–12	75–85	80–140	74/112	82/118	20–40
3–5 yr	0.54–0.68	15–20	90–108	80–120	76/116	84/124	20–40
6–9 yr	0.68–0.85	20–28	122–133	75–115	78/122	86/130	16–25
10–12 yr	1.00–1.07	30–40	138–147	70–110	82/126	90/134	16–25
13–15 yr	1.07–1.22	42–50	152–160	60–100	86/136	92/144	16–20
16–18 yr	1.30–1.60	53–60	160–170	60–100	92/142	98/150	12–16
Adult	1.40–1.70	60–70	160–170	60–100	90/140	115/210	10–14

[a]**A child's weight in kg** is about twice the age in years + 8.

[b]**Pulse range** in infancy includes crying vigorously and sound sleep. In general, a heart rate over 160 per minute is of concern when not vigorously crying. Pulse rates **over 220** are usually supraventricular tachycardia in children.

[c]**Blood pressure** (BP): The **childhood formula** for normal 50th percentile systolic systolic BP (SBP) for 2 to 10 years is 90+ (two times the age in years); below the 5th percentile, the lower limit of the SBP is estimated by the formula 70+ (two times the age in years). The diastolic DBP is normally two-thirds of systolic.

[d]Any **respiratory rate** of >60 or <10/min is abnormal at any age. Normal rates: infant rate 25–30/min; preschool 20/min; school child and adult 16/min.

bpm, beats per minute; rpm, respirations per minutes.

Modified from Nadas A. *Pediatric cardiology.* 3rd ed. Philadelphia: Saunders, 1976; Blumer JL, ed. *A practice guide to pediatric intensive care.* St. Louis: Mosby, 1990; AAP and ACEP Respiratory Distress in APLS Pediatric Emergency Medicine Course, 1993; Second Task Force on Blood Pressure Control in Children *Pediatrics* 1987;79:1; Linakis JG. Hypertension. In: Fleisher GR, Ludwig S et al. eds. *Textbook of pediatric emergency medicine.* 3rd ed. Baltimore: Williams and Wilkins, 1993.

TABLE 4-3. *Reed classification of the level of consciousness*

Stage	Conscious level	Pain response	Reflexes response	Respiration	Circulation
0	Asleep	Arousable	Intact	Normal	Normal
I	Comatose	Withdraws	Intact	Normal	Normal
II	Comatose	None	Intact	Normal	Normal
III	Comatose	None	Absent	Normal	Normal
IV	Comatose	None	Absent	Cyanosis	Shock

Modified from Reed CE, Driggs MF, Foote CC. Acute barbiturate intoxication: a study of 300 cases based on a physiologic system of classification of the severity of the intoxication. *Ann Intern Med* 1952;37:290.

    C. Certain aspects of the **pharmacokinetics (toxicokinetics)** of toxic agents should be emphasized.

        1. Drug absorption after a toxic ingestion may be delayed and prolonged.

        2. The half-life and total body clearance is often lengthened

        3. Liver metabolizing enzymes may become saturated slowing hepatic elimination

        4. Drugs with large volumes of distribution are often highly tissue-bound and measures to enhance their elimination are not very effective

        5. Poor perfusion of the liver and the kidneys secondary to the toxic effects of the substance may slow clearance.

    D. Toxic substances have **seven common major pathophysiologic mechanisms** that may produce symptoms

TABLE 4-4. *Glasgow coma scale*

Scale	Adult response	Score	Pediatric 0–1 years[a]
Eye opening	Spontaneous	4	Spontaneous
	To verbal command	3	To shout
	To pain	2	To pain
	None	1	No response
Motor response			
To verbal command	Obeys	6	—
To painful stimuli	Localized pain	5	Localizes pain
	Flexion withdrawal	4	Flexion withdrawal
	Decorticate flexion	3	Decorticate flexion
	Decerebrate extension	2	Decerebrate flexion
	None	1	None
Verbal response			
Adult	Oriented and converses	5	Cries,smiles,coos
	Disoriented but converses	4	Cries or screams
	Inappropriate words	3	Inappropriate
	Incomprehensible sounds	2	Grunts
	None	1	Gives no response
Child	Oriented	5	
	Words or babbles	4	
	Vocal sounds	3	
	Cries or moans to stimuli	2	
	None	1	

[a]Data from Seidel J. Preparing for pediatric emergencies. *Pediatr Rev* 1995;16:470.
  Other data from Teasdale G, Jennett B. Assessment of coma impaired consciousness. *Lancet* 1974;2:83; Simpson D, Reilly P. Pediatric coma scale. *Lancet* 1982; 2:450.

TABLE 4-5A. *Differential of structural from toxic-metabolic coma*

Feature	Structural coma	Toxic-metabolic coma
Pupillary response	Absent	Present (exceptions: atropine, glutethimide, hypoxia, hypoglycemia)
Brain stem compression Cranial nerve palsies	Present	Absent
Ocular-vestibular reflexes (doll's eye and Cold Caloric tests)	Absent	Intact (exceptions: large amounts of sedative-hypnotic, ethanol, anticonvulsants)
Focal signs Asymmetrical findings	Present	Absent
Rostocaudal progression Manifestations	Present	Absent
	Consistent (does not vary with each examination)	Inconsistent (varies with each examination)
Motor response	Spastic (exception: lower pons and medulla	Flaccid (exceptions: stimulants phenothiazines, glutethimide, methaqualone, cyclic antidepressants)
Temporal relationships		
Respirations	Retained until late	Lost early
Light reflex	Lost early	Retained until late

1. They may interfere with the **transport or tissue utilization** of oxygen (carbon monoxide, methemoglobinemia, cyanide) resulting in hypoxia, or decrease of an essential substrate such as glucose
2. They may **depress or stimulate the central nervous system (CNS)** and produce coma (opioids, sedative-hypnotics) or convulsions (sympathomimetics such as cocaine, amphetamines)
3. They may effect the **autonomic nervous system** producing anticholinergic action (belladonna alkaloids) or cholinergic action (organophosphate insecticides)
4. They may effect the **lungs** by aspiration (hydrocarbons) or systemically (paraquat)

TABLE 4-5B. *Rostocaudal progression with right supratentorial mass*

Anatomical level	Respiratory	Pupil	Oculocephalic	Motor
Upper diencephalic	Eupnea Yawns and sighs	Small reactive	Loss of fast nystagmus	R. appropriate L. hemiparesis
Lower diencephalic	Cheyne Stokes (CSR)	Small reactive	Loss of fast nystagmus	L. hemiparesi decorticate
Midbrain mesencephalon	CSR, hyperventilation (CNH)	Midposition fixed (unreactive) (MPF)	Dysconjugate (loss of medial rectus)	Decerebrate
Upper pons	CNH, ataxic	MPF	Dysconjugate	Decerebrate weak
Lower pons	Ataxic, eupnea	MPF/pinpoint	Absent	Flaccid
Upper medulla	Ataxic	MPF	Absent	Flaccid

CNH, central neurogenic hyperventilation.
Modified from References 67 and 68.

TABLE 4-5C. *Confused patient*

	Functional (Psychiatric)		Organic	
Feature	Mood	Schizophrenia	Delirium	Dementia
Focal neurological	No	No	Maybe	No
Asterixis	No	No	Maybe[a]	No
Onset	Gradual	Gradual	Acute	Insidious
Orientation	Normal	Normal	Disoriented	Disoriented
Level of consciousness	Normal	Normal	Fluctuating	Normal (early)
Attention	Normal	Normal	Impaired	Normal (early)
Hallucinations	Rare	Auditory	Visual	None/tactile
Memory deficits				
Short-term	Intact	Intact	Fluctuating	Stable
Long-term	No	No	Impaired	Impaired
Thought process	Grandiose	Complex	Simple rambling	Disorganized less incoherent
Delusions	Deprecatory	Elaborate		

[a] Suggestive toxic-metabolic encephalopathy.

5. They may effect the **heart and vasculature** producing myocardial dysfunction (cyclic antidepressants), dysrhythmias (quinidine) and hypertension (amphetamine, cocaine) or hypotension (calcium channel blockers, beta-adrenergic blockers, and phenothiazines)

6. They may produce **local damage** (caustics and corrosives)

7. They may produce **delayed effects** on the liver (acetaminophen) or the kidneys (heavy metals).

E. **Poisoning exposure routes** may be local, systemic or both.

1. **Local** (skin, eyes, mucosa of respiratory or GI tract) where contact is made with the poisonous substance or systemic where the poison absorbed into the body or both types may occur together. Local effects are nonspecific chemical reactions that depend on the concentration, contact time, and type of exposed surface.

2. **Systemic** effects depend on the dose, the distribution of the poison and the functional reserve of the organ system. Complications from poisons such as shock, hypoxia, chronic exposure and existing illness may also influence toxicity.

F. The patient with exposure to a potential toxin may be **asymptomatic** for several reasons. The substance may be relatively nontoxic; insufficient amount has been involved; or a sufficient amount has not been absorbed to produce toxicity at the time the patient was evaluated.

1. **Absorption** may be significantly delayed and prolonged after an overdose of drugs with **anticholinergic properties** such as antihistamines, belladonna alkaloids, diphenoxylate with atropine (Lomotil), phenothiazines and cyclic antidepressants. This anticholinergic property slows the GI mobility which delays the rate but increases the quantity absorbed and prolongs the effect.

2. **Sustained release preparations** also have delayed and prolonged absorption.

3. **Concretions** may form with certain substances such as salicylates, iron, glutethimide, and meprobamate, which can delay absorption and prolong the action.

4. Patients ingesting substances such as acetaminophen, *Amanita phalloides* type mushrooms, acetonitrile, ethylene glycol, lithium, methanol, methylene chloride, monoamine oxidase inhibitors, oral hypoglycemic agents, parathion, and paraquat may be asymptomatic until the parent compound is **metabolized into its toxic metabolite.**

G. **The asymptomatic patient** who has been exposed to a toxic substance should have decontamination procedures accomplished.

1. In the case of ingestion it is done by the induction of emesis, gastric lavage and the administration of single and multiple doses of activated charcoal (MDAC), or whole bowel irrigation. No procedure is routinely performed but is dependent on potential toxicity, age of the patient, time of ingestion and effectiveness of procedure. **If no attempt is made to decontaminate** the patient, the reason should be clearly documented on the medical record.

2. **Syrup of ipecac-induced emesis** should be tried only if the patient has ingested an agent that does not cause **rapid onset of CNS depression or convulsions** and ingestion has occurred in less than 1 h.

   a. Some of the agents that will produce **rapid onset of CNS depression** are ethanol, short-acting benzodiazepines (BZPs), short-acting barbiturates, short-acting nonbarbiturate sedative-hypnotics, short-acting opioids, tricyclic antidepressants.

   b. Some of the agents that will produce **rapid onset of convulsions** are beta-blockers, camphor, calcium channel blockers, chloroquine, codeine, isoniazid, mefenamic acid, nicotine, propoxyphene, phencyclidine, organophosphate insecticides, strychnine and cyclic antidepressants.

3. Most of the ED physicians prefer gastric lavage and/or activated charcoal (AC) as the major GI decontaminating measures. Inducing emesis is avoided because it removes less of the ingested toxin and interferes with administration of charcoal which adsorbs greater amounts of the ingested susceptible substance.

III. **Identification of patient and the toxic agent**

A. If there are no immediate life-threatening manifestations a careful **history** is obtained. The information obtained from the history is notoriously unreliable in intentional and abuse overdose situations. Corroborative historical information from additional sources is extremely useful and should be sought.

B. The use of the newspaper reporter's questions may provide an easily remembered format—who, what, when, how much, where, and why. The answers to these questions should be **temporally related and documented relative to the time of exposure** (e.g., the symptoms developed at approximately 0600 5/7/96 4 h postingestion). Any management should likewise be temporally related to the time after exposure. The basic information to obtain is **SATS: S** = substance (brand name, trade name, ingredients, regular acting, sustained release, enteric coated); **A** = amount ingested; **T** = time ingested; and **S** = symptoms (relate time ingestion to time of symptoms and what intervention has taken place.

1. **Who.** The first question should be "How is he/she acting now?"

   a. If **symptomatic** immediately send to a health care facility **with the original container.** However, the label may not describe the contents if the material is not in the original container. Multiple medications are frequently stored in the same bottle or in containers different than their original.

   b. If **asymptomatic**, one should obtain information that is **AMPLE: A** = age and allergies; **M** = current or available medications; **P** = past history of medical illnesses, substance abuse or intentional ingestions; **L** = time of last meal which may influence absorption; and **E** = events leading to present condition. Attempt to establish the time of exposure and onset of symptoms.

   c. Ask EMS personnel about the patients's symptoms and history in transport.

   d. If the patient is a female in reproductive years, ask about pregnancy and obtain pregnancy test.

   e. Medical alert bracelets and other indicators of important conditions should be sought.

2. **What** information includes the trade name, generic name, ingredients, formulation (liquid, solid, gas), manufacturer, and intended use of the substance.

   a. Check with pharmacy on the label for other drugs purchased.

   b. If information about the names of the product is unavailable ask about the substance or medications' intended use; the odor and color of the substance, the substance in the vomitus, the bowel movements and the urine and the odor of the patient's breath.

   c. What action has been taken to eliminate the poison?

   d. Ask about occupation and hobbies.

   e. Intentional ingestions are often multiple substances and frequently include ethanol, acetaminophen and aspirin.

   f. Street names and slang expressions are useful only if the name of the substance fits the clinical manifestations.

3. **When** information includes the time of exposure or when the patient was last seen. The time of exposure is important in estimating when the onset of the symptoms would be expected, when the peak action would be reached, and how long it might last. This is important in determining the timing for obtaining a blood sample for quantitative analysis and interpreting the plasma concentrations (see Table 4-29 below). "When" is important in the differential diagnosis. The onset from toxic-metabolic mental status changes is similar to vascular disease and starts in minutes to hours, CNS infectious disease onset is hours to days, compressive masses of the CNS onset is days to weeks and slow tumors and degenerative disease onset is months to years.

4. **How much** should elicit the amount of the exposure (a single swallow in a child is 0.3 mL/kg or approximately 1 teaspoonful, in an adult a tablespoonful or 15 mL) and strength of the poison (9). Container types may help in estimating the amount. The packaging is important. Perfumes come in small bottles and are often released a drop at a time. Sprays put out limited amounts. The estimated toxicity of a substance can be obtained from the Regional PCC.

5. **Where** and what the patient was doing brings into perspective accidental exposure possibilities such as detergents in the kitchen; perfumes (ethanol) in the bedroom, and hydrocarbons in the garage. Recreational substances such as marijuana and

cocaine are usually used in groups, but heroin can be used alone. Information about exposure to environmental hazards and occupational toxins should be sought.

6. **Why** refers to intent—accidental, intentional, therapeutic error, substance abuse. These questions may be delayed until a more appropriate time.

C. **Consult the Regional PCC** for the exact ingredients and the latest in first aid, advanced care, and follow-up management, even if familiar with the substance and its toxicity, because the first aid information on the labels of products are notoriously inaccurate, product ingredients change, and newer methods of management are constantly becoming available. Figure 4-2 is a typical PCC Record for obtaining basic poison information.

D. **In children,** exposures **under 1 year and over 5 years of age** should be viewed with suspicion. Poisoning under one year may be chemical maltreatment or child abuse (11,12). Tables 4-1a and 4-1b are of medication that are extremely toxic to children (10).

1. **"Accidental" ingestions** should be investigated in children, unless there is a reasonable explanation, under the following circumstances: over the age of five years; more than one episode of "accidental" ingestion; bizarre clinical manifestations which suggest "Munchausen by proxy" syndrome; and "accidental" ingestions under one year of age. In addition, necropsy of child abuse cases should include toxicologic analysis. Poisoning in a child over the age of 5 years may be a **"cry for help"** indicating an intolerable home situation (11,12).

2. **"Munchausen by proxy" syndrome"** is a factitious disorder in a child perpetrated by the parent. It has **four features**: illness simulated by parent or caretaker; repeated presentation of child for medical care that results in multiple procedures; denial by parent or caretaker of knowledge about cause of illness; and abatement of symptoms when the child is separated from parent or caretaker (11–14).

```
Name caller_____Age____Weight_____Date_____
Phone number _____
Substance Brand _____Formulation (slow release, enteric
sustained coated)_____
Ingredients _____
Amount _____
Symptoms (onset and progression in relation to time of exposure)
_____
_____
Time of call _____Time/date of Exposure _____
History of ingestion_____
Recent Medication_____
General Health_____
Therapy_____
Followup Times_____
Referral_____
Outcome_____
```

FIG. 4-2. Poisoning control information record.

IV. **Physical findings**. A thorough physical examination can help to confirm the suspected diagnosis and to detect the unsuspected.

   A. The physical assessment must begin with an analysis of the vital functions by means of documenting them (respirations, pulse, perfusion [capillary refill and mental status], blood pressure and core temperature).

   B. The **vital signs evaluation** is not just an analysis of rates and numbers but how effectively these functions are being performed. The examiner must have an understanding of the normal variants. They also may be clues to the diagnosis (Table 4-2). The physical examination focuses on the vital functions, cardiopulmonary function and neurological status. Evaluation of these parameters provides important clues to the toxic agent.

   C. **Document** the exact time of the examination (military time is preferred). The order of the examination may vary with the presentation. Examine clothing, shoes, hat, wallet and look for medical identification bracelets or necklaces.

V. **Guidelines for hospital disposition**

   A. **Classification as "high risk patients"** depends on clinical judgment. Any patient with the need for cardiorespiratory support or persistent altered mental status for 3 h or more should be considered as a candidate for intensive care. Guidelines for admitting patients over 14 years to an ICU, after 2 to 3 h in the ED, include the following (16):

      1. Need for intubation
      2. Seizures
      3. Unresponsiveness to verbal stimuli
      4. Arterial carbon dioxide pressure greater than 45 mm Hg
      5. Any rhythm except sinus arrhythmia
      6. Second or third degree atrioventricular block
      7. QRS greater than 0.12 s, in tricyclic antidepressant poisoning a QRS greater than 0.10 s and signs of toxicity.
      8. Systolic blood pressure less than 80 mm Hg.

   B. **Indications for pediatric intensive care** have been reported in 105 patients with poisoning: coma (n = 55), respiratory insufficiency (n = 15), ingestion of potential lethal dose (n = 13), cardiac monitoring for asymptomatic tricyclic antidepressant overdose or dysrhythmias (n = 6), convulsions (n = 5), shock (n = 1), hepatic failure (n = 1), and extreme agitation (n = 1) (16).

VI. **Definitive assessment of vital functions** (see Differential Diagnosis).

   A. **Respiratory system** (17–23)

      1. Assess the rate (tachypnea is increase in rate), depth (hyperpnea is an increase in tidal volume), pattern, ease of respiration and the presence of upper airway protective reflexes. Take respirations for a full minute unless apneic or ineffective respirations.

      2. In addition evaluate the work of breathing (accessory muscles, head bobbing in children, nasal flaring, retractions, stridor, prolonged respirations), auscultation of the peripheral of the lung fields over the apices and laterally for air entry (tidal volume 5 to 7 mL/kg).

      3. Note chest wall excursion and the presence of central or peripheral cyanosis. Cyanosis is a late sign of respiratory failure.

4. **Tachypnea** without distress ("quiet tachypnea") is usually from nonpulmonary diseases and is often an effort to maintain a normal pH by respiratory compensation. Tachypnea with distress indicates increased work of breathing and may be caused by aspiration pneumonitis, CNS stimulant intoxications, e.g., salicylates, withdrawal states or irritant fumes. Tachypnea and ineffective shallow respirations can coexist producing alveolar hypoventilation.

5. **Bradypnea,** shallow respirations and respiratory failure may be caused by CNS depressant intoxications, and opioids, paralytic agents, e.g., neuromuscular blockers, paralytic plant toxins, botulism, and paralytic shell fish.

6. **Wheezing respirations.** "Not all that wheezes is asthma." Foreign bodies, cholinergic agents, beta-adrenergic blockers, and irritant gases, and occupation hypersensitivity cause wheezing.

B. **Cardiovascular system** (24–33)

1. **Peripheral pulses** are a reflection of peripheral perfusion and allows estimation of the stroke volume, heart rate, heart rhythm, systemic vascular resistance and blood pressure (BP). Hypotension is a late sign of shock and means decompensation. The BP may not fall until more than 25% of the circulating blood volume is lost.

2. Early signs of **shock** are decreased pulse volume, discrepancies between central and peripheral pulse volumes and decreased skin perfusion, narrow pulse pressure, bradycardia and anxiety. A decreased pulse volume may indicate hypothermia, diminished cardiac output or shock.

3. **Skin perfusion** is lost first. This perfusion is evaluated by capillary refill (CRF) which normally is less than 2 s (3 s in adult females and 4.5 s for the elderly) (28,29). CRF does not appear to be as reliable a test in mild and moderate hypovolemia in adults and children (29).

4. **Sinus arrhythmia and extrasystoles** are common in healthy children and young adults.

5. Measure the heart rate a full minute unless absent or weak.

6. All poisoned patients deserve **ECG monitoring** for dysrhythmias initially and as soon as possible a 12 lead ECG is obtained to determine duration of the intervals and waves.

7. **Document** the method used to measure the BP (arm, auscultation, palpation or Doppler) and use the proper size cuff.

8. **Bradycardia** may be produced by excess cholinergic activity or depressed sympathomimetic activity (e.g., carbamates, organophosphate), vagotonic activity (e.g., cardiac glycosides), interference with release or depletion of the catecholamines (e.g., beta-adrenergic blockers, calcium channel blockers), damage or membrane depression of the myocardium (e.g., tricyclic antidepressants, quinidine) or increased intracranial pressure (e.g., vitamin A excess, outdated tetracycline), CNS depressants (e.g., sedative-hypnotic). Reflex bradycardia occurs with alpha-adrenergic agonists (e.g,. phenylpropamine).

9. **Tachycardia** may be produced by excess anticholinergic activity stimulation of release of catecholamines (e.g., amphetamines, cocaine), vasodilation or inadequate volume (e.g., nitrites), hypoxia, and withdrawal from ethanol or sedative-hypnotics.

10. **Dysrhythmias.** The correction of hypoxia and metabolic derangements (electrolytes, hypoglycemia, acid-base disturbances) will spontaneously rectify many dysrhythmias. Dysrhythmias may be due to sympathomimetic effects (e.g., cocaine), anticholinergic effects, CNS altered regulation of peripheral autonomic activity, direct effects on myocardial membrane (e.g., cardiac glycosides, quinidine, tricyclic antidepressants). Some substances lower antidysrhythmic threshold (e.g., halogenated compounds). A very dangerous dysrhythmia **Torsades de pointes** ("Twisting of the points") is dangerous dysrhythmia predisposes to ventricular fibrillation. It has been seen with terfendine and astemizole overdoses and interactions, quinidine and type Ia, Ib, Ic and III antidysrhythmics.

11. **Hypertension** rarely requires vigorous therapy, as it is usually only seen initially, is transient, and is often followed by life-threatening hypotension. **Hypertension with tachycardia** occurs with anticholinergic agents and CNS stimulants (e.g., amphetamines, cocaine). Naloxone has been reported to release catecholamines and produce hypertension. **Hypertension with bradycardia** may be caused by intoxications with agents that increase the intracranial pressure (24–27) (see Differential Diagnosis).

12. **Hypotension with tachycardia** are associated with true vascular volume loss, vasodilation due to loss of vascular tone (e.g., phenothiazine intoxications), depression of cardiac output and dysrhythmias that interfere with cardiac filling. Common intoxications that may cause early **hypotension with bradycardia** (e.g., beta-adrenergic blockers, calcium channel blockers) (26,27,31–33)

C. **Temperature** (34–43). Assess the core rectal temperature with an instrument to detect extremes of hyperthermia and hypothermia (not the classic glass thermometer which is not able to register the extremes of temperature).

1. **Febrile states** are regulated temperature elevations and develop secondary to a physiologic readjustment of the thermoregulatory set-point to a higher level. The most frequent cause is infection. Antipyretic medication acts to inhibit prostaglandin synthesis and reduce the temperature of infections. Antipyretic medications reduce these fevers.

2. **Temperature elevation** associated with toxicologic emergencies is unregulated temperature due to excess muscle activity, impaired thermoregulation, hypermetabolic state, interferences with oxidative phosphorylation, and impaired dissipation of heat. The autoregulatory mechanism is not functioning. This type of temperature elevation is referred to as hyperthermia or heat illness. It also occurs in anticholinergic, sympathomimetic overdoses (cocaine) and ethanol withdrawal. Toxicologic temperature elevations require external cooling measures and control of excess muscular activity such as convulsions. Antipyretics are not useful in these cases (34–41).

3. **Hyperthermia syndromes** are life-threatening elevations of temperatures. The syndromes all have altered mental state, rigidity, acidosis, and temperature elevation except the serotonin syndrome.

   a. A genetic **inborn error** of muscle metabolism on exposure to certain anesthetic agents, e.g., halothane and succinylcholine.

    b. The **malignant neuroleptic syndrome** (MNS), which is an idiosyncratic reaction in patients on neuroleptic medication (phenothiazines and butyro-phenones) (35).

    c. **Malignant hyperthermia** (MH) is associated with drug interactions as when some synthetic opioids narcotics or tricyclic antidepressants are administered to patient receiving monoamine oxidase inhibitors (MAOI) (34,36,37).

    d. The **serotonin syndrome** (SS) may occur with or without hyperthermia. It occurs in patients taking MAOI who take serotonergic drugs (meperidine, clomipramine) or serotonin inhibitors (fluoxetine, sertraline, paroxetine) without a drug-free interval of at least 5 weeks. Parkinson "drug holidays" have caused serotonin like syndromes (37–41).

  4. **Hypothermia** (32,42–475) may occur when the overdoses (e.g., CNS depressants) interfere with physiologic responses (vasoconstriction, muscle activity) when exposed to a cool environment. Hypothermia is frequently associated with **hypo-glycemia.** In severe hypothermia the pulse is often 40 to 50/min and systolic blood pressure 70 to 90 mm Hg. The bradycardia and hypotension should not be treated. They will resolve with rewarming. For a tachycardia disproportionate to the temperature, suspect hypovolemia, hypoglycemia or toxin ingestion. Hypothermia may mimic death and patients are not pronounced dead until they are "warm and dead."

D. **Abbreviated neurological examination**. Always ensure the cervical spine stability or immobilize the neck before proceeding with the examination. This is especially true with alcoholic patients.

  1. **The mental status, level of consciousness and cognitive function** (48–50). The mental status, respiratory pattern, pupillary response, extraocular movements and motor response should be noted and documented including the time of examination.

    a. **Mental status** is evaluated by the responsiveness scale **AVPU: A** = awake and alert; **V** = response to verbal stimuli; **P** = response to pain; and **U** = unresponsive. Later, the Reed Coma Scale may be used (Table 4-3) or the Glasgow Coma Scale (Table 4-4). The latter overestimates the depth of coma in poisoning.

    b. The patient with altered mental status should be classified **psychiatric, neurological-structural or toxic-metabolic,** although sometimes these states coexist.

    c. **Transient reversible neurologic** disease is produced by toxins more commonly than intrinsic brain disease. Toxins produce diffuse and nonfocal manifestations.

    d. **Any focal neurologic defect** must be assumed to be a primary neurologic event rather than a poisoning and a CT scan is indicated as soon as the vital functions are stabilized. Typically with neurological-structural lesions the pupillary light reflex is lost early but the respirations are retained until late in coma, whereas with toxic-metabolic states with patients in coma the respirations are lost early but the light reflex retained. For differentiation of neurological-structural from toxic metabolic coma, see Table 4-5a.

      e. **The odor of ethanol** on the breath does not exclude other causes of altered mental state.

2. **Rostocaudal progression** is a stepwise deterioration in respiratory pattern, pupillary response, oculovestibular reflex and motor response indicating a cephalocaudal progression from the diencephalon to the medulla. It indicates neurological-structural lesions (Table 4-5b).

3. **CNS Respiratory patterns.** The respiratory patterns are useful to determine the areas of CNS dysfunction in the comatose patient (Table 4-5b).

    a. **The diencephalic pattern or Cheyne Stokes** respirations consists of periodic hyperpnea alternating with apnea and correlates with bilateral cerebral cortical dysfunction and implies an intact brain stem.

    b. **The midbrain pattern** is hyperventilation consisting of deep, rapid respirations. Hypoxia, metabolic acidosis, CNS stimulation and pulmonary pathology must be excluded.

    c. **Pontine pathology** produces apneustic breathing with breath holding at the end of each inspiration or ataxic breathing which is irregular chaotic breathing of varying amplitude and rate.

    d. This rostocaudal progression of the breathing patterns indicates neurological-structural lesions.

4. For **pupillary responses,** examine the pupil with a bright light and magnifying glass for size, shape, reactivity to both bright and shaded light, equality, consensual reflex, and corneal reflex. Note nystagmus, ocular movements, deviation of eyes, oculogyric crisis and perform a fundoscopic examination for hemorrhages and papilledema.

    a. Most patients with **toxic-metabolic** coma retain their pupillary responses until late.

    b. **A unilateral dilated pupil,** with a downward, outward deviated eye means immediate treatment from a neurologic-structural lesion, localized trauma to the eye or cataract surgery. Unilateral dilation may occur with glutethimide intoxication or a mydriatic drop in one eye and does not represent a neurosurgical emergency.

    c. **Pupillary size** is dependent on a balance between the sympathetic dilation and parasympathetic constriction.

    d. **Mydriasis** is most often produced by agents listed in the mnemonic **SHAW:** **S** = sympathetic agents; **H** = hallucinogens; **A** = anticholinergic agents; and **W** = withdrawal from opioids, sedative-hypnotics and ethanol (see Differential Diagnosis).

        (1) **Nonreactive mydriasis** may be caused by pure anticholinergic poisoning.

        (2) **Reactive mydriasis** is produced by intoxication with sympathomimetic agents, carbon monoxide, monoamine oxidase inhibitor overdose, and withdrawal.

        (3) **Delayed mydriasis** occurs with methanol intoxication (formate destruction of the retina) and botulism.

e.   **Miosis** is caused most often by intoxications with most opioids, except meperidine (has anticholinergic properties), dextromethorphan (paralysis of the iris). Miosis is often present carbamate and organophosphate poisoning, in phenothiazine, in clonidine, nicotine, and phencyclidine overdoses. Miosis unresponsive to light and naloxone suggests pontine pupillary centers damage (see Differential Diagnosis).

f.   **Nystagmus** suggests overdose from anticonvulsants, opioids, sedative-hypnotics, phencyclidine, and ethanol; however, the absence of nystagmus does not exclude intoxication from these substances (see Differential Diagnosis).

5.   **Extraocular movements** are determined in the comatose patient by the **cold caloric test or doll's eye reflex.** The tests are dangerous to the cervical spine and the cold caloric test is preferred. These oculovestibular brain stem reflexes involve cranial nerves III, IV, VI, medial longitudinal fasciculus, vestibular portion of cranial nerve VIII and the cerebral cortex. After inspecting the auditory canal to exclude perforation of the tympanic membrane and cerumen, ice water at 1°C is introduced into the auditory canal and the eyes are observed for the physiologic response, which is a slow deviation toward the side of the cold water (ipsilateral) injection and a rapid correction nystagmus in the opposite direction contralateral). The mnemonic **COWS** (**c**old **o**pposite, **w**arm **s**ame) refers only to the nystagmus rapid movement.

a.   **Slow deviation movement** indicates an intact brain stem and the rapid correction nystagmus indicates intact cerebral cortex.

b.   **Single eye movement** indicates medial fasciculus (brain stem) pathology.

c.   **No response** occurs with severe hypothermia, drugs and substances producing paralysis or brain death.

d.   **Psychologic "pseudo-coma"** has normal nystagmus which differentiates it from true coma.

e.   **Toxic-metabolic coma** will often have intact eye deviation but without nystagmus, whereas **neurological-structural coma** has no movement or single eye movement without nystagmus.

6.   **Cognitive function** may be assessed by the mnemonic **ROARS: R** = reasoning by the addition of numbers; **O** = orientation by time, place, person (self or recognition of a familiar face); **A** = attention by 5-digit recall; **R** = recent memory by four-item recall in 5 min; and **S** = sensations. In **carbon monoxide exposures** minimally symptomatic patients may require hyperbaric chamber. A careful cognitive examination may help to decide who needs treatment. Testing should include general orientation, memory testing (address, phone number, date of birth), and cognitive testing (serial 7's, forward and backward spelling of three-letter and four-letter words) (52–54).

7.   **Psychiatric patients** often have well articulated speech at normal or rapid speed and are oriented.

a.   With **organic disease** time orientation is the first to be lost, then place, finally the patient's own name.

b.   A patient who knows the time or place and not his/her name has a **psychiatric problem.** Table 4-5c may be useful in differentiating patients with psychiatric problems from patients with organic disease.

     c.   Patients with intact cerebral cortex and psychiatric illness will have nystagmus present on the cold caloric test (note: don't do the cold caloric test on an awake patient); resist eye opening and may not allow their hand to fall and strike their face.

     d.   The **hallmark** of an organic illness is disorientation, and for psychiatric illness is orientation.

8. **The confused patient** may be in the state of delirium, dementia (Table 4-5c), psychosis or anxiety. **Hallucinations** are false perceptions that do not actually occur, **delusions** (false ideas) and **illusions** (false interpretations) without loss of consciousness.

     a.   **Delirium** is an acute confusion state with reduced awareness and reduced higher level of cortical function. The **cardinal feature is reduced alertness.** Illusions and hallucinations are often present. It is usually transient and reversible with global disturbances in the cognitive process and fluctuation in level of consciousness (55). It is usually toxic-metabolic in origin and the common substances include alcohols, anticholinergics, barbiturates, BZPs, hallucinogens, CNS stimulants (amphetamines, cocaine) and withdrawal.

        (1) **Clinically** it is characterized by disturbed arousal (sleep-wake cycle), disorientation, with impaired attention and short memory, slight incoordination, impaired speech, sometimes with anxiety and restlessness. These signs are often accompanied by hallucinations and delusions.

        (2) **Differential diagnosis** is depression (lacks clouding of consciousness), acute psychosis (has auditory hallucination, lacks fluctuating level of consciousness, and anxiety (see Differential Diagnosis).

     b.   **Dementia** is a clinical state characterized by a decline from a previously attained intellectual level involving the memory, cognitive functions, and adaptive behavior **without reduction in arousal and the patient is clinically alert.** It has a gradual onset and persists for more than 1 month. It is usually organic and the commonest form of dementia is Alzheimer disease (see Differential Diagnosis).

9. **Agitated, violent and psychotic: Violence** is aggressive assault or combativeness. **Agitation** is uncontrollable restlessness or excessive excitability. **Psychosis** is a mental derangement which may cause violence or aggression. These patients may harm themselves and others (55–60). For additional causes and the management see section for treatment (67–70) see pp. 115–117, Section 12. See Table 4-6 for classification of the severity.

     a.   The **cause** of violence may be psychiatric, situational frustration, and organic diseases. Most patients labeled as violent are schizophrenic, especially of the paranoid type (30% to 40%) (60). **Organic violent behavior** usually occurs over 40 years of age without a previous psychiatric history. The patients are disoriented, lethargic or stuporous, have visual hallucinations or illusions and abnormal vital signs (55–60).

     b.   **Drugs and chemicals** may produce violence or precipitate a violent psychosis in a patient with underlying psychiatric disorder. The most frequent include amphetamines, anticholinergics (scopolamine, Jimson weed), cocaine, ethanol (intoxication, intolerance and withdrawal), hallucinogens,

TABLE 4-6. *Classification of severity of stimulants*

Severity	Manifestations
Grade 1	Diaphoresis, hyperreflexia, irritability, mydriasis tremors
Grade 2	Confusion, fever, hyperactivity, hypertension, tachycardia, tachypnea
Grade 3	Delirium, mania, hyperpyrexia, tachydysrhythmias
Grade 4	Coma, convulsions, cardiovascular collapse

Modified from Epelin DE, Done AK. Amphetamine poisoning: effectiveness of chlorpromazine. *N Engl J Med* 1968;278:1361.

phencyclidine, sedative-hypnotics (intoxication or withdrawal) and occupational chemical exposures include sulfides, and mercury.

C. **Differential diagnosis** exclude hypoxia, hypoglycemia, electrolyte disturbances, metabolic and endocrine disorders. In one review **hypoglycemia** accounted for 9% of violent patients (60). The **diaphoretic violent patient** is usually organic, i.e., hypoglycemic, sepsis, withdrawal, heat stroke, MI, or pulmonary edema.

D. **Clues** to potentially violent patients are: agitation, loud speech, startles easily, tense posture, sits on edge of chair, paces back and forth, clinched fists, tattoos (prison tattoos are black and fuzzy), tattoo that reads "born to kill."

10. **Motor nerve function**
  a. Apply noxious stimuli.
  b. Observe if patient can localize the source by reaching across the midline, or develops decorticate or decerebrate posturing.
  c. Note involuntary movements, focal weakness, flaccidity, spasticity, convulsions, and fasciculations.
  d. A rostocaudal progression of motor function suggests a neurological-structural lesion.

11. Deep tendon reflexes, superficial, and pathologic **reflexes** may show focality which suggests a neurological-structural lesion.

12. **Meningeal signs** should be sought, although they may be masked in coma. They usually are infectious in origin but aseptic meningitis has been reported with several medications including nonsteroidal antiinflammatory agents (61,62). Subarachnoid hemorrhage may present in a similar manner.

13. **Autonomic nervous system** is evaluated by the assessment of the cardiorespiratory system such as a decline in blood pressure not accompanied by a compensatory increase in pulse or the absence of the normal oscillations of pulse variation (no reduction of pulse rate with inspiration or increase with expiration), bladder function, bowel sounds (parasympathetic system gives excessive peristaltic activity), temperature control and sweating, pupillary responses (parasympathetic system produces miosis and accommodation, and sympathetic system dilation to dim light).

14. **Coma Scales** (67–71)
  a. **AVPU system** is a rapid means of documenting the level of consciousness (A = alert; V = response to verbal stimuli; P = response to painful stimuli; U = unresponsive).

    b. In definitive monitoring of coma due to intoxication some prefer to use the **Reed Coma Scale** (Table 4-3), because the Glasgow coma scale overestimates the degree of impairment.

    c. **Document** the descriptive state of consciousness (not just a score number) with the time and date of assessment. Some institutions have monitoring charts for this purpose.

    d. **Glasgow Coma Scale** (Table 4-4) was originally designed for estimating the prognosis in head trauma. The scale does not distinguish between diffuse and focal impairment. All patients unconscious for 5 min or more should be admitted regardless of score.

        (1) The score utilizes three factors: eye opening, motor and verbal response.

        (2) The best response is 15, the worst is 3, and a score of 8 or less indicates frank coma (67). Alcohol and depressant drugs, however, lower the scores.

        (3) According to Simpson and Reilly (71), scoring each variable is influenced by age. Normal scores are as follows: birth to 6 months is 9; 6 to 12 months is 11; 1 to 2 years is 12; 2 to 5 years is 13; and more than 5 years 14.

    e. **Coma** (67–71) may be produced by hypoxia causative agents that interfere with oxygen transport in blood and/or interfere with tissues utilization of oxygen, CNS depressants, hypoglycemic agents, enzyme inhibitors, hallucinogens or postictal or complications of intoxicant such as intracranial hemorrhage from hypertension or injury (71) (Table 4-7).

15. In toxicologic emergencies examine the **orogastrointestinal tract** for the presence of mouth burns or edema, oral staining, drooling, dysphagia and the presence or absence of bowel sounds.

    a. **Absent bowel sounds** may indicate ileus associated shock, anticholinergic intoxication or secondary to a perforation such as may occur in acid ingestions.

        (1) Absent bowel sounds are a **contraindication** to AC and cathartics.

        (2) Determine by palpation if bladder distention and **urinary retention** exist, such as may occur as with anticholinergic agents.

TABLE 4-7. *Mnemonic for the causes of coma and convulsions*

Metabolic disorders
  A   Alcohol
  E   Endocrine, electrolyte disturbances, epilepsy
  I   Intoxication
  O   Oxygen deprivation
  U   Uremia and metabolic disorders hepatic, hypertension
Other causes
  T   Trauma, tumor
  I   Infection
  P   Psychologic
  S   Shock, strokes (cardiovascular accident)

16. The **body weight** is important, especially in children, for calculating out doses of emergency drugs and antidotes. The **Broselow Pediatric Resuscitative Tape** allows measurement of the child's length to determine emergency drug dose.

17. **Skin appearance** (32,33,72). Examine the skin for needle tracks, particularly in tattoos. The skin should be classified as red (erythematous), white (pale), blue (bruised or cyanotic) warm, cool, dry, or moist. Mark sites of lesions on a body diagram and on the patient. Look for piloerection of opioid withdrawal (72,73). For poisons associated with skin manifestations, see Table 4-8 (see Differential Diagnosis).

18. **Odors** (74-78). Ethanol is ingested with many drugs so its presence does not exclude other drug ingestions or underlying medical and surgical conditions. Large numbers of the population do not have "gifted" olfactory apparatus to detect the odor of cyanide and acetone, therefore the absence of a classic odor does not exclude the presence of a toxin. For list of odors of intoxicants, see Table 4-9 (see Differential Diagnosis).

VII. **Intoxications that produce common clinical disturbances.** These changes may serve as clues to the intoxicating agent; however, the typical clinical findings may be obscured in mul-

TABLE 4-8. *Overdose and poisons that have skin manifestations*

Types of lesions	Potential causative agent
Aciniform	Bromides, dactinomycin, dioxin (245 TCCD), iodides, lithium, polyhalogenated biphenyls, steroids
Alopecia	Alkylating chemotherapeutic agents, androgens, boric acid, burns (caustics, phenol), chloroquine, ergot, heavy metals (especially arsenic and thallium), radiation, selenium
Bulla	Caustics and corrosives, carbon monoxide, insect bites, marine injuries, sedative-hypnotics, snake envenomation
Cyanotic	Carbon monoxide, hypoxia, methemoglobinemia (aniline and azo dyes, dinitrobenzene, local anesthetics, nitrates, nitrites, nitrobenzene, nitrophenol, phenacetin, trinitrotoluene), sulfhemoglobin (hydrogen sulfide)
Desquamation	Arsenic, acrodynia (mercury), boric acid, epidermal necrolysis
Diaphoresis	Amphetamines, carbamates, cocaine, insulin, dinitrophenol cholinergic mushrooms, hypoglycemic producing substances, nicotine, nitrites, opioids, organophosphates, pentochlorophenol, parasympathomimetics, salicylates, withdrawal
Dry and flushed	Anticholinergic, ethanol
Epidermal necrolysis	Allopurinol, barbiturates, hydantoin, phenylbutazone, penicillin, sulfonamides, tetracycline
Erythema multiforme	Barbiturate, chlorpropamide, griseofulvin, hydantoin, penicillin, phenothiazines sulfonamides, thiazides
Flushed	Alcohol, anticholinergic, antihistamines, boric acid, carbon monoxide (rarely), cyanide, disulfiram-ethanol reaction, nicotinic acid, nitrites, scromboid fish poisoning, rifampin, toxic shock syndrome, vancomycin
Jaundice	Acetaminophen (late), antimalarials (G-6-PD deficiency) arsine gas, castor beans, fava beans, hepatotoxic, agents, hemolytic (G-6-PD deficiency), mushrooms, naphthalene (with and without G-6-PD deficiency), heavy metals, phosphorous, solvents
Purpura	Anticoagulants (medical or in rodenticides), envenomations (insects, spiders, snakes), salicylates

Modified from Olsen et al.; Mofenson and Greensher; and Modly et al.

TABLE 4-9. *Odors as clues to intoxications*

Odors	Potential agents or conditions
Acetone	Acetone, isopropanol, metabolic acidosis (salicylate, diabetic ketoacidosis, and other causes)
Airplane glue	Ethchlorvynol, toluene, aromatic hydrocarbon inhalation
Alcohol	Ethanol (no alcohol odor with ethylene glycol or Vodka)
Ammonia	Ammonia or uremia
Bitter almonds (silver polish)	Cyanide (not detectable by 50% of population)
Bleach (hypochlorite)	Hypochlorite
Carrots	Cicutoxin of water hemlock
Coal gas	Carbon monoxide is odorless but mixed with illuminating gas for detection
Disinfectants	Creosote, phenol
Formaldehyde	Formaldehyde, methanol
Foul	Bromides, foreign body in orifice, lithium
Hemp (burnt rope)	Marijuana
Garlic	(Arsenic, dimethylsulfoxide (DMSO), malathion, parathion, yellow phosphorous, selenium, tellurium, zinc phosphide
Mothballs	Camphor, naphthalene, paradichlorobenzene
Peanuts	Rodenticide Vacor (now banned)
Pears	Chloral hydrate, paraldehyde
Rotten eggs	Disulfiram, hydrogen sulfide, hepatic failure, mercaptans, N-acetylcysteine
Shoe polish	Nitrobenzene
Violets (urine-specimen)	Turpentine
Vinyl shower curtain	Ethchlorvynol
Wintergreen	Salicylate

tiple drug overdose or by complications of the original intoxication such as hypoxia and shock. The common clinical presentations are presented in Table 4-10.

A. **Toxic syndromes (Toxidromes).** The identification of various toxic syndromes requires integrating of data provided by both the vital signs and the physical examination to elicit manifestations specific to an intoxicant. This collection of manifestations may assist in the diagnosis when the agent is unknown and may help in anticipating manifestations that will develop.

1. **Anticholinergic** (antihistamines H2 blockers, atropine, belladonna alkaloids, Jimson weed, some mushrooms, tricyclic antidepressants)—**"dry as a bone", "red as a beet", "blind as a bat", "hot as a hare", "mad as a hatter", "the bowel and bladder lose their tone and the heart goes on alone"**), dry skin ("as a bone"), flushed skin ("red as a beet"), mydriasis which may be unresponsive ("blind as a bat"), hyperthermia ("hot as a hare"), hallucinations ("mad as a hatter"), urinary retention, decreased bowel sounds and tachycardia ("the bowel and bladder lose their tone and the heart goes on alone").

2. **Cholinergic** muscaric and nicotinic effects (carbamate insecticides and medications organophosphate insecticides, some mushrooms, nicotine, parasympathetic medications)—**Dumbels: d**efecation, **u**rination, **m**iosis, **b**ronchospasm, **e**xcessive salivation, **l**acrimation, **s**eizures.

TABLE 4-10. *Common clinical presentations and etiologies*

Clinical presentation	Toxic agents	Medical diseases
Acidosis	Alcohols and glycols	Diabetes mellitus
	Cyanide	GI losses
	Iron isoniazid	Lactic acidosis
	Salicylates	Shock
	Stimulants	Renal RTA
		Uremia
Bradycardia	Beta-adrenergic blockers	Increased ICP
	Calcium channel blockers	Structural heart lesions
	Cardiac glycosides	Conduction defects
	Cholinergic agents	Hypothermia
	CNS depressants	Sleep
	Lithium	Athletes at rest
	Opioids	Jaundice
	Organophosphates insecticides	Stokes-Adams syndrome
	Phenylpropanolamine (reflex)	Carotid sinus syndrome
	Quinidine	
	Tricyclic/cyclic antidepressants	
Coma	Alcohols	Hypothyroidism
	Barbiturates	Anoxia
	Benzodiazepines	Encephalopathies
	Carbon monoxide	CVA
	Neuroleptic	Metabolic
	Opioids	Trauma
	Sedative hypnotics	
	Tricyclic antidepressant	
Convulsions	Alcohols/glycols	Anoxia
	Camphor	Febrile (child)
	Carbon monoxide	
	Cyanide	Infectious
	Isoniazid	Metabolic/endocrine
	Hypoglycemia agents	(hypoglycemia)
	Mushroom (Gyromitra)	Neoplastic
	Phenothiazines	Traumatic
	Sympathomimetics (cocaine,	Vascular (CVA)
	amphetamines, PCP)	Idiopathic epilepsy
	Strychnine	
	Salicylates	
	Theophylline	
	Tricyclics/phenothiazines	
	Withdrawal	
	Heavy metals (lead, Li)	
Dysrhythmias	Antidysrhythmics	Electrolyte
	Antihypertensive agents	
	Beta-adrenergic blockers	Hypoxia
	Calcium channel blockers	Idiopathic
	Chloral hydrate	
	Chloroquine	Myocarditis
	Digitalis	Myocardial
	Lithium	infarction
	Neuroleptics	
	Sympathomimetics (cocaine,	
	amphetamine, phencyclidine,	
	phenylpropanolamine,	
	theophylline)	
	Tricyclics	

(continued)

TABLE 4-10. (*continued*)

Clinical presentation	Toxic agents	Medical diseases
Hypertension	Anticholinergic (T)	Carcinoid
	Clonidine (R)	
	Hallucinogens (T)	Essential
	Lead encephalopathy (B)	Pheochromocytoma
	Phenylephrine (R)	Renal disease
	Phenylpropanolamine (R)	
	Sympathomimetics (T)	Increased intracranial
	(amphetamine, cocaine,	pressure
	theophylline)	
	Thyroid (T)	
	Vitamin A excess (B)	
	Withdrawal (T)	
Hypotension	Antihypertensive agents (T)	Anaphylaxis
	Arsenic (T)	Dehydration
	Barbiturates (T)	Heart failure
	Beta-adrenergic blockers (B)	Hemorrhage
	Calcium channel blockers (B)	Hypovolemia
	Carbon monoxide (T)	Sepsis
	Caustics (T)	Shock any cause
	Clonidine (B)	
	Cyanide (T)	
	Cardiac glycoside (B)	
	Disulfiram reaction (T)	
	Iron (T)	
	Opioids (B)	
	Organophosphate insecticides (B)	
	MAOI (T)	
	Neuroleptics (T)	
	Sedative-hypnotics (T)	
	Theophylline (T)	
	Tricyclic antidepressants (T)	
	Vasodilators (nitrites) (T)	
Organic brain	Anticholinergic	Infections
syndrome (toxic	Ethanol	Metabolic
psychosis)	Digitalis	Psychosis
	Hallucinogens	
	Inhalants (solvents)	
	Stimulants (cocaine,	
	amphetamines, phencyclidine)	
	Withdrawal	
Pulmonary edema	*Cardiac*	
	Antidysrhythmics	
	Beta blockers	
	Calcium channel blockers	
	Cyclic antidepressants	
	Noncardiac	Aspiration
	Barbiturates	Fluid overload
	Gases toxic	Heart failure
	Hydrocarbon aspiration	Hypoxia
	Opioids	Near drowning
	Organophosphates	Shock
	Salicylates	
	Neurogenic	
	Sympathomimetics	

(*continued*)

TABLE 4-10. (*continued*)

Clinical presentation	Toxic agents	Medical diseases
Pulmonary edema (*continued*)	*Irritant gases* 　　Smoke 　　Chlorine inhalation	
Tachycardia	Alcohols and glycols (early) Anticholinergics Antihistamines Cardiac glycosides CNS stimulants Hallucinogens Nitrates and nitrites Phencyclidine Phenothiazines Plants Salicylates Sedative-hypnotics (early) Sympathomimetics Thyroid Tricyclic and cyclic 　　antidepressants	Fever Hyperthermia Hyperthyroidism Hypovolemia Shock Dysrhythmia PAT, atrial dysrhythmias Electrolyte Anxiety Carditis CHF
Torsades de Pointes	Amantadine Arsenic Antidysrhythmic agents: 　　Ia, Ib, Ic, III Fluoride Phenothiazines Maprotiline Organophosphates Thallium	Congenital syndromes Electrolyte derangement 　　(decreased Mg^{++}, 　　decreased Ca^{++}) Coronary artery disease
Wheezing	Aspirin Beta-blocker bronchospasm Cholinergic mushroom Cholinergic medications Irritant gases: chlorine, 　　smoke,occupational 　　hypersensitivity	Bronchospasm asthma Cardia asthma Foreign body Cystic fibrosis Pneumonia Anaphylaxis Carcinoid

T, tachycardia (in the clinical presentation of hypotension, tachycardia early later bradycardia); B, bradycardia; R, reflex bradycardia initially.

3. **Hypermetabolic** syndrome (phenol compounds [dinitrophenol, pentachlorphenol herbicides], salicylates]—convulsions, restless, fever, hyperpnea, tachycardia, metabolic acidosis)

4. **Opioid syndrome** (opioids)—miosis, CNS depression (flaccid coma), hypoventilation, hypotension, bradycardia, hypothermia.

5. **Sympathomimetics syndrome** (amphetamines, caffeine, cocaine, phenylpropanolamine, methylphenidate, theophylline)—convulsions, hyperthermia, hypertension, mydriasis, psychosis, tachycardia.

6. **Torsion-head and neck syndrome** (idiosyncratic reaction with extrapyramidal manifestations) (Amantidine, antihistamine H2 blockers, brompheramine, lev-

odopa, meyaclopramide, phenothiazines and butyphenones, sertraline)—dyspho-nia, oculogyric crisis, rigidity, tremor, torticollis.
7.   **Phencyclidine syndrome:** miosis, rotatory nystagmus, combativeness.
B.   **Manifestations by drug category.** List the common intoxicants' effect on the CNS, heart rate, respirations, temperature, blood pressure pupils of the eyes, deep tensor reflexes, skin, muscle tone, bowel sounds. If the feature is in bold it is an important observation in diagnosis and management.

Alcohols, barbiturates, sedative, hypnotics

CNS—depression, lethargy
Heart rate—bradycardia, sometimes tachycardia initially
Respirations—depressed, slow (acidosis—alcohols/glycols hyperventilation)
Temperature—hypothermia
Blood pressure—hypotension with tachycardia
Pupils—pupils vary; horizontal nystagmus; miosis (alcohol, barbiturates); mydriasis (glutethimide)
Reflexes—depressed DTR
Skin—flushed; moist (ethanol)
Muscle tone—decreased and flaccid
Bowel sounds—decreased

Anticholinergic, antihistamines

CNS—delirious, Alice in Wonderland syndrome
Heart rate—tachycardia, dysrhythmias
Respirations—slight tachypnea
Temperature—hyperthermia
Blood pressure—slight hypertension
Pupils—dilated often fixed
Skin—flushed, dry
Muscle tone—usually normal
Bowel sounds—decreased to absent

Antidepressants (rapid onset)

CNS—coma, seizures, hallucinations
Heart rate—dysrhythmias; sinus and superventricular tachycardia initially then wide QRS, QT, and ventricular tachycardia
Respirations—vary
Blood pressure—hypertension early, hypotension later
Temperature—may be elevated
Pupils—dilated early
Reflexes—depressed
Skin—moist
Muscle tone—varies
Bowel sounds—may be decreased

BZPs

CNS—depression, light coma
Heart rate—bradycardia

Respirations—bradypnea
Blood pressure—varies, not usually affected
Temperature—nonspecific
Pupils—vary
Reflexes—DTR intact
Skin—moist
Muscle tone—flaccid
Bowel sounds—may be decreased

Beta-adrenergic blockers
CNS—coma
Heart rate—bradycardia and slowed cardiac conduction; pindolol, oxprenolol tachycardia initially
Respirations—not affected
Temperature—not affected
Blood pressure—hypotension pindolol; oxprenolol hypertension initially
Skin—not affected
Bowel sounds—not affected
Metabolic—hyperglycemia, hypokalemia

Calcium channel blockers
CNS—coma
Respirations—not affected
Heart rate—bradycardia
Blood pressure—hypotension
Pupils—dilated if hypoglycemic
Hypoglycemia
Skin—not affected
Bowel sounds—not affected
Metabolic—hypoglycemia, hyperkalemia

Hypoglycemic agents oral
CNS—seizures or coma
Respirations—not affected
Heart rate—not affected
Temperature—low if hypoglycemia
Pupils—dilated if hypoglycemia
Skin—diaphoretic if hypoglycemia
Bowel sounds—not affected
Metabolic—hypoglycemia

Iron and other heavy metals (arsenic or mercury salts)
CNS—varies
Heart rate—tachycardia
Respirations—vary (tachypnea with acidosis or shock)
Temperature—normal
Blood pressure—hypotension with tachycardia (shock)
Pupils—nonspecific

Skin—nonspecific

Bowel sounds—abdominal pain, vomiting, diarrhea (with blood), radiopaque pills

Metabolic—acidosis, anion gap, hyperglycemia and leucocytosis

Isoniazid

CNS—seizures

Heart rate—increased

Respirations—usually not affected, lactic acidosis compensated by hyperpnea

Temperature—elevated with seizures

Blood pressure—elevated

Skin—not affected

Reflexes—increased

Muscle tone—increased

Bowel sounds—not affected

Metabolic—lactic acidosis, anion gap

Lysergic acid diethylamide

CNS—euphoria, anxiety, panic reaction, hyperalert, time and visual distortions, depersonalization, psychosis, flashbacks

Heart rate—tachycardia

Respirations—not affected

Temperature—not affected

Blood pressure—slightly elevated

Pupils—moderately dilated

Bowel sounds—not affected

Lithium

CNS—confused, tremors, seizures

Heart rate—tachycardia, dysrhythmias

Respirations—not affected

Temperature—normal

Pupils—nonspecific

Skin—not affected unless coagulopathy

Muscle tone—increased reflexes, course tremors

Bowel sounds—increased—diarrhea

Marijuana

CNS—euphoria, anxiety, panic reaction, delirium, rarely hallucinations

Heart rate—tachycardia

Respirations—not affected but may have laryngitis, bronchitis

Temperature—slight elevation

Blood pressure—slight elevation

Eyes—pupils slightly constricted, conjunctival erythema

Bowel sounds—not affected

Neuroleptics (phenothiazine and nonphenothiazine)

CNS—seizures, coma

Heart rate—tachycardia with dysrhythmias

Blood pressure—hypotension
Respirations—bradypnea
Temperature—depressed if in cold environment, hypothermias, hyperthermia in
    neuroleptic malignant syndrome
Pupils—pinpoint
Idiosyncratic reaction—dystonias
Reflexes—hyperactive but varies
Skin—nonspecific
Muscle tone—varies
Bowel sounds—may be decreased

Opioids

CNS—depression, seizures (meperidine, pentazocine, codeine, propoxyphene)
Heart rate—slow, propoxyphene—dysrhythmias
Respirations—bradypnea, pulmonary edema
Temperature—hypothermia
Blood pressure—hypotension
Pupils—miosis (pinpoint pupils); mydriasis (meperidine, dextromethorphan,
    Lomotil)
Reflexes—depressed DTR
Skin—moist, nonspecific
Muscle tone—flaccid
Bowel sounds—decreased

Phencyclidine

CNS—hyperactivity, feelings of invulnerability, violent, bizarre behavior,
    psychosis, slurred speech, ataxia, catatonia, flashbacks
Heart rate—tachycardia
Respirations—not affected
Temperature—elevated, hyperthermia
Blood pressure—elevated
Eyes—pupils usually miotic, rotatory nystagmus
Skin—diaphoresis
Muscle tone—rigidity, rhabdomyolysis, myoglobinuria
Bowel sounds—not affected

Salicylates

CNS—coma, seizures
Heart rate—tachycardia
Respiratory—tachypnea (respiratory alkalosis adult) or metabolic acidosis
    compensation (small child)
Temperature—usually normal or elevated
Blood pressure—varies
Pupils—vary
Skin—moist diaphoretic
Bowel sounds—not affected
Metabolic—anion gap, hypoglycemia, hypokalemia

Stimulants, hallucinogens

   CNS—euphoria, hyperactive, agitation, delirium, psychosis, myoclonus, seizures

   Heart rate—tachycardia, dysrhythmias; sometimes reflex bradycardia

   Respirations—tachypnea

   Temperature—elevated, may be hyperthermia

   Blood pressure—hypertension with tachycardia and dysrhythmias

   Pupils—dilated

   Skin—moist

   Muscle tone—increased muscle tone, rhabdomyolysis, myoglobinuria

   Bowel sounds—vary

VIII. **Hospital preparation procedure for possibly contaminated patients.** A protocol should be prepared as part of the ED policies and procedures on how to handle the possibly contaminated patient, especially from hazardous material incidents. Note: Critically injured patients must be resuscitated first before decontamination.

   A. **Attendants** should wear disposable gowns, gloves (use several layers of latex gloves in hydrofluoric acid exposures), shoe covers and masks. Additional **protective equipment** is determined by the circumstances and the substances involved. Contact Regional PCC and Chemtrec 1-800-424-9300 in hazardous material incidents.

   B. Arrange a **special access route** separate from the usual emergency entrance. Rope off and secure area. Cover pathway floors and floor of working area with disposable nonpenetrable plastic material.

   C. Have **water from shower drain into special tanks** not into the regular sewer system.

   D. If necessary **cover air vents** so contaminated substances will not have access to hospital ventilation system. However, this concentrates the substance where the staff is located.

   E. **Remove the patient's clothes** and place in specially marked plastic bags. Leather goods are irreversibly contaminated and must be abandoned.

   G. **Remove bedding linen at end of procedure** and place in specially marked plastic bags.

IX. **Management of the symptomatic poisoned patient** (79–87)

   A. **The first priority** is to establish and maintain vital functions and to stabilize the cervical spine.

       1. During each stage of resuscitation consider assessment, therapy, monitoring.

       2. After these essentials are established consideration can be given to identification of the toxic substance, prevention of further absorption, administration of an antidote, if available, and enhancement of elimination.

       3. For the patient with depressed mental status and depressed respirations, certain measures should be done routinely: establish an airway; give oxygen by bag-valve mask; establish vascular access; obtain an immediate reagent strip blood glucose value (send a specimen to the laboratory for confirmation) and if necessary administer i.v. glucose, naloxone, thiamine, monitor ECG; obtain arterial blood gases; electrolytes and blood and urine specimens for toxicology as indicated; perform gastric lavage, administer AC and a cathartic unless contraindicated after airway protected and stabilized. The GI decontamination methods may be omitted if excessive time has elapsed depending on the intoxicant (85). Sorbitol is not recommended under 3 years of age)

B. Assessment and maintenance of vital functions:

1. Establish and secure a clear **airway** by the head tilt and chin lift maneuvers (only if there is no cervical neck injury). If this fails or if there is suspicion of neck injury use the jaw thrust. The airway can be maintained by oropharyngeal or nasopharyngeal airways for a brief time. If the patient can tolerate an artificial airway they will probably require endotracheal intubation.

2. Assess the **respiratory status** by evaluation of chest excursions, breath sounds, the work and mechanics of breathing, and pulse oximetry. If respirations are absent or ineffective initiate **ventilation** with bag-valve-mask and **100% oxygen.** Concern over pulmonary damage by excess oxygen has no place in the initial resuscitation. "The brain gets soft long before the lungs get hard." Always hyperventilate and oxygenate with 100% oxygen prior to intubation.

   a. **The** decision for **endotracheal intubation** is determined clinically and does not await blood gas results. The five **indications** for intubation include:

      (1) Central hypoventilation: decreased respiratory rate including apnea, irregular respirations, insufficient respiratory excursions)

      (2) Respiratory failure: inadequate oxygenation or ventilation secondary to airway disease, intrinsic lung disease and fatigue

      (3) Shock with impending respiratory failure

      (4) Lack of protection of the airway with altered mental status (comatose or status epilepticus) required to avoid the consequences of pulmonary aspiration.

      (5) Hyperventilation for increased intracranial pressure.

   b. **Endotracheal** tubes in intoxicated adult patients should be **cuffed. Noncuffed** endotracheal tubes are recommended in children under 8 years. The **pitfalls** are inability to visual the vocal cords or for the cords to relax so repeated attempts were necessary, esophageal intubation, emesis, aspiration, intubation of the right main stem bronchus, trauma to mucosa, air leaks (pneumothorax and pneumomediastinum). The orotracheal is preferred to nasotracheal intubation because it is performed under direct vision. It frequently requires neuromuscular blockers if patient does not have a flaccid jaw and unrestricted neck mobility. However, with possible cervical spine injury, it should be accomplished with cervical spine immobilization (88).

   c. **Rapid sequence intubation**. This sequence is to accomplish endotracheal intubation which will avoid the complication of aspiration, concern about increased intracranial pressure, and interference combativeness, agitation and seizures. It uses potent sedatives, cricoid pressure (Sellick Maneuver) to prevent regurgitation (88–92). See Table 4-11 for the agents used for Rapid Sequence Intubation and Fig. 4-3 for the pediatric algorithm. **Rapid sequence intubation involves the Ps**: **P**reparation, **P**reoxygenation, **P**retreatment, **P**aralysis with anesthesia, **P**ass the tube, **P**ost-intubation (88,91,92).

TABLE 4-11. *Muscle-relaxing agents for rapid sequence induction*

Drug	Dose IV	Onset	Duration
Succinylcholine	1.0–1.5 mg/kg (>10 kg)	30–60 sec	4–10 min
	1.5–2.0 mg/kg (<10 kg)		
Vecuronium	0.2–0.25 mg/kg	60–90 sec	90 min
	0.1 mg/kg (standard)	2–3 min	25–40 min
	0.01 mg/kg (defasciculating)		
Pancuronium	0.1 mg/kg	2–5 min	45–90 min
	0.01 mg/kg (defasciculating)		

Modified from Reference 91.

(1) Adults or children over 10 years

    (a) Preparation. Secure i.v. line, continuous cardiac monitoring, continuous pulse oximeter, assistants assigned tasks, properly working laryngoscope, proper blade size, proper endotracheal tube size and whether or not cuffed. If cuffed, check for leaks, tapes for post-intubation ties, insure proper bag-valve-mask size and in working order, ensure suction is working and instantly available, have all necessary drugs mixed and ready to administer and have cricothyrotomy tray available in case of failure.

    (b) Preoxygenation with **high-flow 12 to 15 L 100% oxygen** using nonrebreathing mask for 5 min if possible (washes out nitrogen

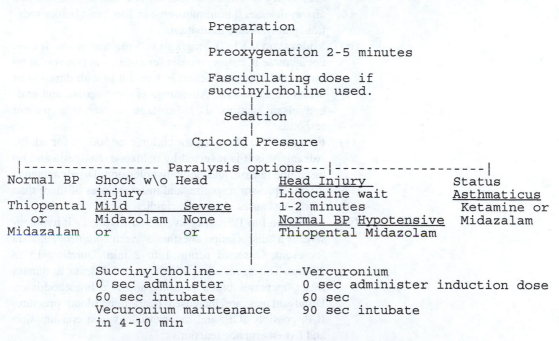

FIG. 4-3. Pediatric rapid sequence intubation (RSI).

and protects from hypoxia) or at least three conscious deep breaths equal to vital capacity may have to make do in an extreme emergency.

(c) **Pretreatment** (92)

   (i) **Nondepolarizing vecuronium** 0.01 mg/kg up to 1 mg i.v. push as "defasciculating dose" (or pancuronium 1 mg i.v. push, or D-tubocurarine 3 mg i.v. push). The choice of the sedative to be administered will be determined by concern about increased intracranial pressure (ICP), intraocular pressure (IOP), interference by seizures, combativeness or agitation (90–92). Some premedications are the following.

   (ii) **Sodium thiopental** 3 to 5 mg/kg i.v. or 250 mg adults. It may rarely cause hypotension if administered rapidly or if the patient is hypovolemic. It can cause bronchospasm and laryngospasm. It is contraindicated in porphyria and asthma. Onset of action is less than 1 min and duration of action 10 to 30 min. Advantage is that it acts rapidly and decreases intracranial pressure (ICP). Disadvantage is that it produces hypotension and histamine release; Therefore, avoid if reactive airway disease.

   (iii) **Lidocaine** 1.5 to 2.0 mg/kg i.v. push. Useful when there is head injury to avoid elevation of ICP and IOP or reactive airway disease. It is administered in 1 to 2 min before sedation, paralysis and intubation.

   (iv) **Midazolam** 0.1 to 0.2 mg/kg i.v. 5 mg maximum. It does not increase ICP, has amnesia for event, and is reversed by flumazenil. Onset of action is 1 to 2 min with duration of action 30 to 60 min. Advantage is short action, and anticonvulsant action. Disadvantage is variable patient response.

   (v) **Fentanyl** 2 to 10 µg/kg for children or 500 µg for adults. Advantage is it is reversed by naloxone, analgesia and no histamine release, and rarely hypotension. Disadvantage is it blunts pressor response, and in large doses of more than 10 mg/kg causes chest wall rigidity.

   (vi) **Ketamine** 1 to 1.5 mg/kg i.v. (0.5 to 1.0 mg/kg if hypotensive) is a "dissociation anesthesia" with complete amnesia for event. Onset of action 1 to 2 min. Duration 15 to 30 min. This agent allows the laryngeal reflexes to remain intact, increases blood pressure and is a bronchodilator. Disadvantages are increased heart rate, blood pressure, ICP, possibly IOP, and myocardial oxygen consumption and has emergence reactions.

(d) **Wait 2 to 3 min.**

(e) **Defasciculating dose** of vecuronium 0.01 mg/kg i.v. given simultaneously with lidocaine if head injury. For other agents used for defasciculating dose and for muscle relaxant doses, see Table 4-11.

(f) **Paralysis.** Administer **succinylcholine** 1.5 mg/kg i.v. push. Continue oxygen administration. In bradycardia patients, administer **atropine sulfate** 0.01 mg/kg up to 0.5 mg and minimum 0.1 mg regardless of size (paradoxical bradycardia).

(g) **Pass the tube. Intubation** is accomplished with patient in "sniffing position" and **apply pressure to cricoid cartilage. Do not use positive pressure with cricoid pressure.**

(vii) **Post-intubation. Immediately after** intubation institute positive pressure ventilation and consider longer term neuromuscular blockade. Verify location of ET tube by auscultation, chest radiograph and end-tidal CO_2 detector.

(2) **Child under 10 years** (88–92) (for the algorithm on pediatric rapid sequence intubation, see Fig. 4-3).

(a) **Preparation**

(b) **Preoxygenation**

(c) **Pretreatment** which may be unnecessary **under 5 years** because they rarely have significant fasciculation. In children **over 5 years** defasciculation with pancuronium, vecuronium for succinylcholine. In children succinylcholine may increase vagal tone causing bradycardia or asystole therefore to administer **atropine sulfate** 0.01 mg/kg up to 0.5 mg and never less than 0.1 mg regardless of size because of paradoxical bradycardia. Use **midazolam** 0.1 to 0.2 mg/kg i.v. as sedating agent. May use pancuronium 0.1 mg/kg i.v. or other agents for paralysis in place of succinylcholine but longer onset of action.

(d) **Wait 2 to 3 min** if possible.

(e) **Paralysis** with **succinylcholine** 1.5 to 2.0 mg/kg i.v. push or pancuronium 0.1 mg/kg i.v. for paralysis. Continue oxygen administration.

(f) **Pass the tube**.

(g) **Post-intubation.**

2. After intubation **suction** secretions. If they are copious consider organophosphate poisoning or pulmonary edema.

3. The **endotracheal tube** will also serve as a **route of access** for certain emergency medications such as epinephrine, lidocaine, atropine, naloxone, and diazepam should venous access be delayed and/or intraosseous infusion not accomplished. Take a roentgenogram to confirm the location of the endotracheal tube.

c. **Mechanical ventilation support** is indicated in acute respiratory failure (hypoxemia with PaO_2 50 to 60 mm Hg despite a high FiO_2 70% to 100%); apnea; and hypoventilation and respiratory acidosis with pH 7.20 to 7.25.

(1) Positive end-expiratory pressure (PEEP) may be used to prevent or treat alveolar collapse and is the most effective respiratory support for patients with adult respiratory distress syndrome (ARDS).

(2) Many poisoned patients require respiratory support until the toxin is eliminated by being metabolized or excreted.

(3) The arterial blood gases are the best objective determination of ventilation but must be interpreted in conjunction with the clinical status. A "normal" PaO_2 in a patient with significant tachypnea is abnormal. Keep the PaO_2 at above 60 mm Hg and more than 90% saturated.

(4) Obtain a follow-up chest and neck roentgenogram.

(5) Types of assisted ventilation are as follows.

(a) **Controlled ventilation** with abolition of spontaneous breathing rapidly leads to atrophy of the respiratory muscles, therefore assisted modes that trigger the patient's inspiratory efforts are preferred.

(b) **Assist-control ventilation** which delivers a breath either when triggered by the patient's inspiratory effort or independently if such effort does not occur within a preselected period. The patient may initiate each breath in the assist mode if his inspiratory effort is strong enough, otherwise the ventilator provides backup.

(c) **Intermittent mandatory ventilation** (IMV) which delivers periodic positive-pressure breaths from the ventilator at a preset volume and rate and spontaneous breathing is allowed. A continuous flow IMV or demand flow IMV exist.

(d) **Pressure-support ventilation** where the physician sets the level of pressure (rather than the volume) to spontaneously augment every spontaneous effort. Airway pressure is maintained at a preset level until the inspiratory flow falls below a certain level (e.g., 25% of peak flow).

(e) If **bronchospasm** is present, after the patient is removed from the exposure, administer supplemental moist oxygen and aerosolized beta-2 adrenergic agonist agent, e.g., albuterol 2.5 mg in a nebulizer. If the patient has been receiving a beta-blocker, discontinue it. Beta-2 adrenergic agonists may not be effective, therefore consider an aminophylline infusion of 6 mg/kg i.v. over 30 to 60 min. For organophosphate or cholinergic bronchospasm crisis, administer atropine.

3. Assess **cardiovascular status** by evaluation of volume, rate and rhythm of the peripheral pulses, skin and brain perfusion and the ECG monitor.

a. **Cardiopulmonary resuscitation** (CPR) is initiated immediately, *if* necessary.

b. **Continuous cardiac monitoring** for dysrhythmias is essential in the comatose patient and patients with cardiotoxic drug exposure, e.g., tricyclic antidepressants and phenothiazines.

c. Obtain and analyze a 12 lead ECG as to duration of intervals and waves.

4. Establish **vascular access,** ensure adequate circulation and perfusion.
   a. In **children** younger than 3 years of age the intraosseous site should be used after 90 to 120 s have elapsed or three unsuccessful i.v. attempts.
   b. In **hemodynamically unstable** patients who do not respond to adequate fluid replacement, central lines or a Swan Ganz Catheter should be established.
   c. **Obtain blood for studies** (glucose, sodium, potassium, chloride, BUN, creatinine, calcium, magnesium, creatine kinase, arterial blood gases, carboxyhemoglobin, liver enzymes, ammonia, coagulation studies, osmolality, blood culture and toxicologic analysis). Therapeutic diagnostic tests are listed in Table 4-12.
      (1) Clinical judgment and the historical information will determine which tests should be done immediately.
      (2) Look at the **color of the blood** obtained (brown suggests methemoglobinemia and bright red venous blood suggest carboxyhemoglobin and cyanohemoglobin).
      (3) Keep one specimen in reserve for additional studies.
   d. **Shock and hypotension** should be managed by correction of hypoxia, volume expansion, correction of acidosis, rewarming in hypothermia, and correction of electrolyte disturbances, treatment of dysrhythmias producing hypotension and vasopressors, if necessary (26,27).
      (1) **Shock:** Administer a bolus of crystalloid solution (0.89% saline or Ringer's lactate) in 5 min of 20 mL/kg in children or 300 to 500 mL in adults and repeat according to response (improvement in mental status, capillary refill, pulse volume, decrease in tachycardia, and blood pressure).
         (a) **Avoid excess fluids** once shock and hypovolemia are stabilized, especially in conditions susceptible to pulmonary edema or cerebral edema, where careful regulation of fluids is required.

TABLE 4-12. *Therapeutic diagnostic tests*

Toxin	Diagnostic	Route	Positive response
Anticholinergic	Physostigmine, 2 mg adult	i.v.	Nonspecific; not recommended
Benzodiazepine	Flumazenil, 0.02 mg/kg	i.v.	Consciousness improves; Caution with patients on BZP and TCAD
Digitalis	FAB antibodies	i.v.	Dysrhythmia improves; hyperkalemia improves
Insulin	Glucose, 1 g/kg	i.v.	Consciousness improves; hypoglycemia improves
Iron	Deferoxamine, 40 mg/kg	i.m.	"Vin rose" color urine; negative does not exclude
Isoniazid	Pyridoxine, 5 g	i.v.	Seizures abate
Opioid	Naloxone, 0.1 mg/kg	i.v.	Consciousness improves; ventilation improves
Phenothiazine idiosyncrasy	Diphenhydramine, 1 mg/kg	i.v.	Dystonia and torticollis resolve

BZP, benzodiazepine dependency or using to control seizures; TCAD, tricyclic antidepressants may cause dysrhythmias or seizures.

(b) **Vasopressors** may be considered earlier in place of excess fluids. **Dopamine,** 2 to 20 µg/kg/min infusion, is the vasopressor usually chosen; however, in agents producing alpha-receptor blockage, such as phenothiazines and tricyclic antidepressants, **norepinephrine,** an alpha-agonist, 4 to 8 µg/min in adults (0.1 to 1.0 µg/kg/min infusion) titrated every 5 to 10 min to desired effect is preferred over dopamine. **Epinephrine** infusion 1 µg/kg/min titrated to desired response may be used. Vasopressors may be used in combination. Norepinephrine and epinephrine are the choice in severe hypotension.

(c) Treat the **cardiac dysrhythmias** that contribute to hypotension and poor perfusion (usually with rates below 40/min or above 180/min in adults). Treat a wide QRS immediately with sodium bicarbonate bolus. For specific agents for intoxicant, see Table 4-13.

(d) **Hypothermic hypotension** does not respond to fluids but does normalize on warming. Hypothermia body temperature of 32°C (90°F) should be expected to have a systolic blood pressure of 70 to 90 mm Hg.

(2) The **specific therapy** (Table 4-13).

(3) An **indwelling catheter** should be inserted to obtain urine for analysis and to monitor output. A **nasogastric** should be inserted and attached to suction to preclude vomiting and aspiration.

e. **Hypertension** in a young person is more significant than in a chronic hypertensive individual.

(1) Hypertension is usually initially transient and does not require therapy.

(2) **Hypertensive crisis** (hypertension associated with heart failure, myocardial ischemia or encephalopathy), is treated nitroprusside, 0.3 to 2 µg/kg/min is recommended. Nitroprusside maximum dose is 2 µg/kg/min and 10 µg/kg/min for no longer than 10 min. Thiocyanate

TABLE 4-13. *Therapeutic diagnostic tests II*

Toxic ingestion	Specific therapy	Vasopressor
Beta-adrenergic antagonist	Glucagon	Epinephrine
	Amrinone	Dobutamine
	Isoproterenol	
Calcium channel blocker	Calcium	Dopamine
	Glucagon	Dobutamine
	Sodium bicarbonate	Isoproterenol
	Amrinone	
Alpha-adrenergic antagonist or phenothiazine	Norepinephrine	
	Phenylephrine	
Cyclic antidepressants	Sodium bicarbonate	Norepinephrine
		Phenylephrine
Cholinergic agents	Atropine	Dopamine
Opioids	Naloxone	Dopamine
Magnesium	Calcium	Dopamine

poisoning has been reported with higher rates of administration. If suspect thiocyanate poisoning from nitroprusside treat with sodium thiosulfate 25% 1.65 mL/kg without sodium nitrite) and without waiting for laboratory confirmation (93). Diazoxide or longer action antihypertensives are usually not recommended because they have too long a duration of action (Table 4-14).

(3) **If focal neurologic signs,** do not treat the mild-moderate hypertension and obtain a CT scan.

f. **Maintain the circulation.** Failure to respond to a fluid challenge with a good urinary output necessitates consideration of a central line to monitor the adequacy of fluid therapy and the competence of the cardiovascular system. This also brings into consideration the possibility of renal failure.

(1) **Early renal failure** is suggested by oliguria, urine specific gravity below 1.010 and urine sodium greater than 30 mEq/L.

(2) Patients in **coma** are predisposed to develop inappropriate secretion of the antidiuretic hormone (SIADH). Therefore, fluid should be administered only to correct the hypovolemia and shock and then limited to maintenance. Fluid and electrolyte status should be carefully and frequently monitored.

g. **Electrolyte and acid-base disturbances** occur in many intoxications.

(1) **Hypokalemia** (salicylate and theophylline intoxications) and disturbances in acid base balance predispose to dysrhythmias.

(2) Life-threatening **hyperkalemia** may be present and is treated by calcium administration (**not used in digitalis intoxications**), bicarbonate, glucose and insulin infusions, and later, sodium polystyrene sulfonate.

5. **Dysrhythmias and conduction blocks.** Contributing factors are hypoxia, acidosis and electrolyte abnormalities, which should be corrected. Periodically a 12 lead ECG should be obtained for details about intervals and wave abnormalities. Table 4-15 gives normal ECG intervals in children.

a. Life-threatening hemodynamically **unstable ventricular dysrhythmias** should receive countershock. **Countershock should be used with caution in digitalis intoxication** because of the tendency to produce ventricular fibrillation. This is an indication for FAB. If countershock is used digitalis intoxications start with the lowest electrical dose.

TABLE 4-14. *Antihypertensive drugs for emergency use*

Adult dose	Pediatric dose
Nitroprusside, 0.3–2 mg/kg/min; 10 µg/kg/min can be given for 10 min only initially	Same
Phentolamine, 2.5–5 mg i.v. slowly	0.02–0.1 mg/kg i.v. slowly
Labetalol, 20 mg i.v. q 10 min	0.5 mg/kg i.v. 0.25 mg/kg q 2 h
Diazoxide, 1–3 mg/kg i.v. max 150 mg, i.v. q 5–15 min until desired effect, repeat q 4–24 h	Same

TABLE 4-15. *ECG finding in children*

Age	Heart rate (bpm)	PR interval (sec)	QRS wave (sec)
Newborn	90–180	0.07–0.16	0.03–0.08
3 mo to 1 yr	80–160	0.07–0.16	0.03–0.08
1–3 yr	70–140	0.08–0.16	0.04–0.08
4–10 yr	60–120	0.09–0,17	0.04–0.07
>10 yr	60–110	0.09–0.20	0.04–0.08

PR interval = time between sinus atrial node and atrial ventricular node. QRS = duration for ventricular depolarization.

    b. For less urgent **ventricular tachycardia,** lidocaine 1 to 3 mg/kg i.v. or phenytoin 5 to 15 mg/kg i.v. with ECG and blood pressure monitoring may be used.

    c. **Tricyclic antidepressant** overdose with evidence of cardiac toxicity, such as wide QRS tachycardia, should be treated by bolus of 2 mEq/kg sodium bicarbonate i.v. (30).

    d. **Torsades de Pointes** may be treated with magnesium sulfate 2 g slowly i.v. as a 20% solution over 1 min followed by an infusion of 1 mg/min. In children the dose is 25 to 50 mg/kg. Overdrive pacing may also be used (94–96).

    e. **Unstable bradycardia** and second and third degree blocks should be managed in an emergency with a transvenous or external pacemaker. For less urgent but **unstable patients with bradycardia** (syncope, hypotension) treat with atropine 0.01 to 0.03 mg/kg i.v. minimum 0.1 mg or isoproterenol 1 to 10 µg/min i.v.

    f. **Hypothermia** with a body temperature of 32°C to 35°C (90°F to 95°F) will have bradycardia of 40 to 50 and will normalize on rewarming.

    g. **Unexplained cardiac arrest** in a young person. Examine for drugs hidden in bowel, vagina or rectum (body packers or stuffers).

    h. **Specific antidotal therapy** for dysrhythmias are listed in Table 4-11b.

  6. **The comatose** or altered mental status patient. If the patient is unconscious always stabilize the cervical spine, if airway protective reflexes are absent, endotracheal intubation, and if ineffective respirations, ventilate with 100% oxygen. If a cyanotic patient fails to respond to oxygen consider cyanide intoxication or methemoglobinemia. Perform a reagent strip test for blood glucose to detect hypoglycemia. Document the time, date, and the depth of the coma (97–99).

    a. **Glucose.** Always **confirm** the glucose reagent strip result with laboratory blood glucose analysis. However, do not delay treatment for the official laboratory confirmation. Administer glucose if the glucose reagent strip visually reads less than 120 mg/dL. Acceptable reagent trip values are within 25% of the laboratory values. Reagent strips are inaccurate at very high or low blood glucose concentrations. It is preferable to use **venous** blood, rather than capillary, for the reagent strip especially if the patient is in shock or hypotensive because capillary blood result may create a false impression of hypoglycemia and mislead into accepting it as a cause of altered mental status (97).

(1) **Hypoglycemia** may be the cause of coma and altered mental status. It accompanies many overdoses (ethanol especially in children, clonidine, insulin, organophosphates, salicylates, and sulfonylureas).

(2) If hypoglycemia is present or suspected immediately administer the following:

    (a) Neonate: 10% glucose (5 mL/kg)

    (b) Children: 25% glucose 0.25 g/kg (2 mL/kg) i.v.

    (c) Adolescents/adults: 50% glucose 0.5 g/kg (1 mL/kg) i.v.

(3) Large amounts of glucose given rapidly to nondiabetic patients may cause a **reactive hypoglycemia** (due to release of insulin) and transient hyperkalemia. Recent evidence suggests that excess glucose may accentuate **damage** in ischemic cerebrovascular and cardiac tissue by providing the fuel for anaerobic metabolism to produce lactic acidosis (97,99–101). However, studies were on chronic models, not acute patients. In patients with hyperosmolar coma, glucose bolus increases the hyperosmolarity (97,100). If the patient has **focal neurological signs** it may be wise to withhold glucose since hypoglycemia causes focal signs in less than 10% of patients (97).

(4) **Indications for i.v. glucose**: all patients with altered mental status (AMS); numerical hypoglycemia on reagent strip; nonfocal neurological exams and borderline glucose levels; and AMS when rapid reactant strip testing is not available (97,102).

(5) **Document** the response to i.v. glucose and if the patient improves, continue infusion of glucose as necessary to keep the blood glucose at 100 to 150 mg/dL.

b. **Thiamine** provides the cofactor for a number of metabolic pathways and may avoid precipitating the thiamine deficiency encephalopathy (Wernicke-Korsakoff syndrome). The overall incidence of thiamine deficiency is 0.8% to 22% of the general population due to malabsorption, malnutrition and 12% of ethanol abusers.

(1) **The classic triad of Wernicke encephalopathy** is global confusion, ophthalmoplegia, and ataxia. The Korsakoff psychosis is a short-term memory disorder that results in confabulation. Wernicke encephalopathy ophthalmoplegia usually responds within 4 h but the other aspects respond slowly if at all (97–99).

(2) **Indications for i.v. thiamine** are if the patient appears malnourished or is a chronic alcoholic. Thiamine 100 mg i.v. at the time of the glucose administration. Theoretically, considerations that thiamine must be administered prior to the glucose are not valid (97,98). The clinician should be prepared to manage anaphylaxis due to thiamine, although reports indicate this is an extremely rare occurrence (97–99). Of 989 consecutive patients administered an i.v. thiamine bolus, only 1 reaction of general pruritic nature occurred.

    c. **Naloxone,** the first pure opioid antagonist, reverses CNS and respiratory depression, miosis, bradycardia, decreased GI peristalsis of opioids acting through mu, kappa, and delta receptors. It also affects the endogenous opioid peptides (endorphins and enkephalins). This accounts for the variable responses (not therapeutically consistently useful) that have been reported from intoxications with ethanol, BZPs, clonidine, captopril and valproic acid, and in head and spinal cord injuries (103). It may precipitate opioid withdrawal, violent behavior and unmask concomitant sympathomimetic intoxication. Its use is reversed for respiratory depression (rate of respirations less than 12 and depth and elevated PCO_2) and consistent opioid intoxication (97).

    (1) If no response to glucose, **administer naloxone** as a diagnostic test or a therapeutic agent to reverse CNS and respiratory depression. The dose is 0.1 mg/kg in a **child** or 2 mg to 20 kg (5 years) in suspected overdose (104). However, there is a risk of withdrawal seizures in respiratory depressed **newborns** whose mother may have been maintained on methadone during pregnancy, therefore the dose should be 0.01 mg/kg (104). In an **adult** the recommended 0.1 to 0.2 mg be administered initially to avoid withdrawal and violent behavior (104) and if no withdrawal or violent behavior, double the dose progressively to a total of 10 mg (104). Other toxicologists administer 2 mg every 2 to 5 min for five doses until a total of 10 mg. If no response by 10 mg, a pure opioid intoxication is unlikely. The **duration** of action is only 30 to 60 min (half-life 20 to 30 min).

    (2) **Nalmefene** (Revex), a longer acting parenteral opioid antagonist is undergoing investigation but its role in opioid overdose is not clear at this time (100).

    (3) **Larger doses** of naloxone may be required for poorly antagonized synthetic opioid drugs: buprenorphine, codeine, dextromethorphan, fentanyl pentazocine, propoxyphene, diphenoxylate, nalbuphine, new potent "designer" drugs or long-acting opioids such as methadone.

    (4) If suspect **opioid addiction** administer a lower dose 0.1 to 0.2 mg (to prevent violent withdrawal), then progress in doubling fashion until 10 mg (100).

    (5) Naloxone should be given with caution in possible combinations of opioid and **sympathomimetics** (cocaine "speedball" or amphetamine overdose because it may counteract the opioid action unmasking hypertension (111–114), dysrhythmias (103), and convulsions from the stimulants (106).

    (6) **Routes.** Naloxone can be administered through the endotracheal tube as a minimum dose of 2 mg, intraosseous (same dose as given i.v.), sublingual, and i.m. The preferred route is i.v.

    (7) **Document** the response: improvement in respiratory rate and depth, dilation of pupils, reversal of hypotension and improvement in level of consciousness.

(8) Complications. Although naloxone is safe and effective (107,108), there are reports of pulmonary edema with naloxone reversal of opioid overdose. For this reason some clinicians start with 0.4 mg in adults and if no reaction give 2 mg every 1 to 2 min to 10 mg (109). Some clinicians have suggested limiting the administration of naloxone to patients with less than 12 respirations/min in adults (80% sensitivity for predicting who will respond), pinpoint pupils, and those with circumstantial evidence of opioid intoxication (i.e., track marks) (110). However, assessment of respiratory effectiveness by rate alone does not ensure adequate ventilation or oxygenation. Other reported complications include seizures (106), hypertension (111–114), cardiac arrest (115), sudden death (119), and patient violence (117). Naloxone has been used in the treatment of shock, stroke, spinal injuries, and overdose without significant complications. The complications rate in 813 patients with prehospital administration was less than 1% and all reactions were inconsequential (108).

(9) If there is a significant response to naloxone a **continuous infusion** has been advocated because many opioids outlast the short half-life of naloxone (20 to 30 min). **Indications** for a continuous infusion in an intensive care setting are as follows:

(a) A second dose is required to produce a response or there is recurrent respiratory or neurologic depression.

(b) There is exposure to poorly antagonized opioid.

(c) A very large overdose has occurred.

(d) Decreased opioid metabolism, e.g., impaired liver function. The naloxone infusion hourly rate is equal to the initially effective amount required to produce an arousal. A repeat dose in 15 to 30 min after the infusion has been started as a bolus may be required. The infusions are titrated to avoid respiratory depression and opioid withdrawal manifestations. Tapering of infusions can be attempted after 12 h of therapy has stabilized the patient's condition (118–121).

d. Flumazenil (Romazicon) is a pure competitive BZP antagonist. It has been demonstrated to be safe and effective for BZP-induced sedation and in patients undergoing short procedures as endoscopy and cardioversion. Flumazenil reverses the sedative, ataxic, muscle relaxant, anxiolytic, and anticonvulsant effects of BZPs (122).

(1) Fumazenil is not recommended to improve ventilation. Its half-life is 0.7 to 1.3 h, which is shorter than most of the BZP. Liver dysfunction decreases clearance by 60% (122).

(2) BZPs are identified in 10% of fatalities caused by drug intoxication; however, a pure BZP overdose rarely results in death (123). Flumazenil's role in coma appears limited and should be clarified. It should not be used routinely and is not an essential ingredient of the coma therapeutic regime (124–134).

(3) Flumazenil should **not be administered** to
   (a) Cyclic antidepressant intoxications
   (b) Patients who may be using long-term BZPs because it may precipitate the life-threatening withdrawal state.
   (c) If BZPs are used to control seizures
   (d) In head trauma
   (e) If BZPs use is anticipated in the near future.

(4) **Dose.** After the airway is secured if necessary, flumazenil is administered 0.2 mg (2l mL) or 10 µg/kg body weight up to 0.2 mg in children, over 30 s, wait 3 min for a response, if desired consciousness is not achieved, administer 0.3 mg (3 mL) over 30 s at 0.2 mg/min, wait 3 min for a response. If desired consciousness is not achieved, administer 0.5 mg (5 mL) over 30 s at 60 s intervals up to a cumulative dose of 3 mg in an hour (30 mL). If no results after 5 mg the diagnosis of BZP toxicity should be questioned (123).

(5) **Complications.** There have been reports of dysrhythmias (135) and death often from seizures (135–138).

7. **Convulsions** (141–154). Exclude other movement disorders, e.g., dystonia and myoclonus. Convulsions may be the direct effect of the toxin, or secondary to hypoxia or other metabolic or electrolyte disturbances.

   a. **Specific therapy** should be administered, e.g., 100% oxygen for carbon monoxide is 100% oxygen, calcium for ethylene glycol produced hypokalcemia, i.v. glucose for intoxications inducing hypoglycemia. Pyridoxine and diazepam for the control isoniazid seizures. Seizures in patients on lithium or salicylates may indicate toxic concentrations in the brain which require hemodialysis.

   b. **Anticonvulsant** may be necessary. Diazepam or lorazepam are the agents of choice but recurrent or persistent seizures require phenobarbital and possibly neuromuscular blockers (as adjuncts) or pentobarbital coma or general anesthesia (Table 4-16).

TABLE 4-16. *Common anticonvulsant therapy in children*

Agent	Dosage	Rate	Duration action
Diazepam i.v.	Initial 0.3 mg/kg Repeat 0.2–0.3 mg/kg	1 mg/min	15 min
Diazepam rectal	Initial 0.5 mg/kg Rectal 0.25 mg/kg[a] or i.v. 0.1 mg/kg		
Phenytoin i.v.	15–18 mg/kg	25 mg/min	
Phenobarbital i.v.	10–20 mg/kg	30 mg/min	
Lorazepam i.v.	Initial 0.05–0.1 mg/kg Repeat 0.05 mg/kg	<2 mg/min	2–12 h

[a]Modified from Siegler PS. The administration of rectal-diazepam for acute management of seizures. *J Emerg Med* 1990;8:155; Albano A, et al. Rectal diazepam in pediatric status epilepticus. *Am J Emerg Med* 1989;70:168.

c. **Diazepam** acts to enhance gamma-aminobutyric acid (GABA), the major inhibitory neurotransmitter and blocks calcium reuptake. It temporarily terminates the seizures 79% of the time. The i.v. preparation contains 5 mg of diazepam in 1 mL of 40% propylene glycol solution. The propylene glycol vehicle has been confused with ethylene glycol on certain laboratory procedures and it may add to the toxicity in ethylene glycol intoxications. Rapid i.v. injection of propylene glycol may cause hypotension and shock. It should be administered at a rate of less than 2.5 mg/min in adults and less than 1 mg/min in children. The doses should be given i.v. in status epilepticus (142,143,146).

(1) **Neonate** 0.1 to 0.3 mg/kg every 15 to 30 min over 2 to 3 min not to exceed 2 mg in 24 h.

(2) **Children** 30 days–5 years 0.2 to 0.5 mg/kg/dose over 2 to 3 min every 2 to 5 min up to maximum total dose of 5 mg.

(3) **Children** older than 5 years **1 mg/dose (total dose)** over 2 to 3 min every 2 to 5 min up to total dose of 10 mg.

(4) **Adults** 5 to 10 mg (total dose) every 10 to 20 min up to 30 mg, may repeat in 2 h if necessary (149).

(5) Diazepam should be administered into an i.v. line as close to the puncture site as possible to avoid absorption by plastic tubing. It enters the brain rapidly and usually acts within s, its half-life is 20 min but its duration is only 20 to 30 min.

(6) Monitor vital signs and ECG during administration and **be prepared with ventilatory support** to treat apnea. Respiratory depression and hypotension may occur in 12% to 13% of patients (145). Phenobarbital enhances diazepam's respiratory depressant effect (141).

d. **Lorazepam** (144,145). The i.v. preparation contains 2.4 mg/mL with 0.18 mL of propylene glycol has actions similar to diazepam.

(1) It has slower onset of action (2 to 3 min versus less than seconds for diazepam), it has longer duration of action than diazepam (3 to 6 h versus 20 to 30 min for diazepam) because of its smaller volume of distribution (12 L/kg versus 133 L/kg for diazepam) and its lower protein binding (85% versus 98% for diazepam) permit higher rate of transfer to the cerebrospinal fluid (CSF) (145,146). The i.v. doses are as follows:

(2) **Neonates:** 0.05 mg/kg/dose over 2 to 5 min, repeat in 10 to 15 min. Contains benzyl alcohol.

(3) **Children:** 0.1 mg/kg/dose at a rate of 1 mg/min, over 2 to 5 min up to maximum 4 mg repeated twice at intervals of 10 to 15 min, if required.

(4) **Adult:** 2.5 to 10 mg/dose repeated twice at intervals of 10 to 15 min, if required. The usual effective dose in adults is 4 to 5 mg, maximum is 8 mg. It should be administered no faster than 1 to 2 mg/min.

e. **Phenytoin** stabilizes neuronal membranes and reduces sodium influx and calcium passage through the membranes. The i.v. preparation contains 1 g phenytoin in 20 mL of 40% propylene glycol as the vehicle. Rapid infusion may cause dysrhythmias, ventricular standstill, hypotension and shock.

Phenytoin is effective as a single agent in termination of 56% to 80% of seizures, but with toxic and metabolic disturbances this rate falls to 40%. Phenytoin does not enhance gamma-aminobutyric acid (GABA) and therefore is not effective against cocaine, isoniazid, gyromitra mushroom, theophylline intoxications that interfere GABA (149).

(1) **The loading dose** i.v. is 15 to 20 mg/kg as a "piggy-back" infusion dilute in 0.9% saline (not glucose because it causes crystallization) to a concentration of 10 mg/mL. A 0.22-um filter should be placed on the i.v. line. The patient should be on a cardiac monitor throughout the infusion and until 60 min after completion (153). It should be administered at a rate of 1 mg/kg/min up to 25 mg/min in children and adults with cardiopulmonary disease and 50 mg/min in adults without cardiac disease (141,143). The maximum dose is 30 mg/kg in the first 8 h and 40 mg/kg in 24 h or 1.5 g as loading dose in adults.

(2) The onset of action may be seen 10 min into infusion with maximum effect within 10 min after completion of infusion. Its half-life is 20 to 36 h.

(3) Therapeutic plasma concentrations 10 to 20 µg/mL are maintained for 6 h. Obtain a serum phenytoin plasma concentration after 30 to 60 min (141,143,146).

f. **Phenobarbital** (141–143) interferes with the transmission of impulses from the thalamus to the cortex by enhancing the effect of GABA. The i.v. preparations are 30, 60, 65, and 130 mg/mL. It should be administered at a rate not to exceed 30 mg/min in children or 100 mg/min in adults. The i.v. doses are as follows:

(1) **Children:** 15 to 20 mg/kg over 20 min initially followed by 5 to 10 mg/kg/dose at interval of 20 min until seizures are controlled or 40 mg/kg is reached.

(2) **Adults:** initial dose 7.5 to 20 mg/kg or about 300 to 800 mg followed by 120 to 240 mg/dose until seizures are controlled or 1.2 g maximum.

(3) **The disadvantages** of phenobarbital is its slow absorption by the brain parenchyma, requiring 10 to 20 min for its anticonvulsive effects. It also has a long half-life of 50 to 100 h and alters the mental status for prolonged periods. It is the drug of choice for barbiturate withdrawal. Obtain serum phenobarbital concentration 30 to 60 min after administration.

g. **Midazolam** depresses all levels of the CNS through increased action of GABA. The half-life is 2 to 4 h and duration of sedation is 30 min to 2 h, although its effects may last 10 h or more after infusion. The dosage is 0.05 to 0.1 mg/kg i.v., maximum 2.5 mg/dose over 2 min. Respiratory arrest may occur if given rapidly or in excessive doses. Although not approved by the FDA, it has been used safely and effectively in status epilepticus refractory to standard anticonvulsant (147,154). Rivera et al. administered a loading dose of 0.15 mg/kg to 24 children with refractory status epilepticus followed by an infusion at rates of 1 to 18 µg/kg/min (0.06 to 1.08 mg/kg/h) and terminated the seizures in all children (147,148,138). It can be given i.m. if there is no venous access.

h. **Neuromuscular blockers or general anesthesia.** If the anticonvulsant fails to control the seizures within 1 h after the onset, the patient may require neuromuscular blockade and assisted ventilation. Neuromuscular agents will facilitate intubation and will abolish motor activity. Refractory convulsions may be managed by pentobarbital coma, or halothane general anesthesia. They are not anticonvulsants and require EEG monitoring for nonmotor brain seizure activity (146–149,154).

i. **Pentobarbital anesthesia** requires intubation, ventilatory support and hemodynamic monitoring preferably with Swan-Ganz catheter and continuous EEG monitoring. The loading dose is 5 mg/kg at an infusion rate of 25 mg/kg/min followed by 2.5 mg/kg/h maintenance to achieve an EEG that shows suppression-burst pattern. Recurrent seizures are treated with a 50-mg bolus followed by an increase in maintenance infusion by 0.5 mg/kg/hr. Tapering is recommended after 12 to 24 h of EEG control at a rate of 0.5 to 1 mg/kg/h every 4 to 6 h (150).

j. Agents reported in the literature **no longer recommended** include lidocaine, chloral hydrate, paraldehyde (i.v. preparation no longer available in United States).

k. **Status epilepticus** (SE) means the seizure episode has lasted over 30 min or a series of seizures when the victim does not regain consciousness between seizures. The **incidence** is about 250,000/year (one in every 1,000 Americans) (151). Ten percent occur in children (151). After 90 min of seizure activity, the CNS neuron damage occurs, electrolyte abnormalities develop, lactic acidosis develops within 30 min (will normalize within 1 h after the seizures cease), and convulsions become more difficult to control (148,149) (Table 4-17).

(1) The cause of SE varies from illicit drugs, alcohol, and trauma in the adolescent to stroke, tumor and infection in the elderly and, in children, fever, infection, and lead encephalopathy. **Substances that cause refractory seizures** include alcohol, amphetamines, amoxopine, cocaine, isoniazid, chronic lead encephaloathy, theophylline.

(2) **The complications of prolonged seizures** include, hypoxia, hypoglycemia, hyperthermia, hypotension, dysrhythmias, rhabdomyolysis and myoglobinuria, pulmonary and cerebral edema, and disseminated intravascular coagulation. In addition leukemoid reactions and CSF pleocytosis develop (149).

(3) The **treatment** of status epilepticus in adults includes the following:

(a) Stabilization: Airway and intubate early. Ventilate and oxygenate. Use pulse oximetry to monitor oxygenation.

(b) Monitor vital signs including temperature and use ECG monitor for dysrhythmias.

TABLE 4-17. *Treatment of status epilepticus*

Time	Procedure
0–5 min	Assess cardiorespiratory function, take history, and perform neurologic and physical examination. Obtain blood specimens for anticonvulsant drug levels, glucose, BUN, creatinine, calcium, magnesium, electrolytes, complete blood count, metabolic screen, drug screen, arterial blood gases.
6–9 min	Start i.v. infusion with saline solution. Administer 25 g of glucose, along with B vitamins.
10–45 min	Infuse lorazepam 0.1 mg/kg (4–10 mg total) at <2 mg/min. Begin infusion of phenytoin, 20 mg/kg at 25 mg/min; this may take 20–40 min total; carefully monitor ECG, respiration, and blood pressure. If patients are on phenytoin, give 9 mg/kg. If seizures persist, give additional phenytoin, 5 mg/kg at the same rate and, if needed, another 5 mg/kg until a maximum of 30 mg/kg has been given.
46–60 min	If seizures persist, intubate and give phenobarbital 20 mg/kg at <100 mg/min i.v.
>1 h	If seizures persist, pentobarbital anesthesia 5 mg/kg at 25 mg/min; follow by 2.5 mg/kg/h, or general anesthesia should be implemented. Neuromuscular blockers if needed. Neuromuscular blockers are adjuncts not anticonvulsant.

Modified from Watson C. Status epilepticus. Clinical features, pathophysiology and treatment. *West J Med* 1991; 155; Jagonda A, Riggio S. Refractory status epilepticus in adults. *Ann Emerg Med* 1993; 22:1337–1348.

    (c) Evaluation: Indwelling urinary catheter and monitor urinary output. Insert nasogastric tube in place and monitor output. EEG monitor especially if using neuromuscular blockers or barbiturate anesthesia. Recheck infusion for proper function and drug delivery at frequent intervals.

    (d) Blood studies include blood glucose, electrolytes, CPK, BUN, creatinine, magnesium, calcium, phosphorous, liver function, PT and PTT, ethanol blood concentration, CBC, differential, and anticonvulsant blood level.

    (e) Urine. Toxic screen for substances of abuse, urinalysis, pregnancy test on all females of child-bearing age, and urine for myoglobin.

    (f) Consider a lumbar puncture and computerized tomography of head

    (g) Administer **thiamine** 100 mg i.v. and **magnesium** 1 to 2 g in all patients with alcoholism or malnourished patients. Administer 100 mg pyridoxine i.v.

  8. **Increased intracranial pressure (ICP)** is managed by attempting to control cerebral blood volume to maintain mean arterial pressure (MAP) between 60 to 90 mm Hg and **cerebral perfusion pressure** (CPP) between 50 to 70 mm Hg. The CPP is calculated as the difference between the mean arterial pressure and the ICP (153). Assessment by a neurosurgeon is advised and intracranial pressure monitors are helpful.

a. **Hyperventilation** to a PCO_2 of 25 mm Hg (range 20 to 35 mm Hg). Hypocarbia produces pH mediated cerebrovascular vasoconstriction that decreases the cerebral blood flow 5% for each millimeter fall in PCO_2. However, positive end expiratory pressure (PEEP) may raise the ICP.

b. **Restriction of fluid** if suspect inappropriate secretion of the antidiuretic hormone (ISADH).

c. **Avoid extreme hyperglycemia** because osmotically active glucose especially in ischemic tissue aggravates cerebral edema by producing lactic acidosis.

d. If hyperventilation fails to lower the ICP, **mannitol** is introduced i.v. 0.25 up to 1 g/kg/dose of 20% solution run in over 30 to 60 min (avoid serum osmolality of more than 320 mOsmol/L).

e. **Furosemide** 1 mg/kg up to 40 to 80 mg/dose is given with the first dose of mannitol to reduce the initial paradoxical elevation in ICP.

f. **High-dose corticosteroids.** Methylprednisone 15 to 30 mg/kg or dexamethasone 0.25 to 0.5 mg/kg up to 40 mg a day has been given to inhibit CSF production in acute interstitial edema due to brain tumors and in pseudotumor cerebri, but most current studies demonstrated no improvement in functional outcome in head injury.

g. **Barbiturates**. Pentobarbital 5 to 30 mg/kg i.v. loading dose are given to stabilize the membranes and to decrease neuronal metabolism and to suppress bursts on EEG.

h. **Elevation of head** 30 degrees above the level of the heart (facilitates venous drainage), if vital signs are stable may be helpful but is controversial.

9. **Establish an indwelling urinary catheter** to obtain urine for analysis and monitor urinary output (the average normal output is 1 to 2 mL/kg/h in a child or 60 mL/h in adults).

a. Perform a complete urinalysis and baseline urine culture if catheterized. Obtain 100 mL of urine for toxicologic analysis.

b. Examine the urine for oxalate or monohydrate crystals which may be seen with **ethylene glycol intoxication.** Test the urine for **myoglobin** (positive 3+ or 4+ benzidine or ortho-toluidine test of urine for blood but less than 10 red blood cells and the urine ferroprotein myoglobin of more than 100 mg/dL imparts a brown color to the urine).

c. **Rhabdomyolysis** (155–160) (muscle necrosis) occurs with prolonged immobilization on a hard surface, violent muscle activity, prolonged convulsions, myositis and some metabolic myopathies. Destruction of the muscle membrane causes the lysis or leakage of the muscle cytoplasmic constituents including myoglobin. **Myoglobinemia and myoglobinuria** may occur with or without rhabdomyolysis. The creatine kinase (CK) is often over 10,000 units. Rhabdomyolysis may result in myoglobinemia which can precipitate in the renal tubules and cause renal failure, compartment syndrome (160), disseminated intravascular coagulation and metabolic normalities.

(1) Rhabdomyolysis has **over 150 causes** but occurs most frequently with amphetamines, ethanol, heroin, cocaine and phencyclidine intoxications.

(2) **Management** of myoglobinuria consists of **fluid diuresis** to produce a urine output of 3 to 5 mL/kg/h or 200 to 350 mL/h and **furosemide** 2 to 5 mg/kg up to 200 mg in adults and **mannitol** 0.5 g/kg of 20% solution (25 g in adults) run in over 30 min, if necessary. **Alkalization** of the urine to pH of more than 7.0 by adding sodium bicarbonate to i.v. fluids is controversial but should be considered if acidosis is present or if there are high levels of potassium. Correct and monitor any associated electrolyte abnormalities, metabolic acidosis, and hyperthermia (155–161).

10. **Computerized axial tomography (CAT)** of the head should be considered if:

a. There are **focal** or lateralizing signs such as hemiparesis.

b. The etiology remains unclear. Not all structural lesions produce lateralizing focal signs. "No patient should be denied a CAT study if there is a suspicion of a mass lesion despite the absence of focality."

c. There is **evidence of increased intracranial pressure (ICP)** (papilledema or herniation syndromes). If the signs of increased intracranial pressure are present, reduce the ICP by hyperventilation and mannitol while preparing for computerized axial tomography.

d. The patient has taken substances that may produce an intracranial hemorrhage or other CNS complications.

e. Patient shows evidence of deterioration despite good medical supportive care.

11. **Temperature disturbances.** Only deeply placed flexible probes of the core body temperature should be used (see **VI.12c** and Differential Diagnosis). **Conversion factors:**

$$\text{Centigrade (°C)} \times 1.8 + 32 = \text{Fahrenheit (°F)}$$
$$\text{Fahrenheit (°F)} - 32 \times 0.55 = \text{Centigrade (°C)}$$

a. **Hyperthermia** (79–86)

(1) **Malignant hyperthermia** (MH) (79–86). The Malignant Hyperthermia Association and the North American Hyperthermia Registry have merged and established a **MH Hotline service on treatment:** 1-800-644-9737 (26).

(a) Immediately discontinue all volatile inhalation anesthetics, and succinyl choline. Hyperventilate with 100% oxygen at high gas flows; at least 10 L/min. The circle system and CO_2 absorbant need not be changed.

(b) **Sedation** with a BZP is required to allow the patient to tolerate the ice bath, and it reduces motor activity and muscle tone thereby decreasing heat generation. The BZP will also protect the patient from seizures associated with cocaine and sedative-hypnotic withdrawal.

(c) **Dantrolene sodium** (Dantrium, 20 mg dantrolene lyophilized powder for reconstitution, 3000 mg mannitol and sodium hydroxide in a 70-mL vial). It is a phenytoin derivative that inhibits the calcium release from the sarcoplasm reticulum resulting in decreased muscle contraction, and dopamine agonists such as bromocriptine mesylate or amantadine hydrochloride have been reported to be successful in combination with cooling and good supportive measures in malignant hyperthermia caused by reaction to anesthetic agents (79–84). It does not reverse the rigidity or psychomotor retardation resulting from the central dopamine blockade (79–81). Dantrolene is protein bound and metabolized in liver to less active 5 hydroxy derivatives and excreted in the urine as metabolites. Use with **caution** in patients with cardiac disease, obstructive pulmonary disease or preexisting hepatic disease.

(i)   **Dantrolene** 20 mg (a 70-mL vial) is mixed with 60 mL distilled water for injection without a bacteriostatic agent. The **dose** is 2 to 3 mg/kg i.v. as a bolus 1 mg/kg/min with increments (average dose 2 to 5 mg/kg). Repeat loading dose every 10 min until the signs of MH (e.g., tachycardia, rigidity, increased end-tidal CO_2 and temperature elevation) are controlled, up to a maximum total dose of 10 mg/kg. Hepatotoxicity occurs over 10 mg/kg/dose. Occasionally greater than 10 mg/kg/dose is needed. To prevent recurrence administer 1 mg/kg i.v. every 6 h for 24 to 48 h post episode. After that, oral dantrolene, 1 mg/kg used every 6 h for 24 h as necessary. Watch for **thrombophlebitis** following dantrolene. It is best administered into a **central vein** (81–83). The **critical factor** is to administer enough dantrolene to terminate all signs of MH. Repeat loading dose every 15 min if tachycardia and metabolic acidosis persist.

(ii)   Administer **bicarbonate** to correct metabolic acidosis as guided blood gas analysis. In the absence of blood gas analysis 1 to 2 mEq/kg should be administrated.

(iii)   Simultaneous with above, **actively cool** the hyperthermic patient. Use i.v. cold saline (not Ringer's lacate) 15 mL/kg every 15 min $\times$ 3. Lavage the stomach, bladder, rectum and open with cold saline as appropriate. Surface cool with ice and hypothermic blanket. Monitor closely since over-vigorous treatment may lead to hypothermia.

(iv)   **Dysrhythmias** will usually respond to treatment of acidosis and hyperkalemia. If they persist or are life-threatening, standard antidysrhythmic agents may be used, with the exception of calcium channel blockers (may cause hyperkalemia and cardiovascular collapse).

      (v) **Determine and monitor** every 6 h end-tidal CO_2, arterial, central, or femoral venous blood gases, creatinine kinase serum potassium, calcium, clotting studies, core and central body temperature, serum and urine myoglobin, and urine output.

     (vi) **Hyperkalemia** is common and should be treated with hyperventilation, bicarbonate, i.v. glucose and insulin (10 units insulin in 50 mL 50% glucose titrated to potassium level or 0.15 ug/kg regular insulin in 1 cc/kg 50% glucose). Life-threatening hyperkalemia may also be treated with calcium (e.g., 2 to 5 mg/kg of $CaCl_2$)

    (vii) **Ensure good urine output** of more than 2 mL/kg/h by hydration and/or administration of mannitol or furosemide. Consider central venous or pulmonary artery monitoring because of fluid shifts and hemodynamic instability than can occur.

   (viii) Sudden unexpected cardiac arrest in children less than 10 years old after succinylcholine in absence of hypoxemia and anesthetic overdose treat as acute hyperkalemia first using calcium chloride along with other means to reduce serum potassium.

  (d) **Bromocriptine mesylate** 2.5 to 10 mg orally or through a nasogastric tube three times a day or **amantadine** 100 mg twice a day has been used; however, there is no scientific data on its efficacy, but it seems reasonable. It may be used with dantrolene (79–83).

  (e) **Neuromuscular blockers** may be used to decrease muscular activity. Use *nondepolaring* pancuronium, atracurium or vecuronium but **not** succinylcholine or d-tubocurare. **Do not use** antipyretic medications, phenothiazine (thorazine), butyrophenones (haloperidol) or cooling blankets. Alcohol baths are potentially toxic (79,81).

(2) **Management of other types of drug-hyperthermia consists of the following:**

  (a) Similar to malignant hyperthermia but dantrolene has not been investigated or is not anticipated to be effective.

  (b) **Hypothermia** management depends on body temperature and hemodynamic stability. Normothermia is 36°C to 37.5°C (98°F to 99.5°F) core temperature (26,87–92). Hypothermia is frequently associated with hypoglycemia. Administer glucose if hypoglycemic. Bradycardia 40 to 50/min and hypotension 70 to 90 mm Hg systolic should not be vigorously treated or fluid overload may occur. Rewarming is the management.

    (i) Body temperatures of **32°C to 35°C (89.6°F to 95°F) with stable hemodynamics** are managed by increasing the body heat production with gradual external rewarming at

1°C/h by wrapping in insulated clothing and blankets, offering warm liquids, if alert, and placing in a warm environment. Warming may be difficult to achieve in glycogen depleted or the patient is malnourished or debilitated. If the hemodynamics are unstable heat must be transferred to the patient as for lower temperatures.

(ii) Body temperatures **30°C to 32°C (86°F to 89.6°F) with stable** hemodynamics require the transfer of heat to the patient by heated blankets, warm i.v. solutions (37°C to 43°C) and warm humidified oxygen. Cardiac monitoring is advised.

(iii) Body temperatures of **30°C to 32°C (86°F to 89.6°F) with unstable hemodynamics** require the initiation of active core rewarming in addition to the above measures with warm humidified oxygen (42°C to 45°C), a warming bath (40°C to 41°C), and heated GI irrigation (gastric lavage and colonic enemas).

(iv) Body temperatures **below 30°C (86°F)** should be rewarmed rapidly because of danger of ventricular fibrillation. The methods to be considered in addition to above procedures are peritoneal lavage with heated dialysate (40°C to 42°C), extracorporeal blood rewarming, thoracotomy, and mediastinal lavage with heated fluids.

12. **Management of the agitated, violent, or chemically induced psychotic patient**. These patients may harm themselves and others. The causes of these behaviors were discussed in the previous section.

   a. **Dialogue** used to calm a violent patient may include—"Can I get you a drink of water?" (Never offer hot coffee.) "I see you are upset. Would you tell me why?" "You obviously control yourself well." "I understand how you feel." Specify required behavior in positive terms—"do this" rather than "don't do that." Note the patient's agitation, loud speech, tense posture, and clenched fists. All EDs should develop weapon screening protocols, have furniture and decorations that cannot be used as weapons and have code words to the staff to call for help, e.g., "Need Dr. Armstrong here." Treat violent patients "like a king"—walk in facing him and back out.

   b. If **restraints** are needed, document the reason, e.g., "to facilitate evaluation (organic), or that there is a psychiatric or personality disorder; therefore to administer medication to prevent harm, to himself and/or others."

   (1) **Physical restraints** should be monitored frequently (at least every 15 min and document) to prevent neurovascular sequel and avoid rhabdomyolysis (Fig. 4-4).

   (2) **Pharmacologic restraints**

   (a) **Haloperidol** produces competitive blockade of the postsynaptic dopamine receptors, depresses the cortex, hypothalamus, and has

```
Name of Patient_____ Chart #_____
Date_____Seclusion Time in_____Time out_____
Physician order obtained Dr._____ Date_____
circle 1 2 3 4   Time in _____Time out_____Date____
The following measures to alter the patient's behavior have failed
[ ]  Patient has been removed from stimuli
[ ]  Patient has been encouraged to express feeling in usual manner
[ ]  Staff has been assigned to listen to patient
[ ]  Patient has been offered noncompetitive tasks to complete
[ ]  Patient has been medicated
[ ]  Other Specify _____
Reason for seclusion and restraint explained to patient.
_____

Behavior necessitating restraint _____

Vital signs on admission to seclusion P__R__Temp___BP____Time____
Name of physician (write clearly)_____
Nurse _____
```

Date	Time	Seclusion Room	VS q 15 min	Bath Room	Fluids (cc)	Food	Limb RA LA RL LL Waist	Circu-lation	Range of motion	Staff sign.

FIG. 4-4. Seclusion and restraint record.

strong alpha-adrenergic and anticholinergic blocking activity (63–66). It is not FDA approved for i.v. use. Do not use long-acting deconate salt of haloperidol. The **dose** for young adults varies 0.5 to 5 mg orally three times a day or 2 to 5 mg i.m. every 4 to 8 h, as needed. The doses may be increased rapidly for prompt control 5 to 10 mg and repeated every 30 to 60 min for eight doses. Maximum oral daily dose is 100 mg or 0.1 mg/kg/day i.m. Change to oral as soon as possible. Doses higher than 10 mg do not increase effectiveness (97). Initial dose for the **elderly** should be decreased 0.5 to 2.0 mg (81,87–89). The **side effects** are primarily dystonic reactions, although the neuroleptic malignant syndrome has been described after a single dose. **Avoid haloperidol** in pregnancy, lactation, with lithium (encephalopathic interaction), phencyclidine intoxication, withdrawal syndromes and drug intoxications with anticholinergic properties. Haloperidol and phenothiazine both have undesirable anticholinergic and alpha-blocking effects (63–66,81).

(b)   Alternatives **diazepam** 0.1 to 0.2 mg/kg i.v. slowly 5 mg/min adults and over 3 min in children for anxiety and agitation may repeat every 1 to 4 h as needed, oral dose 0.1 to 0.3 mg/kg or **lorazepam** 2.5 to 10 mg/dose i.v. or i.m. repeated twice at intervals of 15 to 20 min, if required and followed by 0.01 to 0.05 mg/kg i.m., i.v., sublingual or oral every 6 h. **Thiothixene hydrochloride** 4 mg i.m. bid to q.i.d. to 30 mg daily or **fluphenazine** 2.5 to 10 mg oral or i.m. every 6 to 8 h. If extrapyramidal symptoms develop administer benztropine 2 mg i.m. or diphenhydramine 1 mg/kg i.v. followed by oral doses for 5 to 7 days. **Droperidol** 10 mg i.v. or i.m. may be more useful than haloperidol (short i.m. half-life 2.2 h versus i.m. haloperidol 10 to 19 h) but causes hypotension (63,64). **Chlorpromazine** is not advised because of its alpha-adrenergic blocking effects which causes orthostatic hypotension.

(c) **Rapid tranquilization (RT)** (81–92) Explain to the patient the medication will make him or her calm. A combination of antipsychotic medication with lorazepam is more effective than antipsychotic medication alone. Core psychotic symptoms do not respond to a few doses and require weeks of therapy (Table 4-18)

(i) Most patients respond to a combination of haloperidol 5 mg i.m. or thiothixene 10 mg and lorazepam 5 mg i.m. in the same syringe. Some clinicians use haloperidol 5 mg i.m. and lorazepam 10 mg i.m. The medication is administered hourly. Most patients respond to one to three doses. The use of antipsychotic medications i.v. in the ED has not been well studied (81). The dosage should be reduced to half in patients older than 65 years of age.

TABLE 4-18. *Rapid tranquilization of the violent patient*

Type	Tranquilization
Schizophrenia, mania, or other psychosis	Lorazepam 2–4 mg i.m. combined with haloperidol 5 mg i.m. or thiothixene 10 mg i.m. or thiothixene 10 mg i.m. or 20 mg concentrate or haloperidol 5 mg i.m. 10 mg concentrate loxapine 10 mg i.m. or 25 mg concentrate p.o.
Personality disorder	Lorazepam 1–2 mg p.o. every 1–2 h or 2–4 mg (0.5 mg/kg) i.m. every 1–2 h
Alcohol withdrawal	
Agitation, tremors, abnormal VS	Chlordiazepoxide 25–50 mg p.o. q 4–6 h
>65 yr, liver disease	Lorazepam 2 mg p.o. q 2 h
Extreme agitation	Lorazepam 2–4 mg i.m. q h RT if not controlled
Cocaine/amphetamine	
Mild-moderate agitation	Thiothixene 10 mg p.o. every 8 h
Severe agitation	Thiothixine 10 mg i.m. or 20 mg concentrate or loperidol 5 mg i.m. or 10 mg concentrate
Phencyclidine	
Mild hyperactivity, tension, anxiety, excitement	Diazepam 10–30 mg p.o. or lorazepam 2–4 mg i.m. (0.05 mg/kg)
Severe agitation, excitement, hallucinations, bizarre behavior	Haloperidol 5–10 mg i.m. q 30–60 min

All doses given every 30–60 min; half dose for >65 years.
RT, rapid tranquilization.
Modified from Dubin WR, Weiss KJ. *Handbook of psychiatric emergencies.* Springhouse, PA: Springhouse, Corp., 1991.

C. Decontamination

1. **Inhalation exposures** are extremely dangerous since the lung represents such a large surface area for absorption and after absorption the toxin is rapidly circulated to the most vital organs—brain, heart, and liver. The health care providers should protect themselves from contamination. Examples include dermal absorbed insecticides such as organophosphates and inhaled fumes of hydrogen sulfide and cyanide.

   a. **Treatment.** This type of exposure requires immediate cautious removal from the hazardous environment by adequately protected rescuers, administration of 100% humidified oxygen, assisted ventilation, and bronchodilators, if necessary. If the myocardial threshold for dysrhythmias has been lowered by toxins such as chlorine, avoid use of epinephrine, if possible (162,163).

   b. Observe for **edema of the respiratory tract** manifests as stridor, hoarse voice, and later **noncardiogenic pulmonary edema** manifests by dyspnea, tachypnea, increased work of breathing and hypoxemia.

   c. For the **symptomatic patient** requires arterial blood gases, chest roentgenogram and blood tests for the offending substance such as carboxyhemoglobin or cyanide, although treatment should not await laboratory results (162,163).

2. **Dermal exposures**

   a. Attendants should wear protective gear (gloves, gown, goggles, and shoe covers).

   b. Remove contaminated clothes, contact lenses, and jewelry immediately, and place in specially marked plastic bags.

   c. Gently rinse and wash the skin with copious amounts of water for at least 30 min including the hair, fingernails, navel, and perineum. Do not use forceful flushing in a shower which may cause deeper penetration of the toxic substance. Initially the water should be slightly cool to avoid vasodilation and increased absorption. Use soap to remove oily substances. Caustic contamination may require prolonged irrigation. Catch the water in special containers and do not allow this to run into sewers.

   d. There are rare substances which may react with water and should be brushed off, e.g., chlorosulfonic acid, calcium oxide, and titanium tetrachloride.

   e. For certain substances local application of certain chemical compounds applied as soaks may be useful. For hydrofluoric acid use calcium gluconate soaks and gloves, for oxalic acid calcium gluconate soaks, for phenol use mineral oil or Golytely, and for white phosphorous use copper sulfate. Uncovered phosphorous will ignite in air and should be held under water (162,163).

3. **Ocular exposures**

   a. Ocular decontamination consists of at least 15 to 20 min irrigation with fully retracted eyelids. A 1,000-mL bag of sterile 0.9% saline attached to i.v. tubing is useful to direct the stream across the nasal bridge into medial aspect of the eye. Make sure the patient blinks. If eye pain makes irrigation difficult, instill a topical anesthetic agent; however, this eliminates pain as a sign.

    b. If the material is an acid or alkali assess the pH of the tears and continue to irrigate as long as the pH is abnormal. The pH of the eye is the most important factor of toxin-induced eye damage. *Do not instill neutralizing solutions.* Check the ocular pH 10 min after completion of irrigation to ensure it remains within normal. Alkali contamination often requires 3 h of irrigation.

    c. After irrigation examine the eye with a fluorescein stain and Wood's light or slit lamp for corneal damage.

    d. Ophthalmologic consultation should be sought. At this point the ophthalmologist may instill a topical cycloplegic agent, e.g., 5% homatropine or 2% scopolamine to prevent spasm of the ciliary body, and instill a topical antibiotic (sulfisoxazole or gentamicin) and apply a sterile patch.

4. GI decontamination. Nontoxic ingestions are not true poisonings and can be adequately managed by reassurance from a knowledgeable professional.

    a. Nontoxic ingestions (164) (Table 4-19): Criteria for considering ingestions nontoxic are as follows:

TABLE 4-19. *Usually nontoxic ingestion (unless ingested in very large quantity)*

A&D ointment	Corticosteroids and their ointments
Abrasives	Crayola Markers
Adhesives	Crayons (marked AP, CP, CS-140)
Air fresheners	Crazy Glue (cyanoacrylate)
Ajax Cleaner	Cyclamate
Aluminum foil	Dehumidifying packets (silica or charcoal)
Antacids	Deodorants (spray and refrigerator)
Antibiotic ointments	Detergents (phosphate type, anionic)
Antiperspirants	Dishwashing liquid soap (not automatic
Ashes (wood, fireplace)	electric dishwasher) (Mr Clean, Dawn,
Baby products (cosmetics)	Joy, Tide, Wisk)
Baby wipes	Disposable diapers—not aspirated
Ballpoint pen inks	Erasers
Bathtub floating toys	Etch-A-Sketch
Bath oil (castor oil and perfume)	Eye makeup
Battery (conventional type if bitten)	Fabric softener
Bleach (<5%)	Felt-tip markers and pens
Body conditioners	Fertilizer (nitrogen, phosphoric acid, and potash)
Bubble bath (detergents)	Fingernail polish
Calamine lotion	Fish bowl additives
Candles	Fluoride—caries preventive
Caps (for toy pistols)	Glade Plug In
Cat food	Glitter glues and pastes
Caulk	Glowstick/jewelry
Chalk (calcium carbonate)	Golf ball core (may cause mechanical injury)
Charcoal and charcoal briquettes	Grease
Cigarette ashes	Gypsum
Cigarettes (less than one)	Hair products (conditioner, shampoos, not Lindane)
Clay (modelling)	Hand lotions and creams
Cold packs (a swallow)	Hydrogen peroxide 3%
Colognes[a]	Indelible markers
Comet Cleaner	Ink (blue, black)
Contraceptive pills (without iron)	Iodophor disinfectant

(continued)

TABLE 4-19. (*continued*)

Kaolin	Prussian blue (ferricyanide)
Kitty litter	Putty
Lanolin	Rouge
Latex paint	Rubber cements
Laxatives	Rust
Lipstick	Rug cleaners/shampoos (most: Glory,
Lotrimin cream	Resolve, Woolite)
Lubricants	Saccharin
Lysol Disinfectant Spray (70% ethanol)	Sachets (essential oils)
Magic Marker	Shampoo (liquid)
Makeup (eye, liquid facial)	Shaving creams
Mascara (domestic)	Shoe polish
Massengil Disposable Douches	Silica gel
Matches (book type, three books)	Silly putty
Mineral oil	Soaps and soap products
Mineral Gro Plant Food	Soil Shackles
Newspaper	Starch
Nutrasweet	Sunscreen and tan preparations
PAAS Easter egg dyes (after 1980)	Sweetening agents
Paints (indoor latex acrylic)	Teething rings (fluid may have bacteria)
Pencil lead (graphite)	Thermometers (mercury, phthalate alcohol)
Perfumes[a]	Toilet water[a]
Petroleum jelly (Vaseline)	Toothpaste (even fluoride)
Photographs	Vaseline
Plastics	Vitamins (even fluoride), excluding iron
Plaster (non–lead-containing)	Warfarin (single dose)
Play-Doh	Water color paint
Polaroid picture coating	Windex Glass Cleaner With Ammonia D
Porous tip ink marking pens	Zinc oxide
Preparation H suppository/ointment	Zirconium oxide

[a]Depends on the alcohol content.

(1) Absolute identification of the product;

(2) Absolute assurance that a single product was ingested;

(3) Assurance that there is no signal word on the container;

(4) A good approximation of the amount ingested;

(5) The ability to call back at frequent intervals to determine if symptoms have developed.

(6) **Children:** A satisfactory explanation of the circumstances is necessary to exclude chemical maltreatment by the caretaker in children under 1 year of age and to exclude a "cry for help" indicating an intolerable home situation in children over 6 years of age.

b. **Decontamination and the prevention of absorption** (165)

(1) **Controversies**

(a) In the past it has been found that dilution of gastric contents may raise the levels of certain intoxicants; that 25% of gastric lavage fluid passes into the small intestine and is associated with a high complication rate (166); that neutralization may cause an exothermic reaction which may increase the damage of certain caustics and corrosives; and that gastric evacuation may be potentially harmful for alkaline caustics and petroleum distillates. **Critical assessment of emetics** in adults in the ED have convinced some of the poison centers and many EDs to abandon this technique because of poor yield after 30 to 60 min, it interferes with retention of AC and oral antidotes. However, failure to perform GI decontamination has medicolegal implications in certain situations with unreliable historical data, e.g., substance abuse and suicides. Therefore it is important to document on the chart the reason for not providing the procedure, e.g., clinical presentation, time elapsed, interference with AC or oral antidote (167).

(b) In 1985 a study on the management of poisoned patients without gastric emptying but with the use of AC brought to light questions on the **efficacy of gastric emptying procedures** (168). Other studies have questioned the efficacy of the decontamination procedures of the poisoned and overdosed patient. A **randomized study of 808 drug overdose patients** indicated that neither gastric emptying (ipecac-induced emesis in alert patients or gastric lavage in obtunded patients) nor AC treatment affected the outcome in 451 patients who arrived asymptomatic at the hospital. Gastric emptying in 337 symptomatic patients was associated with a higher prevalence of intensive care and aspiration pneumonia. These results suggested that gastric emptying and AC in the asymptomatic patient was unnecessary and that gastric emptying procedures should be performed selectively not routinely in symptomatic patients (169). The study was criticized on the basis of its exclusion criteria.

(c) In England, investigators assessed the gastric residue with a **flexible endoscope** and found residual solid in 5 of 13 patients treated with ipecac-induced emesis and 15 of 17 managed by gastric lavage (170). In a second study **barium impregnated pellets** were swallowed by volunteers. Roentgenogram showed 18 of 20 emesis treated patients retained the pellets and 17 of 20 patients managed with gastric lavage also retained them. In addition they found the pellets in the small bowel suggesting that the gastric emptying procedures may also force the gastric content into the small bowel (171).

(d) Another group of investigators used **radionucleotides** and abdominal scans revealed ipecac-induced emesis retained 37.1% and lavage 65% (172).

(e) **AC studies** of overdose patients appear to indicate no benefit of ipecac-induced emesis (188) or gastric lavage (189) with AC over AC by itself. Another disagreement has developed. The author of a 1991 commentary argues that the efficiency of MDAC for phenytoin, phenobarbital, and theophylline is unproven and supportive care is the choice for the first two and hemoperfusion for the latter (192). Other investigators remind us that the role of MDAC altering the clinical course of intoxications has never been assessed (193,194).

(f)   These controversies should stimulate further investigation of GI decontamination, its risks and benefits, and indicate GI decontamination is no longer routine procedure.

(2)   General statements

(a)   Gastric evacuation for all patients with ingestion overdose should not be routinely performed and is questionable if more than 1 to 2 h after ingestion (167). These procedures carry a morbidity and mortality and should be reserved for patients who are most likely to benefit from them based on their clinical presentation and the time of ingestion (173). Neither of these procedures are completely effective, moving less than 50%.

(b)   **Young children** (younger than 5 years old): Syrup of ipecac induced-emesis administered immediately in the home or AC in the ED orally is preferred to gastric lavage in cases of ingestion of semi-solids or solids because of the difficulty in inserting a large enough orogastric tube to remove these particles. Emesis is also used for substances not absorbed by AC (except acids or alkali); sustained release or enteric coated tablets; and when the material is too large to be removed by an orogastric tube lavage, e.g., mushroom pieces or plant parts.

(c)   **Older children** (older than 5 years of age), adolescents, and adults: Gastric lavage may be preferred, if they are in the medical facility, will not interfere with administration of adsorbents, e.g., AC and oral antidotes, e.g., N-acetylcysteine. Gastric lavage is useful for the removal of liquids and small tablet particles. If the time postingestion is over 1 to 2 h, studies suggest only a small yield (170,172,174).

(d)   **Dysrhythmias and cardiotoxic drug ingestion:** Both emesis and gastric lavage should be used with caution in patients with dysrhythmias or the ingestion of cardiotoxic drugs, since the vagal response may result in serious dysrhythmias or cardiac arrest.

(e)   **AC** appears to be agent of choice for GI decontamination in most instances if the toxin is known to be absorbed and compliance can be assured. Some patients will not take AC orally and a tube will have to be inserted. In these cases, it may be useful to aspirate first and then insert AC in the initial lavage fluid (168,175–177).

(3)   Emesis (165,167–169,177,178,179–181). Recent AAPCC data has shown a decline in the use of Syrup of ipecac from 13.3% in 1986 to 6.1% of exposures in 1990.

(a) **Syrup of ipecac** is the preferred method for the induction emesis. The doses are outlined in Table 4-20. Some researchers have safely used larger doses. The dose may be repeated once if the child does not vomit within 15 to 20 min. The vomitus should be collected and inspected for fragments of pills and possible analysis. The appearance, color, odor of the gastric contents should be noted as they may be clues of the identity of the toxic substance. A single dose induces vomiting with 15 min in more than 60% of patients and more than 90% within 30 min. The yield (amount recovered) ranges from 19% to 62%. After 1 h very little is recovered.

(b) **Never use salt water** (which has produced fatal hypernatremia), or fluid extract of ipecac (which is 14 times as potent and has caused death).

(c) **Mechanical induction** by stimulation of the posterior pharynx with a finger or an object, such as a spoon, is usually ineffective and may cause injury to the victim and the rescuer.

(d) **In an emergency,** hand dishwashing liquid has been used (3 tablespoons in a glass of water) when there would be a long delay in reaching a hospital and ipecac syrup was not available. Do not use electric dishwasher detergent or concentrates of hand dishwashing solutions (9). However, this has not been extensively investigated.

(e) **Infants younger than 1 year of age.** Emesis is not recommended under 6 months of age. For infants 6 months to 1 year, the dose is 10 mL; however, induction of emesis should be performed under supervision probably in a health care facility (9).

TABLE 4-20. *GI decontamination agents*

Medication	Dose	Comments
Ipecac syrup p.o.	10 mL for 6–12 mo 15 mL for 1–12 yr 30 mL for adolescents	Contraindicated for caustics, petroleum distillates, early onset coma, or convulsions. May repeat once if no response in 20 min.[a]
Activated charcoal p.o.	1 g/kg p.o. or via nasogastric tube; repeated doses 4–6 h	Does not adsorb caustics, heavy metals, alcohols, glycols, solvents. Bowel sounds must be present. initial dose with saline cathartic.
Polyethylene glycol–electrolyte solution (GoLytely)	2 L/h for adults and 0.5 L (20–40 mL/kg) for 5 h	Useful in iron overdose, "body packers," some "body stuffers." May be useful in sustained release preparations.

[a]The dose may be repeated once if the child does not vomit within 15–20 min. Studies have investigated a single dose of 30 mL. The side effect profile was similar to the 15-mL dose.

"Body Packer"—ingestion of packages containing drugs for purposes of transporting contraband. The containers are well made and less likely to open in gastrointestinal tract.

"Body Stuffer"—ingestion of packages containing drugs for the purposes of hiding evidence. The containers are more likely to open in the gastrointestinal tract unless they are in plastic vials.

(f) Contraindications and inappropriate use

    (i) **Loss of protective airway reflexes**, e.g., accompanying coma or convulsions. The gag reflex is developed by infants by about 6 months. The gag reflex may be absent in about 25% of normal individuals and does not mean that the airway protective reflexes are lost.

    (ii) Ingestion of a substance with **caustic or corrosive** properties, e.g., alkali or acids. For common caustics found in the home, see Table 4-21.

    (iii) Ingestion of substances that are likely to produce **abrupt depression of consciousness** and impair the protective airway reflexes, e.g., ethanol, ultra-short BZPs, heterocyclic antidepressants, and short-acting barbiturates.

    (iv) Ingestion of substances that are likely to produce an **early onset of seizures** and impair the protective airway reflexes, e.g., amphetamines, camphor, cocaine, ibuprofen of more than 400 mg/kg, isoniazid, nicotine, strychnine, heterocyclic antidepressants (Table 4-22).

    (v) Ingestion of **petroleum distillates** hydrocarbons (kerosene, gasoline or signal oil). Petroleum distillates are not usually removed unless they are ingested in very large 5 mL/kg quantities or are the vehicle for dangerous additives. Mineral seal oil in furniture polish is not removed at all. Hydrocarbons are not synonymous with petroleum distillates and dangerous hydrocarbons such as aromatic hydrocarbons, halogenated hydrocarbons should be removed because of systemic absorption and CNS depression under medical supervision. The mnemonic for dangerous additives that should be removed is **CHAMP**: **C** = camphor; **H** = halogenated hydrocarbon (e.g., trichloroethane); **A** = aromatic hydrocarbons (e.g., benzene); **M** = heavy metals; and **P** = pesticides. Emesis should not be used to remove camphor because of early seizures.

TABLE 4-21. *Common caustic and corrosive materials around the home*

Ammonia	Hydrofluoric acid
Cement and cement cleaners	Lime (calcium oxide)
Clinitest tablets	Lye (K^+ and Na^+ hydroxide)
Coffee pot cleaners	Metal cleaners
Cuticle remover	Mildew removers
Denture cleaners	Oven cleaners
Drain cleaners	Pipe smokers' cleaners
Electric dishwasher detergents	Rust removers
Formaldehyde	Toilet bowl cleaners
Hair bleaches, permanents, straighteners	Wart removers

TABLE 4-22. *Substances ingested where emesis induction should usually be avoided*

Ammonia (caustic)	Isoniazid (seizures)
Amphetamines (seizures)	Isoproterenol (gastritis/coma)
Anesthetics, local (seizures)	Kerosene (aspiration)[a]
Antihistamines (seizures/coma)	MAOI (seizures)
Batteries (aspiration, caustic)	Manganese (not necessary)
Barbiturates, short-acting (coma)	Mercury elemental (not necessary)
Benzene (seizures/coma)[a]	Mercury inorganic salts (caustic)
Benzodiazepine, ultra-short (coma)	Metaldehyde (seizures)
Beta-blockers (CV collapse)	Methylene chloride (coma)
Cadmium (gastritis)	Mineral seal oil (aspiration)
Calcium channel blockers (CV collapse)	Naphtha (aspiration)[a]
Camphor (seizures)	Naphthalene (seizures)
Carbon tetrachloride (coma)	Nicotine (seizures)
Caustic/corrosive (caustic)	NSAIDS (seizures)
Chloroform (coma)[a]	Ibuprofen >400 mg/kg
Chloroquine (seizures/coma)	Organochlorine (seizures)
Chromium (hemorrhagic gastritis)	Organophosphate (seizures)
Clonidine (apnea/coma)	Paint removers (aspiration)
Cocaine (seizures)	Paraquat
Copper (hemorrhagic gastritis)	Pentachlorophenol (seizures)
Corrosives/caustics (caustic)	Petroleum distillates (aspiration)
Cyanide (seizure/coma)	Phencyclidine (seizures)
Cyclic antidepressants (seizures/coma)	Phenol (caustic)
DEET diethyl-m-toluamide (seizures)	Phenylpropanolamine (seizures)
Dextromethorphan	Phenothiazine
Detergents	Phosphorous (caustic)
Anionic (not necessary)	Quinidine (seizures/coma)
Electric dishwasher (caustic)	Quinine (seizures/coma)
Ethanol (seizures/coma)	Selenious acid (caustic)
Ethylene dibromide (caustic/coma)	Signal oil (aspiration)
Fluoroacetate (seizures)	Strychnine (seizures)
Food poisoning (not necessary)	Theophylline (seizures) AC
Formaldehyde (caustic)	Toluene/zylene (coma)[a]
Fluorinated hydrocarbons (coma)[a]	Trichloroethane (coma)[a]
Hexoresorcinol (caustic)	Trichlorethylene (coma)[a]
Hydrocarbons (aspiration, coma)[a]	Turpentine (aspiration)
Hydrogen fluoride (caustic)	Loperamide (coma)
Hydrogen peroxide (caustic)	Opioids (coma)
Iodine (caustic)	

[a]Induced emesis in a hospital setting under medical supervision. The table indicates when emesis is usually avoided because of the danger in parenthesis (aspiration in cases of petroleum distillates, caustic action of substance, abrupt onset of convulsions or coma, a sudden onset of cardiovascular compromise, loss of clue as to toxicity). Emesis may be considered in some cases of less abrupt onset of coma or seizures, if there is a delay of >60 min in reaching a medical facility, and the ipecac syrup can be administered immediately after the ingestion.

CV, cardiovascular; MAOI, monoamine oxidase inhibitor; NSAIDs, Nonsteroidal antiinflammatory drugs; AC, activated charcoal.

   (vi) **Infants** under 6 months of age because of possible immature protective airway reflexes and the lack of data to establish the safe and effective dose of ipecac syrup.

  (vii) Prior significant vomiting or hematemesis.

 (viii) Ingestion of a **foreign body** emesis is usually ineffective and risks aspiration and obstruction of the airway.

(ix) **Neurologically impaired** individuals with possibly impaired airway protective reflexes.

(x) **Absence of bowel sounds.** When no bowel sounds are present, gastric lavage and suction is preferred.

(xi) **Unstable patients** in shock or with respiratory distress

(xii) **In special situations** such as late in pregnancy, in the elderly, in hypertensive crisis, or in increased intracranial pressure.

(g) **Apomorphine** is mentioned only to advise against its use. It may produce prolonged opioid depressant effects that last longer than the action of naloxone and naloxone does not counteract the violent and prolonged emetic effect.

(h) **Anecdotal advice** that additional fluids and keeping the patient in motion will enhance the emesis have not been scientifically supported.

(i) **If emesis does not occur** and removal is still indicated on the basis of the toxicity of the ingested material, gastric lavage is performed. In the above doses, syrup of ipecac usually does not represent a hazard if emesis does not occur.

(4) **Gastric lavage (GL)** (9,167–169,177,178,181) has been described in the medical literature as early as 1819. It is the preferred method of GI emptying in cooperative adolescents and adults that are already in a medical facility. GL usefulness decreases with the time that elapses after ingestion and it removes 10% to 20% of gastric contents 1 h after ingestion (170–172,174). A large enough tube can not be inserted for large pills and plant parts in children. GL is useful for fluid ingestions but they are absorbed rapidly or pass beyond its reach. The best results are obtained with the largest possible orogastric hose that can be reasonably passed. For adolescents and adults, use a no. 42 Fr Lavacuator hose, in children use a no. 22 to 28 Fr orogastric tube. Nasogastric tubes are not large enough for this purpose.

(a) **Amount and composition of fluid** used varies with patient size. Large amounts of fluid may force the substance into the duodenum (173). Aliquots of 10 mL/kg/lavage of 0.9% saline up to 400 mL in adults are used (194). Tap water lavage may produce hyponatremia especially in children. Total lavage is usually 3,000 mL or "till clear" (173).

(b) The **procedure** requires the airway be protected, if necessary. The orogastric tube is passed in a left lateral decubitus position with the head down lower than the hips. Suction should be readily available to clear the secretions and in case of vomiting. Measure the length of tube to be inserted to help confirm its position (measure from glabella to tip of xiphoid process) and mark on tube. Lavage with adequate volumes and continue until clear. In patients with CNS and respiratory depression, loss of protective airway reflexes and respiratory distress require endotracheal intubation before inserting the orogastric tube. The location of the tube is best confirmed by aspiration of gastric contents, injecting air into the tube and feeling the air enter the stomach. Auscultation of air may be misleading. Some clinicians use AC in the initial lavage solution after the initial aspiration of the gastric contents. This has the advantage of adsorbing any toxin and also serves as a marker for completion of lavage "till clear." Attempt to recover as much of the lavage fluid as administered as injected. The gastric contents should be aspirated, inspected, and saved for possible analysis (173).

(c) The **complication rate** of gastric lavage is estimated at 3%. The complications are aspiration pneumonitis, esophageal tears and perforation (183,184), electrolyte imbalance in young children, and cardiovascular dysfunction and arrest. A decrease in PaO_2 has been shown to occur during lavage and transient ECG changes in as many as 40% of patients who had lavage (183,184).

(d) **Contraindications to gastric lavage** (167–169,176,177)

  (i) Caustic or corrosive ingestions because of the danger of perforation.

  (ii) Uncontrolled convulsions because of the danger of aspiration or injury during the procedure.

  (iii) Hydrocarbon and petroleum distillate products without endotracheal intubation. Although this is controversial if only aspiration and a small nasogastric tube is used.

  (iv) Comatose patients or patients with absent airway protective reflexes require insertion of endotracheal tube to protect against aspiration.

  (v) Cardiac dysrhythmias must be controlled before gastric lavage is initiated because the insertion of the tube may create a vagal response and cause a life-threatening dysrhythmia or arrest.

(5) **AC** (192,194,201–203)

(a) The "universal antidote" is neither universal nor an antidote and has been abandoned. The "Black Bottle" was reintroduced into the United States in 1963 (186). AC in sufficient (10:1 ratio) quantities binds many toxins. In the ED where compliance can be assured, AC may be used alone, after emesis and with or after gastric lavage for substances known to be significantly adsorbed by it (202,203). Some EDs use AC as the initial lavage fluid after aspiration. This has the advantage of adsorbing any toxin and also serves as a marker for completion of lavage "till clear." Superactivated charcoals were removed because of impurities (201).

(b) **The initial oral AC dose** 1 g/kg or 15 to 30 g in children and 60 to 100 g in adults. It is administered as a soupy slurry suspension of 25 g in at least 100 mL water (25%) solution, initially with a cathartic, to avoid forming "briquettes" in the bowel. Multiple doses of 0.5 g/kg are administered orally every 2 to 6 h but the cathartic is repeated only daily. If the patient vomits the dose it may be repeated and antiemetic such as metoclopramide used. If AC is used concomitantly with the oral antidote **N-acetylcysteine** (NAC), no change in dosage of NAC is necessary. The substances AC does not adsorb are more easily remembered than the multitude of agents it does (Table 4-23) (165–170,188,203).

    (c) **Additional uses.** AC may also be useful in the following circumstances: ingestion of long-acting sustained release preparations and ingestion of substances with enterohepatic recirculation (Table 4-24); and it serves as a stool marker of intestinal mobility which may indicate the time the initial ingested product has been eliminated from the GI tract.

    (d) **Contraindications**

        (i) Caustics or corrosive—charcoal is ineffective and may obscure or look like a burn.

        (ii) Absence of bowel sounds (adynamic ileus).

        (iii) Signs of intestinal obstruction, perforation or peritonitis.

        (iv) If unable to confirm location of gastric tube.

        (v) Lack of adequate airway protection, e.g., in comatose patients. If necessary, endotracheal intubation should be used.

(6) **GI dialysis** refers to MDAC.

    (a) This facilitates the passage of substances from the plasma into the intestine by presumably creating a concentration gradient between the blood and the bowel fluid resulting in an efflux of the material into the intestinal lumen. There are a number of studies showing repeated doses of oral AC are effective in reducing the nonrenal half-life of substances or their metabolites even when the substances were administered i.v. (186,198). Cathartics should be administered daily not with each dose.

TABLE 4-23. *Substances poorly adsorbed by activated charcoal*

C	Caustics and corrosives, cyanide[a]
H	Heavy metals (arsenic, iron, lead, lithium, mercury)
A	Alcohols (ethanol, methanol, isopropyl) and glycols (ethylene glycols)
R	Rapid onset or absorption cyanide[a] and strychnine
C	Chlorine and iodine
O	Others insoluble in water (substances in tablet form)
A	Aliphatic and poorly absorbed hydrocarbons (petroleum distillates)
L	Laxatives sodium, magnesium, potassium

[a] If ingested, activated charcoal is given in large doses; 1 g of activated charcoal adsorbs 35 mg of cyanide.

TABLE 4-24. *Some substances with enterohepatic recirculation*

Chloral hydrate	Nonsteroidal antiinflammatory agents
Colchicine	Phencyclidine
Digitalis preparations	Phenothiazine
Glutethimide	Phenytoin
Halogenated hydrocarbons	Salicylates
Isoniazid	Tricyclic antidepressants
Methaqualone	

Data from Greensher J, Motenson HC, Picchoni AL, et al. Activated charcoal update. *JECEP* 1979;8:261–263; Mauro LS, Nawarskas JJ, Mauro VF. Misadventures with activated charcoal and recommendations for safe use. *Ann Pharmacother* 1994;28:915; Caldwell JW, Nava AJ, De Haas DD. Hypernatremia associated with cathartics in overdose management. *West J Med* 1987;147:593.

    (b)   Below is a list of some of the **products where repetitive doses of AC have been studied** and recommended as enhancing clearance (Table 4-25). However, current evidence indicates MDAC should be considered in patients ingesting a life-threatening amount of these drugs. Remember the mnemonic **"Pretty Darn Short QTc"**: **P** = phenobarbital; **D** = dapsone; **S** = salicylate; **Q** = quinine; **T** = theophylline; and **C** = carbamazepine (194). The patient should have GI mobility monitored during therapy (194). There is controversy over whether this procedure influences the clinical course (193,194).

    (c)   **The dose** recommended initially is 50 to 100 g in adults followed by not less than 12.5 g/h. In children the initial dose 10 to 25 g. Studies have shown that the administration of hourly dose produced a shorter half-life than less frequent dosing, although the total amount was the same. The AC should be continued until recovery and/or the plasma drug concentration is within therapeutic range (194–196).

    (7)   **Cathartics** (204–210). Despite the lack of scientific data proving that cathartics are useful in poisonings, they continue to be used.

TABLE 4-25. *Substances whose body clearance may be enhanced by MDAC*

Acetaminophen	Disopyramide	Phenytoin
Carbamazepine[a]	Glutethimide	Propoxyphene
Chlordecone	Meprobamate	**Quinine**
Cyclosporin	Methotrexate[a]	**Salicylate**[a,b]
Dapsone[a]	Nadolol	**Theophylline**[a,b]
Digoxin[a]	**Phenobarbital**[a]	Tricyclic antidepressants
Digitoxin	Phenylbutazone	Valproate

[a]May be effective if the agent is administered p.o. or i.v..
[b]One gram of AC adsorbs 300 mg of theophylline and 133 mg of salicylate. In bold are the substances in which MDAC, is proven effective in enhancing clearance.
MDAC, multiple dose activated charcoal.

(a) **The saline type** cathartics are not recommended in children under 5 years of age. Oil-based cathartics are also not recommended. Sorbitol, a very potent osmotic cathartic, is not recommended for children under 5 years of age because of possible severe electrolyte disturbances (204,205,215). Studies have found sorbitol produced little if any benefit (212–214). The suggested dosage for the commonly used cathartics is listed in Table 4-26. AC suspensions come with and without sorbitol. (Actidose contains 0.2 g AC and 0.4 g sorbitol.) Oral hypertonic phosphate enemas as cathartics are no longer recommended.

(b) **Contraindications**
  (i)   Absence of bowel sounds (adynamic ileus)
  (ii) Evidence of intestinal obstruction
  (iii) Preexisting electrolyte disturbances
  (iv) Magnesium sulfate in renal impairment (206–210)

TABLE 4-26. *Cathartic dosage by age*

Cathartic	Synonym	Pediatric	Adolescent/adult
Sodium sulfate	Gauber's salt	250 mg/kg/dose	15–30 g/dose
Magnesium sulfate	Epsom salt	250 mg/kg/dose	15–30 g/dose
10% solution		2.5 mL/kg	150–250 mL/dose
10% solution contains 8.3 mEq	Mg^{2+}/g salt		
Magnesium citrate	Citrate of Mg	4 mL/kg/dose	250 mL (8 oz)/dose
10% contains 16 mEq	Mg^{2+}/g of salt		
Sorbitol concentrate	—	35%	35%
Age		>5 year	
Dose g/kg		1–1.5 g/kg	1–2 g/kg (max 150 g/dose)
Dose mL/kg		3–4 ml/kg	3–6 mL/kg (max 350 mL/dose)
Maximum dose		—	150 g or 350 mL/dose
Frequency		Once only	Once only
Bisacodyl (Dulcolax)	—	0.3 mg/kg	5–15 mg

Modified from Caldwell JW, Nava AJ, De Haas DD. Hypernatremia associated with cathartics in overdose management *West J Med* 1987;147:593; Gazda-Smith E, Synhavsky A. Hypernatremia following treatment of theophylline toxicity with activated charcoal and sorbitol. *Arch Intern Med* 1990;150:689; Smilkstein MJ, Smolinske SC, Kulig KW, et al. Severe hypermagnesemia due to multiple dose cathartic therapy. *West J Med* 1988;148:208; Woodward JA, Shannon M, Lacourture PG, et al. Serum magnesium concentrations after repetitive magnesium cathartic administration. *Am J Emerg Med* 1990;8:297; Weber CA, Santiago RM. Hypermagnesemia: a potential complication during treatment of theophylline intoxication with oral activated charcoal and magnesium containing cathartics. *Chest* 1989;95:56; Gren J, Woolf A. Hypermagnesemia associated with catharsis in a salicylate intoxicated patient with anorexia nervosa. *Ann Emerg Med* 189;18:200; Garrelts JC, Watson WA, Holloway KD, et al. Magnesium toxicity secondary to catharsis during management of theophylline poisoning *Am J Emerg Med* 1989;7:34; Goldberg M, Spector R, Park G, et al. The effect of sorbitol and activated charcoal on serum theophylline concentrations after slow release theophylline. *Clin Pharmacol Ther* 1987;41:108–111; McNamara R, Aaron CK, Gemborys M, et al. Sorbital cathasis does not enhance the efficacy of charcoal simulated acetaminophen overdose. *Ann Emerg Med* 1989;18:934–938; Keller RE, Schwab RA, Krenzelok EP. Effect of sorbital added to activated charcoal in preventing salicylate absorption. *Ann Emerg Med* 1990;19:654–656; Harchelroad F, Cottington E, Krenzelok EP. Gastrointestinal transit times of a charcoal/sorbitol slurry in overdose patients. *Clin Toxicol* 1989;27:91; Sullivan JB, Krenzlok EP. Repetitive doses of the activated-charcoal combination: a word of caution. *Am J Emerg Med* 1988;6:201.

    (v) Sodium sulfate in conditions requiring salt restriction

    (vi) Evidence of GI perforation or peritonitis

    (vii) Evidence of GI bleeding

    (viii) Patients with diarrhea

    (ix) Children under 1 year of age (fluid-electrolyte disturbances) (204,205,214,215)

(8) **Whole bowel irrigation** (WBI) (218–236) consists of using surgical bowel-cleansing solutions polyethylene glycol, 60 g, in a balanced isotonic electrolyte salt solution to be used until the bowel has been cleansed of the intoxicant (218–221).

    (a) **Indications:** Ingestion of substances that are poorly adsorbed by AC (e.g., iron, lead, lithium, zinc) (229,232,233). There are additional implications in other ingestions, i.e., slow-release preparations (221), and asymptomatic "body packers" (222) and "crack vials" ingestion of "body stuffers" of illicit drugs, e.g., cocaine (222,229) and heroin (222,234). Most of the indications are still investigative except for iron intoxication.

    (b) **Procedure:** The procedure is to administer, usually through a 6 to 8 Fr. polyvinyl feeding nasogastric tube because of its unpleasant taste, but occasionally orally, the colonic irrigation solution (GoLytely or Colyte). The rate 40 mL/kg/h in children (0.5 L/h) younger than 5 years of age and 2 L/h in adolescents and adults (218,220).

    (c) **Endpoint** is when the stools are clear and have the appearance of the infusate. This takes approximately 2 to 4 h (218,220), although others have administered it from 6 to 12 h (224). Ideally the tablets or contraband can be identified on radiograph of the abdomen and their removal is the end point.

    (d) **Metoclopramide** may be given orally 0.1 mg/kg before initiating the lavage or if significant vomiting occurs during the procedure give i.v. and slow the rate of administration (218).

    (e) Animal experiments adding **polyethylene glycol to AC**-salicylates and AC-theophylline combinations showed decreased adsorption and desorption of salicylate and theophylline and no therapeutic benefit over AC alone (228,230,233). Polyethylene solutions are bound by AC in vitro decreasing the efficacy of AC. If both are clinically indicated, administer the AC first, and MDAC should not be given (230).

    (f) **Contraindications** include extensive hematemesis, ileus, bowel obstruction, perforation or peritonitis.

(9) **Sodium polystyrene sulfonate** (Caseload, SPS) is a cation exchange resin which releases sodium in exchange for other cations that may prevent the absorption of **lithium.** Available as oral powder 1.25 g/5 mL oral suspension or 1.25 g/5 mL suspension for rectal use. It is administered for hyperkalemia 15 g orally to four times a day or 30 to 50 g as needed as retention enema. It is not absorbed and is excreted unchanged in the feces. Adverse reactions are electrolyte disturbances, ECG abnormalities, hypokalemia, and sodium retention (237).

X. **Laboratory studies** (238–246). Initially obtain an ECG for dysrhythmias or conduction delays (with cardiotoxic medications), a chest radiography for aspiration pneumonia (if history of loss of consciousness or unarousable) and noncardiac pulmonary edema, electrolyte concentrations in the blood and calculate out anion gap, an acid-base and blood gas profile (if respiratory distress or altered mental status). For appropriate testing on the basis of clinical toxicologic presentation, see Table 4-27. All laboratory specimens should be carefully **labeled,** timed, and dated. For potential legal cases a **"Chain of custody"** must be established. In cases of elevation or depression of the **body temperature** the pH and blood gases change. For each degree of temperature of more than $37°C$ ($98.6°F$), the blood pH decreases 0.015, P_{CO_2} increases 4.4%, and Pa_{O_2} increases 7.2%. The opposite occurs for each degree less than $37°C$. **It should be emphasized that there are limitations to using the formulas in the absence of clinical data.**

   A. Obtain **blood specimens** when establishing vascular access. These studies may have to be repeated when the toxins have passed through their distribution phase and are in the elimination phase.

   B. Evaluate and correct **electrolyte and acid-base disturbances.** The causes of a metabolic acidosis and an anion gap are as follows:

   1. **Metabolic acidosis** (low pH with a low Pa_{O_2} and low HCO_3) and **an anion gap (AG).** The AG is calculated from the standard serum electrolytes. Subtracting the total CO_2 (reflects the actual measured bicarbonate) and chloride from the sodium. $(Na - [Cl + HCO_3]) = AG$. The potassium is usually not used in the calculation because it may be hemolyzed and is an intracellular cation.

   2. The AG is an estimate of those anions other than chloride and HCO_3 necessary to counterbalance the positive charge of sodium and potassium (249–253). The AG

TABLE 4-27. *Condition of the patient and appropriate tests*

Condition	Tests
Comatose	Toxicologic tests (acetaminophen, sedative-hypnotic, ethanol, opioids, benzodiazepine), glucose, ammonia, CT scan, CSF analysis
Respiratory toxin	Spirometry, arterial blood gases, chest roentgenogram, O_2 saturation monitor
Cardiac toxin	ECG 12-lead and monitoring, echocardiogram, serial cardiac enzymes, hemodynamic monitoring
Hepatic toxin	Enzymes (AST, ALT, GGT), ammonia, albumin, bilirubin, glucose, PT, PTT, amylase
Nephrotoxin	BUN, creatinine, electrolytes (Na, K, Mg, Ca, Po4), serum and urine osmolarity, 24-h urine for heavy metals, creatine kinase, serum and urine myoglobin, urinalysis, and urinary sodium
Bleeding	Platelets, PT, PTT, bleeding time, fibrin split products, fibrinogen, type and match

serves as clue to etiologies, compensation and complications. The lack of anion gap does not exclude a toxic etiology. The normal gap is 8 to 12 mEq/L by flame photometer. However, there has been a lowering of the normal anion gap to 7 ± 4 by the ion selective electrodes or coulometric titration. The "downward" shift reflects the increase of chloride values. In recent studies the average person could be expected, with newer technology, to have an AG of 7 (range 3 to 11) using ASTRA techniques (255). Some studies have found anion gaps to be insensitive for determining the presence of toxins (239,240,248,249). It is important to recognize salicylates, methanol and ethylene glycol since they have specific antidotes and extracorporeal methods are effective in management. A list of the etiologies of increased anion gap, decreased anion gap and metabolic acidosis with no gap are in Table 4-28. The most common cause of a **decreased anion gap** is laboratory error.

2. Use an **acid-base map** to determine if the disorder is primary or secondary, if compensation is occurring, to estimate the third factor when two factors are known and to determine if the patient is progressing in correct direction.

3. **Other blood chemistry derangements** that suggest certain intoxications (Table 4-29):

4. **Serum osmolal gaps** (255–260). The serum **osmolality** is a measure of the number of molecules of solute/kg of solvent or mOsm/kg of water and the **osmolarity** is solute/L of solution or mOsm/Liter of water at a specified temperature. Osmolarity is usually calculated and osmolality is usually measured. They are considered interchangeable where 1 liter equals 1 kg. The normal serum osmolality is 280 to 290 mOsm/kg or 280 ± 10 mOsm/kg.

    a. The **serum osmolal gap** or delta **osmolality (D-Omol)** is defined as the difference between the measured osmolality (M-Osm) determined by the freezing point method (not by vapor pressure method) and the calculated osmo-

TABLE 4-28. *Etiologies of metabolic acidosis*

Non-gap hyperchloremic	Increased-gap normochloremic	Decreased-gap
Acidifying agents		
Adrenal insufficiency	Methanol	Laboratory error[b]
Anhydrase inhibitors	Uremia[a]	Intoxication—Br, Li
Fistula	Diabetic ketoacidosis[a]	Protein abnormal
Osteotomies	Paraldehyde,[a] Phenformin	Sodium low
Obstr uropathies	Isoniazid	
Renal tubular acidosis	Iron	
Diarrhea uncomplicated[a]	Lactic acidosis[b]	
Dilutional	Ethanol,[a] ethylene glycol[a]	
Sulfamylon	Salicylates, starvation	
	Solvents	

[a] Indicates hyperosmolar situation. Recent studies have found the anion gap may be relatively insensitive for determining the presence of toxins.
[b] Lactic acidosis (carbon monoxide, cyanide, hydrogen sulfide, hypoxia, ibuprofen, iron, isoniazid, ischemia, phenformin, salicylates, seizures, theophylline).

TABLE 4-29. *Blood chemistry derangements in toxicology*

Derangement	Toxin
Acetonemia without acidosis	Acetone or isopropyl alcohol
Hypomagnesemia	Ethanol, digitalis.
Hypocalcemia	Ethylene glycol, oxalate, fluoride
Hyperkalemia	Beta-blockers, acute digitalis, renal failure
Hypokalemia	Diuretics, salicylism, sympathomimetics, theophylline, corticosteroids, chronic digitalis
Hyperglycemia	Diazoxide, glucagon, iron, isoniazid, organophosphate insecticides, phenylurea insecticides, phenytoin, salicylates, sympathomimetic agents, thyroid, vasopressors
Hypoglycemia	Beta-blockers, ethanol, insulin, isoniazid, oral hypoglycemic agents, salicylates
Elevated CPK	Amphetamines, ethanol, cocaine, or phencyclidine
Elevated creatinine and normal BUN	Isopropyl alcohol, diabetic ketoacidosis

larity (C-Osm) by the following formula. The serum sodium multiple by 2 plus the BUN divided by 3 (1/10 molecular weight (MW), plus the glucose divided by 20 (1/10th of its MW). This estimate is usually within 10 mOsm of simultaneously measured serum osmolality (245–247). Ethanol, if present, is included in the equation to eliminate its influence by adding ethanol concentration divided by 4.6 (1/10 of its MW) (Table 4-30). Osmolal gap is an increase of the laboratory freezing point osmolality of more than 10 mOsm/kg H2O above the calculated osmolality.

Calc mOsm $= 2(Na^{2+}) + BUN\ mg/dL/3\ (2.8) + blood\ glucose\ mg/dL/20$ (18) + ethanol mg/dL/4.6

The D-Omol value requires a hemodynamically intact individual; therefore it is **not valid in shock and postmortem state.** Metabolic disorders such as hyperglycemia, uremia and dehydration increase the osmolarity but usually do not cause D-Omol greater than 10 mOsmol/kg.

   b. A gap of more than 10 mOml suggests unidentified osmolal-acting substances are present: acetone, ethanol, ethylene glycol, ethchlorvynol, glycerin, isopropyl alcohol, isoniazid, ethanol, mannitol, methanol sodium bicarbonate (1 mEq/kg raises osmolality 2 mOml/L), and trichloroethane. Other alcohols and glycols should be sought when the degree of obtundation exceeds that expected from the blood ethanol concentration (BEC) or when other clinical conditions exist, e.g., visual loss (methanol), metabolic acidosis (methanol and ethylene glycol), and renal failure (ethylene glycol) (257).

   c. **False elevated osmolal gap** (255–260)
      (1) Low molecular weight non-ionized substances—acetone, dextran, dimethyl sulfoxide, diuretics, ethanol, ethyl ether, ethylene glycol, isopropanol, paraldehyde, mannitol, methanol, sorbitol, trichloroethane, and diabetic ketoacidosis.
      (2) Hyperlipidemia
      (3) Specimen tubes with EDTA (lavender), oxalate (grey); citrate (blue) falsely elevate osmolality.

TABLE 4-30. *Alcohol/glycols levels*

Alcohol/glycol	1 mg/dL in blood raises osmolality mOsm/L	Molecular weight	Conversion factor
Ethanol	0.228	40	4.6
Methanol	0.327	32	3.2
Ethylene glycol	0.190	62	6.2
Isopropanol	0.176	60	6.0
Acetone	0.182	58	5.8
Propylene glycol	—	72	7.2

Example: Methanol osmolality. Subtract the calculated osmolality from the measured serum osmolarity (freezing point method) = osmolar gap × 3.2 (one-tenth molecular weight) = estimated serum methanol concentration.

      d.   **False-negatives** (normal osmolal gap in the presence of toxic alcohol or glycol poisoning) (255–260):
          (1)   Parent compound—methanol, ethylene glycol already metabolized to a metabolite which does not increase the anion gap (e.g., acids)
          (2)   The boiling point elevation or vapor pressure was used instead of the freezing point depression method (e.g., methanol will evaporate and not be recognized).
          (3)   Ingestion of a relatively large (less osmotically active) agent (e.g., ethylene glycol) in a patient with a relatively low baseline gap.
      e.   The serum concentration mg/dL = factor*) mOsm gap × molecular weight divided by 10 (Table 4-30).
      f.   Although the value of the test is questioned by some (17,18), the osmolar gap, early in the ingestion, is useful in predicting the degree of toxicity. The freezing point serum osmolarity and the serum electrolytes for calculation should be drawn **simultaneously.** An **early** osmolar gap is due to the parent drug and **delayed** metabolic acidosis and anion gap is due to the metabolites (present within 12 to 24 h).
  C. Obtain **urine** for analysis
     1.   Send a urine specimen (more than 100 mL). Look for crystals of ethylene glycol, bedside test for myoglobin (3+ 4+ blood on reagent strip but less than 10 RBC on microscopic examination), do a bedside ferric chloride test, and send specimen for toxicology. Split the specimen and keep one for reserve should future studies be needed on the initial specimen.
     2.   **Ferric chloride test** is the qualitative test for presence of salicylates or phenothiazines is a nonspecific test with 100% sensitivity for salicylates with accurate negative predictive values but poor sensitivity for phenothiazines. It is useful if the clinician is aware of its limitations. In the presence of phenolic substances the indicator changes color. A positive test for salicylates does not indicate salicylate overdose—just that salicylate or another substance with phenolic properties is present. False-negatives for salicylate have never been reported (261). It is performed by

adding 0.5 mL of 10% ferric chloride to 2 mL of acidified urine. A purple color indicates a positive test. If the color blanches when 20% sulfuric acid is added it suggests phenothiazine was present (262,263) (Table 4-31).

D. Roentgenographic studies

    1. Chest and neck roentgenogram for pathology such as aspiration pneumonia, pulmonary edema, foreign bodies and to determine the location of the endotracheal tube.

    2. Abdominal roentgenogram (264–266) to detect radiopaque substances.

        a. Many of the substances have varying consistency in their degrees of radiopacity and are not always seen. The only consistent ones are calcium carbonate, undissolved or solid ferrous sulfate tablets (ferrous gluconate is weakly visible) and potassium chloride (264).

        b. The mnemonic for radiopaque substances seen on abdominal x-ray is **CHIPES: C** = chlorides and chloral hydrate; **H** = heavy metals (arsenic, barium, iron, lead, mercury, zinc); **I** = iodides; **P** = Play Doh, Pepto-Bismol, phenothiazine (inconsistent); **E** = enteric coated tablets; and **S** = sodium, potassium and other elements in tablet form (bismuth, calcium, potassium) and solvents containing chlorides, e.g., carbon tetrachloride.

E. Toxicologic studies (267–273). For the average laboratory false-negatives occur at a rate of 10% to 30% and false-positive at a rate of 0% to 10%. The **specificity of a test** influences the false-positive rate. A **false-positive** detects a substance that is not there due to cross reactions or interferences (Table 4-32). The **sensitivity of a test** influences the false-negative rate. **A false-negative** is failure to find a drug that is present. **A negative toxicology** does not exclude a poisoning. The negative predictive value of toxicologic screening is about 70%. If the test seeks a metabolite common to that class, agents in that class which metabolize by a different pathway may escape detection. For example the following BZPs are not detected by screening tests: alprazolam, clonazepam,

TABLE 4-31. *Ferric chloride test*

Drug/chemical/disease	Color reaction
Antipyrine	Cherry red
Alcaptonuria	Add to dark urine → turns blue, green fades in seconds
Acetacetic acid	Purple color
Bilirubin	Green stable
Phenylbutazone	Yellow → violet
Carcinoid	Blue-green
Ketosis	Purple fades in seconds
Lysol	Green stable
L-Dopa	Green
Maple sugar urine disease	Green stable
Melanin	Add to dark urine → black or black/gray precipitate
Paraaminosalicylic acid	Red-brown
Phenothiazines	Purple fades with 20 N H_2SO_4
Phenol (Lysol)	Add to brown/black urine → turns violet
Phenylpyruvic acid	Violet color
Salicylate	Purple intensifies with 20 N H_2SO_4

temazepam, and triazolam. **A positive screen predictive value** is about 90%. A positive test does not correlate with mental or physical impairment or under influence, does not indicate route of administration and cannot tell time of use or amount used

1. It is advisable to communicate with the toxicologic analyst exactly what substance is suspected (if known) or at least the category of the possible toxin on the basis of the patient's manifestations. The **"toxic or coma" urine screen** is a qualitative urine test for several common drugs, usually substances of abuse (cocaine and metabolites, opioids, amphetamines, BZPs, barbiturates, and phencyclidine). Since these tests may vary with each hospital and community the physician should determine exactly which substances are included in the screen. It is always advisable to obtain an **acetaminophen level** in overdose situations, since there are no clinical manifestations to guide when the decision for treatment must be started.

2. Ethylene glycol, RBC cholinesterase, serum cyanide, methemoglobin assays are not readily available so therapy must be based on clinical judgment. **Ethylene glycol** may be suspected by oxalate or hempseed crystals in the urine, the presence of metabolic acidosis with anion gap, an osmolar gap and fluorescence of urine or oral mucosa if it were in antifreeze. **Organophosphate poisoning** confirmation may be suspected when a large dose of atropine fails to produce atropinization. **Cyanohemoglobin** may be suspected by bright red venous blood, lactic acidosis, bright red venous blood due to venous hyperoxemia, and decreased arteriovenous oxygen tension difference. **Methemoglobinemia** may be suspected by the presence of cyanosis with chocolate colored lips, a normal PaO_2 early and brown "chocolate colored" blood.

3. For certain ingestions **quantitative blood levels** should be obtained at specific times postingestion to avoid spurious low values in the distribution phase which results from incomplete absorption from the GI tract. Table 4-33 lists the times

TABLE 4-32. *Interferences with common toxicologic testing*

Drug or toxin	Method	False-positives or interferences
Acetaminophen	Spectrochemical	Salicylate, methylsalicylate (can increase level 10% in µg/mL), phenol, salicylamide, bilirubin, renal failure (each 1 mg/dL increase creatinine = 30 µg/mL acetaminophen)
	GC	Phenacetin
	HPLC	Cephalosporins, sulfonamides
	IA	Phenacetin
Amphetamines (d-amphetamines)	GC	Other volatile stimulant amines, meperidine metabolite, antihistamine metabolite
	IA	Phenylpropanolamine, ephedrine, fenfluramine, isomethe-prene, isoxsuprine, phenteramine, phenmetrazine, doxepin,[a] labetalol, L-amphetamine in Vick's inhalers, ranitidine, ritodrine in FPIA. Benzathine penicillin[b]
	TLC	MDA, MDMA and other similar amines, labetalol
Barbiturates	IA	NSAID in FIPA
Benzodiazepines	IA	Oxzepam, temazepam, alprazalam NSAIDs in FIPA
Chloride	SC	Bromide (0.8 mEq Cl = 1 mEq/Br)
Cocaine	AI	"herbal teas" (benzoyylegonine)

(continued)

TABLE 4-32. *Continued*

Drug or toxin	Method	False-positives or interferences
Creatinine	TLC	Urochromes and endogenous acids
	SC	Ketoacidosis may increase creatinine up to 2–3 mg/dL, cephalosporins, creatinine with rhabdomyolysis
Digoxin	IA	Endogenous digoxin-like naturetic substances in newborn (1 ng/mL); renal failure (1 ng/mL); cross-reacting metabolites in renal failure (2 ng/mL); pregnancy; liver disease; oleander and other plant glycosides
		Digoxin binding antibody (FAB)
Ethanol	SC	Other alcohols, ketones (by oxidation methods), isopropanol alcohol (by enzyme methods), *Candida albicans,* and proteus
Ethylene glycol	SC	Other glycols, propylene glycol in i.v. phenytoin, diazepam and others, triglycerides
Isopropanol	GC	Skin disinfectant isopropanol up to 40 mg/dL but usually trival
Iron	SC	Desferoxamine falsely lowers TIBC 15%, lavender-top vacutainer has EDTA, which binds and lowers iron
Lithium	SC	Green-top Vacutainer (heparin) tube; lithium-heparin may elevate Li 6-8 mEq/L
Marijuana (11-nor-9 carboxyltetra hydrocanabinol	IA	Ibuprofen, fenprofen, chronic NSAID
		Melinin, steroids,
	TLC	Metadone, antihistamines
		Passive inhalation 20 ??g/mL
Methemoglobinemia	SC	Sulfhemoglobinemia (10% cross + by co-oximeter), methylene blue (2 mg/kg transient false + 15% methemoglobinemia level) hyperlipidemia (triglyceride 6,000 = methbg 28.6%)
Osmolarity	Osm	Lavender-top (EDTA) 15 mOsm/L, gray top (fluoride-oxalate) 150 mOsm/L, blue top (citrate) 10 mOsm/L
		Falsely normal if vapor methods used because alcohols are vaporized
	VP	Methanol, etrhanol, acetone gap is underestimated
Opioids: morphine/ codeine)	IA	Hydrocodone, hydromorphine, oxycodone, 6-monacetyl-morphine, two poppy seed bagels for 16 h, one lemon poppy seed muffin (18,19) Vick's Formula 44
	TLC	Hydrocodone, dextromethorphan
Phencyclidine	IA	Phencycidine analogs, dextromethorphan, phenothiazines, diphehydramine
	TLC	antihistamines, methadone, meperidine
Salicylates	SC	Phenothiazines, acetaminophen, ketosis, salicylamide, diflunisal, accumulated salicylate metabolites in renal failure (10% increased)
		Decreased or altered salicylate by bilirubin; phenylketones
	GC	Methylsalicylate, eucalyptol, theophylline
	HPLC	Antibiotics, theophylline
Theophylline	SC	Diazepam, caffeine, accumulated theophylline metabolites in renal failure
	HPLC	Acetazolamide, cephalosporins, endogenous xanthines and accumulated theophylline metabolites in renal failure
	GC	Phenobarbital (rare)
	IA	Caffeine, accumulated theophylline metabolites in renal failure

[a] Doxepin gives unconfirmed amphetamine by Abbot Adx test. Test is negative if not confrmed on thin-layer chromatography. N-desmethyldoxepin is structuallly related to methamphetamine in high concentrations and cross reactivity is sufficient to cause false-positive test. (Adapted from Merigen KS, Browning P. Doxepin causing false positive urine test for amphetamine. *Ann Emerg Med* 1993;22:1370.)

[b] Benzathine salt of phenoxypenicillin penicillin with Syva Emit I polyclononal. (Adapted from Berthier M, et al. *J. Pediatr* 1995;127:669–670.) SC spectrochemical; GC, gas chromatography (interferencess more common with older methods); HPLC, high-pressure liquid chromatography; IA immunoassay; TLC thin-layer chromatography; FPIA, fluorescent polarization immunoassay. (Adapted from Olsen KR. *Drug overdose and poisoning.* Norwalk, CT: Appleton & Lange, 1993.)

postingestion when the **quantitative tests** should be obtained (the elimination phase). It is always wise to obtain serial tests of the substance that show a positive serum follows the trend.

4. In general it is wise to **store 10 mL of blood** in two red-topped and **100 mL urine** in the refrigerator for further investigation of toxins not initially suspected. A purple (lavender-topped tube with EDTA preservative is obtained for patients in whom carboxyhemoglobin is suspected. Special (lead-free) tubes are used for cases of suspected lead poisoning.

5. **Cross reactions or interferences** (Table 4-32).

6. **The detection time** is the number of days after intake of a substance that an individual would be expected to excrete detectable levels of the substance or metabolite in urine. Variances are due to such factors as dosage, frequency of use, liquid consumption, and individual metabolic characteristics. In general, urine detection is possible for 1 to 3 days after cocaine exposure, 2 to 4 days after heroin (monoacetylmorphine is diagnostic of heroin use but is only detectable 12 h after use), 2 to 4 days after PCP, and if chronic use, double the time.

XI. **Antidotal therapy.** After the basic life support measures, emergency antidotes can be used to reverse life-threatening manifestations. The emergency antidotes are oxygen, naloxone, atropine, pralidoxime, cyanide kit (nitrites and thiosulfates), FAB digoxin binding antibodies and methylene blue. Only 1% of the 1,280,751 exposure reported to the AAPCC data base received any of the 17 specific antidotes (excepting oxygen). Table 4-34 lists common poisons and their antidotes. Table 4-35 lists antidotes that should be stocked in an ED and their initial dose.

A. **Toxic substances and their emergency antidotes:**

1. **Acetaminophen (APAP)**—The antidote is *N*-**acetylcysteine**, a derivative of the amino acid, cysteine, which constitutes the central portion of the glutathione molecule. The exact mechanism is unclear. Presumably NAC is metabolized by hepatocyte to cysteine, a glutathione precursor, which provides sulfhydryl groups that can readily enter the cells and bind to the reactive toxic metabolite, *N*-acetyl-*p*-benzoquinoneimine (NAPQI). Glutathione can also repair oxidative damage via glutathione peroxidase system (274,275).

   a. The **dose** is 140 mg/kg followed by 70 mg/g every 4 h for 17 doses. It should be diluted from its usual 10% to 20% to a 5% solution. If the dose is vomited within 1 h after administration it should be repeated.

2. **Anticholinergic**—The antidote is **physostigmine**, a tertiary amine that crosses the blood brain barrier producing reversible inhibitor of cholinesterase, the enzyme that degrades acetylcholinesterase. Physostigmine is not routinely used but limited to severe life-threatening anticholinergic manifestations (severe delirium and dysrhythmias) (276–278).

   a. The **dose** 0.5 to 2 mg i.v. (children 0.2 mg/kg) using a cardiac monitor, slowly over 5 min. Do not use in phenothiazine or tricyclic antidepressant overdose.

3. **BZP**—The antidote is **flumazenil,** a highly specific BZP antagonist without agonist properties was marketed in 1991 for reversal of BZP sedation (not hypoventilation). It acts to displace the centrally acting BZP agonists by competitive inhibition at the receptor sites (120–130).

TABLE 4-33. *Substances where quantitative blood values may be necessary*

Substance	Specimen	Time post ingestion to obtain specimen	Toxic concentration
Acetaminophen	Serum	After 4 h	>150 µg/mL at 4 h
Carbamazepine	Serum	Stat steady-state	>12 µg/mL
Carboxyhemoglobin	Blood	Stat	Extrapolate
Digoxin	Serum	6–8 h	>2 ng/mL adult, >4 ng/mL child
Ethanol	Serum	0.5–1 h	>80 mg/dL (800 µg/mL)
Ethylene glycol	Serum	0.5–1 h	>20 mg/dL (200 µg/mL)
Iron			
Liquid	Serum	2 h	>350 µg/dL (3.5 µg/mL)
Tablet	Serum	4 h	>350 µg/dL (3.5 µg/mL)
Isopropanol	Serum	0.5–1 h	>50 mg/dL (500 µg/mL)
Lithium	Serum	8–12 h	>1.5 mEq/L
Methanol	Serum	0.5–1 h	>20 mg/dL (200 µg/mL)
Methemoglobin	Blood	Stat	>30%
Paraquat	Plasma	8 h	>1 µg/mL within 24 h
Phenobarbital	Serum	Stat steady state	>40 µg/mL
Phenytoin	Serum	1–2 h	>20 µg/mL
Primidone	Serum	Stat	>12 µg/mL
Salicylate	Serum	After 6 h	>30 mg/dL (300 µg/mL)
Theophylline	Serum		
Liquid		1 h	>20 µg/mL
Regular tablet		1–3 h	>20 µg/mL
Slow release		3–10 h	>20 µg/mL

a.   The manufacturer and the medical literature have warnings about using flumazenil as an antidote. Do not give if overdose of tricyclic antidepressants, known convulsive disorder or long-term use of BZP (may produce withdrawal). Much higher doses of BZPs are needed to control convulsions associated with flumazenil use. Its use as a diagnostic and therapeutic agent in coma of unknown etiology must await further studies (125,126). Flumazenil may be indicated for reversal of the sedative effect of BZPs after procedures, for pure BZP overdose situations with no history of long-term use (119–130).

b.   **The dose** (first secure airway) is 0.2 mg over 30 s i.v., (child dose 0.01 mg/kg not established), wait 3 min for response, if not 0.3 mg over 30 s, wait 3 min for response if not, 0.5 mg at 60 s intervals up to cumulative dose of 3 mg (1 mg in children). If responds closely monitor for resedation for at least 6 h (119–130).

4.   **Beta-adrenergic blockers**—The antidote is **glucagon,** a polypeptide hormone that stimulates the production of adenyl cyclase to increase intracellular cyclic adenosine monophosphate (cAMP) which elevates the serum glucose by glycogenolysis, causes vascular smooth muscle relaxation, has positive inotropic, chronotropic, and dromotropic activity (279–281).

a.   **The adult dose** is 5 to 10 mg i.v. (child 0.05 to 0.1 mg/kg) titrate to response of normal vital signs. Maintenance dose 2 to 10 mg/hr.

TABLE 4-34. *Common poisons and their recommended antidote*

Toxin	Antidote or Drug Therapy
Acetaminophen (in many analgesics)	N-acetylcysteine
Anticholinergic (antihistamines, plants, GI medications)	Physostigmine (caution)
Anticoagulants (in rodenticides)	Vitamin K_1
Antimony (ant paste)	Dimercaprol (BAL)
	Penicillamine
Arsenic (ant traps)	Dimercaprol (BAL)
	Penicillamine, Succimer
Beta-blockers	Glucagon
Benzodiazepines	Flumazenil
Bismuth (GI medication)	Dimercaprol (BAL)
Botulism	Botulism antitoxin
Carbamate insecticide	Atropine
Calcium channel blockers	Calcium gluconate
Carbon monoxide	100% oxygen, hyperbaric oxygen
Chloroquine (antimalarial)	Diazepam
Cocaine	Labetalol
Cyanide (fruit stone seeds, nitroprusside for hypertension, plastic fires, metal polishes)	Lilly Cyanide Kit contains amyl nitrite, sodium nitrate, sodium thiosulfate
	Investigative Vitamin B_{12a}
Convulsions, refractory	Pancuronium bromide
Digoxin, digitoxin, plants	Fragment antibody (Digibind)
Ethylene glycol (antifreeze)	Ethanol
Fluoride (rodenticides)	Calcium gluconate
Gold (antirheumatoid)	Dimercaprol (BAL)
Heparin	Protamine sulfate
Hydralazine (antihypertensive)	Pyridoxine
Hydrofluoric acid (etching glass)	Local calcium gluconate jelly
	Soak in magnesium sulfate
Iron (dietary supplements)	Deferoxamine (Desferal)
Isoniazid (antituberculous)	Pyridoxine
Lead (old paints and plaster, dust)	Calcium disodium edetate (EDTA)
	Dimercaprol (BAL), Succimer
Mercury (fungicides, thermometers)	Dimercaprol (BAL), Succimer
	Penicillamine
Methemoglobinemia (nitrites, dyes)	Methylene blue
Methanol (antifreeze, dry gas)	Ethanol
Opioids	Naloxone
Organophosphate insecticides	Atropine, pralidoxime chloride
Phencyclidine (abused "Angel Dust")	Ammonium chloride (caution)
Phenobarbital	Sodium bicarbonate
Phenothiazine dystonic reaction	Diphenhydramine
Phenylurea rodenticide (Vacor)	Nicotinamide
Salicylate	Sodium bicarbonate
Snake bite	Antivenom
Spider bite, Latrodectus (Black widow)	Antivenom
Tricyclic and cyclic antidepressants	Sodium bicarbonate

5. **Calcium channel blockers—Calcium** may reverse the negative inotropic effects of calcium channel blockers but is not consistently effective (282,283).
   a. **The dose:** Calcium chloride 10% 0.2 mL/kg up to 1 g over 10 to 15 min i.v. infusion with continuous cardiac monitoring.
   b. Calcium gluconate 10% 0.5 mL/kg of elemental calcium up to 2 g over 10 to 15 min. Repeat if life-threatening.
   c. Determine calcium blood concentration after third dose.

6. **Cyanide**—The cyanide antidote kit consists of amyl nitrite, sodium nitrite and sodium thiosulfates. Nitrites oxidize the hemoglobin to methemoglobin to bind the cyanide and may enhance endothelial detoxification by vasodilation. Sodium thiosulfate is a sulfate donor that converts the cyanide to the less toxic thiocyanate by the enzyme rhodanese. Thiosulfate is relatively nontoxic and may be administered empirically in suspected cyanide poisoning (284–288).
   a. Do not give adult doses to children. **The dose of amyl nitrite** is to crush two ampules in gauze and place under nose, for deep inhalation for 30 s. This phase may be omitted if venous access is available. **Sodium nitrite i.v.,** 10 mL 10% solution over 3 to 5 min (children 0.33 mL/kg if hemoglobin is unknown), if suspect anemia or hypotension start with lower dose and dilute in 100 mL over at least 5 min. **Sodium thiosulfate i.v.** is administered as 12.5 g or 50 mL of 25% solution (children 400 mg/kg or 1.6 mL/kg) at 2 to 5 mL/min. If no response in 30 min repeat 1/2 of sodium nitrate dose.
   b. **Hydroxocobalamin** (vitamin B_{12a}) which converts to cyanocobalamin (vitamin B_{12}) is currently being used in France (289).

7. **Digitalis**—The antidote is **digoxin-specific antibody fragments (FAB) which** are antibodies obtained from digoxin immunized sheep and cleaved so only the fragment binding antibody is administered to bind with the cardiac glycoside (290–292).
   a. **Empiric** dose (40 mg binds 0.6 mg of digoxin). If the ingested amount is divided by three, that equals the approximate number of vials required. If amount unknown and life-threatening dysrhythmias or eminent cardiac arrest, administer 10 vials i.v. through a no. 22 micron filter or as a bolus. The number of vials on the basis of the serum concentration digoxin concentration at steady state at 6 to 12 h postingestion. Number of vials for digoxin = serum digoxin (ng/mL) × body weight (kg)/100. Number of vials for digitoxin = serum digitoxin (ng/mL) × body weight (kg)/1000. On basis of serum digoxin in ng/mL × 5.6 × weight in kg divided by 600 = number of vials.

8. **Ethylene glycol**—The antidote is **ethanol**, a competitive substrate that inhibits the enzyme alcohol dehydrogenase (ADH) and prevents the metabolism of ethylene glycol to toxic metabolites. A blood ethanol concentration of 100 mg/dL is needed to saturate the enzyme. If a patient is on disulfiram, use hemodialysis in place of ethanol. Ethanol therapy is started at blood ethylene glycol of more than 20 mg/dL, and hemodialysis added if level is more than 50 mg/dL (293–295).
   a. The dose of ethanol is listed in Table 4-35.

(Text continues on page 150)

TABLE 4-35. *Initial doses of antidotes for common poisonings*

Antidote	Use	Dose	Route	Adverse reactions (AR)/comments
N-Acetylcysteine (NAC, Mucomyst). Stock level to treat 70-kg adult for 24 h: 7 vials, 20%, 30 ml.	Acetaminophen, carbon tetrachloride (experimental).	140/mg/kg loading, followed by 70 mg/kg every 4 h for 17 doses.	p.o.	Nausea, vomiting.
Atropine. Stock level to treat 70-kg adult for 24 h: 1 g (1 mg/ml in 1.10 ml).	Organophosphate and carbamate pesticides.	Child: 0.02–0.05 mg/kg repeated every 10–15 min to max of 2 mg as necessary until cessation of secretions. Adult: 1–2 mg q 10–15 min necessary. Dilute in 1–2 mL of NS for ET Instillaton. (Consult PCC for details on continuous i.v. infusion).	i.v./ET	Tachycardia, dry mouth, blurred vision, and urinary retention. Ensure adequate ventilation before administration.
Calcium chloride (10%). Stock level to treat 70-kg adult for 24 h: 5–10 vials 1 g (1.35 mEq/ml).	Hypocalcemia, fluoride, calcium channel blockers.	0.1–0.2 mL/kg (10–20 mg/kg) slow push every 10 min up to max 10 ml (1 g).	i.v.	Administer slowly with blood pressure and EKG monitoring and have magnesium available to reverse calcium effects. AR: Tissue irritation, hypotension, dyshythmias from rapid injection. Contraindications: Digitalis glycoside intoxication.
Calcium gluconate (10%). Stock level to treat 70-kg adult for 24 h: 5–10 vials 1 g (0.45 mEq/ml).	Hypocalcemia, fluoride, calcium channel blockers, hydrofluoric acid, black widow envenomation.	0.2–0.3 mL/kg (20–30 mg/kg) slow push; repeat as needed up to max dose 10–20 ml (1–2 g).	i.v.	Same comments in calcium chloride.
Calcium gluconate gel. Stock level: 3.5 g.	Hydrofluoric acid.	2.5-g USP powder added to 100-ml water-soluble lubricating jelly such as K-Y Jelly or Lubifax (or 3.5 g into 150 ml). Some use 6 g of calcium carbonate in 100 g of water-soluble lubricant. Place injured hand in surgical glove filled with gel. Apply q 4 h.	Dermal	Powder is available from Spectrum Pharmaceutical Co. in California: 800-772-8786. Commercial preparation of calcium gluconate gel is available from Pharmascience in Montreal, Quebec: 514-340-1114.

(continued)

TABLE 4-35. (*Continued*)

Antidote	Use	Dose	Route	Adverse reactions (AR)/comments
Infiltration of calcium gluconate.	Hydrofluoric acid.	If pain persists, calcium gluconate injection may be needed (see below). Dose: Infiltrate each square centimeter of the affected dermis and subcutaneous tissue with ~0.5 ml of 10% calcium gluconate using a 30-gauge needle. Repeat as needed to control pain.	Infiltrate	—
Cyanide antidote kit. Stock level to treat 70-kg adult for 24 h: 2 Lilly Cyanide Antidote kits.	Cyanide; hydrogen sulfide (nitrites are given only; do not use sodium thiosulfate for hydrogen sulfide); individual portions of the kit can be used in certain circumstances. (Consult PCC.)	Amyl nitrite: 1 crushable ampule. Use new amp q 3 min. May omit step if venous access established.	Inhalation	If methemoglobinemia occurs, do not use methylene blue to correct this because it releases cyanide.
Cyanide antidote kit. Stock level to treat 70-kg adult for 24 h: 2 Lilly Cyanide Antidote kits.	Cyanide; hydrogen sulfide (nitrites are given only; do not use sodium thiosulfate for hydrogen sulfide); individual portions of the kit can be used in certain circumstances. (Consult PCC).	Sodium nitrite—Child: 0.33 mL/kg of 3% solution if hemoglobin level not known, otherwise based on tables with product. Adult: up to 300 mg (10ml). Dilute nitrite in 100 ml of 0.9% saline, slowly increase rate to as rapidly as possible without fall in BP. Slow infusion if fall in BP.	i.v.	If methemoglobinemia occurs, do not use methylene blue to correct this because it releases cyanide.
	Do not use sodium thiosulfate for hydrogen sulfide; individual portions of the kit can be used in certain circumstances. (Consult PCC.)	Sodium thiosulfate— Child: 1.6 ml/kg of 25% solution. Adult: may be repeated every 30–60 min to a maximum of 12.5 g or 50 mL. Administer over 20 min.	i.v.	Nausea, dizziness, headache, tachycardia, muscle rigidity, and bronchospasm (rapid administration).
Dantrolene, sodium (Dantrium). Stock level to	Malignant hyperthermia.	1–2 mg/kg q 10–15 min. When temperature and heart rate decrease, slow infu-	i.v.p.o.	AR: Hepatotoxicity occurs with cumulative dose of 10 mg/kg; thrombophlebitis

(*continued*)

TABLE 4-35. (*Continued*)

Antidote	Use	Dose	Route	Adverse reactions (AR)/comments
treat 70-kg adult for 24 h: 700 mg from 35 vials (20 mg/vial).		sion rate of 1–2 mg/kg q 6 h until all evidence of syndrome subsides. To prevent recurrence, 1–2 mg/kg i.v. or orally up to 100 mg 4× daily for 2–3 d.		(best given in central line).
Deferoxamine (Desferal). Stock level to treat 70-kg adult for 24 h: 12 vials (50 mg/ampule).	Iron	Infusion (i.v.) of 15 mg/kg/h (3 ml/kg/h of 500 mg in 100 ml of D_5W); or 50 mg/kg i.m. up to 1 g q 4 h.	Preferred i.v.; can also give i.m.	Hypotension (minimized by avoiding rapid infusion rates); deferoxamine challenge test 50 mg/kg is unreliable if negative.
Digoxin-specific Fab antibodies (Digibind). Stock level to treat 70-kg adult for 24 h: 20 vials.	Digitalis glycosides (synthetic or natural).	One vial binds 0.6 mg of digitalis glycoside; ingested dose may be estimated from serum level. (See table with PCC.)	i.v.	Allergic reactions (rare), return of condition being treated with digitalis glycoside.
Dimercaprol (BAL in oil). Stock level to treat 70-kg adult for 24 h: 1,200 mg (4AMPS—100 mg/ml 10% in oil in 3-ml ampule).	Chelating agent for arsenic, mercury, lead, antimony, bismuth, chromium, copper, gold, nickel, tungsten, and zinc.	3–5 mg/kg q 4 h usually for 5–10 d.	Deep i.m.	Local infection site pain and sterile abscess, nausea, vomiting, fever, salivation, hypertension, and nephrotoxicity (alkalinize urine).
Ethanol (ethyl alcohol). Stock level to treat 70-kg adult for 24 h: 3 bottles 10% (1L each).	Methanol, ethylene glycol.	10 ml/kg loading dose concurrently with 1.4 ml/kg (average) infusion of 10% ethanol. (Consult PCC for more details.)	i.v.	Nausea, vomiting, sedation, use 0.22 μm filter if preparing from bulk 100% ethanol.
Flurpazenil (RoMazicon). Stock level to treat 70-kg adult for 24 h: 10 vials (0.1 mg/ml, 10 ml).	Benzodiazepines.	Administer 0.2 mg (2 mL) over 30 sec (pediatric dose not established 0.01 mg/kg). Wait 3 min for a response. If desired consciousness is not achieved, administer 0.3 mg (3 mL) over 30 sec. Wait 3 min for response. If desired consciousness is not achieved, administer 0.5 mg (5 mL) over 30 sec	i.v.	Nausea, vomiting, facial flushing, agitation, headache, dizziness, seizures. *Do not use for unknown or antidepressant ingestions.* May not reverse respiratory depression.

(*continued*)

TABLE 4-35. (*Continued*)

Antidote	Use	Dose	Route	Adverse reactions (AR)/comments
		at 60-sec intervals up to a maximum cumulative dose of 3 mg (30 mL) (1 mg in children). Because effects last only 1–5 h if patient responds monitor carefully closely over next 6 h for resedation. If multiple repeated doses, consider a continuous infusion of 0.2–1 mg/h.		
Folic acid (Folvite). Stock level to treat 70-kg adult for 24 h: 2–100-mg vials.	Methanol/ethylene glycol (investigational).	1 mg/kg up to 50 mg every 4 h for 6 doses.	i.v.	Uncommon.
Glucagon. Stock level to treat 70-kg adult for 24 h: 100 mg (10 vials, 10 U).	Beta-blockers, calcium channel blockers, hypoglycemic agents.	Adult: 5–10 mg, then infuse 1–5 mg/h. Child: 0.05–0.1 mg/kg, then infuse 0.07 mg/kg/h. Large doses up to 100 mg/24 h have been used.	i.v.	Hyperglycemia, nausea, and vomiting. Dissolve in D5W, not in 0.9% saline. Do not use diluent in package because of possible phenol toxicity.
Magnesium sulfate. Stock level to treat 70-kg adult for 24 h: ~25 g (50 ml of 50% or 200 ml of 12.5%).	Torsades de pointes.	Adult: 2 g over 1–2 min. If no response in 10 min, repeat and follow by continuous infusion 1 g/h. Child: 25–50 mg/kg initially, and maintenance is 30–60 mg/kg/24 h (0.25-0.50 mEq/Kg/24 h) up to 1,000 mg/24 h. (Dose not studied in controlled fashion.)	i.v.	—
Methylene blue. Stock level to treat 70-kg adult for 24 h: 5 ampules (10 mg/10 ml).	Methemoglobinemia.	0.1–0.2 mL/kg of 1% solution, slow infusion, may be repeated every 30–60 min.	i.v.	Nausea, vomiting, headache, dizziness.
Naloxone (Narcap). Stock level to treat 70-kg adult for 24 h: 3 vials (1 mg/ml, 10 ml).	Comatose patient; ineffective ventilation or adult respiratory rate of <12; opioids.	Infant/child: 0.1 mg/kg up to 2 mg from birth to 5 yr or 20 kg. Adult: 2 mg q 2–3 min up to 10–20 mg total; may give con-	i.v., ET	Acute withdrawal symptoms if given to addicted patients.

(*continued*)

TABLE 4-35. (*Continued*)

Antidote	Use	Dose	Route	Adverse reactions (AR)/comments
		tinuous infusion. Response dose in mg × 24 is added to maintenance fluid. Infusion rate is one-24th of maintenance in ml/h. Titrate to adequate respirations.		
Physostigmine (Antilirium) Stock level to treat 70-kg adult for 24 h: 10 ampules (2 ml each).	Anticholinergic agents (not routinely used, only indicated if life-threatening complications).	Child: 0.02 mg/kg slow push to max 2 mg q 30–60 min. Adult: 1–2 mg q 5 min to max 6 mg.	i.v.	AR: Bradycardia, asystole, seizures, bronchospasm, vomiting, headaches. *Do not use for cyclic antidepressants.*
Pralidoxime (2-PAM, Protopam). Stock level to treat 70-kg adult for 24 h: 12 vials (1 g/20 ml).	Organophosphates.	Child: <12 yr, 25–50 mg/kg and ≥12 yr: 1–2 g/dose over 15–30 min; then q 6-8 h for 24–48 h. Adult: Max dose 12 g/day. Maintenance i.v. infusion 1 g in 100 ml 0.89% saline at 5–20 mg/kg/h (0.5–12 ml/kg/h) up to max 500 mg/h or 50 ml/h. End point is absence of fasiculations and return of muscle strength.	i.v.	Nausea, dizziness, headache, tachycardia, muscle rigidity, and bronchospasm (rapid administration).
Pyridoxine (Vitamin B6). Stock level to treat 70-kg adult for 24 h: 4 ampules (50 mg in 5 ml or 250 mg in 25-ml vial).	Seizures from isoniazid or gyromitra mushrooms; ethylene glycol (investigational).	Isoniazid (unknown amount ingested): 5 g in 50 ml of D5W over 5 min and diazepam 0.1–0.3 mg/kg i.v. at different site (synergism); may repeat q 5–20 min until seizure controlled; up to 375 mg/kg has been given (52 g). Isoniazid (known amount): 1 g for each g INH ingested over 5 min with diazepam (dose above). Gyromitra mushrooms: 25 mg/kg child or 2–5 g adult i.v. over 15–30 min to max 20 g. Ethylene glycol: 100 mg i.v. daily.	i.v.	Uncommon; for Gyromitra mushrooms, some use p.o. 25 mg/kg/day early when mushroom is suspected.

(*continued*)

TABLE 4-35. (*Continued*)

Antidote	Use	Dose	Route	Adverse reactions (AR)/comments
Sodium Bicarbonate (NaHCO₃). Stock level to treat 70-kg adult for 24 h: 10 ampules or syringes (500 mEq).	Tricyclic antidepressant (TCAD) cardiotoxicity (wide QRS > 0.14 sec, ventricular tachycardia, severe conduction disturbances); or metabolic acidosis; phenothiazine cardiotoxicity.	1–2 mEq/kg i.v. undiluted as a bolus; if no benefit on cardiotoxicity, repeat twice in a few minutes apart. An infusion of NaHCO₃ may follow to keep blood pH at 7.5–7.55 but not higher.	i.v.	Monitor serum sodium, potassium and blood pH because fatal alkalemia and hypernatremia have been reported. Continuous infusion of bicarbonate by itself is of limited usefulness in settings of TCAD intoxication because of delayed onset. Prophylactic NaHCO₃ has not been encouraged.
Sodium Bicarbonate (NaHCO₃). Stock level to treat 70-kg adult for 24 h: 10 ampules or syringes (500 mEq).	Salicylate: to keep blood pH 7.5–7.55 (not >7.55) and urine pH 7.5–8.0.	2 mEq/kg of (NaHCO₃) will raise the blood pH 0.1 U. Alkalinization recommended if salicylate concentration of >40 mg/dL in acute poisoning and at lower levels if symptomatic in chronic intoxication. If acidemia is present with a pH of <7.2, add 2 mEq/kg as a loading dose followed by 2 mEq/kg every 3 to 4 h to keep the pH slightly alkaline at 7.5–7.55. If acidemia, recommend isotonic NaHCO₃: 3 ampules of (NaHCO₃) to 1 L of D5W rate of 10–15 mL/kg/h or sufficient to produce a normal urine flow and a urine pH of ≥7.5. After urine output established, add potassium 40 mEq/L.	i.v.	Monitor *both* the urine and blood pH. Do not use the urine pH alone to assess the need for alkalinization because of the paradoxical aciduria that may occur. Adjust the urine pH to 7.5–8 by (NaHCO₃) infusion.
Sodium Bicarbonate (NaHCO₃). Stock level to treat 70-kg adult for 24 h: 10 ampules or syringes (500 mEq).	Long-acting barbiturates: phenobarbital, mephobarbital metharbital (Gemonil), barbital (Butisol), primidone. Alkalinization is *not* effective for the shorter and intermediate barbiturates.	NaHCO₃: 1–2 mEq/kg or 100 mEq in 1 L of D5W with 40 mEq/L potassium at rate of 100 mL/h in adults. Adequate potassium is necessary to accomplish alkalinization.	i.v.	Additional sodium bicarbonate and potassium chloride may be needed. Adjust the urine pH to 7.5–8 by (NaHCO₃) infusion.

(*continued*)

TABLE 4-35. (*Continued*)

Antidote	Use	Dose	Route	Adverse reactions (AR)/comments
Vitamin K (Aqua Mephyton). Stock level to treat 70-kg adult for 24 h: 100 mg (2–5 ml ampules, 10 mg/ml).	Warfarin, indanedione, and super-warfarin rodenticides.	Therapeutically: (a) If abnormal coagulation studies develop or clinical bleeding, give p.o. 0.4 mg/kg/dose infants and children and 10–25 mg/dose in adults; administer until the PT is normal, then D/C and monitor PT for 5 d. (b) In clinical bleeding, 0.6 mg/kg/dose for <12 yr SQ, i.m., i.v. every 4–4.8 h depending on the severity or 10–50 mg in adults; i.v. rate should be <1 mg/min or 5% of the total dose per minute; i.m. and s.q. administration have not been associated with anaphylaxis but are not as useful in severe bleeding; s.q. route preferred over i.m. because of risk of hematomas. (c) Although package insert for vitamin K_1 states i.v. should not be given, the literature recommends i.v. 1–5 mg in children or 5–10 mg in adults every 6 h for *severe emergency bleeding;* staff must be prepared to manage the rare anaphylactoid reaction and monitor patient in ICU. (d) "Superwarfarin" poisoning may require up to 40 mg/kg i.v.	p.o./s.q./ i.m./i.v.	*Vitamin K_1 is not recommended prophylactically in empiric treatment of anticoagulant ingestion and most do not require any treatment.* Intravenous doses of >1.3 mg/kg/d have been associated with Heinz body hemolytic anemia in animals and anaphylaxis. Oral therapy with vitamin K_1 may be considered for maintenance therapy 1–5 mg in children and 10–25 mg in adults. 50–200 mg may be needed. Monitor by PT. If SQ, 5–10 mg in adults and 1–5 mg in children q 6 h; change to p.o. as soon as possible. Duration of therapy: For warfarin intoxication, vitamin K for 5–7 d. For "superwarfarin" intoxication, may require larger doses of vitamin K up to 2 mg/kg/d initially followed by 1 mg/kg/d for 7 d, then 0.5 mg/kg/d until there is no sign of bleeding for at least 1 week, which usual takes 4–6 weeks. Blood products: Severe bleeding may require emergency infusions of blood products, fresh frozen plasma, and/or packed red blood cells or fresh whole blood transfusions because it may take several hours for vitamin K_1 to be fully effective.

ET, endotracheal tube.

9. **Iron**—The antidote is **deferoxamine** (DO), a relatively specific iron chelator that binds ferric (+3) iron from the mitochondria and cells at the 3 N-OH sites to form ferroxamine (297). About 100 mg DO binds 8.5 to 9.35 mg of free iron in serum thereby reducing the ferritin stores in the liver and spleen.

    a. The **dose i.v. for a continuous infusion** is at a maximum rate of 15 mg/kg/h (3 mL/kg/h). The total amount administered should not exceed 6 g in 24 h in children and 8 g in adults (296,297), although greater than these amounts have been used in serious iron poisoning (298). The manufacturer recommends i.m. administration unless the patient is in shock. Most toxicologists administer DO i.v. if treatment is necessary (299,300).

10. **Isoniazid** (INH) hydrazide, monomethylhydrazine (Gyromitra mushroom—The antidote is **pyridoxine,** a water soluble B complex vitamin which acts as a co-enzyme with L-glutamic acid decarboxylase (GAD) to convert glutamic acid to gamma-aminobutyric acid (GABA), the major inhibiting neurotransmitter. It also enhances the metabolism of glyoxylic acid, the toxic metabolite of ethylene glycol, to glycine (301–304).

    a. In INH poisoning, the **dose** of pyridoxine is 1 g i.v. for each gram of INH ingested; dilute in 50 mL dextrose or saline and administer over 5 min. If the ingested amount is unknown, empirically administer 5 g i.v. Use with diazepam (synergistic). In **ethylene glycol** poisoning, administer 50 mg i.v. every 6 h. In **gyromitra mushroom**, 25 mg i.v. and repeat as necessary. Diazepam works synergistically with pyridoxine to control INH seizures and should be given with pyridoxine.

11. **Methanol**—The antidote is **ethanol**, a competitive substrate that inhibits the enzyme alcohol dehydrogenase (ADH) and prevents the metabolism to the toxic metabolites formaldehyde and formate. A blood ethanol concentration of 100 mg/dL is needed to saturate the enzyme. Ethanol therapy is started at blood methanol levels of more than 20 mg/dL, hemodialysis is added if levels are more than 50 mg/dL. If the patient is on disulfiram, use hemodialysis in place of ethanol. Dose of ethanol is the same as for ethylene glycol poisoning therapy (Table 4-35).

12. **Opioids**—The antidote is **naloxone**, a pure opioid antagonist that competitively blocks mu, kappa and sigma opioid receptors in the CNS. Naloxone acts within 1 to 2 min i.v. and lasts 1 to 4 h, half-life is 30 to 60 min. Anecdotal reports suggest that high-dose naloxone may reverse CNS depression with clonidine, ethanol, BZPs, and valproic acid but the effects are inconsistent (118,119,121,305).

    a. **Naloxone** dose 0.1 mg/kg in child up to 2 mg, in adult 2 mg every 2 to 3 min up to 10 to 15 mg. If no response by 10 to 15 mg, the diagnosis is questioned. If suspect addiction 0.1 mg and double dose (121). Larger doses of naloxone are needed for synthetic opioids, and less in addicts.

13. **Organophosphate and carbamates**—The antidote is **atropine**, a parasympatholytic agent that competitively blocks the action of acetylcholine at the muscarinic receptors (306–310).

    a. Organophosphate poisoning atropine **dose** initially is 2 mg in adults i.v. (children 0.05 mg/kg) and may be repeated every 5 to 10 min until bronchial secretions and bronchospasm are relieved. Atropine is administered in larger increments until all secretions are dry. If the initial dose does not produce atropinization it confirms the diagnosis of cholinergic poisoning organophosphate poisoning. A **continuous atropine infusion** may be needed in severe cases (use preservative free atropine). The infusion consists of 8 mg in 100 mL infused at rate of 0.02 to 0.08 mg/kg/h (0.25 to 1.0 mL/kg/h) 1 to 5 mg boluses can be given as needed to control secretions or severe bradycardia.

   b.   In **drug-induced bradycardia,** administer 0.5 to 1.0 mg i.v. (children 0.01 to 0.05 mg/kg i.v. to maximum dose of 0.5 mg) and 1.0 mg in an adult and repeat as needed. If no response by 3 mg, the fully vagolytic dose in an adult, there is no further benefit to be expected. Repeat every 15 min as needed. **Doses** less than 0.1 mg in a child or 0.5 mg in adults may result in paradoxical slowing of the heart rate.

   c.   **In organophosphate intoxication** follow atropine with **pralidoxime (2-PAM) IV** reverses organophosphate effects by reactivating the phosphorylated cholinesterase enzyme and protecting the enzyme from further inhibition particularly at the nicotinic receptors with reversal of skeletal muscle weakness. **The dose** is 1 to 2 g in adults (children 20 to 50 mg/kg) i.v. not to exceed 200 mg/min in adults (4 mg/kg/min in children). 2-PAM may be administered as continuous infusion in a 1% solution 1 g in 100 mL saline at rate of 200 to 500 mg/h (children 5 to 10 mg/kg/h) and titrate to clinical response.

14. **Salicylate**—The antidote is **sodium bicarbonate** is an alkalinizing agent that reacts with hydrogen ions to correct acidemia and produce alkalemia. Urinary alkalinization with sodium bicarbonate enhances the renal elimination of salicylate and certain other acidic drugs including phenobarbital. Alkalinization also may prevent the intracellular distribution of salicylate. Alkalinization and fluid diuresis may also prevent the deposition of myoglobin in the renal tubules (311–314).

   a.   The **dose** is 1 mEq/kg expected to raise the serum pH 0.1, although this calculation is not a substitute for carefully monitoring the blood and urine pH and the serum sodium. The half-life of $NaHCO_3$ is about 45 min.

   b.   **Sodium bicarbonate may be** needed to correct the serum pH **salicylates, methanol,** and **ethylene glycol.** Hypokalemia and fluid depletion prevent effective urinary alkalinization, therefore, add 40 mEq/L of potassium. Monitor electrolytes and urine pH frequently, and maintain at 7.5 to 8.0.

   c.   **The dose** in cardiotoxic drug intoxication is listed below

15. **Tricyclic antidepressants and membrane depressant effects of other cardiotoxic drugs**—For patients with prolonged QRS interval, ventricular tachycardia and/or severe conduction blocks, the hypertonic sodium may be more important in reversing the cardiac toxicity than changes in the pH. The sodium ion appears to rectify the effect of the drugs on the sodium channel of the Purkinje fibers and also inhibits angiotensin II synthesis which prolongs QRS. Alkalinization has been shown to increase the protein binding of the drugs. Alkalinization

appears to be useful in treating patients with prolonged QRS of more than 0.10 s (when other signs of cardiac toxicity), but has not been shown to be preventative of cardiac toxicity (30,315–318).

  a. The **dose** of sodium bicarbonate is 2 to 3 mEq/kg as a bolus **within 5 min.** If the cardiotoxicity is not improved this dose may be repeated twice. Monitor with repeated serum electrolytes, and pH and maintain the serum pH at 7.4 to 7.5. There is no evidence that continuous infusions are as effective as boluses when given as needed. Table 4-36 contains medications and their dosages used for toxicologic emergencies in children. Table 4-37 contains cardiac medications and their dosages used in children.

XII. **Enhancement of elimination** (319–322). These methods are not ED procedures.

  A. **Indications for enhanced elimination include**

  1. Severe or critical intoxication with deteriorating state despite maximal supportive care, e.g., sedative-hypnotic overdose with refractory hypotension.

  2. The normal route of elimination is impaired, e.g., lithium overdose with renal impairment.

  3. Ingestion of lethal overdose or lethal concentration, e.g., methanol, theophylline, and paraquat.

  4. Patient's medical problems increase the hazards of the toxic substances, e.g., prolonged coma, chronic obstructive pulmonary disease, congestive heart failure, and renal impairment.

  B. **Forced diuresis** increases the glomerular filtration rate used in conjunction with ion trapping to prevent renal reabsorption of poisons. The procedure is to administer enough fluid to establish a renal flow of 3 to 5 mL/kg/h. Forced diuresis may be dangerous because of fluid overload; congestive heart failure, renal failure, electrolyte abnormalities, inappropriate secretion of the antidiuretic hormone, pulmonary edema, and cerebral edema may develop. Establishing an adequate urine flow of 2 mL/kg/h is usually sufficient. **Saline diuresis** may enhance the excretion of bromide, isoniazid, and lithium. Clinical efficacy has not been established.

  C. **Ion trapping**. Alteration of the urine pH may prevent renal reabsorption of poisons that undergo glomerular filtration and active tubular secretion. Many substances are reabsorbed through the renal tubule cells in the nonionized form. Fluid balance, acid-base, and electrolytes must be carefully monitored.

TABLE 4-36. *Ethanol dose in treatment of methanol intoxication[a]*

Dose Concentration	Intravenous 10%[b]	Oral 50%
Loading	10 mL/kg	2.0 mL/kg
Maintenance patient	Rate mL/kg/h	mL/kg/h
Occasional drinker	1.4	0.28
Alcoholic	1.96	0.39
Nondrinker	0.83	0.16
Maintenance during hemodialysis	1.5–2.5, up to 91 ml/h	0.3–0.5, up to 18.2 ml/h

[a]The loading dose and the maintenance dose are administered concomitantly over 30–60 min.
[b]If 5% solution loading dose of 20 mL/kg, maintenance is 2–4 ml/kg 5% solution. Titrate to blood ethanol concentration of 100 mg/dL (322 mmol/L). Double the maintenance dose of ethanol if hemodialysis is used.

TABLE 4-37. *Medications for toxicologic emergencies in children*[a]

Medication	Dose	Comments
Naloxone i.v./ETT	0.1 mg/kg <20 kg 2 mg/dose >20 kg	May follow with continuous infusion of initial response/h. Need 10 mg to exclude opioid etiologic agent.
N-Acetylcysteine p.o.	140 mg/kg loading	Follow with 70 mg/kg for 17 doses.
Pyridoxine i.v.	Gram for gram or 5 g	Synergistic with diazepam 0.3 mg/kg; i.v. administer both.
Cyanide kit		
Amyl nitrite inhaler	Inhalation	Omit if venous access.
Sodium nitrite IV	0.33 mL/kg 3% solution	10 mL 3% diluted 100 mL.
Sodium thiosulfate IV	1.65 mL/kg 25% solution	5 mL/min; some omit this step.
Deferoxamine	50 mg/kg i.m. test dose	Test not reliable.
IM	If symptoms, 15 mg/kg/h and	
IV	monitor BP and respirations	

[a]First Contact Poison Control Center.

1. **Alkalinization of the urine.** Those chemicals having an acid pH, which will not cross the lipid semipermeable membrane when in the ionized form, predominate in an **alkaline urine media** with a pH of 7.5 or greater and are excreted rather than reabsorbed. Alkaline ion trapping and diuresis enhances the elimination of chlorphenoxyacetic acid herbicides, chlorpropamide, phenobarbital, and salicylates.

2. **Acidification of the urine** may enhance the elimination of alkaline substances, including amphetamines, cocaine, phencyclidine, quinine, quinidine, sympathomimetics, and strychnine. It is not often recommended because of the risks of acidosis, and many of these agents may cause rhabdomyolysis and myoglobinuria.

D. **Extracorporeal methods.** These methods (peritoneal dialysis, hemodialysis, charcoal hemoperfusion, hemofiltration, exchange transfusion) are not ED procedures. They should be reserved for the minority of poisons that need more than good medical supportive care. The role of plasmapheresis in poisonings has yet to be defined.

1. **Dialysis** is considered in patients who have been intoxicated by a dialyzable toxin who have not responded or are deteriorating in spite of good medical care. A dialyzable toxin is one whose volume distribution (V_d) is less than 1 L/kg, protein binding is less than 50%, is water soluble, has a small molecular weight less than 500 Daltons, long elimination half-life and the contribution of dialysis to the total clearance will be significant. Drugs with large volume distributions of more than 5 L/kg are antidepressants, digoxin, lindane, opioids, phencyclidine, phenothiazines. Substances with low V_d (less than 1 L/kg) include alcohols and glycols, lithium, phenobarbital, salicylate, and theophylline.

   a. Substances that are **metabolized** to more toxic compounds that are dialyzable should be considered for dialysis depending on their blood concentration and the clinical circumstances.

    b. **Hemodialysis** should be considered immediately if the patient is stable and has a methanol or an ethylene glycol concentration of more than 50 mg/dL, or has neurologic manifestations and a lithium concentration of more than 4 mEq/L. The patient is systemically anticoagulated, requires central venous access (femoral or subclavian vein) and develops transient hypotension. The toxins flow passively across the semipermeable membrane down the concentration gradient into the dialysate solution. There is often a transient hypotension. Flow rates up to 300 to 500 mL/min and clearance rates may reach 200 to 300 mL/min). A mnemonic for dialyzable drugs is **The BAGELS: The** = theophylline; **B** = bromides; **A** = alcohols; **G** = glycols; **E** = electrolytes; **L** = lithium, long-acting barbiturates (phenobarbital); **S** = salicylate.

    c. Dialysis may be indicated as **general supportive** care if the following conditions exist:

        A—acid base disturbances that are unresponsive
        E—electrolyte disturbances that are unresponsive
        I—intensive care without response in cases of a dialyzable toxin
        O—overhydration
        U—uremia

    d. **Peritoneal dialysis** consists of dialysate fluid introduced into the peritoneal cavity through a transcutaneous catheter and then drained off. The peritoneal lining serves as the semipermeable membrane. It is easier to perform and does not require anticoagulants but it is only 10% to 15% as effective as hemodialysis.

2. **Hemoperfusion** uses the same procedure as hemodialysis including anticoagulation, but the blood is pumped directly through a channel containing adsorbent material (either charcoal or resin). Because the toxin is in direct contact with the adsorbent material it may be useful even with highly protein bound substances, with lipid soluble substances, and with high protein binding. It can achieve higher clearance rates than hemodialysis. Charcoal hemoperfusion has proved useful in theophylline intoxication, short-acting barbiturates, and some nonbarbiturate sedative/hypnotics (ethchlorvynol, glutethimide, meprobamate), phenytoin, and theophylline. Thrombocytopenia is a common complication.

3. **Exchange transfusion** removes poisons effecting red blood cells including methemoglobin and arsine-induced hemolysis.

4. **Chelation** techniques for enhanced removal of heavy metals will be discussed under specific heavy metals.

5. **Additional considerations in the intensive care**

    a. Nasogastric tube to avoid distention
    b. Frequent position changes
    c. Administration of antacids every 2 h if gastric pH is less than 1.5
    d. A daily urinalysis and culture if patient is catheterized
    e. Eye care and methylcellulose eyedrops every 4 h
    f. Passive range of motion exercises
    g. Provision for nutritional requirements by the alimentary or parenteral routes.

XIII. **Guidelines for deposition: consult with PCC**

A. **Legal rights of EDs** have to be addressed. Question the right to retain patients against their will in suicidal overdose or after administration of naloxone-induced arousal. Question the right to preform procedures, refused by the patient such as gastric lavage, and diagnostic testing of blood and urine. Question the right of a parent to refuse treatment recommendations for their poisoned child.

B. **Criteria for ED visit include** exposure to caustic/corrosive substance, asymptomatic patient with exposure to an amount sufficient to predict severe life-threatening manifestations, symptomatic patient, asymptomatic patient suspicion of chemical maltreatment in children or intentional overdose in adolescents or unknown or multidrug overdoses in adults.

C. **Asymptomatic nonintentional overdose** patients may be discharged when it becomes apparent that the time of onset and peak action has passed without any manifestations.

D. A history of a predicted potentially serious overdose should be observed for **at least 4 to 6 h** if regular acting medication before transfer to a nonemergency facility such as psychiatric unit or institution or discharged.

E. **Some of the delayed reacting substances** that require **more than 6 h observation** include acetaminophen, acetonitriles (artificial nail remover forms cyanide in vivo within 4 to 12 h), concretion formers (meprobamate, salicylates), enteric coated preparations, methanol, methylene chloride (industrial paint stripper that forms carbon monoxide in vivo), ethylene glycol, lithium, Lomotil in children, monoamine oxidase inhibitors, slow-release preparations (lithium, theophylline), sulfonylureas (delayed onset hypoglycemia), tricyclic antidepressant overdose in children. Some of these substances may need repeated blood concentrations to be certain they are decreasing.

E. Any patient who is **already symptomatic** should be considered for admission, have careful observation of vital functions, cardiac monitoring, and if intentional exposure, one to one suicide precautions. If symptoms are present, the patient can not be discharged until free of toxic effects and is not at risk of sequelae.

F. Patients with **altered mental status or intentional overdose** cannot sign out against medical advice (AMA). Intentional overdoses need suicide precautions and psychiatric clearance for competency before they can be discharged regardless of the amount ingested, even if it was nontoxic. Most states have provisions to place psychiatric patients on involuntary observation for up to 72 h.

E. **Chemical child abuse** must be considered in children, especially under 1 year of age and over 5 years where it may indicate an intolerable home situation. Child abuse and sexual abuse may be associated.

G. **The ICU.** Those with acid-base disturbances, cardiac conduction defects, cardiac dysrhythmias, electrolyte imbalances, need cardiorespiratory support, clinical deterioration, develop hypercapnia, hyperthermias, hypoglycemia, hypothermia, hypoxia, have existing significant medical disorders, require monitoring for antidotal therapy or enhanced elimination procedures, and develop respiratory distress (3,8,15,16).

H. It is important to establish the existence of **pregnancy** in any patient with overdose or intoxication in the reproductive age because of special concerns in management of the pregnant patient including the induction of emesis, x-ray of the abdomen, fetotoxicity, and teratogenicity of toxins and antidotes.

I. **Environmental and occupational exposures.** The appropriate agencies should be notified, e.g., Hazardous Material Management (Hazmat), local and state Health Departments, Office of Occupation Safety and Health and Environmental Protection Agency (EPA).

J. **Discharge and follow-up**

1. Intentional overdose—psychiatric assessment referral and follow-up; limited amount of prescription to 2 weeks.

2. Nonintentional overdose—poison prevention education of parents and instruction on the safe use of drugs and chemicals of adults, assistance in the administration of medications for the elderly or confused.

3. Substance abuse patients—Counselling should be arranged

XXIV. **Summary.** In summary, the approach to the initial evaluation and management of the poisoned patient is assessment of the severity of the exposure, basic and advanced life support, differentiation between neurological-structural and toxic-metabolic and psychiatric pseudo-coma, identification of the toxic substance, and initiation of methods to limit absorption and enhance elimination.

TABLE 4-38.   *Cardiac and vasoactive medication*

Medication	Initial dose	Maximum dose	Comment
Adenosine	50 µg/kg i.v.	Double dose up to 250 µg/kg	Rapid i.v. push
Bretylium	5–10 mg/kg i.v.	30 mg/kg	Rapid i.v. push
Captopril	0.1 mg/kg at <2 mo p.o.	—	—
	0.3 mg/kg at >2 mo p.o.	—	—
Digoxin	PMNB 30 µg/kg/d i.v.	—	Intravenous half total digitalizing dose
	FTNB 60–80 µg/kg/d i.v.	—	
	Child 40–60 µg/kg /d i.v.	—	
Diazoxide	3–5 mg/kg i.v.	May repeat 15–30 min	Hyperglycemia
Furosemide	1–2 mg/kg i.v.	—	Same dose i.v., i.m., p.o.
Hydralazine	0.1–0.5 mg/kg over 12 h i.v.	—	—
Lidocaine	1–3 mg/kg/kg i.v. or ETT	20–50 µg/kg /min by infusion	Use 1 mg/kg for cardioversion
Nifedipine	0.25 mg/kg p.o.	—	Hyperglycemia
Nitroprusside	0.5 µg/kg /min i.v. titrate to response 10 µg/kg/min for 10 min only	—	2 µg/kg/min max cyanide toxicity
Propranolol	1 mg/kg/min i.v. p.o.	—	Not in asthmatics
Verapamil	0.1 mg/kg	May repeat 0.1–0.3 mg/kg, first dose max 10 mg	Avoid under 1 yr of age

References

1. *Cost of injury in the United States. A report to Congress,* 1990 CDC.
2. Hoffman RS, Goldfrank LR. The impact of drug abuse and addiction on society. *Emerg Clin North Am* 1990;8:457–480.
3. Tista KJ, Willbrodt ET, Lankan PN. The frequency of drug-related MICU/INCU admissions [Abstract PIII-31]. *Clin Pharmacol Ther* 1993;53;214.

4. Litovitz TL, Felberg L, Soloway RA, et al. 1994 annual report of the American Association of Poison Control Centers toxic exposure surveillance system (TESS). *Am J Emerg Med* 1995;13:591–597.
5. Plum F, Posner JB. *The diagnosis of stupor and coma*. 3rd ed. Philadelphia, FA Davis Co, 1980.
6. Clotzer D, Sager A, Soclar D, et al. Prior approval in the pediatric emergency room. *Pediatrics* 1991;88:674.
7. Foldes SS, Fischer LR, Kaminsky K. What's an emergency? The judgement of two physicians. *Ann Emerg Med* 1994;23:23–24.
8. American College of Emergency Physicians. Clinical policy for the initial approach to patients presenting with an acute toxic ingestion or dermal or inhalation exposure. Am Coll Emerg Phys: 1995:25:570–585.
9. Rodgers GC Jr, ed. *American Academy of Pediatrics Committee on Injury and Poison Prevention: handbook of common poisonings in children*. Elk Grove Village, IL: American Academy of Pediatrics, 1994.
10. Koren G. Medications which can kill a toddler with one tablet or one teaspoonful. *Clin Toxicol* 1993;31:407–413.
11. McGuire TL, Feldman KW. Psychologic morbidity of children subjected to Munchausen syndrome by proxy. *Pediatrics* 1989;83:289–292.
12. Rogers D, Tripp J, Bentovim A, et al. Non-accidental poisoning: an extension of child abuse. *BMJ* 1976;1:793–796.
13. McClung JB, Murray R, Braden NJ, et al. Intentional ipecac poisoning in children. *Am J Dis Child* 1988;142:637–639.
14. Verity CM, Winckworth C, Burman D, et al. Polle syndrome: children of Munchausen. *BMJ* 1979;18:422–423.
15. Brett AS, Rothchild N, Gray R, et al. Predicting the clinical overdose. *Arch Intern Med* 1987;147:133–137.
16. LaCroux J, Gaudvealt P, Gauthier M. Admission to a pediatric intensive care unit for poisoning. A review of 105 cases. *Crit Care Med* 1989;17:749.
17. Menzel DB, McCellan RO. Responses of the respiratory system in toxicology. In: Doull J, et al., eds. *The basic science of poisons*. New York: Macmillan, 1987 pp 50–100.
18. DaSilvia AMT. Principles of respiratory therapy. In: Haddad LOM, Winchester JF, eds. *Clinical management of poisoning and drug overdose*. Philadelphia: WB Saunders, 1983:198.
19. Garay SM. Pulmonary principles. In: Goldfrank LK, ed. *Toxicologic emergencies*. Norwalk, CT: Appleton-Century-Crofts, 1985:80.
20. Wald PH, Balmes JR. Respiratory effects of short-term high intensity toxic inhalations. Smoke, gases and vapors. *J Intensive Care Med* 1987;2:260.
21. Shanies HM. Noncardiac pulmonary edema. *Med Clin North Am* 1977;61:1319.
22. Armstrong CW, et al. An outbreak of metal fume fever. *J Occup Med* 1983;25:886.
23. Beauchamp RO. A critical review of the literature on hydrogen sulfide toxicity. *CRC Crit Rev Toxicol* 1984;13:25.
24. Benowitz NL, Goldschalger N. Cardiac disturbances in the toxicologic patient. In: Hadad LM, Winchester FJ, eds. *Clinical management of poisoning and drug overdose*. Philadelphia: WB Saunders, 1983:65.
25. Levin RJ. Cardiac principles. In: Goldfrank LK, ed. *Emergency toxicology*. New York: Appleton-Century-Crofts, 1985:86.
26. Tingelstad J. Shock. *Pediatr Rev* 1995;16:347–348.
27. Corneli HM. Evaluation, treatment and transport of pediatric patients in shock. *Pediatr Clin North Am* 1993;40:303–319.
28. Schriger DS, Baraff LJ. Defining normal capillary refill: variations with age, sex and temperature. *Ann Emerg Med* 19988;177:932–935.
29. Scrounger DS, Baraff LJ. Capillary refill—is it a useful predictor of hypovolemia of hypovolemic states? *Ann Emerg Med* 1991;20:601–605.
30. Pentel P, Benowitz NL. Tricyclic antidepressant poisoning: management of arrhythmias. *Med Toxicol* 1986;1:101–121.
31. Balazs T, Hanig JP, Herman EH. Toxic responses of the cardiovascular system. In: Doull J, et al, ed. *Toxicology: the basic science of poisons*. New York: Macmillan, 1985:387.
32. Olsen KR, Pentel PR, Kelley MT. Physical assessment and differential diagnosis of the poisoned patient. *Med Toxicol* 1987;2:52–81.
33. Done AK. Signs, symptoms and sources. *Emerg Med* Jan 1976:15:2–77.
34. Tomarken JL, Britt BA. Malignant hyperthermia. *Ann Emerg Med* 1987;16:1253.
35. Guze BH, Baxter LR. Neuroleptic malignant syndrome. *N Engl J Med* 1985;313:163.
36. Rosenberg J, et al. Hyperthermia associated with drug intoxication. *Crit Care Med* 1986;14:964.
37. Feighhner J, Boyer W, et al. Adverse consequences of fluoxetine and MAOI combination therapy. *J Clin Psychol* 1990;51:222–225.
38. Kline SS, Mauro LS, Scala-Barnett DM, et al. Serotonin syndrome versus neuroleptic malignant syndrome as a cause of death. *Clin Pharmacokinet* 1989;8:510–514
39. Guze H, Baxter LR Jr. The serotonin syndrome. Case responsive to propranolol [Letter]. *J Clin Psychopharmacol* 1986;6:119–120.
40. Sternbach HY. The serotonin syndrome. *Am J Psychiatr* 1991;148:705–713.
41. Ruiz F. Fluoxetine and the serotonin syndrome. *Ann Emerg Med* 1994;24:983.
42. Stine RT. Accidental hypothermia. *JACEP* 1977;59:364.
43. Larach MG. Accidental hypothermia. *Lancet* 1995;345:493–498.
44. Zell SC, Kurtz KJ. Severe exposure hypothermia. A resuscitation protocol. *Ann Emerg Med* 1985;14:339–345.

45. Jolly BT, Ghezzi K. Accidental hypothermia. *Emerg Clin North Am* 1992.10, 311–327.
46. Martin TG. Near drowning and cold water immersion. *Ann Emerg Med* 1984;13:263.
47. Danzl DP, Pozos RS. Multicenter hypothermia survey. *Ann Intern Med* 1987;16:1042–1055.
48. Voelker R. Managing malignant hyperthermia. *JAMA* 1995:294:1902.
49. Henry GL. Neurologic emergencies. 2. Altered mental status. *Emerg Med* 1988; Mar 15:24–57.
50. Sabin TD. The differential diagnosis of coma. *N Engl J Med* 1974;290:1062.
51. Zun L, et al. A survey of the form of mental status examination administered by emergency physicians. *Ann Emerg Med* 1986;15:916–922.
52. Buckley RG, Aks SE, Eshon JL. The pulse oximeter gap in carbon monoxide intoxication. *Ann Emerg Med* 1994;24:252–259.
53. Tomaszewski CA, Thom SR. Use of hyperbaric oxygen in toxicology. *Emerg Clin North Am* 1994;12:437–459.
54. Hampson NB, Dunford RG, Kramer CG, et al. Selection criteria utilized for hyperbaric oxygen treatment of carbon monoxide poisoning. *J Emerg Med* 1995;13:227–233.
55. Rummans TA, Evans JM, Krahn LE, et al. Delirium in elderly patients: evaluation and management. *Mayo Clin Proc* 1995;70:989–998.
56. Rice MW, Moore GP. Management of the violent patient. *Emerg Med Clin North Am* 1991;9:13–30.
57. Dubin WR. Overcoming danger with violent patients: guidelines for safe and effective management. *Emerg Med Rep* 1992;13:106–112.
58. Dubin WR, Weiss KJ. *Handbook of psychiatric emergencies.* Springhouse, PA: Springhouse Corp, 1991.
59. Wasserberger J, Ordog GJ, Hardin E, et al. Violence in the emergency department. *Top Emerg Med* 1992;14:71–78.
60. Tintinalli J. Violent patients and the prehospital provider. *Ann Emerg Med* 1993;22:1276–1279.
61. Carasiti ME. Drug-induced aseptic meningitis. *Resident Staff Physician* 1988;43:11–17.
62. Widener HL, Littman BM. Ibuprofen-induced meningitis in systemic lupus erythematosus. *JAMA* 19772:230:1062.
63. Clinton JE, Sterner S, Stelmackers Z, et al. Haloperidol for sedation of disruptive emergency patients. *Ann Emerg Med* 1987;16:319.
64. Thomas H, Schwartz E, Petrilli R. Droperidol versus haloperidol for chemical restraint of aggitative and combative patients. *Ann Emerg Med* 1992;21:407–413.
65. Ayd FJ. Haloperidol: twenty years clinical experience. *J Clin Psychiatr* 1988;39:807.
66. Dubin WR, Feld J. Rapid tranquilization of the violent patient. *Am J Emerg Med* 1989;7:313–320.
67. Jennett B, et al. Assessment of outcome after severe brain damage. A practical scale. *Lancet* 1975;1:480–484.
68. Teasdale G, Jennett B. Assessment of coma and impaired consciousness: a practical scale. *Lancet* 1974;2:81–84.
69. Levy DE, et al. Predicting the outcome from hypoxic-ischemic coma. *JAMA* 1985;253:1420–1427.
70. Strickbine-Van Reet P, et al. A preliminary prospective neurophysiological study of coma in children. *Am J Dis Child* 1984;138:492–495.
71. Simpson D, Reilly P. Pediatric coma scale. *Lancet* 1982;2:450.
72. Mofenson HC, Greensher J. The unknown poison. *Pediatrics* 1974;54:336–342.
73. Modly CE, et al. Evaluation of alopecia; a new algorithm. *Cutis* 1989;43:148–152.
74. Cone TE. Diagnosis and treatment: some diseases, syndromes and conditions associated with an unusual odor. *Pediatrics* 1968;41:993–995.
75. Mace JW, et al. The child with an unusual odor. *Clin Pediatr* 1976;15:57–62.
76. Shelley ED, et al. The fish odor syndrome. *JAMA* 1984;251:253–256.
77. Schiffman SS. Taste and smell. *N Engl J Med* 1983;308:1275–1279,1337–1342.
78. Goldfrank L, et al. Teaching the recognition of odors. *Ann Emerg Med* 1982;11:684–666
79. Haddad LM, Roberts JR. A general approach to the emergency manmagement of poisoning. In: Haddad LM, Winchester JF, eds. *Clinical management of poisoning and overdose.* 2nd ed. Phildelphia: WB Saunders, 1990.
80. Ellenhorn MJ, Barceloux DG. Gut decontamination. In: *Medical toxicology: diagnosis and treatment of human poisoning.* New York: Elsevier Science, 1988.
81. Rumack BH, ed. *Poisondex information system.* Denver: Micromedex, 1991.
82. Olsen KR, ed. *Poisoning and drug overdose.* Norwalk, CT: Appleton & Lange, 1994.
83. Goldfrank LR, et al. *Goldfrank's toxicologic emergencies.* Norwalk, CT: Appleton & Lange, 1994.
84. Oderda G, Klein-Shwartz W. General management of the poisoned patient. *Crit Care Q* 1982;4:1–18.
85. Saxena K, Kingston R. Acute poisoning—management protocol. *Postgrad Med* 1982;71:67–77.
86. Sullivan J, Rumack B, Peterson RG. Management of the poisoned patient in the emergency department. *Top Emerg Med* 1979;1:1–12.
87. Kulig K. Initial managemenbt of ingestions of toxic substances. *N Engl J Med* 1992;326:1677–1681.
88. Walls RM. Rapid sequence intubation in head trauma. *Ann Emerg Med* 1993;22:1003–1013.
89. Walls RM. Rapid sequence intubation in head trauma. *Ann Emerg Med* 1993;22:1003–1013.
90. Aimed G, et al. Rapid sequence anesthesia for emergency intubation. *Pediatr Emerg Care* 1990;6:200.
91. Walker LA, et al. Using rapid sequence induction to facilitate tracheal intubation. *Emerg Med Rep* 1993;14:126–132.
92. Luten R. *APLS instructor manual: the pediatric emergency medicine course testbook.* 2nd ed. Dallas: American Academy Pediatrics/American College Emergency Physicians, 1993.
93. Gelb LN. New labelling for sodium nitroprusside emphiasizes risk of cyanide toxiciy. *FDA Med Bull* 1991;21:3–4.

94. Tzivoni D, et al. Magnesium therapy for torsades de points. *Circulation* 1988;77:392.
95. Piccone G, et al. Magnesium infusion in treatment of torsades de pointes. *Am Heart J* 1986;112:847.
96. Stratmann HGG, Kennedy HL. Torsades de pointes associated with drugs and toxins: recognition and management. *Am Heart J* 1987;113:1470–1482.
97. Hoffman RS, Goldfrank LR. The poisoned patient with altered conscious. Controversies in the use of a "coma cocktail." *JAMA* 1995:277:562–567.
98. Wrenn KD, et al. A toxicity study of parenteral thiamine hydrochloride. *Ann Emerg Med* 1989;18:867–869.
99. Stephen JM, et al. Anaphylaxis from the administration of thiamine. *Am J Emerg Med* 1992;10:61.
100. Browning RG, Olson DW, Stueven HA, et al. 50% glucose antidote or toxin? *Ann Emerg Med* 1990;17:683–687.
101. Hoffman JR, Schriger DL, Votey SR, et al. The emperic use of hypertonic dextrose in patients with altered mental status: a reapprasil. *Ann Emerg Med* 1992;21:21–24.
102. Atkin SH, Dasmahapatra A, Jaker MA, et al. Fingerstick glucose determination in shock. *Ann Intern Med* 1991:114:1020–1024.
103. Azar I, Turndorf H. Severe hypertension and multiple atrial premature contractions following naloxone administration. *Anesth Analg* 1979;58:524–525.
104. Committee on Drugs American Academy of Pediatrics: Emergency drug dosages for infants and children. Naloxone use in newborn. Clarification. *Pediatrics* 1989;83:803.
105. Kaplan JI, Mars JA. Effectiveness and safety of intravenous nalmefene for emergency department patients with suspected narcotic overdose; a pilot study. *Ann Emerg Med* 1993;22:187–190.
106. Mariani PJ. Seizure associated with low dose naloxone. *Am J Emerg Med* 1989;7:127–129.
107. Kaplan JI, Mars JA. Effectiveness and safety of intravenous nalmefene for emergency department patients with suspected narcotic overdose: a pilot study. *Ann Emerg Med* 1993;22:187–190.
108. Yearly DM, Paris PM, Kaplan RM, et al. The safety of the prehospital naloxone administration by paramedics. *Ann Emerg Med* 1990;19:902–905.
109. Schwarl JA, Koenigsberg MD. Naloxone-induced pulmonary edema. *Ann Emerg Med* 1987;18:1294.
110. Hoffman JR, Schriger DL, Luo JS. The emperic use of naloxone in patients with altered mental status: a reapprasal. *Ann Emerg Med* 1991;20:246–252.
111. Wasserberger J, Ording GJ. Naloxone-induced hypertension in patients on clonidine. *Ann Emerg Med* 1988;17:557.
112. Levin ER, Drayer JI, Weber MA. Severe hypertension induced by naloxone. *Am J Med Sci* 1985;290:70–72.
113. Tanka GY. Hypertensive reaction to naloxone. *JAMA* 1974;228:24–26.
114. Manelli M, Maggi M, Defeo ML, et al. Naloxone administration releases catecholamines. *N Engl J Med* 1983;308:654–655.
115. Cuss FM, Colaco CB, Baron JH. Cardiac arrest after reversal of effects of opiates with naloxone. *BMJ* 1984;4:363–364.
116. Andree RA. Sudden death following naloxone administration. *Anesth Analg* 1980;59:782–784.
117. Gaddis GM, Watson WA. Naloxone-associated patient violence: an overlooked toxicity? *Ann Pharmacother* 1982;26:196–198.
118. Goldfrank L, Weisman RS, Errick JK, et al. A dosing nomogram for continuous infusion IV naloxone. *Ann Emerg Med* 1986;15:566–510.
119. Tenenbein M, et al. Continuous naloxone infusion for opiate poisoning in infancy. *J Pediatr* 1984;105:645.
120. Lewis JM, et al. Continuous naloxone infusion in pediatric narcotic verdose. *Am J Dis Child* 1984;136:844–846.
121. Mofenson HC, Caraccio TR. Continuous infusion of intravenous naloxone. *Ann Emerg Med* 1987:3:374.
122. Fiser DH, Moss MM, Walker W. Critical care for clonidine poisoning in toddlers. *Crit Care Med* 1990;18:1124–1128.
123. Brogden RN, Goa KL. Flumazenil: a preliminary review of its benzodiazepam antagonist properties, intrinsic activity and therapeutic use. *Drug* 1988;35:448–467.
124. Finkle BS, McClosky KL, Goodman LS. Diazepam and drug associated deaths:a survey in the United States and Canada. *JAMA* 1979:242:429–434.
125. Sugarman JM, Paul RI. Flumazenil: a review. *Emerg Pediatr Care* 1994;10:37–43.
126. Knudsen L, et al. Benzodiazepine intoxication treated with flumazenil (Anexate, RO 15-1788). *Anesthesia* 1988;43:274–276.
127. Hojer J, Baehrendtz S. The effect of flumazenil (Po15-1788) in the management of self-induced benzodiazepine poisoning in a double-blind study. *Acta Med Scand* 1988;224:357–365.
128. O'Sullivan GF, Wade DN. Flumazenil in the management of drug overdose with benzodiazepines and other agents. *Clin Pharmacol Ther* 1987;42:254–259.
129. Burkhart KK, Kulig KW. The diagnostic utility of flumazenil (a benzodiazepine antagonist) in coma of unknown etiology. *Ann Emerg Med* 1990;19:319–321.
130. Spivey WH, Roberts JR, Derlet RW. A clinical trial of escalating doses of flumazenil for reversal of suspected benzodiazepine overdose in the emergency department. *Ann Emerg Med* 1993;22:1813–1821.
131. Kulka PJ, Lauven PM. Benzodiazepine antagonist: an update of their role in emergency care of overdose patients. *Drug Safety* 1992;7:381–386.
132. Geller E, Crome P, Schaller MD, et al. Risks and benifits of therapy with flumazenil (anexate) in mixed drug intoxications. *Eur Neurol* 1991;31:241–250.

133. Chern T, Hu S, Lee C, et al. Diagnostic and therapeutic utility of flumazenil in comatose patients with drug overdose. *Am J Emerg Med* 1993;11:122–124.
134. Winkler E, Almog S, Kriger, et al. Use of flumazenil in the diagnosis and treatment of patients with coma of unknown etiology. *Crit Care Med* 1993;21:538–542.
135. Short T, Maling T, Gallently D. Ventricular arrhythmia precipitated by flumazenil. *BMJ* 1988;296:1070–1071.
136. Burr W, Heniger K, Heninger G. Death after flumazenil. *BMJ* 1989;298:1713.
137. Lopez A, Robollo J. Benzodiazepine withdrawal syndrome after a benzodiazepine antagonist. *Crit Care Med* 1990;18: 1480–1481.
138. Lim AG. Death after flumazenil. *BMJ* 1989;299:858–859.
139. Ronald OK, Dahl V. Flunitrazepam intoxication in a child treated with the benzodiazepine antagonist flumazenil. *Crit Care Med* 1989;17:1335–1356.
140. Spivey WH. Flumazenil and seizures. Analysis of 43 cases. *Clin Ther* 1992;14:293–305.
141. Delgado-Escueta AVC, Westerlain C, Treiman DM, et al. Current concepts: management of status epilepticus. *N Engl J Med* 1982;306:1058.
142. Vinning EPG. Use of barbiturates and benzodiazepines in treatment of epilepsy. *Neurol Clin* 1986;4:617.
143. Freeman JM, Vinning EPG. Status epilepticus. *Pediatr Ann* 1985;14:764–770.
144. Deshmulch A, et al. Lorazepam in the treatment of refractory neonatal seizures. *Am J Dis Child* 1986;140;1042.
145. Lacey DJ, Singer WD, et al. Lorazepam in the therapy of status epilepticus in children and adolescents. *J Pediatr* 1986;108:771.
146. Bleck TP. Status epilepticus. *Clin Neuropharmacol* 1991;14:191–199.
147. Rivera R, Segnini M, Baltodano A, et al. Midazolam in the treatment of statius epilepticus in children. *Crit Care Med* 1993;21:991–994.
148. Bleck TP. Advances in the management of refractory status epilepticus. *Crit Care Med* 1993;21:955–956.
149. Jagoda A, Riggio S. Refractory status epilepticus in adults. *Ann Emerg Med* 1993;22:1332–1348.
150. Van Ness P. Pentobarbital and EEG burst suppression, in the treatment of status epilepticus. refractory to benzo-diazepines and phenytoin. *Epilepsia* 1990;37:464–471.
151. Maytal J, et al. Low morbidity and mortality of status epilepticus in children. *Pediatrics* 1989;83:323.
152. Hauser WA. Status epilepticus: epidemiologic considerations. *Neurology* 1990;40:2:9–13.
153. Popper AH, Kennedy SF. *Neurological and neurosurgical intensive care.* Rockville, MD: Aspen, 1988.
154. Kumar A, Bleck TP. Intravenous midazolam for the treatment of refractory status epilepticus. *Crit Care Med* 1992;20: 483–488.
155. Curry SC, et al. Drug- and toxin-induced rhabdomyolysis. *Ann Emerg Med* 1989;18:1068–1084.
156. Koppel C. Clinical features, pathogensis and management of drug-induced rhabdomyolysis. *Med Toxicol Adverse Drug Exp* 1989;4:108–126.
157. Marks EA, Arsura EL. Cocaine-induced rhabdomyolysis. *Emerg Med* 1990;Aug 15:79–82.
158. Patel R, et al. Myoglobinuric renal failure in phencyclidine overdose. Report of 8 cases. *Ann Emerg Med* 1980;9:549–553.
159. Wrenn KD, et al. Sorting through the rhabdomyolysis: an enigma made manageable. *Emerg Med Rep* 1987;8:163.
160. Qwen CA, Mubanak SJ, Hargens AF, et al. Intramuscular pressures with limb compression: clarification of pathogen-esis of the drug-induced muscle compartment syndrome. *N Engl J Med* 1979;300:1169–1172.
161. Sinert R, Kohl L, Rainone T, Scalea T. Exercise-induced rhabdomyolysis. *Ann Emerg Med* 1994;23:1301–1304.
162. Robinson MD, Stewart PN. Hazardous material exposure in children. *Pediatr Emerg Care* 1987;3:179.
163. Plante DM, Walker JS. EMS response at a hazardous material incident: some basic guidelines. *J Emerg Med* 1989;7:55–64.
164. Mofenson HC, Caraccio TR, Greensher J. Ingestions that are considered nontoxic. *Emerg Clin North Am* 1984;2:159.
165. Chaffee-Bahanon C, Lacouture P, Lovejoy FH Jr. Risk assessment of ipecac in the home. *Pediatrics* 1984;75:1108.
166. Harchelroad F, Cottington E, Krenzelok EP. Gastrointestinal transit times of a charcoal/sorbitol slurry in overdose patients. *Clin Toxicol* 1989;27:91.
167. Olsen KR. Is gut emptying all washed up? *Am J Emerg Med* 1990;8:560–561.
168. Kulig K, Bar-Or D, Cantril SV, et al. Management of acutely poisoned patients without gastric emptying. *Ann Emerg Med* 1985;14:562–567.
169. Merigian KS, et al. Prospective evaluation of gastric emptying in the self-poisoned patient. *Am J Emerg Med* 1990;8:479–483.
170. Saetta JP, Quintion DN. Residual gastric content after gastric lavage and ipecacacuanha-induced emesis in self poi-soned patients: an endoscopic study. *J R Soc Med* 1991;84:35–38.
171. Saetta JP, et al. Gastric emptying procedures in the self-poisoned patient: are we forcing gastric contents beyond the pylorus? *J R Soc Med* 1991;84:274–276.
172. Young WF Jr, Bivins HG. Evaluation of gastric emptying using radionucleotides: gastric lavage versus ipecac-induced emesis [Abstract]. *Ann Emerg Med* 1991;20:952.
173. Tandberg D, Troutman WG. Gastric lavage and the poisoned patient. In: Roberts JR, Hedges JR, eds. *Clinical proce-dures in emergency medicine.* 2nd ed. Philadelphia: WB Saunders, 1991:655–662.
174. Harstad E, Mollen KO, Simesen MH. The value of gastric lavage in the treatment of acute poisoning. *Acta Med Scand* 1942:112:478–484.

175. Tandberg D, et al. Ipecac-induced emesis versus gastric lavage: a controlled study in normal adults. *Am J Emerg Med* 1986;4:205–209.
176. Albertson TE, et al. Superiority of activated charcoal alone compared with ipecac and activated charcoal for acute drug overdose. *Ann Emerg Med* 1989;18:56–59.
177. Cupit GC, Temple AR. Gastrointestinal decontamination in the management the poisoned patient. *Emerg Med Clin North Am* 1984;2:15–28.
178. Rodgers GC, Matyunas NJ. Gastrointestinal decontamination for acute poisoning. *Pediatr Clin North Am* 1986; 33:261–285.
179. Czajka PA, et al. Nonemetic effects of syrup of ipecac. *Pediatrics* 1985;75:1101–1104.
180. Auerbach PS, et al. Efficacy of gastric emptying: gastric lavage versus induced with ipecac. *Ann Emerg Med* 1986;15:292–301.
181. Tenenbien M, Cohen S, Sitar DS. Efficacy of ipecac-induced emesis, orogastric lavage, and activated charcoal for acute drug overdose. *Ann Emerg Med* 1987;16:838–841.
182. Winter ML, Snodgrass R. 3% hydrogen peroxide (H_2O_2) emesis: a possible alternative if ipecac is not available. *Vet Hum Toxicol* 1991;33:352.
183. Askenasi R. Esophageal perforation: an usuasual complication of gastric lavage. *Ann Emerg Med* 1984;13:146.
184. Wald PH, Stern J, Weiner B, et al. Esophageal tear following forceful removal of an impacted oral-gastric lavage tube. *Ann Emerg Med* 1985;15:80–82.
185. Holt LE, Holz PH. The black bottle. *Pediatrics* 1963;63:306–314.
186. Neuvonen PJ, Olkkola KT. Oral activated charcoal in the treatment of intoxications. Role of the single and repeated doses. *Med Toxicol* 1988;3:33–58.
187. Jones DV, Work CE. Volume of a swallow. *Am J Dis Child* 1964;102:427.
188. Neuvonen PJ, Vartiasnen M, Tokola O. Comparison of activated charcoal and ipecac syrup in prevention of drug absorption. *Eur J Clin Pharmacol* 1983;24:557–562.
189. Watson WA, Leighton J, Guy J, et al. Recovery of tricyclic with gastric lavage. *J Emerg Med* 1989;7:373–377.
190. Elliott CG, et al. Charcoal lung. Bronchiolitis obliterans after of activated charcoal. *Chest* 1989;96:672–674.
191. Dockstader L, Wrenn K, Roderwald L, et al. Inappropriate use of syrup of ipecac [Abstract]. *Vet Hum Toxicol* 1991;33:368.
192. Tennenbein M. Multiple doses of activated charcoal: a time for reappraisal? *Ann Emerg Med* 1991;20:529–531.
193. Pond SM. Role of repeated oral doses of activated charcoal in clinical toxicology. *Med Toxicol* 1986;1:3.
194. Bradberry SM, Vale JA. Multiple dose activated charcoal: a review of relevant clinical studies. *Clin Toxicol* 1997 33:407–416.
195. Park GD, Radmonski L, Goldberg MJ, et al. Effects of size and frequency of oral doses of activated charcoal on theophylline clearance. *Clin Pharmacol Ther* 1983;34:663–666.
196. Ilkhanipour K, Yearly DM, Krenzelok EP. The comparative efficacy of various multiple-dose activated charcoal regimes. *Am J Med* 1992;10:298–300.
197. Donavan PJ, Cline DC. Phenytoin administration by a constant intravenous infusion: selective rates of administration. *Ann Emerg Med* 1991:20:139–142.
198. Goldberg M, Spector R, Park G et al. The effect of sorbitol and activated charcoal on serum theophylline concentrations after slow release theophylline. *Clin Pharmacol Ther* 1987;41:108–111.
199. McNamara R, Aaron CK, Gemborys M, et al. Sorbital cathasis does not enhance the efficacy of charcoal simulated acetaminophen overdose. *Ann Emerg Med* 1989;18:934–938.
200. Keller RE, Schwab RA, Krenzelok EP. Effect of sorbital added to activated charcoal in preventing salicylate absorption. *Ann Emerg Med* 1990;19:654–656.
201. Fine JS, Goldfrank LR. Update in medical toxicology. *Pediatr Clin North Am* 1992;39:1031–1049.
202. Greensher J, Mofenson HC, Picchoni AL, et al. Activated charcoal update. *JECEP* 1979;8:261–263.
203. Mauro LS, Nawarskas JJ, Mauro VF. Misadventures with activated charcoal and recommendations for safe use. *Ann Pharmacother* 1994;28:915.
204. Caldwell JW, Nava AJ, De Haas DD. Hypernatremia associated with cathartics in overdose management. *West J Med* 1987;147:593.
205. Gazda-Smith E, Synhavsky A. Hypernatremia following treatment of theophylline toxicity with activated charcoal and sorbitol. *Arch Intern Med* 1990;150:689.
206. Smilkstein MJ, Smolinske SC, Kulig KW, et al. Severe hypermagnesemia due to multiple dose cathartic therapy. *West J Med* 1988;148:208.
207. Woodward JA, Shannon M, Lacourture PG, et al. Serum magnesium concentrations after repetitive magnesium cathartic administration. *Am J Emerg Med* 1990;8:297.
208. Weber CA, Santiago RM. Hypermagnesemia: a potential complication during treatment of theophylline intoxication with oral activated charcoal and magnesium containing cathartics. *Chest* 1989;95:56.
209. Gren J, Woolf A. Hypermagnesemia associated with catharsis in a salicylate intoxicated patient with anorexia nervosa. *Ann Emerg Med* 1989;18:200–203.
210. Garrelts JC, Watson WA, Holloway KD, et al. Magnesium toxicity secondary to catharsis during management of theophylline poisoning. *Am J Emerg Med* 1989;7:34.

211. Goldberg M, Spector R, Park G, et al. The effect of sorbitol and activated charcoal on serum theophylline concentrations after slow release theophylline. *Clin Pharmacol Ther* 1987;41:108–111.
212. McNamara R, Aaron CK, Gemborys M, et al. Sorbital cathasis does not enhance the efficacy of charcoal simulated acetaminophen overdose. *Ann Emerg Med* 1989;18:934–938.
213. Keller RE, Schwab RA, Krenzelok EP. Effect of sorbital added to activated charcoal in preventing salicylate absorption. *Ann Emerg Med* 1990;19:654–656.
214. Harchelroad F, Cottington E, Krenzelok EP. Gastrointestinal transit times of a charcoal/sorbitol slurry in overdose patients. *Clin Toxicol* 1989;27:91.
215. Sullivan JB, Krenzlok EP. Repetitive doses of the activated-charcoal combination: a word of caution. *Am J Emerg Med* 1988;6:201.
216. Tennenbein M. Whole bowel washout in iron poisoning. *J Pediatr* 1987;111:142–147.
217. Sullivan JB, Krenzlok EP. Repetitive doses of the activated-charcoal combination: a word of caution. *Am J Emerg Med* 1988;6:201.
218. Sandheimer JM, Sokol RJ, Taylor SF, et al. Safety, efficacy and tolerance of intestinal lavage in pediatric patients undergoing diagnostic colonoscopy. *J Pediatr* 1991;119:148–152.
219. Ingebo KB, Heyman MB. Polyethylene glycol-electrolyte solution for intestinal clearance in children with refractory encopresis: a safe and effective therapeutic program. *Am J Dis Child* 1988;142:340–342.
220. Tennenbein M, et al. Whole bowel irrigation in ironpoisoning. *J Pediatr* 1987;111:142–147.
221. Kirschenbaum LA, Matthews RN, Sitar DS, et al. Whole bowel irrigation vs. activated charcoal in sorbitol for the ingestion of modified release pharmaceuticals. *Clin Pharmacol Ther* 1989;46:264–271.
222. Hoffman RS, Smilkstein MJ, Goldfrank LR. Whole body irrigation and the cocaine body packer. A new approach to a common problem. *Am J Emerg Med* 1990;8:523.
223. Posthuma R. Whole body irrigation in pediatric patients: a comparison of irrigating solutions. *J Pediatr Surg* 1988;23:769.
224. Palatnick W, Tennenbein M. Safety of treating poisoning patients with whole bowel irrigation. *Am J Emerg Med* 1986:2005.
225. Mann KV, Picotti MA, Spevack TA, et al. Management of acute iron overdose. *Clin Pharmacol* 1989;8:428.
226. Burhart KK, Kulig KW, Rumack BH. Whole bowel irrigation as treatment for zinc sulfate overdose. *Ann Emerg Med* 1990;19:1167.
227. Hoffman RS, Chiang WK, Weisman RS, et al. Prospective evaluation of "crack vial" ingestions. *Vet Hum Toxicol* 1990;32:164.
228. Rosenberg PJ, Livingston DJ, McLellan BA. Effect of whole-bowel irrigation on the antidotal efficacy of oral activated charcoal. *Ann Emerg Med* 1988;17:681
229. Kirshbaum LA, Sitar DS, Tennenbein M. Interaction between whole-bowel irrigation solution and activated charcoal: implications for the treatment of toxic ingestions. *Ann Emerg Med* 1990;19:1129.
230. Hoffman RS, Chang WK, Howland MA, et al. Theophylline desorption from activated charcoal caused by whole bowel irrigation solution. *Clin Toxicol* 1991;29:191.
231. Burkhart K, Wuerz R, Donovan JW, et al. Whole body irrigation as adjunctive treatment for sustained-release theophylline poisoning [Abstract 7]. Presented at the AACT/AAPCC/ABMT/CAPCC, Toronto, Canada, September 30 to October 4, 1991.
232. Roberge RJ, Martin T, Michelson EA, Schneider SM, et al. Whole bowel irrigation in acute lead ingestion [Abstract 5]. Presented at the AACT/AAPCC/ABMT/CAPCC, Toronto, Canada, September 30 to October 4, 1991.
233. Murphy DG, Gerace RV, Peterson RG, et al. The use of whole body irrigation in acute lead ingestion [Abstract 6]. Presented at the AACT/AAPCC/ABMT/CAPCC, Toronto, Canada, September 30 to October 4, 1991.
234. Betzelos S, Mueller P. Whole bowel irrigation in a heroin body packer [Abstract 8]. Presented at the AACT/AAPCC/ABMT/CAPCC, Toronto, Canada, September 30 to October 4, 1991.
235. Brown CR, Becker CE, Osterloh JD, et al. Whole gut lavage in simulated drug overdose. *Vet Hum Toxicol* 1987;29:492.
236. Rosenberg PJ, Livingston DJ, McLellan BA. Effect of whole-bowel irrigation on antidotal efficacy of oral activated charcoal. *Ann Emerg Med* 1988;17:681–683.
237. Tomaszewski C, Musso C, Pearson JR. Prevention of absorption of lithium by sodium polystyrene sulfonate in volunteers. *Vet Hum Toxicol* 1990;32:351.
238. Kellermann A, Fihn S, LoGeorgo J, et al. Impact of drug screening in suspected overdose. *Am J Emerg Med* 1987; 1988;6:14–20.
239. Bailey D. The role of the laboratory in the treatment of the poisoned patient: laboratory perspective. *J Anal Toxicol* 1983;7:136–141.
240. Brent J, Wang R, Foley M, et al. Anion gap is not sensitive in diagnosis of toxic metabolic acidosis [Abstract]. *Ann Emerg Med* 1991;20:195.
241. Helper B, Sutheimer C, Sunshine I. The role of the toxicologic laboratory in suspected ingestions. *Pediatr Clin North Am* 1986;33:245–260.
242. Weisman R, Howland M. The toxicology laboratory. *Top Emerg Med* 1983;5:9–15.
243. Winter SD, et al. The fall of the anion gap. *Arch Intern Med* 1990;150:311–313.

244. Oh MS, Carrol HJ. The anion gap. *N Engl J Med* 1977;279:814.
245. McCarron MM. The role of the laboratory in the treatment of the poisoned patient: clinical perspective. *J Anal Toxicol* 1983:7:142–145.
246. Kaye S. Bedside toxicology. *Pediatr Clin North Am* 1970;17:518.
247. Gabow P. Disorders associated with altered anion gap. *Kidney Int* 1985;27:472.
248. Dinuble MJ. The increment in the anion gap: overextension of a concept? *Lancet* 1988;1:951–952.
249. Winter SD, Pearson R, Gabow PA, et al. The fall of the anion gap. *Arch Intern Med* 1990;150:311–313.
250. Emmett M, Narins RG. Clinical use of the anion gap. *Medicine* 1977;56:38–54.
251. Oh MS, Carroll HJ. The anion gap. *N Engl J Med* 1977;297:814–817.
252. Gabow PA, Kaehny WD, Fennessy PV, et al. Diagnostic importance of the anion gap. *N Engl J Med* 1980;303: 854–858.
253. Mizock BA, Falk JL. Lactic acidosis in critical illness. *Crit Care Med* 1992;20:80–93.
254. Badrick T, Hickman PE. The anion gap—a reappraisal. *Am J Clin Pathol* 1992;98:249–252.
255. Lund ME, Banner W, Finley PR, et al. Effects of alcohols and selected solvents on serum osmolaity. *J Clin Toxicol Clin Toxicol* 1983;20:115–132.
256. Walker JA, Schwartzbard A, Krause EA, et al. The missing gap: a pitfall in the diagnosis of alcohol intoxication by osmometry. *Arch Intern Med* 1986;146:1843–1844.
257. Snyder H, Williams D, Zink B, et al. Accuracy of blood ethanol determination using serum osmolality. *J Emerg Med* 1992;10:120–133.
258. Robinson AG, Loeb JN. Ethanol: the commonest cause of elevated plasma osmolality. *N Engl J Med* 1971;284: 1253–1255.
259. Galvan LA, Watts MT. Generation of an osmolality gap-ethanol nomogram from routine laboratory data. *Ann Emerg Med* 1992;21:1443–1448.
260. Browning RG, Curry SC. Effect of glycol ethers on plasma osmolality. *Hum Exp Toxicol* 1992;11:488–490.
261. Foni M, Tomaszewski C, Kerns W, et al. Bedside ferric chloride urine tests to rule out salicylate intoxication. *Vet Hum Toxicol* 1994;35.
262. Blanke RV, Decker WJ. Analysis of toxic substances. In: Tietz NW, ed. *Textbook of clinical chemistry*. Philadephia: WB Saunders, 1986:1670–1744.
263. Kaye S. *Handbook of emergency toxicology*. 3rd ed. Springfield, IL: Charles C. Thomas Publisher, 1970:48.
264. Savitt DL, Hawkins HH, Roberts JR. The radiopacity of ingested medications. *Ann Emerg Med* 1987;16:331–339.
265. Handy CA. Radiopacity of oral nonliquid medications. *Radiology* 1971;98:525–533.
266. Greensher J, Mofenson HC, Gavin WJ. Usefulness of abdominal x-rays in diagnosis of poisoning. *Vet Hum Toxicol* 1979;211:45–46.
267. Osterloh J. Utility and reliability of emergency toxicologic testing. *Emerg Med Clin North Am* 1990;8:693–723.
268. Synder JW, Vlasses PD. The role of the laboratory in the treatment of the poisoned patient. *Arch Intern Med* 1988;146:297.
269. Bailey DM. The role of the laboratory in treatment of the poisoned patient. Laboratory perspective. *J Anal Toxicol* 1983;7:136–141.
270. Helper B, Sutheimer C, Sunshine I. Role of the laboratory in suspected ingestions. *Pediatr Clin North Am* 1986; 33:245–260.
271. Weissman R, Howland MA. The toxicology laboratory. *Top Emerg Med* 1983;5:9.
272. Wiley JF. Difficult diagnosis in toxicology: poisons not detected by the comprehensive drug screen. *Pediatr Clin North Am* 1991;38:725–737.
273. McCarron MM. The role of the laboratory in the treatment of the poisoned patient: clinical perspective. *J Anal Toxicol* 1983;7:142.
274. Mitchell JR, et al. Acetaminophen-induced hepatic injury: protective role of glutathione in man and rationale for therapy. *Clin Pharmacol Ther* 1974;18:676–684.
275. Holdiness MR. Clinical pharmacokinetics of *N*-acetylcysteine. *Clin Pharmacokinet* 1991;20:123–134.
276. Duvoisin RO, Katz R. Reversal of central anticholinergic syndrome in man with physostigmine. *JAMA* 1968;206:1963.
277. Rumack BH. Anticholinergic poisonings: treatment with physostigmine. *Pediatrics* 1973;52:449–451.
278. Pentel P, Peterson CD. Asystole complicating the treatment of tricyclic antidepressant overdose. *Ann Emerg Med* 1980;9:588–590.
279. Peterson CD, Leader JS, Steiner S. Glucagon for beta blocker overdose. *Drug Intell Clin Pharmacol* 1984;18:394–398.
280. O'Malhony D, O'Leary P, Molloy MG. Severe oxprenolol poisoning: the importance of glucagon infusion. *Hum Exp Toxicol* 1990;9:101–103.
281. Perkins CM. Serious verapamil poisoning: treatment with intravenous calcium gluconate. *BMJ* 1978;21:1127.
282. Lipman J, Jardine I, Roos C, et al. Intravenous calcium chloride as an antidote to verapamil-induced hypertension. *Intensive Care Med* 1982;8:55–57.
283. Henry M, Kay MM, Viccellio P. Cardiogenic shock associated with calcium channel and beta blocker reversal with intravenous calcium chloride. *Am J Emerg Med* 1985;3:334–336.
284. Kulig K. Cyanide antidotes and fire toxicology. *N Engl J Med* 1991;325:1801–1806.
285. Chen KK, Rose CL, Cloves GHH. Amyl nitrite and cyanide poisoning. *JAMA* 1933;100:1920–1922.

286. Way JL, Sylvester D, Morgan RL, et al. Recent perspectives on toxicologic basis of cyanide antagonism. *Fundam Appl Toxicol* 1984;4:S231–S239.

287. Berlin CM. Treatment of cyanide poisoning in children. *Pediatrics* 1970;46:793.

288. Mofenson HC, Greensher J, et al. Cyanide poisoning in children. *Pediatrics* 1971;47:1093.

289. Hall AH, Rumack BH. Hydroxocobalamin/sodium thiosulfate as a cyanide antidote. *J Emerg Med* 1987;5:115–121.

290. Smith TW, Haber E, Yeatman L, et al. Reversal of advanced digoxin intoxication with FAB fragments of digoxin-specific Fab fragments of digoxin-specific antibodies. *N Engl J Med* 1976;294:797–800.

291. Smith TW, Butler VP Jr, Haber E, et al. Treatment of life threatening digitalis intoxication with digoxin specific FAB antibody fragments: experience with 26 cases. *N Engl J Med* 1982;307:1357–1362.

292. Antman EM, Wenger TL, Butler VP Jr, et al. Treatment of 150 cases of life-threatening digoxin intoxication with digoxin-specific FAB antibody fragments. Final report on multicenter study. *Circulation* 1990;81:1744–1752.

293. Burkhart KK, Kulig KW. The other alcohols. *Emerg Med Clin North Am* 1990;8:913–928.

294. Becker CE. The alcoholic patient as a toxic emergency. *Emerg Clin North Am* 1984;2:47–60.

295. Hall AH. Ethylene glycol and methanol: poisons with toxic metabolic activation. *Emerg Med Rep* 1992;13:29–38.

296. Whitten CF, Chen YC, Gibson GW. Studies in acute iron poisoning. II. Further observations of desferrioxime in the treatment of acute experimental iron poisoning. *Pediatrics* 1966;38:102–110.

297. Westlin WF. Deferoxamine as a chelating agent. *Clin Toxicol* 1971;4:597–602.

298. Lovejoy FH Jr. Chelation therapy in iron poisoning. *Clin Toxicol* 1983;1a:871–874.

299. Tenenbein M, Kowalski S, Sienko A, et al. Pulmonary toxic effects of continuous desferrioxamine administration in acute iron poisoning. *Lancet* 1992;339:699–771.

300. Cheney K, Gumbiner C, Benson B, et al. Survival after a severe iron poisoning treated with intermittent infusions of deferoxamine. *Clin Toxicol* 1995;33:61–66.

301. Wason S, Lecoutuer P, Lovejoy FH Jr. Single high-dose pyridoxine treatment for isoniazid overdose. *JAMA* 1981;940:1120.

302. Brown A, Mallett M, Fiser D, Arnold WC. Acute isoniazid intoxication: reversal of central nervous system symptoms with large doses of pyridoxine. *Pediatr Pharmacol* 1984;4:199–202.

303. Yardbrough BE, et al. Isoniazid overdose: treatment with high doses of pyridoxine. *Ann Emerg Med* 1983;12:303.

304. Chin L, Sievers ML, Laird HE, et al. Evaluation of diazepam and pyridoxine as antidotes to isoniazid intoxications in rats and dogs. *Toxicol Appl Pharmacol* 1978;45:713.

305. Chamberlain JM, Klein BL. A comprehensive review of naloxone for the emergency physician. *Am J Emerg Med* 1994;12:650.

306. Namba T, Nolte CT, Jackrel J, et al. Poisoning due to organophosphates insecticides. *Am J Med* 1971;50:475–492.

307. Du Toit PW, et al. Experience with intensive care management of organophosphate insecticide poisonings. *S Afr J* 1981;60:227.

308. Farar HC, Wells TG, Kearns T. Use of continuous infusion of pralidoxime for treatment of organophosphate poisoning in children. *J Pediatr* 1990;114:658–661.

309. Le Blance FN, et al. A severe organophosphate poisoning requiring the use of an atropine drip. *Clin Toxicol* 1986;24:69–76.

310. Bardin PG, van Eeden SF, Moolman JA, et al. Organophosphate and carbamate poisoning. *Arch Intern Med* 1994;154:1433.

311. Temple AR. Acute and chronic effects of aspirin toxicity and their treatment. *Arch Intern Med* 1981;141:364–369.

312. Hill H. Current concept: salicylate intoxication. *N Engl J Med* 1973;288:1110–1112.

313. Done AK. Salicylate intoxication: significance of measurements of salicylate in blood in cases of acute ingestion. *Pediatrics* 1960;26:800.

314. Winter RW. *The salicylate poisoned patient.* New York: Medical Programs Inc, 1969.

315. Fromer DA, Kulig K, Marx JA, et al. Tricyclic antidepressant overdose: a review. *JAMA* 1987;257:521–526.

316. Walsh DM. Cyclic antidepressant overdose in children: a proposed treatment protocol. *Pediatr Emerg Care* 1986;2:28–35.

317. Pentel P, Benowitz NL. Efficacy and mechanism of action of sodium bicarbonate in the treatment of desipramine toxicity in rats. *J Pharmacol Exp Ther* 1984;230:12–19.

318. Slovis CM. Emergency management of cyclic antidepressants overdose: an effective and organized approach. *Emerg Rep* 1993;14;116–124.

319. Blyte C, Lorch J, Cortell S. Extracorporeal therapy in the treatment of intoxications. *Am J Kidney Dis* 1984;3:321.

320. Pond SW. Diuresis, dialysis and hemoperfusion. *Emerg Clin North Am* 1984;2:29–45.

321. Balsam L, Cortitsidis GN, Fienfeld DA. Role of Hemodialysis and hemoperfusion in the treatment of intoxications. *Contemp Management Crit Care* 1990:61–71.

322. Winchester JF. Fluid and electrolyte balance. In: Haddad LM, Winchester JF, eds. *Clinical management of poisoning and drug.* Philadelphia: WB Saunders, 1990:148–167.

Emergency Toxicology, Second Edition,
edited by Peter Viccellio.
Lippincott–Raven Publishers, Philadelphia © 1998.

5

Enhancement of Elimination

†Clark S. Homan and °James G. Ryan

†Department of Emergency Medicine, State University of New York at Stony Brook, Stony Brook, New York 11794-7400; °Department of Emergency Medicine, North Shore University Hospital, Manhasset, New York 11030

I. **pH alteration and forced diuresis**
  A. **Mechanism of action**
    1. **pH alteration**
      a. Objective is to alter the pH, thereby making the toxin predominantly polar or ionic.
      b. Ion trapping occurs when the induced polar form is unable to be reabsorbed back across the cells of the renal tubule (Table 5-1).
      c. Ionic or polar toxins have difficulty crossing cell membranes, resulting in:
        (1) Decreased reabsorption and enhanced excretion in the renal tubule
        (2) Decreased absorption in the gut (Table 5-1)
      d. Nonionic or nonpolar toxins easily cross cell membranes, resulting in:
        (1) Increased reabsorption and decreased excretion in the renal tubule
        (2) Increased absorption in the gut (Table 5-1)
      e. Alkalinization of the urine has a limited role in treatment of weak acids and is usually reserved for phenobarbitol (1), salicylates (2), and 2,4 dichloro-phenoxyacetic acid (3).
        (1) The slightly alkalotic serum pH of 7.4 causes the acidic toxin to be polar.
        (2) The polar acidic toxin is much less likely to cross the cell membrane, leaving the serum and entering the cells.
      f. Acidification of urine is not recommended by many poison centers, as this has not been proven to be clinically effective and may result in metabolic acidosis. Weakly alkaline toxins are much less effectively treated with ion trapping by pH alteration for several reasons.
        (1) Alkaline toxins leave the serum and enter the cells.
          (a) The slightly alkalotic serum pH of 7.4 causes the alkali toxin to be nonpolar.
          (b) The nonpolar alkali leaves the serum and enters the cell.
          (c) Once in the cell, the acidic intracellular pH causes the alkaline toxin to become polar.
          (d) The polar alkali then become ionically trapped within the cell.

TABLE 5-1. *Principles of ion trapping*

Toxin	Solution	Charge/polarity	Clinical effect
Acid	Alkalotic	Ionized	Excretion increased Absorption decreased
Alkali	Acidotic		
Acid	Acidotic	Nonionized	Excretion decreased Absorption increased
Alkali	Alkalotic		

2. **Forced diuresis**
   a. Increased urinary output results in enhanced elimination of some toxins.
   b. Urine output should be 5 ml/kg to obtain a significant effect.
   c. Toxins that are effectively eliminated by forced diuresis are usually dialyzable.
   d. Forced diuresis is much less effective than hemodialysis.
   e. Hemodialysis should be used for serious or potentially fatal toxic absorption.
B. **Therapeutic regimen**
   1. **Baseline laboratory evaluation**
      a. Electrolytes
      b. BUN/creatinine
      c. Serum toxin concentration
      d. Arterial blood gases (ABGs) to assess acid-base status
      e. Urine pH
   2. **Alkalinization of the urine**
      a. $NaHCO_3$ 1 to 2 mEq/kg body weight is mixed in 5% dextrose/0.5 N saline 15 ml/kg.
      b. Infuse i.v. over 3 to 4 h.
      c. Check urine pH every hour and maintain at pH 7.5 to 8.
      d. Urine volume should be maintained at a minimum of 3 to 6 ml/kg/h. Many physicians use only alkalinization and avoid alkaline diuresis because of the danger of pulmonary and cerebral edema, especially with salicylate intoxication (4).
      e. Additional i.v. boluses of $NaHCO_3$ at 0.5 mEq/kg may be administered.
      f. A maintenance i.v. infusion may be started instead of serial bolus therapy.
         (1) Diuretic therapy with furosemide or mannitol may be initiated at this point.
         (2) Solution is made by mixing 50 to 100 mEq $NaHCO_3$ in 1 L of 0.45% saline. It is administered at a rate of 250 to 500 ml/h, which promotes diuresis.
      g. ABGs should be checked for extreme elevations in blood pH.
      h. Potassium and electrolytes must be closely monitored and corrected if necessary; severe abnormalities may require an ICU setting.
   3. **Acidification of the urine**
      a. **Diuresis** may be obtained by administering i.v. saline and a diuretic (mannitol or furosemide).

b. **Goal** of the therapy is a urinary pH of 4.5 to 6.0 and urine output of 3 to 6 ml/kg/h.

c. **Ammonium** chloride is the preferred agent.

    (1) Dose: 75 mg/kg/24 h given either i.v. as a 2% solution or p.o. in four to six divided doses.

    (2) ICU monitoring is mandatory to monitor and correct:

        (a) Electrolyte status

        (b) Acid-base status

        (c) Development of complications, e.g., ammonia encephalopathy (5)

d. **Hydrochloric acid** is an alternative agent.

    (1) Dose: 0.1 M HCl solution 0.2 mEq/kg/h i.v.

    (2) Administration must be through a **central venous line.**

e. **Absorbic acid** (controversial)

    (1) Several authors have stated that absorbic acid effectively acidifies urine (6), but others refute these claims (7).

    (2) Evidence suggests that absorbic acid is only effective in decreasing urinary pH by inhibiting the enzyme urease in patients with concurrent urinary tract infections (8). Therefore, its clinical usefulness is limited.

    (3) Dosage: 2 g i.v. (9) or 6 g p.o. (6) are recommended but controversially effective in acidifying the urine of human volunteers.

C. Indications

  1. Toxins are more effectively treated by urinary pH alteration and diuresis if they possess the following characteristics.

    a. Renal elimination as a primary route of excretion

    b. Significant renal tubular reabsorption of the toxin

    c. Small volume of distribution

    d. Low protein binding

  2. **Specific indications**

    a. **Alkaline diuresis** to promote elimination of weak acids

      (1) **Phenobarbital**

        (a) Severe poisoning is best treated by hemodialysis, which avoids complicating pulmonary edema.

        (b) Alkalinization effectively increases elimination of phenobarbital (1) and is warranted for significant but not severe poisoning.

      (2) **Salicylates**

        (a) Severe poisoning is best treated by hemodialysis, which avoids the complications of noncardiogenic pulmonary (10) and cerebral (11) edema.

        (b) Salicylate excretion is dependent on pH alteration, and diuresis has only a small effect (3).

      (3) **2,4-Dichlorophenoxyacetic acid:** Severe poisonings may be effectively treated with urinary alkalinization (3).

(4) Tricyclic antidepressants
  (a) Alkalinization of the serum is indicated to decrease the cardio-toxic effects, which are greater with acidosis.
  (b) Indicated for cardiotoxicity even without acidosis (QRS > 0.1 s, ventricular tachycardia, or severe conduction disturbances). The salt loading appears to improve cardiotoxicity (12–14).
  (c) Alkaline diuresis does not effectively enhance elimination.
(5) Methotrexate
  (a) May assist in the maintenance of renal excretion (15).
b. Acidic diuresis to promote elimination of weak alkalis
  (1) Amphetamines
    (a) Beckett and Rowland showed that 57% to 66% of amphetamine was recovered unchanged in the urine within 6 h when the urinary pH ranged between 4.80 and 5.15 (16); (less than 5% of amphetamine was recovered when the urinary pH was 7.6 to 8.3).
    (b) Acid diuresis not recommended for amphetamine toxicity which may cause rhabdomyolysis, resulting in myoglobinuria-induced acute tubular necrosis and renal failure rendering acidic diuresis ineffective.
    (c) pH changes may enhance the cardiotoxicity observed with amphetamine poisoning.
  (2) Phencyclidine (PCP)
    (a) Severe cases are often associated with marked elevations in serum creatinine, metabolic acidosis, hyperkalemia, and hyper-uricemia, which compromise renal function and necessitate hemodialysis.
    (b) Acidic diuresis is not a particularly efficient therapy because PCP has a large volume of distribution and less than 10% of PCP is excreted by the kidneys.
    (c) PCP-induced rhabdomyolysis results in myoglobinuria, which may cause acute tubular necrosis, rendering acidic diuresis ineffective.
  (3) Strychnine
    (a) Acidification of the urine has been shown to enhance renal elimination of this weak base.
    (b) Elimination of this toxin by acidic diuresis requires far more time than onset of the serious, often fatal toxic effects of this agent.
  (4) Quinidine and quinine
    (a) Urinary acidification has not been shown to greatly increase renal elimination.
    (b) Use of this therapeutic modality is not presently recommended.
D. Contraindications
  1. General factors
    a. Renal dysfunction
    b. Cardiac insufficiency

       c. Uncorrected fluid deficits
       d. Uncorrected electrolyte abnormalities
       e. Inability to closely monitor fluid, electrolyte, and hemodynamic status
    2. **Specific factors**
       a. Acidic diuresis: rhabdomyolysis or myoglobinuria
       b. Ammonium chloride: hepatic insufficiency
 E. **Complications**
    1. **General complications**
       a. Fluid overload
       b. Cerebral edema
       c. Pulmonary edema
       d. Acid-base abnormalities
       e. Electrolyte abnormalities
         (1) Hypokalemia
         (2) Hypernatremia
         (3) Hypocalcemia
         (4) Hypomagnesemia
    2. **Specific complications**
       a. Acidic diuresis
         (1) Rhabdomyolysis
         (2) Myoglobinuria
       b. Ammonium chloride
         (1) Ammonia encephalopathy

II. **Activated charcoal**
 A. **Mechanism**
    1. Serial doses of activated charcoal have been reported to interrupt the enterogastric and enterohepatic circulation of toxic metabolites.
    2. Optimal doses have not been established, but recommendations are as follows.
       a. Single dose: 1 g/kg. Pediatric dose: 15 to 30 g. Adult dose: 60 to 100 g.
       b. Multiple-dose therapy: 10 g q1h to 40 g q4h. Dose for activated charcoal is 0.25 to 0.5 g/kg every 1 to 4 h. The optimum dose not established.
       c. Continuous nasogastric tube infusion: 0.25 to 0.50 g/kg/h (may decrease nausea and vomiting)
       d. Recent study suggests multiple-dose activated charcoal may be only effective with phenobarbital, dapsone, salicylates, quinidine, theophylline, and carbamazepine (17).
    3. **Gastrointestinal (GI) dialysis** has been used to describe the process of diffusion of the toxin from a high level in the serum to lower levels within the gut mucosa cells. Subsequently the toxin diffuses from the mucosal cells back into the GI lumen, where the concentration of toxin has been significantly lowered by intraluminal charcoal adsorption.
    4. **Activated charcoal** also works to decrease serum levels of toxin by binding to the agent prior to absorption in the gut, resulting in enhanced elimination via the GI tract.

   5. Toxic agents are more efficiently eliminated by **serial charcoal therapy** if they have:

     a. Significant enterohepatic or enteroenteric circulation (18)

     b. Lower volume of distribution

     c. Decreased protein binding

   6. Adsorbability of charcoal may be diminished by concurrent administration of other agents. Examples:

     a. Saline cathartics (routinely added to activated charcoal so this is not considered to be a clinically significant interaction)

     b. Ethanol

     c. Cocoa powder

     d. Ice cream

     e. Milk

B. Indications

   1. Charcoal effectively adsorbs most agents. New indications, e.g., for valproic acid (19) are continually being recommended in the literature. Recent experimental data has shown charcoal to be effective in adsorbing botulinum toxin (20) and parathion (21).

   2. A list of agents adsorbed by charcoal would be too exhaustive for this text. A more clinically useful approach is outlined in Table 5-2, where toxins not effectively adsorbed by charcoal are listed. Substances poorly adsorbed by activated charcoal are listed in Table 5-3.

   3. Some studies have shown that charcoal alone effectively induces emesis (22,23).

C. Contraindications

   1. For caustic ingestions

     a. Ineffective adsorption

     b. May induce vomiting

     c. Induction of complications if perforation has occurred, i.e., mediastinitis

     d. Limitation of visual field during endoscopy

   2. For comatose patients without first securing the airway

   3. For acetaminophen ingestions (relative)

     a. The antidote *N*-acetylcysteine is actively adsorbed to charcoal (24).

     b. Some studies indicate that the adsorption of *N*-acetylcysteine is not significant (25). Others disagree and report a reduction of up to 39% of *N*-acetylcysteine absorption when it is given 30 min after administration of charcoal (26).

TABLE 5-2. *Toxins not effectively adsorbed by charcoal*

Acids	Ipecac
Alkalis	Lithium
Bromide	Malathion
Cyanide	Methanol
DDT	*N*-Methylcarbamate
Ethanol	Potassium
Ethylene glycol	Tobramycin
Ferrous sulfate	Tolbutamide
Iodide	

    c. The activated charcoal does not have to be retrieved via the NG tube prior to administration of *N*-acetylcysteine. There is no dose adjustment required even if the activated charcoal and *N*-acetylcysteine are given concurrently despite reduction of *N*-acetylcysteine absorption. Separating activated charcoal and *N*-acetylcysteine by 1 to 2 h is recommended to decrease the risk of vomiting (27–29).

D. Complications
1. Adsorption of antidotes
2. Adsorption of other therapeutic medications (30)
3. Pulmonary aspiration (31,32) resulting in bronchiolitis (33), pneumonitis, death
4. Empyema
5. Vomiting
6. Constipation
7. GI obstruction typically occurs with repeated dosing in patients with decreased GI motility (34).
8. Perforation (35)
9. Hypermagnesemia as a result of concurrent administration of magnesium-containing cathartics (36)
10. Corneal abrasions secondary to charcoal introduced into patient's eyes during vomiting (37).

III. Hemodialysis

A. Mechanism of action
1. Blood is circulated past a semipermeable membrane via an extracorporeal method. Substances in the blood are removed by diffusion down a concentration gradient. Anticoagulation with heparin is necessary.
2. The drug or substance being eliminated should have the following characteristics for dialysis to be effective (38).
   a. Low molecular weight (500 Daltons or less)
   b. Low plasma protein binding
   c. Low lipid solubility
   d. High water solubility
   e. Easily diffusible across dialysis membrane
   f. Low volume of distribution
   g. High plasma concentration

B. Indications for dialysis are present in the following patient-and drug-related aspects. Institution of dialysis in the clinical situation is not a common event. Refer to Table 5-4 for a list of agents that are dialyzable.
1. Clinical deterioration in the face of maximum supportive therapy.
2. Strong clinical evidence of toxicity accompanied by cardiopulmonary or thermal instability.
3. Laboratory confirmation of lethal blood level of the toxic agent.
4. Presence of renal compromise.
   a. When the toxic substance is metabolized or excreted by the kidneys.
   b. When chelating agents are indicated for heavy metal intoxications.

TABLE 5-3. *Substances poorly adsorbed by activated charcoal*

C—Caustics and corrosives, cyanide*
H—Heavy metals (arsenic, iron, lead, lithium, mercury)
A—Alcohols (ethanol, methanol, isopropyl) and glycols (ethylene glycols)
R—Rapid onset or absorption (cyanide* and strychnine)
C—Chlorine and iodine
O—Others insoluble in water (substances in tablet form)
A—Aliphatic and poorly absorbed hydrocarbons (petroleum distillates)
L—Laxatives (sodium, magnesium, potassium)

*If cyanide ingested activated charcoal (AC) is given in large doses. 1 gram AC adsorb 35 mg cyanide.
  Latest information has indicated AC recommended for use in cyanide ingestions (Kulig, Ref 23) and AC adsorbs N-methylcarbamate.

    5. Poisoning with an agent known to produce delayed toxicity (39).
    6. Poisoning with a drug which is metabolized into a more toxic form (39).
    7. Presence of significant hepatic compromise when the toxic agent is metabolized by the liver.
    8. Presence of prolonged coma (40).
    9. Strong history of absorption of a lethal dose of a toxic substance, i.e., methanol and ethylene glycol.
    10. Hemodialysis is preferred to hemoperfusion to remove several toxins, including methanol (41), ethylene glycol (42), salicylates (43), and lithium (44).

C. Contraindications
    1. The toxic agent is not effectively dialyzable (Table 5-5).
    2. Use in the presence of available therapeutic modalities that are more effective, i.e., true antidotes, as in opiate toxicity
    3. Presence of shock, which renders the patient hemodynamically unstable
    4. Presence of coagulopathy because of the subsequent heparinization required

D. Complications
    1. Spontaneous hemorrhage
    2. Venous thrombosis
    3. Hypotension
    4. Infection
    5. Hepatitis
    6. Electrolyte dysequilibrium
    7. Anaphylaxis due to hemodialyzing agents (45)
    8. Air embolism
    9. Blood leak from equipment
    10. Death secondary to equipment malfunction or failure
    11. Platelets can decrease
    12. Removal of therapeutic medications

IV. Peritoneal dialysis
    A. Mechanism of action
        1. Eliminates toxic metabolites from the blood by utilizing the peritoneum as the membrane for dialysis.

TABLE 5-4. *Commonly encountered dialyzable agents*

Acetaminophen	Ergotamine	Paraquat
Acetone	Ethanol	Penicillin
Alcohol	Ethylene glycol	Phenacetin
Amikacin	Fluoride	Phenobarbital
Aminophylline	5-Fluorouracil	Phenytoin
Ampicillin	Folic acid	Phosphate
Analgesics	Gentamicin	Plants, animals,
Antimicrobials/anticancer	Halides	herbicides, insecticides
drugs	Iodide	Potassium
Atenolol	Isoniazid	Procainamide
Azathioprine	Isopropanol	Propranolol
Bacitracin	Kanamycin	Quinidine
Bromide	Lead	Quinine
Camphor	Lithium	Salicylate
Carbenicillin	Mannitol	Salicylic acid
Carbon monoxide	MAO inhibitors	Sodium
Cardiovascular drugs	Meprobamate	Solvents, gases
Cefamandole	Metals, inorganics	Streptomycin
Cephalothin	Methanol	Strychnine
Chloral hydrate	Methyldopa	Sulfonamide
Chloramphenicol	Methylprednisolone	Tetracycline
Chloride	Methylsalicylate	Theophylline
Chloroquine	Nafcillin	Tobramycin
Colchicine	Neomycin	Vancomycin
Cycloserine	Paraldehyde	

2. Useful for toxins that are water soluble, are poorly protein bound, have low molecular weight, and have a low volume of distribution (46).
3. Clearance of toxins is determined by the dialysate flow rate, molecular weight of the toxin, and surface area of the peritoneum (46).
4. Rate of toxin removal is much slower than hemodialysis and hemoperfusion. Peritoneal dialysis should only be implemented if these other faster modalities are not available.

B. Procedure
1. A catheter is inserted through the anterior wall of the abdomen under local anesthesia.
2. Dialysis fluid is then instilled into the peritoneal cavity in allocations of 1 to 2 L.
3. The dialysis fluid is allowed to equilibrate for 30 to 260 min and then is drained.

C. Advantages over hemodialysis
1. Complications less severe
2. Easier to initiate owing to lack of technologically sophisticated equipment
3. May be implemented much faster

D. Disadvantages
1. Only 10% to 20% as effective as hemodialysis for the elimination of toxins, which results in a limited role for the treatment of poisoning (47).
2. Effectiveness may be decreased by:
   a. Poor return of dialysate
   b. Poor catheter placement
   c. Inappropriate patient positioning

    3. Effectiveness may be increased by certain drugs, e.g., dipyridamole, that increase vascular permeability and may increase peritoneal clearance (48).

E. Indications. May be used for essentially the same toxins as hemodialysis (Table 5-5).

F. Contraindications

    1. Severe or life-threatening absorption of toxin for which peritoneal dialysis would be too slow and inefficient.

    2. The presence of significant hypotension or vasoconstriction because these conditions greatly diminish the effectiveness.

    3. The toxic agent is not effectively dialyzable (see Table 5-5).

G. Complications

    1. Infection, e.g., peritonitis

    2. Catheter placement, e.g., perforation or hemorrhage

    3. Decreased elimination of toxin due to ineffective instillation and drainage

    4. Pleural effusion

    5. Electrolyte imbalance

    6. Arrhythmias

    7. Perforation of intestine, bladder, liver, spleen

V. Hemoperfusion

A. Mechanism of action and physiology

    1. Hemoperfusion acts as the parenteral analogue of oral activated charcoal.

    2. Blood is routed from an outflow arterial catheter and returned via a venous catheter. Full anticoagulation with heparin is necessary.

        a. The blood is circulated extracorporeally through a filter.

        b. Toxic substances in the blood are removed by adsorptive materials, i.e., resin or charcoal present in the filter.

    3. High blood charcoal flow rates (300 ml/min) through the filter should be utilized to make efficient use of the high charcoal or resin adsorbent rates. Glucose, calcium, albumin, CBC, platelets, electrolytes, and urine and serum osmolarity must be monitored closely, as adsorption to charcoal may alter these parameters.

B. Advantages over hemodialysis

    1. Obviates the need for a membrane

    2. Diminishes the role of toxin permeability

    3. Is not limited by low water solubility or high molecular weight

    4. Is not as greatly limited by increased protein binding

C. Factors limiting clearance of toxins

    1. Adsorbability of resin or charcoal for the toxic substance involved.

    2. Volume of distribution (V_d): not effective for $V_d > 400$ L, e.g., tricyclic antidepressants (49)

    3. Plasma concentration of toxin

    4. Rate of blood flow through the filter (typically 150 to 300 ml/min)

D. Indications

    1. The decision to institute hemoperfusion can be made based on the same criteria used for initiating hemodialysis (see **III.B**).

    2. Hemoperfusion is helpful for clearing toxic substances that are poorly eliminated by hemodialysis because of high lipid solubility or high protein binding.

3. Appropriate institution of hemoperfusion for the management of toxic absorption is not commonly indicated in clinical practice.

4. Limited data are available as to which toxins are best treated by hemoperfusion. Table 5-6 lists the agents for which hemoperfusion has been shown to be effective. Method of choice for phenytoin, phenobarbitol and theophylline (50).

5. Hemoperfusion may be recommended in combination with hemodialysis for patients with electrolyte disturbance (51).

6. Hemoperfusion may be used in both children (52) and adults (53).

E. **Contraindications** are similar to those for hemodialysis.

1. Toxic agent is not effectively eliminated by hemoperfusion.

2. Other modalities are available that are more effective, e.g., *N*-acetylcysteine for acetaminophen toxicity.

3. There is hemodynamic instability.

4. Coagulopathy is present because heparinization is required.

F. **Complications**

1. Hemorrhage (54), which may be secondary to (**a**) heparinization, (**b**) thrombocytopenia (55), or (**c**) a reduction of clotting factors.

2. Platelet dysfunction (56)

3. Hypotension (57)

4. Hypothermia (58)

5. Infection

6. Leukopenia (59)

7. Depressed phagocytic activity of granulocytes (60)

8. Decreased immunoglobulin levels (61)

9. Hypoglycemia

10. Hypocalcemia (62)

11. Noncardiogenic pulmonary edema [63]

12. Rebound elevation in blood level of toxin secondary to redistribution from other body compartments

13. Air or charcoal embolism

14. Mechanical failure of apparatus (charcoal columns should be changed every 4 h)

VI. **Plasmapheresis and plasma exchange**

A. **Mechanism:** A volume of blood is removed, and all blood components except the plasma are returned to the circulation. Plasmapheresis replaces the extracted plasma with a crys-

TABLE 5-5. *Agents not responding to dialysis*

Aluminum	Diphenylhydantoin	Ouabain
Benzodiazepines	Glutethimide	PCP
Carbon tetrachloride	Hallucinogens	Phenothiazines
Chlordiazepoxide	Iron	Procainamide
Chlorpropamide	Isoniazid	Quinidine
Cocaine	Magnesium	Secobarbital
Copper	Mercury	Tin
Cyanide	Methaqualone	Tricyclic antidepressants
Cyclophosphamide	Methotrexate	Zinc
Diazoxide	Narcotics	
Digoxin	Organophosphates	

talloid solution, and plasma exchange replaces the plasma with a protein solution. Limited clinical data are available delineating the efficacy of these techniques and guidelines for management.

B. Procedure

1. Blood is removed via a cannula, mixed with heparin and citrate, and pumped through a cell separator.

    a. Centrifugal cell separators separate cellular elements based on their increased density. Platelets are lost with this method because they have a density close to that of plasma.

    b. Membrane-based plasmapheresis separates the cellular components by passing the blood through a membrane with 0.2- to 0.6-μm pores.

       (1) This method separates water, electrolytes, and proteins.

       (2) Platelets are conserved and returned to the circulation.

2. Cellular components are mixed with a crystalloid or protein solution.

3. This cellular solution is then reinfused into the patient.

C. Advantages over hemodialysis and hemoperfusion

1. More effective for toxins that have high protein binding

2. Useful for toxins that are not filtered well by hemodialysis or hemoperfusion (Table 5-7)

D. Disadvantages

1. It is much less efficient than hemodialysis and hemoperfusion because it clears much smaller plasma volumes.

2. Often 10% or less of the total body load of highly protein-bound toxins are removed.

3. **Hemodialysis and hemoperfusion are preferred to plasmapheresis and plasma exchange for toxins that are dialyzable.**

E. Indications

1. Specific indications exist for a class of toxins that are highly protein bound but poorly dialyzed or filtered (64) (Table 5-7).

    a. One report showed that plasma exchange was two or three times more effective than hemodialysis or peritoneal dialysis for removing phenytoin (65), but total body phenytoin was decreased by only 10%.

TABLE 5-6. *Toxins shown to be eliminated by hemoperfusion*

Amanita mushrooms	*Gyromitra* mushrooms	Phenothiazines
Amobarbital	Hexobarbital	Phenytoin
Carbromal	Lidocaine (resin)	Primidone
Carbon tetrachloride	Meprobamate	Procainamide
Chloral hydrate	Methaqualone	Quinidine
Colchicine	Methotrexate	Secobarbitol
Cortinarius mushrooms	Methsuximide	Theophylline
Digitoxin	*N*-Acetylprocainamide	Thallium
Diquat	Oxychlorodone	Trichloroethanol
Ethchlorvynol (resin)	Paraquat	Tricyclics (resin)
Glutethimide	Phenobarbitol	

    b. Removal of 30% of total body toxin has been reported for propranolol (66) and L-thyroxine (67).

    c. Removal of 10% of total body toxin has been reported for salicylate (68).

    d. Other toxins listed in Table 5-7, including phenobarbitol, digoxin, tobramycin, and prednisone, have been reported to have less than 10% of total body burden removed (69).

  2. Plasmapheresis is theoretically able to eliminate any toxin located primarily within the circulation (70).

  3. Nontoxic indications are multiple and varied, and include myeloma, idiopathic thrombocytopenic purpura, systemic lupus erythematosus, rheumatoid arthritis, herpes, and hepatitis B (71).

F. Contraindications

  1. Toxins for which more effective therapy exists

  2. Significant bleeding disorders

G. Complications

  1. Infection

  2. Allergic reactions

    a. Anaphylactic shock

    b. Angioedema

    c. Urticaria

  3. Hemorrhagic disorders

    a. Disseminated intravascular coagulation

    b. Thrombocytopenia

    c. Increased coagulation times

  4. Increased coagulation

    a. Pulmonary embolus

    b. Cerebral thrombosis

    c. Myocardial infarction

  5. Hypervolemia

    a. Congestive heart failure

    b. Hypertension

  6. Hypovolemia

  7. Citrate toxicity

    a. Arrhythmias

    b. Syncope

    c. Tetany

    d. Paresthesias

  8. Pneumothorax

  9. Adult respiratory distress syndrome

 10. Cardiac arrhythmias

 11. Seizures

VII. Hemofiltration

A. Background and availability

  1. Relatively recent experimental technique

TABLE 5-7. *Agents eliminated with plasmapheresis*

Amanita mushrooms	Prednisone
Digitoxin	Propranolol
Digoxin	Quinine
L-Thyroxine	Salicylate
Paraquat	Tobramycin
Phenytoin	

   2. Not readily available in most centers

   3. May be used for adults and children (72)

B. Mechanism and procedure

   1. Uses the same principals of hemodialysis

   2. Blood passes through thousands of hollow bored fiber filters.

   3. The patient's arterial pressure can be used to create flow and obviate the need for an external pump.

C. Indications:

   1. Toxins with low volume of distribution

   2. Molecular weight between 10,000 to 40,000 (depends on filter)

D. Advantages over hemodialysis

   1. Can remove molecules with a large molecular weight (>500)

   2. Effective for aminoglycosides (73,74)

   3. Treatment can be continuous

   4. Hemofiltration can be used after hemodialysis or hemoperfusion to minimize the risk of rebound from tissue bound stores (75)

References

1. Linton AL, Luke RG, Briggs JD. Methods of forced diuresis and its application in barbiturate poisoning. *Lancet* 1967;2:7512.
2. Morgan AG, Polak A. The excretion of salicylate in salicylate poisoning. *Clin Sci* 1971;41:475–484.
3. Prescott L, Park J, Darrien I. Treatment of severe 2,4-D and mecaprop intoxication with alkaline diuresis. *J Clin Pharmacol* 1979;7:111.
4. Yip L, Dart RC, Gabow PA. Concepts and controversies in salicylate toxicity. *Emerg Clin North Am* 1994;12:351–364.
5. Warren SE, Swerdlin ARH, Steinberg SM. Treatment of alkalosis with ammonium chloride: a case report. *Clin Pharmacol Ther* 1979;25:624–627.
6. Nahata MC, Cummins BA, McLeon DC. Effect of absorbic acid on urine pH. *Am J Hosp Pharm* 1981;38:33.
7. Murphy FJ, Zelman S, Mau W. Absorbic acid as a urinary acidifying agent. II. Its adjunctive role in chronic urinary infection. *J Urol* 1965;94:300.
8. Axelrod DR. Absorbic acid and urinary pH [Letter]. *JAMA* 1985;254:7310.
9. Barton CH, Sterling ML, Thomas R, et al. Ineffectiveness of intravenous abscorbic acid as an acidifying agent in man. *Arch Intern Med* 1981;141:211–212.
10. Heffner JE, Sahn SA. Salicylate induced pulmonary edema. *Ann Intern Med* 1981;95:405.
11. Buchanan N, Kundig H, Eyberg C. Experimental salicylate intoxication in young baboons. *J Pediatr* 1975;86:225.
12. Pentel P, Benowitz NL. Tricyclic antidepressant poisoning: management of arrhythmias. *Med Toxicol* 1986;1:101–121.
13. Pentel P, Benowitz NL. Efficacy and mechanism of action of sodium bicarbonate in the treatment of desipramine toxicity in rats. *J Pharmacol Exp Ther* 1984;230:12–19.
14. McCabe JL, Cobaugh DJ, Mengazzi J, et al. A comparison of hypertonic saline, sodium bicarbonate and hyperventilation in severe tricyclic overdose in swine. *Vet Hum Toxicol* 1993;35:367.

15. Chan H, Evans WE, Pratt CB. Recovery from toxicity associated with high dose methotrexate: prognositc factors. *Cancer Treat Rep* 1977;61:797–804.
16. Beckett AH, Rowland M. Urinary excretion kinetics of amphetamine in man. *J Pharm Pharmacol* 1965;17:628.
17. Bradberry SM, Vale JA. Multiple dose activated charcoal: a review of the revelant clinical studies. *Clin Toxicol* 33: 407–416.
18. Huang J. Stereoselective gastrointestinal clearance of disopyramide in rabbits treated with activated charcoal. *J Pharm Sci* 1988;77:959.
19. Alberto G, et al. Central nervous system manifestations of a valproic acid overdose responsive to naloxone. *Ann Emerg Med* 1989;18:889.
20. Gomez HF, Johnson R, Guven H, et al. Adsorption of botulinum toxin to activated charcoal with a mouse bioassay. *Ann Emerg Med* 1995;25:818–822.
21. Guven H, Tuncok Y, Gidener S, et al. In vitro adsorbtion of dichlorvos and parathion by activated charcoal. *Clin Toxicol* 1994;32:157–163.
22. Albertson TE, et al. Superiority of activated charcoal alone compared with ipecac and activated charcoal in the treatment of acute toxic ingestions. *Ann Emerg Med* 1989;18:56–58.
23. Kulig K, et al. Management of acutely poisoned patients without gastric emptying. *Ann Emerg Med* 1985;14:562.
24. Rumack BH, et al. Acetaminophen overdose: 662 cases with evaluation of oral acetylcysteine treatment. *Arch Intern Med* 1981;141:380.
25. Renzi FP, et al. Concomitant use of activated charcoal and *N*-acetylcysteine. *Ann Emerg Med* 1985;14:568.
26. Ekins BR, et al. The effect of activated charcoal on *N*-acetylcysteine absorption in normal subjects. *Am J Emerg Med* 1987;5:483.
27. Chamberlain J, Gorman R, Odera GM, et al. Use of activated charcoal in a simualted poisoning with acetaminophen: a new loading dose for *N*-acetylcysteine. *Ann Emerg Med* 1993;22:1398–1341.
28. Brent J. Are activated charcoal and *N*-acetylcysteine interactions of clinical significance? *Ann Emerg Med* 1993; 22:1900–1903.
29. Spiller HA, Krenzelok EP, Grande GA, et al. A prospective evaluation of the effect of activated charcoal before oral *N*-acetylcysteine in acetaminophen overdose. *Ann Emerg Med* 1994;23:519.
30. Torre D, et al. In vitro influence of charcoal on ciprofloxacin activity. *Drugs Exp Clin Res* 1988;14:333.
31. Harsh HH. Aspiration of activated charcoal. *N Engl J Med* 1986;314:318.
32. Harris CR, Filandrinos D. Accidental administration of activated charcoal into the lung: aspiration by proxy. *Ann Emerg Med* 1993;22:1470–1473.
33. Elliott CG, et al. Charcoal lung: bronchiolitis obliterans after aspiration of activated charcoal. *Chest* 1989;96:672.
34. Atkinson SW, Young Y, Trotter GA. Treatment with activated charcoal complicated by gastrointestinal obstruction requiring surgery. *Br Med J* 1992;305:563.
35. Gomez HF, Brent JA, Munoz DC. Charcoal stercolith with intestinal perforation in a patient treated for amitriptyline ingestion. *J Emerg Med* 1994;12:57–60.
36. Weber CA, Santiago RM. Hypermagnesemia: a potential complication during treatment of theophylline intoxication with oral-activated charcoal and magnesium-containing cathartics. *Chest* 1989;95:56.
37. McKinney PE, Phillips S, Gomez HF, et al. Corneal abrasions secondary to activated charcoal. *Am J Emerg Med* 1993; 11:562.
38. Gibson TP, Nelson HA. Drug kinetics and artificial kidneys. *Clin Pharmacokinet* 1977;2:403.
39. de Broe ME, Bismuth C, de Groot et al. Haemoperfusion: a useful therapy for a severely poisoned patient? *Hum Toxicol* 1986;5:11–15.
40. Winchester JF, et al. Dialysis and hemoperfusion of poisons and drugs-update. *Trans Am Soc Artif Intern Organs* 1972;23:762.
41. McCoy HG, et al. Severe methanol poisoning: application of pharmacokinetic model for ethanol therapy and hemodialysis. *Am J Med* 1979;67:804.
42. Parry MF, Wallach R. Ethylene glycol poisoning. *Am J Med* 1974;57:143.
43. Hill JB. Salicylate intoxication. *N Engl J Med* 1973;21:1110.
44. Clendeninn NJ, et al. Potential pitfalls in the evaluation of the usefulness of hemodialysis for the removal of lithium. *J Toxicol Clin Toxicol* 1982;19:341.
45. Daugirdas JT, et al. Severe anaphylactoid reactions to cuprammonium cellulose hemodialysis. *Arch Intern Med* 1985; 145:489–494.
46. Golper TA. Drugs and peritoneal dialysis. *Dial Transplant* 1979;8:41–43.
47. Simon NM, Krumlovsky FA. The role of dialysis in the treatment of poisonings. *Ration Drug Ther* 1971;3:1.
48. Maher JF, et al. Enhanced peritoneal transport with dipyridamole. *Trans Am Soc Artif Intern Organs* 1977;23:219.
49. Heath A, et al. Treatment of antidepressant poisoning with resin hemoperfusion. *Hum Toxicol* 1983;1:361.
50. Park GD, Spector R, Roberts RJ, et al. Use of hemoperfusion for treatment of theophylline intoxication. *Am J Med* 1983;74:961–966.

51. Bently C, Kjellstrnad CM. The treatment of severe drug intoxication with charcoal hemoperfusion in series with hemodialysis. *J Dialysis* 1979;3:337.
52. Chabers BM, Kjellstrand CM, Weigand C, et al. Techniques for use of charcoal hemoperfusion in infants: experience in two patients. *Kidney Int* 1980;18:386–389.
53. Cutler RD, Forland SC, St. John PG, et al. Extracorporeal removal of drugs and poisons by hemodialysis and hemoperfusion. *Ann Rev Pharmacol Toxicol* 1987;27:169–191.
54. Sangster B, van Heyst ANP, Sixma JJ. The influence of haemoperfusion on haemostasis and cellular constituents of the blood in the treatment of intoxications. *Arch Toxicol* 1981;47:269–278.
55. Chang TMS. Microencapsulated absorbent hemoperfusion for uremia, intoxication and hepatic failure. *Kidney Int* 1975;7:387.
56. Peerschke EIB. Ca^{+2} mobilization and fibrinogen binding of platelets refractory to adenosine diphosphate stimulation. *J Lab Clin Med* 1985;106:111–122.
57. Papadopoulou ZL, et al. The use of charcoal. *Int J Pediatr Nephrol* 1980;1:187.
58. Gelfand MC, et al. Charcoal hemoperfusion in severe drug overdosage. *Trans Am Soc Artif Intern Organs* 1977;23:599.
59. Kolthammer JC, Watson PA, Lang SA, Fennimore J. The safety assessment in the dog of a charcoal haemoperfusion column. *Clin Soc Mol Med* 1976;51:515–524.
60. Vanholder R, Ringoir S. Biocompatibility: an overview. *Int J Artif Organs* 1989;12:356–365.
61. Rommes JH, Sangster B, Gmelig Meyling FHJ, Daha MR, van Heyst ANP. The influence of hemoperfusion on white cells, immunoglobulin concentrations, and the complement system in the treatment of intoxications. *Arch Toxicol* 1983;52:149–156.
62. Pond S. Diuresis, dialysis, and hemoperfusion. *Emerg Med Clin North Am* 1984;2:29–45.
63. Engstrom JW, et al. Noncardiogenic pulmonary edema after charcoal hemoperfusion. *South Med J* 1985;78:611.
64. Seyffart G. Plasmapheresis in treatment of acute intoxications. *Trans Am Soc Artif Intern Organs* 1982;28:673.
65. Liu E, Rubenstein M. Phenytoin removal by plasmapheresis in thrombotic thrombocytopenic purpura. *Clin Pharmacol Ther* 1982;31:762.
66. Talbert RL, Wong YY, Duncan DB. Propranolol plasma concentrations and plasmapheresis. *Drug Intell Clin Pharm* 1981;15:993.
67. Ashkar FS, et al. Thyroid storm treatment with blood exchange in normal volunteers. *Clin Pharm* 1984;3:396.
68. White RL, et al. Salicylate removal during plasma exchange in normal volunteers. *Clin Pharm* 1984;3:396.
69. Matzke GR. Does plasma exchange alter drug therapy? *Clin Pharm* 1984;3:421.
70. Hamblin T. Where now for therapeutic apheresis. *Br Med J* 1984;289:779.
71. Silvergleid AJ. Applications and limitations of hemopheresis. *Annu Rev Med* 1983;34:69.
72. Zobel G, Trop M, Beitzke A, et al. Vascular access for continuous arteriovenous hemofiltration of infants and young children. *Artif Organ* 1988;12:16–19.
73. Matzke GR, O'Connell MB, Collins AJ, et al. Disposition of vancomycin during hemofiltration. *Clin Pharmacol Ther* 1986;40:425–430.
74. Golper TA, Bennett WM. Drug removal by continuous arteriovenous hemofiltration: a review of the evidence in poisoned patients. *Med Toxicol* 1988;3:341–349.
75. Pond SM, Johnston SC, Schoof DD, et al. Repeated hemoperfusion and continuous hemofiltration in a paraquat poisoned patient. *J Toxicol Clin Toxicol* 1987;25:305–316.

Emergency Toxicology, Second Edition,
edited by Peter Viccellio.
Lippincott–Raven Publishers, Philadelphia © 1998.

6

Toxicology Screening

Role of the Clinical Laboratory

†Kathleen A. Leonard and °Jay L. Bock

†Blood Bank and Transfusion Service, The New York Hospital, New York, New York 10021;
°Department of Pathology, State University of New York at Stony Brook, Stony Brook,
New York 11794-7300

I. Introduction

A. Background (1–3)

1. **Clinical toxicology** involves the detection and treatment of poisonings caused by a wide variety of substances, including household and industrial products, animal poisons and venoms, environmental agents, pharmaceuticals, and illegal drugs. The toxicology laboratory must provide appropriate testing in three general areas: (a) identification of agents responsible for acute or chronic poisoning; (b) detection of drugs of abuse; and (c) therapeutic drug monitoring. Increasingly sophisticated analytic methods are available to accomplish these tasks, but it is imperative that they be used judiciously.

2. The number of compounds for which true emergency laboratory results are needed to guide therapy are still relatively few. For most potentially lethal intoxications, the **patient must be treated empirically** before the laboratory results are known. It is especially true in the case of toxicology screens, where the turnaround times vary considerably but are often significantly longer than for specific quantitative drug levels.

B. Clinical context (4–7)

1. Although laboratory results can be helpful in the diagnosis and management of poisoning and overdoses, the importance of the **clinical history and physical examination** cannot be overemphasized. Placing undue importance on toxicology results can be misleading, particularly with regard to qualitative drug "screening" for a large number of compounds.

2. A widely held misconception is that the laboratory can routinely detect any of the thousands of potential drugs or toxins that may be present in a sample. Because the financial and personnel resources required for such complete "screens" would be prohibitive, clinical laboratories must employ **selective procedures** suitable for the patient population in question. Therefore in most cases in clinical or hospital based settings, tests are done for only a finite number of compounds, generally the more common drugs of abuse. Ideally, a diagnosis of poisoning would be made

clinically, with the laboratory playing a confirmatory role. However, an adequate clinical history obviously may be unobtainable from the obtunded or uncooperative patient, and in certain situations toxicologic data may be essential for management. A positive finding, even if it does not necessitate specific therapy, may preclude the need for more extensive testing, whereas a negative result engenders further evaluation (Table 6-1).

C. Laboratory utilization

1. **Effective utilization** of the toxicology laboratory requires that the clinician be familiar with the extent of its services and routine availability. There may be wide variations in service between a community hospital and a tertiary care facility, and the clinician should know (a) the tests that are available, (b) during which hours of the day they are done, and (c) the turnaround time. For tests not available on site, the clinician should be familiar with the capabilities of local reference laboratories and arrangements for specimen transport.

2. **Turnaround time** and **off-hours availability** of toxicology screens vary considerably, from 1 h to several days, depending on where the test is run and what contractual arrangements have been made. Traditional toxicology screen methods, primarily chromatographic techniques, are time-consuming, labor-intensive, and highly dependent on technician interpretation. Tests using automated immunoassay kit methodology have made it possible to shorten turnaround time considerably: to within 60 to 90 min plus collection and transport time. Although turnaround time is improved, these kits can test for only a limited number of drugs. In addition, as discussed later, there are a number of cross-reacting substances, including cough and cold preparations, which cause false-positive results on immunoassay. More elaborate confirmatory methods, generally not required for emergency toxicology, may significantly lengthen turnaround time for the final results.

II. Information necessary for the laboratory (6). Close communication between clinical and laboratory personnel is essential. At a minimum, the ordering requisition for a toxicology screen should contain the following information.

TABLE 6-1. *Caveats*

The content of toxicologic "screens" varies among institutions: ordering physicians must know which drugs are tested by their particular laboratory.

A widely held misconception is that the laboratory can *routinely* detect any of the thousands of potential drugs or toxins that may be present in a sample. Some of the more common drugs and toxins that cannot be detected by routine toxicology screens include digoxin, lithium, methanol, isopropranol, acetone, ethylene glycol, iron, carboxyhemoglobin, methemoglobin, cyanide, and heavy metals. All must be ordered as a specific test level.

Generally, hallucinogenic and "designer" drugs are not easily detected and require further discussion with the clinical toxicology consultant.

A negative toxicologic screen only signifies that the *specific drugs tested for* in the *particular specimen type* at the *time the specimen was obtained* were not detectable. It does not rule out a toxic ingestion.

A single quantitative level may be misleading and must be correlated with the time of ingestion. Repeat levels will document that the concentration has peaked and that absorption is fully or nearly completed.

No single specimen type is universally appropriate for identification of drugs or toxins. When in doubt, obtain as many as possible: urine, serum, whole blood, gastric contents, and nonbiological material (i.e., tablets, injectables).

A. **Suspected agent(s).** The content of toxicology screens varies among laboratories. Although a standard screen may not include the suspected agent, if alerted beforehand the laboratory may be able to modify procedures as needed in order to search for the suspected agents first.

B. **Suspected dose.** Analytic sensitivities vary among laboratories, and some facilities may not be able to detect therapeutic concentrations of certain drugs in their routine screens. Knowledge of the approximate dose ingested is important because in certain cases the use of more sensitive analytic methods designed for therapeutic monitoring, *not* screening, may be necessary.

C. **Time of ingestion and sampling.** Knowledge of both the ingestion and sampling time is necessary to determine the degree of drug absorption; with serial determinations, knowledge of sampling times is critical, as a single quantitative level may be misleading and must be correlated with the time of ingestion. Serial levels, timed appropriately with respect to the pharmacokinetics of the agent, document that the concentration has peaked, which helps to guide further therapy.

D. **Clinical presentation.** Knowledge of the clinical presentation helps the laboratory select the most appropriate screening procedures. The appropriate screen for a patient with a depressed level of consciousness is entirely different from the appropriate screen for a patient with bizarre behavior.

E. **Location of the patient**

III. **Choice of specimen** (8)

A. **Qualitative versus quantitative tests.** No single specimen type is universally appropriate for identification of toxic agents. The selection of specimen type is based on both the pharmacokinetics of the suspected agent and laboratory methodology. Because of this variation in laboratory methods, the exact specimen type required may vary slightly from institution to institution. In general, **quantitative tests** are performed on serum or whole blood, and **qualitative tests** are performed on urine and gastric contents. The major exception to this rule is **quantitation of heavy metals,** generally performed on urine, which must be collected in acid-washed, metal-free containers. When in doubt, obtain as many specimen types as possible and forward to the laboratory, where the most appropriate specimens can be selected. For the broadest possible screening (which, again, is rarely needed, especially in emergency toxicology), **minimally, blood and urine** should be sent.

B. **Specimen characteristics**

1. **Whole blood.** Collect with oxalate anticoagulant and fluoride preservative (typically a "gray-top" collection tube—but note that the tube tops are not always the same). Whole blood is sometimes used for volatile agents (ethanol, methanol, isopropanol, ethylene glycol).

2. **Serum** (red-top tube). Used for most other quantitative determinations.

3. **Urine.** Collect 50 to 75 ml in a plastic container with no preservative. Urine is well suited to toxicologic analysis for a number of reasons. It can be noninvasively collected in large quantities, and most drugs are concentrated in urine, particularly the opiates, phenothiazines, and phencyclidine. Frequently, both parent drug and the characteristic metabolite(s) are present in urine, aiding in qualitative identification. As an aqueous, protein-free solution, it is well suited to chemical analysis.

4. **Gastric contents.** Collect 50 to 75 ml in a plastic container with no preservatives. Depending on the degree of drug absorption, gastric fluid may contain high concentrations of unmetabolized drugs.

5. **Nonbiologicals.** Nonbiologicals, such as pills, contain higher concentrations of the suspected agent and may be simpler to analyze than body fluids. Hospital laboratories, however, are often unfamiliar with the analysis of such specimens. In such cases, the material may be sent to a local reference laboratory.

IV. **Selection of test panels** (6,8–13)

A. **Use of routine laboratory tests.** Before considering sophisticated toxicology analyses, clinicians should glean as much information as possible from more routine laboratory tests. Particularly important is a **standard chemistry panel,** including electrolytes, calcium, glucose, BUN, and creatinine.

1. **Hypoglycemia** can explain CNS depression and may be due to intoxication with ethanol, insulin, or other hypoglycemic agents.

2. **Metabolic acidosis,** indicated by low serum bicarbonate with an elevated anion gap and low arterial blood pH, may result from intoxication with salicylate, methanol, or ethylene glycol.

3. Measurement of **serum osmolality** by freezing-point depression, together with the standard chemistry panel, allows identification of an **osmolal gap** (see Chapter 14), which may indicate intoxication with ethanol or other alcohols.

4. If arterial blood gas measurement is performed, **direct measurement of oxygen saturation** with a CO-oximeter allows detection of methemoglobin, resulting from intoxication with various oxidizing drugs (see Chapter 13), or CO-hemoglobin.

5. **Urinalysis** may disclose oxalate crystals, consistent with ethylene glycol poisoning.

6. Many other abnormalities in standard laboratory tests may aid in the initial diagnosis of poisoning.

B. **Screens versus specific assays.** Effective selection of toxicology tests always involves both clinical and laboratory considerations, necessitating close collaboration between the respective departments. Unlike most divisions of the clinical laboratory, where clinicians usually specify individual assays, in clinical toxicology the choice of assays is less well defined.

1. Depending on the institution, it is possible to order specific quantitative assays for suspected agents, or a **toxicology screen,** which consists of a battery of usually qualitative tests. Although the screen often has a slower turnaround time and higher cost, physicians tend to order such a panel, particularly when faced with a patient with a suspected drug ingestion or overdose and an inadequate clinical history.

2. Although routine comprehensive toxicology screening has been shown frequently to identify unsuspected drugs, it has been suggested that a more selective use of laboratory tests would not substantially alter therapy or outcome.

C. **"Standard" toxicology screens**

1. No standard toxicology screen exists. Although certain drugs are almost universally tested for, the drugs chosen for a screening panel vary significantly among institutions. The drug list is generally specified with the test ordering information,

test results, or both. The choice is influenced by a variety of factors, including the geographic location of the institution, the patient population, local drugs of abuse, individual physician preferences, and laboratory method capabilities.

2. **A "negative" screen** therefore can rule out only the finite number of compounds tested for at concentrations above the threshold of detection for the particular method used. It is important to note that inclusion of drugs in a screening panel is generally governed by methodologic as well as clinical considerations. Thus a **typical serum "tox screen"** might test for a variety of alkaloid drugs, which can be readily extracted from serum at alkaline pH and then identified by chromatography (see below). Volatile agents such as ethanol and methanol require a different technical approach and hence might have to be separately specified by the clinician; similarly, many other agents have entirely different analytic requirements and are not generally included in "tox screens." The clinician must specify individual assays for such agents if intoxication is suspected. Some of the more common of the compounds in this category are lithium, digoxin, methanol, isopropanol, acetone, ethylene glycol, iron, carbon monoxide, cyanide, heavy metals, and organophosphate insecticides.

D. **Interpretation of toxicology screen results.** Toxicology screen results are usually reported with a list of the drugs tested for and a comment regarding detection or presence of the drug.

1. **Positive screens:** The notation "drug detected" is entered next to the particular drug found. As discussed below, if no confirmatory method is used, the possibility of a false-positive test should be considered (see **V.B.1.a–d**).

2. **Negative screens:** The notation "drugs tested for not detected" or similar comment is made. Negative toxicology screen results in the face of strong clinical suspicions to the contrary may occur for a number of reasons.

   a. Drugs clinically suspected and in fact present in a patient are **not tested for.** Thus, a seemingly negative toxicology screen result is misleading. If laboratory personnel are notified of the suspected agents, they can generally either modify the existing screen or suggest alternative test strategies.

   b. The toxicology screen is performed on a specimen collected at a time **outside the detection period** for a particular drug. Most of the common drugs of abuse are detectable in urine for 48 to 72 h after ingestion, e.g., amphetamines, opiates and derivatives, intermediate-acting barbiturates, benzodiazepines, and cocaine. Short-acting barbiturates are cleared within approximately 24 h. Long-acting barbiturates and phencyclidine are detectable for 7 to 8 days. Note that in chronic, heavy smokers cannabinoids may be detectable for up to 1 month after cessation of use.

   c. The drug may be present in concentrations **below the limits of detectability** for the method used.

3. In general, when faced with an unresponsive patient and an incomplete clinical history, **minimum testing** should include quantitation of ethanol, acetaminophen, salicylate, and barbiturates. A broader toxicology screen may be requested, but it is essential to know in advance the expected turnaround time. Testing for acet-

aminophen is particularly important, as it may lead to delayed, possibly severe toxicity that can be prevented by a specific antidote. Barbiturates are often quantified as a class ("total" barbiturate), but a significant level may necessitate that the specific agent be identified, as short-acting barbiturates are much more potent than long-acting ones.

V.   **Analytic methods in toxicology** (4,8,14–25)

   A.   In general, the methods used for particular toxicologic tests or panels are a well established part of the laboratory routine, and information about them is available on request. As such, there is no need for clinicians to specify methods. However, in order to interpret toxicology results properly, the clinician should have a rudimentary familiarity with the analytic methods employed. Several methods exist, varying in sensitivity, specificity, assay time, and cost; the choice depends on the size and budget of the institution, the types of patients served, the proximity to more elaborate toxicology facilities, and other factors.

   B.   Methods can generally be classified as either screening or confirmatory.

   1.   **Screening methods** are generally qualitative, relatively simple and inexpensive, and designed to maximize sensitivity, possibly with some sacrifice of specificity. Currently the most widely used screening tests are based on immunoassay methods, such as the EMIT dau kit system (Enzyme Multiplied Immunoassay Technique, Syva Corp., Palo Alto, CA). Screening methods, given the emphasis on maximizing sensitivity, may produce significant numbers of false-positive results. There are a wide variety of cross-reacting substances, including both prescription and non-prescription medications, particularly cough and cold preparations. Some of the more common cross-reactivities are listed below (21). Because of the inherent limitations of screening tests, definitive results must be based on a second procedure, a confirmatory test such as gas chromatography and/or mass spectrometry.

   a.   **Amphetamines:** A false-positive result for amphetamines may be obtained due to cross reactivity with dopamine, ephedrine, fenfluramine, methylphenidate, phentermine, phenylephrine, phenylpropanolamine, propylhexedrine, and pseudoephedrine.

   b.   **Barbiturates:** A false-positive result for barbiturates may be obtained due to cross reactivity with phenytoin and glutethimide.

   c.   **Opiates:** A false-positive result for opiates may be obtained due to cross reactivity with chlorpromazine, dextromethorphan, and diphenoxylate. A number of prescription pain medications may also be detected as opiates, including codeine, hydromorphone, meperidine, oxycodone, and *d*-propoxyphene.

   d.   **Phencyclidine:** A false-positive result for phencyclidine may be obtained due to cross reactivity with chlorpromazine, dextromethorphan, diphenhydramine, doxylamine, meperidine, and thioridazine.

   2.   **Confirmatory methods** are designed to have near-perfect specificity and tend to be technically much more complex and demanding. Confirmatory methods are of relatively little importance in the context of emergency toxicology. Their principal use is in legal situations, where it must be established beyond a reasonable doubt

that a particular drug was present. In these cases, integrity of specimen handling (chain of custody) becomes as important as the analytic procedure itself in order to rule out the possibility of specimen tampering or substitution.

C. It should be noted that occasionally a "false-positive" may result from innocent exposure to the agent being tested for. In such a case, confirmatory tests are generally positive as well. An instance that has received wide publicity is ingestion of poppy seeds (as in a roll or bagel), which contain small amounts of morphine, causing a positive urine test for opiates. Even sophisticated confirmatory tests cannot identify the source of an individual's exposure nor whether that exposure is related to clinical symptoms. The "poppy seed defense," however, may be foiled by identification of 6-monoacetylmorphine by gas chromatography/mass spectrometry, which would prove exposure to heroin (22).

D. Spot tests, the most rudimentary toxicology tests, are generally performed on urine. In its simplest form, this test only involves adding a reagent to the urine and looking for a color change. Spot tests are available for a number of compounds, including salicylate, acetaminophen, phenothiazines, iron, carboxyhemoglobin, halogenated hydrocarbons, ethchlorvynol, and heavy metals. The tests are rapid and convenient; but sensitivity and specificity are generally poor, and accurate quantitation is virtually impossible. Because of improvements in other technologies, spot tests now have a rather limited role in emergency toxicology.

E. Ultraviolet spectroscopy. Many drugs have characteristic ultraviolet spectra, but they must be extracted from body fluids in order to measure these spectra. For some drugs (e.g., barbiturates, benzodiazepines, methaqualone, glutethimide, and theophylline), the method offers reasonable sensitivity and specificity, but it is much less powerful and versatile than chromatographic methods (see **V.G.**).

F. Immunoassays

    1. Immunoassays are based on recognition of particular drugs by specific **antibodies.** Many types of immunoassay configuration can be devised. Those not involving radioactivity or separation steps (homogeneous immunoassays) can be automated on routine clinical chemistry instruments, making them convenient for laboratories of all sizes. Immunoassays can be made highly sensitive and quite specific, but their specificity is never absolute. Molecules with a similar structure generally cross-react to some degree, and occasionally substances interfere with the assay in some other fashion. For example, it is frequently impossible to distinguish between a drug and its metabolites (for urine screening, this characteristic may be an advantage) or among several closely related drugs, e.g., the family of tricyclic antidepressants. Immunoassays also have the drawback that each analyte must be individually assayed using an available antibody reagent. Nevertheless, some of the more modern, discrete analyzers can readily perform multiple homogeneous immunoassays with minimal operator intervention, so a panel of commonly abused drugs (e.g., barbiturates, cocaine, opiates, phencyclidine, methaqualone, cannabinoids, amphetamines, propoxyphene, benzodiazepines, methadone) can be readily tested.

    2. Immunoassay techniques have also been modified for **on-site testing** in the emergency department and other outpatient settings. These tests are known as **drug**

dipsticks; and they utilize paper strips impregnated with drug-specific antibody, e.g., to theophylline. The specimen is applied to the paper, and reagents causing a color development are added. Again, there are variations among commercial brands, but generally the color intensity or size of the color band is proportional to the drug concentration. A chemical dipstick test for ethanol in saliva, which also detects methanol, is available (20): Alco Screen Saliva Dipstick, Chem-Elec, North Webster, IN. Although when properly performed methods for on-site testing can yield useful results quickly, issues of cost, accuracy, quality control, and regulatory requirements may limit their application. In general, the clinical laboratory should be involved in decisions to establish on-site testing or should provide alternative means for achieving an acceptably rapid turnaround time.

G. **Chromatography** is a powerful technique for separating substances based on slight differences in chemical properties. Different drugs have different characteristic mobilities in a particular chromatographic system, allowing fairly confident identification. In contrast to immunoassays, small chemical changes (e.g., addition or removal of a methyl group), commonly cause substantial changes in chromatographic mobility. Thus the parent drug can usually be distinguished from its metabolites. Many chromatographic techniques are available.

   1. **Thin-layer chromatography** (TLC) has been widely used for urine toxicology. It does not require special equipment, is suitable for analysis of large batches of samples, is available in commercial kit form (Toxi-Lab, Marion Laboratories, Laguna Hills, CA), and allows use of various color reagents in addition to chromatographic mobilities to aid in drug identification. TLC, however, is too slow and cumbersome to be readily applied to emergency toxicology, and it is generally not quantitative. Its sensitivity is relatively poor.

   2. **Gas chromatography** (GC) and **high-performance liquid chromatography** (HPLC) are powerful techniques requiring dedicated equipment and skilled operators, but they can be adapted to a wide range of screening or quantitative assays.

      a. **GC** is the technique of choice for volatile agents (ethanol, methanol, isopropanol, ethylene glycol) but, especially with the use of derivatization techniques, can be adapted to most drugs. Use of open tubes (capillaries) allows rapid, high-resolution separations. Many detection methods can be applied, some with high sensitivity; and definitive drug identification is possible by coupling the GC with mass spectrometry (see below).

      b. **HPLC,** which was developed more recently than GC, is a more natural technique for the analysis of nonvolatile compounds. Modern columns perform highly efficient separations, although resolution is not as good as that of GC. Detection is usually by ultraviolet spectrophotometry, which in its most sophisticated form (diode-array detection) permits spectral scanning of each eluting peak to aid in identification.

H. **Mass spectroscopy and other specialized techniques.** When mass spectroscopy (MS) is coupled to gas chromatography (GC-MS), nearly foolproof drug identification is possible because substances are identified from both their retention time measured by GC and their characteristic fragmentation pattern on MS. Using computer-based libraries of fragmentation patterns, GC-MS can be used to screen a wide variety of drugs simultaneously. Despite the availability of affordable bench-top instruments, however, GC-MS remains too sophisticated for routine application in clinical toxicology, although it has tremendous importance as the essential confirmatory technique in forensic toxicology.

I. **Nuclear magnetic resonance** (NMR) is another technique that can perform both definitive substance identification and screening of body fluids, albeit at a much lower sensitivity than GC-MS. The technique, however, is even more expensive than GC-MS. Toxic metals, for which most of the previously discussed methods do not apply, can be analyzed by sophisticated spectroscopic techniques, including atomic absorption, plasma emission, neutron activation, and x-ray fluorescence.

References

1. Flanagan RJ, et al. Analytical toxicology. *Hum Toxicol* 1988;7:489.
2. Hepler BR, Suthelmer CA, Sunshine I. The role of the toxicology laboratory in emergency medicine. *J Toxicol Clin Toxicol* 1982;19:353.
3. McCarron MM. The role of the laboratory in the treatment of the poisoned patient: clinical perspective. *J Anal Toxicol* 1983;7:142.
4. Epstein FB, Hassan M. Therapeutic drug levels and toxicology screen. *Emerg Med Clin North Am* 1986;4:367.
5. Epstein FB, Ellers MA. Poisoning. In: Rosen P, ed. *Emergency medicine: concepts and clinical practice*. 2nd ed. Washington, DC: Mosby, 1988.
6. Balley DN. The role of the laboratory in treatment of the poisoned patient; laboratory perspective. *J Anal Toxicol* 1983;7:136.
7. Welsman RS, Howland MA, Verebey K. The toxicology laboratory. In: Goldfrank LR, et al., eds. *Goldfrank's toxicologic emergencies*. 5th ed. Norwalk, CT: Appleton & Lange, 1994.
8. Poklis A. Drugs of abuse: an integrated approach to urine screening. *Lab Management* 1986;24:49.
9. Walber CB. Comprehensive approaches to emergency toxicology. *J Anal Toxicol* 1983;7:146.
10. Balley D, Manoguerra AS. Survey of drug abuse patterns and toxicology analysis in an emergency room population. *J Anal Toxicol* 1980;4:199.
11. Brett AS. Implications of discordance between clinical impression and toxicology analysis in drug overdose. *Arch Intern Med* 1988;148:437.
12. Rygnestad T, Berg KJ. Evaluation of benefits of drug analysis in the routine clinical management of acute self poisoning. *Clin Toxicol* 1984;22:51.
13. McCarron MM. The use of toxicology tests in emergency room diagnosis. *J Anal Toxicol* 1983;22:51.
14. Burtis CA, Ashwood ER, eds. *Tietz textbook of clinical chemistry*. Philadelphia: W.B. Saunders, 1994.
15. Bock JL. A look at toxicology's powerful new techniques. *Diagn Med* 1984;7:45.
16. Peat MA. Analytical and technical aspects of testing for drugs of abuse: confirmatory procedures. *Clin Chem* 1988; 34:471.
17. McBay AJ. Drug analysis technology—pitfalls and problems of drug testing. *Clin Chem* 1987;33:33B.
18. Pippenger CE, Galen RS. Drug dipsticks: what do they do? how do they work? *Diagn Med* 1985;8:38.
19. Hurley WT, et al. Evaluation of a rapid theophylline test strip assay in the emergency department setting. *Ann Emerg Med* 1988;17:1029.
20. Schwartz RH, et al. Evaluation of colorimetric dipstick test to detect alcohol in saliva: a pilot study. *Ann Emerg Med* 1989;18:1001.
21. Council report. Scientific issues in drug testing. *JAMA* 1987;257:3110.
22. Mule SJ, Casella GA. Rendering the "poppy seed defense" defenseless: identification of 6-monoacetylmorphine in urine by gas chromatography/mass spectroscopy. *Clin Chem* 1988;34:1427.
23. Bailey DN. Results of limited versus comprehensive toxicology screening in a university medical center. *Am J Clin Pathol* 1996;105:572–575.
24. Kelly KL. The accuracy and reliability of tests for drugs of abuse in urine samples. *Pharmacotherapy* 1988;8:263–275.
25. Lehrer M. Application of gas chromatography/mass spectrometry instrument techniques to forensic urine drug testing. *Clin Lab Med* 1990;10:271.
26. Aziz K. Drugs-of-abuse testing: screening and confirmation. *Clin Lab Med* 1990;10:493.

Emergency Toxicology, Second Edition,
edited by Peter Viccellio.
Lippincott–Raven Publishers, Philadelphia © 1998.

7

Electrocardiographic Manifestations of Toxic Agents

Judd E. Hollander

Villanova, Pennsylvania 19085

Cardiovascular sequelae account for a large percentage of the morbidity and mortality associated with drug overdoses and toxin-related fatalities. Toxicity from specific cardiovascular drugs is dealt with in Section IV, Medical Toxicology. This chapter focuses on the electrocardiographic manifestations of the poisoned patient.

Toxins can result in electrocardiographic derangements through one of the following routes: (a) they can have peripheral effects on the sympathetic or parasympathetic nervous system which modify systemic vascular resistance through effects on peripheral blood vessels (for example, vasodilation with a rebound tachycardia or ischemia) with secondary electrocardiographic effects; (b) toxins can have centrally mediated effects on the sympathetic or parasympathetic nervous system which result in hemodynamic derangements, and the secondary electrocardiographic effects; and (c) they may also have direct cardiac effects which can result in changes in cardiac output or altered electrical conduction.

I. **Rate disturbances.**
   A. **Sinus Tachycardia.** Sinus tachycardia is the most common electrocardiographic manifestation of toxic agents.
   1. **Direct effects.** Effects on neuronal transmission can directly result in an increased heart rate. Toxins can cause tachycardia through direct stimulation of beta-1 adrenergic receptors or by decreasing the degradation of norepinephrine. Indirectly, toxins can result in tachycardia through increased release of norepinephrine from the presynaptic adrenergic neurons, decreased reuptake of norepinephrine into the presynaptic neurons, increased release of epinephrine from the adrenal gland, and decreased vagal tone from anticholinergic agents.
   2. **Decreased peripheral vascular resistance.** Peripheral vascular resistance may be decreased through drug-induced vascular relaxation, blockade of alpha adrenergic receptors, central depression of vascular tone, or true hypovolemia. A rebound tachycardia can occur in response to each of these causes of decreased systemic vascular resistance.
   3. **Depressed cardiac output.** Drug-induced myocardial depression may result in a compensatory tachycardia.

TABLE 7-1. *Common toxins that result in sinus tachycardia*

Amphetamines	Lithium
Angiotension converting enzyme inhibitors	Metaraminol
Anticholinergic agents	Monoamine oxidase inhibitors
Antihistamines	Mushrooms
Arsenic	Nicotine
Caffeine	Norepinephrine
Carbon monoxide	Oxymetazolone
Cocaine	Phenothiazines
Disulfuram	Phenylephrine
Diuretics	Phenylpropanolamine
Dopamine	Pseudophedrine
Ethanol and other toxic alcohols	Salicylates
Ephedrine	Theophylline
Epinephrine	Thyroid hormones
Hypoglycemic agents	Tricyclic antidepressants
Iron	Withdrawal states

4. **Other.** Any clinical condition that results in hypoxia, or acidosis, in addition to the above processes can further influence the likelihood of developing sinus tachycardia.

5. **Common toxins that cause sinus tachycardia** are shown in Table 7-1.

B. **Sinus bradycardia.** Bradycardic rhythms can occur early in some overdose situations, but they may also occur as pre-terminal events in massive overdoses of any drug. Metabolic changes may result in electrolyte imbalances that can result in bradycardic rhythms. At the terminal stage, the presence of bradycardia will not be helpful in formulating a differential diagnosis. In the absence of terminal events, toxins can induce bradycardia through central nervous system effects, agonism of peripheral alpha-1 adrenergic receptors, antagonism of beta adrenergic receptors and calcium receptors, enhanced vagal tone from digoxin, organophosphates or cholinergics agents, or direct effects on the cardiac conduction system. Common toxins that result in sinus bradycardia are shown in Table 7-2.

TABLE 7-2. *Common toxins that result in sinus bradycardia*

Antiarrhythmic agents
    Type 1a: Disopyramide, procainamide, quinidine, cyclic antidepressants
    Type 1b: Lidocaine, phenytoin, mexiletine, tocainide
    Type 1c: Encainide, flecainide, lorcainide
    Type 2: Beta-adrenergic antagonists
    Type 3: Amiodorone, bretylium, sotalol
    Type 4: Calcium channel antagonists
Alpha-adrenergic agonists:
    Clonidine, guanabenz, alpha-methyldopa, yohimbine
Cardiac glycosides: Digoxin, digitoxin
Opioids
Organophosphates or carbamates
Sedative-hypnotics: Benzodiazepines
Terminal phases of any massive ingestion resulting in cardiovascular compromise

1. **Central mediated bradycardia.** Drugs that cause central nervous system sedation may slow cardiac output and typically produce a mild sinus bradycardia. Examples of such agents are sedative-hypnotic agents and opioid antagonists.
2. **Adrenergic agonists.** Alpha agonists lead to vasospasm and reflex bradycardia. Central alpha agonists like clonidine or guanabenz can cause a centrally mediated bradycardia. Toxins that decrease beta-1 stimulation to the heart can result in bradycardia.
3. **Effects on the cardiac conduction system.** Direct effects on the cardiac conduction system or pacemaker cells may result in the most severe bradycardias. Beta-antagonists, calcium antagonists, and antiarrhythmic agents can result in severe bradydysrhythmias through this mechanism.

II. **Cardiac conduction**
   A. **Normal cardiac conduction.** Some understanding of the normal action potential and the generation of the electrocardiogram is essential to a complete understanding of toxin generated arrhythmias (Fig. 7-1). The action potential can be thought of as occurring in five phases. In phase 0, the cell becomes depolarized with fast inflow of sodium. During phase 1, inward sodium channels begin to close while the change in membrane potential opens calcium channels. This slow inward flow of calcium is responsible for the increased intracellular calcium that results in phase 2 activation of the Purkinje cell. In phase 3, the membrane permeability to sodium and potassium returns to normal and the cell becomes repolarized. In the phase 4 resting state, there is active transport of sodium, potassium and calcium to reestablish the resting membrane potential below the depolarization threshold. It is during this phase 4 resting state that stimulation may cause depolarization that reaches the threshold to fire an action potential. The electrocardiogram that results from myocardial electrical stimulation is shown below the action potential in Fig. 7-1.
   B. **Abnormal cardiac conduction.** Arrhythmias can result through three different mechanisms: abnormal impulse formation, abnormal impulse conduction, or triggered automaticity.
      1. **Abnormal impulse formation.** The intrinsic firing rate of automatic impulses is related to the slope of phase 4 depolarization. Toxins that increase the rate of rise of phase 4 depolarization, lower the threshold potential toward the resting membrane potential, or increase the resting membrane potential so that it approaches the threshold for depolarization will result in increased firing of the tissue.

         On the other hand, toxins that decrease the rate of rise of phase 4 depolarization, raise the threshold potential away from the resting membrane potential, or decrease the resting membrane potential further away from the threshold for depolarization which will result in decreased firing of the tissue.
      2. **Abnormal impulse conduction or reentry.** When impulses encounter refractory tissue (phases 1 and 2 of the action potential) through which they cannot propagate, they travel down alternate more slowly conducting pathways. After traveling down the slow pathway they may return to the area that was originally refractory. This area may now be able to carry an electrical impulse. As a result a reentry pathway with conduction down the slow pathway and retrograde conduction up the fast pathway may occur. This reentry is the cause of some arrhythmias.

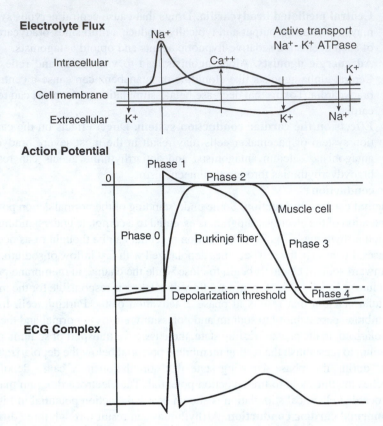

FIG. 7-1. Relationship of electolyte flux across the cell membrane, the myocardial cell action potential and the electrocardiogram complex. Reproduced with permission from Goldfrank's Toxicologic Emergencies. (Appleton and Lange).

   3. **Triggered automaticity.** Certain cardiac tissue do not typically develop spontaneous phase 4 depolarization; however in the presence of certain toxins they may be prone to depolarization for short periods of time. If these depolarizations reach threshold, these normally inactive cells may result in excitation.

III. **Common toxins and related electrocardiographic changes (including arrhythmias).**
   A. **Type 1 Antiarrhythmic agents.** Type 1 antiarrhythmic agents are membrane stabilizing or local anesthetic agents that reduce conductivity, excitability, and automaticity. As such, type 1a, 1b, and 1c antiarrhythmic agents increase the PR, QRS and QTc intervals (1). In therapeutic doses, type 1a agents may cause notching or widening of the p-waves; decrease the amplitude of the T-waves (flatten or invert); cause prominent u-waves; and cause a nonspecific ST segment depression through an effect on repolarization (2). These agents can result in intraventricular conduction delays, ventricular fibrillation, ventricular tachycardia, atrioventricular blocks, and asystole.

B. **Stimulants.** Sympathetic stimulation may result in sinus tachycardia, supraventricular tachycardia, or ventricular tachycardia, in addition to hypertension, hyperthermia, increased muscle activity, seizures, and mental status alterations. Cardiovascular collapse and respiratory arrest may be the end result. In some animal models, cocaine has resulted in prolongation of the PR, QRS, QTc intervals (3). Low doses of cocaine did not alter electrocardiographic intervals when administered to humans in a controlled setting (4). Clinically, a prolonged QTc interval has been observed in patients with recent cocaine use (5).

C. **Digitalis and related compounds.** After an overdose, the inhibition of the sodium-potassium ATP-ase dependent cell membrane pump results in depressed conduction velocity. In addition, digoxin enhances triggered automaticity, and increases sympathetic activity further enhancing automaticity. Digoxin-related increases in parasympathetic activity further decrease conduction velocity. As a result of both triggered automaticity and decreased conduction velocity, digoxin can result in dangerous brady-dysrhythmias and tachydysrhythmias. Atrial tachycardia with atrioventricular block is almost pathognomonic for digitalis toxicity. Bradydysrhythmias include sinus bradycardia, sinoatrial block, atrioventricular block, atrial fibrillation (or flutter) with a slow ventricular response, idioventricular rhythms, and asystole (6). Inhibition of the sodium-potassium exchange may result in hyperkalemia, further exacerbating bradydysrhythmias. Tachyarrhythmias include junctional tachycardia, ventricular tachycardia, and ventricular fibrillation (6). Typical electrocardiographic changes include ST segment depression, decreased amplitude of the T-wave (or biphasic T-waves), shortening of the Q-T interval, and an increased U-wave amplitude (2).

D. **Beta-antagonists.** Beta adrenergic antagonists reduce heart rate and prolong the PR interval. There is no change in the QRS interval; the QT interval may shorten (1). Slight peaking and a large amplitude T-wave may occur (2). Beta adrenergic antagonists usually result in sinus bradycardia or first degree atrioventricular block. In patients with underlying cardiovascular disease or large ingestions, more severe heart block may occur. In addition to the direct membrane depressant effects (type 2 antiarrhythmic effects), beta antagonists have central nervous system depressant effects and block peripheral sympathetic stimulation. They also have negative inotropic effects through interference with the effects of catecholamines on the heart. The hypotension that results from decreased ejection fraction and bradydysrhythmias can be very difficult to treat.

E. **Calcium channel antagonists.** Calcium channel antagonists prolong the PR interval, A-H interval, and both the AV nodal effective and functional refractory periods (7). Calcium antagonists do not influence the QRS or QTc intervals (1). Clinically, these effects result in sinus bradycardia, junctional rhythms, first, second, and third degree atrioventricular blocks (8). Patients may also experience sinus tachycardia, possibly in response to the negative inotropic effects of calcium antagonists. Atrial and ventricular dysrhythmias have also been noted.

F. **Anticonvulsants.** Intravenous administration of phenytoin can result in decreased myocardial contractility with secondary hypotension and rebound tachycardia. A prolonged atrioventricular conduction time with a resultant PR prolongation and a prolonged QRS complex can occur. These electrocardiographic effects are the result of the carrier, propylene glycol, and not phenytoin itself. As a result, these effects are only seen with intravenous administration. Oral ingestion of phenytoin may result in PR and QTc interval shortening; the QRS interval is not altered. ST segment and T-wave changes are unusual (2). Most commonly, oral phenytoin does not produce significant electrocardiographic effects and arrhythmias are rare. Carbamazepine may also cause atrioventricular block.

G. **Psychotropic medications.** Tricyclic antidepressants can result in prolonged PR, AV, QRS, and QTc intervals. Through these mechanisms tricyclic antidepressants can result in supraventricular tachycardia, ventricular tachycardia, and ventricular fibrillation. Various degrees of heart block, junctional rhythms, and asystole can also occur. A QRS interval greater than 0.10 has been associated with seizures and a QRS or more than 0.16 or an R wave of more than 3 mm in aVR have been associated with ventricular dysrhythmias (9,10). Tricyclic antidepressants may result in a right axis deviation for the terminal 40 millisec of the frontal plane QRS (11,12). Newer heterocyclic antidepressants have less of an effect on the conduction system and are considerable less likely to result in dysrhythmias.

Phenothiazines prolong the PR, QRS, and QTc intervals through type 1a antiarrhythmic effects. They may also cause wide, flat, notched or inverted T-waves, prominent u-waves, and ST segment depression. Atrioventricular blocks and life threatening ventricular dysrhythmias may occur, most commonly with thioridazine and mesoridazine. Lithium use may result in nonspecific electrocardiographic ST-T wave abnormalities and prolonged QT interval, as seen in hypokalemia. Rhythm disturbances as a direct result of lithium are less common except in cases of pre-existing cardiovascular disease or acute cardiovascular collapse. Arrhythmias secondary to monoamine oxidase inhibitors are generally late premorbid sequelae.

H. **Antibiotics.** Several classes of antibiotics have been implicated in the genesis of dysrhythmias (13). Torsades de pointes has occurred in patients on pentamidine, amantadine, and erythromcin. Pentamidine has structural similarity to procainamide. It prolongs the QTc and also may also cause ST-T wave changes. Amantidine has structural similarity to the tricyclic antidepressants, and has been reported to cause a wide-complex tachycardia. Erythromycin may result in torsades de pointes in patients with a long QT syndrome. In combination with second generation antihistamines, erythromycin results in QTc prolongation similar to class 1a antiarrhythmics. Trimethoprim-sulfamethoxasole and chloroquine have also been reported to result in ventricular dysrhythmias.

I. **Antihistamines.** High doses of H1 receptor antagonists may have quinidine like effects with QRS widening and QT interval prolongation (14). Torsades de pointes has occurred and is commonly associated with combined use of macrolide antibiotics or imidazole antifungals and second generation antihistamines (15), which through inhibition of the cytochrome p-450 enzyme system results in increased levels of H1 receptor antagonist.

J. **Sensitizing agents.** Some toxins may sensitize the myocardium or cardiac conduction system to endogenous catecholamines. For example, chloroflourocarbons and butane may potentiate the effects of epinephrine, resulting in dysrhythmias. Thyroid hormone ingestion may also result in dysrhythmias, in a similar manner.

K. **Electrolyte altering medications with secondary conduction abnormalities.** Toxins or medications that affect electrolytes resulting in hypo- or hyperkalemia, hypomagnesemia, or hypocalcemia may result in electrocardiographic abnormalities and dysrhythmias secondary to the electrolyte abnormalities. Hyperkalemia may result in peaked T-waves, intraventricular conduction defects, small or absent p-waves, and ST segment elevations. Hypokalemia may result in ST segment depression, decreased T-wave amplitude, prominent U-waves, and prolongation of the QTc. Hypocalcemia may result in QTc prolongation (as a result of lengthening of the ST segment) and T-wave changes. Although hypocalcemia may decrease the QRS duration, these changes are usually small and clinically insignificant. P-waves, PR intervals, and U waves are not affected.

IV. **Myocardial Ischemia.** Toxins can precipitate myocardial ischemia through hypertension and tachycardia, thereby increasing myocardial oxygen demand, coronary artery vasoconstriction, platelet aggregation, and enhanced thrombus formation. The most common toxin to result in myocardial ischemia is cocaine; however, other sympathomimetic agents (amphetamines, etc.) may also result in ischemia. The typical electrocardiographic manifestations of ischemia can be seen in the setting of toxin induced ischemia. They include ST segment elevation, T-wave flattening or inversion, and development of Q-waves in the distribution of one or more epicardial vessels. Due to the young age of many patients who use recreational drugs, they may have electrocardiographic benign early repolarization. The J-point elevations and ST segment elevations can be confused with ST segment elevations secondary to myocardial ischemia (5).

References

1. Podrid PJ. Antiarrhythmic drug therapy. Benefits and hazards. *Chest* 1985;88:452–459.
2. Chou TC. *Electrocardiography in clinical practice.* 2nd ed. Philadelphia: W. B. Saunders, 1986.
3. Kloner RA, Hale S, Alker K, Rezkalla S. The effects of acute and chronic cocaine use on the heart. *Circulation* 1992;85:407–419.
4. Daniel WC, Pirwitz MJ, Horton RP, et al. Electrophysiologic effects of intranasal cocaine. *Am J Cardiol* 1995;76:398–400.
5. Hollander JE, Lozano M Jr, Fairweather P, et al. "Abnormal" electrocardiograms in patients with cocaine-associated chest pain are due to "normal" variants. *J Emerg Med* 1994;12:199–205.
6. Woolf AD, Wneger T, Smith TW, Lovejoy FH. The use of digoxin-specific Fab fragments for severe digitalis intoxication in children. *N Engl J Med* 1992;326:1739–1744.
7. Singh BN. Antiarrhythmic actions of calcium antagonists. *Coron Artery Dis* 1994;5:27–36.
8. Ramoska EA, Spiller HA, Winter M, Borys D. A one year evaluation of calcium blocker overdoses: toxicity and treatment. *Ann Emerg Med* 1993;22:196–200.
9. Boehnert MT, Lovejoy FH. Value of the QRS duration versus the serum drug level in predicting seizure and ventricular arrhythmias after an acute overdose of tricyclic antidepressants. *N Engl J Med* 1985;313:474–479.
10. Liebelt EL, Francis PD, Woolf AD. ECG lead aVR versus QRS interval in predicting seizure and arrhythmias in acute tricyclic antidepressant toxicity. *Ann Emerg Med* 1995;26:195–201.
11. Niemann JT, Bessen HA, Rothstein RJ, Laks MM. Electrocardiographic criteria for tricyclic antidepressant cardiotoxicity. *Am J Cardiol* 1986;57:1154–1159.
12. Wolfe TR, Caravati EM, Rollins DE. Terminal 40-ms frontal plane QRS axis as a marker for tricyclic antidepressant overdose. *Ann Emerg Med* 1989;18:348.
13. Martyn R, Somberg JC, Kerin NZ. Proarrhythmia of nonantiarrhythmic drugs. *Am Heart J* 1993;126:201–205.
14. Clark RF, Vance MV. Massive diphenhydramine poisoning resulting in a wide complex tachycardia: successful treatment with sodium bicarbonate. *Ann Emerg Med* 1992;21:318–321.
15. Honig PK, Woosley RL, Zamami K, Conner DP, Cantilena LR. Changes in the pharmacokinetics and electrocardiographic pharmacodynamics of terfenadine with concomitant administration of erythromycin. *Clin Pharmacol Ther* 1992;52:231–238.

Emergency Toxicology, Second Edition,
edited by Peter Viccellio.
Lippincott–Raven Publishers, Philadelphia © 1998.

8

Special Considerations in Pregnancy

Jeffrey L. Margulies

Stony Brook, New York 11790

The pregnant patient presents a unique challenge to the emergency physician, both in managing a potential poisoning and in preventing an iatrogenic problem. There are **two patients to consider.** As a normal pregnancy progresses, specific hemodynamic and cardiovascular changes occur in the mother. The usual pathophysiology of the poisoning is superimposed on this patient, as are the potential sequelae of therapeutic interventions. In addition, the implications for the fetus must be considered separately, in relation to its unique physiology and its stage of development. Finally, psychosocial factors must also be recognized.

I. **Physiologic considerations**

  A. In a normal pregnant woman at term, **cardiac output** may have increased to as much as 40% above normal nonpregnant levels. Pregnancy may thus be considered a natural state of volume overload. In a third-trimester pregnant female, about 10% of cardiac output goes to the uteroplacental unit. Normally, uterine blood flow is directly related to maternal cardiac output. As a pregnancy progresses, other adjustments that are necessary to the development of the fetus occur, along with an increase in blood flow from placenta to fetus

   1. In the normal cardiovascular system, there is a linear inverse relationship between cardiac output and systemic vascular resistance. In pregnancy, cardiac output is increased largely because of an **increase in stroke volume,** with a normal or slightly increased heart rate. Systemic vascular resistance, if measured, is normal to low.

   2. There appears to be little or **no specific autoregulation in the uterine vascular bed.** The circulatory resistance of the uteroplacental unit is one part of the total systemic vascular resistance of the mother. The fetus depends on a maternal mean arterial pressure adequate for uteroplacental perfusion.

   3. The altered hemodynamic status of the pregnant woman is often unappreciated in the uncomplicated patient because it is tolerated so well. This is because of the large cardiovascular reserves found in the normal healthy system.

  B. Normal **maternal arterial oxygen tension** is about 100 mm Hg, and its O_2 content is about 16.1 ml/100 ml of blood. The placental exchange of oxygen extracts about 5 ml of O_2 per 100 ml of blood, producing in the mother a uterine-mixed venous oxygen tension of about 34 mm Hg. This is consistent with the critical, relatively horizontal part of the normal oxyhemoglobin dissociation curve.

1. The **oxygen affinity of fetal blood** is greater than that of maternal blood, so its oxyhemoglobin saturation curve is relatively to the left. Fetal blood has a greater oxygen carrying capacity than maternal blood, with a fetal hemoglobin content of 16.3 g/dl, as compared to a maternal hemoglobin content of 12 g/dl. Normal fetal arterial oxygen tension is about 20 mm Hg (relatively low), and its oxygen content is about 12 ml per 100 ml of blood. Because of the different shape and position of the fetal oxyhemoglobin dissociation curve, a relatively small drop in fetal arterial oxygen tension can severely and dangerously lower oxygen content.

C. **The binding affinity of plasma protein for many drugs is decreased** in pregnant women. The larger volume of distribution due to expanded intravascular space in a pregnant woman may cause lower serum levels than would otherwise be predicted.

D. **Other relevant changes associated with pregnancy** include
   1. Increased tidal volume, resulting in a resting pCO_2 lower than normal
   2. Increased potential for regurgitation and aspiration, due to pressure on hollow abdominal viscera
   3. Inability to concentrate urine
   4. Decreased serum albumin
   5. Relative anemia
   6. Changes in absorption due to decreased gut motility, changes in hepatic metabolism, or changes in excretion due to increased glomerular filtration rate may also alter drug levels from those that would be expected in the nonpregnant state.

      Some of the physiologic changes that occur in the mother during the course of pregnancy are summarized in Table 8-1.

E. For practical purposes, **the fetus is exposed to most chemicals to which the mother is exposed,** and the greater the dosage to the mother, the greater will be the exposure for the fetus.
   1. Although **the placenta** is a barrier for many purposes, it should not be considered a toxicologic barrier with respect to many common drugs in use. The lipid membranes of the placenta are relatively permeable to substances having a molecular weight less than 1,000 Daltons, although several larger molecules have been identified as reaching the fetus. Protein-bound, highly ionized drugs do not cross the placenta well.
   2. **The passage of substances across the placenta increases with increased placental blood flow.** A role for metabolism by the placenta has not been identified. However, due to differences in fetal circulation and metabolism at different stages of development, toxic exposure in a fetus may exhibit different levels of that agent during the exposure, equilibration, and elimination phases of its kinetics.

II. **Consideration of agents**. All manner of toxicologic possibilities exist during pregnancy. **The average woman is exposed to three to six drugs during the course of pregnancy.** This creates concern, whether these are drugs of abuse or drugs taken for legitimate medical indications. Estimates of the number of mothers who have medications prescribed for them during pregnancy range from 10% to 45%, and this does not include self-administered over-the-counter medications While overdoses in pregnant women may represent a low percentage of calls to poison control centers, the agents involved in these calls run the entire gamut of tox-

TABLE 8-1. *Some physiologic changes during pregnancy*

		Pregnant		
	Nonpregnant	First trimester	Second trimester	Third trimester
Cardiac output (1/min)	4–6	↑	6–7	6–7
Heart rate (beats/min)	60–80	↑	↑	80–95
Systolic BP (mm Hg)	90–120	↓0–15	↓0–15	normal
Diastolic BP (mm Hg)	60–90	↓10–20	↓10–20	normal
HCT (%)	37–47%	38%	34–39%	34–39%
Peripheral WBC (m²)	4.7–10.6	5–12	12–18	12–18
Polymorphonuclears (%)	55	66	69	60
Sed. rate (mm/hr)	20	↑	↑	↑
Fibrinogen (mg/dl)	200–400	200–286	286–315	353–410
BUN (mg/dl)	10–16	7–10	7–10	7–10
Creatinine (mg/dl)	0.5–1.5	0.4–0.8	0.4–0.8	0.4–0.8
pCO₂	35–45	32–34	32–34	32–34
Systemic vascular resistance (dynes/cm³)	1743	979	1277	1224
Blood volume (ml)	2600	3150	3850	3950

↑ = increasing, ↓ = decreasing

icologic problems. The effects of maternal use of cigarettes, alcohol, and drugs of abuse are increasingly being documented and publicized. In addition, the literature describes many incidents of environmental toxic exposures in pregnant women, ranging from carbon monoxide poisoning to snakebite.

A. Determination of potential teratogenicity in an individual mother for a particular exposure depends on many factors, only some of which are understood. The duration and level of exposure may vary. The developmental age at which the fetus is exposed to an agent, as well as its genetic predisposition, may determine whether a problem will ensue and what the nature of it may be. The nature of the agent, its ability to cross the placenta, and its metabolism are all variables to be considered in assessing the implications to the fetus of an exposure of its mother.

B. More than 80% of all drugs approved and on the market are not officially approved by the Food and Drug Administration (FDA) for use during pregnancy. Although there is much animal and human research given to determination of teratogenicity, an FDA statement that a substance is safe for use during pregnancy is usually won only after long empiric experience, and is not often given.

    1. The FDA classification system, established in 1977, offers an approach to prescribing drugs based on a characterization of the substance's potential for teratogenicity. When faced with a question of potential teratogenicity in a particular patient, standard references should be consulted.

        a. Class A. Controlled human studies have not shown a risk to the fetus. The risk of fetal harm seems remote.

        b. Class B. Either animal studies indicate no fetal risk but there are no controlled human studies, or animal studies indicate an adverse effect on the fetus but well-controlled human studies do not show a risk to the fetus.

      c.   **Class C.** Either teratogenic or embryocidal effects have been shown in animal studies but there are no controlled studies in humans, or studies in humans or animals are not available.

      d.   **Class D.** Positive evidence of human fetal risk exists, but benefits may outweigh risks in certain situations.

      e.   **Class X.** Studies or experience have shown fetal risk that clearly outweighs any possible benefits.

  2. Application of the FDA classification system for a particular patient demands an **individualized risk-benefit assessment for mother and fetus.** In general, a drug should not be used if there are no toxicity data available about it. If therapy is indicated for the mother, it should be accomplished with the fewest possible agents, with the lowest possible dosage, and for the shortest possible period of time. Where applicable, hospital emergency department (ED) therapeutic protocols for pregnant patients should be developed in conjunction with the institution's obstetric service. For the individual patient, if the clinical situation allows time for consultation, it is often prudent to consult with the mother's obstetrician before recommending any medication.

III. **Specific therapeutic considerations. Ideally, the pregnant woman should take no medications at all during pregnancy,** other than those associated with routine prenatal care and prescribed by her obstetrician. There are many ED situations involving pregnant women where nonspecific or symptomatic treatment might be used, such as for colds, flu, simple headaches, or minor trauma. Often, the emergency physician can easily gain the agreement of the pregnant woman not to use medications for problems that are self-limited and can be managed with other supportive measures. If minor medical therapy does seem warranted, however, the emergency physician may consider involving the patient's obstetrician in making the decision.

    With the caveat to avoid medications in the pregnant patient wherever possible, this section will consider some situations that may require active intervention by the emergency physician.

  A. **Analgesia.** Acetaminophen is the analgesic and antipyretic of choice during pregnancy. Aspirin and other nonsteroidal antiinflammatory agents should generally be avoided. If use of one of these drugs becomes necessary, ibuprofen may be the safest. Of the narcotic analgesics, experience suggests it is safe to use meperidine or morphine sulfate where indicated. As always, respiratory depression in the mother—or in the newborn—is managed with appropriate doses of naloxone.

  B. **Asthma.** The prevention of fetal hypoxia must be a primary consideration in the risk-benefit assessment of drug therapy in the pregnant patient presenting with an acute exacerbation of asthma. In general, therapy is identical to that in the nonpregnant asthmatic. Epinephrine is relatively contraindicated and should not be used when other adrenergic modalities will suffice. Aerosolized metaproterenol is acceptable first-line therapy. Terbutaline and other selective alpha-2 agents are also acceptable, but these agents may be theoretically contraindicated at or near term, since they have also been administered to arrest premature labor. Theophylline is considered relatively safe in pregnancy and is therefore a mainstay of therapy. Intravenous aminophylline may be used acutely, and oral forms may be used for therapy after discharge, with the caution that every effort should be made to assure that serum levels are not above the therapeutic range. Corticosteroids may be used when indicated. Methylprednisolone and prednisone are the preferred i.v. and p.o. forms, respectively. Dosage and duration of therapy should be limited when possible.

C. **Cardiac arrhythmias.** Lidocaine remains the drug of choice for treatment of ventricular arrhythmias during pregnancy. Procainamide, quinidine, atropine, and isoproterenol have also been used safely. Phenytoin, generally not a first-line drug in any case, should be avoided as much as possible. Experience with verapamil for supraventricular tachycardias is limited but, thus far, favorable. Digoxin has been used safely for this purpose, and propranolol may also be considered.

D. **Hypertension.** Discussion of the management of eclampsia or pre-eclampsia is beyond the scope of this section. Nevertheless, pregnant patients may present to the ED with hypertensive emergencies or urgencies. Maintenance of adequate intravascular volume and avoidance of iatrogenic hypotension are key to preventing hypoperfusion of the uteroplacental unit. Nitroprusside provides rapid onset of action and the ability to finely control therapy, and there is some successful experience with its use during pregnancy. It should be reserved for the most severe of hypertensive emergencies, however, since the drug and its toxic metabolite, cyanide, do cross the placenta. Diazoxide has less predictable effects and, if used, should be administered by a small bolus regimen of 30 or 60 mg every 2 to 3 min, rather than by a 150- or 300-mg bolus. Hydralazine is generally considered to be the drug of choice for many acute hypertensive problems during pregnancy, although it is not generally recommended for chronic use. An initial i.v. test bolus of 5 mg should be used 10 to 15 min before more aggressive therapy, to minimize the chance for undue lowering of blood pressure.

By virtue of long experience, alpha-methyldopa is considered relatively safe in pregnancy, and therefore useful for a hypertensive urgency or chronic therapy Clonidine and ACE inhibitors are generally not recommended in pregnancy. There is limited but optimistic experience with calcium channel blockers, including nifedipine and verapamil, although they cannot yet be routinely recommended for hypertensive emergencies in pregnancy. There is some experience with the use of selective alpha-blocking agents such as metoprolol and labetalol for management of chronic hypertension during pregnancy, but experience in the ED setting is limited. The use of diuretics is controversial because of the potential for intravascular depletion and therefore is generally not advised.

E. **Infections.** Penicillins, including semisynthetic derivatives, are generally considered safe in the pregnant patient. First-and second-generation cephalosporins are also generally considered safe. Experience with newer synthetic penicillins and later-generation cephalosporins is too limited for them to be readily recommended. Nitrofurantoin has generally been considered safe. Aminoglycosides may be used for specific indications, including sepsis; therapy should be followed closely. Clindamycin may be used in the treatment of anaerobic infections. An erythromycin base may be used for penicillin-allergic patients, although erythromycin estolate is to be avoided.

Sulfonamides, including such combinations as trimethoprim-sulfamethoxazole, are contraindicated in the last trimester of pregnancy. Tetracyclines and metronidazole are not recommended in pregnancy.

F. Radiology. As with other emergency therapeutics, a risk-benefit assessment must be made. The radiation from diagnostic plain films used in the ED is exceedingly low, but even this level of radiation should be avoided when possible. If the study is essential to the mother's well-being, however, it usually must be done. A pregnant woman who has neck pain after an auto accident, for example, needs a study done of her cervical spine. But if an x-ray is not likely to change the management of the presenting problem, as may be the case with a twisted ankle, then a more conservative approach may be warranted. When feasible, the mother, her family, and her obstetrician should participate in the decision.

G. Rapid Sequence Intubation should be used when indicated in resuscitation efforts. The one-time use of sedatives, such as midazolam or short-acting barbiturates, should pose no problem, although if delivery is imminent, respiratory depression in the newborn is a theoretic consideration to be anticipated and managed. Pretreatment with lidocaine, if indicated, is also appropriate. Succinylcholine and nondepolarizing agents such as atracurium or vancuronium appear to be safe.

H. Seizures. Therapy of status epilepticus is unchanged by pregnancy. The risks to the fetus of hypoxia and acidosis outweigh the risks of therapy in the acute situation. This applies to the use of phenytoin, diazepam or lorazepam, and phenobarbital. The potential for respiratory depression in the newborn should be recognized.

On the other hand, therapy for a "first seizure" in a pregnant woman who is otherwise well should be discussed with the patient and her obstetrician, as maintenance therapy with all antiepileptics may carry some risk for the developing fetus and for the delivery.

I. Wounds. There are no contraindications specific to pregnancy for the use of local cleansing agents and local anesthetics for management of superficial wounds. It should be emphasized that the management of tetanus immunoprophylaxis does not change with pregnancy, and there is no contraindication to the use of adult tetanus-diphtheria toxoid or tetanus immune globulin where they are indicated by the nature of the wound and the patient's previous immune status. Although there is only very limited experience with the management of rabies in pregnancy, the extremely lethal nature of the disease warrants the usual immune therapy, if indicated, during pregnancy.

Needle-stick exposures of pregnant health care professionals is a common problem in the ED. In general, the management of potential hepatitis exposure is not altered by pregnancy. Gamma globulin, hepatitis B hyperimmune globulin, or inactivated-virus hepatitis B vaccine may be used when indicated for acute exposure.

IV. Approach to overdose/exposure management. The overwhelming principle for acute management of an overdose or other potential toxic exposure in a pregnant woman is that **optimal fetal outcome is dependent on optimal maternal treatment.**

A. The basics of emergency management apply, and the approach and initial evaluation are not essentially changed because of the pregnant state. The use of $D_{50}W$, thiamine, and naloxone are not contraindicated by pregnancy. Aggressive use of oxygen therapy is certainly appropriate. If gastric emptying is indicated, syrup of ipecac or lavage may be used as appropriate. Activated charcoal and magnesium sulfate cathartic may be used, if needed. If there is need for a specific antidote, the usual risk-benefit decision about prescribing in pregnancy must be made. In general, however, a theoretical risk to the fetus is not a reason to withhold a treatment truly needed by the mother.

B. There are **additional specific considerations for the emergency physician** to remember.

   1. **The age of the fetus should be estimated.** This can be done by dates; by history of other evaluation, such as ultrasound, done during prenatal care; and by physical exam when possible.

   2. **The pregnancy should be initially evaluated.** Fetal heart-rate recording should be taken with initial vital signs and repeated regularly. The mother should be asked about awareness of fetal movements, and these can be noted on exam. Symptoms of abdominal cramping or pain and vaginal leakage, spotting, or bleeding should be elicited.

   3. **Placing the patient in the left lateral decubitus position** prevents impairment of systemic venous return by the gravid uterus. Most patient care maneuvers, including transfer by ambulance and gastric lavage, can be done with the patient in this position.

   4. Particular attention must be made to **preserving adequate perfusion pressure to maintain uteroplacental blood flow,** recognizing that because of the normal physiologic changes of pregnancy, signs of hypoperfusion may be apparent later than expected.

   5. It must be recognized that **toxicology studies** on the mother do not give a reliable picture of what is happening to the fetus.

   6. **Therapeutic interventions** may have effects on the pregnancy. For instance, premature labor may be part of a narcotic withdrawal syndrome induced by naloxone in a heroin addict. A bolus of $D_{50}W$ at the time of delivery may affect neonatal glucose control.

   7. The emergency physician should expect to **work closely with the obstetrician,** and early notification is important. In the most extreme of presentations, premature labor or other complications such as abruptio placentae may have to be managed. A decision about delivery may have to be made. Even in the mildest of potential overdose situations, an obstetrical consult should be considered before discharge from the ED.

   8. The role of **psychiatric evaluation** before discharge from the ED is not changed by pregnancy.

   9. **The emergency physician should not expect to make any specific predictions or reassurances** to the pregnant mother about potential consequences to her baby of an exposure for which she is being seen. Rather, all available information about the exposure should be well documented. This should include the nature of the exposure, timing in relation to the pregnancy, duration of the exposure, and observed course of the patient during emergency management. The patient may be referred to her obstetrician for counseling about possible outcomes of the pregnancy.

C. **Common Poisonings in Pregnancy**

   1. **Acetaminophen** is the most common overdose in pregnancy. The disease course, evaluation and management are the same as in the nonpregnant patient. The potential for hepatic toxicity in the fetus is also similar, and is greatest in the third trimester. While *N*-acetylcysteine should be used in a standard protocol for the mother, it probably does not cross the placenta enough to be of benefit to the fetus.

2. **Salicylates** are also a common consideration in any overdose. The toxicity and management in the mother are similar to that in the nonpregnant patient. Since salicylate crosses the placenta and the fetus has decreased ability to metabolize it, the effects on the fetus can be significant, with toxic levels and stillbirth reported.

3. Since **iron** is used frequently as a dietary supplement in pregnant women, the potential for overdose is common. The effects on the mother are not changed in pregnancy. Deferoxamine should be used as indicated. There is conflicting data on the ability of iron to cross the placenta, and little evidence of fetal toxicity due to iron overdose.

4. **Opiate abuse** presents the potential for many complications. In a mother who has overdosed on an opiate, naloxone should be used when indicated for respiratory depression in the mother. Naloxone crosses the placenta, and heroin withdrawal in the fetus has been induced, with complications including spontaneous abortion or fetal death. In general, withdrawal should be avoided during pregnancy. If methadone maintenance is used, the pregnant women may require higher doses than one who is not pregnant.

5. **Cocaine abuse** may also cause myriad complications. In the first trimester, teratogenicity, and an increased rate of spontaneous abortions have been reported. At the end of pregnancy, cocaine may induce increased uterine contractility, with premature labor, abruptio placenta, or stillbirth.

6. If acute **carbon monoxide** poisoning occurs in pregnancy, the presentation may be similar to that in the nonpregnant woman. Since CO crosses the placenta and has a strong affinity for fetal hemoglobin, the complications may be greater in the fetus than in the mother. The usual indications for 100% oxygen therapy and for hyperbaric oxygen therapy in the mother should be followed. There appear to be no contraindications to use of HBO in the pregnant woman. Fetal distress in the setting of CO poisoning, after successful treatment in the mother, may be an indication for repeat HBO therapy.

V. **The nursing mother.** The approach to prescribing medication for the nursing mother is similar to that taken when she was pregnant. **Medications should be avoided except when a specific therapeutic indication is present, and a risk-benefit assessment is always made.** Every attempt should be made to avoid any medication with known toxicities, or for which no toxicity data are available; these would necessitate cessation of nursing.

A. **Most agents that are present in the mother's serum will be rapidly present in her breast milk.** The level in the breast milk will parallel the serum level, and will clear with approximately the same half-life. Agents that are less lipid soluble, more protein bound, and more acidic, and have a higher molecular weight will achieve lower levels in breast milk, and where possible a suitable substitute may be sought. Drugs not absorbed from the gastrointestinal system into the mother's serum will not be present in the milk. Reports of effects in nursing infants due to maternal ingestions are limited.

1. If possible, **dosing regimens** should be tailored so that a dose of medication is taken right after the conclusion of one feeding and hours before the next. If possible, a delay of 4 h is desirable.

2. The **mother should be cautioned to report any changes** in her child that might signal toxicity. These changes might include subtle alterations in behavior, sleep patterns or feeding.

B. Where applicable, **therapeutic protocols** for ED patients who are nursing mothers should be developed **in conjunction with the institution's pediatric service.** For the individual patient, consultation with the child's pediatrician may be advised.

C. **Common Drugs Contraindicated in Breast Feeding**

1. **Radioactive substances,** used for diagnostic or therapeutic reasons, usually will require temporary cessation of breast feeding. Technetium-99m may be found in breast milk 3 days after use. Iodine-131 and gallium-67 may each be found in milk up to 15 days after use. If such agents are necessary, it may be prudent to consult with the Radiation Physicist.

2. **Drugs of abuse** are always contraindicated in breast feeding, and may be hazardous to the nursing infant as well as harmful to the well-being of the mother. Amphetamine is known to concentrate in breast milk. Cocaine intoxication, opiate withdrawal symptoms or PCP hallucinations have been reported to have been passed on to infants. Prolonged or high level nicotine use may induce symptoms in infants; this may be related to cigarettes or substitutes used with the intention of aiding cessation of smoking. Alcohol in large amounts may affect the behavior and feeding of infants.

3. **Psychotropic agents** may pose some concerns. Lithium is strongly contraindicated, as significant blood levels may be found in the infant of a nursing mother on lithium. Although there is little experience with most antipsychotic, antidepressant or antianxiety agents, they do appear in breast milk and it is recommended that they be used only with great caution.

4. **Ergotamines,** used for the treatment of migraines, will induce serious side effects in nursed infants, and are therefore contraindicated.

5. Among commonly used antibiotics, use of **metronidazole** is of serious concern, because of its potential mutagenic effects. If used in a single dose regimen, breast feeding should be interrupted for 24 h. Use of **chloramphenicol** is also of concern, because of its potential for bone marrow suppression.

6. The commonly used **antiepileptics,** phenobarbital and primidone, may cause feeding problems and sedation in infants, and should therefore be used with caution.

VI. **Psychosocial considerations**

A. **Pregnancy is not considered to precipitate suicidal gestures or successful suicide attempts.** The vast majority of pregnant women making suicidal gestures are doing so for the first time in their lives. Peak frequency occurs when the pregnancy is diagnosed and during the seventh month. A single agent is usually used, and the gesture is often considered impulsive. The incidence of psychiatric illness in pregnant patients is not different from that in the nonpregnant population. **Neurotic depression is the most common psychiatric diagnosis.** Nevertheless, a psychiatric consultation should be done before the pregnant overdose patient is discharged from the ED.

B. **Social disorders** in the pregnant patient touch a nerve, and present particular problems for the health care system. Problems of **homelessness and poverty** manifesting in the

ED mean there are two patients in need. **Drug abuse,** alcohol use and abuse, and cigarette use are often cited in relation to pregnancy. Untoward negative effects from exposure to the myriad **chemicals** in modern industrial society are only partially understood.

Problems of prematurity, congenital and developmental defects, withdrawal syndromes in infants, nutrition, and long-term care for these children all make demands that can scarcely be met.

Society wants a perfect baby. Every parent wants—and demands—a perfect baby. When managing a pregnant woman who has had a potentially toxic exposure, the emergency physician should be aware of this psychological overlay in the patient. Where there are few answers, sensitivity and rational advice are key.

Selected Readings

Berkowitz RL, Coustan DR, Mochizuki TK. *Handbook for prescribing medications during pregnancy.* 2nd ed. Boston: Little, Brown, 1986.

Briggs GG, Freeman RK, Yaffe SJ. *Drugs in pregnancy and lactation.* 4th ed. Baltimore: Williams & Wilkins, 1994.

Dalessio DJ. Seizure disorders and pregnancy. *N Engl J Med* 1985;312:559–563.

Kamrin MA, Carney EW, et al. Female reproductive and developmental toxicology: overview and current approaches. *Toxicol Lett* 1994;74:99–119.

Key TC, Resnik R. Maternal changes in pregnancy. In: Danforth, Scott, eds. *Obstetrics and gynecology.* 5th ed. New York: Lippincott, 1986.

Lee SR. Psychiatric disorders during pregnancy. *AFP* 1983;28:187–194.

Nissen JC. Treatment of hypertensive emergencies of pregnancy. *Clin Pharmacy* 1982;1:334–343.

Pregnancy labeling. *FDA Drug Bull* 1977; Sept:23–24.

Rayburn W, Aronow R. Drug overdose during pregnancy: an overview from a metropolitan poison control center. *Obstet Gynecol* 1984;64:611–614.

Rayburn WF, Lavin JP. Drug prescribing for chronic medical disorders during pregnancy: an overview. *Am J Obstet Gynecol* 1986;155:565–569.

Schwartz R, Retzke U. Cardiovascular effects in pregnant women. *Acta Obstet Gynecol Scand* 1983;62:419–423.

Turner ES, Greenberger PA, Patterson R. Management of the pregnant asthmatic patient. *Ann Intern Med* 1980;6:905–918.

Whipkey RR, Paris PM, Stewart RD. Drug use in pregnancy. *Ann Emerg Med* 1984;13:346–354.

Whittle MJ, Hanretty KP. Prescribing in pregnancy. *BMJ* 1986;293:1485–1488.

Emergency Toxicology, Second Edition,
edited by Peter Viccellio.
Lippincott–Raven Publishers, Philadelphia © 1998.

9

Pediatric Poisonings

†Philip I. Hubel, *David Barlas, °Thomas R. Caraccio, and °Howard C. Mofenson

†*Department of Emergency Medicine, North Shore Long Island Jewish Health System, Great Neck,
New York 11021; *Department of Emergency Medicine, North Shore University Hospital,
Manhasset, New York 11030; °Department of Emergency Medicine, Long Island Regional Poison
Control Center, Winthrop University Hospital, Mineola, New York 11501*

I. Introduction

    A. For epidemiologic purposes, toxic exposures during childhood can be divided into two types: accidental (unintentional) and suicidal (intentional) (1). In one study, 39% of exposures were in children younger than 3 years of age. More than half (53%) were in children under the age of 6 year, and fatalities in this group comprised 2.8%. Accidental exposures accounted for 59% of cases. Suicidal poisonings, on the other hand, tended to occur in older children, who usually ingested multiple substances, particularly prescribed or over-the-counter medications and common household substances such as alcohol; it took longer for them to receive medical attention than those with accidental poisonings. Because poisonings in older children and adolescents are managed similar to adult poisonings, only issues relevant to infants and young children are considered in this chapter.

    B. **Curious youngsters explore their surroundings with their mouths.** The Poisoning Prevention Packaging Act of 1970 mandated child-resistant containers, and since its adoption, mortality from childhood poisonings has been decreasing (2). In 1995, common household products (cosmetics, personal care products, and cleaners) and plants accounted for 30% of all reported pediatric exposures, and pharmaceutical agents, most commonly analgesics, accounted for 33% (3).

    C. **Neonates** are exposed to a growing list of potentially toxic environmental and therapeutic agents. Such exposure may be through misjudgment of both drug dosage and route of administration, misuse of medications, or improper baby care. Medications given to the pregnant mother cross the placenta, thereby affecting the fetus before or during labor and delivery. In addition, the newborn may have been exposed to a variety of drugs in utero and hence show signs of adverse reactions. Because of the immaturity of the neonate's liver, lungs, kidneys, and CNS, the process of metabolizing and eliminating drugs and poisons is delayed. Moreover, the clinical signs and symptoms of poisoning are not always immediately recognized (4). Therefore when poisoning is suspected in a neonate, the patient requires close monitoring as well as careful attention when calculating doses.

II. Pediatric pharmacokinetics. Age-related variations in absorption, distribution, metabolism or excretion in children may influence the effects of a drug or toxin.

    A. **Absorption.** Gastrointestinal absorption is influenced in the first few weeks of life by relative achlorhydria, delayed gastric emptying time, and unpredictable intestinal mobility. Acidic drug absorption may be decreased. The gastric pH soon after birth is between 8 to 6 and falls rapidly after several hours to between 3 and 1.5. There is considerable heterogenicity, however, and about 19% of infants exhibit achlorhydria until the end of the first week. It isn't until the first month that all infants have normal gastric acidity.

1. **Dermal absorption** in infants and children is greater than adults due to the higher surface area-to-body weight ratio which enhances percutaneous absorption. Severe dermal intoxications from dermal absorption have resulted from aniline dye clothing markers, diphenhydramine (Caladryl), boric acid used on diaper rashes, chronic 3% hexachlorophene applications in premature infants for treatment of staphylococcal infections, naphthalene for de-mothing clothes in infants with glucose-6-phosphate dehydrogenase deficiency, pentochlorophenol in laundry detergents, and phenyl mercury used as a fungicide in diaper rinse (5).

B. **Distribution.** An important aspect of drug distribution is total body water (TBW). At 75% of body weight, TBW is highest in the term newborn, with extracellular fluid (ECF) 35 to 44% and intracellular fluid (ICF) 33%. By 6 months of age, TBW declines to 60% of body weight with ECF 23% and ICF 47%. The blood brain barrier is incomplete in newborns, resulting in increased permeability to lipid-soluble drugs.

C. **Protein binding.** Infants and young children will display less protein binding than adults, leaving more free drug available for distribution and interaction with protein receptors.

1. **Acidic drugs.** Infants and children have less plasma protein than adults, and their serum albumin is qualitatively different with a lower capacity for binding acidic drugs. This results in more free drug with enhanced potential for toxicity.

2. **Alkaline drugs.** The binding of alkaline drugs to alpha-1-glycoprotein does not reach adult capacity until 7 to 12 years.

D. **Drug metabolism.** Changes in hepatic blood flow and enzymatic activity also influence drug metabolism during childhood.

1. The rates of **oxidative metabolism** (hydroxylation) of acetaminophen, phenobarbital, phenytoin, diazepam, lidocaine and nortriptyline, and of **glucuronidation** of chloramphenicol, salicylic acid and nalidixic acid are reduced in newborns and have played a part in tragic intoxications such as the "gray baby syndrome" associated with chloramphenicol toxicity. After 1 month of age there is a dramatic increase in these enzymes' efficacy and they approach adult levels at 1 year of age.

2. **Sulfonation** and **demethylation** in the newborn are at adult levels.

3. Differences in **acetaminophen metabolism** in children younger than 9 years of age with increased sulfonation rather than glucuronidation may be responsible for reduced hepatotoxicity.

E. **Elimination.** Renal function is incomplete in newborns, who have a glomerular filtration rate only 35% to 50% of adults. Renal function comparable to adults is not reached until 6 months to 1 year of age.

F. **Pharmacogenetic differences** such as glucose 6-phosphate dehydrogenase deficiency and pseudocholinesterase deficiency may also play a role in certain intoxications (e.g., cocaine, organophosphates).

III. **Approach to the poisoned child**
  A. **Historical information.** If the patient demonstrates no life-threatening manifestations, a focused history is obtained by asking the reporter's questions: **Who, what, when, how much,** and **why.** An **"AMPLE"** history should also be obtained: *A*llergies, *m*edications, *p*ast medical history, *l*ast meal, and *e*vents surrounding the exposure. Because most young children come to the emergency room (ER) with a caretaker, there is someone on hand who knows or can speculate what the child may have ingested. If possible, the **remaining ingested substance and its container** should be secured. For further details on the history see Chapter 4.
    1. Because of their relatively smaller size, children can exhibit severe and possibly fatal toxicity with a small amount of some medications (for examples, see Table 9-1). In evaluating the amount of a potentially toxic liquid agent that has been ingested it is helpful to know that the **volume of a swallow** is 0.3 ml/kg in a child and 15 ml in an adult (6).
    2. The literature from poison control experience suggests that **"accidental" ingestions in some children deserve investigation of the circumstances.**
      a. Ingestions in children older than 5 years of age may be a "cry for help" indicating an intolerable home circumstance.
      b. More than one episode of "accidental" ingestion.
      c. Bizarre manifestations may indicate "Munchausen by proxy" syndrome.
    3. Necropsy of suspected child abuse cases should include toxicologic analysis.
  B. The **physical examination** of children reveals classic **toxidromes** similar to those in adults in relation to normal **vital signs** for age. Table 9-2 lists age-appropriate values. The physician should look to other causes when there is a discrepancy between the physical examination and the symptoms expected from the history. With children it is particularly vital to know the approximate **height** and **weight** (which can be estimated as 2 × age in years + 8). See also Table 4-2 in Chapter 4.

IV. **General management.**
  A. **Basic and advanced life support with attention to airway, breathing, and circulation** are essential elements to the management of any poisoning. The reader should be familiar with the principles and details of a pediatric resuscitation that are available in PALS and APLS courses and texts (see also Chapter 4).
  B. **Emesis,** when it occurs early, can reduce toxin absorption (7,8). However, the effectiveness of emesis in the emergency department (ED) if more than 1 h has transpired from the time of ingestion has been questioned with children as well as with adults. Aside from the usual contraindications to emesis (caustic substances, hydrocarbons, decreased level of consciousness, and materials likely to produce rapid onset of neurologic symptoms, e.g., cyclic antidepressants), infants younger than 6 months old and debilitated patients should not vomit because of the likelihood of aspiration (9).
    1. The benefits of keeping **syrup of ipecac** in the home appear to outweigh the risks (10). Home administration has been associated with decreased time from ingestion to therapy (with presumably decreased morbidity) and fewer ER visits for ingestions. Mothers from a variety of socioeconomic backgrounds were found capable of using ipecac appropriately. Giving ipecac without professional consultation

TABLE 9-1. *Selected medications with small potentially fatal doses in a 10-kg toddler*

Medication	Minimum potentially fatal dose	Maximum unit available	Amount potentially fatal
Methyl salicylate	200 mg/kg	1.4 g/ml	<1 tsp
Camphor (Campho-Phenique)	100 mg/kg	1 g/5 ml	1 tsp
Theophylline	8.4 mg/kg	500 mg	1 tablet
Thioridazine	15 mg/kg	200 mg	1 tablet
Chlorpromazine	25 mg/kg	200 mg	1–2 tablets
Chloroquine or hydroxychloroquine	20 mg/kg	500 mg	1 tablet
Imipramine	15 mg/kg	150 mg	1 tablet
Desipramine	15 mg/kg	75 mg	2 tablets
Codeine	15 mg/kg	60 mg	3 tablets
Diphenhydramine (Benadryl)	25 mg/kg	50 mg	5 tablets
Pentazocine (Talwin)	45 mg/kg	50 mg	9 tablets
MAOI	25 mg/kg	15 mg	15 tablets
Dimenhydrinate (Dramamine)	25 mg/kg	10 mg	25 tablets

From ref. 42, with permission.

seems to be uncommon; and in instances where no advice was obtained, contraindications existed in 4% of cases. Because of the impressive safety record of ipecac, physicians should encourage its availability in households as part of a strong injury prevention program. However, **parents should be instructed to call a poison control center before administering syrup of ipecac.**

   2. **Ipecac dose by age**
      a. 6 to 9 months: 5 ml
      b. 9 to 12 months: 10 ml
      c. 1 to 6 years: 15 ml
      d. Over 6 years: 30 ml

C. **Activated charcoal (AC)** will adsorb many toxins. Lithium, heavy metals, caustics, alcohols, and petroleum distillates are exceptions. The dose of AC is 1 g/kg orally, with a minimum of 15 g. Optimum dosage has not been established, but ideal therapy allegedly is a 10:1 ratio AC to toxin. It is administered as a slurry mixed with water given

TABLE 9-2. *Vital signs: normal values for children*

Age	Weight (kg)	Pulse (per min)	Systolic BP (mm Hg)	Respiratory rate (per min)
Newborn	3.5	94–175	60 ± 10	30–60
1 mo	4.0	100–190	80 ± 10	30–60
6 mo	7.0	111–179	90 ± 30	24–30
1–2 yr	10–12	98–163	96 ± 30	20–24
3–5 yr	14–18	65–132	99 ± 25	16–22
6–9 yr	20–28	60–115	105 ± 13	14–20
10–12 yr	32–34	50–110	112 ± 19	12–20
12–14 yr	34–40	50–105	120 ± 20	12–20
15–16 yr	50	50–100	120 ± 20	12–20
>16 yr	60–70	50–100	120 ± 20	10–20

orally or by nasogastric or orogastric tube provided bowel sounds are present. **Be certain that the tube is in the stomach before administering AC.** Deposition into the airway has resulted in "charcoal lung" with a 70% mortality in reported cases. AC is usually administered initially with a cathartic, but cathartics are not necessary in children.

1. **Multiple-dose activated charcoal (MDAC).** Repeated administration of AC decreases the half-life and increases the clearance of phenobarbital, dapsone, salicylate, quinidine, theophylline, and carbamazepine (11). Subsequent cathartics should only be given every 24 h, not with each AC dose, in order to prevent electrolyte abnormalities and osmotic diuresis. At present there are no controlled studies that demonstrate that MDAC alters the clinical course of an intoxication (11–13). The dose of MDAC varies from 0.25 to 0.50 g/kg every 1 to 4 h, and continuous nasogastric tube infusion of 0.25 to 0.5 g/kg/h has been used to decrease vomiting.

D. **Cathartics.** Are felt by many toxicologists to be unnecessary and potentially harmful in young children (especially sorbitol).
   1. **Magnesium sulfate:** 250 mg/kg
   2. **Magnesium citrate:** 4 ml/kg
   3. **Sodium sulfate:** 250 mg/kg
   4. **Sorbitol** 70% (w/v) solution
      a. Children over 3 years: 2.8 to 4.3 ml/kg with AC
      b. Children 1 to 3 years: 1.4 to 2.1 ml/kg, but dilute to 35%.
      c. Children under 1 year: do not use

E. **Whole-bowel irrigation (WBI).** Osmotic bowel-cleansing solutions of polyethylene glycol (PEG) with balanced electrolytes are used to avoid changes in body weight or electrolytes (14,15).
   1. **Indications (not FDA approved) and potential indications:**
      a. **Substances that are poorly absorbed by AC** such as iron, other heavy metals, and lithium. WBI has been used successfully in iron overdose when abdominal radiographs reveal incomplete emptying of excess iron (15).
      b. **Sustained-release preparations.**
      c. **Asymptomatic "body packers"** of contraband. (16).
   2. **Procedure.** Administer the PEG solution (GoLytely or Colyte) orally or by nasogastric or orogastric tube at a rate of 0.5 L/h in children younger than 5 years of age and 2 L/h in adolescents and adults for 5 h. The end point is reached when the rectal effluent is clear or radiopaque materials can no longer be seen in the GI tract on abdominal radiograph (16).

E. **Altered level of consciousness.** All patients whose mental status is less than their usual baseline should receive a standard intravenous cocktail of naloxone, thiamine, and glucose. Reagent strip glucose determination may be performed but should always be confirmed by the clinical laboratory result. There is a concern about hyperglycemia increasing cerebral and myocardial ischemia but this is rare in children.
   1. **Glucose**
      a. Neonates: 5 ml/kg as 10% dextrose
      b. Children: 2 ml/kg as 25% dextrose
      c. Adolescents: 1 ml/kg as 50% dextrose

    2. Naloxone:
      a. Children: 0.1 mg/kg (up to 2 mg)
      b. Adolescents: 2 mg q 1 to 2 min up to 10 mg
    3. Thiamine: 25 to 50 mg

F. Flumazenil may be selectively used to reverse the sedative and respiratory depressant effects of pure benzodiazepine overdose. However, seizures may be precipitated in certain settings: (a) benzodiazepine-dependent patients, (b) epileptics who are controlled with benzodiazepines or other medications, and (c) patients who have co-ingested toxins which can themselves cause seizures. Dosage: 0.01 mg/kg q 1 to 2 min up to 1 mg (17).

G. Alkalinization with or without diuresis with sodium bicarbonate 1 to 2 mEq/kg in 15 ml/kg of D5W q 1 to 2 h is used in the therapy of weak acid intoxications such as salicylates, long acting barbiturates such as phenobarbital, 2,4 dichlorophenoxyacetic acid, chlorpropamide, methotrexate, and methanol. Additional boluses of 0.5 mEq/kg may be administered to maintain the pH between 7.45 and 7.55. Many clinicians employ alkalinization without diuresis because of the possibility of fluid overload. The hemodynamic status, fluids, blood gases and electrolytes, and glucose must be very closely monitored during these procedures.

V. Management of specific poisons. Issues pertinent to the pediatric patient are discussed here, whereas in-depth discussions of specific toxins are reviewed elsewhere in the book.

A. Acetaminophen. Adolescent suicide attempts tend to be more severe than childhood accidental ingestions, resulting in toxic blood levels and hepatotoxicity two to six times higher than in younger children (18). The metabolism in children under 9 years of age is mainly by sulfonation, which carries a lower risk of hepatic injury (19). Studies have indicated that the toxic level in children is 200 µg/ml, which is higher than the accepted level of 140 µg/ml in adults (20). The management is the same as for adults with oral N-acetylcysteine.

B. Cyanide. Two cases of pediatric accidental ingestion of an acetonitrile-containing cosmetic have been reported, and the product was mistakenly assumed by the physician to be an acetone-containing nail polish remover (21). Both children had blood cyanide levels in the potentially lethal range. The observed delayed onset of severe toxic reactions supports the proposed mechanism of acetonitrile conversion to inorganic cyanide via hepatic microsomal enzymes. Physicians and poison centers should be alerted to the existence of this highly toxic product, which is sold for removal of sculptured nails. It is likely to be confused with the less toxic acetone-containing nail polish removers. The management of cyanide poisoning produced by acetonitrile is treated with sodium thiosulfate and the nirite portion of the cyanide kit is not used. See antidote table in Chapter 4.

C. Disc batteries represent a distinct type of pediatric foreign body because of their potential for severe morbidity and mortality. Button batteries are being used with increasing frequency in a variety of devices, including hearing aids, watches, and calculators. Most contain a heavy metal such as mercury and an alkaline electrolyte. Injury may occur by four mechanisms: (a) electrolyte leakage from batteries; (b) alkali produced from external currents; (c) mercury toxicity; and (d) pressure necrosis. Emesis is ineffective and unsafe. Chest radiograph and observation for symptoms can detect those at risk of complications (22). An external metal detector has been used successfully in detecting the location of metallic objects in the gastrointestinal tract (23).

   1. **Esophageal impaction** can result in corrosive esophagitis and perforation. Early diagnosis and urgent removal are required.
   2. **Complications** are less frequent if the battery has passed distal to the esophagus. These patients can be managed conservatively, with spontaneous passage occurring in most cases.

D. **Ethanol** is found in beverages and a variety of personal care products. An especially troublesome toxin that smells pleasant, looks colorful, and is readily accessible to young children is mouthwash, which is 15% to 28% ethanol. Hypoglycemia is a common finding in pediatric ethanol ingestions because hepatic metabolism inhibits gluconeogenesis by reversing the NAD/NADH ratio. When glycogen stores are depleted several hours postingestion, hypoglycemic neurologic injury may occur (24). Hence, the ingestion of products containing ethanol requires careful and frequent monitoring of the blood glucose in the first 3 h following exposure. Blood ethanol concentrations (BEC) greater than 50 mg/dl have been associated with hypoglycemia. On rare occasions BEC below this level have produced hypoglycemia and rarely the hypoglycemia has been delayed. Management with intravenous glucose may be required (25).

E. **Hydrocarbon** ingestion is primarily a toxicologic problem of pediatric patients, with up to 84% of all cases occurring in those under 3 years old (most being between ages 1 and 3) (26). Hydrocarbons are found in many readily accessible household products like gasoline, kerosene, lighter fluid, mineral spirits, fuel oil, lubricating oil, and furniture polish that may be enticing because of their smell and color. Fortunately, children rarely ingest large amounts, and if they do they frequently vomit soon afterward. Gastric decontamination should only be attempted if very large amounts are ingested (more than 20 ml/kg), if aromatic, halogenated, or heavy metal-containing hydrocarbons are ingested, or if the hydrocarbon is a vehicles for other dangerous toxins. Mineral seal oil in furniture polish should be removed by gastric emptying (27). Gastric decontamination of hydrocarbons may produce significant complications, and should be performed with appropriate airway protection. Hydrocarbon pneumonitis is the primary morbidity, and children who remain asymptomatic with a normal chest radiograph after 6 to 8 h of observation may be discharged (28,29).

F. **Iron** was the most common cause of fatalities in children in 1993 (30). Children's chewable vitamins are rarely a cause of iron intoxication since they contain only 15 to 18 mg of iron. They are rarely radiopaque on radiograph. Most severe poisonings are from adult iron preparations (31). Iron is not adsorbed by activated charcoal, but decontamination can be accomplished by whole bowel irrigation with polyethylene glycol electrolyte lavage solution. Gastrotomy has been successfully performed to remove bezoars seen on abdominal radiograph (14,32–34).

   1. **Deferoxamine should be given to patients with iron levels of more than 500 mcg/dl**, dosage of 40 mg/kg i.v. (preferred) or i.m. unless hypotension is present. With hypotension, a second intravenous line is needed for volume expansion, and intravenous deferoxamine is given via continuous infusion at a rate of 15 mg/kg/h.

2. When iron levels are **less than 500 mcg/dl,** the level at which treatment with defer-oxamine should begin is controversial and can be based on the following situations.
   a. Systemic signs of toxicity.
   b. Mild to moderate symptoms with radiopaque material on abdominal radio-graph, leukocytosis of more than 15,000/mm^3 within 6 h after ingestion, and glucose of more than 150 mg/dl.

G. **Organophosphate insecticides.** Atropine is both a diagnostic and therapeutic antidote. The initial dose is 0.02 to 0.05 mg/kg intravenously in children, and further administration every 10 to 15 min may be titrated to drying of the bronchial secretions. The end point of atropine administration is not development of anticholinergic signs (drying of secretions, dilation of pupils, etc.). If the signs of atropinization develop the patient does not have organophosphate poisoning. See antidote table in Chapter 4. Pralidoxime (2-PAM) is an enzyme regenerator used in irreversible organophosphate acetylcho-linesterase poisoning but not in mild cases of reversible acetylcholinesterase poisoning caused by carbamates. In severe carbamate poisoning, however, many toxicologists would administer it. In the past it was believed that "aging" of the phosphate on the esteric site of acetylcholinesterase rendered pralidoxime ineffective, however studies show it is now effective even after 24 h. (35,36) When treatment is indicated, the dose is 25 to 50 mg/kg in 5% dextrose, with 0.45 N saline administered intravenously over 10 to 30 min.

H. **Salicylate** intoxication has declined steadily since the late 1970s with improved packaging and concern over the association of aspirin with Reye's syndrome. As a result, severe salicylate poisoning has shifted toward very young children, with more than 50% of pediatric deaths due to salicylates occurring in those younger than 1 year old (37). Most poisonings are due to orally ingested aspirin, but methylsalicylate as candy flavoring may contribute to salicylate poisoning. Percutaneous absorption and toxicity can result from application of the keratolytic agent salicylic acid or oil of wintergreen (methylsalicylate, containing 1.4 g/ml or 7 g/tsp of salicylate) (38). In children under 4 years of age, salicylism results in metabolic acidosis or a mixed disturbance within 4 h, rather than the respiratory alkalosis seen in adults. Hypoglycemia may be found more frequently in children than in adults. The management is similar to adults with ion trapping by alkalinization of the urine. Most toxicologists use alkalinization without diuresis (39).

VI. **Disposition.** Current literature supports the hypothesis that the clinical course of patients with drug overdose can be adequately predicted during the first few hours of observation (40). The following general guidelines, in conjunction with toxin-specific information found elsewhere in this text and through the regional poison control center, should be helpful in making disposition decisions:

A. **The asymptomatic patient.** Onset and peak time of absorption of the toxin should be determined. The peak time would help determine how long the patient with an unintentional ingestion should be observed in the ED or inpatient unit, and when they could be safely discharged to a reliable caretaker.

B. **The symptomatic patient.** The severity of the symptoms and toxicity of the agent (including its peak and duration of action) are helpful to determine where the patient should be admitted and observed (i.e., medical unit, telemetry unit, or ICU). For example, prolonged toxicity occurs with ingestions of oral hypoglycemics, methadone, diphenoxylate (in children), severe mushroom poisoning, and substance withdrawal.

C. **Be aware of "delayed toxic time bombs"** such as acetaminophen, carbon tetrachloride, ethylene glycol, mercury, methanol, toxic mushrooms (*Amanita phalloides, Gyromitra, and Orellanine*), organophosphates, paraquat, and thallium.

D. **Indications for pediatric intensive care.** One study of patients with intentional ingestions attempted to define a subgroup of patients who would require an ICU or monitored bed. Patients in this "high-risk" subgroup had at least one of the following criteria: intubation in the ED, hypercarbia, QRS greater than or equal to 0.12 s, cardiac dysrhythmias other than sinus tachycardia, hypotension (systolic BP of less than 80), unresponsiveness to verbal stimuli, or seizures. Of 209 patients, 151 did not display any high-risk complications while in the ED for 2 to 3 h and went on to have a benign hospital course with standard detoxification and supportive treatment alone (40). Of note, patients with tricyclic antidepressant overdose may develop sudden cardiac dysrhythmias and probably warrant cardiac monitoring. The decision to admit the patient to an intensive care setting should be individualized based on the initial presentation, any comorbidities, the nature and number of the involved agents, and the potential for delayed toxicity.

E. **Precautions** regarding the general care of the patient should be specified on the basis of the patient's intention, medical history, and actions of the drug. For example, seizure and suicide precautions should be ordered as indicated.

F. **Discharge** from the hospital or ED generally requires the patient to be asymptomatic at the time of discharge. Discharge instructions should include clear guidelines for seeking medical attention and to return to the ED in the event of a sudden change in the condition of the patient. Follow-up plans should be made with the patient or caretaker.

G. Appropriate **psychosocial intervention** is indicated in cases of child abuse and neglect, substance abuse, and suicidal gestures.

H. The caretakers of children with accidental ingestions must be educated in poison prevention measures (See below).

VII. **Prevention**

A. No chapter on pediatric toxicology would be complete without a developmentally appropriate discussion of **preventive care.** Parents of children encountered in the ED for suspected poisoning are receptive to poison prevention education. One of every two children who has ingested a poison does so again within a year (41). Poison prevention techniques should be reviewed, e.g., "poison proofing" the home and posting local poison control center telephone number stickers by telephones throughout the home.

B. Parents and children should be made aware of the **inherent toxicologic dangers** at that child's developmental stage. The fetus and breast-fed newborn are exposed to all maternal ingestants and inhalants via the placenta and breast milk. The 6-month-old can grasp small objects and put them in his or her mouth. At 12 to 15 months, children walk independently, open doors, and feed themselves. The 1- to 3-year-old toddlers are at greatest risk for poisoning, as they are capable of getting into closets and drawers and reaching and climbing onto tabletops and counters.

C. Parental advice should include the following **principles,** which, if practiced, would prevent morbidity and mortality among thousands of children annually.

1. Keep household cleaning products in a high, locked cabinet rather than under the sink. Place safety latches on all kitchen and bathroom cabinets and drawers that contain potentially hazardous substances. If locks are impractical, place the most toxic substances on the highest shelves. Always keep household poisons separate from food.

2. Lock all reachable medicine cabinets and always keep medications and other toxic substances in their original containers. Buy and store them only in childproof containers (e.g., blister packaging). Dispose of unused prescription medications by flushing them down the toilet.

3. Medication should be considered medicine, not a plaything—certainly not candy. Avoid administering medication to others in front of children; They might try to imitate this activity with a younger sibling. Parents should instruct grandparents that a significant number of childhood toxic exposures result from medication accessible to the child at the grandparents' home. For this reason, grandparents must take care to make their environment poison-proof when grandchildren are visiting.

4. Syrup of ipecac should be readily available in the home for use with medical direction.

References

1. Fazen LE, Lovejoy FH, Crone R. Acute poisoning in a children's hospital: a 2-year experience. *Pediatrics* 1986; 77:144–151.
2. Walton WW. An evaluation of the Poison Prevention Packaging Act. *Pediatrics* 1982;69:363–370.
3. 1995 annual report of the American Association of Poison Control Centers Toxic Exposure Surveillance System. *Am J Emerg Med* 1996;13:551–597.
4. Elhassani SB. Neonatal poisoning: causes, manifestations, prevention, and management. *South Med J* 1986;79: 1535–1543.
5. Mofenson HC, Caraccio TR. General principles of pediatric pharmacology. *Med Times* 1984;Feb:6–26.
6. Jones DV, Work CE. Volume of a swallow. *Am J Dis Child* 1964;102:427.
7. Bond GR. Home use of ipecac syrup is associated with a reduction in pediatric emergency department visits. *Ann Emerg Med* 1995;25:338–343.
8. Amitai Y, Mitchell AA, McGuigan A, Lovejoy FH. Ipecac induced emesis and reduction of plasma concentration of drugs following accidental overdose in children. *Pediatrics* 1987;80:364–367.
9. Rodgers GC, Matyunas NJ. Gastrointestinal decontamination for acute poisoning. *Pediatr Clin North Am* 1986; 33:261–285.
10. Steinhart CM, Pearson-Shaver AL. Poisoning. *Crit Care Clin* 1988;4:845–872.
11. Bradberry SM, Vale JA. Multiple dose activated charcoal: a review of relevant clinical studies. *Clin Toxicol* 1996; 33:407–416.
12. Tenenbein M. Multiple doses of activated charcoal: a time for reappraisal. *Ann Emerg Med* 1991;20:529–531.
13. Pond SM. Role of repeated oral doses of activated charcoal in clinical toxicology. *Med Toxicol* 1986;1:3.
14. Tenenbein M. Whole bowel irrigation in iron poisoning. *J Pediatr* 1987;111:142–147.
15. Mofenson HC, Caraccio TR. Gastrointestinal decontamination and the prevention of absorption. *Curr Opin Pediatr* 1992;4:279–290.
16. Hoffman RS, Smilkstein MJ, Goldfrank LR. Whole bowel irrigation and the cocaine "body packer." *Vet Hum Toxicol* 1989;31:374.
17. Sugarman JM, Paul RI. Flumazenil: a review. *Pediatr Emerg Care* 1994;10:37–43.
18. Rumack BH. Acetaminophen overdose in young children—treatment and effects of alcohol and other additional ingestants in 417 cases. *Am J Dis Child* 1984;138:428.

19. Miller RP, Roberts RJ, Fisher LJ. Kinetics of acetaminophen elimination in newborns, children and adults. *Pharmacol Ther* 1976;19:284.
20. Gorman RL, Klein-Schwartz W, Oderda G. Pediatric acetaminophen ingestions—when is health care referral necessary? Abstract presented at the 23rd Annual Meeting of the AACT/AAPCC/ABMT/CAPCC, Toronto, Canada, October 11–14, 1991.
21. Caravati EM, Litovitz TL. Pediatric cyanide intoxication and death from an acetonitrile-containing cosmetic. *JAMA* 1988;260:3470–3473.
22. Litovitz T, Schmitz BF. Ingestion of cylindrical and button batteries: an analysis of 2382 cases. *Pediatrics* 1992; 89:747–757.
23. Shaikh A. Button battery ingestion in children. *Pediatr Emerg Care* 1993:9:224–229.
24. Weller-Fahey ER, Berger LR, Troutman WG. Mouthwash—a source of acute ethanol intoxication. *Pediatrics* 1980; 66:302.
25. Vogel C, Caraccio TR, Mofenson HC, Hart S. Alcohol intoxication in young children. *Clin Toxicol* 1995;33:25–33.
26. Anas N, Namasonthi V, Ginsburg CM. Criteria for hospitalizing children who have ingested products containing hydrocarbons. *JAMA* 1981;246:840.
27. Victoria MS, et al. Hydrocarbon poisoning: a review. *Pediatr Emerg Care* 1987;3:184–186.
28. Truemper E, Santiago R, Atkinson S. Clinical characteristics, pathophysiology, and management of hydrocarbon ingestion: case report and review of the literature. *Pediatr Emerg Care* 1987;3:187–193.
29. Victoria MS, Nangia BS. Hydrocarbon poisoning: a review. *Pediatr Emerg Care* 1987;3:184–186.
30. Litovitz TL, Holm KC, Bailey K, Schmitz BF. 1991 annual report of the American Associatiopn of Poison Control Centers Toxic Exposure Surveillance System. *Am J Emerg Med* 1992;10:452–505.
31. Banner WJ, Tong TG. Iron poisoning. *Pediatr Clin North Am* 1986;33:393–409.
32. McCarthy T, Olson KR, Spangler S. Documentation with serial radiographs of successful whole bowel irrigation with GoLytely in a massive iron ingestion. *Vet Hum Toxicol* 1989;31:333.
33. Tenenbein M, Wiseman W, Yatscoff RW. Gastrotomy and whole bowel irrigation in iron poisoning. *Pediatr Emerg Care* 1991;7:286–288.
34. Peterson CD, Fifield GC. Emergency gastrotomy for acute iron poisoning. *Ann Emerg Med* 1980;9:262–264.
35. De Silva JH, Wijewickrema R, Senenayake N. Does pralidoxime affect the outcome of the management in acute organophosphate poisoning? *Lancet* 1992;339:1136–1238.
36. Amos RG, Hall A. Malathion poisoning treated with protopam. *Ann Intern Med* 1965;62:1013–1016.
37. Snodgrass WR. Salicylate toxicity. *Pediatr Clin North Am* 1986;33:381.
38. Davis M, Labadanis D, Greaves M. Systemic toxicity from topically applied salicylic acid. *BMJ* 1979;1:661.
39. Prescott L, Balali-Mood M, Critchley JAJH. Diuresis or urinary alkalinization for salicylate poisoning? *BMJ* 1982;285:1383–1386.
40. Brett AS, Rothchild N, Gray R, Perry, M. Predicting the clinical overdose. *Arch Intern Med* 1987;147:133–137.
41. Bernstein J, et al. Prevention and the role of the poison control center. In: Goldfrank LR, et al., eds. *Goldfrank's toxicologic emergencies*. 3rd ed. East Norwalk, CT: Appleton-Century-Crofts, 1986:149–158.
42. Koren G. Medications which can kill a toddler with one tablet or one teaspoonful. *Clin Toxicol* 1993;31:407–413.

Emergency Toxicology, Second Edition,
edited by Peter Viccellio.
Lippincott–Raven Publishers, Philadelphia © 1998.

10

Special Considerations in the Geriatric Patient

†Nina Mazur and °Adam L. Church

*†Deceased; °Department of Emergency Medicine, North Shore University Hospital,
Manhasset, New York 11030*

Emergency treatment of the poisoned geriatric patient presents unique dilemmas based on demographics, medication usage, physiology of aging, and clinical presentation.

I. **Demographics.** The "graying" of the United States reflects the growth of the aging segment of our population, currently numbering more than 25 million retirees, with a projected population of 39 million people over age 65 by the year 2010 (1,2). Hidden within those figures is a dramatic increase in the 85 age group—the frail elderly or "old old"—projected to double during the 20-year period of 1980 to 2000. At least 15 million people will be 85 years old or older by the year 2050 (3). Historically, elderly patients use emergency departments (EDs) far more than expected based on their representation in the community. In the United States, each decade past age 65 not only accounts for a greater proportion of hospitalizations and rehospitalizations, but some reports indicate a difference of as much as 100% from one decade to the next (4).

II. **Medication usage**

A. **Iatrogenic drug-induced disease** is common in the elderly. Every ED physician is familiar with the "shopping-bag-full-of-multicolored-pills" syndrome. Drug reactions are responsible for 3% to 10% of elderly hospital admissions (5).

B. **Polypharmacy** in the elderly is very common, resulting from increased prevalence of chronic disease, somatic complaints, and overdiagnosis, which translates into overtreatment. Common conditions reported as being overdiagnosed are hypertension, congestive heart failure, dementia, and diabetes. Patients with these conditions often receive three or more drugs per visit to a primary physician (2). Nearly one quarter of community-dwelling elderly are prescribed potentially inappropriate medications (6–10).

C. The elderly use more than 30% of all prescribed medications, accounting for 40% of all adverse drug reactions (11,12). More than 80% of geriatric patients are taking three or four drugs a day, often including psychotropic agents. The percent of patients on potentially toxic agents increases with age and hospitalization, and the number of adverse reactions increases with the number of medications. It is not unusual to find elderly hospitalized patients on 10 or more drugs. In the case of outpatient treatment, the effects of polypharmacy are compounded by compliance problems secondary to confusing regimens, as well as by the significant addition of over-the-counter medications by many elderly patients (13).

D. Suicide of elderly patients is often accomplished via ingestion of analgesics, benzodiazepines, and barbiturates that had been prescribed for symptomatic relief of depressive symptoms masquerading as somatic complaints and sleep disorders. From 1980 to 1992, the number of suicides in the >65 age group increased by 36% (14). In 1992, this group accounted for 13% of the U.S. population but nearly one-fifth of the suicides.

III. **Physiology**

A. There is a **decline in organ and tissue function** with age. However, age-related physiologic changes are not uniform among individuals, and indeed different organ systems age at different times within the same individual. These changes may be reflected in altered pharmacokinetics of drugs and lowered thresholds for organ damage.

B. Aging is associated with an increased gastric pH, decreased intestinal blood flow, and increased gastric emptying time. These factors may be responsible for gastric bleeding that occurs with NSAID use. Increased gastric emptying is particularly important for patients on anticholinergics and cyclic antidepressants. Despite the **gastrointestinal tract changes,** the absorption of drugs remains relatively unchanged in the elderly. Rather, it is the decreased capacity to eliminate drugs, either through metabolism or excretion, that accounts for the increased plasma concentration of many drugs in elderly patients. There are exceptions of course. For example, the bioavailability of digoxin has been shown to decrease in the elderly (15).

C. Decreased **hepatic blood flow** and decreased hepatic metabolic activity can result in toxic levels of drugs, depending on hepatic elimination. The impact of physiologic changes depends on whether the drug is taken orally or parenterally and whether the drug is highly or poorly extracted (16).

1. Highly extracted drugs are flow-limited and are affected by alterations in hepatic flow, which can be 12% to 40% less in the elderly. Such drugs are dextropropoxyphene (Darvon), nortriptyline (Aventyl), morphine, lidocaine, propranolol, and labetalol.

2. Poorly extracted drugs are more sensitive to changes in the metabolic capacity of the liver. Included in this category are phenytoin, diazepam, warfarin, chlorpromazine, quinidine, digoxin, theophylline, acetaminophen, and others (Table 10-1). Unfortunately, from a clinical point of view, liver function tests are not directly correlated with drug-metabolizing capacity and therefore are not helpful for determining the best dosage regimen for elderly patients. There is little guidance in the *Physician Desk Reference* (PDR) specific to geriatric patients, as clinical trials of pharmaceuticals, prior to revised 1983 U.S. Food and Drug Administration testing requirements, often did not include the age 65+ population.

D. **Renal function** is generally 40% less than in young adults.

1. Creatinine clearance in young subjects ranges between 80 and 120 ml/min, whereas healthy octogenarians may clear only 20 to 40 ml/min.

2. This marked loss of renal function increases levels of drugs that are partly or entirely eliminated by renal excretion: cimetidine, lithium, procainamide, digoxin, chlorpropamide, and most of the commonly used antimicrobial agents.

3. There are several formulas and nomograms for quickly estimating creatinine clearance for patients that take into consideration age, weight, sex, and serum creatinine. Cockcroft and Gault's (17) formula is frequently used.

Table 10-1. *Drugs affected by age-related physiologic changes*

Highly extracted drugs affected by hepatic flow	Poorly extracted drugs affected by changes in metabolic capacity of liver
Dextropropoxyphene	Phenytoin
Nortriptyline	Diazepam
Morphine	Warfarin
Propranolol	Chlorpromazine
Labetalol	Quinidine
Chlormethiazole	Digitoxin
Lidocaine	Theophylline
Meperidine	Acetaminophen
	Tolbutamide

Drugs affected by changes in renal function	Drugs affected by changes in protein levels
Cimetidine	Warfarin
Lithium	Theophylline
Procainamide	Salicylates
Digoxin	Phenylbutazone
Chlorpropamide	Sufadiazine
Gentamicin	Phenytoin

Creatinine clearance (males) = $[140 - \text{age (years)}] \times [\text{body wt. (kg)}]$ divided by $72 \times$ serum creatinine (mg/dl). For females, the result is multiplied by 0.85.

It should be noted that due to much smaller muscle mass in the elderly, the diminished serum creatinine may make this estimate unreliable.

E. There are still other **age-related changes** that can increase drug availability and drug effect. The distribution of a drug in the body depends on body composition, plasma protein binding, and blood flow to the organs.

    a. Age-related changes in **body composition** have been well described. There is a decrease in total body water, a decrease in lean body mass, and an increase in body fat. The volume of distribution (V_d) of water-soluble drugs is smaller in the elderly with increased plasma concentrations; and the V_d of water-soluble drugs (e.g., ethanol, digoxin, antipyrine, and cimetidine) is smaller in the elderly with increased plasma concentrations. Notable exceptions are pancuronium and tobramycin (18). There can be a 50% increase in the free fraction of drugs, e.g., acetazolamide, valproate, diflunisal, salicylate, and naproxen (19).

    Alterations in body fat may result in prolonged action of highly lipid-soluble drugs. The half-life of diazepam can be 75 to 80 h in the elderly compared to 20 h in a 20-year-old (20).

    b. **Lowered albumin levels** typically seen in the elderly—3.5 g/dl, compared to 4.0 to 4.5 g/dl in younger people (21)—can result in a significantly increased percentage of unbound drug for *acidic* drugs that are usually protein-bound. Basic drugs are bound to alpha 1-acid glycoproteins, which are usually not decreased in the elderly (19). Wallace and Whiting (22) demonstrated that the decreased albumin concentration in the elderly significantly increased the percentage of unbound salicylate, phenylbutazone, and sulfadiazine. Other protein-bound drugs that are similarly affected are warfarin, meperidine, theophylline, and phenytoin. Phenytoin has 1.2 to 3.0 times higher free fraction in the elderly.

  c. Pulmonary function declines with age. A healthy 90-year-old has approximately half the function of a young adult. It follows, then, that drug reactions with pulmonary effects are more likely to result in morbidity or mortality.

IV. **Clinical presentation.** The elderly, particularly the very old, are difficult to evaluate in the ED. Obtaining the all important clinical history is hampered not only in elderly patients with identified causes of cognitive loss (Alzheimer's disease, cerebrovascular accident, organic brain syndrome) but is also made more difficult by subtle memory loss and decreased visual and auditory acuity. Patience and a quiet, nonstressful environment (facilitating the interview process) are in short supply in most EDs. Older patients tend not to follow the classic disease presentations.

  A. Unintentional **salicylate intoxication** in the elderly has been reported as going undetected for up to 3 days after admission. Patients may present with neurologic findings, confusion, shortness of breath, and perhaps pulmonary edema and acidosis. Typically, an effort is made to find one unifying diagnosis that ties all the symptoms together. Unfortunately in the elderly, multiple diseases and drug effects may be present concomitantly, masking each other and attenuating the time needed to diagnose and treat the presenting complaint.

  B. **Alcoholism** in the elderly is drastically underdetected (23). The elderly alcoholic may present with memory or behavior changes, falls, sleep disturbance, or cardiac arrhythmias. For a given amount of alcohol, a 60-year-old has a higher (20%) blood alcohol concentration than a younger person because of decreased total body water (24).

  C. **Falls** rank in the top two causes for injury-related death among older U.S. residents (14). Benzodiazepines and neuroleptics have been found to be potent risk factors for falls and fall-related fractures. The relative risk of a serious fall is increased by a factor of 2.5 when long half-life sedatives are used (25,26).

V. Evaluation of the elderly patient should include careful review of all medications the patient is receiving, both prescription and nonprescription. Arterial blood gas assays evaluate for the possibility of toxins associated with acidosis. An ECG may demonstrate drug-related arrhythmias. Results from a CBC and assays for electrolytes, glucose, and BUN usually do not uncover the drug responsible for the patient's symptoms, but they do prevent the physician from overlooking accompanying medical problems and help guide supportive care. Whenever the etiology of a symptom or constellation of symptoms is unclear in the geriatric age group, drugs should always be high on the list of the differential diagnosis.

References

1. Eliastam M. Elderly patients in the emergency department. *Ann Emerg Med* 1989;11:1222.
2. Michocki RJ, Lamy PP, Hooper FJ, Richardson JP. Drug prescribing for the elderly. *Arch Fam Med* 1993;2:441–444.
3. Suegak JS, Taeuber CM. Demographic perspectives of the long-lived society. *Daedalus* 1986;115:77–115.
4. Baum SA, Rubenstein LZ. Old people in the emergency room: age related differences in emergency department use and care. *J Am Geriatr Soc* 1987;35:398–404.

5. Nolan L, O'Malley K. Prescribing for the elderly. I: Sensitivity of the elderly to adverse drug reactions. *J Am Geriatr Soc* 1988;36:142–149.
6. Wilcox SM, et al. Inappropriate drug prescribing for the community-dwelling elderly. *JAMA* 1994;272:292–296.
7. Gosney M, Tallis R. Prescriptions of contraindicated and interacting drugs in elderly patients admitted to hospital. *Lancet* 1984;2:564–567.
8. Adams K, et al. Inappropriate prescribing in the elderly. *J R Coll Phys Lond* 1987;21:39–41.
9. Browne M, et al. A computer-assissted survey of contraindicated and interacting drugs in long stay geriatric patients. *Br J Pharm Prac* 1987;9:250–254.
10. Gosney M, et al. Inappropriate prescribing in Part 3 residential homes for the elderly. *Health Trends* 1989;21:129–131.
11. Baum C, et al. Drug use in the United States in 1981. *JAMA* 1984;241:1293.
12. Nolan L, et al. Adverse drug reactions in the elderly. *Br J Hosp Med* 1989;41:446.
13. Stoller EP. Prescribed and over the counter medicine use by the ambulatory elderly. *Med Care* 1988;26:1149–1157.
14. Center for disease control and prevention. Suicide among older persons—United States, 1980–1992. 1996; 45(1):3–6.
15. Lamy PP. Comparative pharmacokinetic changes and drug theory in an older population. *J Am Geriatr Soc* 1982; 30 (11 Suppl):511–9.
16. Tsujimoto G, et al. Pharmacokinetics and pharmacodynamic principle of drug therapy in old age. Part I. *Int J Clin Pharmacol Ther Toxicol* 1989;27:13–26.
17. Cockcroft DW, Gault MH. Prediction of creatinine clearance from serum creatinine. *Nephron* 1976;16:31–41.
18. Montamat SC, et al. Management of drug therapy in the elderly. *N Engl J Med* 1989;321:303–309.
19. Wallace SM, et al. Plasma protein binding of drugs in the elderly. *Clin Pharmacokinet* 1987;12:41–72.
20. Stein BE. Avoiding drug reactions: seven steps to writing safe prescriptions. *Geriatrics* 1994;49:28–36.
21. Annesly TM. Special considerations for therapeutic drug monitoring. *Clin Chem* 1989;35:1337–1341.
22. Wallace S, Whiting B. Factors affecting drug binding in plasma of elderly patients. *Br J Clin Pharmacol* 1976;3: 327–330.
23. Rose J. The "other drug problem." *Am. Fam. Physician* 1988;38:90.
24. Scott RB. Alcohol effects in the elderly. *Comp Ther* 1989;15:8–12.
25. Tinetti ME, Speechley M, Ginter SF. Risk factors for falls among elderly persons living in the community. *N Engl J Med* 1988;319:1701–1707.
26. Ray WA, Griffin MR, Downey W. Benzodiazepines of long and short elimination half-life and the risk of hip fracture. *JAMA* 1989;262:3303–3307.

Emergency Toxicology, Second Edition,
edited by Peter Viccellio.
Lippincott–Raven Publishers, Philadelphia © 1998.

11

Hemoglobin Toxins

James G. Ryan

*Department of Emergency Medicine, North Shore University Hospital,
Manhasset, New York 11030*

Toxins can cause alterations in hemoglobin structure, rendering hemoglobin incapable of performing its primary function of oxygen transport. Three induced hemoglobinopathies have been described as clinically relevant: carboxyhemoglobin, methemoglobin, and sulfhemoglobin. Since carbon monoxide poisoning is discussed separately in Chapter 74, only the last two disorders will be discussed here.

I. Methemoglobinemia

A. Properties

1. Pathophysiology and pharmacokinetics

a. Normally in the erythrocyte, 99% of the **iron component** of hemoglobin is present in the reduced (Fe^{2+}) state and approximately 1% is in the oxidized (Fe^{3+}) state. Maintenance of this equilibrium is important because hemoglobin with Fe^{3+} (methemoglobin, or met-Hgb) is unable to bind oxygen.

b. This **normal Hgb/met-Hgb ratio** is maintained by two enzyme systems. The primary enzyme, met-Hgb reductase, accounts for 95% of this reaction and is dependent on NADH to function. The secondary system is also a met-Hgb reductase but is dependent on NADPH, which in the red blood cell is a product of the G6PD-dependent hexose monophosphate shunt. This secondary system accounts for only 5% of normal activity but is important because it may be induced to remove met-Hgb more rapidly. This equilibrium may be shifted owing to structurally abnormal (congenital) hemoglobins, enzyme deficiencies, or increased production of met-Hgb by various toxins.

c. **Congenital methemoglobinemia** may be due to an abnormal hemoglobin or to a relative or total enzyme deficiency. Abnormal M hemoglobins are usually due to a single amino acid substitution that yields hemoglobins that contain an iron moiety permanently in the Fe^{3+} state. This condition has been described in the heterozygous state with met-Hgb levels of 25% to 30%. The homozygous state has not been described, as it is probably inconsistent with life. Congenital (primary) met-Hgb reductase deficiencies have been described as well. Homozygotes for this deficiency have been described as having 10% to 50% met-Hgb levels and are asymptomatic except for cyanotic discoloration. Heterozygotes have minimally increased met-Hgb levels (in the 2% to 3% range) and are not usually symptomatic. Both homozygotes and heterozygotes are more sensitive to toxins that induce met-Hgb formation. Patients with a deficiency of the secondary (NADPH-dependent) system do not exhibit an increased met-Hgb level owing to the small role this enzyme usually plays, but they may not respond to treatment of induced methemoglobinemia, as discussed later.

d. Methemoglobinemia may also be **induced** by drugs or **chemicals** that can oxidize Hgb directly or by forming other oxidizing agents during their metabolism. Some agents produce methemoglobinemia without predisposing factors, but patients with a met-Hgb reductase deficiency or infants (due to decreased activity of met-Hgb reductase and the increased sensitivity of Hgb F) are at increased risk (1–4).

2. Sources of induced methemoglobinemia. A large number of substances have been noted to induce methemoglobinemia (Table 11-1), several of which are commonly used drugs. Among the more common are nitrites, nitrates, aniline products, and local anesthetics.

a. **Nitrites** are strong oxidizing agents and can easily induce methemoglobinemia. They are even used for the treatment of cyanide poisoning to induce methemoglobinemia, although this mechanism of action has been questioned.

b. **Nitrates** comprise a more frequently used class of drugs but cannot induce methemoglobinemia directly. They have been found to be converted to

TABLE 11-1. *Etiology of acquired methemoglobinemia*

Medications	Chemical agents
Acetanilid	Aniline dyes
Aminosalicylic acid	Bromates
Benzocaine	Chlorates
Bismuth	Chlorobenzene
Dapsone	Chromates
Lidocaine	Naphthalene
Lignocaine	Nitrates
Mafenide	Nitrites
Methylene blue	Nitrobenzene
Metoclopramide	Nitroethane
Nitrates	Nitrophenol
Nitrites	Nitrous gases
Nitrofurantoin	Trinitrotoluene
Nitroprusside	
Phenacetin	Household products
Phenazopyridine	Air fresheners
Phenelzine	Artificial nail glues and removers
Phenobarbitol	Cleaning products
Phenytoin	Dyes
Prilocaine	Inks (especially indelible inks)
Quinolones	Paints
Resorcin	Shoe polish
Sulfonamides	Solvents
Tetracaine	Varnishes
Trimethoprim	Well water
Vitamin K	Young infants with diarrhea

nitrites by bacteria in the GI tract or on the skin. Intravenous injection of nitrates has not been noted to cause methemoglobinemia. Infants who have ingested nitrate-contaminated well water (3,5) and infants treated for burns with silver nitrate-containing creams have developed this disorder because of this conversion on the skin or in the gut (6,7).

    c. **Local anesthetics** are commonly used by many practicing physicians but only rarely produce significant methemoglobinemia. Most cases have been noted in infants, owing to their increased susceptibility, as noted earlier. Methemoglobinemia has even occurred with the use of topical anesthetic preparations, especially when applied to mucous membranes or abraded or injured skin (8,9).

    d. **Other drugs.** Many commonly used drugs have caused met-Hgb formation (Table 11-1), although infrequently. The drugs on this list include such commonly used agents as phenytoin, sulfonamides, and phenazopyridine (urinary anesthetic) as well as some antimalarial agents. The minimal frequency with which methemoglobinemia has been reported suggests that only susceptible individuals (met-Hgb reductase deficiency) develop problems with these drugs.

    e. **Aniline and nitrobenzene** are found in many common household products, such as shoe polish, ink, paints, varnishes, and cleaning products. Unlike many of the other agents mentioned above, these substances are strong inducers of methemoglobinemia and can produce met-Hgb in the absence of any predisposing factors.

    f. **Artificial nail products** have been noted to contain many toxic substances. Some nail glue removers contain acreonitrile which may cause cyanide poisoning. *N,N*-dimethyl-*p*-toluidine is used to make artificial fingernails and nitroethane is used in some artificial fingernail removers. Both of these substances may cause methemoglobinemia. Nitroethane may produce a delayed and prolonged methemoglobinemia, since it is metabolized to nitrite before producing its toxicity (10).

    g. **Young infants with diarrhea** have been found to have significant methemoglobinemia. The etiology of the methemoglobinemia in these patients is unclear, but should be considered in this clinical setting.

  3. **Mechanism of action.** The toxicity of met-Hgb is a function of its inactivation of hemoglobin, making it unable to carry oxygen. This action causes a relative anemia that, if of sufficient degree, deprives the tissues of oxygen. The effects of met-Hgb may be worsened by an underlying anemia. In addition to the reduced oxygen-carrying capacity of the blood, met-Hgb increases the affinity of Hgb for oxygen, thereby decreasing oxygen delivery to the tissues. Because Hgb molecules consist of tetramers, a small amount of met-Hgb is divided among a large number of molecules. Therefore, even a small amount of met-Hgb can affect a significant amount of the total Hgb molecules, decreasing oxygen delivery by all the affected Hgb (11,12).

B. **Clinical presentation**

  1. **History.** Deriving a proper and precise history is important and can often lead to the diagnosis. The patient may have a wide, nonspecific array of complaints; and detailed questioning about any possible exposure to an offending agent listed above can lead to the diagnosis. Potential exposures from drinking water, medicines, home remedies, foods, hobbies, and occupations should be included. Information about other family members with similar symptoms or diarrhea in infants would also be helpful.

   a. met-Hgb has a brownish blue color, and a **low level** often produces noticeable cyanotic skin discoloration without symptoms (Table 11-1).

   b. At **higher levels,** patients complain of nonspecific symptoms such as weakness, fatigue, dizziness, headache, dyspnea, and palpitations.

   c. With **severe toxicity** patients can exhibit an altered mental status, seizures, and cardiac arrest.

  2. **Physical examination** is not very helpful in the evaluation of methemoglobinemia. The only specific finding is a brownish blue cyanotic discoloration of the skin, which may be present at levels at which patients are asymptomatic. A met-Hgb level as low as 10% to 15% (approximately 1.5 g/dL) is required to produce cyanosis (13). Blood from these patients does not turn red when exposed to air as does blood from a patient with cyanosis due to hypoxia. The remainder of the physical examination is often normal or nonspecific and therefore not helpful except for disclosing other possible etiologies for the cyanosis and symptoms.

  3. **Course.** Because methemoglobinemia is not caused by a single toxin but is a syndrome, the clinical course is not as easily predictable as those caused by other toxins. Many cases are asymptomatic except for cyanosis, but some substances produce severe, rapidly progressing symptoms. Most drugs used in clinical practice are not strong met-Hgb inducers and therefore do not produce rapidly progressive courses, but other agents used in household products and industrial products can produce a severe, rapidly progressive course.

C. **Differential diagnosis.** Because the presenting complaints are often vague and the physical examination is nonspecific, determining the diagnosis of a patient with methemoglobinemia can be difficult and challenging. The true incidence of this syndrome is unknown, as it is frequently asymptomatic or minimally symptomatic and thus missed by the clinician. In order to avoid missing these cases, a thorough clinical and laboratory evaluation should be undertaken in patients with symptoms possibly referable to met-Hgb.

  1. The most common and striking finding in these patients is a **brownish cyanosis** with discoloration of the lips, nail beds, ear lobes, and mucosa. This chocolate brown discoloration may be present in the absence of any other complaints. This cyanosis differs from that caused by hypoxia in several ways. Cyanosis caused by hypoxia is usually accompanied by evidence of severe cardiopulmonary disease and frequently responds to oxygen. The cyanosis of methemoglobinemia may be present in a patient who otherwise appears well; it is due to the low level of met-Hgb (1.5 g/dL) required to cause a visible cyanosis (13), in contrast to the deoxygenated Hgb level (4 g/dL) in the Fe^{2+} state. The cyanosis—if of hypoxic etiology— would be expected to respond to administration of oxygen, assuming the underlying problem is not so severe that the arterial PO_2 (PaO_2) cannot be elevated by oxygen administration.

2. Patients may also present with symptoms referable to the **CNS or cardiopulmonary system** or vague complaints referable to a **viral syndrome.** If the met-Hgb level is high enough to cause symptoms, cyanosis should be present, providing an important clue to the diagnosis. If the cyanosis goes undetected or is ignored because of normal PaO$_2$, however, the diagnosis may be elusive. Any patient with cyanosis but a normal PaO$_2$ should have a measured (not calculated; see **D.1** below) oxygen saturation assay and a met-Hgb level.

3. Patients with signs or symptoms that may be referable to **hypoxia but without evident cyanosis** present a more difficult situation. In these patients other substances such as carbon monoxide and sulfhemoglobin (rarely), as well as met-Hgb, may interfere with tissue oxygenation. The true or measured oxygen saturation is decreased if any of these toxins is the cause. If the oxygen saturation is decreased, more specific tests can be performed to confirm the diagnosis. Studies have suggested that some patients with symptoms suggestive of viral syndromes have an elevated carboxyhemoglobin level. The finding of hemoglobin toxins in frequently unsuspected settings suggests that measured oxygen saturations may be a useful adjunct to blood gas analyses in many if not all settings.

D. **Laboratory analysis**

1. **General considerations**

   a. **Routine laboratory tests** are not helpful for determining the diagnosis of methemoglobinemia. The CBC is usually normal, and chemistry analyses may yield a nonspecific anion gap lactic acidosis in the presence of severe toxicity.

   b. **Arterial blood gas** (ABG) analyses may yield varying results but are most helpful for excluding a hypoxic cause of cyanosis. Early in the course these patients may hyperventilate, yielding respiratory alkalosis. As the tissues become deprived of oxygen, metabolic acidosis develops, followed eventually by respiratory acidosis as respirations slow and cardiopulmonary arrest ensues. The PaO$_2$ should be normal in these patients until terminal stages unless an underlying pathologic situation exists. Despite the normal PaO$_2$ in these patients, the actual amount of oxygen in the blood is low, as evidenced by the decreased oxygen saturation.

      (1) True oxygen saturation as measured by **co-oximetry** is not equivalent to the calculated oxygen saturation derived from the PaO$_2$ as traditionally reported with ABG results. This calculated SaO$_2$ gives a falsely normal oxygen content when toxins that inactivate Hgb but do not affect oxygenation are present. Therefore oxygen saturation should be measured in any patient in whom hemoglobin toxins are in the differential diagnosis.

      (2) Oxygen saturation measured by **pulse oximetry** is altered by the presence of met-Hgb. Pulse oximetry measures oxygen saturation by measuring the absorption of light at wavelengths of 660 and 940 nm. The absorptions at these wavelengths are different for oxygenated and deoxyhemoglobin. The ratio of these absorptions can be calculated to

yield a percentage of oxygenated hemoglobin or oxygen saturation. The presence of met-Hgb, which has different absorption qualities, alters this ratio and causes a decrease in the calculated oxygen saturation. This decrease in the pulse oximeter reading does not correlate with the true met-Hgb content and should be quantified by specific met-Hgb levels (14).

c. **Several bedside screeening tests** may suggest the presence of methemoglobin and provide usefel information while confirmatory tests are pending. If a drop of blood is placed on filter paper it will yield a deep brown color if methemoglobin is present. Similarly, a test tube filled with blood will not turn red when shaken with cyanide or oxygen is bubbled through it. However, with the rapid availability of blood gas analysis and co-oximetry in most emergency departments, these tests are rarely necessary.

2. **Toxin-specific tests.** Methemoglobin levels are generally measured using spectrophotometric techniques via an instrument called a co-oximeter. The co-oximeter measures light absorption of the blood specimen at various wavelengths, usually four, and can calculate the presence of different hemoglobins based on the results. The hemoglobin species usually measured are oxyhemoglobin, deoxyhemoglobin, carboxyhemoglobin, and methemoglobin. These results are then combined to yield the total hemoglobin, and the percentages of the various hemoglobins are calculated. Methemoglobin produces an absorption peak at 620 to 630 nm and can be used to quantitate the amount present.

a. The results of this analysis can be altered by substances that have similar absorption spectra or that can alter these spectra. **Sulfhemoglobin** has an absorption peak in the same range as that of methemoglobin and must be considered when an elevated methemoglobin level is reported by a co-oximeter. The presence of sulfhemoglobin can be determined by adding carbon monoxide or cyanide to the mixture (15). Carbon monoxide binds readily to sulfhemoglobin, but not to methemoglobin, and forms carboxysulfhemoglobin, which augments the absorption peak at this wavelength. Cyanide binds methemoglobin readily but not sulfhemoglobin. The elimination of this peak after the addition of cyanide suggests that the responsible agent is methemoglobin (15). **Hyperlipidemia** has also been reported to cause falsely elevated methemoglobin levels by interfering with light absorption (16). Elevated lipid levels may yield a falsely elevated methemoglobin level but do not produce cyanosis as would be expected with significant levels of the other mentioned substances.

b. Sample collection and storage procedures may alter methemoglobin levels in specimens. Freezing blood specimens may induce methemoglobin formation or increase the amount already present. Specimens should be collected into heparin- or EDTA-containing tubes, as fluoride/oxalate tubes have been noted to increase methemoglobin levels (16).

c. **Range of toxicity** (8,17,18). Because methemoglobin causes a relative anemia by inactivating hemoglobin, the symptoms are proportional to the percent of methemoglobin as well as the total hemoglobin content of the blood: 1% to 3%, none; 10%, cyanosis, but no complaints; 30%, mild, nonspecific symptoms of headache, fatigue, dizziness, dyspnea, palpitations; 50%, altered mental status, worsening symptoms, metabolic acidosis, dysrhythmias, convulsions; 70%, may be lethal if untreated (cardiovascular collapse). Note that anemic patients may display symptoms at lower Met-Hgb levels.

E. Management

    1. General considerations

        a. ABCs

            (1) Evaluate adequacy of airway.

            (2) Assess adequacy of oxygenation and ventilate.

                (a) Administer high-concentration oxygen.

                (b) Intubate if necessary.

            (3) Maintain blood pressure via fluids and pressor agents as necessary, however, vasoconstrictors may only have limited benefit.

        b. Seizures: Administer diazepam (Valium) and phenytoin (Dilantin) as per standard seizure protocol.

        c. Arrhythmias

            (1) Supraventricular: Sinus tachycardia is expected; treat other arrhythmias as per standard protocols.

            (2) Ventricular: Treat malignant ventricular arrhythmias as per standard protocols. One should remember that lidocaine can induce methemoglobin formation and may be contraindicated if a local anestheitc is the cause of the methemoglobinemia.

        d. Oxygen therapy is generally recommended but has not been evaluated in controlled studies. Hyperbaric oxygen has been shown to improve or worsen the methemoglobinemia depending on the substance inducing it (19–21).

        e. Detoxification

            (1) Dermal. Wash offending agent from the skin with soap and water.

            (2) Oral

                (a) Emesis or **lavage** may be useful during the first hour. If an aniline dye is the offending agent, 5% acetic acid may be administered to remove this toxin.

                (b) Charcoal should be administered, as it binds most agents.

                (c) One dose of **cathartic** may be administered with the charcoal.

    2. Toxin-specific treatment. The treatment of choice is **methylene blue,** which acts as a cofactor to induce the secondary or NADPH-dependent methemoglobin reductase system. Once induced, this system rapidly converts methemoglobin to hemoglobin, with effects being seen within minutes. Patients who are deficient in this enzyme or who have insufficient quantities of NADPH (G6PD deficiency) may not respond to this form of treatment, and alternate forms of therapy are used (see **I.E.3**).

        a. Methylene blue is generally well tolerated but may produce dizziness, tremors, confusion, precordial chest pain, vomiting, and apprehension, especially at high doses. The urine may have a blue discoloration due to renal excretion, and dysuria may accompany this change. A mild hemolytic anemia may occur, and more severe anemias have been reported, especially in G6PD-deficient individuals and neonates. If a hemolytic reaction occurs, this should be treated with the same regimen as hemolysis from other causes: hydration, alkalinization of the urine, and transfusion as necessary.

b. Because methylene blue has potential toxicity, not all patients with methemoglobinemia should be treated. Patients with methemoglobin **levels <30% who are asymptomatic** require only procedures that prevent further absorption of the offending agent and observation to ensure that the levels are declining. **Symptomatic patients** (other than cyanosis) should be treated with decontamination procedures and methylene blue. Patients who have **no symptoms but methemoglobin >30%** may either be treated with methylene blue or be observed closely for worsening toxicity while decontamination procedures are instituted. Patients who maintain an oxyhemoglobin level of greater than 5 g/dL usually do not require treatment with methylene blue. If signs of toxicity develop, specific therapy should be instituted.

c. The **dose** of methylene blue is 1 to 2 mg (0.1 to 0.2 mL/kg) of a 1% solution. This dose may be administered intravenously over 5 min and may be repeated in 1 h if symptoms have not resolved. Methylene blue may itself produce a bluish discoloration of the skin (22), which alone should not be used as a criterion for more aggressive therapy. Repeat methemoglobin levels should be obtained and the clinical examination and symptoms used to guide treatment. The maximum dose of methylene blue is 5 to 7 mg/kg.

d. Patients who do not respond to initial therapy should be evaluated for sulfhemoglobinemia, G6PD deficiency, and NADPH methemoglobin reductase deficiency (11,23).

3. **Treatment failures.** Patients who have significant symptoms and fail to respond to therapy comprise a difficult and controversial group. These patients should be considered to have sulfhemoglobinemia, G6PD deficiency, or NADPH methemoglobin reductase deficiency (11,23). No specific treatment exists for any of these problems, and various therapies have been suggested including transfusions, exchange transfusions, and hyperbaric oxygen. **Hyperbaric oxygen** has been shown in some studies to worsen the methemoglobinemia (19–21) induced by certain agents, but it was not associated with increased mortality. With other agents methemoglobin formation has decreased when hyperbaric oxygen was administered. The current role for hyperbaric oxygen is undetermined, but theoretically it seems appealing as a possible temporizing measure, as significant amounts of oxygen may be dissolved in the blood, diminishing the need for hemoglobin for oxygen transport. It may provide time, in a critically ill patient, to replace the altered hemoglobin with normal hemoglobin via transfusions (11,21).

F. Disposition and follow-up. Patients who have ingested a significant amount of a methemoglobin-forming agent should be observed until it can be determined that absorption is complete and the methemoglobin levels are declining. This observation period should probably last 12 to 24 h owing to the possibility of delayed absorption of some substances. Patients with minimal evidence of toxicity generally have no sequela and do not require specific follow-up. Patients who have severe toxicities (e.g., cardiopulmonary arrest, coma) may develop encephalopathy due to hypoxia and may require neurologic follow-up, but most survivors have minimal if any long-term sequela.

II. Sulfhemoglobinemia

A. Properties

1. Sulfhemoglobin is a hemoglobin molecule altered by the addition of a sulfur atom in the porphyrin ring, making it incapable of carrying oxygen. Unlike methemoglobin, there is no enzyme capable of converting sulfhemoglobin to normal hemoglobin, and so it persists for the life of the red blood cell. Whereas methemoglobin causes an increased affinity of the hemoglobin molecule for oxygen in the neighboring porphyrin rings, sulfhemoglobin decreases this affinity, allowing easier release of oxygen to the tissues (15). It results in less severe toxicity with equivalent levels of methemoglobin and sulfhemoglobin.

2. Phenacetin, acetanilid, sulfonamides, metoclopramide, and dapsone have been implicated in the formation of sulfhemoglobin. Hydrogen sulfide, which is clearly toxic, may be an occupational cause, but the ability of hydrogen sulfide to form sulfhemoglobin is controversial. Toxic gases from the combustion of products containing sulfur groups have also been implicated as a cause of sulfhemoglobinemia.

B. Clinical presentation

1. **History.** Sulfhemoglobin, like methemoglobin, at a low level produces noticeable cyanotic skin discoloration without symptoms. At higher levels, patients complain of nonspecific symptoms, such as weakness, fatigue, dizziness, headache, dyspnea, and palpitations. With severe toxicity patients may exhibit an altered mental status, seizures, and cardiac arrest.

2. **Physical examination** is not helpful when evaluating sulfhemoglobinemia. The only specific finding is a cyanotic discoloration of the skin that may be present at low levels. A sulfhemoglobin level as low as 2% to 3% (approximately 0.5 g/dL) may produce noticeable cyanosis (13). Blood extracted from these patients does not turn red when exposed to air as does blood from a patient with cyanosis due to hypoxia.

3. **Course.** Sulfhemoglobinemia, unlike methemoglobin, is not converted to normal hemoglobin and persists until the red blood cells involved are broken down by the reticuloendothelial system. Because the life of a red blood cell is approximately 100 days, the time course of a significant poisoning can be prolonged without treatment.

C. Differential diagnosis

1. The most common and striking finding in these patients is **cyanosis,** which may be present in the absence of any other complaints. This cyanosis differs from that of hypoxia by several features. Cyanosis caused by hypoxia is usually accompanied by evidence of severe cardiopulmonary disease, and it frequently responds to oxygen. The cyanosis of sulfhemoglobinemia may be present in a patient who otherwise appears well owing to the low level of sulfhemoglobin (0.5 g/dL) required to cause a visible cyanosis, in contrast to the level of deoxygenated Hgb (4 g/dL) or

methemoglobin (1.5 g/dL). This cyanosis, if of hypoxic etiology, would be expected to respond to administration of oxygen, assuming that the underlying problem is not so severe that the PaO_2 cannot be raised by oxygen administration.

2. Patients may also present with symptoms referable to the **CNS** or **cardiopulmonary system,** or vague complaints referable to a **viral syndrome.** If the level of sulfhemoglobin is high enough to cause symptoms, cyanosis should be present, providing an important clue to the diagnosis. If the cyanosis goes undetected or is ignored owing to a normal PaO_2, however, the diagnosis may be missed. Any patient with cyanosis but a normal PaO_2 should have the oxygen saturation measured (not calculated; see **D.2**). The patient with signs or symptoms that may be referable to hypoxia but without evident cyanosis presents a more difficult situation. In these patients other substances, e.g., carbon monoxide and methemoglobin, as well as sulfhemoglobin, may interfere with tissue oxygenation. True (measured) oxygen saturation is decreased if any of these toxins is the cause. If the oxygen saturation is decreased, more specific tests can be performed to confirm the diagnosis. Some studies have even suggested that patients with symptoms suggestive of viral syndromes have an elevated carboxyhemoglobin level. The findings of hemoglobin toxins in frequently unsuspected settings suggests that measured oxygen saturations may be a useful adjunct to blood gas analyses in many if not all settings.

D. **Laboratory analysis**

   1. **General considerations**

      a. **Routine laboratory tests** are not helpful for diagnosing sulfhemoglobinemia. The CBC is usually normal, and chemistry analyses may yield a nonspecific anion gap lactic acidosis with severe toxicity.

      b. **ABG analyses** may yield varying results but are probably most helpful for excluding a hypoxic cause of cyanosis. Early in the course these patients may hyperventilate, yielding respiratory alkalosis. As the tissues become deprived of oxygen, metabolic acidosis develops, followed eventually by respiratory acidosis as respirations slow and cardiopulmonary arrest ensues. The PaO_2 should be normal in these patients until terminal stages, unless an underlying pathologic situation exists. Despite the normal PaO_2 in these patients the actual amount of oxygen in the blood is low, as evidenced by the decreased oxygen saturation. The true oxygen saturation, measured by a co-oximeter, is not equivalent to the calculated oxygen saturation derived from the PaO_2, as traditionally reported with ABG results. This calculated SaO_2 gives a falsely normal oxygen content when toxins that inactivate hemoglobin but do not affect oxygenation are present. Therefore oxygen saturation should be measured in any patient in whom hemoglobin toxins are in the differential diagnosis.

   2. **Toxin-specific tests**

      a. **Sulfhemoglobin levels** are generally measured using spectrophotometric techniques via the co-oximeter (see **I.D.2**) Sulfhemoglobin produces an absorption peak at 620 to 630 nm, which is in the same range as that of methemoglobin (15) and is reported as methemoglobin by most co-oximeters. Some co-oximeters, depending on the wavelengths measured, can differentiate sulfhemoglobin from other abnormal hemoglobins.

b. Sulfhemoglobin can be **differentiated from methemoglobin** by adding carbon monoxide or cyanide to the mixture. Carbon monoxide binds readily to sulfhemoglobin but not to methemoglobin, forming carboxysulfhemoglobin, which augments the absorption peak at this wavelength (15). Cyanide binds methemoglobin readily but not sulfhemoglobin. The elimination of this peak after the addition of cyanide suggests that methemoglobin is the responsible agent.

c. **Isoelectric focusing** (15) has been described as an accurate and reliable technique for differentiating various altered hemoglobins, but the technique is not as readily available as co-oximetry.

d. **Range of toxicity** for sulfhemoglobin would be expected to be fairly similar to or less severe than that of methemoglobin at equivalent levels owing to sulfhemoglobin's effect of lowering the oxygen affinity of hemoglobin. Levels in the range of 5% to 15% would be expected to cause cyanosis without additional symptoms. Slightly higher levels cause nonspecific symptoms, e.g., nausea, headache, and palpitations. With 50% to 60% sulfhemoglobin, the patient would experience worsening cardiopulmonary symptoms and possible obtundation, with the possibility of death at 70% to 80%. The symptoms of sulfhemoglobinemia may appear at lower levels if any underlying disease exists, most notably anemia.

E. **Management**
  1. **General therapy**
     a. Same as for methemoglobinemia in terms of the ABCs of treatment, seizures, and arrhythmias (see **I.E.1.a–c**).
     b. **Oxygen**
        (1) Therapy with oxygen is generally recommended, but it has not been examined in controlled studies.
        (2) Hyperbaric oxygen is theoretically appealing to temporize in severely toxic patients, but few scientific data exist to document its efficacy.
     c. **Detoxification**
        (1) **Respiratory exposure.** The patient should be removed from the source of exposure by rescuers wearing masks or other devices to protect them from exposure.
        (2) **Oral exposure**
           (a) **Emesis or lavage** may be useful during the first hour.
           (b) **Charcoal** should be administered, as it binds most agents.
           (c) One dose of **cathartic** may be administered with the charcoal.
  2. **Toxin-specific treatment.** Until recently, sulfhemoglobinemia has not been well delineated, and the literature contains few case reports about its treatment. There is no specific antidote to convert sulfhemoglobin to normal hemoglobin, and the only currently available therapy is to replace the damaged hemoglobin with func-

tioning red blood cells via **transfusion.** Theoretically, **hyperbaric oxygen** may provide temporary relief through its ability to add significant amounts of oxygen to the plasma even in the absence of red blood cells. This measure may provide temporary relief to the patient until a transfusion can be performed. Because therapy for sulfhemoglobinemia is not well tested and invasive, it should be reserved for patients with severe or life-threatening intoxication.

References

1. Dolan M, Luban N. Methemoglobinemia in two children. *Pediatr Emerg Care* 1987;3:171.
2. Lanir A, Borochowitz, Kaplan T. Transient methemoglobinemia with acidosis and hyperchloremia in infants. *Am J Pediatr Hematol Oncol* 1986;8:353.
3. Lukens J. The legacy of well water methemoglobinemia. *JAMA* 1987;257:2793.
4. Yano S, Danish E, Hsia Y. Transient methemoglobinemia with acidosis in infants. *J Pediatr* 1982;100:415.
5. Comly H. Cyanosis in infants caused by nitrates in well water. *JAMA* 1945;129:112.
6. Cushing A, Smith S. Methemoglobinemia with silver nitrate therapy of a burn. *J Pediatr* 1969;74:613.
7. Stauch B, et al. Successful treatment of methemoglobinemia secondary to silver nitrate therapy. *N Engl J Med* 1969;281:157.
8. Dinneen S, Mohr D, Fairbanks V. Methemoglobinemia from topically applied anesthetic spray. *Mayo Clin Proc* 1994;69:886–888.
9. Eldadah M, Fitzgerald M. Methemoglobinemia due to skin application of benzocaine. *Clin Pediatr* 1993;32:687–688.
11. Curry S. Methemoglobinemia. *Ann Emerg Med* 1982;14:214.
12. Darling R, Roughton F. The effect of methemoglobin on the equilibrium between oxygen and hemoglobin. *Am J Physiol* 1942;137:56.
13. Finch C. Methemoglobin and sulfhemoglobin. *N Engl J Med* 1948;239:470.
14. Eisenkraft J. Pulse oximeter desaturation due to methemoglobinemia. *Anesthesiology* 1988;68:279.
15. Parks C, Nagel R. Sulfhemoglobinemia: clinical and molecular aspects. *N Engl J Med* 1984;310:1579.
16. Murray K, Meth B. Methemoglobin, Medline, and hyperlipemia. *Crit Care Med* 1987;15:797.
17. Done A. The toxic emergency. *Emerg Med* 1976;8:283.
18. Green E, et al. Phenazopyridine hydrochloride toxicity: a cause of drug induced methemoglobinemia. *JACEP* 1979;8:426.
19. Goldstein G, Doull J. Effect of hyperbaric oxygen of *p*-aminopropiophenone and sodium nitrite induced methemoglobinemia. *Pharmacologist* 1970;12:242.
20. Goldstein G, Doull J. Treatment of nitrite induced methemoglobinemia with hyperbaric oxygen. *Proc Soc Exp Biol Med* 1971;138:137.
21. Smith R, Olson M. *Drug-induced methemoglobinemia.* Orlando, FL: Grune & Stratton, 1973.
22. Goluboff N, Wheaton R. Methylene blue induced cyanosis and acute hemolytic anemia complicating the treatment of methemoglobinemia. *J Pediatr* 1961;58:86.
23. Rosen P, et al. Failure of methylene blue in toxic methemoglobinemia. *Ann Intern Med* 1971;75:83.

Selected Reading

Potter L, et al. Methemoglobinemia due to ingestion of *N.N*-dimethyl-*p*-toluidine. *Ann Emerg Med* 1988;17:1098.

Emergency Toxicology, Second Edition,
edited by Peter Viccellio.
Lippincott–Raven Publishers, Philadelphia © 1998.

12
Anion and Osmolar Gaps

Jonathan Borak

Department of Internal Medicine, Yale Medical School, New Haven, Connecticut 06510

The anion gap (AG) and osmolar gap (OG) are arithmetic calculations derived from routinely available serum electrolyte measurements. They provide insight into the causes and severity of intoxications and acidosis. The AG and OG serve as powerful informational tools that can assist the diagnostic reasoning of clinicians caring for victims of toxic ingestions and exposures. AG and OG are also useful for clarifying the mechanisms underlying clinical acid-base disorders. Moreover, these two relatively simple measures may suggest the presence of other important disturbances unrelated to either toxins or acidosis. The usefulness of the AG and OG stems in part from their ready availability. Both are based primarily on calculations made from the serum electrolytes, values that are rapidly determined and routinely obtained for nearly all unstable emergency patients. Because the information needed to calculate the AG and almost all that needed for OG calculations are part of standard patient evaluations, both measures can be regarded as useful data that are readily available and practically "free."

I. Anion gap
A. Definition
1. **Physiologic solutions,** e.g., serum and extracellular fluid (ECF), exist in a state of electroneutrality where the sum of positive charges is exactly balanced by the sum of negative charges. The concentrations of individual cations and anions (expressed as milliequivalents per liter) may vary, but the sums of cations and anions remain equal.

2. Routine laboratory techniques do not demonstrate this equality, however, because some cations and anions go unmeasured. Typically, serum **electrolyte determinations** consider only sodium, potassium, chloride, and bicarbonate. Sodium and potassium, the most important of serum cations, represent about 95% of total serum cationic components. Chloride and bicarbonate, on the other hand, account for only about 85% of serum anions. As a result, routine determination of serum electrolytes usually indicates an inequality between the sums of measured cations and measured anions. This inequality, as presented in Eq. 1, is often referred to as the AG:

$$AG = (Na^+ + K^+) - (Cl^- + HCO_3^-) \qquad (1)$$

Equation 1 can be further simplified in light of the fact that potassium concentration is generally low (about 4.5 mEq/L) and stable. As a result, variations in potassium concentration contribute little to the AG and can be systematically ignored. Accordingly, the AG can be redefined:

$$AG = Na^+ - (Cl^- + HCO_3^-) \tag{2}$$

Alternatively, the AG can be defined in terms of the electrically charged entities that are not routinely measured by clinical laboratory testing: the serum's unmeasured cations (UC) and unmeasured anions (UA). This definition of the AG derives from the principle of electroneutrality and Eq. 2. It defines the AG as the difference between the unmeasured anions and unmeasured cations:

$$Total\ serum\ cations = total\ serum\ anions$$
$$Na^+ + UC = Cl^- + HCO_3^- + UA$$
$$Na^+ - (Cl^- + HCO_3^-) = UA - UC \tag{3}$$
$$AG = UA - UC$$

B. Unmeasured cations and anions

    1. UCs. A number of electrically charged entities contribute to the pools of unmeasured cations and anions in serum and ECF. The most important of the UCs are calcium, magnesium, and potassium. Normally, calcium contributes about 5 mEq/L, magnesium about 1.5 mEq/L, and potassium about 4.5 mEq/L. Accordingly, the UC level has a normal value of about 11 mEq/L. Rarely, proteins contribute to UCs—proteins that have isoelectric points in excess of 7.4 and therefore are positively charged in physiologic solutions. In general, however, proteins have low isoelectric points, carry net negative charges in serum or ECF, and contribute to the pool of UAs.

    2. UAs include proteins, phosphates, sulfates, and organic acids. In the absence of disease, proteins represent the largest proportion of UAs, about 15 mEq/L. The most important anionic protein is albumin, which contributes about 11 mEq/L to the UAs in individuals with normal albumin levels (about 4 g/dL). Other important components of UAs are organic acids, representing about 5 mEq/L, phosphates about 2 mEq/L, and sulfates about 1 mEq/L. There are normally about 23 mEq of UAs per liter in healthy individuals.

C. Normal AG values. When determined according to Eq. 2 in essentially normal individuals, AG values have generally been reported in the range of 11 to 13 mEq/L with SDs of 1.9 to 2.5 mEq/L. The traditionally accepted normal value for the AG (± 2 SD) is 12 ± 4 mEq/L. Newer laboratory methods, particularly ion-selective electrode assays, report higher values for serum chloride and lower AG values than do older methods using colorimetric and flame photometry assays. In laboratories using this newer method, the normal AG range is 7 ± 4 mEq/L.

D. Abnormal AG values are most commonly associated with the presence of metabolic acidosis. Acidotic states are often classified according to the presence or absence of an abnormal (i.e., elevated) AG. However, an elevated AG can be associated with an assortment of nonacidotic conditions, and decreased AG levels are also encountered. Clinicians should use a systematic approach to determine the underlying cause when an abnormal AG is found. Always consider the possibility that apparently abnormal AG values are due to errors in laboratory measurement or reporting.

1. **Elevated AG values**
   a. Most often associated with acidosis due to accumulation of organic acids.
   b. Elevated AG acidosis can be caused by endogenous or exogenous acids (see **I.E**).
   c. AG elevations may result from accumulation of unmeasured anions that do not cause acidosis.
      (1) Large amounts of penicillin and carbenicillin cause an increased AG.
      (2) Infusions of albumin can produce transient hyperalbuminemia and short-lived elevations of the AG.
   d. Decreased UCs, due to a decreased concentration of potassium, calcium, or magnesium, cause the AG to increase.
      (1) The concentration of no one of these three cations can fall enough to produce significant AG elevation without also causing lethal effects.
      (2) The concentrations of all three cations can be simultaneously depressed, thereby causing an elevated AG: Hypomagnesemia may lead to a secondary decline in calcium and potassium concentrations.
   e. The AG can increase with some forms of alkalosis owing to production of lactic and other organic acids to offset the alkalosis.
      (1) AG rarely increases more than 5 mEq/L in these cases.
      (2) It is most often noted with chronic hypocapnia and after gastric drainage.

2. **Decreased AG values**
   a. Decreased AG is less common than an elevated AG.
   b. Systematic laboratory measurement errors are among the most common causes of measured low AG values.
      (1) High-viscosity serum, as occurs with hyperlipemia, is associated with a falsely low AG. Generally, only grossly lipemic serum causes these effects.
      (2) Automated laboratory devices obtain serum samples with too small a volume from viscous specimens, which leads to falsely low calculated values for the serum sodium concentration. Use of those sodium values yields a falsely low AG.
   c. Hypoalbuminemia is the most common cause. A 50% fall in albumin levels (to about 2 g/L) leads to a 5.5 mEq/L decrease in the AG.
   d. Decreased levels of sulfate or phosphate alone do not significantly contribute because their concentrations are normally low.
   e. Accumulations of UCs result in a lowered AG, e.g., with multiple myeloma, when paraproteins with isoelectric points of more than 7.4 accumulate.
      (1) AG in myeloma patients is generally below normal values, and as many as one-third of these patients have an AG less than 6 mEq/L.
      (2) AG is inversely related to the height of the paraprotein spike.
      (3) Because of its higher isoelectric point, IgG myeloma protein causes this effect more often than other forms of myeloma.
   f. Chronic users of bromides and victims of acute bromide poisoning can have falsely low AG values.

(1) Autoanalyzers do not differentiate between chloride and bromide ions. Results of electrolyte determinations may indicate high chloride levels, which actually represent the sum of chloride and bromide concentrations.

(2) Use of those chloride concentrations to calculate the AG yields falsely low AG values.

E. Elevated AG acidosis

1. Toxins and disease states that can cause an elevated AG acidosis are listed in Table 12-1.

2. **Endogenous causes** occur more frequently than exogenous ones. Most common is uremic acidosis associated with retention of sulfates, phosphates, and other organic acids. Other common causes of elevated AG acidosis include ketoacidosis and lactic acidosis. Production of excessive lactic acid can result from endogenous insults, such as hypoxia and hypoperfusion of tissues, or exogenous ones such as toxic exposures to catecholamines, cyanide, alcohol, or phenformin. In either case, the body produces lactate, which accumulates and leads to both the AG and pH changes.

3. **Exogenous causes** of elevated AG acidosis primarily involve toxic ingestions and exposures.

   a. Methanol poisoning is an important cause of elevated AG acidosis.

   (1) Methanol itself does not affect either the pH or AG; however, it is converted to formic acid which does.

   (2) Profound acidosis and markedly elevated AG occur with formate levels exceeding 20 mEq/L.

   (3) Accumulation of formate, even in the absence of acidosis, has been implicated as the cause of methanol-induced toxicity.

   b. Salicylates provoke both respiratory alkalosis and metabolic acidosis.

TABLE 12-1. *Toxins and disease states leading to elevated anion gap acidosis*

Endogenous causes
  Alcoholic ketoacidosis
  Diabetic ketoacidosis
  Lactic acidosis
  Uremia

Exogenous causes
  Arsenic
  Ethanol
  Ethylene glycol
  Iron
  Isoniazid
  Methanol
  Paraldehyde
  Phenformin
  Salicylates
  Strychnine
  Toluene

      (1)   Acidosis is due to accumulation of salicylate as well as to salicylate-induced production of endogenous organic acids.

      (2)   Both mechanisms contribute to the increased AG.

      (3)   In victims with serum salicylate levels of 75 mg/dL, salicylic acid accounts for about 5 mEq/L of the elevated AG, and endogenous organic acids account for the rest.

  c. **Ethylene glycol** is metabolized to several organic acids, notably glycolic, oxalic, and hippuric acids, which lead to pH and AG abnormalities.

      (1)   Glycolic acid is the most important cause of acidosis, and levels of more than 10 mEq/L occur in severe exposure victims.

      (2)   Ethylene glycol exposure is also associated with endogenous production of lactic acid, which contributes to acidosis and AG elevation.

  d. **Paraldehyde** abuse has been correlated with metabolic acidosis and elevated AG values, particularly in chronic alcoholics. The specific metabolite or endogenous acid leading to high AG and acidosis have not been determined.

  e. **Toluene** exposure results in acidosis and elevated AG due to the production of hippuric acid. Up to 7 g of hippuric acid is excreted in the urine following inhalation exposure to 600 ppm for 8 h.

  f. **Other causes** of elevated AG acidosis are listed below. Generally, they interfere with cellular metabolism and cause the production and accumulation of excessive amounts of lactic acid.

      (1)   Isoniazid

      (2)   Iron

      (3)   Arsenic

      (4)   Phenformin

      (5)   Cyanide

F. **Assessment of acidosis.** If an acid-base disturbance is suspected, either because of an elevated AG or for other clinical reasons, the patient is assessed using arterial blood gas (ABG) determinations. That test measures the blood pH and $Paco_2$ levels, which are then used to determine the nature of the disturbance.

  1. **Acid-base disorders** are classified according to the direction of pH disturbance (acidosis or alkalosis), the underlying mechanism (respiratory, metabolic, or mixed), and the duration (acute or chronic). For each set of classifications, there is an expected range of pH and $Paco_2$ values.

  2. **Expected pH and $Paco_2$ ranges** are presented in Fig. 12-1 in the form of an acid-base map. Empirically derived significance bands for each of six "simple" acid-base disturbances are found on that map (metabolic acidosis, metabolic alkalosis, acute and chronic respiratory acidosis, acute and chronic respiratory alkalosis). For patients suffering any of these six simple disturbances, there is a 95% probability that the measured pH and $Paco_2$ will fall inside the respective significance band.

  3. The map can be used to confirm clinical impressions and to indicate situations in which more complex mixed acid-base disturbances may be present. For example, consider a patient found to have an elevated AG. ABG determinations are then performed. If the pH and $Paco_2$ levels fall within the significance band for metabolic

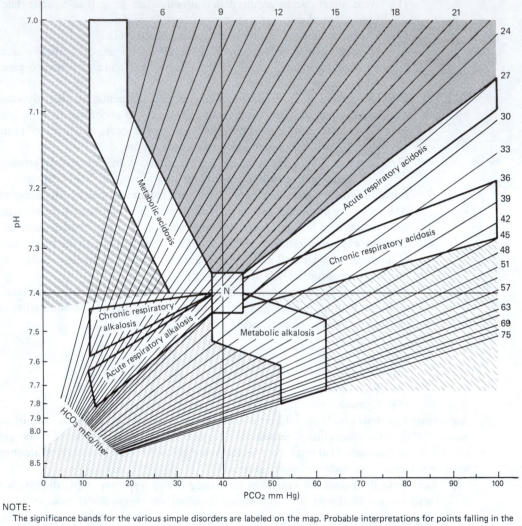

NOTE:

The significance bands for the various simple disorders are labeled on the map. Probable interpretations for points falling in the cross hatched areas between are:

- mixed respiratory and metabolic acidosis
- mixed metabolic acidosis and respiratory alkalosis
- mixed respiratory and metabolic alkalosis
- mixed respiratory acidosis and metabolic alkalosis

The lines that fan diagonally from the lower left-hand corner represent serum bicarbonates corresponding to the values given across the bottom and down the left side within the diagram.

FIG. 12-1. Nomogram for the solution of acid-base interrelations. Carbon dioxide tension (PaCO₂) is shown on the horizontal axis and pH on the vertical axis. (From N. Flomenbaum. Acid-base disturbances. *Emerg. Med.* 1984;16(3):65; adapted from M. Goldberg et al. Computer based instruction and diagnosis of acid-base disorders. *JAMA* 1973;223:269; also F. J. Myers, and B. E. Pennock. The acid-base map—an additional tool for dealing with a difficult problem. *Res Staff Phys.* 1979; 25:45. With permission.)

acidosis, simple acidosis is likely. On the other hand, if the results do not fall within that band, there is a high probability that the patient is suffering from a mixed disturbance.

G. **Acid-base effects on electrolytes.** As the calculated AG depends on measured levels of serum electrolytes, it is also relevant to consider the effects of that acid-base disturbances effect on measured electrolyte levels. It has been known for many years that alterations of systemic acid-base balance significantly affect renal potassium handling and systemic potassium levels.

   1. **Acidosis** is associated with **hyperkalemia.** The mechanisms of this serum potassium increase are two fold: potassium shifts from intra- to extracellular compartments to compensate for the cellular uptake of hydrogen ions; and, inhibition of Na^+/K^+ ATPase activity leading to decreased renal tubular secretion of potassium.

   2. **Alkalosis** can result in the opposite metabolic perturbations resulting typically in **hypokalemia.**

   3. Such electrolyte alterations may lead to slight understatement of calculated AG, but they are not likely to significantly alter the meaning of the calculated AG.

II. **Osmolar gap**

   A. **Definition**

      1. **Osmolality** is a reflection of the number of solute particles in a solution. Numerical measures of osmolality express the number of particles present in a given *weight* of solvent. Only the total number of particles and their concentration are important. It does not matter whether solute particles are large or small, electrically charged or neutral.

      2. **Osmolarity** is a similar measure that expresses the number of solute particles present in a given *volume,* rather than a given weight, of solvent. Because clinical laboratory determinations of serum and ECF solutes are expressed in terms of solvent volumes rather than weights, the osmolarity is a measure of greater clinical usefulness than osmolality. Fortunately, there is little difference between values of osmolality and osmolarity when determined for solutes at concentrations normally found in physiologic solutions. Accordingly, the two can be used interchangeably for clinical applications without need for corrections.

         a. Serum osmolarity can be **measured directly,** as described below, *or calculated* from readily available laboratory data:

         $$\text{Osmolarity} = 2(Na^+) + \text{glucose} \div 18 + \text{BUN} \div 2.8 \tag{4a}$$

         If the serum ethanol level is also known, then the following equation is the preferred approach for calculating serum osmolarity:

         $$\text{Osmolarity} = 2(Na^+) + \text{glucose} \div 18 + \text{BUN} \div 2.8 + \text{ethanol} \div 4.6 \tag{4b}$$

         Equations 4a and 4b incorporate generally accepted, mutually offsetting approximations. For calculation purposes, the osmolarity of serum electrolytes is estimated by doubling the serum sodium concentration. However, sodium chloride has an osmotic coefficient of only 1.86 and is incompletely dissociated in physiologic solutions. Accordingly, Eq. 4 tends to overestimate the osmolarity due to sodium chloride. On the other hand, osmolarity values are calculated for serum but measured for water. Because the water content of serum is about 93% (depending on the concentration of serum proteins and lipids), Eq. 4 tends to understate osmolarity. Fortunately, these two opposing errors tend to cancel out and allow the simplified equation to be used.

   b. Under normal conditions, there is a relatively small difference between the serum osmolarity value that is determined by direct measurement and that calculated using Eqs. 4a or 4b. With some disease states and following certain toxic exposures and ingestions, however, the difference between measured and calculated osmolarity can be large. That difference is the OG.

B. Osmolality measurements

   1. Dissolved solutes affect four physicochemical properties of solvents: boiling point, freezing point, vapor pressure, and osmotic pressure. Effects on those properties, which are known as *colligative properties,* are directly related to the number of particles in solution. Addition of 1 g molecular weight (MW) of solute, which contains 6.023×10^{23} particles (Avogadro's number), to 1 kg of water causes the following alterations to water's physicochemical properties: boiling point increased by 0.52°C; freezing point decreased by 1.86°C; vapor pressure decreased by 0.3 mm Hg; and osmotic pressure increased by 17,000 mm Hg.

   2. Theoretically, serum osmolality (and osmolarity) can be determined by assessing alterations of any of these four colligative properties.

   a. In practice, most clinical laboratories use **freezing point** determinations as the method of choice for measuring serum osmolality.

   b. **Boiling point** determinations can be problematic because they require correction for barometric pressure and denaturation of serum proteins. Moreover, volatile substances, such as methanol and ethanol, may go undetected because they vaporize from solution at temperatures below water's boiling point and therefore fail to contribute to boiling point elevations.

   c. **Vapor pressure** measurements are unable to detect the presence of volatile compounds because those compounds do not proportionately affect water's vapor pressure: The decreased vapor pressure of water is offset by the increased vapor pressure of the volatile substances in water solution. In addition, vapor pressure determinations are upwardly biased when lipemic serum is tested.

C. Normal OG values. The measured osmolality in normal, healthy adults is 285 to 286 ± 4.2 to 4.3 mOsm/kg (SD) with a range of 275 to 300 mOsm/kg. The calculated osmolarity is normally less than the measured value. The generally accepted normal value for the OG is generally regarded as less than 10 mOsm/L, but a recent study found that normal values ranged from +15 mOsm/L to −5 mOsm/L. Thus, a negative OG may be normal.

D. Abnormal OG values are most common when large amounts of low–molecular-weight solutes are dissolved in the serum and ECF. The OG depends on the number of particles present as solute, not the size or weight of those particles. Only a limited number of substances are compatible with life at concentrations causing significant elevations of OG. Clinicians should use a systematic approach to determine the underlying cause when an abnormal OG is found. Always consider the possibility that apparently abnormal OG values are due to errors in laboratory measurement or reporting.

1. **Elevated OG value**
   a. Most often occurs with increased measured osmolality and normal calculated osmolality due to accumulation of large amounts of osmotically active solutes not normally included in the osmolality calculation.
      (1) A limited number of toxins can cause significant elevation of OG without also causing lethal effects.
      (2) The most common toxic cause of an elevated OG is ethanol. Other toxic substances that elevate the OG and their osmolal effects at lethal blood levels are listed in Table 12-2.
      (3) Nontoxic solutes that elevate the OG are sorbitol, mannitol, glycerin, and diatrizoate sodium.
   b. OG elevations with a normal measured serum osmolality suggest decreased serum water content.
      (1) Conditions that lead to significant decreases of serum water are hyperlipidemia and hyperproteinemia.

TABLE 12-2. *Contributions of toxic substances to serum osmolality at potentially lethal levels*

Substance	MW (kDa)	Lethal level (mg/dl)	Osmolality (mOsm/kg H_2O)
Ethanol	46	350	80.0
Ethyl ether	26	180	70.0
Isopropanol	60	340	60.0
Methanol	32	80	27.0
Acetone	58	55	10.0
Trichloroethane	133	100	9.0
Paraldehyde	132	50	4.0
Ethylene glycol	62	21	3.5
Chloroform	119	39	3.5
Salicylate	180	50	3.0
Chloral hydrate	165	25	1.6
Ethchlorvynol	144	15	1.1
Meprobamate	218	30	1.0
Phenobarbital	232	15	0.7
Barbital	184	10	0.6
Glutethimide	217	10	0.5
Diphenylhydantoin	252	10	0.4
Dinitro-O-cresol	198	7.5	0.4
Methamphetamine	149	4	0.3
Meperidine	247	3	0.1
Methaqualone	250	3	0.1
Secobarbital	238	3	0.1
Toluene	92	1	0.1

Modified from Glasser et al. (1973).

(2) Abnormally high levels of plasma solids displace serum water and cause falsely low serum sodium determinations. Use of those sodium values yields falsely low calculated osmolality and a falsely elevated OG.

(3) Usually serum must be grossly lipemic before decreased serum water is detected. Only a severe dysproteinemia causes an elevated OG, e.g., multiple myeloma with a total protein concentration more than 10 g/dL.

(4) Proteins and triglycerides are such large molecules that, even at high blood levels, they add little to the measured osmolality.

2. **Negative OG values**

a. They do not occur physiologically.

b. If the calculated osmolarity is greater than the measured osmolality, laboratory or arithmetic error should be suspected.

E. OG and calculation of blood alcohol

1. The most common **exogenous causes** of increased OG are alcohols, particularly ethanol, methanol, and isopropanol. When direct measurement of the blood alcohol level is not rapidly or readily available, the osmolar effects of these substances can be used to estimate their blood levels. This estimate can be useful for the management of trauma victims and other comatose patients when directly measured levels of blood alcohol are delayed.

2. **Calculation.** The blood level of an alcohol known (or suspected) to have been ingested is estimated by multiplying the OG by the MW of that particular alcohol and dividing by 10: Blood level nearly equal to (OG × MW of alcohol) divided by 10 (5) where MW of ethanol = 46; MW of methanol = 32; and MW of isopropanol = 60.

F. **Summary.** The AG and OG are simple to derive and useful clinically for evaluating acidotic patients and those with suspected intoxications. In addition, the AG and OG provide insights into the presence of other potentially important clinical conditions. In light of the ease with which they are calculated and their general applicability, all clinicians should be familiar with their computation and use.

Selected Readings

Barlow WK. Volatiles and osmometry. *Clin Chem* 1976;22:1230.

Bradbury SM, Vale JA. Disturbances of potassium homeostasis in poisoning. *J Toxicol Clin Toxicol* 1995;33:295.

Champion HR, et al. Alcohol intoxication and serum osmolality. *Lancet* 1975;1:1402.

Emmett M, Narins RG. Clinical use of the anion gap. *Medicine (Baltimore)* 1977;56:38.

Field MJ, et al. Regulation of renal potassium metabolism. In: Narins RG, ed. *Maxwell and Kleeman's clinical disorders of fluid and electrolyte metabolism.* New York: McGraw-Hill, 1994.

Fischman CM, Oster JR. Toxic effects of toluene; a new cause of high anion gap metabolic acidosis. *JAMA* 1979;24:1713.

Flomenbaum N. Acid-base disturbances. *Emerg Med* 1984;16:65.

Gennari FJ. Serum osmolality. *N Engl J Med* 1984;310:102.

Glasser L, et al. Serum osmolality and its applicability to drug overdose. *Am J Clin Pathol* 1973;60:695.

Goldberg M, et al. Computer-based instruction and diagnosis of acid-base disorders. *JAMA* 1973;223:269.

Hoffman RS, et al. Osmol gaps revisited: normal values and limitations. *Clin Toxicol* 1993;31:81.

Jacobsen D, et al. Anion and osmolal gaps in the diagnosis of methanol and ethylene glycol poisoning. *Acta Med Scand* 1982;212:17.

Levin-Scherz JK, et al. Acute arsenic ingestion. *Ann Emerg Med* 1987;16:702.

Martin-Amat KE, et al. Methanol poisoning: ocular toxicity produced by formate. *Toxicol Appl Pharmacol* 1978;45:201.

Murphy JE, Preuss HG, Henry JB. Evaluation of renal function and water, electrolyte, and acid-base balance. In: Henry JB, ed. *Clinical diagnosis and management by laboratory methods*. 17th ed. Philadelphia: WB Saunders, 1984.

Murray T, Long W, Narins RG. Multiple myeloma and the anion gap. *N Engl J Med* 1975;292:574.

Myers FJ, Pennock BE. The acid-base map—an additional tool for dealing with a difficult problem. *Resident Staff Physician* 1979;25:45.

Oh MS, Carroll HJ. The anion gap. *N Engl J Med* 1977;297:814.

Pappas AA, Gadsden RH, Taylor EH. Serum osmolality in acute intoxication: a prospective clinical study. *Am J Clin Pathol* 1985;84:74.

Sejersted OM, et al. Formate concentrations in plasma from patients poisoned with methanol. *Acta Med Scand* 1983;213:105.

Smithline N, Gardner KD. Gaps—anionic and osmolal. *JAMA* 1976;236:1594.

Winter SD, et al. The fall of the serum anion gap. *Arch Intern Med* 1990;150:311.

Emergency Toxicology, Second Edition,
edited by Peter Viccellio.
Lippincott–Raven Publishers, Philadelphia © 1998.

13

Nontoxic Ingestions

†Adam L. Church and °Nina Mazur

*†Department of Emergency Medicine, North Shore University Hospital,
Manhasset, New York 11030; °Deceased*

There were more than 1.9 million human exposure cases reported by the 65 poison centers of the Association of Poison Control Centers in 1994. A total of 42.4% of these exposures had no effects or were deemed nontoxic by the poison information specialists. More than 85% of all exposures had minimal or minor effects that required no follow-up. The ability to determine if an exposure is toxic or not is a tremendously important and valuable skill. It is very difficult to separate toxic and nontoxic by mere list alone as most of the substances on the earth are potentially toxic given the right circumstances. Toxicity is dependent on the amount, route, inherent toxicity, host (allergies, liver or kidney problems, pregnancy, etc.), and time of exposure (acute versus chronic). To evaluate if an exposure is nontoxic, the health care worker must take all of these factors into account. Histories must be done carefully and diligently to assess the following criteria, which have been modified from Mofenson et al.:

1. **Absolute identification of product.** Ability to reference ingredients per manufacturer. Labels must be read carefully and completely. (a) Name spelled correctly: packaging may be very similar. Clorox contains sodium hypochlorite, while Clorox 2 contains sodium carbonate. (b) Year of manufacture. Formulations change without trade name changes. (c) Form: liquid versus crystal. Crystals usually are more concentrated. Drano liquid contain sodium hydroxide and 1,1,1-trichloroethane. Drano granules contain NaOH.
2. **Route of exposure** identified.
3. Absolute assurance that only a **single product** was involved in the exposure.
4. No Consumer Product Safety Commission **signal word** on container (see Table 28-2).
5. Good approximation of **amount exposed/ingested,** i.e., container size. Children swallow approximately 1 tsp. Adults swallow approximately 3 to 4 tsp. Males move slightly bigger boluses than females.
6. Presence of **symptoms** and ability to call back frequently to assess for change.
7. **Ingestions in children:** <1 or >5 years old should be viewed as suspicious. An in depth social situation review is required. Repeated ingestions or adult ingestions usually require hospital evaluation to assess intent. If every substance on the earth is potentially toxic, it is our job to determine if a particular exposure will have no adverse effects. Toxicologic publications are more frequently using the terms no observed effect level (NOEL) or no observed adverse effect level (NOAEL). Reporting centers may use these terms interchangeably. These terms represent the maximum dose that produces no significant adverse effects. We as health care practitioners by taking a careful history try to determine if the NOEL or NOAEL

has been surpassed. Since 1983, data for clinical toxicology of commercial products have been computerized as part of the National Institutes of Health, Environmental Protection Agency, Chemical Information System (NH-EPA-CIS) and are available worldwide.

I. **Nontoxic substances.** Table 13-1 lists many substances that are generally considered nontoxic. Further information on some specific substances follows.

    A. Most of the **nontoxic arts and crafts products** are specifically made for children. The art and craft products that are made for industrial or professional use can be toxic because of appreciable amounts of pigment. Examples highlight the dangerous ingredients:

TABLE 13-1. *Nontoxic substances*

A&D ointment	Disposable diapers	Mineral oil
Abrasives (silicates)	Douches	Miracle Gro Plant Food
After-shave powders	Easter egg dyes	Newspaper
Air fresheners	Erasers	Nutrasweet
Ajax Cleaner	Etch-A-Sketch	Paste, library type
Aluminum foil	Eye makeup	Pastels
Antacids	(pencil, shadow, mascara)	Pencil lead (graphite)
Antibiotic ointments	Fabric softener	Petroleum jelly
Ashes (wood)	Felt-tip markers and pens	Photographs
Baby preparations	Fertilizer (without herbicides	Plaster (non–lead-containing)
Cream	or insecticides)	Plastics
Oil	Finger paint	Play Doh
Powder	Fingernail polish	Preparation H
Soap	Fish bowl additives	(suppository/ointment)
Shampoo	Fluoride—caries preventive	Prussian blue (ferricyanide)
Bleach (<5% hypochlorite)	Glade Plug In	Rouge
Body conditioners	Glitter	Rubber cements
Bubble bath	Glowstick (dibutyl phalate)	Rug cleaners
Calamine lotion	Glues and pastes	(most: Glory, Resolve, Woolite)
Candies	(if nontoxic label)	Rust
Caps (chlorates)	Golf ball components	Sachets (essential oils)
Cat food	Grease	Shaving cream
Cat litter	Gypsum	Shoe polish
Chalk	Hair products (not Lindane,	Silica gel
Chapstick	alcoholic, or straighteners)	Silly putty
Charcoal	Hand lotions and creams	Soaps and soap products
Cigarette ashes	Hydrogen peroxide (3%)	Soil spackles
Clay (modeling)	Indelible markers	Starch
Cleansing creams and lotions	Ink	Sunscreen and suntan
Comet Cleaner	Incense	preparations
Contraceptive pills (without iron)	Iodophor disinfectant	Teething rings
Corticosteroid ointments	Kaolin	Thermometers
Corticosteroids	Lanolin	(mercury, phalthalates, alcohol)
Cough drops	Latex paint	Toilet water
Crayola products (all)	Laxatives	Toothpaste
Crazy Glue (cyanoacrylate)	Lipstick	Vitamins (without iron)
Cyclamate	Lotrimin cream	Warfarin (single dose, <0.5%)
Dehumidifying packets	Lubricants	Water color paint
(silica or charcoal)	Lysol disinfectant (70% ethanol)	Windex Glass Cleaner With
Deodorants (underarm)	spray (not toilet bowl cleaner)	Ammonia D
Detergents (anionic)	Makeup (eye, liquid facial)	Zinc oxide
Dishwashing liquid soap	Mascara (domestic)	Zirconium oxide
(not automatic dishwasher)	Matches (book type, ≤3 books)	

cadmium sulfate in yellow, arsenic in violet, and copper in green. It should be noted that flake white paint for preparing canvas for oil painting contains lead and is exempt from the lead in paint ban under the U.S. Consumer Product Safety Act. However, it must contain appropriate warning labels. The presence of the Art & Creative Materials Institute, Inc. (ACMI) seals (Fig. 13-1) **certified product** (CP) or **approved product** (AP) seal on a crayon, watercolor, or craft product easily identifies nontoxic varieties. Crayons and pastels are grouped into two major categories: children's and industrial/professional. Children's crayons are further subdivided into wax and pressed crayons, both of which are nontoxic. Finger paints also carry the CP or AP seal. It should be noted that some imported crayons were recently found to contain lead. Industrial crayons and artist's pastels may be highly toxic because of lead chromate, organic, or inorganic contents.

B. **Glues.** There are many available that are rated as nontoxic. Stick glues and children's glues that are nontoxic carry the AP or CP label. All the other glues (e.g., model, rubber, contact, waterproof) may be considered toxic.

C. **Pencil lead** provokes frequent worried inquiries from parents for both ingestion and superficial puncture wounds and foreign body incidents. Pencil lead is graphite, not lead, and is relatively biologically inert. Inhalation of graphite powder has caused allergic symptoms and benign pneumoconiosis. Failure to completely remove any remnants of pencil lead embedded in the skin leaves a permanent "tattoo." Though cosmetically unaesthetic, there are no medical sequelae.

D. **Petroleum jelly** (Vaseline) can produce a mild laxative effect not requiring treatment.

E. **Candles** (paraffin waxes) are not digested or absorbed and so pass through the system unchanged. Decorative candles may contain a variety organic or inorganic matter which may be toxic if ingested or burned.

F. **Starch** (amylum) is used for starching and sizing fabrics. Amylophagia, the eating of starch, particularly during pregnancy, is recognized as a common form of pica in certain localities. In one review, the incidence was as high as 35%. Some women retain the habit for years and may ingest several pounds of starch daily. Because starch accounts for the bulk of the diet, the commonly observed iron deficiency anemia may be the result of the practice, not its cause.

G. **Talcum powder** is worth considering separately. Though it is completely harmless and inert when ingested, it can be **hazardous when inhaled.** The hazard is both acute and chronic: acute in cases of massive aspiration by infants and chronic in cases of industrial exposures in talc miners. Infants have died from pulmonary edema and pneumonia within hours after inhaling talcum powder. The powder dries the mucous membranes of the bronchioles, disrupts pulmonary clearance, and clogs small airways. Victims usually display dyspnea, tachypnea, tachycardia, cyanosis, and fever. Bronchopulmonary lavage is not effective because talc is insoluble in water. One child who survived a massive aspiration of baby powder later developed progressive diffuse pulmonary fibrosis. This fact brings us back to the concept that it is not only the product, but the quantity and the mode of exposure, that determine toxicity.

H. **Pepper,** the common household spice, is lethal to rats at a dose of 12.5 g/kg. In an unusual homicide, a mother poured the entire contents of a pepper shaker into the mouth of her 4-year-old daughter, and the child died of asphyxiation.

I. **Thermometers** employ a number of fluids, depending on the intended use. Clinical thermometers usually contain about 0.1 ml of mercury, an amount that presents no ingestion hazard. In general, the toxicity of metallic mercury and most mercury compounds depends on in vivo release of the mercuric ion. It should be noted that mercury has increased toxicity in the vapor form, thus spills should not be cleaned up with a vacuum cleaner. Thermometers used to measure for ambient temperatures, indoor and out, may contain triethyl phosphate, toluene, xylene, or one of several alcohols. These thermometers contain 0.3 to 0.5 ml, never more than 1 ml. Thermometers for Arctic weather measurements contain pentane. Cooking thermometers contain methylbenzoate. All these thermometers have two factors in common: The amount of liquid in any thermometer is small, and the liquids are not highly toxic. Thus thermometers do not represent a severe toxic hazard.

J. **Symptomatic tobacco** ingestions commonly produce vomiting and sometimes lethargy or irritability. Tobacco ingestions can be fatal and are addressed in the nicotine chapter. According to the AAPCC there were no fatalities in 8,758 tobacco product exposures in 1994. However, five cases were noted to have major detrimental outcomes.

K. **Cured plastics** are nontoxic except for hypersensitivity reactions. These reactions have been attributed to small amounts of hardener remaining with the finished product. Non-cured plastics and some glues contain hardeners which are strongly alkaline, pH 13 to 14, and may produce chemical burns.

L. **Hair spray** although considered nontoxic may cause chronic lung changes similar to sarcoid (thesaurosis).

M. **Confirmed nonexposures** are difficult to establish with certainty. Nationally, in 1994, there were 6,115 cases where reliable evidence indicated that exposure never occurred.

Selected Readings

Art & Creative Materials Institute. *What you need to know about the safety of art & craft materials.* Boston: Art & Creative Materials Institute, 1994.

Finkel AJ, Hamilton A, Hardy H. *Hamilton and Hardy's industrial toxicology.* 4th ed. John Wright PSG Inc., Littleton, MA, 1983.

Goldfrank L. *Goldfrank's toxicologic emergencies.* 5th ed. East Norwalk, CT: Appleton & Lange, 1994.

Gosselin R. *Clinical toxicology of commercial products.* 5th ed. Baltimore: Williams & Wilkins, 1984.

Litovitz TL, et al. *1994 annual report of the American Association of Poison Control Centers toxic exposure surveillance system.* Amer J Emerg Med 1995; 551–597.

Mofenson HC, Greensher J, Caraccio TR. Ingestions considered to be nontoxic. *Emerg Med Clin North Am* 1984;2:159–174.

Mofenson HC, Greensher J. The non-toxic ingestion. *Pediatr Clin North Am* 1970;17:583–590.

Rosen P. *Emergency medicine concepts and clinical practice.* 2nd ed. St. Louis: Mosby, 1988.

Seiler HG, Sigel H, Sigel A. *Handbook on toxicity of inorganic compounds.* New York; Marcel Dekker Inc, 1988.

Tardiff RG, Rodricks J. *Toxic substances and human risk: principles of data interpretation.* New York: Plenum Publishing, 1987.

Tintinalli J. *Emergency medicine: a comprehensive study guide.* 2nd ed. New York: McGraw-Hill, 1988.

Additional information may be obtained from the Center for Safety in the Arts/NYFA (CSA), which is the only national resource center for information on health and safety in the visual and performing arts. CSA, 155 Avenue of the Americas, New York, NY 10013. (212) 366-6900.

Emergency Toxicology, Second Edition,
edited by Peter Viccellio.
Lippincott–Raven Publishers, Philadelphia © 1998.

14

Chemical Warfare Agents

Frederick R. Sidell

Bel Air, Maryland 21014

Chemical warfare agents have long been considered compounds of military interest only. However, the release of the nerve agent sarin in Tokyo subways in March 1995 called attention to this group of compounds as possible terrorist weapons. The major chemical warfare agents are the nerve agents and the vesicant, sulfur mustard. Cyanide was used unsuccessfully in World War I and was allegedly used against the Kurds by Iraq in March 1988; its precursors were found in Japanese subway stations after the nerve agent attack. It is discussed elsewhere in this volume. Phosgene and chlorine, other World War I agents, are also covered in other chapters. The riot control agents ("tear gas"), used by law enforcement officials and by the military in training, are briefly discussed below.

I. **Nerve agents** are the most toxic chemical warfare agents. They were developed pre–World War II by Germany; their only known battlefield use was by Iraq against Iran. They were used twice by terrorists in Japan: the first was in Matsumoto in June 1994, where there were about 600 casualties and seven deaths, and the second was in the Tokyo subways in March 1995, which caused 5,510 people to seek medical attention and 12 deaths. Nerve agents are identical in their biological activity to organophosphorus insecticides, e.g., Malathion; to carbamate insecticides, e.g., carbaryl; and to carbamate medications, e.g., pyridostigmine, neostigmine, and physostigmine.

   A. **Properties:** The nerve agents are esters of phosphoric acid. The major nerve agents are GA (tabun; ethyl *N,N*-dimethylphosphoroamidocyanidate), GB (sarin; isopropyl methylphosphonofluoridate), GD (soman; pinacolyl methyl phosphonofluoridate), and VX (*O*-ethyl-*S*-(2-isopropylaminoethyl)methyl phosphonothiolate). Under temperate conditions, they are clear, colorless liquids. (The commonly used term "nerve gases" is incorrect; the agents are liquids.) Several (GA, GD) have faint odors, but these are not distinctive enough for detection. Their freezing points range from −30°C to −56°C, and their boiling points from 158°C to 298°C. Their volatilities range from about the volatility of water (GB) to that of light motor oil (VX). Their vapors are heavier than air, so they tend to sink into valleys, trenches, and basements.

   B. **Pathophysiology:** Nerve agents exert their biological effects by **inhibition of the enzyme acetylcholinesterase.** Normally this enzyme hydrolyzes, or breaks down, the neurotransmitter acetylcholine at those structures having cholinergic receptor sites. In the presence of an inhibitor (nerve agents and their close relatives the organophosphate and carbamate insecticides and carbamate drugs) acetylcholine is not destroyed and continues to stimulate the structure causing hyperactivity of the muscle, gland, or nerve. These structures include those with muscarinic receptor sites (exocrine glands and smooth muscles) and with nicotinic receptor sites (primarily skeletal muscles and autonomic ganglia). Hyperactivity of these structures causes the signs and symptoms of nerve agent poisoning (and the signs and symptoms of poisoning by organophosphate insecticides and carbamates).

1. Cholinesterase, in a slightly different form, is found on the red cells (where it is known as erythrocyte-, red cell-, or acetyl-cholinesterase) and in the plasma (where it is known as plasma-, serum-, or butyryl-cholinesterase); this latter enzyme preferentially hydrolyzes butyrylcholine). These enzymes are routinely monitored in people who work with nerve agents or organophosphate insecticides. Different cholinesterase inhibitors preferentially inhibit one or the other blood enzyme. Nerve agents preferentially inhibit the red cell enzyme; many insecticides preferentially inhibit the plasma enzyme. Even with a compound that preferentially inhibits the plasma enzyme, acute clinical effects correlate better with red cell cholinesterase inhibition (1).

C. The **initial clinical effects** from a sublethal amount depend on the route of exposure and the amount of exposure. Most human exposures to these agents, both from accidents in the U.S. development and production program many decades ago and from the Japanese experiences, have been by vapor exposure. A sublethal droplet on the skin causes a different clinical presentation.

1. **Vapor**

   a. Exposure to a small amount of vapor causes effects in the sensitive organs of the face. Eyes: miosis with size of the pupil decreasing as amount of exposure increases; conjunctival injection with possible subconjunctival hemorrage; pain in or around the eye or head; nausea and vomiting (thought to be a reflex action); and complaints of "dim vision" (from miosis and possibly disruption of cholinergic pathways in the CNS) and "blurred vision." Nose: rhinorrhea. Mouth: salivation. Airways: bronchoconstriction and bronchosecretions with complaints ranging from "my chest is tight" to obvious severe dyspnea (after a small exposure the airway effects may reverse within 15 to 30 min).

   b. Exposure to a large amount of vapor will cause loss of consciousness within seconds, followed several minutes later by convulsions. These stop within minutes as muscles become flaccid and breathing stops.

   c. Vapor alone, i.e., no associated liquid exposure, causes almost immediate effects; these effects reach maximal intensity within minutes and do not worsen significantly once the patient is out of the contaminated atmosphere.

2. **Liquid on skin**

   a. A very small droplet on the skin (estimates of the LD_{50} on skin range from 10 mg for the nonvolatile VX to 1,700 mg for the volatile GB; the higher estimates for the G-agents are because these agents tend to evaporate rather than to penetrate the skin) may cause muscular fasciculations and sweating at the site, but these are rarely noticed. A larger, but nonlethal amount, will cause gastrointestinal (GI) effects—nausea, vomiting, cramping, and diarrhea—along with complaints of muscular weakness. The onset of these effects may be as long as 18 h after contact, and they may occur even if the site were decontaminated soon after exposure.

b. A large amount on skin, the LD_{50} or greater, will cause a precipitate cascade of events starting within 30 min of contact, which may occur even though decontamination occurred shortly after contact. This sequence, following an asymptomatic interval, consists of sudden loss of consciousness, followed by convulsions, muscular flaccidity, and apnea, all occurring within minutes of onset.

c. After skin contact with liquid, there is usually an asymptomatic interval of several minutes to many hours before the sudden onset of effects; these effects may worsen as more agent enters the circulation from the layers of the skin.

D. The **diagnosis** is made by the history, symptoms, physical examination, and laboratory findings.

1. **History.** The patient may be able to relate that he was on or near a military installation where nerve agent is stored and started to have dim vision, rhinorrhea, and/or difficulty breathing ("tightness in my chest"). Or he may say that he was in a public place and people around him were clutching their chests and falling down, some perhaps convulsing. If the patient is unconscious, the rescuers may provide a history that he was found unconscious, gasping for air, with copious salivations, and possibly bleeding from the mouth from having convulsed.

2. **Initial symptoms** of vapor exposure are dim vision ("like putting on sunglasses"), rhinorrhea, and some degree of dyspnea. After a sublethal amount of liquid on the skin, the initial symptoms are GI: vomiting, cramps, and diarrhea.

3. **Physical examination** varies depending on route and amount of exposure. A small amount of vapor will usually cause miosis, rhinorrhea, and abnormal chest sounds. A sublethal droplet may produce signs of increased GI activity. (A person exposed to liquid usually will not have miosis unless the exposure was severe.) A severely exposed casualty will be convulsing or flaccid, will be gasping for air (with abnormal breath sounds) or apneic, will have miosis, will have copious secretions from the mouth and nose, and, very characteristically, will have generalized muscular fasciculations.

4. **Laboratory**

a. The most characteristic laboratory finding is an **inhibition of red blood cell cholinesterase** (RBC-ChE). There is a large variation in the activity of this enzyme in a normal population, and a marginal decrease from a normal mean may not be diagnostic. A person severely symptomatic (as described above) will have an enzyme activity close to 0% of the average normal activity (2). The person with systemic effects from liquid on the skin will also have a decrease of under 30% of the normal average (3). However, a person with mild to moderate effects from vapor exposure may have normal RBC-ChE activity or may have a markedly inhibited enzyme activity (3). There is no correlation between these vapor effects (which are "local" or "topical") and the systemic enzyme activity. Plasma cholinesterase activity is affected to a lesser degree by these agents and it will be markedly inhibited in a severe exposure, but it is a less useful measure than the RBC-ChE.

b. Prolonged **hypoxia** from seizure activity will cause a decreased arterial content of oxygen and a metabolic acidosis.

c. The **EKG** is generally unremarkable. Sinus tachycardia is usually present in less severe exposures and is often present in severe exposures. These agents can produce various degrees of heart block, but these are usually transient. ST-T wave changes may follow hypoxia. (Torsade de pointes has been described after OP insecticide poisoning.)

d. **Electrolytes** are generally normal until hypoxia and acidosis occur.

e. **Chest x-ray** is normal in the acute state; infectious complications with accompanying x-ray signs may occur after intubation and prolonged ventilation.

E. **Differential diagnosis.** The full-blown clinical presentation of a person severely intoxicated with a cholinesterase inhibitor is characteristic: miosis, increased secretions, convulsions or flaccidity, marked breathing difficulty or apnea, generalized muscular fasciculations, and loss of consciousness.

1. **Other cholinesterase inhibitors:** OP or carbamate insecticides and carbamate drugs cause the same effects.

2. The **incomplete syndrome** may present problems in diagnosis: difficulty in breathing may be caused by many airway irritants, and often the patient will give a history of previous episodes; and GI symptoms may be caused by common causes of gastroenteritis.

F. **Management**

1. **Self-protection:** The most important aspect of managing a patient from any type of chemical exposure is for the medical care provider to protect himself. Otherwise, there will be one more casualty and one less care provider. This is done by wearing appropriate protective mask (filtration mask approved for these agents or SCBA), gloves, rubber apron, and boots; or insuring that the casualty has been thoroughly decontaminated if he was exposed to a liquid. (Much experience has shown that patients exposed to vapor only do not need to be decontaminated after they have had a period of exposure to fresh air, e.g., during transport; this was confirmed by the Tokyo subway experience.)

2. **Standard life support measures:** Generally, the most important of these (unless there are traumatic injuries also) is ventilation. In an unconscious patient, an endotracheal tube should be inserted as soon as possible both to assist in providing ventilation and to make suction of secretions easier. Assisting ventilation may be difficult initially because of the high resistance from the intense bronchoconstriction; intramuscular atropine (not intravenous atropine in a hypoxia patient) will soon decrease the resistance.

3. **Decontamination:** Clothing removal is adequate for patients exposed to vapor only who have been in fresh air. Patients with liquid exposure should be totally stripped, and their skin should be throughly flushed with soap and water or hypochlorite (bleach). If hypochlorite is used, it should be followed by a water wash.

4. **Antidotes**

   a. **Atropine:** Atropine is the mainstay of therapy. It is a competitive antagonist of acetylcholine at muscarinic sites and will reduce the effects of intoxication at the smooth muscles and glands. Airway constriction, GI effects, and secretions will decrease after an adequate amount of atropine. Atropine can be given i.m., i.v., or into an endotracheal tube; intravenous administration in a hypoxic patient may precipitate ventricular fibrillation. Atropine given by other than the topical route will have little effect on pupil size, and pupil size should not be used as an indication of an adequate amount of atropine.

   (1) The initial dose for mild to moderately exposed patients (patients who are conscious) is 2 mg, i.m. or i.v. Generally symptoms will improve in 5 to 10 min; if not, another 2 mg should be administered. Administration of atropine at 5 to 10 intervals should continue until secretions are diminishing and the patient is breathing comfortably.

   (2) The initial dose for a severely exposed patient (unconscious) is 6 mg which should be given i.m. because these patients usually have some degree of hypoxia. After ventilation has begun, subsequent doses may be given i.v. following the guidelines above.

   (3) Maximal amounts of atropine that have been required in severely exposed patients have been 15 to 20 mg, mostly in the first several hours. This is in contrast to the doses of 100 to 1,000 mg/day reported to be necessary for OP insecticide patients (4).

   (4) Pediatric doses have not been established, but 0.03 to 0.05 mg/kg is recommended. During the Gulf War, many Israeli children accidently injected themselves with atropine via an automatic injector containing 2 mg. Although they had many of the side effects of atropine—tachycardia, dryness of secretions, mydriasis, sedation—none of the effects was serious, and all the children recovered fully (5).

   (5) Atropine is available in an automatic injector containing 2 mg (Survival Technology Institute, Rockville, MD)

   b. **Pralidoxime chloride (2-PAMCl; Protopam):** This quarternary oxime attaches to the nerve agent on the cholinesterase and removes the agent from the enzyme. One agent, GD, quickly forms an irreversible bond with the enzyme, and the oxime is ineffective. This process, by which the agent-enzyme complex becomes refractory to oxime reactivation of the enzyme, is known as "aging." The enzyme complexes formed with other agents age also, but this aging does not take place for many hours, long after the acute effects and therapy. Although an oxime reactivates cholinesterase, the clinical benefit is primarily in those structures with nicotinic receptor sites, the skeletal muscles. Fasciculations decrease and strength improves. The oxime is synergistic with atropine in elevating the LD_{50}.

   (1) The standard adult dose of pralidoxime chloride is 1 to 2 g administered i.v. over 20 to 30 min. Faster administration in normal humans causes a prolonged hypertension; this can transiently be reversed by 5 mg of

phentolamine, i.v. (3). This amount should be repeated once or twice at hourly intervals. Pralidoxime chloride is also available in an automatic injector containing 600 mg for emergency use (Survival Technology Inc., Rockville, MD).

    (2) A pediatric dose has not been established, but a starting dose might be 15 mg/kg given very slowly i.v.

  c. **Diazepam:** The anticonvulsant diazepam should be administered to all severely exposed patients whether they are convulsing or not. In nonconvulsing patients, it might prevent convulsions or might reduce CNS seizure activity in a seizing patient without peripheral signs. The dose is 10 mg, i.m., or 2 to 5 mg, i.v. Other anticonvulsants, e.g., phenytoin, barbiturates, have not been shown to be beneficial against these agents.

  5. **Eyes:** Treatment of miosis is not indicated routinely. Most drugs that might be used, e.g., atropine or homatropine topically, cause visual blurring, whereas vision with miosis is usually adequate except in dim light. Topical therapy will relieve eye pain, nausea and vomiting, or headache and should be administered for these complaints, but not routinely to reverse miosis.

G. **Clinical course**

  1. A conscious patient should recover shortly after administration of one or more doses of atropine and 2-PAMCl unless there is continuing absorption of agent, e.g., from clothing or through skin layers.

  2. If adequately treated before hypoxia has caused CNS damage, the unconscious patient will recover with spontaneous respiration, consciousness, and voluntary muscular movement in 2 to 3 h. He will be weak, unsteady, and possibly mildly stuporous for the next 12 to 24 h, but recovery will continue.

  3. G-agent inhibited RBC-ChE will recover with the production of new red blood cells, at about 1% per day. VX-inhibited RBC-ChE recovers at about 0.5% to 1% per hour for the first day or two, then at about 1% per day.

  4. After vapor exposure, breathing will stop in 6 to 8 min and death will occur shortly thereafter. Most of the deaths in the Tokyo subway incident occurred before assistance could arrive. Similar effects will occur shortly after the onset of effects from a lethal amount on the skin.

H. **Further effects:**

  1. **Eyes:** The ability of the pupil to dilate completely in dim lighting or darkness may not return to normal for about 6 weeks, even though the pupil appears normal under room lighting (2,6).

  2. **CNS:** Minor and often subtle CNS effects may linger for 6 weeks or longer after any degree of exposure. These include irritability, forgetfulness, sleep disturbances, and inability to think clearly and to make decisions. In one case they were reversed by scopolamine (2).

  3. **Delayed peripheral neuropathy** seen after insecticide exposures has not been seen in humans after nerve agent exposure. It has been seen experimentally in animals given huge doses of nerve agents kept alive by heroic measures, including pretreatment with atropine and oximes (7,8).

4. The **intermediate syndrome** reported after insecticide exposures has been seen neither in man nor animals after nerve agent poisoning.

5. **Minor EEG changes** have been reported in averaged groups of people who had been exposed to nerve agents. Changes in individuals' records could not be detected (9).

6. **Long-term behavioral effects** (psychological testing) have not been reported after nerve agent exposure.

II. **Vesicants** (blister-causing agents) may belong to the plant (poison ivy), animal (some sea creatures), or mineral (some chemicals) kingdom. The chemical vesicant of concern as a warfare agent is **sulfur mustard. Lewisite** and **phosgene oxime** are agents developed for warfare purposes, but have seen little use. An analog of sulfur mustard, **nitrogen mustard**, was developed in the World War II era, but was found to be unsuitable for munitions. As Mustargen®, it became a useful chemotherapeutic agent. Sulfur mustard was first used on the battlefield in World War I, and although it was introduced late in that war it produced more casualties than all the other agents. Iraq used this agent extensively against Iran during the Iran-Iraq war.

A. **Mustard**

1. **Properties:** Sulfur mustard (known as H for the impure substance and HD for the almost pure material) is an oily liquid with a high freezing/melting point (57°F) and a relatively low volatility. It ranges from light yellow to dark brown in color, its vapor is heavier than air, and the liquid is heavier than water. It has the odor of onions, garlic, or mustard (hence its name).

2. **Pathophysiology:** The exact mechanism by which mustard produces cellular damage is unknown. After passing through the cellular membrane it rapidly cyclizes, and the cyclic compound reacts with enzymes, proteins, DNA, and other substances. According to one theory (10), damage results from DNA alkylation and crosslinking in rapidly dividing cells such as basal keratinocytes, mucosal epithelium, and bone marrow stem cells. This leads to cellular death, inflammatory reaction, and, in the skin, protease digestion of anchoring filaments at the epidermal-dermal junction to produce blisters. Three points are important: mustard rapidly passes through the outer layers and into cells of the skin and mucous membranes, and once in these cells decontamination does nothing; although mustard damages cells within minutes of contact with the outer layer of the skin, clinical effects do not appear until hours later; and intact mustard is not present in body fluids, including blister fluid.

3. **Clinical effects:** In addition to causing damage by topical contact to the skin, the eyes, and the airways, mustard absorbed in large amounts can damage other cells including those of the bone marrow and the mucosal cells of the GI tract.

   a. **Skin:** The characteristic lesion of mustard is erythema followed by blisters. Erythema begins 2 to 24 h after vapor contact (the time may be shorter after liquid contact). Within the area of erythema small vesicles form, and these gradually coalesce to form the characteristic blister. If the amount of agent is high (liquid exposure) there may be a central area of coagulation necrosis. Warm, moist areas are most sensitive to mustard (e.g., axilla, perineum).

   b. **Eyes:** Eyes are the most sensitive organ to mustard. The lesion ranges from mild conjunctivitis, to corneal edema and clouding, and to corneal destruction and perforation. The latter occurs only with large liquid doses. Associated with eye damage are blepharospasm, lid edema and inflammation, and photophobia which may linger for weeks. Severe damage is rare, and most World War I casualties with eye damage recovered completely.

c. **Airways:** Mustard causes necrosis of the mucosa of the airways, and its effects descend in a dose-dependent manner from the nares to the terminal bronchioles. Initially, or perhaps the only effect, is pain or discomfort in the nose or sinuses; larger amounts of vapor will cause laryngeal damage (voice changes or aphonia) and damage to upper and medium sized airways (nonproductive cough). After a very large amount of vapor there will be damage to the terminal airways with dyspnea, productive cough, and possibly hemorrhage into the alveoli; pulmonary edema is otherwise not a feature of mustard poisoning. Necrosis of the mucosa with associated inflammation can lead to pseudomembrane formation at any level; these may obstruct the airway or break off to obstruct lower airways.

d. **GI tract:** Many mustard casualties have a transient period of nausea and vomiting in the first 24 h of exposure; this is thought to be a reflex activity and does not implicate damage to the GI mucosa. The signs of GI mucosa damage begin days after exposure, and this damage causes the loss of large volumes of fluid and electrolytes.

e. **Bone marrow:** Leukocytosis is common within the first several days after mustard exposure. If the exposure was large the stem cells are destroyed, and a decrease in leukocytes begins around 3 to 5 days post-exposure (11,12). This leukocytopenia is followed by a decrease in erythrocytes and thrombocytes. If the decreases are not marked, i.e., if there are remaining stem cells, recovery will take place as the patient recovers.

f. **Central nervous system:** Mustard has few acute CNS effects, although large amounts given i.v. cause convulsions in animals. Casualties from World War I (11) and from the Iraq-Iran conflict (13) were noted to have mild, very nonspecific effects, such as listlessness, apathy, and lethargy, for as long as a year after exposure.

4. **Management:** There is no antidote for mustard poisoning. Management consists of supportive care and in keeping the damaged organs free of infection.

a. **Skin:** The pain and discomfort of erythema can be managed by soothing lotions, e.g., calamine lotion. Small blisters should be left intact. Large blisters should be unroofed and the denuded area irrigated several times daily followed by liberal application of a topical antibiotic. Systemic analgesics should be used liberally. Fluid loss is not of the magnitude seen after thermal burns, and one must be careful not to overhydrate. Nonetheless, fluid balance must be monitored.

b. **Eyes:** Mild to moderate conjunctivitis can be managed with any of a number of ophthalmic solutions after the eyes are irrigated. After more severe injury a mydriatic (atropine or homatropine ophthalmic ointment) should be applied several times daily to reduce or prevent future synechiae; a topical antibiotic should be applied several times a day; and vaseline or similar substance should be regularly applied to lid edges to prevent them from sticking together during healing. A topical analgesic should be used for examination, but should not be applied regularly. Topical steroids are not of proven value, but their use during the first day might reduce subsequent inflammation. Sun glasses will reduce discomfort from photophobia.

c. **Airways:** Mild to moderate upper airway symptoms will usually respond to steam inhalation and cough suppressants. Cough, fever, leukocytosis, and x-ray changes within the first two days suggests a chemical pneumonitis; antibiotics should not be used. Infection, usually beginning on about the third day, will cause an increased fever and leukocytosis and a change on x-ray; antibiotics should be started only after the organism is identified. In a severely exposed casualty, i.e., one whose airway symptoms begin within 6 h after exposure, intubation should be performed early before laryngeal spasm and edema made it difficult. Oxygen will be needed, and early use of PEEP or CPAP may be of benefit. Bronchospasm will generally be controlled with bronchodilators; if not, steroids may be of value, but there is no evidence that the routine use of steroids is useful.

d. **GI:** Atropine or other antiemetic is useful for the early nausea and vomiting. The later diarrhea and massive fluid loss suggests widespread tissue damage by the agent.

e. **Bone marrow:** Nonabsorbable antibiotics should be considered to reduce the possibility of sepsis from enteric organisms. Cellular replacement (bone marrow transplants or transfusions) has not been attempted, but may be successful.

f. **Other:** In animal studies, sulfur donors, such as sodium thiosulfate, decreased systemic effects and reduced mortality when given preexposure or within 20 min after exposure (14). They do not change the topical effects (skin, eyes, airways). Orally administered activated charcoal and hemodialysis have been of no benefit (12).

g. **Death:** After vapor exposure, death often occurs between the fifth and 10th day after exposure and is due to airway damage with superimposed infection and sepsis in the absence of an immune response. After liquid exposure (no vapor inhalation), death is from tissue damage, similar to radiation effects (mustard has been called a radiomimetic).

5. **Long-term effects:**

a. Mustard may cause **scarring** on the skin after a severe lesion and may lead to cicatrix in airways after infection.

b. **Cancer:** Mustard has caused an increased incidence of upper airway cancer in people repeatedly exposed to it over a period of time (production workers) (15). There is no good evidence that one or two exposures lead to cancer. Mustard is classified as a carcinogen based on laboratory studies.

c. **Eye:** Chronic conjunctivitis and delayed keratitis (20 to 30 years later) have been reported after mustard exposure (16,17).

    d. Reproduction: Mustard is classified as a mutagen based on laboratory studies. There are no data to implicate mustard as a reproductive toxin in man.

B. Lewisite

1. Lewisite is an oily liquid that smells like geraniums, and which is more volatile than mustard.
2. **Pathophysiology:** Lewisite contains arsenic and damages cells. Its mode of activity is unknown.
3. **Clinical effects:** Lewisite damages skin, eyes, and airways and also causes an increase in capillary permeability. There are few human data on Lewisite.
   a. In contrast to mustard, which causes no immediate effects, the effects of Lewisite liquid or vapor are immediate with pain or irritation upon contact with skin, eyes, and upper airways.
   b. Tissue damage occurs almost immediately; skin will be grayish and necrotic within minutes of contact with liquid Lewisite.
   c. Lesions from Lewisite are more severe and are more difficult to treat than those of mustard.
   d. Lewisite does not damage bone marrow. However, it damages capillaries, and the resulting fluid loss may lead to hypovolemia, hypotension, and subsequent organ damage.
   e. Although the closely related arsines cause hemolysis, there are no data that Lewisite does.
4. **Management:** Immediate decontamination will reduce the injury, and since Lewisite causes pain the casualty is more likely to immediately decontaminate himself than after mustard. The antidote BAL (British-Anti-Lewisite; Dimercaprol) given i.m. may reduce systemic effects; it also decreases the severity of skin and eye lesions when applied topically, but these preparations are no longer available. Management of the lesions is otherwise similar to management of mustard lesions.

C. Phosgene oxime: Phosgene oxime is a corrosive substance. Human exposures have been rare, and there are few animal data.

1. Phosgene oxime produces urticaria, not true fluid-filled blisters.
2. Both the vapor and liquid cause irritation or pain on contact.
3. Tissue damage is almost immediate, with blanching and erythema in about 1 min after skin contact.
4. Phosgene oxime causes pulmonary edema after inhalation and after skin exposure.
5. Management is supportive.

III. Riot Control Agents are also known as **tear gas**, irritants, lacrimators, and sternutators. Many of these were used in World War I, but only two are of concern today: orthochlorobenzylidene malononitrile (CS), used by law enforcement agencies and the military, and CN (Mace), available in devices used for self-protection. The two are very similar in their biological effects and will be discussed together.

A. Characteristics: CS and CN are solids dispersed in an aerosol of either powder or in liquid. They have a low effective Ct (Concentration of exposure times the $time$ of exposure) and a high LCt_{50} (the Ct that is lethal for 50% of the population). Their effects begin within seconds after exposure, and usually the effects have gone by 15 to 30 min.

B. Pathophysiology: The mechanism of their biological activity is not well characterized.

C. Clinical effects: These compounds cause pain or irritation to the exposed eyes, nasal area, oral cavity, skin, and airways.

    1. Eyes: Burning, stinging, or pain; conjunctivitis; tearing; and blepharospasm.

    2. Nose and mouth: Burning, stinging or pain; increased secretions.

    3. Skin: Burning, stinging, or pain particularly if the skin is abraded (freshly shaven) or warm and moist. Erythema may develop and usually lasts about 1 h.

    4. Airways: Burning and irritation, with increased secretions and coughing. Although there is a feeling of "tightness in the chest, pulmonary function studies performed very shortly after exposure have shown minimal changes (18,19).

    5. Other

        a. GI: Occasionally nausea and vomiting may follow a large exposure.

        b. An **"alarm reaction"** with tachycardia and hypertension has been reported in people immediately before they were exposed to CS. Both the heart rate and blood pressure returned to normal during the exposure (18).

        c. Ingestion: Occasionally, people eat CS powder or pellets. The LD_{50} is high and the risk of death is low. Animals fed the LD_{50} had some gastric mucosa changes. Effects in humans have been intermittent bouts of cramps and diarrhea, probably from the cathartics and antacids used as therapy (S. Pace, personal communication).

        d. Metabolism: Increased blood concentrations of thiocyanate (cyanide is a metabolite of CS) have been reported after i.v. administration and after very large aerosol exposures of animals to CS (20). Deaths occurred days later because of lung damage, not within minutes from cyanide poisoning. The amount of cyanide liberated from an "intolerable" exposure to CS has been compared to the amount of cyanide liberated from two puffs on a cigarette (21).

        e. Tolerance: People who work around these agents, e.g., in manufacturing, may become tolerant to their effects. Motivated people may tolerate moderate concentrations if an initial low concentration is gradually increased.

D. Management: After exposure to riot control agents improvement is usually rapid, and people rarely seek medical attention.

    1. Eyes: A particle may impact in the conjunctiva or cornea. Thorough flushing of the eye or manual removal (preferably by an ophthalmologist) may be necessary.

    2. Airways: These agents may trigger a bronchospastic reaction in one with reactive airways, but despite large scale use of these agents this has rarely been reported. Bronchodilators, assisted ventilation, and oxygen may be required.

    3. Skin: After exposure to a large concentration in a hot, humid environment, a delayed dermatitis may occur (22). This begins 4 to 8 h after exposure, and erythema may be followed by blister formation. This can be treated with soothing lotions and blister care as described above for mustard.

E. Death: Death has been reported after CN use in enclosed spaces. In all cases an individual refused to exit an enclosed space, and larger amounts of the agent were inserted. There have been no reported deaths from CS or CN from use in the open air.

References

1. Grob D, Lilienthal JL Jr, Harvey AM, Jones BF. The administration of diisopropyl fluorophosphate (DFP) to man. I. Effect on plasma and erythrocyte cholinesterase; general systemic effects; use in study of hepatic function and erythropoieses; and some properties of plasma cholinesterase. *Bull Johns Hopkins Hosp* 1947;81:217–244.
2. Sidell FR. Soman and sarin: clinical manifestations and treatment of accidental poisoning by organophosphates. *Clin Toxicol* 1974;7:1–17.
3. Sidell FR. Clinical considerations in nerve agent intoxication. In: Somani SM, ed. *Chemical warfare agents*. San Diego: Academic Press, 1922:155–194.
4. LeBlanc FN, Benson BE, Gilg AD. A severe organophosphate poisoning requiring the use of an atropine drip. *Clin Toxicol* 1986;24:69–76.
5. Amitai Y, Almog S, Singer R, Hammer R, Bentur Y, Danon YL. Atropine poisoning in children during the Gulf crisis: a national survey in Israel. *JAMA* 1992;268:630–632.
6. Rengstorff RH. Accidental exposure to sarin: vision effects. *Arch Toxicol* 1985;56:201–203.
7. Willems JL, Nicaise M, Bisschop HCD. Delayed neuropathy by the organophosphorus nerve agents soman and tabun. *Arch Toxicol* 1984;55:76–77.
8. Crowell JA, Parker RM, Bucci TJ, Dacre JC. Neuropathy target esterase in hens after sarin and soman. *J Biochem Toxicol* 1989;4:15–20.
9. Duffy FH, Burchfiel JL, Bartels PH, Gaon M, Sim VM. Long-term effects of an organophosphate upon the human electroencephalogram. *Toxicol Appl Pharmacol* 1979;47:161–176.
10. Papirmeister B, Gross CL, Meier HL, Petrali JP, Johnson JB. Molecular basis for mustard-induced vesication. *Fund Appl Toxicol* 1985;5:S134–S149.
11. Vedder EB. The vesicants. In: Vedder EB. *The medical aspects of chemical warfare*. Baltimore: Williams & Wilkins, 1925:125–166.
12. Willems JL. Clinical management of mustard gas casualties. *Ann Med Milit Belg* 1989;3S:1–61.
13. Balali-Mood M. First reports of delayed toxic effects of Yperite poisoning in Iranian fighters. In: *Proceedings of the Second World Congress on New Compounds in Biological and Chemical Warfare*. Ghent, Belgium: University of Ghent, 1986, pgs. 489–495.
14. Vojvodic V, Milosavljevic Z, Boskovic B, Bojanic N. The application of different drugs in rats poisoned by sulfur and nitrogen mustards. *Fund 5* S160–S168.
15. Watson AP, Jones TD, Griffin GD. Sulfur mustard as a carcinogen: ??? relative potency analysis to the chemical warfare agents H, HD, and HT. *Regul Toxicol Pharmacol* 1989;10:1–25.
16. Mann I. A study of eighty-four cases of delayed mustard gas keratitis fitted with contact lenses. *Br J Ophthalmol* 1944;28:441–447.
17. Blondi FC. Mustard gas keratopathy. *Int Ophthalmol Clin* 1971;11:1–13.
18. Bestwick FW, Holland P, Kemp KH. Acute effects of exposure to orthochlorobenzylidene malononitrile (CS) and the development of tolerance. *Br J Indust Med* 1972;29:298–306.
19. Punte CL, Owens EJ, Gutentag PJ. Exposures to ortho-chlorobenzylidene malononitrile. *Arch Environ Health* 1963;6:72–80.
20. Cucinell SA, Swentzel KC, Biskup R, et al. Biochemical interactions and metabolic fate of riot control agents. *Fed Proc* 1971;30:86–91.
21. Himsworth H. *Report of the enquiry into the medical and toxicological aspects of CS (orthochlorobenzylidene malononitrile)*. London: Her Majesty's Stationery Office, 1971.
22. Weigand DA. Cutaneous reaction to the riot control agent CS. *Milit Med* 1969;134:437–440.

Suggested Reading

Somani S, ed. *Chemical warfare agents*. San Diego: Academic Press, 1992.
Marrs TC, Maynard RL, Sidell FR. *Chemical warfare agents*. New York: John Wiley and Sons, 1966.

PART III

Industrial and Household Toxicology

Emergency Toxicology, Second Edition,
edited by Peter Viccellio.
Lippincott–Raven Publishers, Philadelphia © 1998.

15

Ethylene Glycol, Methanol, and Isopropyl Alcohol

Frederick M. Schiavone, Francine D. Cantor, Gerard X. Brogan, and Amy S. Baruch

Department of Emergency Medicine, State University of New York at Stony Brook, University Hospital, Stony Brook, New York 11794-7400.

ETHYLENE GLYCOL

Ethylene glycol is an alcohol similar in structure to ethyl alcohol but with the addition of a hydroxyl group on each carbon. A common and potentially lethal poison, it is most often ingested as a suicide gesture, accidentally, or as a substitute for alcohol by chronic alcohol abusers.

I. **Sources and forms.** Ethylene glycol may be found in a variety of substances, most notably in antifreeze preparations used in car radiators, deicers, and coolants. It is common in many industrial solvents, detergents, corrosives, paints, lacquers, and pharmaceuticals; and has been noted to be used improperly in juices and some European wines (1) (Table 15-1).

II. **Physical and clinical properties.** Ethylene glycol is a colorless, odorless liquid that has a pleasant, warm, but somewhat bittersweet taste. There is an exothermic reaction when it is mixed with water. It is a nonvolatile liquid that is miscible with water, and it has a low freezing point and a boiling point of 197°C (2). The first cases of ethylene glycol intoxication were reported in 1930 (3), and it may be responsible for 40 to 60 deaths a year.

III. **Mechanism of action.** The toxicity of ethylene glycol poisoning is due to its metabolites rather than to ethylene glycol itself. To better understand the toxicity of ethylene glycol and the treatment rationale, a discussion of its metabolism is warranted. Ethylene glycol usually is ingested but can be inhaled or absorbed through the skin. Once ingested, it is rapidly absorbed and distributed throughout the body, with peak serum levels seen within 1 to 4 h. The initial step in the metabolism of ethylene glycol is oxidation to glycol aldehyde by alcohol dehydrogenase, the same enzyme needed to oxidize ethanol, methanol, or isopropanol. Glycol aldehyde is rapidly oxidized to glycolic acid, which is further oxidized to glyoxylic acid. Glyoxylic acid has a short half-life with several metabolic pathways, as seen in Fig. 15-1.

A. The major product of metabolism is formic acid.

B. Glyoxylic acid may be converted to glycine and then, in the presence of folate, converted to carbon dioxide and water.

C. It can conjugate to alphahydroxybetaketoadipate with the help of thiamine and magnesium.

269

Table 15-1. *Sources and forms of ethylene glycol*

Antifreeze preparations
Detergents, cosmetics
Brake fluids and hydraulic fluid
Paint solvents
Softening agent for cellophane
Inks
Synthesis of resins
Floor polishes and waxes
Cleaning compositions for leather, upholstery, and glass
Wines

D.   It may oxidize to oxalic acid and then convert to calcium oxalate, with formation of oxalate crystals in the urine.

E.   Calcium oxalate with dehydrate crystals (envelope-shaped octahedral) and monohydrate (spindle-shaped) crystals are seen in the urine (4). Studies have shown the major acid metabolite to be glycolic acid (5), with smaller contributions from the other metabolites (6). Lactic acid has been shown to increase with the use of ethanol during the treatment of ethylene glycol intoxication seen when large amounts of reduced nicotinamide adenine dinucleotide (NADH) are present (7).

F.   Ethylene glycol and its metabolites are **excreted** by the kidney, differing from methanol, which is much more volatile and may be excreted through the lungs. Renal impairment delays excretion of these compounds. Renal failure is seen with prolonged or untreated ethylene glycol toxicity as a result of direct renal toxicity by the ethylene glycol metabolites. Oxalate crystalluria may cause an obstructive uropathy (4).

G.   The **hallmark of toxicity** is a severe anion gap metabolic acidosis. The **anion gap** is defined as the difference of the serum cations (made up essentially of sodium and potassium) and the serum anions (made up essentially of the serum bicarbonate and chloride) reflected in the following formula:

$$(Na^+ + K^+) - (HCO_3^- + Cl^-)$$

The "gap" represents those anions that are not normally measured in routine electrolyte determinations. They are primarily represented by sulfate, phosphate, and serum proteins. The upper limit of the normal value of the gap is 12 ± 4 mEq/L. When any acid is added to the body (i.e., glycolic, glyoxylic, oxylic, or lactic) the hydrogen ion (H^+) is buffered by bicarbonate to form carbonic acid, which is converted to carbon dioxide and water. These acids cause bicarbonate molecules to be lost from the equation with the addition of unmeasurable anions (8).

H.   Ethylene glycol is also an osmolar active substance. The **serum osmolality** is almost entirely accounted for by the sodium (Na), urea (BUN), glucose, and ethanol (ETOH) concentrations and therefore can be calculated using the following formula (9):

Calculated serum osmolality = 2 Na + BUN/2.8 + serum glucose/18 + ETOH/4.6

1.   The normal serum osmolality is 285 to 295 mOsm/kg. A measured serum osmolality that is more than 10 mOsm above the calculated osmolality suggests the pres-

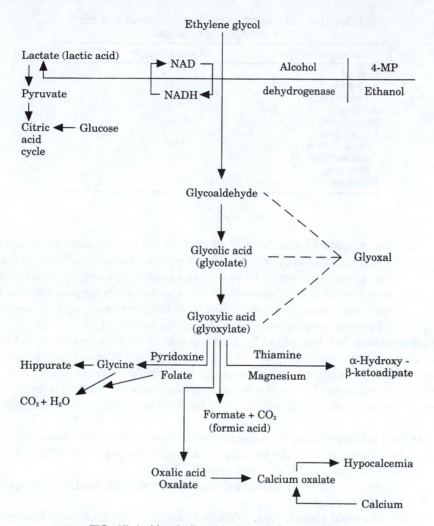

FIG. 15-1. Metabolic pathways of glyoxylic acid.

ence of unmeasured osmolar active particles. Several substances may elevate the serum osmolality, including ethanol, methanol, isopropanol, mannitol glycolate, glyoxylate, formate, formaldehyde, and of course ethylene glycol (8) (Table 15-2). The accuracy of measured osmolality predicting the quantity of unmeasured osmoles appears to be variable, limiting its use.

2. In the clinical setting, where ethanol and ethylene glycol may have been consumed together, the calculated osmolality associated with ethanol may be predictable. Each 100 mg/dL dose of ethanol adds 22 mOsm/kg to the osmolar gap (10). Using the above formula, one may account for the added osmoles per kilogram contributed by the ethanol.

Table 15-2. *Molecular weight of toxic agents that may increase the osmolar gap*

Substance	Molecular weight
Ethanol	46
Methanol	32
Ethylene glycol	62
Acetone	58
Isopropanol	60
Paraldehyde	132
Chloral hydrate	165
Trichlorethane	133
Chloroform	119
Salicylate	180

3. The **minimum lethal level** of ethylene glycol concentration of 21 mg/dL yields 3.4 mOsm/kg. Thus, a *normal osmolar gap does not exclude the diagnosis of ethylene glycol intoxication.* However, *an elevated osmolar gap in the setting of a severe metabolic acidosis with an anion gap strongly suggests ethylene glycol or methanol intoxication.* Other osmolar active substances, such as isopropanol or ethanol, do not generate a severe metabolic acidosis (11).

IV. **Pathophysiology.** Ethylene glycol by itself has mild to no toxic properties. When initially consumed it may produce mild euphoria, similar to ethanol. The most frequent organ systems affected by ethylene glycol intoxication are the CNS and the cardiopulmonary and genitourinary systems. Autopsies have shown that generalized edema and hyperemia involve the brain, lungs, kidneys, and liver (1). Small petechiae and focal hemorrhages are widespread throughout the body.

A. **Diffuse calcium oxalate crystal** deposit may be seen within brain tissue, leptomeninges, choroid plexus, perivascular spaces, and the renal collecting system. Crystallization may occur as early as 1 to 3 h after ingestion.

B. Also noted is a pattern of **diffuse pulmonary edema,** with focal hemorrhagic bronchopneumonia developing.

C. Within the **renal parenchyma,** pathologic findings are bilateral focal hemorrhagic cortical necrosis with dilated proximal tubules filled with yellow birefringent calcium oxalate crystals. These crystals may mimic hippurate crystals in shape and form, but no evidence of hippurate crystals is found despite earlier claims with ethylene glycol toxicity (11).

D. Other pathologic findings may include fatty degeneration and focal necrosis of the liver and striated muscle along with inflammation of the pancreas.

V. **Clinical presentation** of ethylene glycol was described by Berman et al. (12) in three successive stages. The severity and timing depends on the amount of toxin ingested and the timing of treatment. The clinical presentation may also be delayed by concomitant ethanol consumption.

A. The **first stage** occurs 30 min to 12 h after ingestion and may resemble ethanol intoxication, but there is an absence of alcohol on the breath.

1. This clinical stage is characterized by depressive CNS disturbances associated with cerebral edema and calcium oxalate deposition (oxalosis). It may also be characterized by nausea, vomiting, abdominal cramps, and possibly hematemesis.

2. High doses of ethylene glycol may cause neurologic manifestations characterized by severe confusion, hallucinations, and coma, with nuchal rigidity, seizures, hypotonia and hyperreflexia, tremors, and tetany. Cerebral oxalosis with crystallization may be seen within the leptomeninges, accompanied by diffuse capillary compromise, cytotoxic damage, and cerebral edema. Seizures may be intractable and difficult to control. A lumbar puncture may reveal cloudy cerebrospinal fluid (CSF) consistent with a chemical meningitis. A computed tomography (CT) scan at this stage is usually normal but may show cerebral edema with complete obliteration of the lateral and third ventricles. Coma may last a week or more, and the patient may exhibit signs of meningoencephalitis.

3. Patients may also exhibit findings similar to those seen with methanol intoxication (see below) with ocular findings, including decreased pupillary reflexes, nystagmus, decreased visual acuity, optic disk blurring, papilledema, ophthalmoplegia, strabismus, color blindness, and optic atrophy. An elevated osmolar gap, a high anion gap, lactic acidosis, and hypocalcemia are usually noted during this stage. **Urinalysis** may show proteinuria and calcium oxalate crystalluria. An **ECG** may be normal or may show hyperacute T waves consistent with hyperkalemia if a severe metabolic acidosis exists.

B. The **second stage** occurs 12 to 48 h after ingestion and involves primarily the cardiopulmonary system. The patient may develop tachypnea, tachycardia, cyanosis, hypertension, and inspiratory rales. Cardiac and noncardiac pulmonary edema has been reported along with bronchopneumonia, cardiac dilatation, and arrhythmias, usually leading to death if left untreated (13).

C. The **third stage** of ethylene glycol intoxication occurs 24 to 72 h after ingestion and is characterized by acute renal failure. Acute tubular necrosis, renal edema, and renal deposition of oxalate crystals contribute to the subsequent renal failure. The patient may develop costovertebral angle tenderness. Laboratory results may reveal a mild to marked azotemia (12). Radiographs may suggest perirenal edema, and ultrasonography or abdominal CT scans have also reported enlarged kidneys (14).

D. Factor and Lava (15) postulated that a **fourth "neurologic" stage** may be evident, appearing days after the initial ingestion. In a report of four cases, patients were found to have bilateral facial diplegia, with the CSF demonstrating an elevated protein level but no pleocytosis.

VI. **Differential diagnosis.** An unexplained osmolar gap and anion gap acidosis suggest the diagnosis of ethylene glycol poisoning. The development of acidosis may be delayed, particularly in patients who have also ingested alcohol. The differential diagnosis of osmolar and anion gaps is discussed in Chapter 12. Other clues leading to the diagnosis of ethylene glycol poisoning include the development of hypocalcemia, as well as the appearance (usually several hours after ingestion) of oxalate crystals in the urine. Heckerling (16) reported ethylene glycol poisoning with a normal anion gap metabolic acidosis secondary to occult bromide intoxication and hyperchloremia (15). In addition, Leon recently reported a severe ethylene glycol poisoning and coingestion of lithium carbonate in which severe acidosis was not present. It was postulated that the lithium carbonate provided bicarbonate which acted as a buffer combining with glycolic acid as it was formed (43).

VII. Laboratory analysis

   A. Laboratory studies

1. **Arterial blood gases** (ABGs) to determine the presence of a metabolic acidosis, which may be delayed several hours, especially if there is ethanol in the blood.

2. **Serum electrolytes** to calculate an anion and osmolar gap. An anion gap metabolic acidosis may not be present initially where significant coingestion with ethanol may prevent ethylene glycol's hepatic metabolism to organic acids. Serum osmolality measurements and calculation of the osmolol gap may prove to be the clue to the diagnosis (44).

3. **Serum osmolarity** measured by freezing point depression to compare the measured to the calculated serum osmolarity. Determination of an osmolar gap may be inaccurate. An accurate serum osmolality frequently cannot be obtained in the laboratory. Separately, there is variability in the calculated osmolality depending on the calculation used. Since ethylene glycol has a high molecular weight, the contribution to the overall osmolality may be small even when levels are toxic. Lastly, when ethylene glycol is metabolized, the osmolar gap decreases. Toxic metabolites subsequently increase, reflecting a worsening metabolic acidosis (45).

4. **Urinalysis** is helpful to look specifically for calcium oxalate crystals. The presence of calcium oxalate crystals is suggestive of ethylene glycol ingestion, but toxicity can occur in the absence of crystalluria (46). Sodium fluorescein, a fluorescent dye, is present in many antifreeze products. Examination of the urine, as well as mucous membranes, skin, clothing, gastric contents using a Wood's lamp, may confirm a suspected ethylene glycol ingestion early in the clinical presentation when levels are not available (47).

5. **Complete blood count.**

6. **Serum calcium level** (severe hypocalcemia may develop).

7. **Blood ethanol level.**

8. **Serum and urine ketones**—to help exclude other diagnoses (i.e., diabetic ketoacidosis, alcoholic ketoacidosis, starvation ketoacidosis).

9. It is helpful to obtain an urgent **ethylene glycol level.** It is essential that the laboratory use mass spectrometry or gas chromatography with OV1 columns to properly identify the ethylene glycol molecule (17). Other common ingestions that present with a somewhat similar picture (i.e., salicylates and methanol) should also be assayed in the blood. Hewlett et al. (5) advocated the use of **glycolic acid** determination to follow the patient's status or for diagnostic purposes once all the ethylene glycol is metabolized (16).

10. **Electrocardiogram.**

11. **Lactic acid level.**

12. These tests should be repeated as needed to follow the clinical course of the patient (18).

B. Range of toxicity. The minimum lethal dose of ethylene glycol is approximately 1.4 to 1.6 mL/kg, or approximately 100 mL for a 70-kg adult, which may not produce an osmolar gap (3,19), although survival has been reported with ingestions of up to 970 mL (20). There is also a report of an ingestion of 2 L that was successfully treated within 1 h (21).

VIII. Treatment

    A. General treatment for ethylene glycol includes the ABCs of resuscitation and removal of the offending toxin.

        1. In an **alert, awake patient,** emesis may be induced with ipecac. An **obtunded patient** should be intubated and then lavaged via a gastric tube. Charcoal absorbs ethylene glycol poorly, but it is reasonable to administer a charcoal slurry with a saline or sorbitol cathartic if there is any suspicion of multiple ingestion. Fluid balance must be maintained to avoid contributing to acute pulmonary edema or electrolyte abnormalities.

        2. **Seizures** are common with severe ethylene glycol intoxication and should be treated aggressively with diazepam 5 to 10 mg i.v. over 2 to 3 min. This dose may be repeated every 10 min to a maximum does of about 30 mg. If seizures cannot be controlled, check the serum calcium and magnesium levels. Administer a loading dose of phenytoin 15 to 20 mg/kg i.v. at a rate not to exceed 50 mg/min. Stop phenytoin infusion if an arrhythmia or severe hypotension occurs, or when seizure activity stops (17).

        3. Treatment of **severe metabolic acidosis** may be difficult. A pH of less than 7.0 and a serum bicarbonate of less than 7 mL/dL are common with severe ethylene glycol intoxication. Liberal use of sodium bicarbonate solution is appropriate to correct the acidemia (22).

    B. Toxin-specific treatment

        1. **Ethanol.**

        A key step in treating ethylene glycol and methanol intoxication is the use of ethanol. The metabolism of ethylene glycol depends on alcohol dehydrogenase, and ethanol competitively inhibits this enzyme and prevents the formation of toxic metabolites. The affinity of ethylene glycol for alcohol dehydrogenase appears to be similar to that of ethanol (23). The patient may be given alcohol orally, by nasogastric tube, or intravenously. The patient who has been given ipecac/charcoal combination cannot tolerate oral alcohol loading.

            a. **Intravenous loading** of ethanol is best accomplished by administering 10% ethanol solution in D_5W (7.6 to 10.0 mL/kg) over 30 to 60 min (assuming the patient does not have ethanol in his or her system). The goal of the loading dose is to produce a serum ethanol level of approximately 100 to 150 mg/dL. To maintain this serum level, the average person requires a 10% ethanol solution (1.39 mL/kg/h). In patients who are chronic ethanol abusers, a higher level of 1.95 mL/kg/h is necessary to obtain the same serum ethanol levels. The range suggested during hemodialysis is 250 to 350 mg/kg/h (3.2 to 4.4 mL/kg/h when using a 10% solution of ethanol) (24).

            b. **Oral loading** may be done with a 20% ethanol solution (800 mg/kg). The aim again is to produce a serum ethanol level of 100 to 150 mg/dL (17). Chronic alcoholics may require as much as 50% higher doses of ethanol. By treating initially with ethanol, no toxic intermediate metabolites form, and the ethylene glycol is excreted by the kidneys. It is imperative to begin ethanol therapy early in order to maintain a nontoxic state. The serum glucose level should also be followed, especially in children, so as to avoid alcoholinduced hypoglycemia.

   c. One should start ethanol treatment immediately and *not* wait for confirmation of the diagnosis. **Indications** for immediate ethanol therapy are:

     (1) Any suspicion, by the history, of significant ethylene glycol or methanol ingestion.

     (2) Any obtunded or comatose patient with an unexplained osmolar gap, an unexplained severe anion gap metabolic acidosis, or oxalate crystalluria.

     (3) Serum ethylene glycol levels of more than 20 mg/dL (with or without symptoms).

2. **Hemodialysis.** The only definitive therapy for removing ethylene glycol and its metabolites is hemodialysis. Once a metabolic acidosis is present, hemodialysis must be considered. Ethanol therapy should continue throughout dialysis. Hemodialysis decreases the ethylene glycol half-life to 2.5 h when used concurrently with ethanol therapy, whereas the half-life is approximately 17 h with ethanol alone (25).

   a. **Indications for hemodialysis are:**

     (1) Severe metabolic acidosis

     (2) Severe electrolyte abnormality

     (3) Pulmonary edema

     (4) Renal failure

     (5) Blood ethylene glycol levels of more than 50 mg/dL (with or without symptoms)

   b. **Peritoneal dialysis and charcoal hemoperfusion** have been used but are less effective and are undesirable because acidbase disturbance, electrolyte abnormalities, and uremia are left untreated.

   c. **Continuous arteriovenous hemofiltration dialysis (CAVH-D)** may be an effective alternative in cases of hemodynamic instability or in situations where hemodialysis is not available. Christiansson et al. from Sweden reported a severe case of ethyleneglycol poisoning with cardiovascular failure, respiratory distress and oliguria where the patient had a favorable outcome using CAVH-D. Further studies are needed to determine the efficacy of this method (48).

3. **Thiamine and pyridoxine** are necessary to convert glyoxalic acid to glycine and alphahydroxybeta ketoadipate, thereby decreasing the amount of oxalic acid. Thiamine and pyridoxine should be given in doses of 100 mg I.V. q6h until the ethylene glycol level is zero.

4. **Leucovorin (folinic acid) and folic acid** are needed for the conversion of formic acid to carbon dioxide. The recommended dose is leucovorin 1 mg/kg up to 50 mg/dose I.V., followed by folic acid 1 mg/kg and then 50 mg I.V. q4h (26).

> 5. **4-Methylpyrazole (4-MP)** is a strong inhibitor of alcohol dehydrogenase and has been used successfully in human and animal studies with relatively few side effects when used early for ethylene glycol intoxication (27). It is now available in the U.S.A. (called fomepizole) and is given as a 15 mg/kg–10 mg/kg infusion.

C. Disposition. Currently, all patients suspected of ethylene glycol ingestion must be admitted and monitored. Patients who have ingested toxic levels of ethylene glycol may be asymptomatic on initial presentation.

METHANOL

I. **Sources.** Methanol is a common component of gasoline, gasohol, antifreeze, windshield washer fluid, photocopying fluid, perfume, wood alcohol, paint solvents, household cleaners, and various other industrial products (Table 15-1).

II. **Physical and clinical properties**

A. Methanol is a colorless liquid, with molecular structure CH_3OH, that is volatile at room temperature. Its vapor pressure is 100 mm Hg at 21.2°C. It has a boiling point of 64.7°C and a flash point of 12°C. Its specific gravity is 0.81. Methanol itself is harmless, but its metabolites are toxic. When ingested, it is rapidly absorbed from the gastrointestinal (GI) tract, with peak blood levels seen at 30 to 60 min after ingestion, depending on the presence or absence of food (23). Poisoning is usually characterized by a latent period (40 min to 72 h) (17), during which no symptoms are observed. This phase is followed by the development of an anion gap acidosis and visual symptoms. These phenomena are observed only in humans, primates, and some folate-deficient nonprimates.

B. The **metabolism** of methanol involves the formation of formaldehyde by an oxidation catalyzed by alcohol dehydrogenase. Formaldehyde is 33 times more toxic than methanol and was once believed to be the cause of clinical symptoms. Formaldehyde, however, is rapidly converted to formic acid, which is six times more toxic than methanol. The half-life of formaldehyde is 1 to 2 min, so no accumulation is detectable. Furthermore, formic acid levels correlate with the degree of acidosis and the magnitude of the anion gap. Mortality and visual symptoms have been shown to correlate with the degree of acidosis (28).

C. During the conversion of methanol to carbon dioxide and water, there are two rate-limiting steps. The first is the reaction that converts methanol to formaldehyde, which is described above. The second is a folate-dependent mechanism that converts formic acid to carbon dioxide and water (29).

III. **Mechanism of action/pathophysiology**

A. The volume of distribution of methanol is 0.6 L/kg. Methanol is distributed in body water and is practically insoluble in fat. The liver slowly metabolizes it; 3% to 5% is excreted via the lungs and up to 12% via the kidneys (23). The **half-life** of methanol is 12 h, which can be reduced to 2.5 h by dialysis.

B. Formic acid is thought to be responsible for the ocular toxicity associated with methanol poisoning. It inhibits cytochrome oxidase in the optic nerve, disturbing the flow of axoplasm (26). Both formic acid and lactic acid appear to be responsible for the metabolic acidosis and decrease in plasma bicarbonate.

C. It has been proposed by Smith et al. (7,30) that lactic acid is generated by the lowering of hepatic NAD/NADH ratios. Palmisano et al. (29) reported a case of the absence of anion gap metabolic acidosis following ingestion of a potentially lethal dose of methanol along with ethanol, and they also reviewed four similar cases. They attributed this finding to the efficacy of ethanol in preventing metabolism of methanol. The alternative explanation is an enhanced rate of folate-dependent formic acid metabolism in some individuals, preventing formic acid accumulation. The conclusion to be drawn is that, although methanol ingestion is usually characterized by an anion gap acidosis, the absence of an anion gap does not exclude the diagnosis.

D. Methanol mainly affects the CNS with symptoms of inebriation, drowsiness, obtundation, seizure, and coma. It also targets the optic nerve and basal ganglia. Brain hemorrhage was reported by Phang et al. in six of 45 patients (31), though it was unclear whether methanol alone was responsible for these events. All of the patients described underwent heparinization during dialysis, and it is possible that the heparin was at least partially culpable.

IV. Clinical presentation

A. **History.** Methanol poisonings frequently occur as epidemic outbreaks. Often bootleg liquor is implicated. Methanol is sometimes ingested as a substitute for ethanol, when ethanol is either too expensive or unavailable. A case of pediatric poisoning occurred when methanol was mistaken for distilled water and was mixed with formula (28). Methanol poisoning has also occurred by cutaneous absorption and by inhalation. Recent report of methanol toxicity occurred in two firefighters transiently exposed to vaporized methanol and presented with only mild headache (49). Methanol also may be derived from endogenous production and dietary sources. In addition, large amounts of wine or liquor can result in detectable methanol levels due to their methanol content (50). A strong clue to the presence of methanol poisoning is a report of cloudy or misty vision, sometimes described as a snowstorm. Headache, dizziness, nausea, vomiting, epigastric pain, and weakness are early symptoms.

B. **Physical examination**

1. **Decreased visual acuity,** optic disk hyperemia, and peripapillary edema may be present. Vertical and rotatory nystagmus are also reported (17). Later in the course, optic disk pallor and decreased pupillary response to light may be seen but are poor prognostic indicators. The patient may develop irreversible visual loss or blindness.

2. **Breathlessness,** when seen early, is related to unmetabolized methanol. Subsequent tachypnea develops as a compensation for metabolic acidosis. Sudden respiratory failure may be the terminal event.

3. **Severe abdominal pain,** anorexia, nausea, and vomiting may be present. The absence of these symptoms does not rule out a serious ingestion.

4. The spectrum of **neurologic symptoms** is broad, ranging from a mild "hangover-like" feeling to seizures, coma, and basal ganglia infarct. It should be recalled that it is possible for the patient to be completely asymptomatic during the latent period as well as when latency should have ended.

5. **CNS depression,** coma, confusion, slurred speech, and seizures may be present.

6. **Bradycardia, myocardial depression,** and **hypotension** signal severe intoxication.

7. **Nuchal rigidity** and **meningeal signs** have been reported and may be correlated with hemorrhage.

V. Differential diagnosis. Without a history of methanol ingestion, the differential diagnosis is broad. It includes diabetic ketoacidosis, pancreatitis, nephrolithiasis, meningitis, subarachnoid hemorrhage, and retinal detachment. Other toxic ingestions must be considered as well. The differential diagnosis of osmolar gaps and anion gap acidosis is covered in Chapter 12.

VI. Laboratory analysis
  A. Laboratory studies
    1. **Arterial blood gases** (ABGs) to determine if the patient is acidotic.
    2. **Serum electrolytes** to calculate an anion gap.
    3. **Complete blood count** to check mean corpuscular volume and hemoglobin concentration. The work of Swartz et al. (32) suggests that mean corpuscular volume was significantly lower in those patients who were severely poisoned. The mechanism is unexplained.
    4. **Urinalysis** to determine specific gravity and the presence of crystals signaling other toxic ingestions.
    5. **Serum osmolarity** can only be measured by freezing point depression to compare measured and calculated osmolarity. An accurate serum osmolality frequently cannot be obtained in the laboratory. Separately, there is variability in the calculated osmolality depending on the calculation used. Lastly, when methanol is metabolized, the osmolar gap decreases (45). Therefore, the reliability of osmolar gaps to make the diagnosis is poor.
    6. **Serum and urine ketones** to help exclude other diagnoses (i.e., diabetic ketoacidosis, alcoholic ketoacidosis, starvation ketoacidosis).
    7. **Blood alcohol level**
    8. **Blood levels of methanol** and of other common ingestions that present a similar picture (e.g., salicylates and ethylene glycol). Note: The serum methanol level should be measured by gas chromatography, as other methods may fail to detect its presence.
  B. Range of toxicity. A lethal dose is considered to be 1 to 2 mL/kg (24), or 80 mg/dL. Death has also been reported with ingestion of as little as 15 mL of a 40% solution (or 6 g of pure methanol), and survival has been reported after ingestion of 500 to 600 mL of a solution of the same concentration (17). The lowest dose reported to be associated with toxicity is 4 mL of absolute methanol (23,28). Dietary and endogenous sources may account for as much as 1.5 mg/L(26).

VII. Management. The initial management of methanol poisoning is the same as for any other ingestion or injury: Secure an airway and check for breathing and circulation. Outcome appears to depend on the length of the interval between the ingestion and the initiation of specific therapy. It is also dependent on the degree of acidosis (17), which may in part be a function of time. Treatment consists in preventing further absorption by induced emesis or lavage (the latter is preferable) and charcoal for possible coingestions. Ethanol infusion to block conversion of methanol to formate by competitive inhibition of alcohol dehydrogenase forces the elimination of unmetabolized methanol by extrahepatic routes. Fluid replacement is needed for dehydration (and inhibition of antidiuretic hormone). Bicarbonate should be used to correct acidosis (17). Folate enhances formate oxidation to carbon dioxide and water.

Hemodialysis removes both methanol and formate (33). Seizures may be controlled with diazepam and phenytoin.

A. **Ethanol and 4-mp.** See Ethylene Glycol, **VIII.B.1.**

B. **Bicarbonate.** The amount of bicarbonate required may be substantial and depends on the amount of alcohol already metabolized to formic acid. Initially 1 to 2 mEq/kg may be given (17). The goal is to normalize the pH by keeping formic acid in its unprotonated (anionic) form, thereby limiting its entry into the CNS. Frequent ABG determinations are advised (24).

C. **Diazepam and phenytoin.** If seizures develop, initial control may be obtained using **diazepam** 5 to 10 mg i.v. over 2 to 3 min initially for adults, repeated every 10 to 15 min as needed, to a maximum of 30 mg. For children 30 days to 5 years old give 0.25 to 0.40 mg/kg to a maximum dose of 5 mg. In children older than 5 years of age, the maximum dose is 10 mg (17). **Phenytoin** may then be loaded at a dose of 15 to 20 mg/kg i.v. infused at a rate not to exceed 50 mg/min. The patient should be monitored for hypotension and bradycardia (34).

D. **Hemodialysis**

1. There is some disagreement about the blood methanol level that indicates a need for hemodialysis. The more stringent level suggested is 25 mg/dL (24), but others suggest 50 mg/dL (17,26). There have been no controlled studies to establish either recommendation as superior.

2. Aside from a measured blood level of 25 mg/dL or more, the other indications for dialysis are severe acidosis, persistent fluid and electrolyte disturbances despite treatment, visual symptoms, or renal failure. *In the face of any of the above, hemodialysis is warranted regardless of the methanol level* (17,24).

3. Osterloh (33) considered blood methanol levels to be an unreliable indicator of methanol toxicity and the need for hemodialysis. He proposed the use of formate levels. His study and review of the work of others indicate that formate levels more than 20 mg/dL may be expected to produce ocular injury and acidosis. Endogenous formate concentrations are less than 1.2 mg/dL (33).

4. Phang et al. (31) suggested that heparinization during dialysis be avoided, as it may have been a contributory factor in the necrosis and hemorrhage they observed in six of 45 patients. They proposed the use of an artificial kidney with a biocompatible membrane, such as polymethylmethacrylate, with an albumin coating prime.

5. Goldfrank et al. (24) stated that there is no role for peritoneal dialysis or hemoperfusion in the management of methanol poisoning.

6. More recently, Palatnick et al. (51) proposed that hemodialysis be considered for all methanol-poisoned patients who are treated with ethanol infusion because of the increased risk of toxicity and complications during ethanol monotherapy. Unfortunately, the study was small (six patients), retrospective, ethanol levels were not consistently maintained throughout the therapy, and there was no control group. The study also failed to demonstrate any worse outcome with monotherapy. The study, however, did emphasize that hemodialysis will shorten the half-life of methanol, and thus decrease ICU stay and ultimately cost (51).

E. Folic acid

1. Leucovorin (folinic acid) and folic acid are needed for the conversion of formic acid to carbon dioxide and water. The recommended dose initially is leucovorin 1 mg/kg i.v. up to 50 mg/dose, followed by folic acid 1 mg/kg up to 50 mg/dose.

2. Leucovorin is the active form of folic acid. It does not require reduction by the enzyme dihydrofolate reductase to provide one carbon moiety. In asymptomatic patients it is possible to use folic acid alone, as the body has time to perform the necessary conversion (17). Becker (26) suggested folic acid 50 mg i.v. q4h.

F. 4-Methylpyrazole (4-MP) is a competitive inhibitor of alcohol dehydrogenase. The effect of 4-MP on ocular toxicity was investigated by Blomstrand et al. in cynomolgus monkeys with promising results. The advantage of 4-MP over ethanol is the lack of a CNS depressant effect (27). More recently, several patients with a toxic methanol ingestion was successfully treated with 4-MP (54).

G. Disposition. Any patient who has ingested more than an accidental sip of methanol requires treatment and monitoring. The long latency period reported to be between 40 min and 72 h may cause a severely poisoned patient to appear asymptomatic. Methanol has a long half-life of elimination with wide individual differences. Depending on the size of the ingestion and the treatment modalities required, treatment may take several days.

ISOPROPYL ALCOHOL

I. Sources

A. Isopropyl alcohol (molecular weight of 60) is an aliphatic alcohol used widely in industry, medicine, and the home.

B. Home sources include rubbing alcohol, skin lotion, hair tonics, aftershave lotions, and window cleaning fluids. Most "rubbing alcohol" contains 70% isopropyl alcohol.

C. Isopropyl alcohol, like methanol, is ingested by the compromised or misguided alcoholic because it is often less expensive than ethanol.

D. Isopropyl alcohol may be identified by other names, such as isopropanol, secondary propyl alcohol, propan-1-ol, and 2-propanol.

II. Pharmacokinetics and toxicity

A. Isopropyl alcohol is readily absorbed from the GI tract, with peak plasma levels occurring 1 h after ingestion. Clinically significant dermal absorption occurs (35). Coma has been reported in children following dermal exposure (36).

B. Accidental inhalation of isopropanol vapor during massage or alcohol sponging in poorly ventilated areas has been reported to produce deep coma (37).

C. The volume of distribution is 0.6 to 0.7 L/kg. The compound is excreted by first order kinetics with a half-life of 2.5 to 3.2 h. Isopropyl alcohol has a pulmonary alveolar clearance of 8 L/min.

D. Isopropyl alcohol appears to be more toxic then ethyl alcohol but less toxic than methanol. Isopropyl alcohol is metabolized at a slower rate than ethanol.

E. Ketonuria is seen in isopropyl alcohol ingestion because approximately 15% of the ingested dose is metabolized to acetone.

F. The lethal dose in adults is approximately 240 mL of isopropyl alcohol. Patients have exhibited intoxication after doses as low as 20 mL.

G. Rectal absorption may reach blood levels similar to those seen with ingestions.

H. Three ounces of 70% isopropyl alcohol can produce blood levels of 100 mg/dL in a 70-kg person if rapidly absorbed.

I. There appear to be instances of alcoholics tolerant to ethanol exhibiting some degree of crosstolerance to isopropyl alcohol.

J. Blood isopropanol levels of 150 mg/dL are frequently associated with coma. Levels of more than 200 mg/dL have been associated with death in those not undergoing intensive medical treatment.

K. Hemodialyzed patients have survived levels of up to 500 mg/dL.

L. Serum levels around 50 mg/dL indicate mild intoxication. Serum levels of 128 to 200 mg/dL have been associated with deep coma and death.

M. The oxidation of isopropanol to acetone most likely involves the enzyme alcohol dehydrogenase (although ethanol administration has not been used clinically to treat this condition).

N. About 20% to 50% of unchanged isopropanol excretion occurs through the kidney.

O. There is evidence that isopropanol enhances the toxicity of hydrocarbons (38,39).

P. A retrospective review of acetonemic patient suggests that acetone may be converted to detectable amounts of isopropanolunder physiological conditions where reduced NAD is elevated. All five patients with detectable levels were insulin dependent diabetics in diabetic ketoacidosis without any history suggestive of isopropanol ingestion (52).

III. **Clinical manifestations**

  A. **General signs.** A seemingly intoxicated patient with an odor of acetone or "rubbing alcohol" on the breath.

  B. **Cardiovascular signs**
    1. Tachycardia is common.
    2. Hypotension occurs because of peripheral vasodilation.
    3. Bradycardia has been reported.
    4. Like ethanol, chronic use of isopropyl alcohol can cause cardiomyopathy, which may manifest as an arrhythmia.

  C. **Respiratory signs**
    1. Respiratory failure occurs with large ingestions and may appear within 23 h of ingestion.
    2. Aspiration secondary to CNS depression may occur.

  D. **GI signs**
    1. Hemorrhagic gastritis
    2. Vomiting
    3. Hepatocellular damage (sometimes)

  E. **Renal signs**
    1. Renal failure secondary to severe hypotension has been reported.
    2. Myoglobinuria may occur in severe cases.

  F. **Dermoregulatory signs.** Hypothermia may occur secondary to vasodilation and CNS depression.

  G. **CNS signs**
    1. Headache
    2. Dizziness

3. Inebriation
4. Ataxia
5. Coma
6. Nystagmus

H. Other signs. Hemolysis and myopathy (with myoglobinuria) have been reported.

IV. **Laboratory investigation**

A. **Blood/serum**

1. **Osmolal gap.** Usually there is evidence of an osmolal gap. For every 1 mg/dL of isopropanol, there is an osmolal gap of 0.17 mOsm/L. An elevation in osmolal gap of 1 mOsm/L represents an isopropanol level of 6 mg/dL. Levels of ethyl alcohol, methanol, and ethylene glycol should be obtained in addition to isopropanol levels. The presence of other alcohols affects the osmolal gap, and their relative contributions must be considered.

$$\text{Osmolar conc. (mOsm/L)} = \text{concentration (mg/L)/molecular weight}$$

2. **Gas-liquid chromatography** should be employed to determine serum isopropyl alcohol levels. Other methods may be inaccurate.

3. **Acetone levels** are present 0.5 to 1.0 h after ingestion. As the level of isopropyl alcohol drops, the acetone level rises. As acetone may contribute to the CNS depression, this level should be ascertained as well as an isopropyl alcohol level.

4. **Ketosis** characterizes isopropyl alcohol intoxication. Metabolic acidosis, when present, tends to be mild. Ketonemia was not detected in a recent isopropanol ingestion by a Japanese man. This lack of ketonemia was attributed to a failure of the patient's liver to convert isopropanaol to acetone either from an anomalous or deficient alcohol dehydrogenase or inhibition of alcohol dehydrogenase activity by substances ingested by the patient (53).

5. **Both hyperglycemia and hypoglycemia** have been reported (40). Hypoglycemia is by far the more common of the two, but either is an inconsistent finding. It is of special note that the onset of hypoglycemia may be delayed up to several hours after ingestion.

6. There may be **serologic evidence** of renal failure, renal tubular acidosis, or hepatic dysfunction.

7. **Pseudoelevation of serum creatinine**

B. **Urine**

1. **Acetone** is detectable in the urine approximately 3 h after ingestion.
2. **Glycosuria** is typically absent.

C. **Cerebrospinal fluid.** Isolated reports of increased CSF protein have been recorded (41). The pathophysiology is not known.

V. **Treatment**

A. **Emesis** is not suggested, as the onset of CNS depression may occur within 30 min after the ingestion.

B. **Gastric lavage** is most important within the first 2 h after ingestion, but large amounts of isopropyl alcohol can be recovered even if attempted after this 2-h period (42). As CNS depression is a common feature of significant ingestions, particular attention must be paid to airway protection during lavage even in the alert patient. Intubation is recommended for any patient with a compromised mental status or those who by history have ingested an amount of isopropyl alcohol likely to cause CNS depression.

C. Isopropyl alcohol is not absorbed well by activated **charcoal.** Isopropanol is absorbed at an approximate proportion of 500 mg/g carbon. A cathartic should be used when administering the activated charcoal.

D. If **hypotension** develops, treat with intravenous fluids and place the patient in the Trendelenburg position. If no response, dopamine or norepinephrine is indicated.

E. **Hemodialysis** is indicated for patients exhibiting marked symptomatology unresponsive to the above measures. Early hemodialysis is also useful in the patient who by history has ingested a lethal or near-lethal dose. Blood isopropanol levels may fall from 440 mg/dL to 100 mg/dL in as short an interval as 5 h with hemodialysis.

F. **Peritoneal dialysis** is not as effective as hemodialysis but is recommended if symptomatology warrants dialysis. There has been a report of a successful outcome in a patient who underwent peritoneal dialysis for an acetone level of 1,878 mg/dL.

G. **Forced diuresis** is not regarded as effective.

H. **Ethanol administration** has not been used clinically for isopropyl alcohol ingestions as it is for methanol or ethylene glycol poisoning. This difference in treatment may be related to differences in kinetics of elimination between isopropanol and ethanol or methanol as demonstrated in animal studies.

I. **Disposition.** All patients who are symptomatic should be admitted and treated. Asymptomatic patients may be discharged with close follow-up. Since there are no current recommendations for the duration of time a patient should be observed prior to discharge, we suggest adhering to the standard 6-h observation period.

References

1. Verrilli MR, et al. Fatal ethylene glycol intoxication. *Cleve Clin J Med* 1987;54:289.
2. Turk J, Morrell L, Avioli LV. Ethylene glycol intoxication. *Arch Intern Med* 1986;146:1601–1603.
3. Beasley V, Buck W. Acute ethylene glycol toxicosis: a review. *Vet Hum Toxicol* 1980;22:255–263.
4. Cadnapaphornchai P, et al. Ethylene glycol poisoning: diagnosis based on high osmolal and anion gaps and crystalluria. *Ann Emerg Med* 1981;10:94–97.
5. Hewlett TP, et al. Ethylene glycol poisoning: the value of glycolic acid determinations for diagnosis and treatment. *J Clin Toxicol* 1986;24:389–402.
6. Clay KL, Murphy RC. On the metabolic acidosis of ethylene glycol intoxication. *Toxicol Appl Pharmacol* 1977;39:39.
7. Smith SR, et al. Lactate and formate in methanol poisoning. *Lancet* 1982;1:561.
8. Jacobsen P, et al. Ethylene glycol intoxication: evaluation of kinetics and crystalluria. *Am J Med* 1988;84:145–152.
9. Tintinalli J. Of anions, osmols, and methanol poisoning. *JACEP* 1977;6:417–421.
10. Brown CG, et al. Ethylene glycol poisoning. *Ann Emerg Med* 1983;12:501–506.
11. Jacobsen D, Ostby N, Bredesen E. Studies on ethylene glycol poisoning. *Acta Med Scand* 1982;212:11–15.
12. Berman LB, Schreiner GE, Feys J. The nephrotoxic lesion of ethylene glycol. *Ann Intern Med* 1957;46:611–619.
13. Catchings TT, et al. Adult respiratory distress syndrome secondary to ethylene glycol ingestion. *Ann Emerg Med* 1985;14:594–596.
14. Walker JT, et al. Computed tomographic and sonographic findings in acute ethylene glycol poisoning. *J Ultrasound Med* 1945;2:429–431.
15. Factor SA, Lava NS. Ethylene glycol intoxication: a new stage in the clinical syndrome. *NY State J Med* 1987;179–180.
16. Heckerling PS. Ethylene glycol poisoning with normal anion gap due to occult bromide intoxication. *Ann Emerg Med* 1987;16:1384–1386.
17. Rumack BH. *Poisondex toxicologic management (vol. 59).* Denver: Micromedex, 1989.
18. Gabow PA. Ethylene glycol intoxication. *Am J Kidney Dis* 1988;11:277–279.

19. Anonymous. Possible death from drinking ethylene glycol (Prestone): queries, and minor notes [Letter]. *JAMA* 1930;94:1940.
20. Scully R, Gababini J, McNeely B. Case records of the Massachusetts General Hospital, case 38-1979. *N Engl J Med* 1979;301:650–657.
21. Stokes J. Prevention of organ damage in massive ethylene glycol ingestion. *JAMA* 1980;243:2065–2066.
22. Peterson CD, et al. Ethylene glycol poisoning. *N Engl J Med* 1987;304:21–23.
23. Kulig K, et al. Toxic effects of methanol ethylene glycol and isopropyl alcohol. *Top Emerg Med* 1984;1:14.
24. Goldfrank LR, et al. Methanol, ethylene glycol and isopropanol. In: *Goldfrank's toxicologic emergencies*. 4th ed. Norwalk, CT: Appleton & Lange, 1990:481–497.
25. Cheng JT, et al. Clearance of ethylene glycol by kidneys and hemodialysis. *Clin Toxiciol* 1987;25:15–108.
26. Becker C. Methanol poisoning. *J Emerg Med* 1983;1:51.
27. Blomstrand R, et al. Studies on the effect of 4-methylprazole on methanol poisoning using the monkey as an animal model: with particular reference to the ocular toxicity. *Drug Alcohol Depend* 1984;13:343.
28. Litovitz T. The alcohols: ethanol, methanol, isopropanol, ethylene glycol. *Pediatr Clin North Am* 1986;33:311.
29. Palmisano J, et al. Absence of anion gap metabolic acidosis in severe methanol poisoning: a case report and review of the literature. *Am J Kidney Dis* 1987;9:441.
30. Smith SR, et al. Combined formate and lactate acidosis in methanol poisoning. *Lancet* 1982;1:561.
31. Phang PT, et al. Brain hemorrhage associated with methanol poisoning. *Crit Care Med* 1988;16:137.
32. Swartz RD, et al. Epidemic methanol poisoning; clinical and biochemical analysis of a recent episode. *Medicine (Baltimore)* 1981;60:373.
33. Osterloh J. Serum formate concentration in methanol intoxication as a criterion for hemodialysis. *Ann Intern Med* 1986;104:200.
34. Rosen P. *Emergency medicine*. 2nd ed. St. Louis: Mosby, 1988.
35. Martinez TT, et al. A comparison of the absorption and metabolism of isopropyl alcohol by oral, dermal and inhalation routes. *Vet Hum Toxicol* 1986;28:233–236.
36. McFadden SW, Haddow JE. Coma produced by topical application of isopropanol. *Pediatrics* 1969;43:622–623.
37. Gosselin RE, Smith RP, Hodge HC, eds. Isopropyl alcohol. In: *Clinical toxicology of commercial products*. 5th ed. Baltimore: Williams & Wilkins, 1984:111–217.
38. Cornish HH, Adefuin J. Potentiation of carbon tetrachloride toxicity by aliphatic alcohols. *Arch Environ Health* 1967;14:447.
39. Traiger GJ, Plaa GC. Chlorinated hydrocarbon toxicity: potentiation by isopropyl alcohol and acetone. *Arch Environ Health* 1976;28:276.
40. Kelner M, Bailey DN. Isopropyl ingestion: interpretation of blood concentrations and clinical findings. *J Toxicol Clin Toxicol* 1983;20:497.
41. Visudhiphan P, Kaufman H. Increased cerebrospinal fluid protein following isopropyl alcohol intoxication. *NY State J Med* 1971;71:887–888.
42. Light FB, Marx GF. The value of gastric aspiration in a comatose child. *Anesthesiology* 1969;31:478–480.
43. Leon M, Graeber C. Absence of high anion gap metabolic acidosis in severe ethylene glycol poisoning: a potential effect of simultaneous lithium carbonate ingestion. *Am J Kidney Dis* 1994;23:313–316.
44. Ammar KA, Heckerling PS. Ethylene glycol poisoning with a normal anion gap caused by concurrent ethanol ingestion: importance of the osmolol gap. *Am J Kidney Dis* 1996;27:1.
45. Glaser DS. Utility of the serum osmol gap in the diagnosis of methanol or ethylene glycol ingestion. *Ann Emerg Med* 1996;27:343–346.
46. Haupt, et al. Poisindex (R) Editorial Staff. *Poisondex toxicologic management (vol. 88)*. Englewood, Colorado. Micromedex, 1996.
47. Winter, et al. Poisindex (R) Editorial Staff. *Poisondex toxicologic management (vol. 88)*. Englewood, Colorado. Micromedex, 1996.
48. Christiansson LK, et al. Treatment of severe ethylene glycol intoxication with continuous arteriovenous hemofiltration dialysis. *Clin Toxicol* 1995;33:2, 267–270.
49. Aufderheide TP, White SM, Brady WJ, Stueven HA. Inhalation and percutaneous methanol toxicity in two firefighters. *Ann Emerg Med* 1993;22:12.
50. Tintinalli JE. Serum methanol in the absence of methanol ingestion [Letter]. *Ann Emerg Med* 1995;26:393.
51. Palatnick W, Redman LW, Sitar DS, Tenebein, M. Methanol half-life during ethanol administration: implications for management of methanol poisoning. *Ann Emerg Med* 1995;26:202–207.
52. Bailey DN. Detection of isopropanol in acetonemic patients not exposed to isopropanol. *Clin Toxicol* 1990;28:459–466.
53. Chan KM, Wong ET, Matthews WS. Severe isopropanolemia without acetonemia or clinical manifestations of isopropanol intoxication. *Clin Chem* 1993;39:9.
54. Jacobsen D, Sebastian LS, Barron SK, Carriere EW, McMartin KE. Effects of 4-Methylpyrazole, methanol/ethylene glycol antidote, in healthy humans. *The Journal of Emergency Medicine* 1990;8:455–461.

Selected Readings

Arena JM, Drew RM. *Poisoning: toxicology, symptoms, treatments*. Springfield, IL: Charles C. Thomas Publisher, 1986.

Done A. Signs, symptoms and sources. *Emerg Med* 1982;Jan. 15:42.

Goldfrank LR. *Toxicologic emergencies*. 4th ed. Norwalk, CT: Appleton & Lange, 1990.

Haddad L, Winchester J. *Clinical management of poisoning and drug overdose*. Philadelphia: WB Saunders, 1983.

Johns Hopkins Hospital. *The Harriet Lane manual*. Chicago: Year Book Medical Publishers, 1987.

Klassen CD, Amdur MO, Doule J. *Casarett and Doules toxicology*. New York: Macmillan, 1986.

Mattheus SJ, Schneiweiss F, Cersosimo RJ. *A clinical manual of adverse drug reactions*. Norwalk, CT: Appleton-Century-Crofts, 1986.

Noj EK, Kelen GD. *Manual of toxicologic emergencies*. Chicago: Year Book Medical Publishers, 1989.

Rosen P, et al. *Emergency medicine: concepts and clinical practice*. St. Louis: Mosby, 1983.

Emergency Toxicology, Second Edition,
edited by Peter Viccellio.
Lippincott–Raven Publishers, Philadelphia © 1998.

16

Aldehydes, Ketones, Ethers, and Esters

†Stephen R. Hayden, °Lester Kallus, and *Charles F. McCuskey

*†Department of Emergency Medicine, University of San Diego Medical Center, San Diego, California 92103; °Setauket, New York 11733; *New York, New York 10029*

Aldehydes and ketones are produced by oxidation of primary and secondary alcohols, respectively. Generically, aldehydes are represented by the formula RCHO, and ketones RCR'O, the carbonyl group (C=O) being the common structural unit. Many are naturally occurring intermediates in biologic metabolism and are ubiquitous as components of industrial solvents, antiseptics, preservatives, adhesives, and cosmetics. Toxicologic exposure may occur via inhalation, by ingestion, or topically. It produces a wide variety of symptoms and effects.

ALDEHYDES

I. **Formaldehyde (methanal)**

    A. **Sources and available forms.** Formaldehyde is available in many forms, including formaldehyde-urea resins used in the manufacture of adhesives for plywood, veneers, particle board, plastics, and rubber products. It is also found as formalin solution, commonly used as a preservative (1). It can be found as a product of combustion in cigarette smoke and automobile exhaust, and as a component of cosmetics, deodorants, detergents, dyes, and permanent press clothing (2). Health care workers will be most familiar with the use as a tissue fixative.

    B. **Physical and clinical properties.** Formaldehyde is structurally the simplest aldehyde; its chemical formula is HCHO. It is a colorless gas, boiling point (b.p.) 19°C, and has a pungent odor; it is soluble in aqueous solution, producing formalin. Formalin comes in solutions of 37% to 50% formaldehyde, often with 10% to 15% methanol to prevent polymerization. Formalin is a powerful bactericidal agent and is consequently used as a preservative and antiseptic.

    C. **Pharmacology and metabolism.** Upon oral ingestion, absorption of formaldehyde is rapid, and is oxidized to formic acid in the liver by alcohol dehydrogenase with an estimated half-life in plasma of approximately 1.5 min. Formic acid is then metabolized to carbon dioxide and water by a slower folate-dependent enzymatic pathway. The estimated plasma half-life of formic acid is 90 min (3).

    D. **Clinical effects**

        1. **Ingestion** of aqueous formalin

            a. **Local effects.** Formaldehyde is a strong mucosal irritant that produces a severe corrosive gastritis following significant ingestions (4). Erosion, ulceration, hemorrhage, frank coagulation necrosis, and even perforation may occur. The oropharynx and esophagus may develop similar lesions; however, the squamous epithelium of the esophagus seems more resistant to such injury than the columnar gastric epithelium (4).

    b. **Systemic effects** include CNS depression, coma, and severe anion gap metabolic acidosis due to the rapid accumulation of formic acid (3). Death has resulted in one case from ingestion of as little as 30 mL of a 37% solution (5).

  2. **Inhalation exposure.** Inhalation of vapors containing 2 to 5 ppm or more has a direct irritant effect on the respiratory mucosa and nasopharynx (6). Formaldehyde is thought to act as a hapten, although it is currently unproved, that formaldehyde can actually cause immunologically mediated asthma (7). It is known to produce bronchoconstriction directly and a decreased 1-s forced expiratory volume/forced vital capacity ($FEV_{1.0}/FVC$) ratio.

  3. **Dermatologic** effects. Formaldehyde is a potent dermal sensitizer. The response may be immediate and is characterized by drying, erythema, urticaria, desquamation, and hyperesthesias, or a delayed contact dermatitis may develop.

  4. **Ears, nose, and throat.** The oropharyngeal mucosa and conjunctivae similarly become irritated upon exposure to formaldehyde at exposures as low as 0.5 to 1.0 ppm (8). Note that the odor threshold is also 0.5 to 1.0 ppm.

  5. **Hepatotoxicity** has been reported following ingestion of formaldehyde (9).

  6. **Carcinogenicity.** Formaldehyde has been labeled by the U.S. Environmental Protection Agency (EPA) as a probable human carcinogen, producing nasopharyngeal squamous cell cancer in rodents (10).

E. **Signs and symptoms** vary depending on the route and concentration of the exposure. In milder cases, where symptoms are nonspecific (e.g., conjunctivitis, headache, sore throat, fatigue, bronchoconstriction), information should be obtained regarding type of housing (mobile home, urea-formaldehyde resin insulation, particle board) or use of various consumer products (cosmetics, adhesives, detergents) that may contain formaldehyde. If exposure appears to be originating at home or work, air samples may be obtained for measurements.

F. **Diagnostic tests.** Currently, there are no laboratory analyses that are specific for formaldehyde ingestion/exposure (11). Serum levels are not useful owing to their short half-life in plasma, and urine formic acid levels have not been found to be a good index of exposure (12). It is recommended, however, that blood gases should be monitored for the development of acidosis. Serum electrolytes, glucose, BUN, and creatinine should be assayed, liver function tests are obtained, as is the serum methanol level in the event of formalin ingestion.

G. **Therapeutic intervention**

  1. **Oral ingestion.** No specific antidote is available. Follow general principles of treatment of ingestions.

    a. **Dilute** immediately with 100 to 250 mL of water or milk. Emesis should be induced following dilution if it is less than 30 min after ingestion.

    b. **Gastric lavage** should be performed in the emergency department if ingestion occurred within 1 h. A small-bore nasogastric (NG) tube and saline or tap water should be used. Care should be taken when inserting the NG tube to avoid perforation through an area of coagulation necrosis. If mental status is impaired, the patient should be placed in the left lateral decubitus position or intubated prior to lavage in order to prevent aspiration.

 c. **Activated charcoal** 1 g/kg should follow lavage. A cathartic (e.g., magnesium citrate or sorbitol) may be mixed with the charcoal or administered separately.

 d. **Acidosis** should be treated by first correcting any concomitant hypotension or hypoxemia that might lead to lactate formation. If acidosis is severe (pH less than 7.2), sodium bicarbonate 1 mEq/kg i.v. is given as the initial dose; further doses should be administered based on the repeated measurement of blood pH. Hemodialysis may be required for severe acid-base aberrations (pH less than 7.2 refractory to sodium bicarbonate therapy) or other disturbances not resolved by conventional treatment.

 e. **Esophagoscopy** is indicated to assess the severity of tissue damage (13).

 2. **Inhalation exposure.** Remove patient to fresh air and administer supplemental. Treat bronchospasm with nebulized bronchodilators, assist ventilation as necessary, and assess the need for endotracheal intubation.

 3. **Dermal exposure** should be treated with thorough cleansing of the affected area with soap and water.

 4. **Eye/mucous membrane** exposure. Eyes and mucous membranes exposed to formaldehyde should be irrigated copiously with saline or water for at least 15 min. Altered visual acuity, lacrimation, or photophobia that persists may require ophthalmologic evaluation.

 H. **Disposition.** Owing to an elimination half-life of approximately 90 min in plasma, patients who display no signs of serious toxicity or acidosis at 4 to 6 h after exposure may be considered for discharge.

II. Acetaldehyde (ethanal)

 A. **Sources and available forms.** Acetaldehyde is a reagent used in the production of acetic acid, acetic anhydride, *N*-butanol, explosives, varnishes, photographic chemicals, and numerous other compounds. It is a normal product of ethanol metabolism, is a normal result of the combustion of tobacco smoke, and is emitted from automobiles (14). Commercial grades include a 50% aqueous solution or 99% solution in small steel cylinders (15).

 B. **Physical and chemical properties.** Acetaldehyde is a colorless liquid, with the chemical formula CH_3CHO, molecular weight of 44.05, and b.p. 20.2°C. The compound is volatile; exhibits a pungent, fruity odor; and is freely soluble in water, alcohol, ether, gasoline, and acetone. In addition, acetaldehyde is flammable and can react explosively with a variety of substances (16).

 C. **Pharmacology and metabolism.** Acetaldehyde is a normal product of ethanol metabolism. H_3C-CH_2OH is converted to H_3C-CHO by the action of alcohol dehydrogenase. This reaction takes place by first order kinetics, reducing serum ethanol concentration at a constant rate of 15 mg/dL/h. Acetaldehyde is then further oxidized to acetic acid by aldehyde dehydrogenase, which then enters the Krebs cycle. Disulfiram competes for aldehyde dehydrogenase, increasing the serum level of acetaldehyde and leading to the symptoms associated with the disulfiram reaction (17). Acetaldehyde is readily absorbed on inhalation, ingestion, or dermal exposure.

D. **Clinical effects**
1. **Inhalation/exposure to vapors**
    a. **Respiratory** irritation has been demonstrated at 134 ppm, leading to bronchitis and even delayed pulmonary edema, often the cause of acetaldehyde-related deaths (18).
    b. **Ears, nose, and throat.** Acetaldehyde is a mucous membrane irritant.
    c. **Eye** irritation may occur at exposures of 50 ppm, with higher concentrations resulting in photophobia and persistent lacrimation (15). Direct splash injury can produce superficial corneal injury, which usually heals rapidly (19).
2. **Ingestion,** though rare, often produces abdominal pain and cramping, as well as emesis. If significant absorption occurs, symptoms may include headache, diaphoresis, tachypnea, tachycardia, and hypertension, with bradycardia and hypotension as levels rise (15). At high concentrations, CNS depression occurs (18).
3. **Dermatitis** occurs after prolonged contact.
4. **Carcinogenicity.** There is evidence to suggest that acetaldehyde produces squamous carcinoma and adenocarcinoma in laboratory animals (16).

E. **Diagnostic tests.** It is possible to measure acetaldehyde in the blood (11); however, this process has many inherent artifactual errors, levels often do not correlate with clinical symptoms and hence are not routinely recommended (17). Measurement of serum electrolytes, liver function tests, and renal function evaluation should be performed.

F. **Therapeutic intervention.** No specific antidote is available. Treatment should proceed as outlined for formaldehyde (see **I.G**).

III. **Paraldehyde**
A. **Sources and available forms.** Paraldehyde is a cyclic trimer of acetaldehyde used primarily as a sedative/hypnotic and anticonvulsant. It is available as a liquid in 30-mL ampules for oral, rectal, or parenteral use (20).

B. **Physical and clinical properties.** Paraldehyde exists as a liquid at room temperature, with a molecular weight of 132.16. It has a characteristic aromatic odor and an unpleasant taste. On exposure to air and light, it decomposes readily to acetaldehyde; and it is soluble in water.

C. **Pharmacology and metabolism.** Paraldehyde has a rapid absorption phase and a slow elimination phase (21). After oral ingestion peak serum levels occur within 30 min (22), and an elimination half-life of 7.4 h (23). It is estimated that approximately 95% of the oral dose is absorbed (24). Paraldehyde is metabolized to acetaldehyde in the liver, which undergoes further transformation as previously described (see **II.C**).

D. **Clinical effects.** Paraldehyde has a depressant action on the cerebral cortex, markedly decreasing electrical activity. The therapeutic serum range is 150 to 200 mg/L; however, there is considerable variability in the dose required to produce toxicity in different individuals (22). The toxic effects of paraldehyde include severe CNS depression, respiratory depression, and pulmonary edema; hemodynamic compromise is seen infrequently. The hallmark of paraldehyde toxicity is the development of lactic acidosis (20).

E. Diagnostic tests. Serum paraldehyde levels should be determined. There is, however, considerable variability in individual susceptibility to the toxic effects of paraldehyde. Arterial blood gases (ABGs) should be monitored for the development of acidosis and serum lactate levels determined.

F. Therapeutic intervention. No specific antidote is available. Therapeutic efforts are directed at correcting the respiratory depression and pulmonary edema if present, including intubation and positive end-expiratory pressure if necessary. Intervention proceeds in the manner described in I.G., with the exception that emesis is not recommended owing to the rapid absorption of paraldehyde. Like formaldehyde, hemodialysis would be indicated for severe acidosis (pH less than 7.2) that did not respond to conventional sodium bicarbonate therapy.

KETONES

Ketones comprise a broad class of solvents. With the exception of acetone, which is discussed in a subsequent section, they possess similar chemical properties and produce similar ranges of toxicity.

A. Sources and available forms. The common ketone solvents include methyl ethyl ketone, methyl propyl ketone, methyl butyl ketone, ethyl butyl ketone, cyclohexanone, acetophenone, and diethyl ketone. All are commercially available as liquid solvents.

B. Pharmacology and metabolism. These agents in general are rapidly absorbed through the skin and gastrointestinal (GI) mucosa. They are reduced in vivo to their secondary alcohols and are then eliminated as the glucuronide conjugate (25). The ketones are excreted via urine and expired air, and the rate of such elimination varies with the volatility of the individual compound.

C. Clinical effects. Exposure to ketone solvent must be differentiated from exposure to ketone peroxide, which is highly caustic. The numerous ketones may be absorbed by ingestion, inhalation, or dermal contact.

    1. Inhalation/exposure to vapors causes irritation of mucous membranes, especially of the nasopharynx and upper airways, leading to sore throat, cough, and salivation. Conjunctivitis, lacrimation, and corneal damage may occur (26). Inhalation of highly concentrated vapors has produced respiratory depression, dyspnea, headache, dizziness, incoordination, and syncope (26).

    2. Ingestion of these solvents produces a metabolic acidosis in high concentration (27). CNS depression, tachycardia, and aspiration pneumonia have all been reported.

    3. Dermatologic exposure has resulted in urticaria, local erythema, and paresthesias (28).

D. Diagnostic tests. Determination of serum levels is generally not helpful, as serum levels do not correlate with the severity of symptoms. Urine may be tested for an increase in conjugated glucuronic acid (11). Blood pH should be monitored owing to the lactic acidosis that occurs with many of the ketones (29).

E. Therapeutic intervention. No specific antidotes are available, and treatment should follow the general principles outlined in **I.G.**

    1. Acidosis (pH less than 7.20) should be treated by intravenous infusion of sodium bicarbonate 1 mEq/kg, as discussed previously for formaldehyde, and further directed by monitoring the serum pH.

2. **Aspiration pneumonia** that fails to improve with standard therapy might be considered for extracorporeal membrane oxygenation (ECMO), which has been reported useful in refractory cases of hydrocarbon aspiration (30).

F. **Disposition.** Elimination half-life in these compounds varies as a function of their volatility, with the more volatile compounds eliminated more rapidly, therefore requiring less observation time. In general, patients who are asymptomatic at 4 to 6 h may be considered for discharge.

II. Acetone (2-propanone)

A. **Sources and available forms.** Acetone is the primary ingredient in fingernail polish remover. It is a volatile solvent widely used in various glues, varnishes, and rubber cements.

B. **Physical and clinical properties.** Acetone is a colorless liquid, chemical formula $H_3C\text{-}CO\text{-}CH_3$. It is volatile and flammable, and has a characteristic sweet odor. This agent has a specific gravity of 0.79. The odor threshold is 100 ppm (31).

C. **Pharmacology and metabolism.** Acetone is produced in the body by the action of alcohol dehydrogenase on isopropyl alcohol. Acetone is rapidly absorbed through the lungs and GI tract, and more slowly through the skin. It is excreted unchanged primarily through the respiratory mucosa and in urine. The half-life in plasma is approximately 19 to 31 h (32).

D. **Clinical effects.** Toxicity may occur subsequent to ingestion, inhalation, or dermal absorption.

1. **Neurologic manifestations** include CNS depression, ranging from sedation to coma (33). Acetone has effects similar to those of ethanol but more potent anesthetic effects. In addition, ataxia, paresthesias, and seizures have been reported (34).

2. **Respiratory effects.** Depressed respiratory effort may result as well as bronchial irritation. The characteristic sweet odor of acetone on a patient's breath is unmistakable.

3. **GI effects.** Vomiting and hematemesis sometimes occur after ingestion (35).

4. **Renal effects.** Acute tubular necrosis has occurred after exposure.

5. **Metabolic effects** include hyperglycemia, ketosis, and acidosis much like diabetic ketoacidosis (33).

6. **Eye, ear, nose, and throat.** Minor epithelial damage to the cornea occurs upon splash injury, but it resolves quickly.

E. **Diagnostic tests**

1. **Urine** may be tested for acetone.

2. **Serum levels** are useful for determining the extent of exposure. Blood glucose, ABGs, electrolytes, and liver function tests should be monitored. Acetone may interfere with determination of serum creatinine resulting in falsely elevated levels (36).

F. **Therapeutic intervention.** No specific antidote is available. Treatment is based on the severity of symptoms. Generally, ingestions of small amounts of acetone produce little in the way of clinical effects and require little in the way of treatment. As presenting symptoms increase (i.e., CNS/respiratory depression, acidosis, hyperglycemia) therapy should follow the standard guidelines as outlined in **I.G** for formaldehyde. Because of the prolonged elimination half-life, patients with significant ingestions may require observation for up to 30 h.

ETHERS
Ethyl ether

A. Sources and available forms. Ethyl ether is used as an organic solvent and as a reaction medium in many manufacturing processes. It is also used as a surface antiseptic and for cleaning agents and engine-starting fluids. It was used as a general anesthetic for many years until replaced by less flammable agents. Ether is also sniffed as a substance of abuse.

B. Physical and chemical properties. Ethyl ether is formed by the catalytic dehydration of ethyl alcohol. Its chemical formula is $(CH_3CH_2)_2O$. It is a clear, colorless liquid at room temperature and has a sweet, pungent odor. Its boiling point is 35°C. It is flammable; and if exposed to air or light it slowly forms ether peroxides, which are unstable and may cause spontaneous combustion. When mixed with air, oxygen, or nitrous oxide, ether is explosive even at low concentrations. It is nonpolar, lipid-soluble, and slightly soluble in water.

C. Pharmacology and metabolism. Ether rapidly crosses the GI mucosa when ingested orally and immediately passes into the bloodstream when inhaled (37). Absorption across the skin is minimal (38). The serum half-life is short (less than 20 min) and is a function of minute ventilation. The lungs account for 90% of excretion (37). The kidneys, skin, and sweat glands excrete a portion of the remaining ether. The liver oxidizes a small percentage of the ether to acetaldehyde and carbon dioxide (39). Ether readily diffuses into fatty tissues and brain, where it can be detected at elevated levels even after serum levels have declined (38).

D. Clinical effects

 1. **Ingestion**

    a. **Local effects.** When ingested, ether is rapidly absorbed. Concentrated ether causes mucosal necrosis, vomiting, and anorexia (40).

    b. **Systemic effects** mimic those seen with ethanol ingestion, with similar euphoria and CNS depression. Death has occurred following ingestion of as little as 30 mL (41).

 2. **Inhalation exposure.** The most common route of exposure is via inhalation. Detection threshold is 1 ppm; however, chronic exposure elevates this figure up to 2,000 ppm (38). Anesthesia is induced by 100,000 ppm and maintained with 50,000 ppm (42). The limit of exposure set by the Occupational Safety and Health Administration (OSHA) is 400 ppm (43). Ether irritates the respiratory mucous membranes at 200 ppm, and cough and laryngeal spasm are common (42).

 3. **Dermatologic effects.** Ether defats the skin with repeated exposures; however, systemic effects are rarely observed with topical exposure (38). One patient who was being treated with ether to the scalp under an occlusive wrap for seborrheic dermatitis died (44).

 4. **Ears, nose, and throat.** Both the liquid and vapor forms are strong irritants. Superficial epithelial injury may occur, but recovery is usually rapid.

 5. **Ophthalmologic exposure.** Ether may cause superficial injury that heals rapidly without sequelae (19).

 6. **Genitourinary effects.** Ether has been used to unclog the balloon of Foley catheters with subsequent exposure of the bladder mucosa to ether. Hemorrhagic cystitis has occurred, and surgical intervention has been necessary (45).

    E. **Signs and symptoms** of ether ingestion are similar to those seen with acute ethanol ingestion but with quicker onset and shorter duration. Vital signs may reveal hypothermia, bradycardia, and irregular breathing (38). Significant respiratory depression is rare and dose-related. Blood pressure usually is stable (38). Exposure to vapors causes an increase in salivation. Cough and laryngospasm may occur (42). Neurologic manifestations include exhaustion, depression, dizziness, coma, euphoria, headache, hallucinations, and seizures (46). Vomiting is common with ingestion and inhalation exposures (40). Ingestion may also cause gastric distention (40). Long-term sequelae are rare. Minor transient elevations of liver enzymes, especially SGOT and alkaline phosphatase, may occur (38). Transient hypoalbuminemia and albuminuria have also been observed (38). Hyperglycemia is common using anesthetic doses, with an increase in serum glucose of up to 60 mg/dL reported (42). Renal injury with resultant uremia has been reported with intravenous administration, and nephritis has occurred with inhalation anesthesia (38).

    F. **Diagnostic tests.** Blood levels of ether are not commonly obtained. Blood glucose levels, liver function tests, and renal function tests are warranted.

    G. **Therapeutic intervention.** No specific antidote exists. Enhanced elimination is not indicated, as ether has such a short half-life.

        1. **Oral ingestion.** Ether is rapidly absorbed; and emesis, lavage, and charcoal are of little benefit. Dilution with 4 to 8 oz of milk or water may decrease gastric irritation.

        2. **Respiratory exposure.** Remove the patient from further exposure and administer supplemental oxygen. Evaluate for respiratory tract irritation, bronchitis, or pneumonitis. Intubation may be necessary.

        3. **Dermal exposure.** Systemic effects are unlikely to occur, but local decontamination with soap and water is indicated. If clothing is saturated with ether, remove affected items and keep them in a well-ventilated area away from flames.

        4. **Ocular exposure.** If eyes are exposed, lavage with saline or water for at least 15 min. If pain or other symptoms persist, consult an ophthalmologist.

        5. **General management.** Regardless of route of exposure, patients must be observed for evidence of respiratory failure, which may require intubation. Seizures may occur and should be initially treated with lorazepam 5 mg i.v., which may be repeated in 15 min if necessary or diazepam 5 to 10 mg i.v. q 15 min to a maximum dose of 30 mg. If the seizures persist or return, consider phenobarbital or phenytoin.

ESTERS

Esters are carboxylic acid derivatives. The hydrogen in the hydroxyl group is replaced by an alkyl or an aryl group. The structure of the ester can be easily derived from its name. The "ic" of the carboxylic group is replaced by "ate." Thus methyl acetate is the ester formed by combining methanol with acetic acid. Most of the simpler esters are volatile and fragrant. In an acidic environment (e.g., the stomach) esters are hydrolyzed to their carboxylic acid and alkyl or aryl components. Consequently, when managing the patient who has ingested esters, we must be concerned with the potential toxicity of the components as well as that of the ester itself. Thus with esters such as methyl carboxylate, the practitioner must be wary of the potential for methanol intoxication. Two commonly available esters are ethyl acrylate and ethyl acetate.

I. **Ethyl acrylate** is the most commonly available toxic ester. It is widely used in industry, notably in the production of acrylic paints as well as surgical prostheses. Ethyl acrylate is colorless and volatile. As is the case with most simple esters, it is highly volatile and highly fragrant. It may be detected at levels as low as 1 ppm.

A. Because of its volatility, the **most common exposure** is respiratory. Initial exposure causes lacrimation, tachypnea, nausea, lethargy, drowsiness, and headache. Prolonged high concentration may result in corneal burns, pulmonary edema, and seizures. Although cyanosis has been reported in animals, it has not been reported in humans. Highly concentrated exposures may result in seizures.

B. **Treatment.** The first and most important step is removing the victim from the toxic surroundings. The patient should be managed with 100% oxygen. If the patient shows signs of CNS depression, ventilatory support may be temporarily necessary. Management of seizures is discussed below (see **I.B.4**).

1. **Topical exposure** should be managed with generous irrigation.

2. **Oral exposure.** Because the patient may be (or may become) obtunded, emesis should not be induced. If it is believed that exposure was substantial and recent, a wide-bore gastric tube may be passed (after ensuring airway protection). The stomach can then be lavaged with saline until the returning fluid is clear.

3. **Charcoal** should be administered at the standard dose of 1 to 2 g/kg. The charcoal treatment may be repeated in 2 h. A cathartic such as magnesium sulfate (dose), magnesium citrate (4 mL/kg), or sorbitol (1 to 2 g/kg) may be added to the first dose of charcoal.

4. **Seizures** should be treated via standard protocols with diazepam, lorazepam, or phenobarbital.

II. **Ethyl acetate** is widely used in the production of artificial fruit essences. It is also used as a solvent. The compound is of low toxicity. Exposure by inhalation or ingestion is unlikely to require any management. One must remember, however, that the compound is rapidly hydrolyzed in the stomach to form ethanol and acetic acid. The ethanol, once absorbed, could reach toxic levels, especially in children. For this reason, substantial, recent oral ingestion may be managed with gastric emptying (ensuring adequate airway support) followed by charcoal and a cathartic as per the usual protocols.

References

1. National Research Council, Committee on Aldehydes, Board on Toxicology and Environmental Health Hazards. Health effects of formaldehyde. In: *Formaldehyde and other aldehydes*. Washington, DC: National Academy Press, 1981.
2. Feinman SE. *Formaldehyde sensitization*. Draft report prepared by the Consumer Product Safety Commission, 1984.
3. Ells JT, et al. Formaldehyde poisoning: rapid metabolism to formic acid. *JAMA* 1981;246:1237.
4. Bartone NF, Grieco RV, Herr BS. Corrosive gastritis due to ingestion of formaldehyde without esophageal impairment. *JAMA* 1968;203:50.
5. Kline BS. Formaldehyde poisoning with report of a fatal case. *Arch Intern Med* 1975;11:357.
6. Loomis TA. Formaldehyde toxicity. *Arch Pathol Lab Med* 1979;103:321.
7. Patterson R, et al. Formaldehyde reactions and the burden of proof. *J Allergy Clin Immunol* 1987;79:705.
8. Bernstein RS, et al. Inhalation exposure to formaldehyde: an overview of its toxicology, epidemiology, monitoring, and control. *Am Ind Hyg Assoc J* 1984;45:778.
9. Beall JR, Ulsamer AG. Formaldehyde and hepatotoxicity: a review. *J Toxicol Environ Health* 1984;14:1.

10. Squire RA, Cameron LL. An analysis of potential carcinogenic risk from formaldehyde. *Regul Toxicol Pharmacol* 1984;4:107.

11. Duffy JP. *Poisindex system. Commercial, pharmaceutical, biologic substance identification and management (vol. 68).* Denver: Micromedex, 1990.

12. Gottschling LM, et al. Monitoring of formic acid in urine of humans exposed to low levels of formaldehyde. *Am Ind Hyg Assoc J* 1984;45:19.

13. Allen RE, et al. Corrosive injuries of the stomach. *Arch Surg* 1970;100:409.

14. Sittig M. *Handbook of toxic and hazardous chemicals and carcinogens.* 2nd ed. Park Ridge, NJ: Noyes Publications, 1985.

15. *HSDB: Hazardous substance data book (CD-ROM version).* Denver: Micromedex, 1989.

16. Sax NI, Lewis RJ. *Dangerous properties of industrial materials.* 7th ed. New York: Van Nostrand Reinhold, 1987.

17. Eriksson CJP. Human acetaldehyde levels: aspects of current interest. *Mutat Res* 1987;186:235.

18. Proctor NH, Hughes JP. *Chemical hazards of the work place.* 2nd ed. Philadelphia: JB Lippincott Co, 1988.

19. Grant WM. *Toxicology of the eye.* 2nd ed. Springfield, IL: Charles C. Thomas Publisher, 1974.

20. Olin BR. *Drug facts and comparisons.* St. Louis: Mosby, 1990.

21. Anthony RM, et al. Paraldehyde pharmacokinetics in ethanol abusers. *Fed Proc* 1977;36:285.

22. Bostrum B. Paraldehyde toxicity during treatment of status epilepticus. *Am J Dis Child* 1982;136:414.

23. Thurston JH, et al. New enzymatic method for measurement of paraldehyde: correlation of effects with serum and CSF levels. *J Clin Lab Med* 1968;77:699.

24. De Elio T, et al. Some experimental and clinical observations on the anticonvulsant action of paraldehyde. *J Neurol Neurosurg Psychiatry* 1949;12:19.

25. Browning E. *Toxicity and metabolism of industrial solvents.* Amsterdam: Elsevier Science, 1956.

26. Parmeggiani L, ed. *Encyclopedia of occupational health and safety (vol. 1).* 3rd ed. Geneva: International Labour Office, 1983.

27. Burkhart KK, et al. Formate levels following a formalin ingestion. *Vet Hum Toxicol* 1990;32:135.

28. Vavigos GA, Nurse DS. Contact urticaria from methyl ethyl ketone. *Contact Dermatitis* 1986;15:259.

29. Kopelman PG, Kalfoyan PY. Severe metabolic acidosis after ingestion of butanone [Letter]. *Br Med J* 1983;286:21.

30. Jaeger RW, Scalzo AS, Thompson MW. ECMO in hydrocarbon aspiration. Presented at AACT/AARCC/ABMT/CABCC Annual Scientific Meeting, Vancouver, British Columbia, Canada, 1987.

31. Cliris. *Cliris hazardous chemical data.* Washington, DC: U.S. Dept. of Transportation, U.S. Coast Guard, 1985.

32. Ramu A, Rosenbaum J, Blaschke TF. Disposition of acetone following acute acetone intoxication. *West J Med* 1978; 129:429.

33. Gitelson S, et al. Coma and hyperglycemia following drinking of acetone. *Diabetes* 1966;15:810.

34. Gamis AS, Wasserman GS. Acute acetone intoxication in a pediatric patient. *Pediatr Emerg Care* 1988;4:14.

35. Harris LC, Jackson RH. Acute acetone poisoning caused by setting fluid for immobilizing casts. *Br Med J* 1952;2:1024.

36. Hawley PC, Falko JM. "Pseudo" renal failure after isopropyl alcohol intoxication. *South Med J* 1982;75:630.

37. Haggart HW. The absorption, distribution and elimination of ethyl ether. *J Biol Chem* 1924;59:737.

38. Kirwin CJ Jr, Sandmeyer EE. Ethers. In: Clayton GD, Clayton FE, eds. *Patty's industrial hygiene and toxicology (vol. 2a).* 3rd ed. New York: Wiley-Interscience, 1981.

39. Price HL, Dripps RD. General anesthetics. In: Goodman LS, Gilman A, eds. *The pharmacological basis of therapeutics.* 5th ed. New York: Macmillan, 1975.

40. Gosselin RE, Smith RP, Hodge HC. *Clinical toxicology of commercial products.* 5th ed. Baltimore: Williams & Wilkins, 1984.

41. Baselt RC. *Disposition of toxic drugs and chemicals in man.* 2nd ed. Davis, CA: Biomedical Publication, 1982.

42. Knape H. General anesthetics and therapeutic gases. In: Dukes MNG, ed. *Side effects of drugs: an encyclopedia of adverse reactions and interactions.* 9th ed. Amsterdam: Excerpta Medica, 1980.

43. OSHA, Department of Labor, Occupational Safety and Health Administration. 29CFR part 1910; air contaminants; final rule. *Fed Register* 1989;54:2332.

44. Burnett HW, et al. An unfortunate complication of self therapy for seborrheic dermatitis. *Cutis* 1988;41:284.

45. Gattegno B, Michel F, Thibault P. A serious complication of vesical ether instillation: ether cystitis. *J Urol* 1988; 139:357.

46. Wilford BB. *Drug abuse: a guide for the primary care physician.* Chicago: American Medical Association, 1981.

Selected Readings

ACGIH. Threshold Limit Values and Biological Exposure Indices for 1989–90. Presented at the American Conference of Government Industrial Hygiene Inc., Cincinnati, 1989.

Anderson KE, Maibach HI. Multiple application delayed onset contact urticaria: possible relation to certain unusual formalin and textile reactions? *Contact Dermatitis* 1984;10:227.

Borzelleca JF, et al. Studies on the chronic oral toxicity of monomeric ethyl acrylate & methyl methacrylate. *Toxicol Appl Pharmacol* 1964;6:29–36.

DeBethizy JE, et al. The disposition and metabolism of acrylic acid and ethyl acrylate in male Sprague Dawley rats. *Fundam Appl Toxicol* 1987;8:549–561.

Department of Transportation. *1987 emergency response guidebook: guide for hazardous material incidents.* Washington, DC: U.S. Department of Transportation, 1987.

Ghanazim BL, Maronpet RR, Mathews HB. Ethyl acrylate-induced gastric toxicity. I. Effect of single and repetitive dosing. *Toxicol Appl Pharmacol* 1985;80:323–335.

Ghanazim BI, Maronpet RR, Mathews HB. Ethyl acrylate-induced gastric toxicity. III. Development and recovery of lesions. *Toxicol Appl Pharmacol* 1986;83:576–583.

Horvath EP, et al. Effects of formaldehyde on the mucous membranes and lungs: a study of an industrial population. *JAMA* 1988;259:701.

Josselin RE, Smith RP, Hodge HC, eds. *Clinical toxicology of commercial products.* 5th ed. Baltimore: Williams & Wilkins, 1984.

Lederer WH. *Regulatory chemicals of health and environmental concern.* New York: Van Nostrand Reinhold, 1985:131.

Proctor N, Hughes JP. *Chemical hazards of the workplace.* Philadelphia: JB Lippincott Co, 1978.

Emergency Toxicology, Second Edition,
edited by Peter Viccellio.
Lippincott–Raven Publishers, Philadelphia © 1998.

17

Hydrocarbons

†Monica Parraga and °James M. West

†*Department of Emergency Medicine, Metropolitan Hospital, New York, New York 10028;*
°Santa Fe, New Mexico 87501

I. Definitions

   A. Most compounds referred to as **hydrocarbons** are derivatives of petroleum distillation. They compose a group of organic compounds that contain hydrogen and carbon atoms only.

      1. Hydrocarbon exposures accounted for approximately 3% of the 2,155,952 human exposures reported, in 1996, to poison control centers in the United States. The overall fatalities from hydrocarbon exposures were 0.015%. Children under the age of 6 were responsible for 52.8% of the total reported exposures, of which 2.4% of exposure (27,362) involved hydrocarbons (1).

      2. Hydrocarbons are found singly or incorporated with others in a wide variety of commercial products ubiquitous around the home or workplace. Lighter fluid, paint thinners and removers, some furniture polishes, cleaning agents, solvents, various automotive products, and ordinary fuels are common examples.

      3. Exposure to hydrocarbons may be chronic or acute, accidental or intentional via inhalation, ingestion or cutaneous contact. Most cases of exposure involve accidental ingestion by young children. Abuse by inhalation is generally seen in male adolescents and young adults. Substances commonly inhaled include adhesive compounds, nail polish products, aerosols, and typewriter correction fluids. Intentional ingestion is reported in the young and older adult population. The most common substances reported in toxic ingestions are kerosene, gasoline, turpentine, mineral seal oil preparations, and lighter fluid.

   B. **Petroleum distillates**, which are a result of petroleum cracking and fractionation, produce compounds that may be subdivided into three major classes.

      1. The aliphatic hydrocarbons which are the straight saturated and unsaturated compounds.

      2. The halogenated hydrocarbons or the chlorinated hydrocarbons which are usually chlorine substituted aliphatics.

      3. The aromatic (cyclic) hydrocarbons that contain a benzene ring as their central structure.

   C. **Turpentine and pine oil** are products of wood distillation that usually fall under hydrocarbon compounds.

D. Insecticides, heavy metals, and other toxic chemicals are often mixed with petroleum derivatives, and it should be noted that these additives can be more dangerous than the petroleum distillate itself. In addition, the clinical presentation and management of these agents may differ significantly from that of other hydrocarbons. This chapter concentrates on the more commonly ingested "pure" hydrocarbons.

II. Properties of agents
A. Sources
1. Aliphatic hydrocarbons include benzene, gasoline naptha, mineral spirits, kerosene, mineral seal oil. Used as solvents, fluid degreasers, furniture polish, etc.
2. The halogenated (chlorinated) hydrocarbons include substances such as methylene chloride, carbon tetrachloride, trichloroethylene and tetrachloroethylene. These compounds are found in solvents, paint-strippers, degreasers, typewriter correction fluid, and paint/spot removers.
    a. The freons (fluorocarbons, chlorofluorocarbons) are employed as propellants and refrigerants.
3. The aromatic hydrocarbons, benzene, toluene, xylene are found in solvents for paint, lacquers, adhesives, and degreasers.
4. Turpentine and pine oil are also found in solvents, household cleaners, and disinfectants.

B. Physical properties
1. The principal pathologic findings in hydrocarbon ingestions are consistent with respiratory tract injury due to aspiration and spread of the liquid in the lung. The risk for aspiration is determined by the physical properties of viscosity, surface tension, and volatility.
    a. **Viscosity,** the tendency to resist flow or change form is the best estimate of aspiration potential (2). The lower the viscosity the more likely the substance is to penetrate the distal airways. It is measured in efflux time in seconds, or Saybolt Seconds Universal (SSU). Viscosity is also an indirect measure of molecular size. It is the single most important physical property influencing the aspiration tendency of a liquid. The viscosity of a substance determines not only the likelihood of its entry into the trachea but also the rate and extent of its penetration into the terminal bronchioles and alveoli. Products with a lower viscosity (less than 60 SSU) constitute a high risk for aspiration. At more than 60 SSU, hydrocarbons are too viscous to present a significant hazard. Because SSU measurements are often omitted from product labels, the clinician should be generally familiar with the viscosity rating of each agent (Table 17-1).
    b. Surface tension is defined as the cohesiveness of molecules along a liquid surface. A reduced surface tension results in rapid movement from mouth to trachea (3).
    c. Volatility describes the ability of a liquid to vaporize. Highly volatile hydrocarbons will displace alveolar oxygen resulting in hypoxia.
2. Hydrocarbons can be conveniently divided into various simple but overlapping categories according to their physiochemical characteristics.

TABLE 17-1. *Hydrocarbon characteristics*[a]

Product	Synonyms	Industrial availability	Composition, viscosity
Benzin or benzine (not benzene)	Petroleum ether (petroleum ether is *not* an ether)	Dry cleaning solvents, paints	Low boiling point fractions, i.e., pentanes, hexanes, heptanes; SSU < 35
Benzene	Benzol	Paint thinners, varnish removers	C_6H_6; SSU < 35
Gasoline	Petroleum spirit	Fuel	Heptanes, octanes, nonanes; may contain lead; SSU < 35
Naphtha (not naphthaline)	—	Paint and glue thinner, racing fuel, lighter fluid	SSU < 35
Turpentine	Pine oil	Paint thinner, textile cleaning, shoe polish	Cyclic turpentines, wood distillate; SSU < 35
Petroleum spirits	Mineral spirits, stoddard solvent, white spirits	Paint solvent, dry cleaning agent, degreasing agent	Turpentine substitute; SSU < 35
Kerosene	Coal oil, kerosine, jet aviation fuel, no. 1 heating oil	Heating, cooking, jet aviation	Decane to hexadecane; SSU < 35
Diesel oil	—	Engine fuel, home heating	$C_{20}H_{42}$ and heavier; SSU < 60
Mineral seal oil	Signal oil, polish (red)	Furniture polish (red)	Called "seal oil" originally from seals; attractively colored (red); other important additives: turpentine, camphor, lemon, cedar, wintergreen; SSU < 60
Petrolatum	Ingredient in petroleum jelly (Vaseline)	Laxatives, creams, ointments	SSU > 70
Lubricating oil	3-in-One Oil, auto engine oil	Machine lubricant	SSU > 100
Paraffin wax	—	Emollient hydrocarbon, candies, dental molds, tissue embedding	SSU > 100

[a] From top to bottom, the table shows decreasing volatility and increasing viscosity.
Adapted from ref. 30.

a. **High volatility, minimal viscosity:** simple gases such as methane or butane. The inhalation of these substances can rapidly replace alveolar gas, causing hypoxia. In addition, they can easily cross the alveolar-capillary membrane and cause CNS symptoms. The lung is spared injury, but cardiotoxic effects have been reported (4). Aromatic hydrocarbons such as benzene and some chlorohydrocarbons are other examples. Benzine, or "petroleum ether," may also fall into this class. Gastrointestinal (GI) absorption of these agents can be significant.

b. **Intermediate volatility, low viscosity:** examples are gasoline, turpentine, and naphtha. The primary problem with these agents is aspiration; however, they may cause CNS depression when inhaled. Effects from GI absorption are not significant.

    c. **Low volatility, low viscosity:** petroleum spirits, kerosene, mineral seal oil. Pulmonary complications dominate. GI absorption is minimal. Mineral seal oil, the main component of furniture oil, has been implicated as the most commonly aspirated agent (5). Although its SSU rating is somewhat higher than the aforementioned agents, colorizing and odorizing additives may add to its toxicity.

    d. **Minimal volatility, high viscosity:** lubricating oils, mineral oil, asphalt. These materials are highly viscous, essentially nontoxic, but may cause lipoid pneumonias in cases of direct aspiration.

III. Pathophysiology. The pathophysiologic effects of ingested petroleum distillates and turpentine are primarily reflected in pulmonary toxicity. Significant complications of other organ systems are uncommon. Massive ingestions, inhalation of volatile agents, and poisoning by aromatic, camphorated, or halogenated hydrocarbons may present exceptions.

  A. General

    1. It is apparent from the available data that the **pulmonary pathology** following intoxication is not due to GI absorption but to direct effects. Several lines of evidence support this conclusion.

      a. It has been demonstrated that aspiration hazard increases with decreasing viscosity, even when small volumes were placed on the tongues of test animals (6).

      b. Based on animal studies, the LD_{50} oral/intratracheal kerosene ratio is approximately 140:1, suggesting that large amounts must be swallowed and absorbed to produce systemic toxicity (2).

      c. Hydrocarbon pneumonitis is commonly seen in young children who rarely ingest large quantities. Furthermore, a study using a radiolabeled hydrocarbon showed some uptake from the gut, but the amount detected was small (7). Thus, although it appears that some GI absorption may occur (perhaps related to the molecular weights of individual hydrocarbon components), the extent is minimal.

    2. Other investigations have offered further insight. Bratton and Haddow found that large amounts of naphtha instilled into the stomach of rats produced no pulmonary pathology, whereas small amounts instilled directly into the trachea caused severe pneumonitis. Moreover, small amounts injected into a tail vein caused severe lung damage. The results suggested that either naphtha is poorly absorbed from the GI tract, or it is absorbed but rendered less toxic by the liver. To distinguish between these alternatives, a small amount of naphtha was injected directly into the portal vein. It caused severe liver necrosis but no lung damage. As no liver damage was found when 40 times this amount was placed in the stomach, the authors concluded that naphtha is not significantly absorbed from the GI tract. Because lung involvement was noted after intravenous injection but not after portal vein instillation, they further concluded that the organ bearing the first capillary or sinusoidal system through which the material passes is the one injured.

    3. In a more recent study, Dice et al. (9) performed gastrostomies and esophageal transections on dogs and then administered large amounts (20 mL/kg) of kerosene intragastrically. No clinical or radiographic evidence of pneumonitis was found. On necropsy no pulmonary histologic changes were noted.

4. The **CNS toxicity** occasionally observed following hydrocarbon ingestion appears to be indirect and secondary to the pulmonary involvement. Wolfsdorf (10), using baboons, injected kerosene into the portal vein, carotid artery, and left ventricle, as well as intratracheally. Liver injury occurred in the portal vein group, but the lungs and brain were spared. The intratracheal group demonstrated significant pulmonary pathology due to the acute production of aspiration pneumonitis. All animals in this group experienced transient convulsions, apparently due to acute hypoxia with cyanosis. Although modest degrees of cerebral edema were measured (via brain weight ratios) in the intraventricular and intracarotid groups, only one animal in the latter group exhibited serious CNS manifestations. Interestingly, no CNS pathology was noted microscopically in any group. It was concluded that the primate brain is resistant to the direct effects of kerosene; and hypoxia secondary to pneumonitis appears to be the most potent cause of CNS abnormality.

B. **Organ systems**
   1. **Pulmonary injury** is reflected by development of chemical pneumonitis. Initial cyanosis is thought to be caused by displacement of oxygen from alveoli by petroleum distillates.
      a. As the substance spreads to lower airway, bronchospasm reflected by wheezing can occur, resulting in a ventilation perfusion mismatch, more hypoxia and eventually increased CNS depression.
      b. Atelectasis and interstitial inflammation necrotizing bronchopneumonia can result from direct destruction of airway epithelium, aveolar septae and pulmonary capillaries. The latter finding may be due to an alteration of surfactant caused by the lipid solubilization properties of hydrocarbons (11). The resultant increase in minimal surface tension can lead to alveolar instability and collapse as well as distal airway closure. These abnormalities can also cause ventilation-perfusion mismatches resulting in hypoxia. Whether the pulmonary effects are due more to surfactant impairment or to direct parenchymal injury is unclear.
   2. **Neurologic injury**
      a. Following ingestion and aspiration, symptoms of **CNS depression** are primarily due to hypoxia. The more volatile and aromatic compounds, which are more readily absorbed by either the oral or inhalational route, may cause direct CNS effects. Hypoxia may still be a factor, however, as the latter substances may suppress the central ventilatory drive if a sufficient CNS concentration is attained.
      b. Mechanism for toxicity of the central nervous system, although not fully understood, is thought to be based on the fact that neural tissue has a large lipid component and hydrocarbons are effective lipid solvents (12). **Peripheral neuropathy** has been associated with the abuse and industrial exposure of *n*-hexane. Focal axonal swelling and degeneration has been

consistently demonstrated histologically in humans and test animals exposed to this agent (13).

3. **Cutaneous injury** appears to be due to irritant effects and fat solvency properties of hydrocarbons. Dehydration of the skin probably contributes to the damage. The depth of injury is related to the duration of exposure and concentration of the agent, with most wounds being superficial. Cutaneous absorption of these products may occur, but with acute episodes its clinical significance is probably negligible.

4. **Other organ systems**
   a. **GI effects** are generally minimal and result from direct local irritative action on the pharynx, esophagus, stomach, and small intestine. Small areas of fatty infiltration and congestion of the liver have been described, but major hepatic injury has not been reported with petroleum distillate exposure. (Halogenated hydrocarbons, such as carbon tetrachloride, may cause severe hepatic and renal injury.)
   b. **Glomerulonephritis,** renal tubular acidosis, and chronic tubulointerstitial nephritis have been associated with long-term hydrocarbon contact.
   c. **Intravascular hemolysis** following gasoline aspiration has been reported in a small number of cases. Damage to the RBC membrane and induction of lysis by lipid solubilization was a suggested mechanism (14).

IV. **Clinical presentation.** Although studies differ on reported incidences of pulmonary complications after hydrocarbon ingestions, it is clear that nonpulmonary manifestations are distinctly uncommon. The bulk of the medical literature comes from studies or reports of accidental ingestions by young children. Although it is unlikely that the basic clinical picture varies significantly in other groups, it has been shown that with most poisonings more severe outcomes are associated with older age populations and with intentional exposures (1).

A. **Pulmonary signs**
   1. Most patients will become symptomatic within thirty minutes of ingestion. Almost immediately upon aspiration there are signs of oral mucosa and tracheobronchial irritation, manifested as burning of the mouth, coughing, and choking. Gasping, coughing, and choking are signs that aspiration has occurred. Those signs may be transient due to the initial volatization of the petroleum distillates. Prolonged cough is more supportive of aspiration.
   2. Signs and symptoms may progress over the first 24 h. Nasal flaring, intercostal retractions, dyspnea, tachypnea, and varying degrees of cyanosis may follow. If severe injury occurs, pulmonary edema and hemoptysis or pink frothy sputum may be evident later leading to shock and cardiorespiratory arrest. If death is to occur, it usually does so within the first 24 h. (15). Otherwise, pulmonary symptoms plateau in about 48 h, with complete resolution in 3 to 5 days.
   3. Auscultation may demonstrate rales, rhonchi, wheezing, and diminished breath sounds, but abnormal findings are often absent. It is important to understand that lower airway involvement may be present in the face of a normal chest examination. A typical hydrocarbon odor is often detected in these patients but is not a reliable indicator of significant ingestion.

4. Intravenous exposure, though rare, usually causes a chemical pneumonitis, occasionally hemorrhagic in nature.

5. Moderate fever often present does not always correlate with clinical symptoms thought to be a result of direct pulmonary parenchymal damage. Generally, it is not related to bacterial superinfection early on after exposure. Fever may later be an indication of infection.

B. **GI signs.** GI symptoms following hydrocarbon ingestion are frequent, but usually are minor. There is local irritation of mouth and pharynx. Hydrocarbons can cause nausea, vomiting, and abdominal pain and distention. Diarrhea, hematemsis, and melena rare.

1. Capacity of hydrocarbons to produce spontaneous vomiting is related to high risk of developing aspiration pneumonitis.

2. GI symptoms are more commonly associated with turpentine and pine oil (16).

C. **Neurologic signs.** Inhalation and or ingestion of hydrocarbons is invariably associated with central nervous system toxicity. Hydrocarbon exposure results in CNS depression; somnolence, dizziness, hyporeflexia rarely, convulsions, and coma.

1. Unlike the aliphatics, systemically absorbed aromatic and halogenated compounds may have marked initial excitatory effects leading to euphoria, agitation, delerium, hyperreflexia and seizure.

D. **Cutaneous signs**

1. **Contact** with petroleum distillates can cause a variety of skin manifestations ranging from mild erythema to full-thickness skin loss. Features of eczematoid dermatitis such as redness, itching, and inflammation may be seen. A clinical picture resembling toxic epidermal necrolysis with areas of bullae and denuded skin has been described. Compared to thermal and other chemical burns, the latency of the signs and symptoms may be longer.

2. **Subcutaneous injections** of these substances may result in cellulitis and abscess formation. High-pressure injection injuries are particularly dangerous, though initially there may be no signs or symptoms. Significant swelling and pain can develop after a few hours. Ischemic insults, sterile abscess formation, and chronic bone and connective tissue injuries have been reported.

3. **Ocular exposure** generally causes little or no injury. Slight discomfort, photophobia, redness, and transient corneal irritation may be present.

E. **Cardiac signs**

1. Myocardial involvement is rare after acute ingestion. However during solvent abuse, sudden death secondary to dysrythmias can occur. Mechanism by which dysrythmias occur is believed to be a result of hydrocarbon sensitization of myocardium to endogenous catecholamines (17). Sudden death has been reported, especially with abuse of chlorinated and fluorinated (freons) hydrocarbons (18).

F. **Other organ systems**

1. Transient hepatosplenomegaly and urinary and hematologic abnormalities have been rarely noted.

2. Petroleum distillates occasionally serve as vehicles containing anticholinesterase pesticides. A cholinergic crisis must be considered in patients with hydrocarbon

pneumonitis who also display profuse salivation, lacrimation, diarrhea, bronchorrhea, cramps, miosis, and urinary incontinence.

G. Chronic exposure

1. Benzene is considered a human carcinogen. Aplastic anemia and myelocytic and monocytic leukemia, have been reported with chronic benzene exposure
2. Toluene inhalation over long periods of time has been associated with renal tubular acidosis and peripheral sensorimotor neuropathy.

V. Ancillary studies

A. Routine studies

1. **Routine studies** are of little value for purposes of screening patients for admission. Once the need for admission has been determined, various laboratory tests may be done. Arterial blood gases (ABGs) must be measured in all patients with respiratory symptoms. Varying degrees of hypoxia without hypercarbia are the most common findings. Occasionally a metabolic acidosis is seen (e.g., with toluene). The CBC may show a leukocytosis, often with a shift to the left. This finding may be present early after ingestion and persist for several days.
2. Serum electrolytes, coagulation studies, urinalysis, and renal and liver function tests are usually normal shortly after acute ingestions and generally remain so. Chronic exposures or systemically absorbed toxins may represent exceptions.
3. Blood hydrocarbon levels are not readily available and have little diagnostic, prognostic, or therapeutic value. Qualitative testing is occasionally needed for forensic or medicolegal purposes. The toxicologic laboratory may be helpful if concomitant ingestion or toxic additives (e.g., lead) are suspected.
4. An ECG should be performed and continuous monitoring done as indicated. Pulmonary function testing, although impractical in the acutely ill patient, may be useful for following the patient's respiratory status.

B. Radiologic studies

1. Chest x-ray abnormalities correlate poorly with clinical symptoms. Asymptomatic patients may have abnormal chest x-rays (15).
2. Abnormalities appear within thirty minutes but may develop up to 24 h after exposure. Up to 75% of patients hospitalized for suspected hydrocarbon aspiration have chest x-ray abnormalities (19).
3. Most common positive findings are increased bronchovascular markings and bilateral basal infiltrates. Upper lobe infiltrates are uncommon. Infiltrates usually reach their maximum in 3 to 4 days. They generally clear within 2 weeks of onset.
4. Other findings include pleural effusions, pneumothorax, pneumomediastinum, and pneumatoceles. Pneumatoceles usually appear 1 to 3 weeks after ingestion, generally after 1 week of serious respiratory illness. They often demonstrate air-fluid levels on roentgenographic examination. Resolution may take months with no residual disease apparent.

VI. Management.
General measures. Initial therapy is dependent on severity of illness and extent of airway compromise. Therefore evaluate for signs of respiratory distress such as cyanosis, tachypnea, and retractions. Make sure the airway is patent and free of secretions. Nebulized treatments of cardioselective bronchodilators should be given to all patients. Initial manage-

ment includes supportive therapy, close monitoring, pulse oximetry, physical examination, and laboratory values. In more severe exposures, cardiac monitoring and i.v. access is necessary. Patients with significant airway compromise need a chest x-ray. It is recommended that less seriously ill patients wait up to 6 h to see if chest x-rays are indicated (15). Patients with altered mental status should receive narcan, glucose, and thiamine.

1. Initially, most patients with significant exposure become hypocapneic from hyperventilation. But as CNS depression ensues, patients become hypoxenic and hypercapnec. Strongly consider intubation in these patients.

2. Derangement of normal pulmonary surfactant properties by aspirated hydrocarbons has led to suggestions that the early use of **continuous positive-airway pressure** (CPAP) or **positive end-expiratory pressure** (PEEP) is beneficial in severely compromised patients. If selected, such therapy must be used with caution, as these patients are prone to develop lesions leading to pneumatoceles and pneumothoraces; increased airway distending pressures could contribute to these complications and even result in a tension pneumothorax.

3. Note that cyanosis may occur due to methemoglobinemia from products that contain aniline and nitrobenzene. Therefore, treat accordingly.

4. In rare instances where exposure has occurred to methylene chloride or carbon tetrachloride, the treatment of choice is oxygenation or hyperbaric oxygen therapy which has proven to be effective in experimental studies and anecdotal case studies.

5. Drugs such as epinephrine and isoproteronal should be avoided. They may precipitate dysrythmias in hydrocarbon sensitive myocardium. Use the drugs if necessary for resuscitation.

6. After **skin spills,** contaminated clothing should be removed and the affected area copiously irrigated with soap and water. Accurate assessment of the burn surface area and proper fluid management may be required. In the setting of contact burns secondary to motor vehicle accidents, the possibility of petroleum distillate inhalations and associated traumatic injuries should be considered. If ocular exposure has occurred, prolonged irrigation with sterile solutions is indicated.

7. There is no specific treatment for persons found impaired as a result of petroleum distillate inhalation. (Chelation therapy may be indicated if significant organic lead exposure is diagnosed.) If **CNS depression** is pronounced, supportive therapy may be necessary. The emphasis is on adequate oxygenation to prevent or reverse CNS anoxia.

8. Following hydrocarbon injection, treatment consists of cleansing the wound area, tetanus prophylaxis and using x-rays to determine location of material. Surgical debridement and irrigation is highly recommended. It is imperative to recognize the potential seriousness of these exposures (infection and gangrene) and to request immediate surgical evaluation.

B. **Elimination of toxin**
   1. **Gastric emptying.** The issue of gastric evacuation in hydrocarbon ingestions has provoked a great deal of discussion and debate over the years. The two main questions raised are whether to empty the stomach at all and, if so, what methods

should be utilized. In order to answer the first question, the results of several studies must be reviewed and a few clinical assumptions made.

a. First, most ingestions are **accidental,** and up to 90% of them occur in children younger than 4 years old (15,20). The average volume of a child's swallow is small (4.5 mL in 2-year-olds), and many of the products used are bad-tasting. These factors serve to limit the amount ingested. Thus, even when volumes are unknown or if one prudently assumes that dosage information is unreliable, small quantities are generally involved.

b. Second, though some studies have suggested that pulmonary symptoms better correlate with amounts ingested, no reliable data support these claims. Some articles and texts have recommended gastric evacuation for amounts of more than 1 oz or 1 mL/kg. Again, this "toxic" dose has no solid foundation in the literature. Several reviews of human ingestions have, in fact, found no correlation between volumes ingested and the presence or severity of aspiration pneumonitis.

c. More fundamental to the question are the results of various studies and observations (see **III**) that strongly support the view that pulmonary pathology and major CNS toxicity do not result from GI absorption. Emptying the stomach to prevent these complications is rarely worthwhile.

d. Gastric emptying is, however, usually indicated for aromatic hydrocarbons or those containing dangerous additives. These systemically absorbed agents are best recalled by the mnemonic CHAMP: camphor, halogenated products, aromatic compounds, heavy metals, and pesticides (Table 17-2). Ingestions of these substances are approached more aggressively, although small volumes may be inconsequential and not warrant removal. Camphorated agents are rapidly absorbed and may cause seizures. **Benzene** is particularly worrisome, as aplastic anemia and acute myeloblastic leukemia have been strongly associated with exposure. It is the most toxic of the aromatic compounds and is well absorbed from the GI tract—even small quantities must be removed. Small amounts of **parathion** and **carbon tetrachloride** can also be toxic.

e. Recommendations have been made in the past that gastric evacuation may also be indicated if **large amounts** of petroleum distillates or turpentine have been ingested, as with suicide attempts. Although no data exist, these incidents are rare, and most patients vomit spontaneously if large quantities are involved. Simple observation may be preferable.

TABLE 17-2. *Hydrocarbons: indications for gastric evacuation (systemically absorbed agents; additives)*

C	Camphorated products
H	Halogenated products (e.g., methylene chloride, carbon tetrachloride)
A	Aromatic hydrocarbons (e.g., benzene, toluene); aniline
M	Heavy metals (e.g., arsenic, mercury, iron, lead)
P	Pesticides

f. The second major question pertains to **methods of gastric evacuation.**

(1) Some studies have suggested that ipecac-induced emesis is superior to gastric lavage in reducing the incidence and severity of pneumonitis (20a,21). However, problems related to clinical criteria, study design, and methodologies serve to limit these conclusions. On the other hand, no studies have demonstrated the superiority of gastric lavage, and others have found no difference between the two modalities.

(2) From a more practical standpoint, **emesis** has several advantages over lavage. Alert patients seldom aspirate from spontaneous or induced emesis. Lavaging an awake and frightened child can be difficult, and introduction of the tube itself may induce vomiting. If prophylactic intubation is used in an awake patient, further problems are often encountered. Aside from the technical difficulties of intubating small children, the attendant risks of sedation and anesthetization for such a procedure must also be weighed. Cuffed tubes are not always available in small sizes and may be hazardous. Uncuffed tubes may not provide a 100% seal unless carefully chosen and placed.

(3) In summary, gastric evacuation for "pure" petroleum distillate or turpentine ingestions is not recommended. When toxic additives or concomitant ingestions requiring gastric emptying are present, ipecac-induced emesis is preferred over lavage.

(a) **Emesis** is contraindicated if CNS depression or seizures are present or anticipated prior to ipecac's onset of actions (e.g., camphorated products), if antecedent vomiting has occurred, or if respiratory symptomatology is apparent.

(b) **Gastric lavage** is indicated when removal of a substance is necessary but emesis is contraindicated. These situations are uncommon. Use of an endotracheal tube is recommended. Because the smallest diameter of the airway in young children is at the cricoid ring, a proper size uncuffed tube should adequately seal the larynx and prevent aspiration.

2. Other modalities

a. The use of *activated charcoal* for hydrocarbon absorption is limited, however it may have some effect especially in situations with mixed overdoses. A cathartic may be given simultaneously as in other clinical settings (22).

b. Hemodialysis and hemoperfusion are of no value for petroleum distillates.

c. High-frequency jet ventilation has been reported to be beneficial in cases of severe hydrocarbon pneumonitis and adult respiratory distress syndrome. It should be considered as a treatment option especially in children with severe pulmonary complications. This treatment modality appears to decrease barotrauma, air leaks, and ultimately decreases morbidity (23).

d. Extracorporeal membrane oxygenation (ECMO) is a modified cardiac bypass procedure utilized in a patient with a closed chest. It is utilized to support patient oxygenation while allowing lung tissue to heal, therefore minimizing barotrauma from assisted ventilation. The use of ECMO in patients seriously ill from hydrocarbon pneumonitis has been shown to be beneficial in some cases. However, further research is necessary to fully understand its benefit. Careful consideration and consultation with your local poison control center is imperative before implementing ECMO (24).

C. Drug therapy

1. Several studies have demonstrated that corticosteroids are ineffective for preventing or altering the course of hydrocarbon pneumonitis. After intratracheal instillation of kerosene in primates, Wolfsdorf and Kundig (25) could demonstrate no difference in pulmonary pathology between untreated groups and groups treated with dexamethasone. Marks et al. (26) studied children in a double-blind fashion and could show no difference between placebo and steroid-treated groups when comparisons of various clinical parameters and radiographic features were made. The use of antibiotics was not controlled in the latter study.

2. Other animal studies have **combined steroids and antibiotics.** One study reported no difference in clinical, radiographic, laboratory, or postmortem findings between control and treatment groups (27). Another study demonstrated impairment of the host's immune response to inflammatory kerosene pneumonitis and suggested that bacterial colonization was promoted by administration of corticosteroids (28). This study failed to demonstrate a significant role for bacteria in the pathogenesis of experimental chemical pneumonitis and further suggested that alterations of respiratory flora may occur with antibiotic use.

3. Because fever and leukocytosis are common findings in hydrocarbon pneumonitis, it may be difficult to determine when a bacterial **superinfection** has intervened. However, this complication is uncommon, especially in children. Careful serial microbiologic studies may be needed. Although it is clear that prophylactic antibiotics should not routinely be prescribed, some clinicians believe that their use may be justified in patients who are markedly debilitated or who have preexisting pulmonary disease.

4. Because bronchospasm may play a role in the respiratory distress, and some patients present with significant wheezing, the clinician may be prompted to initiate **bronchodilator therapy.** The use of sympathomimetic agents such as epinephrine and isoproterenol could precipitate fatal dysrhythmias, especially in those patients exposed to halogenated hydrocarbons, and should therefore be avoided. Selective beta-2 agonists would be preferred in this setting, but clinical reports of their use are lacking. Theophylline derivatives have not been studied.

VII. Disposition and follow-up

A. Triage

1. Most patients who ingest hydrocarbons have no immediate symptoms and remain **asymptomatic.** These patients require no physician intervention and can be managed at home or over the phone. This strategy assumes that the history is reliable (no toxic additives involved), capable observers are present, and transportation to the hospital is readily available in the unlikely event of delayed symptoms.

2. Patients who had symptoms immediately following ingestion suggestive of **aspiration** (choking, coughing, gagging) should be evaluated in the emergency department. Most present asymptomatically and remain so. The need for obtaining chest roentgenograms in this group is debatable, as the clinical picture is much more predictive of outcome, and delayed symptoms rarely occur. As noted, however, a significant percentage of asymptomatic patients who had initial postingestion symptoms demonstrate radiographic abnormalities. A safe course would be patient observation for 6 h and discharge if the chest films are negative at that time. Unless close, reliable follow-up can be arranged, asymptomatic patients with positive films should probably be admitted for a longer period of observation, even though their course is generally benign.

3. Any patient with **fever, lethargy,** or **respiratory signs or symptoms** should be admitted. These symptoms are usually evident early after ingestion. A few of these patients have normal chest roentgenograms.

4. Patients who have ingested substances that may be systemically absorbed with potential for **delayed organ system toxicity** also require admission. In addition, any patient with well documented massive ingestions or **suicidal attempts** should be held for evaluation and prolonged observation or admitted. The emergency physician should also remember that toxic ingestions can be an early sign of **child abuse** or neglect, and appropriate intervention may be necessary.

B. **Long-term effects.** Full recovery after hydrocarbon pneumonitis is expected. However, some researchers have suggested that minor abnormalities may persist. Foley et al. (29) reevaluated 30 of 101 children who had aspirated kerosene and reported an increased incidence of respiratory infections. Gurwitz et al. (30) studied pulmonary functions of 17 asymptomatic patients 8 to 14 years after an episode of hydrocarbon pneumonitis. (Controls were normal, matched children with no history of lower respiratory tract disease.) Eighty-two percent of these patients had one or more pulmonary function abnormalities. The authors attributed this incidence to small airway obstruction or loss of elastic recoil (or both). The significance of these findings remains unclear.

C. **Prevention.** As for other toxic ingestions, the most effective management measures are those that prevent the condition before it occurs. Parents should be educated to keep potentially toxic materials out of the reach of children. Familiar bottles or containers should not be used for storage of these products. Gasoline siphoning by mouth should be discouraged. Manufacturers of hydrocarbon products for home use should be encouraged to increase the viscosity of such materials when possible and to provide proper labeling. The use of safety closures for these products should also be promoted. Workplace standards must be enforced and, in some cases, expanded.

Acknowledgment: I am greatly indebted to Candice Zemnick for her significant contribution to the successful completion of this chapter.

References

1. Litovitz TL, Smilkstein M, Felberg L, Klein-Schwartz, Berlin R, Morgan JL. 1996 annual report of the American Association of Poison Control Centers toxic exposure surveillance system. *Am J Emerg Med* 1997;15:447–492.

2. Gerarde HW. Toxicological studies on hydrocarbons. V. Kerosene. *Toxicol Appl Pharmacol* 1959;1:462.
3. Ellenhorn MJ. The hydrocarbon products. In: Ellenhorn MJ, et al., eds. *Ellenhorn's medical toxicology diagnosis and treatment of human poisoning.* Baltimore: Williams & Wilkins, 1997:1420–1447.
4. Wason S, Gibler WB, Hassan M. Ventricular tachycardia associated with non-freon aerosol propellants. *JAMA* 1986;256:78.
5. Kulberg AG, Goldfrank LR, Bresnitz EA. Hydrocarbons. In: Goldfrank LR, et al., eds. *Goldfrank's toxicologic emergencies.* 3rd ed. Norwalk, CT: Appleton-Century-Crofts, 1986.
6. Gerarde HW. Toxicological studies on hydrocarbons. IX. The aspiration hazard and toxicity of hydrocarbons and hydrocarbon mixtures. *Arch Environ Health* 1963;6:35.
7. Mann MD, Pirie DJ, Wolfsdorf J. Kerosene absorption in primates. *J Pediatr* 1977;91:495.
8. Bratton L, Haddow JE. Ingestion of charcoal lighter fluid. *The Journal of Pediatrics* 1975;87:633–636.
9. Dice WH, et al. Pulmonary toxicity following gastrointestinal ingestion of kerosene. *Ann Emerg Med* 1982;11:138.
10. Wolfsdorf J. Kerosene intoxication: an experimental approach to the etiology of the CNS manifestations in primates. *J Pediatr* 1976;88:1037.
11. Giammona ST. Effects of furniture polish on pulmonary surfactant. *Am J Dis Child* 1967;113:658.
12. Prockop L. Neurotoxic volatile substances. *Neurology* 1979;862–865.
13. Baker EL, Fine LJ. Solvent neurotoxicity: the current evidence. *J Occup Med* 1986;28:126.
14. Stockman JA. More on hydrocarbon-induced hemolysis [Letter]. *J Pediatr* 1977;90:848.
15. Anas N, Namasonthi V, Ginsburg CM. Criteria for hospitalizing children who have ingested products containing hydrocarbons. *JAMA* 1981;246:840.
16. Jacobziner H, Raybin HW. Activities of the Poison Control Center: turpentine poisoning. *Arch Pediatr* 1961;357–364.
17. Bass M. Sudden sniffing death. *JAMA* 1970;212:2075–2079.
18. Taylor GJ, Harris WS. Cardiac toxicity of aerosol propellants. *JAMA* 1970;214:81–85.
19. Eade NR, Taussiag LM, Marks MI. Hydrocarbon pneumonitis. *Pediatrics* 1974;54:351–357.
20. Machado B, Cross K, Snodgrass WR. Accidental hydrocarbon ingestion cases telephoned to a regional poison center. *Ann Emerg Med* 1988;17:804.
20a. Ng RC, Darnish H, Stewart DA. Emergency treatment of petroleum distillate and turpentine ingestion. *Can Med Assoc J* 1974;111:537.
21. Molinas S. A note on the use of syrup of ipecac by poison control centers. *Natl Clearinghouse Poison Control Center Bull* 1966;10:4.
22. Goldfrank LR. Hydrocarbons. In: Goldfrank LP, et al., eds. *Goldfrank's toxicologic emergencies.* 5th ed. Norwalk, CT: Appleton-Century-Crofts, 1994:1231–1244.
23. Bysani GK, Rucoba RJ, Noah ZN. Treatment of hydrocarbon pneumonitis. *Chest* 1994;106:300–303.
24. Chyka PA. Benefits of extracorporeal membrane oxygenation of hydrocarbon pneumonitis. *Clin Toxicol* 1996;34357–363.
25. Wolfsdorf J, Kundig H. Dexamethasone in the management of kerosene pneumonia. *Pediatrics* 1974;53:86.
26. Marks MI, et al. Adrenocorticosteroid treatment of hydrocarbon pneumonia in children—a cooperative study. *J Pediatr* 1972;81:366.
27. Steele RW, Conklin RH, Mark HM. Corticosteroids and antibiotics for the treatment of fulminant hydrocarbon aspiration. *JAMA* 1972;219:1434.
28. Brown J, Burke B, Dajani AS. Experimental kerosene pneumonia: evaluation of some therapeutic regimens. *J Pediatr* 1974;84:396.
29. Foley JC, et al. Kerosene poisoning in young children. *Radiology* 1954;62:817.
30. Goldfrank L, Kirstein R, Bresnitz E. Gasoline and other hydrocarbons. *Hosp Physician* 1979;9:32–38.

Selected Readings

Aviado DM, Belej MA. Toxicology of aerosol propellants on the respiratory and circulatory systems. I. Cardiac arrhythmia in the mouse. *Toxicology* 1974;2:31.

Banner W Jr. Risks of extracorporeal membrane oxygenation: is there a role for use in the management of the acutely poisoned patient. *Clin Toxicol* 1996;34:365–371.

Belej MA, Smith DG, Aviado DM. Toxicity of aerosol propellants in the respiratory and circulatory systems. IV. Cardiotoxicity in the monkey. *Toxicology* 1974;2:381.

Burkhart KK, Hall AH, Rocco G, Rumack BH. Hyperbaric oxygen treatment for carbon tetrachloride poisoning. *Drug Safety* 1991;6:332–338.

Flanagan RJ, Ruprah M, Meredith TJ, Ramsey JD. An introduction to the clinical toxicology of volatile substances. *Drug Safety* 1990;5:359–383.

Gurwitz D, et al. Pulmonary function abnormalities in asymptomatic children after hydrocarbon pneumonitis. *Pediatrics* 1978;62:789.

Hansbrough JF, et al. Hydrocarbon contact injuries. *J Trauma* 1985;25:250.

King GS, Smialek JE, Troutman WG. Sudden death in adolescents resulting from the inhalation of typewriter correction fluid. *JAMA* 1985;253:1604.

Mivos R, Dean BS, Krenzelok EP. High-pressure injection injuries: a serious occupational hazard. *Clin Toxicol* 1987;25: 297–304

Nierenberg DW, Horowitz MB, Harris KM, James DH. Mineral spirits inhalation associated with hemolysis, pulmonary edema, and ventricular fibrillation. *Arch Intern Med* 1991;151:1437–1440.

Poklis A, Burkett CD. Gasoline sniffing: a review. *Clin Toxicol* 1977;11:35.

Reihardt CF, Azar A, Maxfield ME, Smith PE, Mullin LS. Cardiac arrhythmias and aerosol sniffing. *Arch Environ Health* 1971;22:265–279.

Rinsky RA, Smith AB, Hornung R, et al. Benzene and leukemia: an epidemiologic risk assessment. *N Engl J Med* 1987;316: 1044–1050.

Truss CD, Killenberg PG. Treatment of carbon tetrachloride poisoning with hyperbaric oxygen. *Gastroenterology* 1982;82:767.

White JF, Carlson GP. Epinephrine-induced cardiac arrhythmias in rabbits exposed to trichloroethylene: role of trichloro-ethylene metabolites. *Toxicol Appl Pharmacol* 1981;60:458.

Wolfe BM, Brodeur AE, Shields JB. The role of gastrointestinal absorption of kerosene in producing pneumonitis in dogs. *J Pediatr* 1970;76:867.

Emergency Toxicology, Second Edition,
edited by Peter Viccellio.
Lippincott–Raven Publishers, Philadelphia © 1998.

18

Nitrates and Nitrites

Paula Jane Barclay

Outpatient Family Medicine & Internal Medicine, Allergy & Immunology, Minor Emergencies, X-Ray, & Lab, Basalt, Colorado 81621

I. **Properties of nitrates and nitrites**
   A. **Sources and forms**
      1. **Inorganic nitrates**
         a. **Sodium nitrate and potassium nitrate**
            (1) **Potassium nitrate**—formerly used as a diuretic when taken in a dilute solution.
            (2) Sodium nitrate—used to preserve the color of meat in the pickling or salting process.
            (3) High concentrations of these substances **occur naturally** in spinach, beets, carrots, and cabbage (less than or equal to 1,000 ppm). The toxic nitrites form after the substance is cooked and then allowed to stand at room temperature.
         b. **Bismuth subnitrate**—used as an antidiarrheal agent in the past, it is currently used as an antacid in the United Kingdom (commercial names: Roter Tablets, Stomach Dellipsoids). A paste form is used for treatment of radiation burns (commercial name: Compound Bismuth Subnitrate Cream).
         c. **Silver nitrate**—used for its caustic, astringent, and disinfectant properties. It is used to destroy warts and other small skin growths; to cauterize small blood vessels; as prophylaxis of ophthalmia neonatorum. It is also applied to burns to reduce infection.
      2. **Organic nitrates**—antianginal drugs (generic names, with commercial names in parentheses)
         a. Glyceryl trinitrate (Nitroglycerin)
         b. Isosorbide dinitrate (Isordil, Dilatrate, Isobid, Sorbitrate)
         c. Pentaerythritol tetranitrate (United States: Antime, Duotrate, Mertanil, Pentafin, Peritrate; United Kingdom: Myocardol; France: Nitrodex; Germany: Dilcoran; Switzerland: Dilcoran, Nitrodex; The Netherlands: Pentrit; Sweden: Nitropent; South Africa: Cardilate)
         d. Erythrityl tetranitrate (Cardilate)
         e. Ethyl nitrate (Nitrous Ether Spirit)
         f. Mannitol hexanitrate (Germany: Moloid)

    g. Trolnitrate phosphate (Belgium, Denmark: Anatrit; Australia: Praenitron; Sweden: Nitroduran)

  3. **Inorganic nitrites**

    a. Amyl nitrate—used to treat industrial cyanide poisoning and to diagnose cardiac murmurs; formerly used as an antianginal drug; currently used as a drug of abuse (street name: Mama Poppers).

    b. Isobutyl nitrite—technically a room deodorizer. It is sold for recreational use as an aphrodisiac, abused by some adolescents to "get high," and may be used by some male homosexuals to relax the anal sphincter during intercourse (street names: Rush, Bolt, Hardware, Quicksilver, Satan's Scent, Climax, Oz, Locker Room, Bank, Hiball, Discorama, Bullet, Thrust, Lightning Bolt, Snappers, Flash, Sweat).

    c. Sodium nitrite—principally used for the treatment of cyanide poisoning in conjunction with sodium thiosulfate.

  4. **Organic nitrites**

    a. Bismuth subnitrate in contaminated well water may be converted by intestinal bacteria to nitrites.

    b. Nitrates in contaminated water in the presence of *Bacillus subtilis* spores in dried milk powder are transformed to nitrites.

B. **Physical and chemical properties**

  1. **Inorganic nitrates**

    a. Sodium nitrate and potassium nitrate—white crystalline salts, with a cool saline taste, water-soluble

    b. Bismuth subnitrate—white powder insoluble in water

    c. Silver nitrate (pure form)—colorless, odorless crystals or white crystalline powder with a bitter, metallic taste

  2. **Organic nitrates**

    a. Glyceryl trinitrate—colorless, odorless, volatile, oily liquid with a sweet, aromatic, pungent taste in pure form; usually in pill form

    b. Isosorbide dinitrate—white crystalline powder, water-soluble

    c. Pentaerythritol tetranitrate—white odorless powder

    d. Erythrityl tetranitrate—white tasteless crystals

    e. Ethyl nitrate—clear, faint yellow volatile liquid with an apple-like odor

    f. Mannitol hexanitrate—white crystalline powder with a faint odor

    g. Trolnitrate phosphate—white crystalline odorless powder

  3. **Inorganic nitrites**

    a. Isobutyl nitrite—colorless to yellowish volatile flammable liquid with an unpleasant odor

    b. Amyl nitrite—clear yellow volatile flammable liquid with a fragrant odor

C. **Mechanism of action and pathophysiology**

  1. Nitrates, organic nitrites and nitroso-compounds activate guanylate cyclase and increase synthesis of guanosine $3',5'$-monophosphate (cyclic GMP). Cyclic GMP-dependent protein is stimulated with alteration of phosphorylation of the various proteins in smooth muscle, eventually leading to the dephosphorylation of the light chain of myosin and causing smooth muscle relaxation; all smooth muscle structures are affected. It results in arteriolar and venous smooth muscle relaxation and compensatory tachycardia and vasoconstriction. In the gastrointestinal (GI) tract, these effects cause nausea, vomiting, abdominal pain, and diarrhea.

2. A significant effect of nitrates and nitrites is **methemoglobinemia**. Nitrates and nitrites oxidize hemoglobin to methemoglobin by oxidizing iron from the ferrous (Fe^{2+}) to the ferric (Fe^{3+}) state. Iron in the ferric state is incapable of binding oxygen. The conformity of the methemoglobin causes the affinity of the remaining hemes to be increased, which causes a shift to the left of the oxyhemoglobin curve (similar to carbon monoxide poisoning) and consequently impairs unloading of oxygen to tissues. Infants younger than 6 months of age have a relative lack of the enzyme that converts methemoglobin to hemoglobin (cytochrome-5-reductase = methemoglobin reductase). Patients with G6PD deficiency and NADH-methemoglobin reductase deficiency, infants, pregnant women, and patients with malignant disease are more susceptible to developing methemoglobinemia after exposure to nitrites.

D. **Pharmacology and pharmacokinetics**
   1. **Inorganic nitrates**
      a. Sodium and potassium nitrate—rapidly absorbed through gastric mucosa and excreted unchanged in urine. As little as 1 g of sodium nitrate may be fatal, although doses as high as 30 g have been taken without adverse effects.
      b. Silver nitrate—absorbed through the skin and the GI tract. Silver ion is precipitated by chloride of tissues. Nitrate is converted to nitrite by intestinal bacteria.
      c. Bismuth subnitrate—absorbed through intestinal mucosa. The nitrate is converted to nitrite by intestinal bacteria.
   2. **Organic nitrates.** In general, the nitrates are rapidly absorbed from the GI tract and skin. Nitrates undergo first-pass hepatic denitration by hydroxylation into mononitrates and dinitrates; this denitration markedly reduces their activity. When given orally, high doses are needed to saturate the liver's capacity for degradation, or not enough nitrate would reach the circulation.
      a. **Glyceryl trinitrate**
         (1) Sublingual form—half-life is 1 to 3 min, peaking at 4 min. The dinitrate metabolites (which are 10 times less potent as vasodilators) have a half-life of 40 min.
         (2) Oral form—high doses (e.g., 6.5 mg) are needed to achieve a vasodilatory effect. With a slow onset of action, it peaks at 60 to 90 min and lasts 3 to 6 h.
         (3) Ointment—slow onset of action peaking at 1 to 2 h and lasting 4 to 8 h.
         (4) Transdermal patch—peaks at 1 to 2 h and lasts up to 24 h.
      b. **Isosorbide dinitrate**—denitrated at one-sixth the rate of glyceryl trinitrate. Sublingual form—peak concentration at 6 min with a half-life of 45 min. The major metabolites (isosorbide-2-mononitrate and isosorbide-5-mononitrate) have half-lives of 2 to 5 h and are responsible for the major vasodilatory effects.

    c. Erythrityl tetranitrate—degraded three times faster than glyceryl trinitrate; well absorbed from oral and GI mucosa.

      (1) Sublingual form—5 min to onset of action, peaks in 15 min, and lasts about 3 h.

      (2) Oral form—15 to 30 min to onset of action, peaks in 60 min, lasts 6 h.

    d. Pentaerythritol nitrate—used for prophylaxis. It is denitrated at one-tenth the rate of glyceryl trinitrate. It is well absorbed from the GI tract but is poorly absorbed from oral mucosa; therefore, it is not given sublingually. Its peak effect occurs in 1 h and lasts 5 h. About 40% is excreted unchanged in the feces, and 60% is excreted in the urine as pentaerythritol and pentaerythritol mononitrate.

  3. **Inorganic nitrites**

    a. Amyl nitrate—absorbed into the circulation from mucous membranes, most rapidly by the lungs; it is inactivated by hydrolysis. It is inactive when taken by mouth, as it is rapidly hydrolyzed in the GI tract.

    b. Isobutyl nitrite—rapidly absorbed into the circulation through mucous membranes. It is rapidly hydrolyzed.

II. **Clinical presentation**

  A. **History**

    1. **Oral ingestion of nitrates and nitrites**

      a. **Unintentional versus intentional ingestions**

        (1) **Unintentional ingestion**

          (a) Babies given vegetable juice concentrates (e.g., spinach purees, carrot juice) or well water may develop cyanosis from methemoglobinemia (1). Those who develop cyanosis have usually ingested water containing nitrates in a concentration of more than 10 to 100 ppm. Public Health Service drinking water standards set the limit of nitrate ion at 45 mg/L in drinking water to avoid infant methemoglobinemia. No case reports have occurred when ingestion levels are less than the maximum contaminant level (MCL). Lactating women who consume water with nitrate concentration of 100 mg/L (more than twice the MCL) do not produce breast milk with elevated nitrate levels and no cases of infant methemoglobinemia have been reported to occur via mother-infant transmission. Dairy cows ingesting up to 180 mg/L (four times the MCL) of nitrate in polluted drinking water have been shown to have elevated levels of nitrate in milk produced.

          (b) Chronic ingestion of nitrates at more than 5 mg/kg/day can cause methemoglobinemia; ingestion of large amounts of nitrates on a chronic basis may be associated with development of stomach cancer.

          (c) Epidemics of isolated episodes of intoxications have occurred when sodium nitrate was mistaken for sodium chloride in the preparation of food or when sodium nitrate was used heavily in meat products;

additionally, unintentional use of sodium nitrate in oral laxatives instead of sodium sulfate has resulted in fatal methemoglobinemia.

(2) Intentional ingestion. Suicide attempts with oral antianginal drugs or ingestion of as little as 10 mL of amyl nitrite or isobutyl nitrite can produce methemoglobinemia and death. Ingestion of 2 to 10 g of silver nitrate may be fatal.

b. Symptoms

(1) Infants who have inadvertently been fed high concentrations of nitrates are usually brought in by the family because they are cyanotic and may be lethargic.

(2) Rheumatic symptoms after exposure to nitrates has been documented by double-blind, controlled food challenge studies but have not been associated with methemoglobinemia.

(3) Patients who are on nitrate therapy for angina and ingest more than 5 mg/kg/day usually present with signs of circulatory demise; they are much less likely to show signs of methemoglobinemia.

(4) Patients who attempt suicide with nitrates may be brought in lethargic, disoriented, seizing, or comatose with cyanosis. Ingestion of silver nitrate is associated with black vomitus.

(5) Patients may have methemoglobinemia (less than 5%) without signs or symptoms. Usually a level of 1.5% methemoglobin must be present for a patient to be cyanotic.

2. Inhalation

a. Unintentional versus intentional inhalation

(1) Unintentional inhalation. Exposure limit for glyceryl trinitrate is 0.05 ppm, but concentrations of more than 0.02 ppm can cause headache. Workers bottling isobutyl nitrate developed asymptomatic methemoglobinemia averaging 5%. Ambient air isobutyl concentration was found to be 25 to 155 ppm (2).

(2) Intentional inhalation. Amyl nitrate and isobutyl nitrates are abused for recreational purposes. They are abused by some adolescents for "getting high." In a 1984 survey, 10% of 17,000 teens surveyed admitted to using volatile nitrates at least once (3). Used as an aphrodisiac and to enhance and prolong sexual orgasm, these nitrates are also used by some homosexual men to relax the anal sphincter during intercourse. Epidemiological evidence has shown that the use of nitrite inhalants is an independent risk factor in couples having unprotected anal intercourse in increasing the risk of HIV infection. Acute inhalation of nitrites has been shown to reduce erythrocyte and leukocyte counts and depress natural killer (NK) cell activity, which ultimately play a role in a person's susceptibility to the HIV virus. Because of their volatility (they must be contained in small dark brown bottles) and their use as a sexual accelerant, their presence must be considered in any patient brought in after a fire that occurred during sexual intercourse (4).

b. Symptoms

(1) Patients complain of dizziness, light-headedness, heart pounding, feeling warm, and blurred vision; they also develop headaches, nausea, vomiting, diarrhea, and crampy abdominal pain. Burning in the nose and eyes, cough, and eye pain are not uncommon; pain and itching in areas of local exposure (nose and upper lip) have been reported (5). The "high" is usually described as unpleasant (3).

(2) These patients may be brought in by friends after a "party" or by emergency medical service personnel when they develop more severe symptoms and collapse at parties or discotheques. The history is usually nonspecific, but concomitant ingestion of multiple drugs (cocaine, alcohol, marijuana) is frequent.

B. Physical examination. After oral ingestion, depending on the degree of severity, the patient may be alert, with or without agitation, and may progressively deteriorate to a state of combativeness, lethargy, or coma. Patients develop seizures in more advanced cases. With any significant ingestion the patient is usually afebrile, tachycardic, and hypotensive with an elevated respiratory rate. The skin may be flushed with mild intoxication, but cyanosis with warm skin is an important finding and is associated with methemoglobinemia. The patient may have erythematous conjuctivae, increased intraocular pressure, and yellow, crusting lesions on the nose and upper lip after inhalation. Chronic abusers may have telangiectasias. Vomiting and diarrhea are commonly present with acute intoxication; black vomitus is associated with silver nitrate intoxication.

C. Course

1. With mild cases (methemoglobin of more than 30%), symptoms resolve in several hours if circulatory support is given.

2. If patients with methemoglobinemia of 30% are not diagnosed and treated, they deteriorate after a few hours and ultimately develop hypotension, seizures, and cardiopulmonary arrest secondary to asphyxiation.

III. Differential diagnosis

A. Cardiovascular collapse

1. Cardiac disease
2. Infections with sepsis
3. Dehydration
4. Drugs

B. Cyanosis

1. Cardiopulmonary disease
2. Methemoglobinemia
   a. Hereditary
   b. Acquired
      (1) Nitrates and nitrites
      (2) Aniline dyes
      (3) Sulfonamides
      (4) Acetanilid

          (5) Phenacetin

          (6) Lidocaine, chlorate, phenazopyridine

  C. Seizures

    1. Metabolic

    2. Infectious

    3. Mass lesions

    4. Cerebrovascular accidents

    5. Drug-induced

IV. Laboratory analysis

  A. General tests

    1. In patients with signs of mild toxicity (e.g., cardiovascular signs only), arterial blood gases (ABGs) and electrolytes are normal, and the ECG shows nonspecific changes.

    2. Patients with signs of methemoglobinemia have brownish or chocolate-colored arterial and venous blood that does not turn red when exposed to oxygen. These patients develop an anion gap acidosis with a normal serum potassium and glucose. The ABGs show an acidotic pH, normal Po_2, and decreased Pco_2. The ECG reflects various degrees of hypoxemia, beginning with a tachycardia with nonspecific changes, advancing to bradycardia, ventricular rhythms, and ultimately asystole.

    3. Toxicology screens frequently show the presence of cocaine, ethanol, and marijuana in patients intentionally abusing nitrites.

    4. Ingestion of silver nitrate can cause hypochloremia and hyponatremia.

  B. Specific tests

    1. Serum methemoglobin levels should be measured, but many hospitals do not have the capacity for their immediate determination. If the blood is not assayed within a few hours using endogenous methemoglobin reductase, the methemoglobin value will be falsely low.

      a. If the level of methemoglobin is expressed in grams, the percentage of methemoglobin can be calculated. Express it as the methemoglobin/hemoglobin ratio (e.g., if metHgb = 4 g/dL blood and Hgb = 12 g/dL of blood, then 4/12 = 33% methemoglobinemia exists).

      b. A good, rapid, rough test for methemoglobinemia consists in placing a drop of blood on filter paper. If the blood remains brown compared to a control sample, the patient has a methemoglobinemia of more than 15%. Comatose patients usually have levels of at least 30%.

    2. Gastric nitrate/nitrite and gastric isobutanol (product of hydroxylation of isobutyl nitrite) contents can be analyzed by commercial laboratories in cases of oral ingestion.

    3. Quantitative measurement of glyceryl trinitrate can be performed using high performance liquid chromatography.

V. Management

  A. General measures

    1. Ventilatory support/oxygen as needed

    2. Cardiovascular support

    a. Keep patient warm and recumbent.

    b. Use intravenous saline to support the blood pressure.

    c. Avoid epinephrine and vasoconstrictor drugs.

    d. Use atropine for bradycardia.

  3. Induce emesis with ipecac if the patient is alert enough, followed by activated charcoal; use gastric lavage with intubation if the patient is not alert.

  4. Follow lavage with magnesium or sodium sulfate or sorbitol as a cathartic.

  5. Treat seizures with diazepam or phenytoin.

B. Toxin-specific measures

  1. If the methemoglobinemia is more than 30%, inject **methylene blue** (1 to 2 mg/kg). It can rapidly reverse a methemoglobinemia of moderate degree (30% to 50%).

  2. **Exchange transfusions** should be used for infants, patients who do not respond to methylene blue within 30 to 60 min, patients with G6PD deficiency, and those with methemoglobin levels of more than 70%.

C. Complicating factors and controversies

  1. **Methylene blue** becomes an **oxidizing agent** in high concentrations and actually can cause methemoglobinemia if too much is given. (There is a case report of methemoglobinemia after 500 mg of methylene blue was given to diagnose a fistula.)

  2. **Methylene blue** should not be used for **cyanide poisoning** following accidental overdose with sodium nitrate, as release of cyanide occurs. Exchange transfusion is the treatment of choice in this situation.

VI. Disposition and follow-up. If patients are treated rapidly and complications of shock are avoided (anoxic brain damage, renal failure, and myocardial infarction), there are no long-term sequelae from methemoglobinemia.

References

1. Laaban JP, Bodenan P. Amyl nitrate poppers and methemoglobinemia. *Ann Intern Med* 1985;103:804–806.
2. Nickerson M, et al. *Isobutyl nitrite and related compounds*. San Francisco: Pharmex, 1979.
3. Schwartz RH, Peary P. Abuse of isobutyl nitrite inhalation (Rush) by adolescents. *Clin Pediatr* 1986;25:308–309.
4. O'Toole JB III. Ingestion of isobutyl nitrite, a recreational chemical of abuse, causing fatal methemoglobinemia. *J Forensic Sci* 1987;32:1811.
5. Fisher A, et al. Facial dermatitis in men due to inhalation of butyl nitrite. *Cutis* 1981;27:146–147.

Selected Readings

Arena JM. *Poisoning: toxicology, symptoms, treatments*. 5th ed. Springfield, IL: Charles C. Thomas Publisher, 1986.

Braunwald E, et al. *Harrison's principles of internal medicine*. 11th ed. New York: McGraw-Hill, 1987.

Dax EM, et al. Amyl nitite alters human in vitro immune function. *Immunopharmacol Immunotoxicol* 1991;13:577–587.

Dreisbach RH. *Handbook of poisoning: prevention, diagnosis and treatment*. 12th ed. Norwalk, CT: Appleton & Lange, 1987.

Ellis M, et al. Fatal methemoglobinemia caused by inadvertent contamination of laxative solution with sodium nitrite. *Isr J Med Sci* 1992;28:289–291.

Fan AM, et al. Health implications of nitrate and nitrite in drinking water: an update on methemoglobinemia occurrence and reproductive and developmental toxicity. *Regul Toxicol Pharmacol* 1996;23:35–43.

Goodman LA, et al., eds. *Goodman and Gilman's pharmacological basis of therapeutics*. 7th ed. New York: Macmillan, 1985.

Gosselin RE. *Clinical toxicology of commercial products.* 5th ed. Baltimore: Williams & Wilkins, 1984.

Horne K III. Methemoglobinemia from sniffing butyl nitrite. *Ann Intern Med* 1979;91:417–418.

Kammerer M, et al. Content of nitrate in milk. Relationship with its concentration in the water supply for livestock. *Ann Rech Vet* 1992;23:131–138.

Kaye S. *Handbook of emergency toxicology.* 4th ed. Springfield, IL: Charles C. Thomas Publisher, 1980.

Keating JP, Lell ME. Infantile methemoglobinemia caused by carrot juice. *N Engl J Med* 1973;288:824–826.

Knight TM, et al. Nitrate and nitrite exposure in Italian populations with different gastric cancer rates. *Int J Epidemiol* 1990;19:510–515.

La Vecchia C, et al. Nitrosamine intake and gastric cancer risk. *Eur J Cancer Prev* 1995;4:469–474.

Panush RS, et al. Food induced ("allergic") arthritis: clinical and serologic studies. *J Rheumatol* 1990;17:291–294.

Pobel D, et al. Nitrosamine, nitrate and nitrite in relation to gastric cancer: a case-control study in Marseille, France. *Eur J Epidemiol* 1995;11:67–73.

Reynolds JE. *Martindale: the extra pharmacopoeia.* 28th ed. London: Pharmaceutical Press, 1982.

Rogers MA, et al. Consumption of nitrate, nitrite, and nitrosodimethylamine and the risk of upper aerodigestive tract cancer. *Cancer Epidemiol Biomarkers Prev* 1995;4:29–36.

Seage GR III, et al. The relation between nitrite inhalants, unprotected receptive anal intercourse, and the risk of human immunodeficiency virus infection. *Am J Epidemiol* 1992;135:1–11.

Smith M, Stair T. Butyl nitrite and a suicide attempt. *Ann Intern Med* 1980;92:719–720.

Shesser R, Mitchell J. Methemoglobinemia from isobutyl nitrite preparations. *Ann Emerg Med* 1981;10:262–264.

Soderberg LS, et al. Acute inhalation exposure to isobutyl nitrite causes nonspecific blood cell destruction. *Exp Hematol* 1996;24:592–596.

Walker R, et al. Nitrates, nitrites and N-nitrosocompounds: a review of the occurrence in food and diet and the toxicological implications. *Food Addit Contam* 1990;7:717–768.

Xu G, et al. The relationship between gastric mucosal changes and nitrite intake via drinking water in a high-risk population for gastric cancer in Moping county, China. *Eur J Cancer Prev* 1992;1:437–443.M

Emergency Toxicology, Second Edition,
edited by Peter Viccellio.
Lippincott–Raven Publishers, Philadelphia © 1998.

19

Hydrogen Fluoride

†Carol Barsky and °Fred Landes

†*New York, New York 10014;* °*Department of Emergency Medicine, Berkshire Medical Center, Pittsfield, Massachusetts 01201*

I. **Sources.** Toxic exposures to fluoride compounds during the 20th century have commonly been of three types: ingestions of fluoride-containing insecticides and rodenticides; dietary supplements and fluoridated water; and exposure to hydrofluoric acid compounds in industrial and home products.

  A. Sodium fluoride **pesticides** containing more than 30% NaF are dangerous when ingested. This agent was the one involved in the most serious recorded fluoride ingestion: 261 patients at a state hospital were fed NaF mistaken for powdered milk, and 47 of them died (1). Fluoride-containing insecticides came into use as a replacement for arsenical insecticides when NaF was found to be a stomach poison for cockroaches. Although the use of fluoride insecticides and pesticides has decreased as a result of their relative ineffectiveness, they are still commercially available.

  B. The greatest source of fluoride is **fluoridated water.** Although errors in fluoridation have taken place, there have been no resultant serious toxic effects. Similarly, toothpastes (Crest, Aim, and Colgate) and dietary supplements (Polyviflor) contain fluorides in low concentrations or use compounds that dissociate fluoride in small amounts (e.g., SnF_2 or $NaFPO_4$). Toothpastes are allowed to contain only 120 mg of fluoride per tube (264 mg NaF). Although it is unlikely to cause serious toxicity, the dose of fluoride (milligrams per kilogram) should be calculated for ingestions in order to assess potential pathology.

  C. **Hydrogen fluoride** (HF) is the most commonly used fluoride compound in industry. It is obtained by the action of sulfuric acid on the mineral fluorspar. Industrial uses include the production of plastics, rocket fuels, and silicon chips; aluminum purification; the cleansing of iron, brass, copper, and masonry; the frosting and etching of glass and enamel; as an alkylating agent in the production of high octane gasolines; and in the brewing of beer. Products found in the home that contain HF include erusticators such as Whink Rust Stain Remover, enamel cleaners, and aluminum siding and trailer cleaners. Given the increasing use of HF in industry and the increasing frequency of toxic patients presenting to emergency departments, this chapter focuses on this means of exposure to fluoride compounds.

II. **Physical and chemical properties, and pathophysiology**

  A. HF is a colorless gas that is highly corrosive in liquid and gaseous forms or in solution with water. Its toxicity is based on its physical properties as an acid that dissociates fluoride ion. The acidic component causes the coagulative necrosis of organic tissue that is typical of all acids; the degree is determined by its concentration, duration of exposure, thickness of the skin or tissue exposed, and the organ system involved in the burn. The concentrations of aqueous HF compounds range from 0.5% to 70%; products likely to be found in the home are overwhelmingly in the lower concentration ranges, i.e., less than 15%.

B. Hydrofluoric acid, like other compounds that dissociate fluoride, is distinguished by the *rapid tissue penetration* of the fluoride moiety and absorption by the skin, lungs, and GI tract. Fluoride has been described as a "general protoplasmic poison" (2), that causes inhibition of cellular respiration and glycolytic pathways. The clinical phenomenon of hyperkalemia seen in some patients with fluoride toxicity, postulated to be due to failure of the energy requiring a sodium-potassium pump, has been cited as evidence (2). Tissue destruction continues until free fluoride is bound with tissue cations (e.g., magnesium or calcium). This process can continue for days, in contrast to the rapid neutralization of most acids (3).

C. The **plasma half-life** of fluoride has been reported to be 1.4 h (4). After oral ingestion, fluoride is rapidly deposited in bone or renally excreted. In a case report, an anuric patient was found to have a fluoride half-life of 8 h, with clearance due overwhelmingly to deposition in bone. Serum fluoride levels are therefore diagnostic of toxicity only for the first several hours after exposure, whereas urine fluoride levels remain elevated for days to weeks. Postmortem evaluation of bone is positive for fluoride deposition after acute or chronic exposure (5). The slow release of fluoride from bone after its deposition there has not resulted in toxic effects.

D. The **minimum toxic or lethal dose** of fluoride has not been established. Only large volumes of toothpaste or mouthwash are potentially hazardous. Alternatively, ingested fluoride 3 to 5 mg/kg induces GI toxicity, and more than 5 mg/kg may induce systemic toxicity. Ingestions of more than 30 mg/kg are likely to be fatal.

III. **Clinical presentation** of HF toxicity depends on the type of exposure and physical form of the agent.

   A. **Integument.** The most common type of exposure is after skin contact with aqueous HF in the home or industrial setting. The severity of the burn depends on the strength of the acid, the duration of exposure, and the susceptibility of the involved tissue. Contact with concentrations above 14.5% causes immediate and excruciating pain (6), whereas concentrations of 12% cause symptoms within 1 h, and skin contact with concentrations of 7% become symptomatic one to several hours afterward.

   1. With **high-concentration exposure,** the skin may rapidly progress from normal to becoming erythematous and edematous, followed by a pasty white appearance, the formation of vesicles containing necrotic tissue, and finally ulceration and full-thickness loss. In a case report involving contact with 70% aqueous HF, this entire process took 48 h (7). In some cases, an apparently stable eschar forms with progression of injury underneath it. Burns to the head, face, neck, or chest are at high risk of inhalation, with resultant pulmonary and systemic toxicity.

   2. If the concentration of the acid is low, the patient may complain of severe and increasing pain, with normal-appearing skin, as long as 36 h after contact with the acid. As the upper extremity is frequently involved, subacute digital tissue loss is a common sequela of untreated HF exposure. Symptomatic patients, even in the absence of physical findings, require treatment.

B. Cardiovascular system

1. The cardiovascular complications of acute fluoride toxicity comprise its most dramatic aspect; ventricular arrhythmias and congestive heart failure are the most common causes of precipitous death during the first 6 h after exposure. In one case report, a 23-year-old man with a 10% body surface area burn to the anterior thighs caused by 70% HF acid died after intractable ventricular arrhythmias (8). Postmortem examination revealed extensive areas of necrotic myocardium characterized by hypereosinophilia, clumping of sarcoplasm, loss of nuclei and striations, and a prominent extravascular polymorphonuclear infiltrate and phagocytosis. This case, marked by the absence of inhalation or GI burns (common to many fatal exposures to fluoride) suggests a cardiotoxic effect of HF independent of fluid and electrolyte loss, hypoxia, burns to the GI tract, and other factors seen with fluoride toxicity that may contribute to cardiovascular collapse.

2. Although victims sustaining ventricular arrhythmias have responded to lidocaine and cardioversion, recurrence of ventricular ectopy is the rule. A report of 45 recurrences of ventricular fibrillation is not unique in the literature. There have, however, been survivors among these patients, and aggressive management is warranted.

C. Eye exposure. As with dermal exposure, eye pain may be immediate or delayed depending on the concentration of the hydrofluoric acid solution or gas. With a **strong solution** there may be immediate pain, scarring of the corneal stroma, erosion of the corneal epithelium, and progressive vascularization that may result in blindness. If the concentration of the solution is dilute, eye complaints may begin days after contact with the chemical.

D. Inhalation of gaseous HF, as well as splash burns to the face, neck, and chest, have resulted in serious inhalation injury. Autopsy studies have revealed upper airway erythema and obstruction, epithelial sloughing, uncontrolled bronchiolar bleeding and obstruction, and hemorrhagic pulmonary edema. Respiratory failure has developed unexpectedly in burn patients within the first 24 h after the injury. One 37-year-old man who presented with facial and scalp burns exhibited no respiratory distress on presentation to a hospital, but he became dyspneic 2.5 h after the burn and died 4 h after the accident. Postmortem examination revealed an inflamed bronchial mucosa with tenacious, bloody mucus and severe hemorrhagic (noncardiogenic) pulmonary edema (9). In other case reports, such delays of several hours with normal initial chest roentgenograms are not uncommon (10). Patients with potential inhalation injury require observation and supportive care.

E. Ingestions of aqueous HF or other fluoride compounds that dissociate fluorides are especially toxic to the GI tract. Sodium fluoride is metabolized to HF in the stomach. Hemorrhagic gastritis is frequently the result, with hyperemia and edema of the small bowel. The clinical course of these oral ingestions is stormy: Oral burning and dysphagia are followed by hematemesis, melena, multisystemic involvement, and death. Hemorrhagic pancreatitis has been reported (11), as has fluoride deposition in the liver, with hepatocellular swelling and transamylasemias. The fatal dose of fluoride has been reported to be 30 mg/kg, and as little as 1.5 g has been fatal.

F. Renal involvement. Fluorides cause proteinuria, hematuria, renal cortical necrosis, and azotemia. It is unclear to what extent other factors, such as toxic burn products, fluid third spacing, and hypotension, contribute to renal failure. There is evidence that chronically or acutely oliguric patients may benefit from hemodialysis, and that peritoneal dialysis may be ineffective (4,12). Tubular reabsorption is the dominant process of fluoride excretion; although it can be augmented by osmotic diuresis, the latter has not been of proved value for the treatment of fluoride toxicity.

G. CNS involvement. Fluoride has been associated with a wide variety of neurotoxicity, ranging from confusion to coma, that may result in a critical delay in the patient's seeking medical attention. Headache, pupillodilation, nystagmus, and seizures have been reported as well. Deposition of fluoride in the brain has also been found on autopsy.

H. Systemic and electrolyte effects. Other characteristics of acute fluoride toxicity include hypocalcemia and hyperkalemia.

1. With serious fluoride ingestion, **hypocalcemia** is frequently seen within 1 h of exposure. Ionized calcium levels as low as 1.7 mg/dL were reported during the era of poisoned patients. Clinically, it may result in tetany or widening of the QT interval; these two phenomena are indications for calcium replacement. Tetany is most commonly seen to involve the distal extremities. It is an inconsistent finding, however, even in cases of cardiovascular collapse and severely lowered calcium.

   a. The hypocalcemia has been explained by the formation of insoluble CaF_2 and MgF_2, inaccessible to the intravascular pool. It has also been theorized that the deposition of fluoride in bone results in the formation of new fluoroapatite matrices, which become calcified.

   b. The hypocalcemia seen with fluoride intoxication has been an intense focus of therapeutic intervention. Although early intravenous calcium replacement is indicated, it does not alone (as had been theorized) prevent arrhythmias; several reports have documented cardiac-related deaths with normal or mildly elevated calcium levels after calcium replacement.

2. **Hyperkalemia** and T wave peaking have been reported as preterminal events with fluoride exposures, and hyperkalemia has been induced when sodium fluoride was given intravenously in dogs (13). In vitro studies have shown that potassium effluxes from erythrocytes in contact with fluoride, and that the resultant elevated serum potassium is not reversed by the usual methods of treatment, i.e., glucose and insulin, bicarbonate, or calcium. Hyperkalemia after fluoride intoxication has been postulated to be "more closely related to cardiotoxicity than the change in serum calcium" (14). In many reported cases of fatal fluoride exposure, however, serum potassium has been normal, and the relation between fluoride toxicity and potassium requires further exploration. Similarly, hypomagnesemia has been reported in this clinical setting, but the clinical import of this finding is unclear.

I. Chronic effects. Chronic exposure to gaseous HF has been implicated in a wide spectrum of slowly developing symptoms including obstructive and restrictive lung disease, constipation alternating with diarrhea, kidney and liver pathology, headache, tinnitus, intellectual impairment, and an array of rheumatologic symptoms.

IV. Diagnosis and appropriate workup

   A. When the diagnosis is not obvious, **clinical suspicion** is essential in the diagnosis of fluoride toxicity, given the lack of commonly available laboratory studies to make the diagnosis and the specific therapeutic interventions required for its treatment. A detailed
   occupational history or assessment of accessible chemicals to the suicidal patient may
   suggest the diagnosis.

   B. Cases where the diagnosis has been missed include situations where the patient has presented with pain and a normal physical examination or when the patient is treated as a
   victim of routine acid burn, without recognition of the specific agent. One reported pediatric case involved a 2.5-year-old girl who presented with coma of unknown etiology,
   respiratory failure, hyperkalemia, and QT prolongation. Ultimately, the child was found
   to have ingested a commercial laundry powder containing sodium silicofluoride
   (Na_2SiFl_6.). This patient survived after eight cardioversions, calcium replacement, and
   lavage with 0.1% calcium hydroxide (12).

V. Laboratory analysis and diagnostic studies

   A. Fluoride levels

   1. Serum fluoride levels are elevated for the first 24 h after exposure but correspond
   poorly to the degree of toxicity in the individual patient. This test is rarely immediately available. Normal fluoride levels range from 0.01 to 0.20 mg/L. The lethal
   level is reportedly 3 mg/L, but this point has not been extensively studied.

   2. Urine fluoride levels are elevated for as long as 10 years after chronic fluoride
   exposure owing to back-diffusion from bone. It is also elevated for at least several
   days after acute fluoride exposure.

   3. Serum and urine studies are valuable in the rare instance when it is uncertain that
   the patient has been exposed to fluoride; in the known case, levels are of academic
   interest only.

   B. Other diagnostic studies

   1. Minor fluoride burns, i.e., localized burns involving less than 12% HF, involving
   areas with less than 25 cm^2, and in areas of the body far from the respiratory and
   GI tract do not require laboratory studies for management. **High concentration
   burns,** burns with large areas of involvement, or burns with possible systemic
   effects require monitoring and further diagnostic studies. When the concentration
   of fluoride is unknown, the following guidelines can be followed.

      a. If the chemical is a readily available home use product, the concentration is
      probably low.

      b. If the product originated in an industrial setting, it may have been of a much
      higher concentration and the risk of systemic injury is high.

      c. If the patient complains of pain immediately or within 1 h of exposure, the
      chemical may have been highly concentrated.

   2. Exposure to high concentrations, all ingestions, and possible all inhalation injuries
   require observation and further diagnostic studies. Necessary **diagnostic studies**
   include:

      a. Cardiac monitoring and an ECG to evaluate for arrhythmias and evidence of
      hyperkalemia and hypocalcemia.

    b. Serum electrolytes, BUN, and creatinine.

    c. Ingestions require baseline hematocrits, as well as stool hemoccult examination.

    d. Potential inhalations require arterial blood gases (ABGs) and chest roentgenograms to monitor for pulmonary decompensation and metabolic acidosis. Pulse oximetry is also desirable in this setting.

    e. Swan-Ganz monitoring should be considered with potentially serious systemic toxicity.

VI. **Management and complicating factors**

   A. **Minor burns**

     1. Remove all clothing in the involved area, and lavage copiously with running water or saline for 15 min.

     2. In the industrial setting or for minor burns seen in the emergency department, topical calcium gluconate can be applied to the burn. This agent can be prepared from 3 g of crushed calcium gluconate tablets, liquefied with 5 mL of normal saline, and mixed into 100 g of surgical lubricant (K-Y Jelly). Isolated reports have advocated the addition of dimethylsulfoxide (DMSO) as a penetrant carrier, if available. The use of previously recommended topical agents, such as quaternary ammonium gel, aloe gel, or A&D ointment has been abandoned.

     3. HF burn patients with persistent pain and failure of lavage and gel to relieve symptoms or significant tissue loss have benefited from subcutaneous injections of **10% calcium gluconate** into the burn.

       a. In a study of 85 patients treated with this modality, only one was found to have progression of injury; and it was in a case where therapy had been delayed for 48 h after injury.

       b. The recommended dosage is 0.5 mL of 10% calcium gluconate per square centimeter of involved tissue injected subcutaneously through a 27- or 30-gauge needle.

       c. Serum calcium and QT intervals should be monitored during this therapy. If pain recurs after subcutaneous injection, the procedure can be repeated.

       d. Relief of pain has been used as an endpoint to titrate the injection of calcium gluconate.

       e. Disadvantages of this technique relate to the mechanical trauma and pain of multiple injections, which in the fingers can result in vascular compromise. The latter consideration is significant, as the upper extremity is the most frequent area of exposure to HF. Hence intraarterial calcium gluconate has been recommended for digital involvement.

     4. **Intra-arterial calcium gluconate** has been found to be effective for the treatment of fingers and toes and for upper extremity burns unrelieved by subcutaneous infiltration, with prompt pain relief and improved tissue salvage. The radial artery has been preferentially used, with the brachial artery used if there is incomplete anastomotic flow between the radial and ulnar circulations. Arteriography has been used to demonstrate arterial patency and completeness of the superficial transverse arterial arch.

a. Under the optimal circumstances, treatment is begun within 2 h of the burn, but this modality has been effective 24 h after exposure.

b. The **initial dosage** recommendation is as follows: 10 mL of 10% calcium gluconate diluted with 40 mL D_5W given intraarterially over 4 h. If pain is unrelieved, 20% concentrations have been used. After the first ampul, the infusion can be stopped with the arterial line maintained, observing for recurrence of pain, in which case a second infusion is begun. This dose is repeated until the patient is pain-free for 4 h with the infusion stopped, after which the catheter is removed (15). Although local or field block anesthesia can be used, it invalidates pain relief—a titration endpoint for effective treatment.

c. Practitioners have increased the administered 10% calcium gluconate to as much as 1 ampule/h with good results, but controlled studies have not documented the safety of this therapy (S. Samson, *personal communication*).

d. In a study involving 10 patients (using the lower dose), the side effects of this therapy were limited to local arterial spasm secondary to percutaneous cannulation. In this case, cannulation of the patients' more proximal (brachial) artery was successful, and satisfactory results were attained. A theoretic concern is the potential irritative effects of calcium on the artery, but this point has not been documented.

e. An advantage to the use of intraarterial treatment is elimination of the need to remove the nail if that area is involved; removal is universally recommended if subcutaneous therapy alone is given for burns involving the nail. The disadvantage of this procedure is the risk associated with an invasive vascular procedure. In the absence of a physician comfortable with performing it, subcutaneous therapy and transfer to a specialized center, when appropriate, should be pursued.

5. After calcium injections are completed, the burn site requires **débridement,** as for other burns. Eschars that may hide areas of continued injury should be removed and the area then irrigated, cleaned, and covered with a calcium gluconate or magnesium oxide gel.

6. A burn specialist or plastic surgeon should be consulted early in the treatment of fluoride burns.

B. Inhalation

1. Inhalation victims are administered humidified oxygen after room-air ABGs are assayed, if appropriate. The patient should have a baseline chest roentgenogram and be placed on a cardiac monitor. Patients with burns of the face, neck, or chest, especially with high concentrations of HF, should be admitted to a monitored setting and observed for pulmonary decompensation.

2. If the patient develops pulmonary edema, endotracheal intubation and positive end-expiratory pressure (PEEP) may be used. If there is bronchospasm, beta-adrenergic agents, aminophylline, or epinephrine may be administered. The use of steroids is questionable in the setting of chemical pneumonitis. Pulmonary edema can be delayed for up to 24 h after exposure to HF.

  3. Patients who have inhaled HF are susceptible to all of the systemic effects of fluoride toxicity.

C. Oral ingestion

  1. The patient should be administered a diluent—either milk or water. Milk is theoretically preferable, as it can supply calcium to bind the fluoride ion.

  2. Vomiting is not induced if the ingested compound is caustic (e.g., HF). Unless the patient has been vomiting extensively, nasogastric suction or lavage can be employed shortly after ingestion; the possibility of gastric perforation is balanced by the potential elimination of systemic fluoride toxicity (16). There are few data as to whether charcoal is effective after fluoride poisoning. As endoscopy may be indicated, charcoal should not be given. After lavage, milk of magnesia can be given to soothe the stomach. Shock should be treated aggressively.

  3. These patients are at risk for all of the systemic effects of fluoride toxicity. An endoscopist should be consulted early to evaluate the digestive tract, and a surgeon should be consulted for known or suspected GI injury. All patients who have ingested caustic fluoride compounds or other fluoride compounds in sufficient quantity require admission for observation and a thorough evaluation.

D. Cardiotoxicity

  1. Patients with major HF burns should undergo cardiac monitoring and electrocardiography. The QT interval can be used to evaluate for hypocalcemia, and the complexes can be evaluated for signs of hyperkalemia.

  2. Dysrhythmias are treated as per routine protocols, bearing in mind the negative prognostic implications of ventricular arrhythmias and the likelihood of repeat episodes.

E. Electrolyte disturbances

  1. Tetany and prolonged QT intervals are indications for calcium replacement. **Hypocalcemia** is corrected with 10% calcium gluconate using doses of 0.1 to 0.2 mL/kg i.v. up to 10 mL. The dose can be repeated as necessary; calcium levels should be repeated hourly. Chvostek and Trousseau signs as well as tetany are insensitive indicators of hypocalcemia, and their absence should not be construed as evidence of normal serum levels.

  2. **Hypercalcemia** should be treated as in other settings. If the patient has renal failure, hemodialysis should be considered. Magnesium can be replaced with 2 to 4 mL of 50% $MgSO_4$ i.v. over 40 min.

F. Eye contact. If the eye is exposed to HF, copious irrigation with 2 L of water or normal saline is indicated. Irrigation with $MgCl_2$ or isotonic NaCl have been recommended, but reports of results and toxicity are insufficient to recommend it. Subconjunctival injections of calcium gluconate or calcium chloride are toxic to the eye (16). After irrigation, pH testing of the eye is beneficial. Immediate consultation with an ophthalmologist is indicated.

VII. Disposition

  A. All patients with major burns, systemic fluoride toxicity, suspected ingestion or inhalation, cardiac or neurologic findings, or hypocalcemia should be admitted to an intensive care setting.

B. Burns in specialized areas (e.g., the face, hands, and genitalia) and large burns should be evaluated by a burn specialist.

C. Burns of less than 25 cm^2, that are painless after therapy and are due to low concentration HF can be treated in the emergency department with instructions to return for recurrence of pain and with arrangements for follow-up with an appropriate specialist.

D. The suicidal patient requires psychiatric referral.

References

1. Lidbeck WL, et al. *JAMA* 1943;121:826–827.
2. Hodge HC. *JAMA* 1961;177:313–316.
3. Dibbell DG, et al. *J Bone Joint Surg* 1970;52A:931–936.
4. Berman LB, Taves DR. Fluoride excretion in normal and uremic humans. *Clin Res* 1973;21:100.
5. Hodge HC. *JAMA* 1961;177:109–112.
6. Velvart J. Arterial perfusion for hydrofluoric acid burns. *Hum Toxicol* 1982;2:233–238.
7. Shewmake SW, Anderson BG. Hydrofluoric acid burns. *Arch Dermatol* 1979;115:595–596.
8. Mayer TG. Fatal systemic fluorosis due to hydrofluoric acid burns. *Ann Emerg Med* 1985;14:149–153.
9. Greendyke RM, Hodge HC. Accidental death due to hydrofluoric acid. *J Forensic Sci* 1964;9:383–390.
10. Chan KM, et al. Fatality due to acute hydrofluoric acid exposure. *Clin Toxicol* 1987;25:333–339.
11. Menschel SM, Dunn WA. Hydrofluoric acid poisoning. *Am J Forensic Med Pathol* 1984;5:245–248.
12. Yolken R, et al. Acute fluoride poisoning. *Pediatrics* 1976;58:90–93.
13. Baltazar RF, et al. Acute fluoride poisoning leading to fatal hyperkalemia. *Chest* 1980;78:660–663.
14. McIvor ME, et al. The manipulation of potassium efflux during fluoride intoxication: implications for therapy. *Toxicology* 1985;37:233–239.
15. Vance MV, et al. *Ann Emerg Med* 1986;15:890–896.
16. *Poisindex*. Denver: Micromedex, 1989.

Emergency Toxicology, Second Edition,
edited by Peter Viccellio.
Lippincott–Raven Publishers, Philadelphia © 1998.

20

Acids and Alkalies

Clark S. Homan

*Department of Emergency Medicine, State University of New York at Stony Brook,
Stony Brook, New York 11794-7400*

I. Properties of agents

    A. Sources and forms

        1. Alkalies are present in many household preparations (Table 20-1).

            a. Household bleaches usually cause esophageal irritation but rarely cause strictures or serious injury such as perforation. The active ingredient is usually sodium hypochlorite in concentrations of 3% to 6%. Commercial bleaches may have higher concentrations and are more likely to penetrate the submucosa, causing the development of esophageal strictures. Metabolic acidosis is rare but has been reported following the ingestion of household bleach.

            b. Detergents that contain sodium tripolyphosphate may produce serious tissue injury. Nonphosphate detergents usually carry a low risk of injury. Other agents include sodium silicate and sodium carbonate, which have a pH range of 10 to 13. Usually mild ulcerations without strictures occur. Liquid automatic dishwashing detergents have been associated with toxicity (1).

            c. Thermal burns. Clinitest tablets contain sodium hydroxide and sodium carbonate. Tissue damage occurs secondary to the heat of hydration generated, as well as by direct caustic action. The proximal esophageal mucosa is damaged more frequently than the gastric and duodenal mucosa. These tablets may lodge at the carina in children and cause penetrating injuries (2).

            d. Drain cleaners. Sodium hydroxide is commonly found in drain and oven cleaners, the pH of which is often greater than 12, making them highly corrosive (3). Liquid drain cleaners often cause extensive damage to the esophagus owing to their highly viscous nature. Greater damage also occurs to the stomach than with granulated products because of the liquid vehicle.

            e. Ammonia compounds. The active ingredient ammonium hydroxide may be present in concentrations of 3% to 10% with a pH of up to 12.5. Industrial solutions may have concentrations of 28% with a pH of 13. Agents with 3% concentration usually cause minor irritation, but higher concentrations can cause severe injury to the esophagus and stomach (4). Respiratory tract injury that may be fatal has been reported (5).

TABLE 20-1. *Common household alkalies*

Product	Ingredient
Acetest tablets	Sodium borate 37%
Calgonite Dishwasher Detergent	Sodium phosphates <50%
Cascade Dishwasher Detergent	Phosphates 25–50%
Clorox Liquid	Sodium hypochlorite 5.25%
Clinitest reagent tablets	Sodium hydroxide 50%
Comet Cleanser	Trisodium phosphate 14.5%
Crystal Drano (granular)	Sodium hydroxide 54%
Dow Oven Cleaner (liquid)	Sodium hydroxide 4%
Drano (crystalline)	Sodium hydroxide 50%
Drano (liquid)	Sodium hydroxide 2–10%
Drano Professional (liquid)	Sodium hydroxide 32.0%
Efferdent	Potassium monoperborate
Electrasol Dishwasher Detergent	Sodium tripolyphosphate 20–40%
Liquid Plumber	Sodium hydroxide 0.5–2.0%; sodium hypochlorite 5–10%
Lysol Deodorizing Cleaner	Ammonium chloride 2.7%
Minute Mildew Remover	Calcium hypochlorite 48%
Mr. Clean Liquid	Sodium carbonate
Oxydol Laundry Detergent	Sodium tripolyphosphate 25–49%
Peroxide	Hydrogen peroxide 3.0%
Polident Powder	Sodium tripolyphosphate <15%
Purex	Sodium carbonate 15–25%
Red Devil Drain Opener	Sodium hydroxide 96–100%
Swish Toilet Bowl Cleaner	Ammonium chloride 1.25%
Tide	Sodium silicate 4%
Tilex Instant Mildew Remover	Sodium hypochlorite 5%; sodium hydroxide 1%
Top Job	Sodium carbonate/ammonia

    f. **Cement** is composed of 60% CaO, 17% SiO_2, and 3% Al_2O_3. These materials impart a strong alkalinity that may be directly caustic. Such injuries occur most commonly in home "do-it-yourself" projects. Full-thickness burns may occur especially with prolonged exposure.

    g. **Cosmetics:** The ingestion of hair relaxers that contain alkali materials have been recently reported as a new source which can cause serious injury (6,7).

    h. **Automobile airbag deployment** has been reported to cause alkaline chemical keratitis (8).

  2. **Acids**

    a. **Household products**

    b. **Industrial uses**

      (1) **Acetic acid:** printing, rayon manufacturing, dyeing, disinfectants, hair-wave neutralizers

      (2) **Carbolic acid:** pharmaceuticals, dyes, disinfectants

      (3) **Chromic acid:** cement manufacturing, plating, leather tanning, photography

      (4) **Formic acid:** glue manufacturing, tanning processes, tissue preservative

      (5) **Hydrochloric acid** (muriatic acid): dye manufacturing, bleaching agents, metal refining, plumbing, soldering

(6) **Hydrofluoric acid:** pharmaceutic synthesis, gasoline manufacturing, petroleum refining, metal and glass etching, tanning processes, rust removers

(7) **Nitric acid:** electroplating, engraving, metal refining, fertilizer manufacturing

(8) **Oxalic acid:** leather processing, tanning, chemical manufacturing

(9) **Phosphoric acid:** metal cleaning, disinfectants, rust proofing

(10) **Sulfuric acid:** explosive productions, chemical and fertilizer synthesis

B. **Pathophysiology**

1. **Mechanism of injury**

   a. **Alkaline agents** produce tissue injury by liquefaction necrosis, which may be devastating and difficult to treat. Fats and proteins are saponified, resulting in deep tissue destruction. Further injury is caused by the thrombosis of blood vessels. The penetrating nature of alkalies limits the effectiveness of surface irrigation.

   b. **Acids** cause damage to tissue by coagulation necrosis, which results in a protective eschar.

      (1) The coagulation of tissue impedes the penetration of acid to deeper layers. Damage is primarily superficial, which may result in sloughing of extensive areas of the stomach lining with resultant perforation. Perforation may result in mediastinitis, sepsis, shock, and death.

      (2) Despite the eschar, the acid can be absorbed resulting in systemic acidosis, hemolysis, and decreased cardiac output. Elevated chloride or phosphate may be seen with hydrochloric and phosphoric acid ingestions which may result in their own toxicities.

      (3) Hydrofluoric acid is unusual in that it causes liquefaction necrosis. The fluoride anion binds to calcium and magnesium present in tissue, causing a deep injury much like that seen with alkaline substances. Refer to Chapter 20 for a detailed description.

2. **Factors contributing to injury**

   a. **pH and concentration.** Extremes of pH are associated with greater tissue injury. The esophagus begins to ulcerate at pH 12. Acids with pH 2 or less cause significant injury. Higher concentrations also cause greater damage, making the pH a relative factor. It is possible for a weaker acid to result in greater tissue injury if it is present in high molar concentrations.

   b. **Volume of caustic ingested.** Large volumes result in greater direct injury and potential for perforation and injury to other organ systems. Gastric, pyloric, duodenal, and intestinal exposure to the substance ingested is increased proportionally with increased volumes. High volumes also enhance the risk of emesis, causing further damage.

   c. **Titratable acid/alkali reserve (TAR).** Defined as the number of milliliters of 0.1 M solution of Hcl or NaOH required to titrate 100 mL of a 1% solution of offending caustic to a pH of 8 (9). TAR was found by this study to be a more reliable predictor of alkali injury than pH.

    d.   Contact time

    (1)   Acids and alkalies with high viscosity have prolonged tissue contact time and amplification of injury.

    (2)   The passage of caustic through areas of normal anatomic narrowing increases contact time in these areas. The esophagus in the region of the cricoid cartilage, pharynx, aortic arch, and diaphragm have greater risk of injury and subsequent perforation. The pylorus is at particularly high risk during acid ingestion because of the absence of buffers in the stomach and the pronounced sphincteric spasm due to acid exposure.

    (3)   Crystal or particulate formulation result in penetrating injury that remains localized. The risk of injury is less for crystal formulations than liquid caustics but still has the potential to cause significant injury (10).

    (4)   Liquid formulation increases the contact time of the stomach. The advent of liquid lye preparations resulted in far more serious gastric injuries and perforations that had been observed with granular lye ingestions (Table 20-2).

    e.   Preexisting state of the stomach. The presence of fluid in the stomach affords an immediate dilutional effect on the ingested caustic. The presence of solid food in the stomach imparts an immediate buffering effect on acids or alkalies and helps to prevent damage that is believed to occur early after tissue contact. The magnitude of protection varies with the amount of liquid or solid food present as well as the pH, strength, and volume of caustic ingested.

    (1)   Ingestions of acid on an **empty stomach** often result in damage to the lower two-thirds of the stomach, sparing only the fundus (Fig. 20-3).

    (2)   Ingestions of acid on a **full stomach** have a tendency to cause harm only to the pylorus and lesser curvature (Fig. 20-2).

C.   Time course of injury (Table 20-3)

    1.   Acute inflammatory stage occurs during the first 4 to 7 days. Perforation and acidosis may occur at this early stage of injury. Edema and erythema develop first, followed by thrombosis and cellular necrosis (coagulation or liquefaction necrosis). These changes peak at 48 h after ingestion. Early endoscopy is recommended within 24 to 48 h prior to increased risk of perforation.

    2.   Granulation stage starts at about day 4 and ends approximately 7 days after ingestion. Fibroplasia results in the formation of granulation tissue with the laying down of collagen over the denuded areas of mucosal sloughing.

TABLE 20-2. *Alkali preparations*

Type	Ingestion	Location of injury	Degree of injury
Granular	Not swallowed, spit out	Mouth, pharynx, upper esophagus	Localized; penetrating, less severe; not circumferential
Liquid	Swallowed	Distal esophagus, stomach, duodenum	Generalized; deep; circumferential; more severe

TABLE 20-3. *Time course of injury*

Stage	Day	Pathology
Acute	0–4	Rapid liquefaction necrosis Vascular thrombosis Tissue necrosis Bacterial colonization
Granulation	4–7	Sloughing of mucosa Proliferation of fibroblasts Initial collagen synthesis
Perforation	7–21	Muscularis, mostly fibrous tissue Single layer of epithelium Esophageal wall (weakest) Perforation, causing mediastinitis, peritonitis, sepsis
Stricture	3 weeks to years	Closing of defect by scar Strictures Esophageal obstruction

3. **Perforation** most often occurs between days 7 and 21 but may occur earlier (acute stage). It is during this period that the tissue is the weakest and the risk of perforation highest.

4. **Cicatrization stage** starts at 3 weeks and may persist for years. Dense fibrous tissue formation occurs at variable rates. Overproduction of scar tissue results in stricture formation, which may necessitate treatment with dilation therapy or surgery.

D. **Location of injury**

1. **Alkaline agents** have a predilection for injury to the esophagus. Gastric injury often occurs (11), but it is more common with liquid lye ingestions. The areas of injury at greatest risk are the points of anatomic narrowing, i.e., cricopharyngeus, aortic arch, and diaphragmatic hiatus.

   a. The site and extent of the injury are directly related to the pH and volume of substance ingested.

   b. Granular alkali preparations usually cause local tissue damage. These products tend to be expectorated because of the intense local pain to the oropharyngeal mucosa. Consequently, accidental ingestion and gastric injury are less common with these formulations.

   c. Liquid alkali preparations tend to cause less damage to the oropharynx and esophagus and more damage to the stomach. The liquid vehicle affords more rapid transit through the pharynx and esophagus, thus decreasing the amount of direct contact exposure. The contact time is a direct function of viscosity. The faster transit time of liquid alkalies enables a greater volume and concentration to reach the stomach, which results in greater gastric tissue injury.

2. **Acidic agents** tend to cause their greatest damage to the stomach and pylorus.

   a. The oropharynx and esophagus usually have minimal involvement. However, one series reported esophageal injury in 87.8% of acid ingestions (12). These injuries rarely perforate, and they respond well to supportive care. The lack

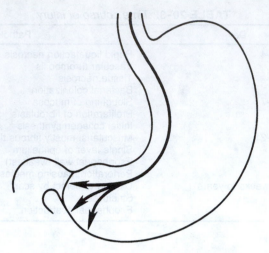

FIG. 20-1. Magenstrasse is the term applied to the pathway acidic agents follow.

of penetration of acids and the rapid transit time appear to account for the minimal extent of these injuries.

b. Figure 20-1 depicts the pathway acidic agents follow in food-filled stomachs (13). It starts along the lesser curvature of the stomach and leads to the pylorus, which explains the location of greatest damage in food-filled stomachs (Fig. 20-2). Stomachs without food tend to have significant injury in the

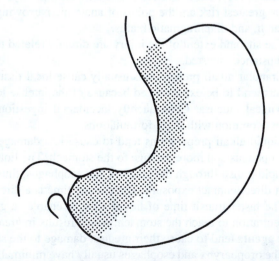

FIG. 20-2. Shaded region indicates the area of greatest injury caused by acid ingestion in a food-filled stomach.

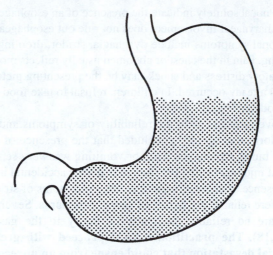

FIG. 20-3. Shaded region indicates the area of greatest injury caused by acid ingestion in an empty stomach.

lower half to two-thirds and may have sparing of the fundus (Fig. 20-3). Initial exposure of the pylorus to acid causes severe spasm, which promotes injury at this site. After several minutes, the pylorus relaxes and allows the gastric contents to move forward, which may result in duodenal and small bowel damage.

II.   Clinical presentation

A.   History

1.   After initial patient stabilization, certain inquiries should be made for all patients.
    a.   Type and concentration of caustic ingested
    b.   Time of ingestion
    c.   Quantity of agent ingested
    d.   If accidental versus intentional
2.   It should be determined if:
    a.   Vomiting has occurred
    b.   A diluent has been previously administered
3.   Attempts should be made to obtain the product container. Information from the labels regarding the specific substance ingested and the pH should be sought. The pH of the substance may be determined in the hospital using pH paper or urine dipstick.

B.   Symptoms

1.   **Pharyngeal pain** is the most common presenting symptom. However, as many as 17% of all significant esophagogastric injuries may not have oral involvement (13). In these cases and particularly in children, clinical suspicion may be enhanced by the presence of a strong alkaline odor on the patient. Burns of the mouth and phar-

ynx do not absolutely indicate the presence of an esophageal burn, and the absence of oropharyngeal involvement does not rule out esophageal injury (14).

2. Additional symptoms include dysphagia, stridor, drooling, and odynophagia, and vomiting. Pain in the chest or abdomen usually reflects more severe tissue damage. Respiratory distress and shock may be the presenting picture if severe tissue damage has already occurred. In children, refusal to take food or drink liquid may represent odynophagia.

3. Controversy exists as to the reliability of symptoms and signs of caustic ingestion. Gorman et al. (15) concluded that the presence of two or more symptoms of oral burns, dysphagia, pain, or vomiting was very sensitive in predicting significant injuries. Crain (16) studied pediatric accidental ingestions and found that the presence of at least two of the three symptoms of stridor, drooling, and vomiting were reliable predictors of esophageal burns. Several other series state that there are no reliable predictors of injury to the gastrointestinal (GI) tract (11,17,18). **The practitioner must proceed with great caution due to the potential devastation that could ensue from an unrecognized and significant caustic ingestion.**

4. Symptoms in children are typically due to unintentional ingestions unless abuse is involved. Evaluation of children may be more difficult owing to lack of a specific history. The child may only be seen near the caustic product and often is not observed actually ingesting the substance. However, the injuries tend to be less severe than in adults because of their unintentional nature. Ingestion should be suspected in a child if there is drooling, dysphagia, refusal to eat, or stridor.

5. a. Caustic ingestion in **adults** is usually intentional and more severe. Mixed drug ingestions should be suspected in all adults. Depression, suicidal, impaired or intoxicated patients make predicting injuries more difficult. Unintentional caustic ingestions in adults tend to have more reliable symptoms.

C. **Physical examination**

1. Erythema, edema, and erosions of the oropharynx are the most common findings on physical examination.

2. Pseudomembrane formation may be present over the mucosa.

3. Hypotension, tachycardia, and changes in mental status signify shock secondary to systemic toxicity.

4. Respiratory distress may be caused by aspiration and mediastinitis as well as acute upper airway obstruction. Although uncommon, glottic and subglottic edema may be present and manifest as stridor and dyspnea. Adult respiratory distress syndrome may develop with massive injury, shock, and sepsis. A late and rare complication, fibrosis of the cricoarytenoid muscle, may cause vocal paralysis and resultant airway obstruction.

5. Sepsis may develop shortly after the initial presentation secondary to bacterial colonization of devitalized tissue. Fever has been reported in as many as 41% of patients with significant esophageal injuries.

D. The **course** of asymptomatic acid and alkali burns is highly variable. The clinical presentation does not reliably predict the occurrence or severity of an esophageal injury (17).

1. **Acute complications**
   a. Upper airway obstruction and injury (19)
   b. GI hemorrhage
   c. Esophageal and gastric perforation
   d. Sepsis
   e. Tracheobronchial necrosis (20), atelectasis (21), and obstructive lung injury (22,23)
2. **Periesophageal complications** secondary to perforation
   a. Mediastinitis
   b. Pericarditis
   c. Pleuritis
   d. Tracheobronchoesophageal fistula
   e. Esophagoaortic fistula
3. **Chronic complications**
   a. Esophageal obstruction
   b. Pyloric stenosis
   c. Squamous cell carcinoma of the esophagus
   d. Vocal cord paralysis with consequent airway obstruction

III. **Laboratory analysis**
   A. **Serologic testing** has been found to be of limited utility during initial management of the caustic ingestion (24).
   B. With significant ingestions, the following studies should be obtained.
      1. CBC, electrolytes, BUN, creatinine, prothrombin time (PT), partial thromboplastin time (PTT), platelet count, and type and crossmatch
      2. Arterial blood gases (ABGs)
      3. Stool for hemoccult blood
      4. Methemoglobin level—in instances where a strong oxidizing agent has been ingested. Refer to Chapter 11 for detailed discussion.
      5. Roentgenograms
         a. Chest film to rule out aspiration pneumonia and mediastinitis
         b. Upright chest film to rule out acute esophageal or gastric perforation
         c. Abdominal films to rule out free air or ascites if perforation has occurred

IV. **Management**
   A. **Stabilization**
      1. Secure the patient's airway.
         a. Oxygen and ventilatory support are provided as indicated.
         b. Orotracheal intubation may be attempted only if it can be performed under complete visualization. Consideration should be given to fiberoptic intubation.
         c. Cricothyroidotomy or tracheostomy should be performed if unable to visualize.
         d. Blind nasotracheal intubation is contraindicated because there may be necrotic tissue proximal to the larynx.
      2. Establish an i.v. line.
      3. Monitor vital signs closely.
      4. Perforation warrants preparation of the patient for emergency surgery.

5. Serologic testing (see **III.A**).
6. Monitor fluid and electrolyte status and pH closely.
7. Patient is to be kept fasting (npo) until endoscopy is performed, with the exception of dilutional therapy.
8. Serial evaluations are performed to monitor for complications such as perforation, upper airway obstruction, aspiration pneumonitis, sepsis, mediastinitis, and GI hemorrhage.

B. **Initial management**
1. **Dilution therapy** is believed to minimize damage to oral, esophageal, and gastric tissue by decreasing concentration. Dilution may also benefit by washing the caustic away from more sensitive tisuues as the upper airway. Opponents argue that the tissue damage occurs immediately after the ingestion and vomiting is increased by dilution therapy (25). Presently, there is no objective evidence in the literature giving evidence to preclude the use of water or milk dilution. Homan has shown in animal studies that the use of saline (26), water and milk dilution therapy have decreased the amount of esophageal tissue injury secondary to both alkali (27) and acid exposure (28).
    a. General, accepted recommendations: One or two glassfuls of milk or water may be administered to the adult patient within 30 min (29); one-half of this dose is usually administered to children. Adults with significant pain and children may be poorly compliant with this regimen.
    b. Diluents are generally believed to be contraindicated in the presence of shock, upper airway obstruction, or in the presence of perforation.
2. **Neutralizing agents** such as weak acids or weak alkalies are controversial.
    a. Many authors feel that these reactions are exothermic in nature, and the heat generated causes additional tissue destruction. This belief is based upon an in vitro beaker study reacting solid caustics with liquid agents (30).
    b. Other studies reacting liquid caustics with liquid neutralizing agents have shown that the heat generated is not great enough to cause a thermal injury (31).
    c. Homan reported animal data using histopathologic outcome parameters gave evidence that neutralization therapy of esophageal alkai exposure with weak acid is effective in decreasing tissue injury (32).
    d. Leape (33) an investigation which evaluated the administration of acetic acid for KOH-induced alkali injuries to the esophagus in cats. This study reported increased survival outcomes with the use of neutralization therapy for alkali esophageal injuries.
    e. Homan conducted additional in vivo animal studies which gave evidence that neutralization therapy for both alkali (34) and acid (35) exposure of the stomach result in temperature changes which would not create a thermal injury.
    f. Inhalation of CO_2 gas as a form of neutralization therapy for treatment of alkali injuries has also been shown to decrease the amount of tissue destruction (36).
    g. Human study is needed before neutralization therapy can be recommended for caustic ingestions.

3. **Blind Passage of a Nasogastric Tube** for gastric lavage is controversial.
    a. Most authors condemn its use for **alkali ingestions.** Some recommend early lavage for **acid ingestion** because of the superficial nature of acidic esophageal injuries and lack of documentation of increased incidence of esophageal perforation. Gastric lavage may be beneficial in cases where strong acids (e.g., sulfuric acid or hydrofluoric acid) are ingested, but there are not enough clinical data to make conclusive recommendations.
    b. Passage of a **nasogastric** tube by endoscopy to act as a stent (37) and facilitate parenteral hyperalimentation is used by some, but has not been studied thoroughly enough to recommend its use. A gastrostomy helps to definitively support nutrition and may also be used for fascilitation of subsequent retrograde balloon dilation (38).
4. **Emesis** is contraindicated.
    a. Additional esophageal injury is caused.
    b. The risk of perforation is increased.
    c. The risk of aspiration is increased.
    d. There may be worsening of glottic edema.
5. **Cathartics** are contraindicated, as they cause a greater amount of damage secondary to the enhanced movement of the caustic substance through the GI tract.
6. **Charcoal** usage is contraindicated because it:
    a. Poorly adsorbs acids and alkalies
    b. Blocks the visual field of endoscopy
    c. May result in chemical mediastinitis if perforation occurs
    d. Use of charcoal for mixed ingestions may be of benefit for the coingested drug but firm recommendations do not exist.

C. **Diagnostic procedures**
    1. **Esophagoscopy.** Direct visualization of the esophagus by esophagoscopy is of primary importance for determining the extent of injury (39,40) All patients who are suspected of having significant caustic ingestions must have early endoscopy within 36 to 48 h (41,42) (Table 20-4). The poor predictability of esophageal injury by signs and symptoms makes this procedure the only method to definitively assess the esophagus (18). Early endoscopy may be important to rule in or out a signifigant injury and guide subsequent management.
        a. There has been some debate regarding the potential danger of the procedure and the risk of iatrogenic perforation of the injured esophageal wall. Use of a flexible endoscope is associated with a lower risk of perforation than the rigid scope (43). Some authorities recommend passage of the scope only to the proximal aspect of the first visualized section of ulceration (44). However, when a flexible pediatric endoscope is passed in a careful manner there is no need to stop at the first burned area because perforation is unlikely.
        b. The esophagus, stomach, and duodenum should be endoscopically evaluated because burns of the esophagus do not correlate with the presence of burns in the stomach.

TABLE 20-4. *Grading of esophageal injury*

Esophageal lesion grade	Endoscopic characteristics	Prognosis
0	No visible lesion	Excellent
1	Edema and erythema limited to intact mucosa; superficial desquamation	Rarely stricture formation
2	Ulceration penetrating beyond mucosal membranes; exudate may be present; may involve muscle	Increased stricture formation
3	Transmural involvement with granulation tissue; total destruction of mucosa	Perforation; frequently more extensive stricture formation

  c. The use of endoscopy in the **asymptomatic patient** is debatable. All of these patients must be evaluated on an individual basis. The quantity and type of caustic substance involved, the reliability of the history, and the presence of signs and symptoms must be considered in the decision to perform esophagoscopy on these patients. Unfortunately, there are no definitive parameters available to make this decision in the asymptomatic patient. Esophagoscopy should be performed during the first 48 h after ingestion if the patient's condition is sufficiently stable. During this time, the risk of perforation is the least. After 48 h, the esophageal wall weakens, and the risk of perforation then increases, making the procedure too risky to perform.

  d. **Indications** for esophagoscopy

   (1) All patients with obvious signs or symptoms

   (2) All lye ingestions regardless of symptoms

   (3) All patients with oral irritation/ulceration

   (4) All children and adults with an unreliable history

  e. **Contraindications** for esophagoscopy

   (1) Unstable patient

   (2) Evidence of perforation

   (3) Upper airway compromise

   (4) More than 48 h after ingestion (greater risk of perforation)

 2. **Barium swallow.** Radiographic contrast studies are usually not indicated for the early diagnostic management of caustic ingestions except when esophagoscopy is incomplete or cannot be performed. These studies are more useful during the follow-up evaluation of these patients to detect such complications as scarring, outlet obstruction, or malignancy (45).

  a. **Esophagography** is usually performed 3 to 4 weeks after injury and at subsequent intervals to evaluate stricture formation in significant esophageal burns.

  b. **Upper GI series** may be particularly valuable for evaluating lesions of the gastric mucosa, pyloris, and duodenum, where severe edema limits the role of endoscopy (46). Water-soluble agents are recommended because of the high rate of perforation (47).

V. Management of complications

   A. Upper airway obstruction may require endotracheal intubation or surgical cricothyrotomy.

   B. Perforation virtually always requires surgical repair (48). Esophagectomy or gastrectomy with colonic interposition are procedures that may be employed (49,50,51). Emergency resection and staged reconstruction are usually undertaken for acute perforations (52,53). Use of a surgical pulmonary patch has been reported for the repair of tracheobronchial necrosis (21).

      1. Complications of perforation, such as GI hemorrhage, sepsis, mediastinitis, and pleuritis, are best managed by treating the underlying cause, i.e., surgical repair of the perforation, which aids in terminating the perpetuation of the disease process. Specific measures (i.e., culture and sensitivity, antibiotic administration, and blood transfusion) must be individualized for each complication.

      2. Clinitest tablets may lodge at the carina in children and perforate the esophagus. These patients can usually be managed with an esophageal end-to-end anastomosis (12).

   C. Inadequate caloric intake

      1. Alkali ingestions may be managed by a feeding gastrostomy.

      2. Feeding jejunostomies may be used for those with acid burns or liquid lye ingestions because of the high incidence of significant gastric burns.

      3. Total parenteral nutrition may be employed as adjunctive therapy.

   D. Stricture formation is usually managed by esophageal dilation. Balloon dilation may be complicated by perforation (53). Retrograde balloon dilation (38) has shown promise for difficult cases. The patient may respond to a single treatment or may require multiple procedures (54). The development of dysphagia, coupled with positive follow-up esophagograms, usually dictates this form of therapy.

   E. Squamous cell carcinoma of the esophagus and pyloric stenosis are chronic complications that usually require surgical intervention. Routine esophagectomy is not recommended for prevention of esophageal carcinoma (55).

   F. Metabolic acidosis

      1. Hypernatremia and hyperchloremic acidosis have been reported after bleach ingestion (56). This complication was believed to be secondary to the high sodium load. The patient was effectively managed by hydration with i.v. 5% dextrose.

      2. Metabolic acidosis following lye ingestion has also been reported (57). The mechanism in this case was reported as a lactic acidosis secondary to inadequate perfusion of injured tissue. This patient was managed aggressively with intravenous sodium bicarbonate and buffer solutions.

      3. Acidemia may develop secondary to absorption of the offending acid agent.

VI. Controversies in management

   A. Neutralizing agents: see **4.b.**

   B. Steroids

      1. Human and animal studies have yielded inconclusive results (18,58). There is some evidence that steroids started within the first 48 h may ameliorate the injury.

If steroids are given, they should be started within 48 h, as they are believed to be ineffective if started later. Several authors have provided evidence that steroids have little effect in preventing stricture formation (59,60). Some studies have shown decreased stricture formation with grade 2 or 3 esophageal injuries.

2. Masking of signs and symptoms of peritonitis, mediastinitis, and sepsis secondary to perforation may occur.
3. Transmucosal injury verified by endoscopy should be present before therapy is initiated.
4. Peptic ulcer or active infection usually precludes steroid therapy.
5. Methylprednisolone 20 mg in patients <2 years of age and 40 mg in patients >2 years of age may be given i.v. every 8 h.

C. **Antibiotics** are recommended to prevent sepsis caused by the proliferation of bacteria, which may gain access to the circulation via damaged tissue (61). There are few data to support this prophylactic indication for antibiotics (62), and patients should probably not be routinely treated with antibiotics (60). Antibiotic therapy should be reserved for specific indications, including:
   1. Perforation
   2. Infection or sepsis
   3. Steroid therapy

D. **Esophageal stenting** by insertion of a nasogastric tube is recommended by some for second and third degree esophageal burns (37,62). The nasogastric tube may be placed only under endoscopic control. The tube may also be utilized for nutrition.

E. **Total parenteral nutrition** may be beneficial by decreasing trauma to the esophagus. Large studies in humans have not been performed to determine its effectiveness (59). However adequate nutrition is important for healing for all burns.

VII. **Disposition and follow-up**

A. Patients with signs of perforation should be considered for **emergency surgery.** The surgical procedure performed is dictated by the organs involved and the degree of tissue damage found on exploration.

B. Admission to the **burn unit** should be considered for all significant epidermal burns.

C. Admission to the **intensive care unit** should be considered for all patients with significant caustic burns to the GI tract. These patients must be monitored closely for subsequent complications, including upper airway obstruction, perforation, and shock.
   1. Patients with caustic ingestions may have clear fluids by mouth. They are started when the patient can swallow saliva, which may be as early as 48 h after a significant GI injury has been sustained. The diet is advanced as tolerated.
   2. Repeat endoscopy and upper GI series may be performed to guide subsequent management and discharge planning.
   3. Upon discharge, all patients are instructed to return immediately if dysphagia develops; as it may signify new stricture formation.
   4. Routine 3-week postingestion esophograms are obtained to detect stricture formation, with follow-up esophograms at regular intervals.
   5. The development of stricture formation usually responds well to esophageal dilation therapy. A few patients who do not respond require surgical lysis of the strictures.

VIII.   Special topics

   A.   Eye injuries

      1.   Symptoms

         a.   Intense pain secondary to tissue damage that varies with the pH, concentration, and contact time.

         b.   With ophthalmic exposure, visual acuity may immediately decrease as a result of corneal epithelium destruction and corneal edema. The degree of severity of ocular burn upon presentation usually predicts the ultimate prognosis of vision (64).

         c.   Forceful rubbing of the eye by the patient secondary to irritation may make examination difficult and cause additional injury.

      2.   Signs

         a.   Lids. Blepharospasm may make examination and treatment difficult. Lid injuries may range from erythema and blister formation to frank necrosis.

         b.   Conjunctiva and cornea. Mild involvement manifests as erythema and small areas of epithelial sloughing on slit-lamp examination. Necrosis and chemosis (conjunctival swelling) develop with more extensive involvement. Serious corneal injury is manifested by corneal clouding progressing to corneal opacity. The intraocular pressure may be elevated (65). Prognosis is related to the amount of avascular necrosis of the conjunctiva and sclera.

         c.   Iris. Injury due to penetrating acid or alkali may result in a severe iritis, resulting in a nonreactive pupil.

         d.   Lens and retina. Injury may result in cataract formation or severe retinitis.

      3.   Treatment

         a.   Irrigation must be undertaken immediately for all acid and alkali eye injuries (66). Normal saline, Ringer's lactate, or D_5W should be instilled into the eye for at least 20 min. Alkali injuries may require longer irrigation owing to their penetrating nature. A suspended i.v. bag that administers low pressure irrigation is ideal. An i.v. bag may be hooked up to a nasal cannula and the prongs placed over the bridge of the nose for continuous irrigation.

         b.   pH of the conjunctiva must be checked every 30 min for 2 h after irrigation is stopped. This is to ensure that the measured pH is that of the tissue and not the irrigating fluid. It should be neutral, or pH 7. If the pH is not normal, an irrigating contact lens should be used to apply continuous irrigation for several h until the pH normalizes (67).

         c.   Exposure of the eye for irrigation may be facilitated by use of:

            (1)   Topical anesthetic

            (2)   Lid speculum for lid retraction

            (3)   Facial nerve block

         d.   Particulate matter, particularly in the conjunctival fornices, must be identified and removed with a cotton swab.

         e.   Anterior chamber paracentesis and irrigation with normal saline is performed by an ophthalmologist. This procedure is recommended if the patient is seen within 2 h after sustaining a severe alkali burn (68).

    f. An ophthalmologist should be consulted for all acid or alkali ophthalmic injuries. The most significant injuries require admission.

    g. **Tissue inhibitor metalloproteinases** offer promise in that they have been shown to decrease the degree of corneal ulceration and perforation in animals (69).

B. Dermal injuries

  1. Signs and symptoms

    a. The patient's complaints and physical findings are similar to those seen with first, second, and third degree thermal burns. However, direct extension may cause damage to deeper dermal tissues and organs than may be apparent on initial observation.

    b. Extensive necrosis may result in significant fluid loss and systemic toxicity.

    c. Initial examination may not detect the extent of tissue injury because tissue response to some chemicals may be delayed for as much as 36 h. pH may be checked. All injuries should be copiously irrigated.

  2. Treatment

    a. Stabilization

      (1) Airway

      (2) Breathing

      (3) Circulation

    b. History

      (1) Type of acid or alkali

      (2) Concentration of the agent

      (3) Duration of exposure

      (4) First aid treatment

      (5) Concurrent injuries

      (6) Prior medical illnesses

    c. All remaining solid or particulate matter should be removed. Medical personnel should wear protective clothing, i.e., protective gloves, gowns, masks, eye gear. Low pressure rather than high pressure irrigation must be used in order to minimize the risk of caustic exposure to health care workers (70).

    d. Contaminated foreign bodies such as clothing, jewelry, and contact lenses must be removed, as these objects perpetuate continued contact with tissue.

    e. Immediate lavage with copious amounts of water decreases the amount of tissue injury. Neutralization of the injured tissue to pH 7 becomes more difficult with increasing delays in lavage.

      (1) With hot metal burns, the elemental sodium, potassium, or lithium combusts spontaneously when exposed to water and is converted to a strong alkali, causing further tissue damage. These burns are best treated by covering with mineral oil to isolate the metal from water.

      (2) Phenol (aromatic acid alcohols) are best lavaged with polyethylene glycol (71).

    f. Woodward (72) has reported on the use of acetic acid for alkali injuries of the skin. He found this form of neutralization therapy to be efficacious for dermal injury caused by strong alkali when irrigation with water is ineffective.

    g. A topical antibiotic cream should be placed over the wound.

    h. Tetanus immunization is provided as needed.

    i. All acid or alkali burns must be closely monitored and reassessed because of the potential delay in tissue injury.

  3. **Disposition and follow-up**

    a. Dermal acid or alkali burns requiring admission

      (1) Second and third degree burns

      (2) First degree burns covering >15% of the body surface area

      (3) Involvement of face, eyes, ears, perineum, hands, or feet

      (4) Patients with other serious underlying illnesses

      (5) Special burns (e.g., with hydrofluoric aid)

    b. Only patients with minor exposures should be considered for discharge, and even these patients warrant close follow-up examinations at 24 and 72 h.

C. **Disk battery injuries**

  1. There has been a significant incidence of caustic GI injuries since the appearance of these batteries on the consumer market (approximately 1980).

  2. Mechanism of injury appears to be from several processes (73).

    a. The electrolyte solution, usually 40% potassium hydroxide or 40% sodium hydroxide, has been shown to cause liquefaction necrosis in animals. Leakage may occur, causing tissue damage.

    b. Hydroxide is generated at the anode, resulting in pH elevation.

    c. If impaction occurs, it may result in local pressure necrosis.

    d. Mercury present in the battery may be absorbed. Only one case of mercury toxicity due to disk battery ingestion has been reported (74).

  3. **Signs and symptoms**

    a. Patient is often asymptomatic.

    b. Most batteries pass through the GI tract without complication.

    c. GI signs and symptoms are the most common presentations of a complicated disk battery ingestion.

      (1) Signs and symptoms of perforation include abdominal pain, nausea, vomiting, and rebound.

      (2) Impaction may present with fever, dysphagia, odynophagia, tachypnea, tenderness, and rebound.

      (3) Battery rupture may present with GI bleeding.

    d. Perforation of the aortic arch may present with hemodynamic instability, and chest pain.

    e. Mercury toxicity has been reported (74).

  4. **Treatment**

    a. Roentgenographic studies from the mouth to the anus should be performed to locate the battery.

    b. Batteries lodged in the esophagus must be removed promptly because the complications due to perforation are grave. Signs and symptoms of perforation and the presence of the battery in the esophagus for more than 24 h are more imminent indications for emergency removal of the battery.

  (1) Intravenous glucagon 0.05 mg/kg may be used to relax the esophageal musculature and promote passage to the stomach.

  (2) A Foley catheter with the patient in a position of the head down to remove the battery has been reported.

  (3) Glucagon or nifedipine to relax esophageal smooth muscle may result in subsequent passage of the foreign body.

  (4) Endoscopy affords removal under direct vision.

  c. Batteries that travel past the esophagus usually are asymptomatically passed per rectum.

  (1) Asymptomatic patients may be managed as outpatients.

  (2) The stool should be checked for the battery, which usually passes within the first week.

  (3) Serial roentgenograms may be used to follow the patient and ensure forward passage of the battery.

  (4) Development of GI signs and symptoms requires immediate reevaluation for a caustic injury secondary to leakage of the disk battery.

  (5) Endoscopy, extraction with a Foley catheter, and surgery have been utilized to remove batteries in symptomatic patients.

References

1. Krenzelok EP. Liquid automatic dishwashing detergents: a profile of toxicity. *Ann Emerg Med* 1989;18:60.
2. Burrington JD. Clinitest burns of the esophagus. *Ann Thorac Surg* 1975;20:400.
3. Howell JM. Alkalinity of non-industrial cleaning products and the likelihood of producing significant esophageal burns. *Am J Emerg Med* 1991;9:560–562.
4. Ernst RW, Leventhal M. Total esophagogastric replacement after ingestion of household ammonia. *N Engl J Med* 1963;268:815.
5. White ES. A case of near fatal ammonia gas poisoning. *J Occup Med* 1971;13:549.
6. Stenson K, Gruber B. Ingestion of caustic cosmetic products. *Otolaryngol Head Neck Surg* 1993;109:821–825.
7. Forsen JW, Muntz HR. Hair relaxer ingestion: a new trend. *Ann Otol Laryngol* 102(10):781–784, 1993 Oct.
8. Smally AJ, Binzer A, Dolin S, Viano D. Alkaline chemical keratits: eye injury from airbags. *Ann Emerg Med* 1992;21:1400–1402.
9. Hoffman RS, Howland MA, Kamerow HN, et al. Comparison of titratable acid/alkaline reserve and pH in potentially caustic household products. *Clin Toxicol* 1989;27:241–261.
10. Neidich GJ. Ingestion of caustic alkali farm products. *Pediatr Gastroenterol* 1993;16:75–77.
11. Zagar SA, Kochhar MD, Nagi B, Mehta S, Mehta SK. Ingestion of strong corrosive alkalis: spectrum of injury to upper gastrointestinal tract and natural history. *Am J Gastroenterol* 1992;87:337–341.
12. Zargar SA, et al. Ingestion of corrosive acids: spectrum of injury to upper gastrointestinal tract and national history. *Gastroenterology* 1989;97:702.
13. Scher LA, Maull KI. Emergency management and sequela of acid ingestions. *JACEP* 1978;7:207.
14. Feldman M, Iben A, Hurley E. Corrosive injury to oropharynx and esophagus. *Calif Med* 1973;18:6.
15. Gorman RL, Therese Khin-Maung-Gyi M, Klein-Schwartz W, et al. initial symptoms as predictors of esophageal injury in alkaline corrosive ingestions. *Am J Emerg Med* 1992;10:189–194.
16. Crain EF, Gershel JC, Mezey AP. Caustic ingestions. *Am J Dis Child* 1984;138:863–865.
17. Gaudreault P, Lovejoy F. Predictability of esophageal injury from signs and symptoms: a study of caustic ingestion in 378 children. *Pediatrics* 1983;71:767.
18. Ferguson MK, Marcello M, Staszak VM, Little AG. Early evaluation and therapy for caustic esophageal injury. *Am J Surg* 1989;157:116–120.

19. Scott JC, Jones B, Eisele DW, Ravich WJ. Caustic ingestion injuries of the upper aerodigestive tract. *Laryngoscope* 1992;102:1–8.
20. Safarti E, Jacob L, Servant JM, et al. Tracheobronchial necrosis after caustic ingestion. *J Thorac Cardiovasc Surg* 1992;103:412–413.
21. Hallagan LF, Smith M. Profound atelectasis following alkaline corrosive airway injury. *J Emerg Med* 1994;12:23–25.
22. Rubin AE, Bentur L, Bentur Y. Obstructive airway disease associated with occupational sodium hydroxide inhalation. *Br J Ind Med* 1992;49:213–214.
23. Hansen KS, Isager H. Obstructive lung injury after treating wood with sodium hydroxide. *Occup Med* 1991;41:45–46.
24. Mansson Jr. Diagnosis of acute corrosive lesions of the esophagus. *Laryngol Otol* 1978;92:499.
25. Knopp R. Caustic ingestions. *JACEP* 1979;8:329.
26. Homan CS, Maitra SR, Lane BP, et al. Effective treatment of acute alkali injury of the rat esophagus with early saline dilution therapy. *Ann Emerg Med* 1993;22:178–182.
27. Homan CS, Maitra SR, Lane BP, Thode HC, Sable M. Therapeutic effects of water and milk for acute alkali injury of the esophagus. *Ann Emerg Med* 1994;24:14–20.
28. Homan CS, Maitra SR, Lane BP, Thode HC, Davidson L. Histopathologic evaluation of the therapeutic efficacy of water and milk dilution for esophageal acid injury. *Acad Emerg Med* 1995;2:587–591.
29. Rumack BH. *Poisindex information system.* Denver: Micromedex 1995.
30. Rumack BH, Burrington JD. Caustic ingestions: a rational look at diluents. *Clin Toxicol* 1977;11:27–34.
31. Maull KI, Osmond AP, Doyle C. Liquid caustic ingestions: an in vitro study of the effect of buffer, neutralization and dilution. *Ann Emerg Med* 1985;14:1160–1162.
32. Homan CS, Maitra SR, Lane BP, Thode HT, Finkelshteyn J, Davidson L. Effective treatment of acute alkali injury to the esophagus using weak-acid neutralization therapy: an ex-vivo study. *Acad Emerg Med* 1995;2:952–958.
33. Leape L. New liquid lye drain cleaners. *Clin Toxicol* 1974;7:109–114.
34. Homan CS, Singer AJ, Henry MC, Thode HC. Thermal effects of neutralization therapy and water dilution for acute alkali exposure in canines [Abstract]. *Acad Emerg Med* 4(1):27–32, 1997 Jan.
35. Homan CS, Singer AJ, Thomajan C, Henry MC, Thode HC Jr. Thermal characteristics of neutralization therapy and water dilution for strong acid ingestion: an in vivo canine model. Accepted for publication to *Academic Emergency Medicine* for 1998; 5 (4).
36. Meyers RL, Glenn L, Orlando RC. Protection against alkali injury to rabbit esophagus by CO_2 inhalation. *Am J Phys* 1993;264:G150–G156.
37. Wijburg FA, Beukers MM, Heymans HS, Bartelsman JF, Hartog Jager FC. Nasogastric intubation as sole treatment of caustic esophageal lesions. *Ann Otol Laryngol* 1985;94:337–341.
38. Davies RP, Linke RJ, Davey B. Retrograde esophageal balloon dilation: salvage treatment of caustic-induced stricture. *Cardiovasc Int Radiol* 1992;15:186–188.
39. Sugawa C, et al. The value of early endoscopy following caustic ingestion. *Surg Gynecol Obstet* 1981;153:553.
40. Lowe JE, et al. Corrosive injury to the stomach; the national history and role of fiberoptic endoscopy. *Am J Surg* 1979;137:803.
41. Vergauwen P, Moulin D, Buts JP, et al. Caustic burns of the upper digestive and respiratory tracts. *Eur J Pediatr* 1991;150:700–703.
42. Zargar SA, Kochhar R, Mehta S, et al. The role of fiberoptic endoscopy in the management of corrosive ingestion and modified endoscopic classification of burns. *Gastrointest Endosc* 1991;37:165–169.
43. Chung RSK, Denbesten L. Fiberoptic endoscopy in treatment of corrosive injury of the stomach. *Arch Surg* 1975;110:725.
44. Kirsch MM, Ritter F. Caustic ingestion and subsequent damage to the oropharyngeal and digestive passages. *Ann Thorac Surg* 1976;21:74.
45. Johns TT, Theoni RF. Severe corrosive gastritis related to Drano: an unusual case. *Gastrointest Radiol* 1983;8:25.
46. Martel WM. Radiologic features of esophagogastritis secondary to extremely caustic agents. *Radiology* 1972;103:31.
47. Han MT. Ileocolic replacement of esophagus in children with esophageal stricture. *J Pediatr Surg* 1991;26:755–757.
48. Curet-Scott MJ, et al. Colon interposition for benign esophageal disease. *Surgery* 1987;102:568.
49. Touloukian RT, Tellides G. Retrosternal ileocolic esophageal replacement in children revisited. *J Thorac Cardiovasc Surg* 1994;107:1067–1072.
50. Gundogdu HZ, Tanyel FC, Buyukpamkcu N, Hicsonmez A. Colonic replacement for the treatment of caustic esophageal strictures in children. *J Pediatr Surg* 1992;27:771–774.
51. Gossot D, Sarfati E, Celerier M. Early blunt esophagectomy in severe caustic burns of the upper digestive tract. *J Thorac Cardiovasc Surg* 1987;84:188.
52. Hugh TB, Meagher AP, Li B. Gastric antral patch esophagoplasty for extensive corrosive stricture of the esophagus. *World J Surg* 1991;15:299–303.
53. Song HY, Han YM, Kim HN, Kim CS, Choi KC. Corrosive esophageal stricture: safety and effectiveness of ballon dilation. *Radiology* 1992;184:373–378.

54. Lahoti D, Broor SL, Basu PP, Gupta A, Sharma R, Pant CS. Corrosive esophageal strictures: predictors of response to endoscopic dilation. *Gastrointest Endosc* 1995;41:196–200.
55. Sarfati E, et al. Management of caustic ingestion in adults. *Br J Surg* 1987;74:146.
56. Ward MJ, Routledge PA. Hypernatraemia and hyperchloraemic acidosis after bleach ingestion. *Hum Toxicol* 1988;7:37.
57. Okonek S, Bierbach H, Atzpodien W. Unexpected metabolic acidosis in severe lye poisoning. *Clin Toxicol* 1981;18:225.
58. Anderson KD, Rouse TM, Randolph JG. A controlled trial of corticosteroids in children with corrosive injury of the esophagus. *N Engl J Med* 1990;323:637–640.
59. Oakes DD, Sherek JP, Mark JBD. Lye ingestion. *J Thorac Cardiovasc Surg* 1982;83:194.
60. Ferguson MK, et al. Early evaluation and therapy for caustic esophageal injury. *Am J Surg* 1989;157:116.
61. Symbas PN, Vlasis SE, Hatcher CR Jr. Esophagitis secondary to ingestion of caustic material. *Ann Thorac Surg* 1983;36:73.
62. Goldman LP, Weigert JM. Corrosive substance ingestion: a review. *Am J Gastroenterol* 1984;79:85.
63. Mills LJ, Estrera AS, Platt MR. Avoidance of esophageal stricture following severe caustic burns by the use of an intraluminal stent. *Ann Thorac Surg* 1979;28:60.
64. Saini JS, Sharma A. Ocular chemical burns—clinical and demographic profile. *Burns* 1993;19:67–69.
65. Paterson CA. Intraocular pressure changes after alkali burns. *Arch Ophthalmol* 1974;91:211.
66. Burns FR, Paterson CA. Prompt chemical eye injuries may avert severe damage. *Occup Health Safety* 1989;58:30.
67. Nelson JD. Chemical injuries to the eyes. *Postgrad Med* 1987;81:62.
68. Grant WM. *Toxicology of the eye* 3rd ed. Springfield, IL: Charles C. Thomas Publisher, 1986.
69. Paterson CA, Wells JG, Koklitis PA, Higgs GA, Docherty AJP. Recombinant tissue inhibitor of metalloproteinases type 1 suppresses alkali–burn–induced corneal ulceration in rabbits. *Invest Ophthalmol Vis Sci* 1994;35:677–684.
70. Jelenko C. Chemicals that burn. *J Trauma* 1974;14:65.
71. Polakoff PL. Treating chemical skin burns varies between acids and alkalies. *Occup Health Safety* 1986;55:24.
72. Woodward D. Irrigation with acetic acid [Letter]. *Ann Emerg Med* 1989;18:911.
73. Litovitz TL. Button battery ingestions: a review of 56 cases. *JAMA* 1983;249:2495.
74. Kulig K, et al. Disc battery ingestion: elevated urine mercury levels and enema removal of battery fragments. *JAMA* 1983;249:2502.

Emergency Toxicology, Second Edition,
edited by Peter Viccellio.
Lippincott–Raven Publishers, Philadelphia © 1998.

21

Phenols

Paula Jane Barclay

Outpatient Family Medicine & Internal Medicine, Allergy & Immunology, Minor Emergencies,
X-Ray, & Lab, Basalt, Colorado 81621

I. Properties
A. Sources and forms
1. **Phenol** (carbolic acid) is a common chemical that is widely available; it is still used in some preparations to treat some skin conditions. It is bacteriostatic at concentrations at more than 0.2%, bactericidal at more than 1%, and fungicidal at more than 1.3%. When applied locally, it exerts a depolarizing anesthetic action. It is frequently used in the production of plastics, disinfectants, and insecticides. Naturally occurring hydroquinones and other phenol derivatives such as ortho-cresol, meta-cresol, para-cresol, and resorcinol are known components of cigarette smoke; the conjugated derivative of free hydroquinone, beta-D-glucopyranoside (arbutrin), occurs naturally in foods such as wheat, pears, coffee, and tea; free hydroquinone occurs naturally in coffee, red wine, broccoli, and wheat cereals; recently, the phenolic compounds in red wine have been shown to inhibit susceptibioity of low-density lipoproteins to oxidation, thereby potentially reducing their atherogenicity. Certain tea phenolics have been shown to inhibit formation of endogenous nitroso-proline (NPRO) when ingested with foods known to produce NPRO, and may exert a protective, anticarcinogenic effect in the stomach.
2. **Phenol derivatives** used for medicinal purposes
   a. **Beta-naphthol.** Formerly used as an anthelmintic for hookworm and tapeworm infections; has been used as an ointment for therapy of scabies, ringworm, and other skin diseases.
   b. **Camphor**. Obtained from distillation of cinnamon camphora wood and purified by sublimation. Camphor is still used in Europe and Asia as a rubefacient and mild analgesic; it is employed in linaments as a counterirritant for fibrositis, neuralgia, and skin conditions.
   c. **Dichlorophen**. Anthelmintic used for therapy of infection due to tapeworms, dwarf tapeworms, and pork tapeworms.
   d. **Guaiacol**. Obtained by liquid or fractional distillation of wood-tar cresote. It is used in expectorants.
   e. **Guaiacyl glyceryl ether**. Reported to reduce the viscosity of tenacious sputum, this derivative is used as an expectorant in capsules, syrups, tablets, and lozenges.

    f.   **Hexylresorcinol**. Used against roundworms, dwarf tapeworms, hookworms, threadworms, whipworms, and giant intestinal flukes; also used as a spermicide in contraceptive creams and in mouthwashes.

    g.   **Hydroquinone**. Used as a depigmenting agent for the skin, e.g., in the treatment for melasma and facial peels.

    h.   **Iodothymol**. Used for therapy of hookworm infections.

    i.   **Monobenzone**. Used as a depigmenting agent in skin creams.

    j.   **Naphthalan liquid**. Used as an emollient and for its antiseptic and analgesic properties in Europe.

    k.   **Prepared coal tar**. Used for the therapy of eczema, psoriasis and other skin problems; found in lotions, ointments, pastes, and solutions.

    l.   **Pyrogallol**. Used as an ointment for treatment of psoriasis, lupus, ringworm; also used as an ingredient in hair dyes.

    m.   **Resorcinol**. Used (as a lotion or ointment) for treatment of acne and seborrheic skin conditions because of its exfoliative, antipruritic, and keratolytic properties; used also in antidandruff shampoos.

    n.   **Tannic** acid. Obtained from wood breakdown, it is used as an astringent for mucous membranes of the mouth and throat; also used for therapy of hemorrhoids in European countries. Formerly used for preparing the colon before barium enemas.

    o.   **Thymol**. Used as a deodorant in mouthwashes and gargles; used in dentistry to prepare cavities before filling; forms a protective cap for dentine.

  3. **Phenol derivatives** used for industrial purposes

    a.   **Chlorocresol**, cresol (Lysol = 50% cresol). Potent disinfectant that is an efficient bactericidal agent against commonplace organisms, including acid-fast bacteria. At 2% concentration, it is used as a handwash; a 1:500 solution is sometimes used as a douche.

    b.   **Chloroxylenol**. Used in dilute solutions as a disinfectant of low toxicity for cleansing wounds, vaginal douching, and disinfection of instruments.

    c.   **Creosote**. Used as a disinfectant; formerly used as an expectorant to treat croup and to fill tooth cavities.

    d.   **Dinitrophenol**. Used as an insecticide; formerly used for weight-reducing purposes. It is highly toxic.

    e.   **Diphenyl**. Fungistatic and effective against molds; it is primarily used for treating wrappers for fruit.

    f.   **Gallic acid**. Used as an antioxidant for oils.

    g.   **Hexachlorophene**. Used as a disinfectant against gram-positive bacteria (less effective against gram-negative bacteria); used as a presurgical scrub; formerly used to bathe infants (now contraindicated for that purpose because of reports of brain damage).

    h.   **Parabens** (methyl, ethyl, propyl, and butyl). With antifungal properties, these compounds are used as preservatives in a variety of pharmaceutical preparations.

    i.   **Pentachlorophenol**. Used as a preservative for a wide range of industrial and agricultural products, including woods, textiles, glues, and starch; used also for control of slime and algae.

    j.   **Tar acids**. Phenolic substances derived from the distillation of coal tar or petroleum; used for disinfectants in hospitals.

B. Physical and chemical properties

  1.   **Phenol derivatives used for medicinal purposes**

    a.   Beta-naphthol. White or almost white crystalline leaflets or powder with a faint phenolic odor and a sharp taste; darkens on exposure to light.

    b.   Camphor. Colorless, transparent or white crystals; crystalline masses with a penetrating aromatic odor and pungent taste.

    c.   Dichlorophen. White or cream-colored powder with a faint phenolic odor; saline and phenolic taste.

    d.   Guaiacol. Colorless oily liquid or crystals with a penetrating aromatic odor and caustic taste.

    e.   Guaiacyl glyceryl ether. White or gray crystals or crystalline aggregates, odorless with a bitter taste.

    f.   Hexylresorcinol. White or yellowish white crystal or crystalline plates or powder with a pungent odor and a sharp, astringent, numbing taste.

    g.   Hydroquinone. Fine white crystals or white crystalline powder that darkens on exposure to light and air.

    h.   Iodothymol. Reddish-brown or buff-colored bulky amorphous powder with an aromatic smell.

    i.   Monobenzone. White, odorless, almost tasteless crystalline powder.

    j.   Naphthalan liquid. Viscous, brown oil-like liquid with a greenish fluorescence and characteristic odor.

    k.   Prepared coal tar. Black, viscous, foul-smelling liquid.

    l.   Pyrogallol. Odorless, colorless or gray-yellow, feathery crystals, or white or yellowish crystalline powder.

    m.   Resorcinol. Colorless or slightly pinkish-gray crystals with a sweet, pungent taste and bitter aftertaste.

    n.   Tannic acid. Yellowish-white or light brown glistening scales; light masses with a characteristic odor and astringent taste.

    o.   Thymol. Colorless crystals or white crystalline powder with a pungent, aromatic odor and taste.

  2.   **Phenols used for industrial purposes**

    a.   Chlorocresol. Colorless crystals with a phenolic odor.

    b.   Chloroxylenol. White or cream-colored crystalline powder with a characteristic odor.

    c.   Creosote. Colorless or pale yellow, highly refractive liquid with a penetrating smoky odor and burning taste.

    d.   Dinitrophenol. Yellow crystals.

    e.   Diphenyl. White crystalline powder.

      f. Gallic acid. White or pale brown, odorless prismatic crystals.

      g. Hexachlorophene. White or pale buff crystalline powder that is odorless or has a slight phenolic odor.

      h. Parabens (methyl). Colorless crystals or a fine, white crystalline powder that is odorless and tasteless but produces a burning sensation on the tongue or mouth followed by local numbness.

      i. Pentachlorophenol. White crystals.

      j. Tar acids. Fluids derived from distillation of coal tar; some are finely dispersed emulsions and others homogeneous solutions.

C. Mechanism of action and pathophysiology

    1. Phenols and phenol derivatives denature all proteins with which they come in contact. Phenol forms a loose complex with protein, acting as a general protoplasmic poison. Because this complex is so loose, phenol is diffusible and penetrates into tissues, even unabraded skin; it is highly toxic, causing extensive tissue necrosis.

    2. When applied locally, phenol itself has a **depolarizing anesthetic action**; it can result in significant injury despite the absence of pain, causing gangrene and sloughing of the affected area.

    3. Phenols **stimulate and then depress the CNS**. In humans, brief stimulation may be related to increased acetylcholine release at the neuromuscular junction, but the prominent effects are CNS depression. They are due to a direct toxic action of phenol on the myocardium and smaller blood vessels. To a lesser degree, as a result of central vasomotor depression, the circulation is depressed.

    4. Phenols have a powerful antipyretic effect, similar to that of salicylates.

    5. Phenols **stimulate respiratory centers** and produce a respiratory alkalosis. Metabolic acidosis follows because of uncompensated renal loss of base during the stage of alkalosis due to renal damage.

    6. Phenol and certain phenol derivatives (hydroquinone, coal tar, resorcinol, and dinitrophenol) cause methemoglobinemia.

D. Pharmacology and pharmacokinetics. Phenol and its derivatives are readily absorbed from the gastrointestinal tract and through skin surfaces. Phenol is largely metabolized by the liver to phenylglucuronide and phenylsulfate, which are excreted through the kidneys. Lesser amounts are oxidized to various catechols and quinols, which are also excreted through the kidneys. A small amount is excreted through the lung.

II. Clinical presentation

  A. History

    1. Local symptoms may develop after application or exposure of skin and mucous membranes to phenol and derivatives. Patients complain of tingling and numbness with mild cases of local exposure; after repeated low-grade exposure, patients experience redness, itching, and burning when they develop contact dermatitis (especially seen with resorcinol, a prominent component of several dermatologic preparations). Full destruction and necrosis of the skin may develop after accidental splashing of the skin with phenol preparations in high concentrations. Exposure of the human eye causes increased lymph production in the conjunctivae, leaving the cornea white and hypesthetic. Eyelids can become severely edematous and scarred, and severe iritis may develop (1).

2. **Systemic symptoms** can occur after local exposure (e.g., accidental industrial exposure or cleansing of extensive burns with phenol preparations), or after accidental or intentional ingestion or inhalation of phenol preparations. Phenol intoxication has been reported after contamination of a community water supply (2).

   a. Common effects experienced after inhalation include headache, nausea, diarrhea, weakness, dizziness, shortness of breath, blurred vision, abdominal pain, vomiting, and rash. Symptoms can occur for up to 6 days after exposure.

   b. After mild ingestion, patients develop abdominal discomfort, nausea, vomiting, and diarrhea. Oral and esophageal burns occur with ingestion of solutions containing more than 5% phenol.

   c. With significant ingestion (as little as 1 g may be lethal), initial transient excitation may occur, quickly followed by convulsions and unconsciousness; cardiovascular collapse, shock, and respiratory failure quickly ensue. Supraventricular and ventricular tachycardia are common and have even been reported in patients undergoing phenol chemexfoliation of the face and neck (3).

3. **Venous thrombosis** has been reported after injections of phenol to produce chemical neurolysis or as motor point blocks in patients with spasticity due to spinal cord injuries, multiple sclerosis, cerebral palsy, brain injuries, or cerebrovascular accidents (4).

4. Industrial inhalation of chlorocresol has been associated with repeated, isolated **facial palsies** that spontaneously reversed after the patient was removed from the source (5).

5. A rare case of toxic shock syndrome after full-face chemical peel with phenol has been reported (6).

B. **Physical examination**

   1. After mild cases of local exposure, examination of the skin may reveal white burns on the skin that are anesthetic; with more severe cases, frank necrosis and sloughing of the skin develops. In cases of chronic exposure, erythema and vesicles develop, leading to contact dermatitis.

   2. Examination of the patient who has developed systemic symptoms initially shows a mildly excited patient who may be profusely sweating and complaining of thirst, abdominal pain, headache, dizziness, and ringing of the ears. The patient is usually diaphoretic and vomiting. A small fraction of phenol may be excreted by the lungs and impart an aromatic odor to the breath.

C. **Course.** If untreated, the patient rapidly deteriorates, developing hypotension, seizures, obtundation, cyanosis (secondary to hypoxia or methemoglobinemia), shallow respirations, fall in body temperature, respiratory failure (sometimes developing frank pulmonary edema), anuria, and death.

III. **Differential diagnosis of unknown exposure/ingestion**

A. Rule out **anticholinesterase poisoning** in an excited, diaphoretic patient with signs of increased GI mobility, hypotension, seizures, and respiratory failure. If the patient has not been exposed to agricultural insecticides, however, this diagnosis is unlikely. The miosis and excessive salivation seen with cholinergic poisoning are not seen with phenol poisoning. An aromatic odor on the breath heightens the suspicion of phenol poisoning. Cyanosis unaccompanied by hypoxia favors methemoglobinemia, which does not occur with cholinergic poisoning.

B. Rule out **cocaine toxicity**, which causes excitation, seizures, hypotension (after initial hypertension normally), and respiratory failure. Marked mydriais, lack of signs of increased GI mobility, and early hypertension help differentiate cocaine toxicity from phenol poisoning.

IV. **Laboratory analysis**

A. **General tests**

1. In patients with signs of mild toxicity, electrolytes are normal; the ECG shows nonspecific changes, and arterial blood gases reflect respiratory alkalosis.

2. As the patient deteriorates, metabolic acidosis develops, and cardiac arrhythmias (supraventricular and ventricular tachycardias) occur; hypoxia develops. In an anuric patient any urine that does pass is smoky-colored and contains albumin, casts, and RBCs.

B. **Toxin-specific tests.** Phenol can be detected in the blood, tissues, and urine.

1. Normal phenol levels in blood
   a. Free phenol: 0 to 4 mg/dL
   b. Conjugated phenol: 0.1 to 2.0 mg/dL
   c. Total phenol: 0.15 to 7.96 mg/dL

2. A rapid method to detect the presence of phenol and phenol derivatives is the **ferric chloride test**: A few drops of ferric chloride turns urine a blue or violet color if phenolic compounds are present. Occasionally, normal urine is positive, however.

3. Workers exposed to phenol in the industrial setting can have their urine phenol monitored. If levels exceed 0.5 to 81.5 mg/L, the patient is receiving toxic doses of phenol.

4. Phenols, cresols, and xylenols can be detected in serum using high-performance liquid chromatography.

V. **Management**

A. **General measures**

1. Ventilatory support/oxygen; intubate as necessary.

2. Cardiovascular support
   a. Keep patient warm and recumbent.
   b. Use i.v. saline and pressors to support the blood pressure.
   c. Use lidocaine for ventricular arrhythmias and bretylium for lidocaine-refractory arrhythmias.

3. Seizures. Administer diazepam i.v. or per rectum; if no response, phenytoin or phenobarbital can be given.

B. **Toxin-specific measures**

1. For dermal exposure, the **skin should be washed with undiluted polyethylene glycol**, a demulcent that is readily available to any emergency department. This agent helps prevent phenol absorption. If polyethylene glycol is not available,

copious amounts of water should be used and the skin washed thoroughly with soap and water for at least 15 min. Systemic effects from absorbed phenol can occur rapidly, so these measures should be instituted quickly.

2. A patient who has had exposure by **inhalation** should be removed from the contaminated area, monitored for respiratory distress (cough, dyspnea), and given 100% humidified oxygen and ventilatory assistance as needed.

3. Because of the potentially **rapid onset of coma and seizures** (within a half-hour for significant ingestions) and because of the corrosive effects of phenol, ipecac for the induction of **emesis is not recommended**. In the absence of esophageal injury, repeated gastric lavage is recommended, followed by administration of **olive oil** or **vegetable oil** to remove surface phenol and prevent deeper penetration; these measures can be followed by a cathartic: castor oil (2 oz) or sorbitol or saline. (Castor oil is purported to delay phenol absorption from the stomach, but the effectiveness of this treatment has not been documented by clinical studies.) If esophageal injury is suspected, endoscopy should be performed to diagnose the extent of injury; lavage is contraindicated.

4. **Treat acid-base disorders**. Dialysis is of no value for the removal of phenol and related compounds but may be needed to support uncontrollable acid-base problems.

5. **Treat methemoglobinemia**. If methemoglobinemia is more than 30%, ingest methylene blue (1 to 2 mg/kg). Exchange transfusion may be needed if methemoglobinemia is more than 70%.

C. **Complicating factors and controversies.** The use of polyethylene glycol versus water for decontaminating the skin is still debated, and no clear advantage of one over the other has been demonstrated. If polyethylene glycol is available, it should be used; the patient's care should not be delayed if it is unavailable, however, and decontamination with water should commence.

VI. **Disposition and follow-up**

A. If patients give a history of significant ingestion but are clinically stable, they should be treated with gastric lavage/cathartics, admitted to hospital, and observed. If the significance of the exposure or ingestion is unclear, there has been several hours' delay between exposure and the seeking of care, and the patient is asymptomatic at the time of evaluation; he or she may be observed for 6 h. At the end of that time, if there are no GI, cardiovascular, or respiratory problems and no CNS compromise, the patient may be discharged. For a patient with local dermal injury (e.g., blanching of the skin with anesthesia in the affected area), the area should be decontaminated extensively; if there are no systemic side effects after 6 h, the person may be discharged with close follow-up, looking for the development of necrosis of the affected area, which could require surgical debridement or skin grafting.

B. Because of its protein-denaturing effects, any patient with significant phenol intoxication can suffer long-term CNS, gastrointestinal (esophageal erosions and scarring, liver failure), cardiac, and renal damage. These patients must be treated aggressively and followed closely.

References

1. Jaeger RW. *Poisoning emergencies: a primer*. St. Louis: Catholic Health Association of the United States, 1987.
2. Jarvis SN, Straube RC. Illness associated with contamination of drinking water supplies with phenol. *BMJ* 1985;290:1800–1802.
3. Lober CW. Chemexfoliation—indications and cautions. *J Am Acad Dermatol* 1987;17:109–112.
4. Macek C. Venous thrombosis results from some phenol injections. *JAMA* 1983;249:1807.
5. Dossing M, Wulff C. Repeated facial palsies after chlorocresol inhalation. *J Neurol Neurosurg Psychiatry* 1986;49: 1452–1454.
6. Dmytryshyn JR. Clinical face peel complicated by toxic shock syndrome: a case report. *J Am Acad Dermatol* 1983;9:163.

Selected Readings

Arena JM. *Poisoning: toxicology, symptoms, treatments*. 5th ed. Springfield, IL: Charles C. Thomas Publisher, 1986.

Balina LM, et al. The treatment of melasma. 20% azelaic acid versus 4% hydroquinone cream. *Int J Dermatol* 1991;30:893–895.

Braunwald E, et al. *Harrison's principles of internal medicine*. 11th ed. New York: McGraw-Hill, 1987.

Brown VK. Decontamination procedures for skin exposed to phenolic substances. *Arch Environ Health* 1975;30:1–6.

Conning DM, Hayes MJ. The dermal toxicity of phenol: and investigation of the most effective first-aid measures. *Br J Ind Med* 1970;27:155–159.

Deisinger PJ, et al. Human exposure to naturally occurring hydroquinone. *J Toxicol Environ Health* 1996;47:31–46.

Dresibach RH. *Handbook of poisoning: prevention, diagnosis, and treatment*. 12th ed. Norwalk, CT: Appleton & Lange, 1987.

Fisher AA. Irritant and toxic reactions to phenol in topical medications. *Cutis* 1980;26:363–364.

Goodman LA, et al., eds. *Goodman and Gilman's pharmacological basis of therapeutics*. 7th ed. New York: Macmillan, 1985.

Gosselin RE. *Clinical toxicology of commercial products*. 5th ed. Baltimore: Williams & Wilkins, 1984.

Grimes PE, et al. Melasma. Etiologic and therapeutic considerations. *Arch Dermatol* 1995;131:1453–1457.

Inhibition of LDL oxidation by phenolic substances in red wine: a clue to the French paradox? *Nutr Rev* 1993;51:185–187.

Kaye S. *Handbook of emergency toxicology*. 4th ed. Springfield, IL: Charles C. Thomas Publisher, 1980.

Langeland T, Braathen LR. Allergic contact dermatitis from resorcinol. *Contact Dermatitis* 1987;17:126.

Miller MA, et al. The treatment of the splitting nail with phenol alcohol partial nail matricectomy. *Dermatol Surg* 1996;22:388–390.

Nanni EJ, et al. Separation and quantitation of phenolic compound in mainstrea cigarette smoke by capillary gas chromatography with mass spectrometry in the selected-ion mode. *J Chromatogr* 19904;505:365–374.

Pifer JW, et al. Mortality study of employees engaged in the manufature and use of hydroquinone. *Int Arch Occup Environ Health* 1995;67:267–280.

Pullin TG, et al. Decontamination of the skin of swine following phenol exposure: a comparison of the relative efficacy of water versus polyethylene glycol/industrial methylated spirits. *Toxicol Appl Pharmacol* 1978;43:199–206.

Reynolds JE. *Martindale: the extra pharmacopoeia*. 28th ed. London: Pharmaceutical Press, 1982.

Soares ER, Tift JP. Phenol poisoning: three fatal cases. *J Forensic Sci* 1982;27:729–731.

Stich HF, et al. Teas and tea components as inhibitors of carcinogen formation in model systems and man. *Prev Med* 1992;21:377–384.

van der Ham AC. et al. The treatment of ingrowing toenails. A randomised comparison of wedge excision and phenol cauterisation. *J Bone Joint Surg [Br]* 1990;72:507–509.

Emergency Toxicology, Second Edition,
edited by Peter Viccellio.
Lippincott–Raven Publishers, Philadelphia © 1998.

22

Lead Toxicity

†Clark S. Homan, †Gerard X. Brogan, and R. Scott Orava

*†Department of Emergency Medicine, State University of New York at Stony Brook,
Stony Brook, New York 11794-7400; Department of Emergency Medicine,
Valley Lutheran Hospital, Mesa, Arizona 85206*

I. **Epidemiology**
   A. Office of Technology Assessment estimates 1.3 million American children deprived of superior function secondary to low lead exposure (1).
   B. About 17% of U.S. children aged 6 months to 5 years (3 to 4 million) children had blood lead levels of 15 µg/dL or higher according to the Third National Health and Nutrition Examination Survey, National Center for Health Statistics (2).
   C. As many as 67.8% of black children in urban, inner-city environments may have levels exceeding 30 µg/dL (3).
   D. Blood levels have recently declined in the United States due to improved awareness and screening programs (4). The use of unleaded gasoline also contributed to this decline.

II. **Sources and forms**
   A. **Oral ingestion**
      1. Children, particularly, ingest leaded paints, pica, or newsprint. (Leaded paint was commonly used in houses built before 1940.)
      2. "Moonshine" whiskey, earthenware, and ceramic food containers have lead-containing glazes.
      3. Water may be supplied via lead pipes, particularly "soft" waters, which are slightly acidic and low in mineral content.
      4. Other sources include fishing weights, shower/window curtain weights, herbal preparations, leaded crystal, solder, plastics, lead pipes, manufactured insecticides, dye, and paint.
   B. **Inhalation** exposure is usually seen in persons involved in welding, battery-recycling plants, demolition, brass foundries, stained-glass window production, burning lead-painted wood, renovation, and firing ranges. Lead is also found in leaded gasoline, motor vehicle exhausts, and industrial emissions,
   C. **Dermal absorption** of inorganic lead occurs infrequently from contact with concentrated aqueous solutions of lead. In contrast to the relative insignificance of skin exposure as a route of inorganic lead absorption, alkyl lead compounds are absorbed more easily. Toxicity among handlers of compounds used for the blending of leaded gasolines has been reported.

    D. Intravenous route

       1. Acute lead poisoning has occurred in i.v. methamphetamine users (5). The suspected source of lead was the lead acetate used as a reagent in the manufacture of phenyl-2-propanone, a precursor of methamphetamine in the amalgam process.

       2. Cases of acute lead poisoning from i.v. exposure to lead in other compounds have also been reported (6–8). One should have a high index of suspicion in any user of illicit i.v. drugs for which inadequate "home processing" is possible and lead-based compounds are involved in the processing. In one series, eight patients initially suspected of having non-A, non-B hepatitis ultimately were diagnosed as having lead poisoning attributed to i.v. methamphetamine use (5).

    E. Serosal and synovial route

       1. Gunshot wounds with deposits in joints, pericardium, peritoneum or other soft tissues may result in lead absorption.

III. Pharmacokinetics

    A. Absorption

       1. Oral exposure. About 300 µg is ingested each day in the normal adult diet, 10% of which is absorbed. Children absorb 50% of ingested lead. However, absorption after ingestion of organolead, such as tetralkyl lead in gasoline, may be as high as 75%.

       2. Inhalation. Absorption is greater and more rapid by the pulmonary route.

       3. Dermal exposure. Absorption is poor except in the case of organic lead.

       4. Dietary deficiencies of calcium, iron, and zinc enhance lead absorption as well as its tissue storage. Iron deficiency associated with lead exposure may complicate treatment with antidotes.

    B. Metabolism

       1. Although poisoning is generally chronic (months to years), symptoms arise acutely. When exposure is by inhalation or the i.v. route, symptoms develop far more quickly than if the lead is ingested.

       2. Half-life: 32 years in bone; 7 years in kidneys.

       3. Once absorbed from the digestive tract, lead is distributed to the viscera, chiefly the kidneys and liver; it is then taken up by the skeletal system and stored as the insoluble, biologically inert tertiary lead phosphate. Lead is also deposited in bone, kidneys, and teeth.

       4. Excretion of lead occurs by way of bile, urine, exfoliation of epithelial tissue, and sweat.

       5. Accumulation and toxicity occur if more than 0.5 mg/day is absorbed.

       6. A dose of 0.5 g of absorbed lead is estimated to represent a fatal dose.

IV. Pathophysiology

    A. On the cellular level, lead reacts with sulfhydryl groups, interfering with enzymes of heme synthesis for hemoglobin and cytochrome production (9). The conversion of delta-aminolevulinic (ALA) acid to porphobilinogen and coproporphyrinogen III to protoporphyrin IX is blocked by lead interfering with delta-ALA dehydratase (10), and coproporphyrinogen decarboxylase. The resultant ALA and coproporphyrin in the urine act as biochemical indicators of lead poisoning. It is of note that ALA and coproporphyrin also accumulate in the urine of patients with hereditary coproporphyria and variegate porphyria. A serum lead level assists the clinician in making the distinction between these porphyrias and lead poisoning. Lead also inerferes with 1,25–vitamin D decarboxylase

(11), brain adenylate cyclase (12), and brain cytochromes (13). Lead also interacts with calcium and may have negative effects upon cellular regeneration (14). Lead blocks ferrochelatase from incorporating iron into protoporphyrin to form heme. This accumulates in the red blood cell chelating zinc to form zinc protoporphyrin.

B. Lead interferes with the sodium-potassium ATPase pump and attaches to the RBC membrane, causing increased fragility and decreased survival of RBCs. Lead also inhibits iron transport across mitochondrial membranes.

C. The bone marrow attempts to compensate for the resultant anemia; RBC production is increased, with immature RBCs being released. Reticulocytes and basophilic stippled cells appear in the peripheral circulation. The basophilic stippling represents abnormally aggregated ribosomes caused by inhibition of 5' pyrimidine nucleotidase resulting in an inability to rid the cell of RNA products.

D. Renal involvement is manifested in acute intoxification by a Fanconi-like syndrome. With prolonged exposure, chronic nephritis is seen. Anemia is related to decreased erythropoieten from proximal tubular damage. Renal colic may result from renal artery spasm. Hypertension may develop secondary to altered renin-angiotensin-aldosterone axis. Altered excretion of uric acid can result in hyperuricemia and gout.

E. Myocarditis and fibrosis occur secondary to lead-induced swelling of myocardial fibers.

F. CNS toxicity is caused by edema and a direct cytotoxic mechanism. Peripheral neuropathies are caused by lead's effect on the myelin sheath. Gamma-aminobutyric acid (GABA)–mediated inhibitory pathways appear sensitive to lead.

G. Lead crosses the placenta and is measurable in umbilical cord blood (15). It had been associated with fetal wastage, premature rupture of membranes, and premature delivery. Although inadequately understood, signs of lead poisoning, particularly neurologic sequelae, have been observed in newborns.

H. Reproductive effects include decreased sperm counts and abnormal sperm.

I. Radiographic lead lines reflect bone arrest, not lead deposition. This is seen only in children.

V. Clinical manifestations are unfortunately nonspecific. Good history-taking with respect to potential exposure may lead the clinician in the right direction when physical findings are nonspecific.

A. GI effects
1. Anorexia
2. Abdominal pain, colic
3. Intermittent vomiting
4. Constipation

B. CNS effects
1. Irritability
2. Learning disability and regression
3. Drowsiness
4. Persistent vomiting
5. Incoordination, weakness, paralysis
6. Headache
7. Peripheral neuropathy—rare in children, but foot drop characteristic; in adults, wrist drop characteristic
8. Stupor
9. Convulsions

      10. Ataxia

      11. Papilledema, optic atrophy, or both

      12. Retinal pigmentation

      13. Cranial nerve paralysis

      14. Encephalopathy (stupor, ataxia, coma, seizures at lead levels greater than 100 (µg/dL)—more common in children than adults

   C. Lead ingestion can be divided into acute and chronic ingestions.

      1. Chronic lead ingestion

         a. Signs and symptoms: nonspecific, vague aches and pains, wrist and ankle drop, chronic nephritis, **blue line** on **gums**

         b. History: environmental source, family history

         c. Laboratory tests: anemia (Hgb of less than 10 g/dL), basophilic stippling, increased urinary ALA, blood level 30 to 60 µg/dL, erythrocyte protoporphyrin less than seven times normal

         d. Radiography: lead lines, opacities on abdominal films

      2. Acute lead ingestion

         a. Signs and symptoms: anorexia, constipation, abdominal pain, behavioral changes, vomiting, lethargy, hyperactivity, clumsiness, ataxia, convulsions, coma (Table 22-1).

         b. History: same as for chronic lead ingestion.

         c. Laboratory tests: same as for chronic lead ingestion; also increased urinary coproporphyrins, blood lead level more than 10 µg/dL, erythrocyte protoporphyrin more than 190 mg/dL or more than seven to 10 times normal.

         d. Roentgenography: same as for chronic ingestion.

   D. Less severe symptomatology may be exhibited in patients who have blood lead levels below the "toxic" level.

   E. The **differential diagnosis** of lead poisoning includes encephalitis, porphyria, peripheral neuropathies (e.g., diabetes mellitus), brain abscess, brain tumor, Reyes syndrome, meningitis (particularly tuberculous meningitis), and other toxic ingestions (e.g., cadmium, zinc, salicylates).

VI. Laboratory findings and Screening

   A. Serum lead level

   Blood lead levels are currently the most widely utilized screening test. Methods employing blood obtained by fingerstick are available. Below are the guidelines from the CDC for interpretation of blood lead levels (16).

      1. A lead level of less than 10 µg/dL is not considered indicative of lead poisoning.

      2. A level of 10 to 14 µg/dL indicates the child is in a border zone. Many of these children have levels less than 10 µg/dL. A detailed environmental history should be taken, and an obvious remediable source of lead may be found. It is unlikely that there is a single predominant source of lead exposure for most of these children. Thus, a full home inspection is not recommended. It is, however, prudent to try to decrease exposure to lead with some simple interventions.

      3. A level of 15 to 19 µg/dL mandates more careful follow-up. The effects of lead at these levels, if persistent, necessitate environmental investigation and remediation.

      4. Levels of 20 to 69 µg/dL call for full medical evaluation, detailed environmental and behavioral history, physical examination, and tests for iron deficiency.

TABLE 22-1. *Acute lead toxicity*

Symptoms	Toddler	Child	Adolescent/adult
Mild	Anorexia, occasional vomiting, irritability, lethargy, refusal to play, weakness	Learning disability or regression; others similar to toddler	Colicky abdominal pain, constipation, limb pain, hypertension
Severe	Slurred speech, anemia, persistent vomiting, peripheral neuropathy, stupor, paralysis, ataxia, convulsions, coma	Similar to toddler	Renal failure, headache, memory loss, tremor, confusion, ataxia, stupor, convulsions, coma

    5. A level greater than 70 µg/dL constitutes a medical emergency that, preferably, should be managed by experienced personnel.

B. Erythrocyte protoporphyrin (EP)

    1. EP is often normal with serum lead levels between 10 and 25 µg/dL and may not detect many patients with serum lead levels greater than 25 µg/dL. EP needs to be performed in conjunction with blood lead levels to obtain a more accurate picture of total body burden (17) of metabolically active lead.

    2. EP accumulates as a result of the lead inhibition of the enzyme ferrochelatase, which binds iron to protoporphyrin, forming hemoglobin. This test is often and incorrectly referred to as FEP, or free erythrocyte protoporphyrin. Protoporphyrin chelates Zinc to Zinc protoporphyrin. Newer technology allows for the specific measurement of all protoporphyrin which is one of the earliest and most reliable indicators of impaired heme synthesis (18). Hyperbilirubinemia interferes with this test.

    3. EP reflects the soft-tissue lead levels and total body lead burden and usually but not always corresponds well with blood lead concentration after the first 2 months of exposure. This lag is due to the time required for ZnP to build up in the erythrocytes after interference with hemoglobin synthesis. Iron deficiency anemia also causes elevation of the EP, but here blood lead levels are normal.

C. CBC

    1. Anemia is not a common finding. Hemoglobin levels of less than 10 g/dL due to lead toxicity are normochromic and normocytic in nature (19), resulting from interference with enzymes responsible for heme synthesis. Bone marrow findings of erythroid hypoplasia and ringed sideroblasts have been reported and are suggestive of interference of RBC synthesis (20). Lead attaches to RBC membranes, causing increased friability and decreased survival time (21). This phenomenon is believed to be due to interference with the RBC membrane sodium-potassium pump. Patients with a predominantly hemolytic pattern are more likely to present with more severe anemias than those with a predominantly hypoproliferative pattern, who usually develop only mild anemia.

    2. Reticulocytosis results from early release of immature RBCs. Myeloid sources attempt to compensate for deceased RBC survival and decreased heme synthesis. Reticulocytosis is not present in iron deficiency anemia and so is valuable for differentiating the two forms of anemia.

    3. Basophilic stippling of erythrocytes on Wright stain of peripheral blood has been observed to be a less frequent occurrence than anemia (22). This finding is also nonspecific to lead poisoning and may be seen with thalassemia and pyrimidine 5′-nucleotidase deficiency.

4. **Eosinophilia** is a more common finding than basophilic stippling but is also nonspecific. It has been shown not to be dose-related (23).

D. Delta-aminolevulinate dehydratase activity (ALA-D)

1. Lead decreases the activity of this enzyme, which is present in the erythrocyte.
2. This test is not as sensitive as blood lead and should only be used in monitoring cases with moderate to severe lead poisoning (24). This test is not as readily available as blood lead.
3. Useful for monitoring of occupational lead exposure (25).

E. Urinary ALA and coproporphyrin III

1. Urinary levels of ALA are increased owing to lead inhibiting the enzyme delta-aminolevulinic acid dehydratase (ALA-D).
2. Lead inhibition of the enzyme coproporphyrinogen oxidase has been proposed as a cause for increased coproporphyrin III.
3. Quantification of urinary ALA and coproporphyrin has been used for surveillance of lead toxicity in exposed individuals. Blood lead levels and EP analysis has largely supplanted ALA and coproporphyrin quantification.

F. Calcium disodium versenate (CaNa$_2$-EDTA) provocation test

1. CaNa$_2$-EDTA mobilization rest has fallen into disfavor as it may dangerously elevate lead levels, is costly, requires parenteral administration by skilled nursing care and is inherently error prone due to the 24-h collection of urine (26).
2. CaNa$_2$-EDTA is administered to evaluate chelatable lead stores. Because serum lead levels may become elevated, it is not recommended for patients who are symptomatic or have blood lead levels more than 70 µg/dL.
3. Patients with lead nephropathy may have falsely low results because urinary lead is the measured parameter (27).
4. This test has been shown to increase CNS lead levels in an animal model (28).
5. Procedure
   a. Administer CaNa$_2$-EDTA 500 mg/m^2 i.m. or dilute this amount in 250 mL D$_5$W and administer i.v. over 1 h.
   b. Copious fluids are encouraged.
   c. Urine is procured for lead analysis: an 8-h specimen from children and a 24-h specimen from adults.
   d. **Lead excretion ratio:** urine lead (µg) divided by CaNa$_2$-EDTA (mg).
      (1) Positive result in children: more than 0.7.
      (2) Positive result in adults: more than 1.0.

G. Indications for serologic evaluation

1. Blood lead level is recommended by the CDC for screening and is the primary test used for surveillance of lead toxicity. Erythrocyte protoporphyrin may be used as a secondary test to evaluate exposure during the previous 3 to 4 months.
2. CBC should be determined for all patients who are being evaluated for lead toxicity. Serum lead determinations help guide subsequent management.
3. ALA-D may also be used for screening, but the test costs more and requires special instrumentation.

4. Urinary ALA and coproporphyrin III may be used for surveillance of continued lead exposure but have largely been replaced by erythrocyte protoporphyrin.

H. Roentgenography

1. **Abdominal flat plate**
   a. May show lead densities in the gastrointestinal (GI) tract if the ingestion was within the previous 36 h. Whole bowel irrigation may be indicated for treatment of this finding.
   b. A negative film does not rule out lead toxicity.
   c. A positive film showing densities in the GI tract gives additional evidence for lead toxicity.

2. **Long bone films**
   a. bone lead measurements may afford improved dosimetry for the purposes of dose-response assessment for chronic exposures and long term outcomes (29).
   b. **Lead lines** are areas of increased density at the distal ends of growing bones, where rapid growth of bone occurs.
      (1) Lead lines are present only if there has been heavy chronic poisoning (minimum 4 weeks).
      (2) The width and density of the lines increase with the duration of the exposure.
      (3) Multiple lead lines indicate repeated episodes of toxicity.
      (4) Lead lines are most commonly seen between the ages of 2 and 5 years when bone is growing rapidly.
   c. Use as a screening test is poor because roentgenograms are usually negative.

I. Hair and tooth lead

1. Not useful for diagnosis and treatment of lead toxicity
2. Best used for population studies (30).
3. Dentine levels indicative of previous exposure to lead (31).

J. Additional testing should be directed to the **specific organs** that may develop pathology as a direct result of lead toxicity.

1. **Neurologic effects**
   a. Intelligence testing
   b. Psychological testing
   c. Motor strength
   d. Lumbar puncture for opening pressure
   e. Cerebrospinal fluid (CSF) for WBCs and protein
   f. Peripheral motor nerve conduction velocity

2. **Renal effects**
   a. Serum creatinine
   b. Urinalysis
   c. 24-h urine for creatinine, protein, and uric acid

3. **Reproductive and endocrine effects**
   a. Decreased sperm counts
   b. Decreased serum testosterone (32)
   c. Metapyrone challenge test (33)
   d. Decreased serum thyroxine
   e. Decreased thyroid-binding proteins (34)

4. GI effects
    a. Elevated SGOT
    b. Elevated SGPT

VII. Treatment

  A. Chelating agents (Table 22-2)

    1. Dimercaprol, BAL (British anti-Lewisite compound)

      a. Mechanism of action

        (1) Sulfhydryl ligands form stable chelate-metal compound intra- and extracellularly.

        (2) Onset of action is 30 min.

        (3) Increases fecal excretion as chelated lead is excreted predominantly in bile within 4 to 6 h (35).

        (4) Increases urinary excretion of chelated lead.

        (5) Chelator of choice in the presence of renal compromise.

      b. Indications

        (1) High lead levels without symptoms

        (2) Acute encephalopathy

        (3) Symptomatic plumbism characterized by

          (a) Abdominal pain

          (b) Anemia

          (c) Headache

          (d) Peripheral neuropathy

          (e) Ataxia

          (f) Memory loss

          (g) Lethargy

          (h) Anorexia

          (i) Dysarthria

          (j) Encephalopathy

      c. Contraindications

        (1) Liver failure, as BAL chelates are excreted primarily in bile.

        (2) Patients with glucose-6-phosphate dehydrogenase (G6PD) deficiency develop hemolysis if BAL is administered.

        (3) Concurrent administration of iron is contraindicated because of the high toxicity of the BAL-iron chelate.

        (4) Contraindicated with a history of peanut oil allergy and in pregnancy.

      d. Adverse reactions include nausea, vomiting, hypertension, tachycardia, headache, lacrimation, salivation, rhinorrhea, anxiety, abdominal pain, and fever. These effects may be mitigated by premedication with diphenhydramine. Elevated liver function tests, and sterile abscesses may also occur.

      e. Administration

        (1) Should be administered as soon as possible to minimize the amount of irreversible cellular damage.

        (2) Dosage of the 10% solution in oil: 50 to 75 mg/m^2 i.m. q4h (36,37).

        (3) The full course is 3 to 5 days as with administration with EDTA. A second course may be indicated after a rest period.

TABLE 22-2. Guidelines for the Use of Various Lead Chelating Agents*

Drug	Route of Administration	Dose	Duration of Treatment	Precautions	Parameters to Monitor
BAL[37]	IM	50–75 mg/m^2 every 4 hours	3 to 5 days	G6PD deficiency† Concurrent iron therapy† Peanut allergy† Ongoing lead exposure†	Hepatic transaminases
CaNa$_2$EDTA[38]	IM/IV	1000 to 1500 mg/m^2/day‡	5 days	Inadequate fluid intake Renal impairment† Ongoing lead exposure†	Urinalysis BUN Creatinine Hepatic transaminases
D-Penicillamine[37,38]	Oral	10 mg/kg/day for 7 days, increase to 10 to 15 mg/kg twice a day over 2 to 4 weeks	6 to 20 weeks	Penicillin allergy† Concurrent iron therapy Ongoing lead exposure† Renal impairment†	Urinalysis BUN Creatinine Complete blood count Hepatic transaminases
DMSA[45]	Oral	10 mg/kg/dose three times a day for 5 days, then 10 mg/kg/dose twice a day for 14 days	19 days	Elevated hepatic transaminases Concurrent iron therapy G6PD deficiency Ongoing lead exposure†	Urinalysis Hepatic transaminases Complete blood count BUN Creatinine

Abbreviations: BAL = dimercaprol, IM = Intramuscular, CaNa$_2$EDTA = calcium disodium ederate, IV = intravenous, G6PD = glucose-6-phosphate dehydrogenase, BUN = blood urea nitrogen, and DMSA = 2,3-dimercaptosucanic acid

*Reprinted with permission from Weitzman M, Glazer D. Lead poisoning. Pediatr Rev. 1992;13:461–468. Copyright © 1992. American Academy of Pediatrics.

†Contraindications.

‡IM dose prepared by mixing EDTA 1:1 by volume with 1% procaine to yield a 0.5% procaine solution. IV dose prepared by mixing full dose of EDTA (1500 or 1000 mg/M^2) in calculated fluid requirement for 24 hours, infused continuously over 24 hours. EDTA may need to be given by IM route, if encephalopathy is present requiring fluid restriction.

2. **Calcium disodium versenate** (CaNa$_2$-EDTA)
   a. **Mechanism of action**
      (1) Works extracellularly to form a stable metal-chelate complex that is excreted by the kidney.
      (2) Increases renal excretion by 20 to 50 times.
   b. **Adverse effects**
      (1) Rash, febrile reaction, fatigue, thirst, myalgias, chills and cardiac dysrhythmias.
      (2) Renal impairment may promote toxicity; urine output must be adequate.
      (3) CaNa$_2$-EDTA should be used together with BAL (4 h after the first dose of BAL) because acute lead encephalopathy may progress if CaNa$_2$-EDTA is given alone secondary to soft tissue lead mobilization resulting in increased blood lead levels.
      (4) Oral administration is ineffective and may actually cause enhanced GI absorption.
      (5) Patients with low zinc stores may be adversely affected because CaNa$_2$-EDTA chelates zinc and reduces total body zinc.
      (6) Other metals are chelated as well. In patients occupationally exposed to cadmium, BAL and EDTA will increase cadmium excretion and result in renal damage. In this situation, both BAL and EDTA are contraindicated.
   c. **Administration**
      (1) CaNa$_2$-EDTA is usually started after the second dose of BAL to avoid an elevation of blood lead.
      (2) Dosage
         (a) Children: 1,000 to 1,500 mg/m^2/24 h (range 50 to 75 mg/kg/24 h) in 0.5% procaine i.m. to avoid fluid overload. The preferred route is i.v. This is given in two, four, or six divided daily doses. Higher doses should be used for encephalopathy. The solution may be diluted in D$_5$W to 2 to 5 mg/mL and given in a slow continuous i.v. infusion (36) (Table 22-2).
         (b) Adults: 1.5 g/24 h i.m. in two divided doses. It may be diluted to a 0.2% to 0.5% solution in D$_5$W and given as a slow continuous infusion.
      (3) A full course is 5 days. Repeat courses may be necessary if the patient is still symptomatic or when lead levels are greater than 50 µg/dL. A 2- to 3-day rest period is recommended between courses.
      (4) Adequate urine output and the BUN, creatinine, and urinary sediment must be monitored closely.

3. **D-Penicillamine**
   a. **Mechanism of action**
      (1) Orally active form lead chelator.
      (2) Exact mechanism is unknown.
      (3) Increases urinary excretion of lead.
      (4) Used to chelate copper in Wilson's disease.

> **b.**   **Adverse reactions**
>> **(1)**   Contraindicated with penicillin allergy because of cross-reactivity with penicillin.
>> **(2)**   Toxic effects may occur in as many as 20% of patients.
>> **(3)**   Adverse effects are similar to those seen with penicillin: rash, fever, anorexia, nausea, vomiting, leukopenia, thrombocytopenia, eosinophilia, hemolytic anemia, Stevens-Johnson syndrome, nephrotoxicity, and proteinuria.
>> **(4)**   Not FDA approved for use in pregnancy.
>> **(5)**   Continued exposure to lead will result in continued absorption of lead at an increased rate.
>
> **c.**   **Administration**
>> **(1)**   Dosage 10 mg/kg/24 h p.o. for 7 days. May increase to 10 to 15 mg/kg q12h over 2 to 4 weeks. Treat for a total of 6 to 20 weeks (36–38).
>> **(2)**   Some recommendations call for initiation of the medication at one-fourth the dosage and gradually increasing to full dosage over 3 to 4 weeks to minimize toxicity.
>> **(3)**   CDC recommendations:
>>> **(a)**   Children: give entire dose on empty stomach 2 h before breakfast.
>>> **(b)**   Adults: give orally in two or three divided doses on an empty stomach 2 h prior to meals.

4.   **Oral dimercaprol analogues:** DMPS (2,3-dimercapto-1-propanesulfonic acid), DMSA (dimercaptosuccinic acid)

> **a.**   **Advantages**
>> **(1)**   Revolutionary therapeutic agent for lead toxicity as it is orally active and can be used with concurrent iron administration.
>> **(2)**   Does not increase lead absorption if there is continuous lead exposure.
>> **(3)**   Has minimal effect on Ca, Fe, Mg, Cu, and Zn.
>> **(4)**   Does not shift lead into the CNS.
>
> **b.**   **Indications**
>> **(1)**   Presently approved for asymptomatic children with blood lead less than 45 µg/dL.
>> **(2)**   Experimental protocol now in use for mild encephalopathy and use in the adult.
>
> **c.**   **Mechanism of action**
>> **(1)**   Similar to BAL
>> **(2)**   Developed as orally active, water-soluble analogues of BAL to reduce toxicity and side effects (39).
>> **(3)**   Shown to be as effective as $CaNa_2$-EDTA in enhancing urinary excretion of lead (40).
>> **(4)**   Demonstrable improvement in neurotoxic effects including clinical depression (41).
>
> **d.**   **Adverse effects**
>> **(1)**   Far less toxic than BAL
>> **(2)**   Minimal adverse effects include anorexia, nausea, vomiting, rashes (42).

        (3) Excretion of Zinc is doubled, but is far less than with other chelating agents (43,44).

        (4) Has minimal effect on Ca, Fe, Mg, Cu, and Zn.

    e. **Administration**

        (1) Dosage of DMSA: 10 mg/kg/dose tid for 5 days, then 10 mg/kg/dose tid for 14 days (36,45) (Table 22-2).

        (2) Liver function tests must be monitored weekly. Mild elevation of liver function tests is not a contraindication for use.

B. **Management of children.** There is no standard method for chelation therapy for lead poisoning (46).

    1. **Symptomatic patient** (Table 22-3)

      a. **Acute lead encephalopathy**

        (1) True emergency requiring immediate treatment.

        (2) Up to 80% of children with encephalopathy develop permanent neurologic damage (47). Early treatment may improve the clinical outcome.

        (3) Chelation therapy is administered as outlined in Tables 22-3 and 22-4.

        (4) Lumbar puncture to rule out infectious etiology. When performed, it should be done with caution as lead encephalopathy may cause elevations in intracranial pressure.

        (5) Seizures may be treated with diazepam, phenytoin, or phenobarbital.

        (6) Status epilepticus may develop and can be treated with sodium amytal or general anesthesia if the above medications are unsuccessful.

        (7) Follow-up blood lead levels after the initial course of therapy are indicated on a regular basis to rule out rebound phenomena and recurrent exposure in the home environment. They should be done for all patients regardless of their initial blood level.

      b. **Without encephalopathy**

        (1) Patient requiring admission

           (a) For chelation therapy

           (b) To ensure removal from the source of exposure

        (2) Chelation therapy is administered as outlined in Tables 22-2 to 22-4.

    2. **Asymptomatic patient** (Table 22-3)

      a. Repeat blood lead levels to eliminate contamination or laboratory error resulting in false positives.

      b. Erythrocyte protoporphyrin levels should be determined at the time the repeat blood lead level is done.

      c. Blood iron levels should also be checked at this time because iron deficiency causes elevated blood protoporphyrin levels.

      d. After these results are confirmed chelation therapy is administered as outlined in Tables 22-2 to 22-4.

      e. Follow-up blood level must be determined at 7 to 10 days after treatment to determine if lead rebound has developed. If the blood lead level is within 5 µ/dL of the initial level and is above 25 µ/dL, a repeat course of therapy is warranted.

C. **Management of adults**

    1. Higher lead levels are required for symptoms to appear in adults than for children.

    2. Chelation therapy for adults is administered as outlined in Tables 22-2 to 22-4.

TABLE 22-3. Suggested Lead Testing and Treatment Protocol*

Class	Blood Lead Concentration (µg/dL)	Regimen
I	≤9	Provide education about lead hazards, cleaning, diet Rescreen according to risk classification
IIA	10 to 14	Provide education about lead hazards, cleaning, diet Rescreen according to risk classification Primary prevention activities according to local public health resources
IIB	15 to 19	Confirm by venipuncture specimen within 1 month if initial sample was capillary specimen Provide education about lead hazards, cleaning, diet Evaluate for iron deficiency, treat if indicated, consider prophylactic doses of iron if currently iron sufficient Consider environmental investigation and lead hazard abatement if venous blood lead levels remain ≥15 µg/dL for 3 months
III	20 to 44	Close surveillance of developmental status Confirm by venipuncture specimen within 1 week if initial sample was capillary specimen Provide education about lead hazards, cleaning, diet Environmental investigation and lead hazard abatement Evaluate for iron deficiency, treat if indicated, consider prophylactic doses of iron if currently iron sufficient Close surveillance of developmental status and possible neuropsychologic evaluation if indicated Consider case management by experienced lead team Consider chelation therapy or EDTA mobilization test if lead level is 25 µg/dL or greater
IV	45 to 69	Confirm by venipuncture specimen within 48 hours if initial sample was capillary specimen Provide education about lead hazards, cleaning, diet Environmental investigation and lead hazard abatement with removal of child from likely source of lead until remediation is satisfactory Chelation therapy within 48 hours Evaluate for iron deficiency, treat if indicated, consider prophylactic doses of iron if currently iron sufficient Close surveillance of developmental status and possible neuropsychologic evaluation if indicated Consider case management by experienced lead team
V	≥70	Confirm by venipuncture specimen immediately if initial sample was capillary specimen Immediate chelation therapy Provide education about lead hazards, cleaning, diet Environmental investigation and lead hazard abatement with removal of child from likely source of lead until remediation is satisfactory Evaluate for iron deficiency; treat if indicated; consider prophylactic doses of iron if currently iron sufficient Close surveillance of developmental status and possible neuropsychologic evaluation if indicated Consider case management by experienced lead team

Abbreviations: EDTA = ethylenediaminetetraacetic acid.
*Adapted from reference 13.

TABLE 22-4. *Chelation Options for Children with Elevated Blood Lead Burdens*

Lead Classification	Treatment Regimen	Comments
Symptomatic		
	• BAL 75 mg/m^2 every 4 hours for 5 days, plus EDTA 1500 mg/m^2/day by continuous IV for 5 days	• BAL given first, followed by EDTA once adequate urine output is documented • EDTA generally given by continuous IV route, can be administered by IV or IM route in two divided doses • Subsequent courses of treatment with same or other drugs is usually indicated depending on posttreatment blood lead level
Asymptomatic		
Blood lead ≥70 μg/dL	• BAL 75 mg/m^2 every 4 hours for 5 days, plus EDTA 1500 mg/m^2/day by IV for 5 days • DMSA 10 mg/kg three times a day for 5 days, then 10 mg/kg twice a day for 14 days	• BAL given first, followed by EDTA once adequate urine output is documented • EDTA generally given by continuous IV route, can be administered by IV or IM route in two divided doses • Subsequent courses of treatment with same or other drugs is usually indicated depending on posttreatment blood lead level
Blood lead 45 to 69 μg/dL	• EDTA 1000 mg/m^2/day by continuous IV infusion for 5 days • DMSA 10 mg/kg three times a day for 5 days, then 10 mg/kg twice a day for 14 days	• EDTA is generally given by continuous IV route, can be administered IV or IM in two divided doses • Subsequent courses of treatment with same or other drugs is often indicated depending on posttreatment blood lead level
Blood lead 25 to 44 μg/dL	• EDTA mobilization test, followed by EDTA 1000 mg/m^2/day by EDTA for 5 days if mobilization test is positive • DMSA 10 mg/kg three times a day for 5 days, then 10 mg/kg twice a day for 14 days • Penicillamine 10 mg/kg/day, increase to 30 mg/kg/day over 2 to 4 weeks, treat for 6 to 20 weeks	• Least consensus regarding management of children with blood lead elevations in this range • Some experts recommend treatment with DMSA or penicillamine for children with negative EDTA mobilization test results • Subsequent courses of treatment with same or other drugs often indicated depending on posttreatment blood lead level
Blood lead 10 to 24 μg/dL		• Chelation not recommended

Abbreviations: BAL = dimereaprol, EDTA = ethylenediaminetetraacetic acid, IV = intravenous, IM = intramuscular, and DMSA = 2, 3-dimercaptosuccinic acid.

D. Supportive management and follow-up care

1. Establish **adequate urine output** prior to administering chelating agents.

   a. A 20-ml per kg fluid bolus may be administered to pediatric patients.

   b. Close fluid monitoring must be employed with encephalopathic patients to avoid worsening of cerebral edema. Intramuscular dosing of CaNa$_2$-EDTA may be used to decrease fluid load.

2. **Dialysis** is required for patients who have significant renal insufficiency.
3. **Renal function** must be monitored daily for patients being treated with chelation therapy.
    a. Urinary protein
    b. Serum creatinine
4. **Blood lead levels** must be checked on a daily basis for patients undergoing chelation therapy. BAL should be discontinued if the blood level drops below 50 μ/dL. Levels above 50 μ/dL is also the level where repeat chelation is indicated.
5. Blood lead levels should be reassessed 10 days after cessation of treatment to rule out lead rebound from lead stores.
6. Follow-up blood lead and ZnP levels should be performed at regular intervals to monitor the patient for recurrent exposure.
7. **Referral to public health and social services** is necessary for all patients with lead intoxication. Restriction or changing of the work environment as well as emergency housing are some aspects of care that may be required (Table 22-3).

References

1. U.S. Congressional Office of Technology Assessment. *Neurotoxicity, identifying and controlling poisons of the nervous system.* Washington, DC, U.S. Government Printing Office, OTA-BA-436, 1990.
2. Brody D, Pirkle J, Kramer R, et al. Blood levels in the U.S. population: phase 1 of the Third National Health and Nutrition Examination Survey (NHANES 3, 1988–91). *JAMA* 1994;272:277–283.
3. Weitzman M, Glotzer D. Lead poisoning. *Pediatr Rev* 1992;13:461–468.
4. Pirkle J, Brody D, Gunter E, et al. The decline in blood levels in the United States (NHANES). *JAMA* 1994;272: 284–291.
5. Chandler DB, et al. Lead poisoning associated with intravenous methamphetamine use—Oregon, 1988. *JAMA* 1990; 263:797–798.
6. Ruttenber AJ, et al. Meperidine analog exposure in California narcotics abusers: initial epidemiologic findings. In: Mrakey SP, et al., eds. *MPTP: neurotoxin producing a parkinsonian syndrome.* Orlando, FL: Academic Press, 1986:339–353.
7. World Health Organization. *Toxic oil syndrome: mass food poisoning in Spain—report of a WHO meeting, Madrid, 1983.* Copenhagen: WHO Regional Office for Europe, 1984:1–2.
8. Allcott JV, Barnhart RA, Mooney LA. Acute lead poisoning in two users of illicit methamphetamine. *JAMA* 1987; 258:510–511.
9. Environmental Protection Agency. *Air quality criteria for lead.* EPA 600/8-83/028. Research Triangle Park, NC: EPA, 1986.
10. Hernberg S, Nikkhanen J, Mellin G, et al. Delta-Aminolevulinic acid dehydratase as a measure of lead exposure. *Arch Environ Health* 1970;21:140–145.
11. Rosen JF, Chesney RW, Hamstra AJ, et al. Reduction in 1,25-dihydroxyvitamin D in children with increased lead absorption. *N Engl J Med* 1980;302:1128–1131.
12. Nathanson JA, Bloom F. Lead-induced inhibition of brain adenyl cyclase. *Nature* 1975;255:419–420.
13. Bull RJ, Lutkenhoff SD, McCarty GE, et al. Delays in the post natal increase of cerebral cytochrome cocncentrations in lead-exposed rats. *Neuropharmacology* 1979;18:83–92.
14. Pounds JG. Effect of lead on calcium homeostasis and calcium- mediated cell function: a review. *Neurotoxicology* 1984;5:295–331.
15. Scanlon J. Umbilical cord lead concentration: relationship to urban or suburban residency during gestation. *Am Dis Child* 1971;121:325–326.
16. Roper WL. *Preventing lead poisoning in young children: a statement by the Centers for Disease Control.* Atlanta, GA: U.S. Department of Health and Human Services, Public Health Service, 1991.
17. Gerson B. Lead. *Clin Lab Med* 1990;10:441–457.
18. Philip AT, Gerson B. Lead poisoning. Effects and assay. *Clin Lab Med* 1994;14:651–670.
19. Granick JL, Sassa S, Kappas A. Some biochemical and clinical aspects of lead intoxication. *Adv Clin Chem* 1978; 20:287.
20. Miwa S, et al. A case of lead intoxication: clinical and biochemical studies. *Am J Hematol* 1981;11:99.
21. Nortier JWR, Sangster B, VanKestern RG. Acute lead poisoning with hemolysis and liver toxicity after ingestion of red lead. *Vet Hum Toxicol* 1980;22:145.

22. Cullen MR, Robins JM, Eskenazi B. Adult inorganic lead intoxication: presentation of 31 new cases and a review of recent advances in the literature. *Medicine (Baltimore)* 1983;62:221.
23. Rosenblatt JS, Marcus SM. Lead poisoning and eosinophilia. *Vet Hum Toxicol* 1985;28:292.
24. Chalevelakis G, Bouronikou H, Yalouris AG, Economopoulos TH, Athanaselis S, Raptis S. Delta-aminolevulinic acid dehydratase as an index of lead toxicity. Time for a reappraisal. *European Journal of Clinical Investigation* 25(1):53–8, 1995 Jan.
25. Hudak A, Naray M, Suveges E. Clinical relevance of urinary delta-aminolevulinic acid/logarithm of creatine ratio in screening for occupational lead exposure. *Am J Ind Med* 1992;21:673–680.
26. Grazanio JH. Validity of lead exposure markers in diagnosis and surveillance. *Clin Chem* 1994;40:1387–1390.
27. Osterloh J, Becker CE. Pharmacokinetics of $CaNa_2$-EDTA and chelation of lead in renal failure. *Clin Pharmacol Ther* 1986;40:686.
28. Chisolm JJ. Mobilization of lead by calaium disodium edetate. *Am J Dis Child* 1987;141:1256–1257.
29. Silbergeld JS, Sauk J, Somerman M, et al. Lead in bone: storage site, exposure source, and target organ. *Neurotoxicology* 1993;14:225–236.
30. Taylor A. Usefulness of measurements of trace elements in hair. *Ann Clin Biochem* 1986;23:364.
31. Needleman HR. The current status of childhood lead toxicity. *Adv Pediatr* 1993;40:125–139.
32. Braunstein GD, Dahlgren J, Loriaux L. Hypogonadism in chronically lead-poisoned men. *Infertility* 1978;1:33.
33. Sandstead HH, et al. Lead intoxication: effect on pituitary and adrenal function in man. *Clin Res* 1970;18:76.
34. Robins JM, et al. Depression of thyroid indices associated with occupational exposure to inorganic lead. *Arch Intern Med* 1983;143:220.
35. Chisolm JJ. Treatment of lead intoxication—choice of chelating agents and supportive therapeutic measures. *Clin Toxicol* 1970;3:527.
36. Glotzer DE. Management of childhood lead poisoning: strategies for chelation. *Pediatr Ann* 23:606–615, 1994 Nov.
37. Piomelli S, Rosen JF, Chisolm JJ Jr, Graef JW. Management of childhood lead poisoning. *J Pediatr* 1984;105:523–532.
38. Shannon M, Graef J, Lovejoy FH. Efficacy and toxicity of D-penicillamine in low level lead poisoning. *J Pediatr* 1988;112:799–804.
39. Aposhian HV. Biological chelation: 2,3-dimercaptopropanesulfonic acid and mesodimercaptosuccinic acid. *Adv Enzyme Regul* 1982;20:301.
40. Graziano JH, LoIacano NJ, Meyer P. Dose response study of oral 2,3-dimercaptosuccinic acid in children with elevated blood lead concentrations. *J Pediatr* 1988;113:751–757.
41. Frumkin H, Gerr F. Dimercaptosuccinic acid in the treatment of depression following lead exposure. *Am J Ind Med* 1993;24:701–706.
42. Jorgensen FM. Succimer: the first approved oral chelator. *Am Fam Physician* 1993;48:1496–1502.
43. Aposhian HV, Aposhian MM. Meso-2,3-dimercaptosuccinic acid: chemical, pharmacological, and toxicological properties of an orally effective chelating agent. *Annu Rev Pharmacol Toxicol* 1990;30:279–306.
44. Graziano JH, Siris ES, LoIacano N, Silverberg SJ, Turgeon L. 2,3-Dimercaptosuccinic acid as an antidote for lead intoxication. *Clin Pharm Ther* 1985;37:431–438.
45. Graziano, JH, LoIacono NJ, Moulton T, Mitchel ME, Slakovich V, Zarate C. Controlled study of meso-2,3- dimercaptosuccinic acid for the management of childhood lead intoxication. *J Pediatr* 1992;120:133–139.
46. Glotzer DE, Bauchner H. Management of childhood lead poisoning: a survey. *Pediatrics* 1992;89:614–618.
47. Benson PF, Chisolm JJ. A reliable qualitative urine coproporphyrin test for lead intoxication in young children. *J Pediatr* 1960;56:759.
48. *Preventing lead poisoning in young children: a statement by the Centers for Disease Control.* Atlanta: USDHEW, PHS, Bureau of State Services, Environmental Health Services, 1978.

Selected Readings

Klassen CD, Amdur MO, Doull J, eds. *Casarett and Doull's toxicology: the basic science of poisons.* 5th ed. New York: McGraw-Hill, 1996.
Goldfrank LR, et al. *Goldfrank's toxicologic emergencies.* 5th ed. Norwalk, CT: Appleton & Lange, 1995.
Hayes AW. *Principles and methods of toxicology.* New York: Raven Press, 1989.
Noji EK, Kelen GD. *Manual of toxicologic emergencies.* Chicago: Year Book Medical Publishers, 1989.

Emergency Toxicology, Second Edition,
edited by Peter Viccellio.
Lippincott–Raven Publishers, Philadelphia © 1998.

23

Cadmium, Mercury, and Arsenic

†Scott T. Elberger and °Gerald M. Brody

*†New York Medical College, Rockville Center, New York 11570; °Department of Emergency
Medicine, Winthrop University Hospital, Mineola, New York 11501*

I. Cadmium

A. **Source and forms.** Cadmium is a nonessential trace metal that has had increasing industrial use during the past 50 years. Its main use is for electroplating metals, especially iron, as rustproofing. Cadmium is also used industrially in pigments and paints, in plastics such as polyvinyl chloride, as cathode material for batteries, in solders, in neutron rods in the nuclear industry, and in fungicides and fertilizers. Environmental exposures to cadmium include cigarette smoking, contaminated foodstuffs such as rice, and exposure during lead and zinc smelting (1).

B. **Pharmacokinetic.** Cadmium is absorbed through the gastrointestinal (GI) and respiratory tracts. Absorption is 30% to 40% by inhalation and about 5% to 10% from the GI tract. Low calcium, protein, and iron increase the absorption (2). Cadmium is transported in the blood by red blood cells and large protein molecules. Lymphocytes synthesize metallothionein, a metal binding protein that concentrates cadmium 3,000 times. The cadmium metallothionein complex accumulates in the kidneys and may produce renal damage (3). Cadmium is cleared by glomerular filtration and urinary levels closely reflect body burden unless renal damage has occurred. Cadmium is not metabolized. About 50% to 75% of the body burden of cadmium is in the liver and kidneys. The body burden of an average person is approximately 30 mg (4). Cadmium does not cross the placenta and is in low concentration in breast milk (5). The elimination half-life is 13-33 years (6).

C. **Clinical presentation**

1. **Acute ingestion** of cadmium usually comes from foods like grains, cereals, and leafy vegetables and is characterized by **abdominal pain, vomiting, and diarrhea**. These symptoms are usually self-limited with no long-term consequences. However, a case of fatal ingestion of 150 g of cadmium chloride has been described (6). **Acute inhalation** of cadmium fumes is characterized by symptoms that develop 4 to 12 h after exposure. **Sore throat, cough, and dyspnea** may be followed by fever, chest pain, and rigors. Progression to pulmonary edema and respiratory failure has been described (7), as has bilateral cortical kidney necrosis (8).

2. **Kidneys and lungs** are the main targets in cadmium toxicity. Chronic cadmium exposure causes the proximal tubular lesion of adult Fanconi syndrome in the kidney (9). Proteinuria, aminoaciduria, glucosuria, and decreased phosphate reab-

sorption may be noted (10,11). These changes are symptom-free. Long-term renal failure may occur.

3. Long-term exposure of the **respiratory system** to cadmium has been associated with the development of chronic obstructive airway disease (12) and possibly an increased risk of developing lung cancer (1). Acute respiratory exposure can produce pheumonitis, pulmonary edema, or both. Olfactory impairment has been found in chronic exposures in smelters (13). In Japan, *itai-itai* (ouch-ouch) disease has been described following the ingestion of cadmium-contaminated rice and is characterized by osteomalacia, fractures, gait disturbance, and the renal abnormalities associated with cadmium described above in **I.C.2** (9).

D. Laboratory analysis

1. Blood work should include a CBC, electrolytes, creatinine, and BUN. Urine should be tested for protein, amino acids, and creatinine. A chest roentgenogram and arterial blood gases (ABGs) should be done as a baseline screen and repeated as clinically indicated.

2. There are no widely accepted criteria for the determination of cadmium toxicity. Blood cadmium levels are unreliable in the acute situation. For chronic exposures, blood cadmium correlates with urine cadmium (13). Whole blood cadmium levels average 0.4 to 1.0 µg/L in nonsmoking, nonexposed adults. Smokers have levels of 1.4 to 4.5 µg/L (14). Urine cadmium levels reflect total body burden and are normally less than 1 µg/L (15). *N*-acetyl-beta-D-glucosaminidose (NAG) with either alpha-1 microglobulin or beta-2 microglobulin have been recommended to assay for low-level exposure (16,17).

E. Management

1. General measures include removal of the patient from further intake of cadmium, either acute or chronic. After ingestion, **GI decontamination** by gastric lavage followed by a demulcent is recommended. Do not use syrup of ipecac. Activated charcoal has not been shown to be effective.

2. **Chelation** has not been demonstrated to have a definite benefit in the treatment of cadmium toxicity. However, it may be useful for treating acute exposures if performed immediately after exposure (18). The chelation agent of choice is EDTA 75 mg/kg/day deep i.m. or slow i.v. in three to six divided doses for 5 days. BAL should not be used, as the combination of BAL and cadmium is nephrotoxic (4). There is no treatment for chronic cadmium exposure except removal from further contamination. Dithiocarbamates, triethylenetetraamine hexaacetic acid (TTHA) encapsulated in liposomes and dimercaptosuccinic acid (DMSA) alone and in liposomes have all been used to some effect in mice (19–23). Extracorporeal complexation, with EDTA and glutathione, combined with hemodialysis have shown promise in a dog model (24). None of these measures are FDA approved.

F. Disposition

1. **Acute inhalation exposure** victims should be admitted for observation and treatment of possible pulmonary complications. Acute ingestions that result in a self-limited gastroenteritis-like picture generally require no treatment.

2. **Chronic exposure victims** require monitoring of renal function, possible renal biopsy, and close observation for any signs of renal failure.

II. **Mercury**

    A. Sources and forms. Mercury is a metal that, in its elemental form, exists as a liquid under normal conditions. There are three types of mercury.

        1. Elemental mercury (Hg) is found in glass thermometers, sphygmomanometers, electrical equipment, scientific instruments, button batteries, paints, and dental amalgams. Dental amalgams cause an exposure of 1.5 to 10 μg/day, and there is no evidence of disease being caused by dental amalgams (25–28). It has been used in felt-making, in the production of caustic soda and disinfectants, as a catalyst in chemical manufacturing, and in the electrolytic production of chlorine from sodium chloride.

        2. Inorganic mercury occurs in divalent (Hg^{2+}; mercuric) or monovalent (Hg^+; mercurous) forms. Mercuric chloride, the most toxic inorganic form, has been used as a disinfectant. Mercurous chloride was once used as a teething powder and laxative (calomel). Mercurous fulminate is an explosive compound (29).

        3. Organic mercury occurs in different forms. The short-chain alkyl compounds (methyl mercury and ethyl mercury) are well known as environmental contaminants that have been incorporated and concentrated in the aquatic food chain. Discharge of contaminated wastes into Minamata Bay in Japan during the 1950s led to an epidemic of neurologic and congenital disease caused by eating contaminated fish (30). Long-chain alkyl and aryl mercurials are used as antiseptics and fungicides.

    B. **Pharmacokinetics**

        1. Elemental mercury most often causes toxicity by absorption after inhalation. It has no toxic effects when swallowed, as it is poorly absorbed. However, in the presence of bowel inflammation or obstruction it reaches higher systemic levels (31). Systemic toxicity has been noted after rupture of a Miller Abbot tube (32). Intravascular injection has caused pulmonary embolization (33).

        2. Elemental mercury is highly lipid-soluble and crosses the blood-brain barrier and placenta easily. On crossing the blood-brain barrier it accumulates in the cerebral and cerebellar cortex, where it is oxidized to the mercuric form. The mercuric ion binds with the sulfhydryl groups of enzymes and cellular proteins, interfering with enzyme and cellular transport functions.

        3. Inorganic poisoning most often occurs via the GI route, although pulmonary and skin absorption can occur. After absorption, inorganic mercury is concentrated in the kidney, where it may cause oliguric renal failure after severe acute exposure. Chronic exposure may lead to proteinuria and nephrotic syndrome. An immunologically mediated nephropathy is also found with chronic low-dose inorganic mercury exposure (34).

        4. Organic mercury toxicity is most often associated with short-chain alkyl mercurials, especially methyl mercury. Degeneration of neurons in the cerebral cortex and cerebellum lead to symptoms of distal paresthesias, ataxia, dysarthria, deafness, and visual field constriction. Methyl mercury crosses the placenta easily and becomes concentrated in the fetus. Increased numbers of stillbirths and children born with cerebral palsy are the outcome of prenatal mercury poisoning (35).

C. **Clinical presentation**
1. **Acute exposure** to elemental mercury vapor may produce a corrosive bronchitis with associated fever, chills, and dyspnea. It may progress to noncardiogenic pulmonary edema and eventually pulmonary fibrosis. Abdominal cramps, diarrhea, and change in vision have been reported (36). CNS damage is manifested as neuropsychiatric disturbances (known as erethism) and intention tremors. Irritability, emotional lability, memory loss, combativeness, anxiety, withdrawal, and depression may be seen (37).
2. **Chronic exposure** to elemental mercury yields a classic triad of gingivitis and salivation, tremor, and neuropsychiatric changes (38). Intention tremors of the muscles that perform fine motor functions may progress to generalized trembling (39).
3. **Acute inorganic mercury exposure** is usually by ingestion. Symptoms caused by mucosal irritation include stomatitis, esophageal erosions, nausea, vomiting, hematemesis, hematochezia, severe abdominal cramping, and cardiovascular collapse. Skin irritation due to mercuric chloride exposure and contact dermatitis due to mercury fulminate and mercuric sulfide can occur. Pink's disease is associated with the use of calomel (mercurous chloride) in children and is characterized by an erythematous rash, fever, splenomegaly, irritability, and hypotonia (40). Acute renal failure may occur within 24 h.
4. **Chronic inorganic mercury exposure** is similar to chronic inhalation exposure (see **II.C.2** above).
5. **Organic mercury toxicity** is a chronic syndrome. Exposure to methylmercury causes paresthesias, ataxia, dysarthria, and deafness. "Tunnel vision" and multiple scotomas may occur, as may erethism. Phenyl mercury and methoxyethyl mercury exposures cause a syndrome similar to that seen with chronic inorganic mercury exposure (see **II.C.4** above).

D. **Laboratory evaluation**
1. Baseline CBC, BUN, creatinine, electrolytes, and urinalysis should be done. ABGs and chest roentgenograms are indicated after exposure to mercury vapor.
2. Whole blood **mercury levels** are reflective of acute inorganic and elemental mercury exposure (41). **Normal levels** are less than 4 µg/dL.
3. Because mercury is excreted in the urine (except for short-chain alkyl organic forms) **24-h urine** specimens for measurement of mercury are helpful.
    a. Levels of less than 10 µg/L are normal.
    b. Levels of more than 100 µg/L in a 24-h collection shows significant exposure.
    c. Levels of more than 300 µg/L are associated with symptoms in the patient (13).
    d. Symptom severity, however, does not correlate with urinary mercury levels.
4. Short-chain alkyl compounds form tight bonds with RBCs, and therefore blood levels correlate accurately with symptoms. Symptoms may appear at whole blood levels of 20 to 50 µg/dL, and fatalities have been reported at 150 µg/dL (42).

E. **Management**
1. **Removal of the patient** from further exposure is important, especially with mercury vapor exposure. Administration of oxygen or assisted ventilation is adminis-

tered as needed. An i.v. infusion with isotonic crystalloid should be available to patients with inorganic mercury ingestion to treat hypotension. However, care should be taken not to overhydrate when mercury vapor exposure occurs, as it may exacerbate noncardiogenic pulmonary edema.

2. Ingestion of inorganic mercury salts requires **cautious gastric emptying**. Do not induce emesis. Milk, egg white, 5% salt-poor albumin, 5% sodium formaldehyde sulfoxylate, or 2% to 5% sodium bicarbonate may be used with gastric lavage to bind the mercury. Activated charcoal is of uncertain benefit and should be avoided if endoscopy is anticipated. Cathartics should not be administered but whole bowel irrigation may be beneficial, especially if x-rays show evidence of radiopaque mercury (43).

3. **Chelation** is useful for treating mercury poisoning (except for short-chain alkyl compounds which are excreted in bile), although no absolute criteria have evolved for its use.

4. **D-Penicillamine** is used for less severe mercury vapor and inorganic mercury poisoning. It cannot be given to penicillin allergic patients. It is given orally at a dose of 100 mg/kg every 6 h (maximum 1 g/day) for 5 days in acute poisoning in children and 250 mg four times a day for 5 days in adults. For chronic poisoning in children 25 to 40 mg/kg/24 h (maximum 1 g/day) divided into twice a day dosing or 250 mg twice a day for adults is given until urine mercury levels are less than 50 μg/L. Fever, rash, leukopenia, and thrombocytopenia may occur and cause discontinuation of therapy. Other adverse reactions include nausea, vomiting, optic neuritis, and lupus syndrome. *N*-Acetyl-D,L-penicillamine has been administered for chronic elemental toxicity and in inorganic mercury neuropathy with partial resolution of symptoms (44–46).

5. **Dimercaprol** (BAL in peanut oil) is used to treat severe inorganic mercury poisoning. It is given as an i.m. injection of a 10% solution in oil (47).

   a. The recommended dose is 3 to 5 mg/kg q4h as a deep i.m. injection × 48 h, followed 2.5 to 3.0 mg/kg q6h for 2 days, then every 12 h for 7 more days. BAL and mercury form a chelate that is water soluble at pH 7.5. Therefore, the urine must be kept alkaline and frequent measures of urinary mercury must be done. Mobilization of mercury may cause renal problems in an already compromised kidney. If there is diminishing urinary output after chelation with BAL, hemodialysis should be considered as the BAL-mercury complex is dialyzable (48).

   b. Adverse reactions to BAL include nausea, vomiting, fever in children, hypertension, tachycardia, lacrimation, salivation, blepharospasm, weakness, paresthesias and transient neutropenia.

   c. With organic methyl mercury poisoning, BAL appears to increase CNS mercury and is contraindicated. BAL and D-penicillamine used in combination may cause formation of a toxic complex and should not be used.

   d. Derivatives of BAL-dimercaptosuccinic acid (DMSA) and 2,3-dimercaptopropane-1-sulfonate (DMSP) are less toxic, more specific therapies but are not yet FDA approved nor readily available. DMSA dosing in elemental mercury poisoning is 10 mg/kg/dose every 8 h for 5 days and 10 mg/kg/dose every 12 h for 2 weeks (49).

6. Ca-EDTA should not be used, as it is nephrotoxic in combination with mercury (29).

F. Disposition

1. Ingestion of elemental mercury requires no follow-up unless the patient has underlying disease that would decrease GI transit time. In that case, abdominal roentgenograms to document the course of the metal within the system is advised. Acute inhalation of mercury fumes requires admission to the hospital to monitor respiratory status.

2. Ingestion of inorganic mercury requires admission to the hospital to monitor volume status and renal function and to observe for significant GI bleeding and cardiovascular collapse.

3. Chronic mercury exposures are basically untreatable at this time. However, as noted above, partial resolution of symptoms has been reported with *N*-acetyl-D, L-penicillamine.

4. In pregnant patients, consider therapeutic abortion as mercury is considered a teratogen.

III. Arsenic

A. Sources and forms

1. **Arsenic** is a metallic compound found in many forms in nature. Its common uses are as pesticides, rodenticides, wood preservatives, herbicides and the manufacturing of glass. The burning of green or pressed wood which contains copper arsenate, for mildew control, has been associated with arsenic toxicity (50). **Arsine gas** (AsH_3) is a byproduct of ore smelting and has been used in the semiconductor industry. Environmental contamination of well water may occur, mainly from occupational waste products (51).

2. Arsenic occurs in both inorganic and organic forms. Inorganic arsenic occurs as a pentavalent form (AS_5 or arsenate) and a trivalent form (AS_3 or arsenite). In general the higher valence compounds are less toxic and the more soluble compounds are more toxic. Arsine gas is the most toxic form of arsenic.

3. Arsenic is well absorbed by **inhalation, ingestion, and dermal exposure**. It is initially bound to the protein portion of hemoglobin in the RBC and then distributed to the liver, spleen, lungs, intestines and skin over the first 24 h. Excretion is mainly renal and arsenic can be detected in the urine up to 10 days after exposure. Arsenic concentrates in hair, nails and skin within 2 weeks of exposure. Estimates of time of exposure can be made by measuring the distance of Mee's lines (transverse white lines in the nail) from the base of the nail or the length of hair from its growth site (52). Hair grows at 0.4 mm/day and nails at 0.1 mm/day.

4. Arsenic does not cross the blood-brain barrier well but inorganic arsenic can cross the placenta. Cord blood arsenic levels have been found to be similar to maternal blood levels. Breast milk does not contain significant amounts of arsenic.

B. Pathophysiology

1. The toxic effects of arsenic are mediated through the trivalent (arsenite) form. Pentavalent forms are believed to be reduced to trivalent forms in vivo. The main

mode of arsenic toxicity is inhibition of enzyme activity by binding to sulfhydryl groups (-SH) (53). It inhibits succinic dehydrogenase activity, uncoupling oxidative phosphorylation. Arsenic is also substituted for phosphorus in the oxidative phosphorylation chain, further increasing the loss of production of high-energy phosphate binds in ATP, which causes widespread multisystem effects.

2. In the **GI tract**, arsenic causes vesicles to form in the submucosa of the splanchnic vessels, producing "rice water" stools, which may be bloody, and possible hematemesis.

3. **Cardiovascular effects** include decreased contractility of the myocardium, prolongation of the Q-T interval, ST-T wave changes, vasodilation and hypotension. Torsade de pointes may be associated with Q-T prolongation (53). Long-term exposure to inorganic arsenic has been implicated as an inducer of hypertension and diabetes mellitus (54).

4. In the **kidneys**, hematuria, proteinuria, acute tubular necrosis and renal cortical necrosis can occur.

5. In the **CNS**, a toxic encephalopathy with seizures and coma may occur. A peripheral neuropathy that is more sensory than motor and appears in asymmetric, distal, stocking-glove distribution can occur after acute or chronic exposures.

6. **Hematologically**, anemia, thrombocytopenia, and leukopenia can occur. Hemolysis after exposure to arsine gas is common.

7. **Hepatic** fatty degeneration and central necrosis followed by cirrhosis can occur.

8. **Skin** desquamation, alopecia, hyperkeratosis of the palms and soles, and fingernail changes all may be seen.

9. Inorganic arsenic has been implicated as a **teratogen** which may produce neural tube defects (55).

C. **Clinical presentation**
1. **Acute ingestion** of arsenic generally produces GI symptoms within 30 minutes but they may be delayed if arsenic is ingested with food.
    a. **Vomiting, severe abdominal pain**, burning in the throat and hematemesis occur, followed by profuse diarrhea within 1 to 3 h. A garlic odor of the breath and feces may be noted. Rapid volume depletion due to vomiting, diarrhea and capillary leakage (causing "third spacing" of fluids) can lead to hypotension. Vasodilation and direct myocardial depression may contribute to shock. A toxic cardiomyopathy may occur and acute CNS manifestations may be seen. Death when it occurs, is usually due to circulatory failure. Acute lethal doses of arsenates are 5 to 50 mg/kg and arsenites less than 5 mg/kg.
    b. **Late sequelae** of acute exposure include hematuria, proteinuria and acute tubular necrosis (56). Anemia, leukopenia and thrombocytopenia can occur. A peripheral neuropathy may be seen 1 to 2 weeks after exposure and subsides slowly if exposure ceases.
2. The patient who has inhaled **arsine gas** presents, after a latent period of 2 to 24 h, with abdominal pain, nausea, vomiting, headache, and shortness of breath. Patients may develop hemolytic anemia, hyperkalemia, and hemoglobinuria. Renal failure may result (57).

3. **Chronic exposure** results in a multitude of complaints: abdominal pain, diarrhea, stomatitis, sensory neuropathy and motor weakness with the lower limbs affected first (58). A Wernicke-type encephalopathy has also been reported as a consequence of chronic arsenic poisoning.

    a. **Dermatologic** features include hyperpigmentation and hyperkeratosis, especially on the palms and soles.

    b. **Hepatic injury** is reflected by jaundice, cirrhosis, and ascites. Portal hypertension with esophageal varices may result (59).

    c. **Peripheral vascular disease** may manifest as acrocyanosis and Raynaud's phenomena, and it may progress to endarteritis obliterans (60).

4. **Carcinogenicity** of chronic arsenic exposure is reflected in increased rates of skin cancer, lung cancer, and angiosarcomas (61,62).

D. **Laboratory evaluation**

1. Initial studies should include a baseline CBC, electrolytes, BUN, creatinine, and liver function tests. Chest roentgenograms and ECGs are appropriate. Abdominal films after ingestions are helpful, as arsenic is radiopaque, and the film can confirm the presence, transport, and removal of the compounds.

2. Because of the short half-life of **arsenic** in the blood, arsenic levels are helpful for acute exposures only. Arsenic is only detectable 2 to 4 after exposure with none detected afterward (63). Exposure to more than 1 mg/L is toxic, and 9 to 15 mg/L is potentially fatal.

3. **Urine levels** are more accurate reflections of recent exposure than are blood levels (64).

    a. Normal levels is less than 25 μg in a 24-h urine specimen.

    b. After seafood, which may be high in organic arsenic, levels can reach 50 to 2,000 μg in a 24-h specimen. The arsenic can be fractionated into inorganic and organic forms by cation exchange cartridge to distinguish poisoning from nontoxic organic exposure.

    c. Toxicity is reflected by levels of 500 to 50,000 μg of arsenic in 24-h urine in the absence of seafood ingestion or after fractionation (63).

4. Hair levels of arsenic may confirm arsenic exposure but may be confusing becasue of external contamination of hair.

E. **Treatment**

1. **GI decontamination** is indicated after acute ingestion. Gastric lavage, not induced emesis, is recommended, as arsenic may cause seizures and coma within a short time. If abdominal roentgenograms reveal a low GI presence of arsenic, whole bowel irrigation is indicated. Activated charcoal and cathartics are of unclear benefit but should be administered.

2. **General supportive measures** for treatment of arsenic poisoning include administration of isotonic i.v. fluids in the face of hypotension. Vasopressors such as dopamine or norepinephrine may be used but only after adequate hydration. Administration of oxygen should be begun and transfusions of blood administered as required. ECG monitoring is essential, and cardiac arrhythmias should be treated as they occur. Monitoring of urine output and renal and liver function is necessary.

3. **Chelation** is best accomplished with BAL (British anti-Lewisite). All serious exposures should be chelated. Indications for treatment include ingestions of unknown amounts, ingestions of more than 120 mg of arsenic trioxide, or a spot urine level of more than 200 µg/L (60). BAL dosage is 2.5 to 5.0 mg/kg/dose i.m. every 4 to 6 h for 48 h, then every l2 to 24 h for 10 days or until the urine arsenic level falls below 50 µg in a 24-h specimen. Actual dosage depends on clinical determination of the severity of exposure. Adverse reactions to BAL include nausea, vomiting, fever in children, hypertension, tachycardia, lacrimation, salivation, blepharospasm, weakness, paresthesias, and transient neutropenia.

4. **Penicillamine** may be used with BAL for severe exposures. The dose is 100 mg/kg/day up to 1 to 2 g for 5 days. It cannot be used in penicillin-allergic patients. Fever, rash, leukopenia, and thrombocytopenia may occur and cause discontinuation of therapy. Other adverse reactions include nausea, vomiting, optic neuritis, and lupus syndrome (65).

5. **Dimercaptosuccinic acid (DMSA)** is under investigation for use in patients with chronic arsenic poisoning and may represent a less toxic alternative for chelation. It is an orally administered agent with rare side effects (66).

6. **Hemodialysis** for acute arsenic exposures has produced unclear results. In the absence of renal failure it has not been shown to be beneficial (67,68).

7. **Arsine gas exposure** is treated initially with removal of the patient from the contaminated environment and removal of all contaminated clothing. Exchange transfusion may be necessary (69).

References

1. National Institute for Safety and Health. Cadmium. *Curr Intell Bull* 1984;42:1.
2. Tandon SK, Khandelwai S, Jain VK, Mathur N. Influence of dietary iron deficiency on acute metal intoxication. *Biometals* 1993;6:133–138.
3. Klaassen CD, Liu J. Role of metallothionein in cadmium-induced hepatotoxicity and nethrotoxicity [Review]. *Drug Metab Rev* 1997;29:79–102.
4. Perry HM, Thind CS, Perry AB. The biology of cadmium. *Med Clin North Am* 1976;60:759.
5. Kowal NE, et al. Normal levels of cadmium in diet, urine, blood and tissues of inhabitants of the United States. *J Toxicol Environ Health* 1979;5:995.
6. Bernard A, Lanwerys R. Cadmium in human population. *Experientia* 1984;40:143.
7. Lucas PA, et al. Fatal cadmium fume inhalation. *Lancet* 1980;2:205.
8. Patwardahan JR, Finickh ES. Fatal cadmium-fume pneumonitis. *Med J Aust* 1976;1:962.
9. Emmerson BT. "Ouch-ouch" disease: the osteomalacia of cadmium nephropathy. *Ann Intern Med* 1970;73:854.
10. Elinder CGT, et al. Assessment of renal function in workers previously exposed to cadmium. *Br J Ind Med* 1985;42:754.
11. Roels H, et al. Evolution of cadmium-induced renal dysfunction in workers removed from exposure. *Scand J Work Health Environ* 1982;8:191.
12. Davidson AG, et al. Cadmium fume inhalation and emphysema. *Lancet* 1988;1:663.
13. Verschoor M, et al. Renal function of workers with low-level cadmium exposure. *Scand J Work Environ Health* 1987;13:232.
14. Friberg L, et al. *Cadmium and health: a toxicological and epidemiological appraisal (vol. 1); Exposure, dose and metabolism (vol. 2).* Boca Raton, FL: CRC Press, 1985.
15. Friberg L. Cadmium. *Annu Rev Public Health* 1983;4:367.
16. Kawada T. Indicators of renal effects of exposure to cadmium: *N*-acetyl-beta-D-glucosaminidase and others [Review]. *Sangyo Eiseigaku Zasshi* 1995;37:69–73.
17. Jung K, Pergande M, Graubaum HJ, Fels LM, Endl U, Stolte H. Urinary proteins and enzymes as early indicators of renal dysfunction in chronic exposure to cadmium. *Clin Chem* 1993;39:757–765.

18. Klaaasen CD, Waalkes MP, Catilena LR. Alteration of tissue deposition of cadmium by chelating agents. *Environ Health Perspect* 1984;54:233.
19. Gupka S, Behari JR, Srivastata S, Misra M, Srivastava RC. Efficacy of liposome encapsulated triethylenetetraamine hexaacetic acid (TTHA) against cadmiumn intoxication: role of lipid composition. *Ind Health* 1995;33:83–88.
20. Srivastava S, Gupka S, Behari JR, Srivastava RC. Mobilization of cadmium by liposome-encapsulated meso-2,3-dimer-captosuccinic acid in pre-exposed mice. *Toxicol Lett* 1991;59:125–131.
21. Basinger MA, Jones MM, Holscher MA, Vaughn WK. Antagonists for acute oral cadmium chloride intoxication. *J Toxicol Environ Health* 1988;23:77–89.
22. Singh PK, Jones MM, Jones SG, et al. Effect of chelating agent structure on the mobilization of cadmium from inter-cellular deposits. *J Toxicol Environ Health* 1989;29:501–518.
23. Behari JR, Gupta S, Srivastava S, Srivastava RC. Influence of size of liposomes in potentiating the efficacy of encap-sulated triethylenetetramine-hexaacetic acid (TTHA) against cadmium intoxication. *Ind Health* 1993;31:29–33.
24. Sheabar FZ, Yannai S, Taitelman U. Extracorporeal complexation haemodialysis for the treatment of cadmium poison-ing. II. In vivo mobilization and removal. *Pharmacol Toxicol* 1989;65:13–16.
25. Iyer K, Goodgold J, Eberstein A, et al. Mercury poisoning in a dentist. *Arch Neurol* 1976;33:788–790.
26. Mantyla DG, Wright OD. Mercury toxicity in the dental office: a neglected problem. *J Am Dental Assoc* 1976;92:1189–1194.
27. Svare C, Peterson L, Reinhardt J, et al: Dental amalgam: a potential source of mercury vapor exposure. *J Dent Res* 1980;59A:391.
28. Lorschieder FL, Vimy MJ. Amalgan and mercury toxicity. *Lancet* 1991;337:851–852.
29. Goldfrank L, Bresnitz E, Weisman R. Mercury poisoning. *Hosp Physician* 1980;5:38.
30. McAlpine D, Araki S. Minamata disease, an unusual neurological disorder caused by contaminated fish. *Lancet* 1958;2:629.
31. Wright GB, Yeoman WB, Cantor CF. Massive oral ingestion of elemental mercury without poisoning. *Lancet* 1980;1:206.
32. Kurt KI. Mercury poisoning from a ruptured Miller-Abbot tube balloon. *Vet Hum Toxicol* 1984;26:405.
33. Celli B, Khan MA. Mercury embolization of the lung. *N Engl J Med* 1976;295:883.
34. Roman-Franco AA, et al. Anti-basement membrane antibodies with antigen-antibody complexes in rabbits injected with mercuric chloride. *Clin Immunol Immunopathol* 1978;9:404.
35. Koos B, Longo L. Mercury toxicity in the pregnant woman, fetus and newborn infant. *Am J Obstet Gynecol* 1976;126:390.
36. Jung RC, Aaronson J. Death following inhalation of mercury vapor at home. *West J Med* 1980;132:539.
37. Smith DL. Mental effects of mercury poisoning. *South Med J* 1978;71:904.
38. Goldwater LJ. *Mercury: a history of quicksilver.* Baltimore: York Press, 1972.
39. Friberg L, Vostal J, eds. *Mercury in the environment—toxicological and epidemiological appraisal.* Cleveland: Chem-ical Rubber Co., 1972.
40. Aronow R, Fleishman LE. Mercury poisoning in children. *Clin Pediatr* 1976;15:936.
41. Gothe DJ, et al. Biological monitoring of exposure to metallic mercury. *Clin Toxicol* 1985;23:381.
42. Hilmy MI, Rahim SA, Abbas AH. Normal and lethal mercury levels in humans. *Toxicology* 1976;5:155.
43. Winthrop University Hospital Long Island Regional Poison Control Center. *Mercury handout.* CAS no. 7439-97-6.
44. Hryhorczuk DO, Meyers L, Chen G. Treatment of mercury intoxication in a dentist with *N*-acetyl-D,L-penicillamine. *Clin Toxicol* 1982;19:401.
45. Kark RAP, et al. Mercury poisoning and its treatment with *N*-acetyl-D,L-penicillamine. *N Engl J Med* 1971;285:10.
46. Markowitz L, Schaumberg NH. Successful treatment of inorganic mercury neurotoxicity with *N*-acetyl-penicillamine despite an adverse reaction. *Neurology* 1980;30:1000.
47. Oehme F. British anti-Lewisite (BAL), the classic heavy metal antidote. *Clin Toxicol* 1972;5:215.
48. Sauder P, et al. Acute mercury chloride intoxication: effects of hemodialysis and plasma exchange on mercury kinetics. *J Toxicol Clin Toxicol* 1988;26:189.
49. Bluhm R, Bobbitt RG, Bonfiglio JF, et al. 2,3-dimercaptosuccinic acid versus *n*-acetyl-penicillamine for the treatment of mercury poisoning. *Ann Emerg Med* 1990;19:631.
50. Peters HA, et al. Seasonal arsenic exposure from burning chromium-copper-arsenate treated wood. *JAMA* 1984;251:2393–2396.
51. Landrigan PJ. Occupational and community exposure to toxic metals: lead, cadmium, mercury and arsenic. *West J Med* 1982;137:536.
52. Gorby MS. Arsenic poisoning. *West J Med* 1988;149:308.
53. Goldsmith S, From AH. Arsenic-induced atypical ventricular tachycardia. *N Engl J Med* 1980;303:1096.
54. Chen CJ, Hsueh YM, Lai MS, et al. Increased prevalence of hypertnsion and long-term arsenic exposure. *Hypertension* 1995;25:53–60.

55. Shalst SL, Walker DB, Finnel RH. Role of arsenic as a reproductive toxin with particular attention to neural tube defects. *J Toxicol Environ Health* 1996;48:253–272.
56. Gernhardt RE, et al. Chronic renal insufficiency from cortical necrosis induced by arsenic poisoning. *Arch Intern Med* 1978;138:1267.
57. Kleinfeld MJ. Arsine poisoning. *J Occup Med* 1980;22:820.
58. Chhuttani PN, Chawla LS, Sharma TD. Arsenical neuropathy. *Neurology* 1967;17:269.
59. Szuler IM, et al. Massive variceal hemorrhage secondary to presinusoidal portal hypertension due to arsenic poisoning. *Can Med Assoc J* 1979;120:168.
60. Tseng WP. Effects and dose-response relationships of skin cancer and blackfoot disease with arsenic. *Environ Health Perspect* 1977;19:109.
61. Ott MG, Holder BB, Gordon HL. Respiratory cancer and environmental exposure to arsenicals. *Arch Environ Health* 1974;29:250.
62. Lee-Feldstein, A. Cumulative exposure to arsenic and its relationship to respiratory cancer among copper smelter employees. *J Occup Med* 1986;28:296.
63. Moyer TP. Testing for arsenic. *Mayo Clin Proc* 1993:68:1210.
64. Valentine JL, Kang HK, Spivey G. Arsenic levels in human blood, urine and hair in response to exposure via drinking water. *Environ Res Arch* 1979;20:24.
65. Petersen RG, Rumack BH. D-Penicillamine therapy of acute arsenic poisoning. *J Pediatr* 1977;91:661.
66. Goldfrank LR, Howland MA, Kirstein RH. Heavy metals. In: Goldfrank LR, et al., eds. *Goldfrank's toxicological emergencies*. 4th ed. Norwalk, CT: Appleton & & Lange, 1990.
67. Vaziri ND, Upham T, Barton CH. Hemodialysis clearance of arsenic. *Clin Toxicol* 1980;17:451.
68. Giberson A, et al. Hemodialysis of acute arsenic intoxication with transient renal failure. *Arch Intern Med* 1976;136:1303.
69. Fowler BA, Weisberg JB. Arsine poisoning. *N Engl J Med* 1975;291:1171.

Emergency Toxicology, Second Edition,
edited by Peter Viccellio.
Lippincott–Raven Publishers, Philadelphia © 1998.

24

Metals: Iron Intoxication

Frederick M. Schiavone

*Department of Emergency Medicine, State University of New York at Stony Brook,
University Hospital, Stony Brook, New York 11794-7400*

I. **Properties of iron**

  A. **Sources.** Iron intoxication remains a common and serious form of accidental poisoning, especially in children. In 1996 approximately 22,000 iron exposures were reported by the American Association of Poison Control Centers (with two deaths reported from these exposures). Fatalities have occurred following pediatric ingestions of 1,200 to 4,500 mg of elemental iron. Adult fatalities have been reported when only supportive care was provided or deferoxamine treatment was delayed.

  1. Iron is a common toxic ingestion for several reasons: Most preparations are over-the-counter vitamins for children and adults and are easily accessible. They come in attractive preparations and are nearly indistinguishable from such candies as Good & Plenty and M&M's, accounting for a high incidence of poisoning in children. They are readily available in the home to young children because of their use during pregnancy and the postpartum period.

  2. Physical and clinical properties Iron is a metallic element with an atomic weight of 55.85, a melting point of 1,530°C, and a density of 7.86 at 20°C. It is the most abundant and important metal used in clinical biochemical reactions. It is essential for the synthesis of hemoglobin, myoglobin, cytochromes, and essential transport proteins. Its content in the body is regulated by changes in absorption, as iron lacks an effective elimination mechanism.

  B. **Pathophysiology.** Most dietary iron consists of ferric salts in either of two valence states: Fe^{2+} (ferrous) or Fe^{3+} (ferric). Normally only about 10% of the 10 to 20 mg of elemental iron a day is absorbed. Gastric acid aids absorption by maintaining iron in a soluble state, in which it is absorbed into the mucosal cells of the duodenum and jejunum in the ferrous form. It is then oxidized to its ferric state and couples to **transferrin**, a serum glycoprotein that delivers iron to tissues throughout the body. Each transferrin molecule can bind two iron atoms. The combined binding sites of all the transferrin in the circulation comprise the **total iron-binding capacity (TIBC)**. Normally, 20% to 45% of the iron-binding sites are filled. Specific receptors on the plasma membranes of target cells recognize transferrin, and iron is released into the cell cytoplasm. Between 80% and 90% of absorbed iron is delivered to the bone marrow for erythropoiesis. Excess iron is stored in the body as ferritin or hemosiderin. Iron toxicity is due to a direct caustic effect on gastrointestinal (GI) mucosa and to the presence of free iron in the circulation directly affecting metabolism and the GI, cardiovascular, hepatic, and central nervous systems (3). In the **acute toxic state** the transferrin becomes saturated (the amount of iron exceeds the TIBC), and the iron molecules distribute themselves into cells. The primary targets are the **Kupffer cells** and the liver parenchymal cells, where iron enters the mitochondria. Iron acts as a potent catalyst of **lipid peroxidation**, causing marked alterations of mitochondrial function. It has been shown that iron can act as an electron sink, shunting electrons away from the electron transport system, thereby causing cellular dysfunction and, ultimately, cell death due to impaired production of adenosine triphosphate (ATP) (4). There exists no significant mechanism for iron excretion except the fixed minimal loss of 1 mg/day from the shedding of cells in the feces (3). Women may excrete up to 2 mg of iron per day during menstruation.

C. **Toxicity**

1. **GI system**. The toxic effects seen are related to iron as direct **corrosive** action on mucosal surfaces. This effect is responsible for hemorrhagic necrosis of the GI wall. Hemorrhage may be severe. Necrosis may lead to perforation and peritonitis (5). A later finding is segmental infarction of the distal small bowel. Survivors of these changes may develop scarring and obstruction 4 to 6 weeks after ingestion (5) along with bezoar formation and obstruction (6).

2. **Cardiovascular system**. There are many factors involved in the decreased cardiac output and shock seen with iron toxicity. With early iron toxicity, the plasma volume drops as a result of a shift of fluid from the vascular compartments to the intracellular space (3). This shift is probably due to a direct effect of iron, or ferritin, causing massive postarteriolar dilatation leading to venous pooling. Simultaneously, blood loss due to hemorrhagic gastroenteritis is worsened by a relative bleeding diathesis secondary to coagulation defects. Tachycardia and compensatory vasoconstriction occur. Further fluid loss results in increased blood viscosity, metabolic acidosis, and severe hypotension (3). Tenenbein et al. (7) reported that iron may also have a direct myocardial depressant effect.

3. **Metabolic effects**. The major metabolic effect seen with iron toxicity is the generation of severe, profound anion gap metabolic acidosis (3). There are several causes of this acidosis. It seems that the conversion of ferrous iron to ferric iron with subsequent release of hydrogen ions plays a major role (8). Acidosis is also secondary to the disruption of mitochondrial function forcing anaerobic respiration; it is enhanced by poor perfusion and the formation of lactic acid and other organic acids. The acidosis may be severe despite bicarbonate and supportive care (3,6). Impaired glucose tolerance leading to hyperglycemia may also be seem in patients with severe toxicity (9).

4. **Hepatic effects**. Pathologic changes in the liver depend on the severity of the toxicity but may range from cloudy swelling of hepatocytes to complete necrosis (5). Late manifestations (after 24 h) of hepatic damage are characterized by a marked coagulopathy that seems to be directly related to iron-induced hepatic damage; it is usually seen in association with elevated serum transaminases and a normal number of platelets, supporting a diagnosis of liver damage rather than consumptive coagulopathy. Tenenbein et al. (10) reported several cases of an early

coagulopathy that was reversible with chelation therapy (deferoxamine) not related to hepatic dysfunction.

5. **CNS effects**. CNS effects vary from depressed sensorium to profound coma. They may be the result of poor perfusion states and concomitant acidosis.

II. **Clinical presentation.** The clinical effects of serious iron poisoning have been described as appearing in stages (11). Such effects correlate with the pathophysiology just described and seem to be related to the level of toxicity found. (All phases may not occur in all cases.)

A. The **first stage** occurs shortly after ingestion and is characterized by a direct corrosive insult to the intestinal mucosa. The patient presents within 6 h with nausea, vomiting, explosive diarrhea (usually bloody), colic, abdominal pain, and upper GI hemorrhage.

1. With severe overdose patients, early onset of shock with a severe anion gap metabolic acidosis may supervene.

2. If no GI symptoms occur within 6 h of ingestion, it is probably not a serious toxic ingestion. However, there have been cases reported of severe shock, coma, and death without GI symptoms (12).

B. The **second stage** has been described as a **quiescent** phase. This poorly described stage has been reported to begin as early as 3 to 4 h after ingestion and to last as long as 48 h (13). It appears that this phase may be masked by initial correction of hypovolemia and other stabilizing measures and so produces no overt clinical signs. It certainly seems possible that despite progressive hypovolemia, hypoperfusion, compensated acidosis, and GI damage, there is little change in mental status, and the patient appears falsely stable for a time. Banner and Tong (12) stated that a period of relative stability or latency may not exist with serious iron intoxication, and careful observation is necessary.

C. The **third stage** is seen 12 to 48 h after ingestion and is characterized by worsening of the **GI hemorrhage**, severe lethargy or coma, shock, **cardiovascular collapse**, and a severe profound metabolic acidosis. Signs of liver damage may become evident with jaundice, hypoglycemia, and coagulation defects. Patients may also demonstrate renal insufficiency secondary to poor perfusion, and it may hinder chelation and elimination of the iron complex (12).

D. A **fourth stage** is commonly described with iron poisoning, associated with **healing** of the GI insult. Late sequelae may occur approximately 2 to 6 weeks after the initial ingestion. Gastric scarring and pyloric and small bowel strictures, with or without obstruction, are the most common lesions. Hepatic damage and cirrhosis are well described with chronic iron ingestions (5).

III. **Diagnosis**

A. The **toxicity** of acute iron ingestion is related to the **total amount** of elemental iron ingested. The elemental iron content can be calculated for any compound from the percentage of iron in each compound; it is determined by dividing the molecular weight of iron by the molecular weight of the compound. Table 24-1 gives some examples of the percent of elemental iron found in the most common iron salt preparations (14).

1. To **calculate the total dose** of elemental iron ingested:

ingested dose (mg/kg elemental Fe) = number of tablets × amount of Fe
× percentage elemental Fe/patient
weight (kg)

2. Table 24-2 lists iron compounds and the total elemental iron per compound (15).

TABLE 24-1. *Total elemental iron in iron compounds*

Compound	Percentage elemental iron
Ferrous sulfate (hydrate)	20
Ferrous sulfate (dried)	37
Ferrous gluconate	12
Ferrous fumarate	33
Ferrous carbonate (anhydrous)	48
Ferric phosphate	37
Ferric cholinate	12

B. The estimated **lethal dose** of elemental iron required for acute iron poisoning is generally accepted to be 200 to 300 mg/kg of elemental iron, although there have been cases of much lower exposure being lethal (14). Although there is no absolute safe lower limit of ingestion, most agree that ingestions of <20 mg of elemental iron/kg are nontoxic. Ingestions of 20 to 60 mg/kg are potentially toxic, and ingestions of 60 mg/kg or more are generally toxic. Any symptomatic ingestion should be evaluated in a health care center or Emergency Department.

C. The most useful **early sign** of iron toxicity is GI irritation with nausea, vomiting, and diarrhea within 6 h of ingestion. If the patient develops GI bleeding, hypotension, acidosis, CNS disturbances, or a coagulopathy, immediate and aggressive therapy is warranted.

D. In cases where it is unknown whether the patient ingested iron, a **rapid qualitative screening test** for the presence of iron in the stomach may be performed. It is done by mixing 2 mL of gastric fluid with two drops of 30% hydrogen peroxide in two disposable test tubes. In a separate container, 4 mL of distilled water is added to a 500-mg ampule of deferoxamine, and 0.5 mL of the deferoxamine-water solution is added to one of the two original tubes. If iron is present, a deferoxamine-iron complex (ferrioxamine) is formed and turns the solution orange-red.

E. In mildly symptomatic or asymptomatic patients, an adjunct for determining iron toxicity in a patient is the **deferoxamine challenge test**. Deferoxamine is a specific iron chelator that binds to iron in serum. The deferoxamine-iron complex forms ferrioxamine, which is water-soluble and forms a vinrose color in solution. The test is performed by giving a single dose of deferoxamine 50 to 90 mg/kg I.M. and observing a light orange to dark reddish-brown color change to the urine. Unfortunately, some patients with high serum iron levels fail to produce a positive result. This test is useful when it is positive, however, and demonstrates that free iron is present in the serum.

IV. Laboratory analysis

A. Laboratory tests that should be done in the overall assessment of the iron-intoxicated patient are serum electrolytes, glucose, BUN, and creatinine. Arterial blood gases (ABGs) and a bicarbonate level are important to assess for metabolic acidosis. It is also important to do a CBC with hematocrit, as well as a type and crossmatch blood test.

B. Although **liver abnormalities** appear later in the course of iron toxicity, liver function tests, transaminases, bilirubin, and coagulation profiles should be done early. Tenenbein and Israels (10) reported several cases of an early coagulopathy associated with a modest hepatic dysfunction that were completely reversed with chelation therapy.

C. Abdominal radiographs should be obtained and may reveal tablets or diffuse densities within the gut. Roentgenograms are not positive with liquid iron preparations. It has

TABLE 24-2. *Products containing iron*

Product	Iron complex	Total elemental iron per unit dose
Chocks Bugs Bunny Plus Iron	Fumarate	18 mg
Chocks Plus Iron	Fumarate	18 mg
Feminis Tablets	Fumarate	18 mg
Femiron With Vitamins	Fumarate	20 mg
Feosol Elixer	Sulfate	44 mg/5 mL
Feosol Plus Capsules	Sulfate	65 mg
Feosol Spansule Capsules	Sulfate	50 mg
Feosol Tablets	Sulfate	65 mg
Fergon Capsules	Gluconate	50 mg
Fergon Elixir 6%	Gluconate	35 mg/5 mL
Fergon Tablets	Gluconate	36 mg
Fer-In-Sol Capsules	Sulfate	60 mg
Fer-In-Sol Drops	Sulfate	15 mg/0.6 mL
Fer-In-Sol Syrup	Sulfate	18 mg/5 mL
Filibon Capsules	Fumarate	30 mg
Filibon OT Tablets	Fumarate	30 mg
Flintstones Plus Iron Mulvit	Fumarate	18 mg
Geriplex Kapseals	Sulfate	6 mg
Gevrabon Liquid	Gluconate	20 mg/30 mL
Golden Bounty Multivitamin	Fumarate	18 mg
Iberet Filmtab	Sulfate	105 mg
Iberet-Liquid	Sulfate	26 mg/5 mL
Iberol Filmtab	Sulfate	105 mg
Monster Vitamins with Iron	Sulfate	30 mg
Natalins Rx Tablets	Fumarate	60 mg
Natalins Tablets	Fumarate	45 mg
One-A-Day Vit Plus Iron	Fumarate	18 mg
One-A-Day Vit Plus Minerals	Fumarate	18 mg
Pals Plus Iron Chewable	Fumarate	12 mg
Poly-Vi-Flor Tab w Iron	Fumarate	12 mg
Poly-Vi-Flor Drops w Iron	Sulfate	10 mg/mL
Poly-Vi-Sol Tablets w Iron	Fumarate	12 mg
Poly-Vi-Sol Drops w Iron	Sulfate	10 mg/mL
Spiderman Vitamins w Iron	Fumarate	18 mg
Stuart Formula (liquid)	Fumarate	5 mg/5 mL
Stuart Hematinic Tablets	Fumarate	22 mg
Stuart Hematinic Liquid	Fumarate	22 mg/5 mL
Stuart Prenatal Tablets	Fumarate	60 mg
Stuartinic Tablets	Fumarate	100 mg
Theragran-M Tablets	Carbonate	12 mg
Tri-Vi-Sol Drops w Iron	Sulfate	10 mg/mL
Unicap M Plus Iron	Sulfate	10 mg
Unicap Plus Iron	Sulfate	18 mg

Adapted from ref. 15.

been shown that positive abdominal radiographs are more likely to be associated with significant symptoms and may help guide management of the patient (16). Repeat abdominal films after gastric lavage may be helpful for determining if any tablets remain. Tablets may become embedded in the GI mucosa and require whole bowel irrigation or gastrotomy for their removal (17,18). Patients should be treated with whole bowel irrigation if pills or tablets are seen beyond the pylorus.

D. The most important laboratory test from a diagnostic and therapeutic perspective is the **serum iron level.**

1. Normal values range from 50 to 175 µg/dL. Peak levels of <350 µg/dL are not considered toxic. However, a patient may be symptomatic and have low serum iron levels due to distribution of iron outside the central compartment. Serum iron levels of >500 µg/dL are definitively toxic and mandate immediate therapy. When the serum iron level falls between 350 and 500 µg/dL, the clinician must look beyond this measurement to determine the course of treatment (4,12,14,19).

2. A single serum iron level is not sufficient, and levels should be obtained at 2-h intervals for the first 6 to 8 h. Although the measurement of serum iron and TIBC is recommended for the evaluation of iron ingestion, it has been shown that the TIBC rises factitiously in the presence of high iron concentrations (20). As such, its usefulness for determining toxicity may be inaccurate. Also, many hospitals cannot do rapid serum iron levels or TIBC. Therefore other historical and clinical considerations should be used to determine toxicity and the need for chelation therapy. Tenenbein and Yatscoff (20) showed that a factitious rise in the TIBC occurs as a result of laboratory error (aberration) in the face of hyperferremia. They further suggested that the TIBC not be used as a clinical parameter when deciding chelation therapy. A high TIBC should not be considered to provide a protective effect with iron toxicity.

E. **Other laboratory tests** that may be useful include a WBC count, serum glucose, and abdominal radiographs. Lacouture et al. (9) reported a significant correlation between these positive laboratory tests and serum iron levels of >300 µg/dL beginning 6 h after ingestion. However, Knasel and Collins-Barrow (21) demonstrated no statistical significance for any of the above parameters. Although these laboratory parameters are helpful in some cases, elevated WBC counts or serum glucose levels are neither sensitive nor specific for determining iron toxicity.

V. **Management**

A. **General measures**. The treatment for iron intoxication includes the ABCs of resuscitation and removal of the offending agent. GI elimination may be effected in several ways.

1. **Ipecac** is a less favored agent because of its delayed onset of action, and it is contraindicated in obtunded patients. However it may be useful in treating patients at home and within 30 min of ingestion. Once the patient is in the Emergency department, **gastric lavage** is the preferred method for GI emptying. After mechanical lavage is performed, radiographs of the abdomen should be obtained to look for pills or any concretion that may have formed (9,14). Several **lavage fluids** have been studied. Bicarbonate, phosphate solution, and deferoxamine solution have been reported to bind the iron salts, making them insoluble and nonabsorbable (bicarbonate, phosphate) or effecting their excretion without further toxicity (deferoxamine).

   a. Bicarbonate solution changes ferrous sulfate to ferrous carbonate, but in what appears to be minimal amounts clinically. Hypernatremia is a potential danger with the use of this solution (22).

   b. In vitro studies have shown hypertonic phosphate solution to be a poor binder of iron, and it can cause serious complications, such as hypocalcemia, hyperphosphatemia, and metabolic acidosis. It is not recommended (22–26).

    c. Neither of the solutions discussed in the two points directly above has been shown to be superior to conventional solutions, i.e., normal saline, and are not recommended.

    d. There are several case reports of successful treatment using **enteral deferoxamine** in severely intoxicated patients (14,27–29). Controversy remains as to whether the iron-deferoxamine complex (ferrioxamine) is absorbed in the GI tract, causing greater toxicity. Westlin (30) demonstrated that massive quantities of deferoxamine would be required to chelate significant amounts of iron. With these considerations in mind, it is recommended that the use of oral deferoxamine be reserved only for those patients demonstrating severe toxic symptoms or serum iron levels exceeding 500 µg/dL. Deferoxamine 2 g/L in a 1.5% bicarbonate solution has been used as a lavage solution with an intragastric bolus of 5 to 10 g of deferoxamine in 25 to 50 mL of water left in place (27).

2. **Whole bowel irrigation** is useful to remove iron tablets from the gut especially in those patients with evidence of pills or tablets beyond the pylorus on radiographs. (31). Several cases have been reported in which polyethylene glycol electrolyte lavage solution (GoLytely) was used, demonstrating its efficiency and safety. As such, whole bowel irrigation may well represent the treatment of choice for eliminating iron from the gut. Patients who demonstrate radiographic evidence of pills or concretions within the GI tract despite aggressive lavage may require a gastrotomy to remove the toxin (17,32).

B. **Toxin-specific measures**

  1. **Deferoxamine**

    a. **Source.** Deferoxamine, produced by the bacterium Streptomyces pilosus, is a specific chelator of ferric iron (29). Poorly absorbed from the GI tract, deferoxamine must be given parentally. However, the iron-deferoxamine complex (ferrioxamine) is absorbed. A dose of 100 mg of deferoxamine binds approximately 9 µg of free circulating elemental iron but does not remove iron from transferrin, hemoglobin, or the cytochrome proteins (12).

    b. **Mechanism of action**

      (1) By binding to the ferric molecule, deferoxamine is effective in the treatment of iron toxicity. It is also believed that deferoxamine, which can pass through the cell membrane, exhibits a protective effect at the cellular level by:

        (a) Limiting the entry of iron into the cell

        (b) Chelating intracellular free iron outside the mitochondria

        (c) Binding intramitochondrial free iron and further preventing lipid peroxidation at the mitochondrial level

      (2) Once absorbed, deferoxamine is distributed in a volume equal to 60% of body weight. Ferroxamine is distributed to a volume of only 20% of body weight, suggesting that deferoxamine does enter the cells (4,29).

    c. **Clinical indications and dosages**

      (1) When do we treat? Specific treatment of iron toxicity usually depends on the history and clinical signs and symptoms of the patient.

(a)   In patients who present totally asymptomatic, the history becomes an important factor when deciding their treatment. If the history suggests an elemental iron ingestion of <20 mg/kg and the patient remains asymptomatic with normal laboratory values, serum iron level of <350 µg/dL, normal TIBC (if available), normal serum glucose, normal WBC count, and normal radiographs, that patient may be discharged.

(b)   In patients with mild to moderate symptoms or who is asymptomatic with possible elemental iron ingestion levels of 20 to 60 mg/kg who may be the most problematic in the emergency department. The patient may become severely intoxicated while being observed. Such patients must be watched for at least 8 h and a serum iron level and TIBC repeated every 3 to 4 h.

(c)   Patients with mild symptoms of nausea, vomiting, or diarrhea and GI bleeding require prompt treatment. For these patients, lavage, administration of a cathartic, and a postlavage radiograph are recommended. If fragments are still present, whole bowel irrigation is recommended. The appropriate laboratory studies should be done along with a 3- to 4-h postingestion stat serum iron level and TIBC. A peak serum iron level of 350 µg/dL or a level greater than the TIBC, an estimated elemental iron ingestion of >60 mg/kg, a positive radiograph demonstrating residual iron in the GI tract, or a positive deferoxamine challenge test would require prompt parenteral deferoxamine treatment. A deferoxamine dose of 90 mg/kg I.M. up to a maximum of 1 g in children or 2 g in adults is appropriate. If the serum iron level does not exceed 500 µg/dL and the patient remains normotensive with no acidosis, the patient should be treated with deferoxamine 90 mg/kg I.M. every 6 to 8 h with a total maximum dose of 6 g.

(d)   Patients who present with severe symptoms of iron intoxication—profound vomiting and diarrhea, hematemesis, melena, shock, or coma—require aggressive treatment.

   (i)   Resuscitative measures include immediate airway control, ventilation, and two large-bore I.V. lines. Gastric lavage with a large-bore orogastric tube may require naso- or orotracheal intubation to protect the airway.

   (ii)   Treatment for the severely toxic patient requires the use of I.V. deferoxamine. The recommended dose is 36 mg/kg/hr with the maximum daily dose up to 36 mg/kg or up to 6 g total in children. It is strongly recommended that the poison center be contacted for adjusting the rate of deferoxamine infusion. These patients require the laboratory tests outlined earlier and prompt admission to the intensive care unit.

d. Side effects

(1) Deferoxamine has been reported to have several adverse effects of which hypotension is the most noteworthy. These effects are dose-dependent and usually respond to a fluid challenge, although occasionally they require vasopressors. A study by Mahony et al. (33) demonstrated that covalently attached deferoxamine to high-molecular-weight carbohydrates such as dextran and hydroethyl starch (hespan) prevented the decrease in blood pressure that may occur with large deferoxamine doses. It is reported that this form of deferoxamine has an unaltered affinity for iron, does not cause detectable hypotension, and is much less toxic when given I.V. in experimental animals than the free drug.

(2) The ferroxamine molecule is excreted by the kidneys. In the presence of renal insufficiency (either caused by iron toxic cardiovascular effects or previous renal failure), the treatment of iron toxicity becomes complicated. Hemodialysis is recommended for use in this clinical setting to remove the ferrioxamine molecule. Another technique tested in animals is the use of continuous arteriovenous hemofiltration (34).

(3) There is little documentation regarding the treatment of pregnant patients. Rayburn et al. (35) reported successfully treating a severely intoxicated pregnant patient without adverse consequences. The only other reported case resulted in a fatal outcome, believed to be due to a delay in deferoxamine therapy (36).

C. Who do you admit?

1. All patients who ingested >60 mg of elemental iron. All symptomatic patients with 20 to 60 mg of elemental iron ingestion. All patients with serum iron levels greater than 500 µg/dL. All symptomatic patients with serum iron levels between 350 to 500 µg/dL. All symptomatic patients with a positive radiograph. All symptomatic patients with TIBC > Serum iron levels.

2. End point of therapy. The total duration of deferoxamine therapy has not been established. However, generally accepted recommendations include continuation of deferoxamine until:

a. Twenty-four hours after the patient's urine has turned clear.

b. Serum iron falls to <100 µg/dL.

c. Patient is asymptomatic.

References

1. Litovitz TL, Smilkstein M, Felberg L, Klein-Schwartz W, Berlin R, Morgan JL. 1996 annual report of the American Association of Poison Control Centers Toxic Exposure Surveillance System. *Am J Emerg Medicine* 1997;15:447–500.
2. Dean BS, Krenzelok EP. Multiple vitamins with iron: accidental poisoning in children. *Vet Hum Toxicol* 1988;30: 23–25.
3. Whitten CF, Brough AJ. The pathophysiology of acute iron poisoning. *Clin Toxicol* 1971;4:585–595.
4. Robotham JL, Lietman PS. Acute iron poisoning. *Am J Dis Child* 1980;134:875–879.
5. Reissmann KR, et al. Acute intestinal iron intoxication. I. Iron absorption, serum iron, and autopsy findings. *Blood* 1955;10:35–45.

6. Ellenhorn MJ, Barceloux DG, eds. Iron. In: *Medical toxicology—diagnosis and treatment of human poisoning.* New York: Elsevier Science, 1988.

7. Tenenbein M, Kopelow ML, Desa DJ. Myocardial failure and shock in iron poisoning. *Hum Toxicol* 1988;7:281–284.

8. Reissmann KR, Coleman TJ. Acute intestinal iron intoxication. II. Metabolic, respiratory, and circulatory effects of absorbed iron salts. *Blood* 1955;10:46–51.

9. Lacouture PG, et al. Emergency assessment of severity in iron overdose by clinical and laboratory methods. *J Pediatr* 1983;99:89–91.

10. Tenenbein M, Israels S. Early coagulopathy in severe iron poisoning. *J Pediatr* 1988;113:695–697.

11. Corey TJ. Ferrous sulfate poisoning: a review, case summaries and therapeutic regimen. *J Pediatr* 1964;64:218–226.

12. Banner W Jr, Tony TG. Iron poisoning. *Pediatr Clin North Am* 1986;33:393.

13. Henretig FM, Temple AR. Acute iron poisoning in children. *Emerg Med Clin North Am* 1984;1:121–131.

14. Rumack BH, ed. *Poisindex information system.* Denver: Micromedex, 1993–1996.

15. Krenzelok EP, Hoff JV. Accidental childhood iron poisoning: a problem of marketing and labeling. *Pediatrics* 1979;63:591–596.

16. Everson GW, et al. Effectiveness of abdominal radiographs in visualizing chewable iron supplements following overdose. *Am J Emerg Med* 1989;7:459–463.

17. Foxforel R, Goldfrank L. Gastrotomy: a surgical approach to iron overdose. *Ann Emerg Med* 1985;14:1223–1226.

18. Peterson CD, Fifield GC. Emergency gastrotomy for acute iron poisoning. *Ann Emerg Med* 1980;9:262–264.

19. Kremzelok EP. Iron poisoning: selected diagnostic, prognostic and therapeutic issues. *Clin Toxicol Forum* 1990;1:5.

20. Tenenbein M, Yatscoff RW. The total iron-binding capacity in iron poisoning: is it useful? *Am J Dis Child* 1991; 145:437–439.

21. Knasel A, Collins-Barrow MD. Applicability of early indicators of iron toxicity. *J Natl Med Assoc* 1986;78:1037–1040.

22. Czajka PA, et al. Iron poisoning: an in vitro comparison of bicarbonate and phosphate lavage solutions. *J Pediatr* 1981;98:491–494.

23. Bachrach L, et al. Iron poisoning: complications of hypertonic phosphate lavage therapy. *J Pediatr* 1979;94:147–149.

24. Dean BS, Krenzelok EP. In vivo effectiveness of oral complexation agents in the management of iron poisoning. *J Clin Toxicol* 1987;25:221–230.

25. Dean BS, et al. A study of iron complexation in a swine model. *Vet Hum Toxicol* 1988;30:313–315.

26. Geffner ME, Opas LM. Phosphate poisoning complicating treatment for iron ingestion. *Am J Dis Child* 1980;134:509–510.

27. Henretig FM, Karl SR, Weintraub WH. Severe iron poisoning treated with enteral and intravenous deferoxamine. *Ann Emerg Med* 1983;12:306–309.

28. Mann KV, et al. Management of acute iron overdose. *Clin Pharm* 1989;8:428–440.

29. Whitten CF, et al. Studies in acute iron poisoning. I. Deferoxamine in the treatment of acute iron poisoning: clinical observations, experimental studies, and theoretical considerations. *Pediatrics* 1985;36:322–325.

30. Westlin WF. Deferoxamine as a chelating agent. *Clin Toxicol* 1971;4:597.

31. Tenenbein M. Whole bowel irrigation in iron poisoning. *J Pediatr* 1987;111:142–145.

32. Venturelli J, et al. Gastrotomy in the management of acute iron poisoning. *J Pediatr* 1982;100:768–769.

33. Mahoney JR Jr, et al. Acute iron poisoning rescue with macromolecular chelators. *J Clin Invest* 1989;84:1362–1366.

34. Banner WJ, et al. Continuous arteriovenous hemofiltration in experimental iron intoxication. *Crit Care Med* 1989; 17:1187–1190.

35. Rayburn WF, Donn SM, Wulf ME. Iron overdose during pregnancy: successful therapy with deferoxamine. *Am J Obstet Gynecol* 1983;Nov 15:717–718.

36. Olenmark, et al. Fatal iron intoxication in late pregnancy. *Clin Toxicol* 1987;25:347–359.

Emergency Toxicology, Second Edition,
edited by Peter Viccellio.
Lippincott–Raven Publishers, Philadelphia © 1998.

25

Insecticides and Pesticides

Michael Osmundson

Department of Emergency Medicine, Swedish Hospital, Seattle, Washington 98104

Insecticides and pesticides are compounds used to eradicate insects and undesirable pests. An estimated 1,000 or more chemicals are currently used as insecticides and pesticides. This chapter deals with those compounds classified as organophosphates, carbamates, pyrethrums/pyrethroids, organochlorines, and the compound *N,N*-diethyltoluamide (DEET). The chemicals are available in a variety of professional exterminating compounds, agricultural chemicals, and nonlicensed preparations available to the general public. A comprehensive list of compounds is beyond the scope of this text, and the reader is referred to standard reference sources, e.g., *Poisindex* (published by Micromedex), for identification of a specific compound.

I. Organophosphates and carbamates

A. Perspective

The terrorist attack in the Tokyo subway using sarin gas (an organophosphate) on March 20, 1995 brought to the forefront these cholinergic toxins. With more than 5,000 injuries and 12 deaths, the potential for major toxicity of these agents was clearly demonstrated (1). The widespread use of organophosphates and carbamates in industrial and agricultural applications accounts for an estimated 25 million poisonings worldwide (2).

B. Properties of agents

1. **Physical and chemical properties.** Organophosphates are esters, amides, or thiol derivatives of phosphoric, phosphonic, phosphorothioic, or phosphonothioic acids. Carbamates are derivatives of carbonic acid.

2. **Mechanism of action/pathophysiology**

   a. Organophosphate insecticides bind to and phosphorylate **carboxylic esterase** enzymes while carbamates inhibit these enzymes by carbamylation. Carboxylic esterases include RBC cholinesterase (acetylcholinesterase or true cholinesterase) and plasma cholinesterase (pseudocholinesterase). The process renders the enzymes incapable of degrading the neurotransmitter acetylcholine. Excessive acetylcholine accumulating at neuroeffector junctions in the skeletal muscle system and in the autonomic and central nervous systems produces first stimulatory and then inhibitory effects on neurotransmission. The inactivation of cholinesterase enzymes by organophosphates occurs in several stages and becomes progressively irreversible after 24 to 36 h (**aging**) (3). The inhibition by carbamates is self-limited. The spontaneous return of cholinesterase activity by carbamates accounts for the less severe intoxication seen with carbamates versus organophosphates. Spontaneous regeneration of enzyme is usually complete by 24 h.

b. The **signs and symptoms** of organophosphate/carbamate poisoning depend on the balance between stimulation of **muscarinic** and **nicotinic** receptors in the autonomic nervous system and skeletal muscle neuroreceptors. The dose received, route and rate of absorption, and other individual factors influence this balance.

(1) Stimulation of **muscarinic receptors** produces a constellation of signs and symptoms best remembered with the mnemonic **DUMBBELS:** **D**efecation, **U**rination, **M**iosis, **B**radycardia, **B**ronchospasm, **E**mesis, **L**acrimation, **and S**alivation. Miosis is a common sign of toxicity, and bradycardia is typically seen as the course of the poisoning progresses.

(2) Stimulation of **nicotinic receptors** causes release of epinephrine and norepinephrine, producing a clinical picture best remembered with the mnemonic **MATCH:** **M**uscle weakness and fasciculations, **A**drenal medulla activity increase, **T**achycardia, **C**ramping of skeletal muscles, and **H**ypertension. Additionally, diaphoresis and mydriasis can be seen, although the latter is distinctly uncommon.

(3) CNS effects of organophosphates are myriad and include anxiety, restlessness, lethargy, confusion, coma, seizures (rarely), and depression of respiratory and cardiovascular centers. Carbamates cause less CNS toxicity as they are less able to penetrate the CNS.

3. **Pharmacology and pharmacokinetics**

a. **Absorption** occurs via the GI, dermal, conjunctival, and respiratory routes. Dermal absorption can be limited by the use of latex or knit cotton gloves (4).

b. **Metabolism** of organophosphates occurs in the liver. Detoxification occurs via the cytochrome P450 monooxygenases. The aryl organophosphates require liver activation to become toxic. Carbamates are spontaneously hydrolyzed from the cholinesterase to regenerate active enzyme.

c. **Excretion** of metabolites occurs in the urine.

d. **Elimination half-life** is unknown for most organophosphate compounds. For malathion the half-life was 2.89 h in one patient, whereas for methylparathion the parathion elimination half-life was 2.1 days (5,6). Hydrolysis of carbamates is usually completed within 24 h.

C. **Clinical presentation**

1. **Signs and symptoms** are usually seen within 12 to 24 h, with many cases manifesting toxic effects within minutes to a few hours of exposure. Carbamate toxicity is seen more quickly than with organophosphates, usually manifest within 15 min to 2 h. Lipophilic organophosphates (e.g., fenthion) may not develop initial signs of poisoning for several days (4).

2. The **diagnosis** can be made using four criteria.

a. Appropriate **history** of exposure to an insecticide or pesticide.

b. Signs and symptoms of excessive **muscarinic and nicotinic stimulation.**

    c. **Depressed plasma and RBC cholinesterase levels.**

    d. Response to **atropine and pralidoxime** therapy. The unresponsiveness of carbamates to pralidoxime is a useful tool to distinguish between these toxins.

3. History. Poisonings usually occur during agricultural applications, accidental exposures, or suicidal attempts. In urban areas suicidal or rarely homicidal intent is the underlying cause for the poisoning. Accidental exposure is more typical for rural and farming areas. Patients may give a history of working with agricultural chemicals in an enclosed space, exposing the skin to these chemicals, or ingesting a compound suspected or known to be an insecticide or pesticide. Epidemics occur with contaminated food products, terrorist activity, or accidental mass release (2).

4. Physical examination. Findings depend on the degree of muscarinic, nicotinic, or CNS stimulation or inhibition as already discussed (see **I.A.2**). Mixed clinical syndromes are common. Miosis and muscle fasciculations are frequent and are reliable indicators of organophosphate toxicity. A **garlic-like odor** may be noted on the breath. Typically, the patient presents anxious and diaphoretic, with tachycardia, miosis, and excessive salivation. Copious vomiting and a profusely watery diarrhea often occur. By systems, signs include the following.

    a. **HEENT:** salivation, miosis, lacrimation, and blurred vision. Parathion poisoning has been associated with mydriasis. Bilateral cranial nerve VI palsies have been reported (7).

    b. **Cardiovascular:** tachycardia or bradycardia, hypotension, arrhythmias, conduction blocks. The initial sinus tachycardia usually evolves into a sinus bradycardia. Ventricular arrhythmias, including torsade de pointes, can occur.

    c. **Respiratory:** dyspnea, tachypnea, increased bronchial secretions, bronchospasm, pulmonary edema.

    d. **Neurologic:** anxiety, tremulousness, ataxia, muscle fasciculations, slurred speech, seizures, choreoathetosis, decreased level of consciousness with confusion, and rarely coma in severe cases. Delayed hallucinations have been reported. Lack of neurologic effects can be presumptive evidence of carbamate poisoning.

    e. **Gastrointestinal:** nausea, vomiting, diarrhea, abdominal cramps.

5. Clinical course

    a. **Duration of symptoms** depends on the severity of the poisoning, the organosphosphate or carbamate compound involved, and the therapeutic interventions.

        (1) **Carbamates.** Toxicity usually abates within 24 h regardless of treatment.

        (2) **Organophosphates**

            (a) Pancreatitis may develop owing to parasympathetically induced ductal obstruction and glandular secretion.

            (b) Temperature elevation may persist as long as a week.

            (c) Unless hypoxic encephalopathy intervenes, survivors are frequently asymptomatic within 10 days, although delayed symptoms of fatigue, lethargy, irritability, and memory impairment have been attributed to persistent organophosphate effect.

(d) Gradual increase in cholinesterase levels generally parallels clinical improvement.

b. **Death** occurs secondary to respiratory arrest caused by respiratory muscular weakness, CNS depression, and excessive bronchial secretions. Bronchospasm is a complicating factor. Cardiovascular function remains intact until near death. Untreated patients usually die within 24 h, and treated patients who die do so within 10 days. **Late death**, as long as 15 days after the acute ingestion, may be caused by ventricular arrhythmias (8,9).

c. An **organophosphate intermediate syndrome** consisting in paralysis of proximal limb muscles, neck flexor muscles, respiratory muscles, and various motor cranial nerves was described in 10 poisoned patients in Sri Lanka (10). The paralytic symptoms began 24 to 96 h after the poisoning and after the resolution of a cholinergic phase. This syndrome lasted 5 to 32 days. Some patients required ventilatory support, and three deaths were due to respiratory failure. Electromyographic findings suggested a postsynaptic neuromuscular junctional dysfunction.

d. **Delayed peripheral neuropathy** can occur 1 to 5 weeks after exposure to certain organophosphate compounds, including *o,o,o*-cresyl phosphate, mipafox, leptophos, trichlorfon (chlorofos or Dipterex), trichloronate (Phytosol), parathion, malathion, and Tamaron (11). A cholinergic toxic phase may or may not precede the peripheral neuropathy; some of the neurotoxic organophosphates are weak acetylcholinesterase inhibitors.

(1) The neuropathy typically begins with paresthesias and pain or cramping in the calves followed by ataxia, weakness, and "toe drop." It rapidly progresses to a flaccid paresis, which can ascend in a manner similar to that seen with Guillain-Barre syndrome. Reflexes are diminished, and there may be some sensory dysfunction. The underlying pathology is a distal (wallerian) degeneration of the long axons of both peripheral nerves and the ascending and descending tracts of the spinal cord. Demyelination occurs secondarily.

(2) This pathologic process is thought to occur when a neurotoxic organophosphate binds to neurotoxic esterase, an enzyme thought responsible for the maintenance of neuronal function (11). After an **"aging"** period, corresponding to the latency period for clinical symptoms, a remaining phosphoryl ester bond is hydrolyzed, leaving the neurotoxic esterase with a charged group that causes axonal degeneration in a manner as yet unknown.

(3) The disease may progress for 2 to 3 months, and muscle wasting occurs.

(4) Recovery of motor function occurs in the reverse order in which the functions were lost. Sensory modalities are recovered early. Patients with severe disorders often do not regain total function.

(5) Treatment with atropine and pralidoxime do not affect the course of the disease.

D. Differential diagnosis

1. **Carbamate versus organophosphate poisoning:** Short-lived toxicity and absence of CNS toxicity favor carbamates.
2. **Nicotinic poisoning** (tobacco/nicotine patch)
3. **Drugs** associated with miosis are opioids, clonidine, guanabenz, phencyclidine, phenothiazines, sedative-hypnotics (ethanol, benzodiazepines, barbiturates, meprobamate).
4. **Pontine hemorrhage** produces miosis
5. **Gastroenteritis** may be confused with mild organophosphate toxicity
6. Poisoning from other **cholinesterase inhibitors** (e.g., neostigmine, pyridostigmine)
7. **Asthma**
8. **Guillain-Barre syndrome:** When delayed, peripheral neuropathy is the primary presentation.
9. **Mushrooms: Clitocybe** and **Inocybe** contain a muscarinic substance. Nicotinic effects are absent.

E. Diagnostic tests

1. **Chemistry**
   a. **Electrolytes:** hypokalemia, hyperglycemia
   b. **CBC:** Leukocytosis with or without a leftward shift may occur secondary to increased catecholamine release from the adrenal medulla.
   c. **Urinalysis:** Proteinuria and glycosuria may occur. The presence of **1-naphthol,** a carbaryl metabolite, indicates carbamate exposure. This test is generally used for monitoring occupational exposure.
   d. Elevated **amylase** is seen with pancreatic injury.
2. The **ECG** may reveal sinus tachycardia initially due to sympathetic stimulation. As increased parasympathetic tone predominates, findings include sinus bradycardia, atrioventricular block, ST and T wave abnormalities, QT prolongation, complete heart block, and asystole. Polymorphous ventricular tachycardia (torsade de pointes) has been reported.
3. **Chest radiograph.** Examine for evidence of hydrocarbon aspiration pneumonitis (some organophosphates are packaged in a hydrocarbon vehicle), noncardiogenic pulmonary edema, and hyperlucency consistent with bronchospasm and air trapping.
4. **Toxin-specific findings. Plasma and RBC cholinesterase** levels are depressed in organophosphate poisoning. Depression of the RBC cholinesterase level is more specific for organophosphate poisoning and parallels the activity of neurosynaptic cholinesterase. However, these levels are not readily obtained. Plasma cholinesterase levels are a less specific but more sensitive measure of toxicity and are readily available in many hospitals. Plasma cholinesterase levels can also be depressed in patients with liver disease, malnutrition, or pregnancy. About 3% of the population carry a genetic trait causing deficiency. A subnormal plasma cholinesterase level due to these conditions does not influence the course of toxicity but may lead

to an erroneous diagnosis of organophosphate poisoning. Carbamates have transient and minimal effects on RBC and plasma cholinesterase measurements; thus, these tests are generally not useful. Depending on the institution, cholinesterase levels may not be immediately available. Thus, their utility is not in directing acute intervention, but in diagnosis and follow up.

   a. Plasma cholinesterase levels usually decline to less than 50% before symptoms are seen. As a rough guide: **20% to 50%** of the normal value are found with mild organophosphate poisoning; **10% to 20%** with moderate organophosphate poisoning; **less than 10%** in cases of severe organophosphate poisoning. These guidelines apply during the acute stage of poisoning. In untreated patients cholinesterase activity remains depressed even after clinical recovery.

   b. In untreated, severely organophosphate poisoned patients plasma cholinesterase levels may require 4 weeks to normalize. RBC cholinesterase regenerates at a rate of **0.5% to 1.0% per day** and may require 5 weeks to 4 months for recovery. In patients treated with pralidoxime, RBC cholinesterase levels usually rise faster than the plasma cholinesterase levels.

F. Management

   1. General measures

   a. Airway management, with frequent suctioning of secretions and respiratory support, is the first priority. Intubation may be required to facilitate control of secretions and for ventilatory support if respiratory failure ensues.

   b. GI decontamination measures are complicated by the rapid onset of toxic symptoms, including copious vomiting, CNS depression, and seizures. Ipecac should not be used. Gastric lavage with a large-bore orogastric tube may be performed, with care taken to prevent aspiration, as many organophosphate compounds are in petroleum distillate vehicles which, if aspirated, may precipitate pneumonitis. Activated charcoal 1 g/kg p.o. is administered unless contraindicated. A cathartic (e.g., sorbitol or magnesium citrate) can be administered once unless diarrhea has occurred.

   c. Dermal decontamination includes removal of clothes by hospital personnel wearing protective gloves and masks. Wash the skin with soap and water, followed by ethanol and water. Contaminated clothes, including leather garments, should be destroyed.

   d. Seizures can be controlled with i.v. diazepam or lorazepam initially. If seizures persist, use i.v. phenobarbital (a loading dose of 10 to 20 mg/kg body weight at a rate of more than or equal to 50 mg/min) or i.v. phenytoin (a loading dose of 18 mg/kg body weight at a rate of more than or equal to 50 mg/min). For status epilepticus uncontrolled by these measures, general anesthesia may be used to control seizure activity.

   e. Ventricular arrhythmias should be treated with lidocaine, procainamide, or defibrillation according to standard advanced cardiac life support protocols. Isoproterenol, overdrive pacing, or i.v. magnesium may be used in cases of polymorphous ventricular tachycardia (torsade de pointes).

f. *Avoid* other acetylcholinesterase inhibitors (e.g., physostigmine and edrophonium chloride), and do not use **succinylcholine** for rapid sequence intubation. Succinylcholine is metabolized by plasma cholinesterase; prolonged paralysis has occurred in cases of organophosphate poisoning in which the plasma cholinesterase levels are depressed.

2. Toxin-specific measures

    a. Atropine is a competitive antagonist of acetylcholine at muscarinic receptor sites. It is a tertiary amine that crosses the blood-brain barrier. Thus, it treats the muscarinic effects and possibly the CNS toxicity of organophosphates.

        (1) After the patient is oxygenated to minimize the risk of **atropine-induced ventricular irritability,** atropine is administered in the following initial doses: adult: 1.0 to 2.0 mg i.v.; pediatric: 0.01 mg/kg i.v. (minimum of 0.1 mg).

        (2) Failure of these doses to reverse the patient's symptoms of excess cholinergic activity provides indirect evidence of organophosphate or carbamate poisoning. Repeat doses of atropine are given as follows: adult: 2.0 mg i.v.: pediatric: 0.05 mg/kg i.v. These doses are **repeated every 15 min** until bronchial secretions are controlled, as this muscarinic receptor-mediated effect poses the greatest life threat. Other parameters, such as pupillary size, should not be used to gauge the therapeutic efficacy of atropine. Once bronchial secretions have been controlled, atropine administration should be repeated whenever the secretions begin to recur.

        (3) **Continuous infusions of atropine** at a rate of 0.02 to 0.08 mg/kg/h have been recommended by some authorities. The average patient poisoned with organophosphates requires 40 mg of atropine per day, but as much as 1,000 mg/day has been used (11). Atropine is the mainstay of carbamate intoxication therapy. Six to 12 h of therapy is usually all that is required.

    b. Oxime Pralidoxime chloride (2-PAM), a quaternary amine oxime, specifically regenerates acetylcholinesterase phosphorylated by organophosphates. It works by attacking the phosphate moiety of the organophosphate-acetylcholinesterase complex, forming an oxime-phosphonate, which lifts off the enzyme, freeing it for normal activity. Thus, 2-PAM reverses both nicotinic and muscarinic effects of organophosphate toxicity. Acute reversal of CNS effects has been observed, although 2-PAM, a quarternary amine compound, theoretically should not cross the blood-brain barrier (7).

        (1) Pralidoxime chloride should be administered in all cases of known or suspected organophosphate poisoning. The drug is more likely to be effective if administered early, although it may have some beneficial effect even when given more than 24 to 36 h after the organophosphate exposure. Doses are as follows: adult: 1.0 g i.v.; pediatric: 25 to 50 mg/kg i.v. The drug should be administered over 30 to 60 min; in a life-threatening situation one-half of the total dose can be given per minute for a total administration time of 2 min.

(2) Onset of action of 2-PAM occurs 10 to 40 min after the initial dose, with improvement in symptoms and a decrease in atropine dosage noted. The 2-PAM dose can be **repeated in 1 h and then every 8 to 12 h until the patient is clinically well and not requiring atropine.** Animal studies suggest that a plasma level of 4 µg/ml may be therapeutic (12). Continuous infusion of 2-PAM at a rate of 500 mg/h in adults to produce a steady-state therapeutic serum level has been advocated, but there are no clinical studies to support this regimen.

(3) Pralidoxime chloride should be used for all organophosphate poisonings, but it is ineffective or minimally effective for treating the following organophosphates: ciodrin, dimefox, dimethoate, methyl-diazenon, methyl-phencapton, phorate, schradan, and Wepsyn (13). Pralidoxime in carbamate poisoning is generally not recommended. Indeed, it may decrease the effectiveness of atropine in carbamate intoxication (14). However, as early differentiation between organophosphate and carbamate toxicity is difficult, it is recommended that pralidoxime be started in any syndrome consistent with these toxins unless organophosphate exposure is ruled out.

(4) Side effects of 2-PAM are negligible when recommended doses are used. In high doses (producing concentrations of 2×10^{-3}) M in humans) 2-PAM may produce a direct neuromuscular blockade and inhibit acetylcholinesterase (15).

(5) As pralidoxime has limited activity against several organophosphates, new oximes have been developed. **HI-6 and Hlo-7** appear to have activity against all known organophosphates. These agents may play a role in military and antiterrorist applications in the future (16).

3. **Complicating factors and controversies.** Alkalinization of the serum to pH 7.5 with sodium bicarbonate may be useful for destroying organophosphate molecules. Organophosphates are esters of phosphoric acid. Hydrolysis of the esteratic portion of the molecule increases as the pH increases. One animal study suggests that sodium bicarbonate therapy favorably affects mortality rates (16); no data for humans exist. Therefore, although this therapy cannot be recommended because of insufficient data, maintenance of a normal serum pH seems desirable and safe.

G. **Disposition and follow-up.** Patients who intentionally ingest organophosphates/carbamates in a **suicide** attempt should undergo psychiatric evaluation and counseling. Follow-up examinations should include evaluation for peripheral neuropathy and for other long-term symptoms, which have been reported sporadically with organophosphate poisoning. These include irritability, nervousness, memory impairment, myalgias, lethargy, headache, and GI complaints. Workers should not be reexposed to organophosphates until acetylcholinesterase levels are more than 75%. Carbamate intoxicated patients should be observed for 24 h following the last dose of atropine. No delayed neurologic syndromes have been reported with carbamate poisoning.

H. Summary of carbamate versus organophosphate poisoning

	Carbamate	Organophosphate
Onset	Rapid (15 min to 2 h)	Slower (hours to days)
Duration	Self-limited (usually completed by 24 h)	Slow recovery (up to 4 weeks in severe cases)
Diagnostic testing	Generally not helpful	Serum cholinesterase levels depressed
Treatment	Atropine	Atropine and pralidoxime
Long-term sequelae	None	Many

II. Pyrethrum, pyrethrins, pyrethroids

A. Properties of agents

1. **Sources and forms of toxins. Pyrethrum** is a natural compound extracted from the chrysanthemum flower. Pyrethrum contains six active components labeled **pyrethrins. Pyrethroids** are synthetic derivatives of the pyrethrins. Many of these compounds are mixed in petroleum distillates, which can produce a hydrocarbon chemical pneumonitis if aspirated.

2. **Mechanism of action/pathophysiology.** In humans these compounds produce cutaneous and inhalational allergic reactions, whereas in insects they prolong nerve sodium channel currents, resulting in repetitive nerve discharges (20).

3. **Pharmacology and pharmacokinetics**
   a. **Absorption.** These compounds are well absorbed from the GI tract. Minimal skin absorption occurs. Little is known regarding subsequent systemic toxicity due to pulmonary absorption.
   b. **Metabolism.** Pyrethrins undergo side-chain oxidation by hepatic microsomal enzymes, whereas the pyrethroids are predominantly metabolized by ester hydrolysis (21). The rapid inactivation of these compounds accounts for their relative lack of systemic toxicity in humans.
   c. **Lethal dose** in humans has been estimated to be 1 to 2 g/kg body weight based on animal data (20).

B. Clinical presentation

1. **History.** Patients may give a history of insecticide exposure followed by symptoms involving the cutaneous, pulmonary, GI, or neurologic systems.

2. **Physical examination**
   a. **Skin.** Erythema, vesiculations, and mild paresthesias have been reported (22). Injection can produce sterile abscesses. Cutaneous reactions are the most common adverse manifestations of pyrethrin exposure.
   b. **Pulmonary.** Upper airway irritation (rhinitis, throat irritation, oral and laryngeal mucosal edema) and lower airway reactions (cough, wheezing, shortness of breath, chest pain) can occur, especially in sensitized patients. Chronic exposure can produce a hypersensitivity pneumonitis with cough, dyspnea, and bronchospasm.
   c. **GI system.** Nausea, vomiting, diarrhea, and abdominal cramping can occur with both oral and inhalational exposures.

    d. Neurologic. CNS excitation, tremors, incoordination, paralysis, or seizures may occur with massive ingestions.

  3. Clinical course. In general, the course is benign, depending on the organ system involved. Cutaneous, GI, and pulmonary reactions usually resolve with symptomatic therapy and withdrawal from exposure, although death secondary to bronchospasm in an asthmatic patient has occurred. One death of a child after oral ingestion and one case of Henoch-Schonlein purpura and death after inhalational exposure have been reported (23,24).

C. Laboratory analysis. No specific laboratory tests are indicated. Because these compounds do not interact with acetylcholinesterases, cholinesterase levels are normal.

D. Management

  1. Supportive therapy should be administered based on the signs and symptoms present. **Vitamin E** oil applied dermally has been reported to relieve cutaneous paresthesias following skin contact (22).

  2. GI decontamination is not indicated unless the patient has **ingested more than or equal to 1 g/kg body weight** of pyrethrum or pyrethrins. At levels below this amount, the risk of aspiration of the hydrocarbon vehicle during GI decontamination outweighs the potential adverse reactions of the insecticide. If GI emptying is indicated, either emesis or lavage after placement of a cuffed endotracheal tube is the preferred method. Patients may be given activated charcoal 1 g/kg body weight, although its efficacy for binding these compounds remains unproved.

  3. Atropine and pralidoxime are of no benefit, as cholinesterases are unaffected.

E. Disposition and follow-up are determined by the patient's symptoms, underlying health problems, and clinical course. In general, most patients exposed to these agents do not require hospitalization.

III. Organochlorines

A. Properties of agents

  1. Sources and forms of toxins. Because of their prolonged storage in animal tissue with resultant deleterious environmental effects, organochlorines (e.g., DDT) have been largely replaced by organophosphates as pesticides. Lindane, used as a pesticide, scabicide, and pediculocide, is the organochlorine pesticide of greatest concern to the clinician. This discussion focuses on the management of lindane poisoning. Permethrin, another commonly used scabicide has a similar toxidrome but is less well absorbed (and presumably less toxic) than lindane via the skin (29).

  2. Mechanism of action/pathophysiology

    a. Organochlorines affect nerve impulse transmission by altering membrane Na^+ and K^+ flux, resulting in CNS hyperexcitability.

    b. Organochlorines produce myocardial irritability, predisposing to cardiac arrhythmias.

    c. Hydrocarbon pneumonitis can occur with aspiration of organochlorines in petroleum distillates.

  3. Pharmacology and pharmacokinetics

    a. Absorption. Lindane is well absorbed via oral and inhalational routes. It is less well absorbed dermally unless prolonged skin contact or repeated applications occur or the skin is abraded.

   b. **Metabolism.** Lindane is partially metabolized in the liver as well as being directly excreted in the urine, feces, and milk.

B. **Clinical presentation**
   1. **History.** Intentional or accidental ingestion, prolonged skin exposure, or multiple repeated dermal applications of lindane can produce clinical problems.
   2. **Physical examination**
      a. **Neurologic.** CNS excitation with tremors, agitation, headache, disorientation, seizures and/or coma can occur. Seizures may be the first manifestation of toxicity.
      b. **Respiratory.** Cough, wheezing, rales, or cyanosis may develop if hydrocarbon aspiration has occurred. Respiratory depression or arrest may occur after seizures.
      c. **GI system.** Nausea, vomiting, and diarrhea may develop.
   3. **Course**
      a. **Symptoms** begin within 30 min to 6 h after ingestion. Nausea, vomiting, and diarrhea may precede CNS irritability, or the latter may occur first. Seizures can occur without prodromal signs of CNS hyperexcitability.
      b. **Seizures** with secondary respiratory depression represent the most significant life-threatening manifestations of lindane toxicity. They are usually self-limited but may be repetitive. Coma can occur.
      c. **Aspiration** of petroleum distillates can cause hydrocarbon pneumonitis.
      d. **Rhabdomyolysis** with myoglobinuria, disseminated intravascular coagulation, and lactic acidosis have been reported after lindane ingestions.
      e. **Aplastic anemia** and **pancytopenia** have been reported with repeated applications or use of more than 1% concentrations of lindane (25).

C. **Laboratory analysis**
   1. CBC, serum electrolytes, glucose, creatinine, and BUN.
   2. Other laboratory analyses are dictated by the patient's clinical condition.

D. **Management.** Efforts should be directed toward respiratory support, control of seizure activity, and dermal and GI decontamination.
   1. **Respiratory support.** Airway management is the first priority. Endotracheal intubation should be performed for respiratory failure and to protect against pulmonary aspiration.
   2. **Seizures**
      a. Seizures can be controlled with diazepam or lorazepam initially. If they persist, use i.v. phenobarbital.
      b. Administer oxygen, i.v. dextrose (1 g/kg body weight to a maximum 50 g in adults) and i.v. thiamine (100 mg).
   3. **Arrhythmias** can be treated with lidocaine (1 mg/kg body weight i.v. bolus followed by a 2 to 4 mg/min constant infusion).
   4. **Intravenous fluids** are given to maintain normal hydration and urinary output, especially in cases of suspected rhabdomyolysis and myoglobinuria.
   5. **Other supportive therapy** is applied as dictated by the patient's clinical condition. Epinephrine should be avoided, as it may exacerbate ventricular arrhythmias in the organochlorine-sensitized myocardium.

E. **Disposition and follow-up.** All patients with a history of lindane ingestion or extensive skin contamination should be observed for 6 h for the development of clinical symptoms. Patients who develop CNS depression, irritability, or seizures or who have known or suspected hydrocarbon aspiration pneumonitis should be admitted to the hospital for further monitoring and treatment. After **6 h** of being asymptomatic, nonsuicidal patients may be discharged home after patient or parental education regarding accidental poisoning. Asymptomatic, suicidal patients should obtain appropriate psychiatric evaluation.

IV. **N,N-Diethyltoluamide (DEET).** Many topical insect repellants contain DEET, a chemical compound readily absorbed after dermal application. Rarely, excessive topical use of this compound has been associated with a toxic encephalopathy, especially in young girls and female infants (26,27,28).

A. **Symptoms** include anxiety, lethargy, involuntary movements of the head, trunk, and limbs (including opisthotonic posturing), athetosis, ataxia, seizures, and coma. Development of the encephalopathy occurs rarely and idiosyncratically, and it may mimic encephalitis of any cause. Oral ingestions of 50 ml of insect repellents containing DEET (47.5% to 95.0% concentrations) have resulted in coma, seizures, and hypotension within 1 h of ingestion, with two deaths reported (27).

B. **Management** includes oral or dermal decontamination; examination for other causes of encephalopathy, coma, seizures, and hypotension; and supportive therapy.

References

1. Yokoyama K. Blood purification for severe sarin poisoning after the Tokyo subway attack. *JAMA* 1995;274:379.
2. Levine RS. Global estimates of acute pesticide morbidity and mortality. *Rev Environ Contam Toxicol* 1992;129:29–50.
3. Murphy SD. Toxic effect of pesticides. In: Klaassen CD, Amdur MO, Doull J, eds. *Casarett and Doulls' toxicology.* 3rd ed. New York: Macmillan, 1986:519–581.
4. Keeble VB. Evaluation of knit glove fabrics as barriers to dermal absoption of organophosphorus insecticides using an in vitro test. *Toxicology* 1993;81:195–203.
5. Lyon J, Taylor H, Ackerman B. A case report of intravenous malathion injection with determination of serum half-life. *Clin Toxicol* 1987;25:243.
6. Gerkin R, Curry S. Persistently elevated plasma insecticide levels in severe methylparathion poisoning [Abstract]. Presented at the AACT/AAPCC/ABMT/CAPCC Annual Scientific Meeting, Vancouver, Canada, 1987.
7. Merrill DG, Mihm FG. Prolonged toxicity of organophosphate poisoning. *Crit Care Med* 1982;10:550.
8. Ludomirsky A, et al. Q-T prolongation and polymorphous ("torsade de pointes") ventricular arrhythmias associated with organophosphorus insecticide poisoning. *Am J Cardiol* 1982;49:1654.
9. Kiss Z, Fazekas T. Arrhythmias in organophosphate poisonings. *Acta Cardiol (Brux)* 1979;34:323.
10. Stuart LD, Oehme FW. Organophosphorus delayed neurotoxicity: a neuromyelopathy of animals and man. *Vet Hum Toxicol* 1982;24:107.
11. Du Toit PW, et al. Experience with the intensive care management of organophosphate insecticide poisoning. *S Afr Med J* 1981;60:227.
12. Sidell FR, Groff LWA, Kaminskis A. Pralidoxime methanesulfonate: plasma levels and pharmacokinetics after oral administration to man. *J Pharm Sci* 1972;61:1136.
13. Package insert. *Protopam (pralidoxime).* New York: Ayerst Laboratories.
14. Dawson RM. Oxime effects on the rate constants of carbamylation and decarbamylation of acetylcholinesterase for pyridostigmine, physostigmine and insecticidal carbamates. *Neurochem Int* 1995;26:643–654.
15. Grob D, Johns RJ. Use of oximes in the treatment of intoxication by anticholinesterase compounds in normal subjects. *Am J Med* 1958;24:497.
16. Lundy PM. Comparison of several oximes against poisoning by soman, tabun, and GF. *Toxicology* 1992;72:99–105.
17. Cordoba D, et al. Organophosphate poisoning: modifications in acid base equilibrium and use of sodium bicarbonate as an aid in the treatment of toxicity in dogs. *Vet Hum Toxicol* 1983;25:1.

18. Sterri S, et al. Effect of toxigonin and P2S on the toxicity of carbamates and organophosphorus compounds. *Acta Pharmacol Toxicol (Copenh)* 1979;45:9–15.

19. Senanayake N, Karalliedde L. Neurotoxic effects of organophosphorus insecticides: an intermediate syndrome. *N Engl J Med* 1987;316:761.

20. Paton DL, Walker JS. Pyrethrin poisoning from commercial strength flea and tick spray. *Am J Emerg Med* 1988;6:232.

21. Abernathy CO, Casida JE. Pyrethroid insecticides: esterase cleavage in relation to selective toxicity. *Science* 1973;179:1235.

22. McCord CP. Pyrethrum dermatitis: a record of the occurrence of occupational dermatoses among workers in the pyrethrum industry. *JAMA* 1921;77:448.

23. Hayes Jr WJ. *Clinical handbook on economic poisons.* USPHS publ. 476. Washington, DC: U.S. Government Printing Office, 1963.

24. Hayes WJ, Vaughn WK. Mortality from pesticides in the United States in 1973 and 1974. *Toxicol Appl Pharmacol* 1977;42:235.

25. Loge JP. Aplastic anemia following exposure to benzene hexachloride (lindane). *JAMA* 1965;193:104.

26. Gryboski J, Weinstein D, Ordway NK. Toxic encephalopathy apparently related to the use of an insect repellent. *N Engl J Med* 1961;264:289.

27. Tenenbein M. Severe toxic reactions and death following the ingestion of diethyltoluamide-containing insect repellents. *JAMA* 1987;258:1509.

28. Aks. Acute accidental lindane ingestion in toddlers. *Ann Emerg Med* 1995;26:647–651.

29. Franz TJ. Comparative percutaneous absorption of Lindane and Permethrin. *Arch Dermatol* 1996;132:901.

Selected Readings

Brill DM, Maisel AS, Prabhu R. Polymorphic ventricular tachycardia and other complex arrhythmias in organophosphate insecticide poisoning. *J Electrocardiol* 1984;17:97.

Davies JE, et al. Lindane poisonings. *Arch Dermatol* 1983;119:142.

De Barbino JP, Laborde A. Toxicity of an insect repellent: *N,N*-diethyltoluamide. *Vet Hum Toxicol* 1983;25:422.

Dressel TD, et al. Pancreatitis as a complication of anticholinesterase insecticide intoxication. *Ann Surg* 1979;189:199.

Du Toit PW, et al. Experience with the intensive care management of organophosphate insecticide poisoning. *S Afr Med J* 1981;60:227.

Kiss Z, Fazekas T. Arrhythmias in organophosphate poisonings. *Acta Cardiol (Copenh)* 1979;34:323.

LeBlanc FN, Benson BE, Gilg AD. A severe organophosphate poisoning requiring the use of an atropine drip. *Clin Toxicol* 1986;24:69.

Lotti M, Becker CE. Treatment of acute organophosphate poisoning: evidence of a direct effect on central nervous system by 2-PAM (pyridine-2-aldoxime methyl chloride). *J Toxicol Clin Toxicol* 1982;19:121.

Merrill DG, Mihm FG. Prolonged toxicity of organophosphate poisoning. *Crit Care Med* 1982;10:550.

Minton NA, Murray VSG. A review of organophosphate poisoning. *Med Toxicol* 1988;3:350.

Morgan DP, et al. Anemia associated with exposure to lindane. *J Clin Endocrinol Metab* 1980;35:307.

Nambe T, et al. Poisoning due to organophosphate insecticides: acute and chronic manifestations. *Am J Med* 1971;50:475.

Paton DL, Walker JS. Pyrethrin poisoning from commercial-strength flea and tick spray. *Am J Emerg Med* 1988;6:232.

Senanayake N, Karalliedde L. Neurotoxic effects of organophosphorus insecticides: an intermediate syndrome. *N Engl J Med* 1987;316:761.

Stuart LD, Oehme FW. Organophosphorus delayed neurotoxicity: a neuromyelopathy of animals and man. *Vet Hum Toxicol* 1982;24:107.

Tafuri J, Roberts J. Organophosphate poisoning. *Ann Emerg Med* 1987;16:193.

Tenenbein M. Severe toxic reactions and death following the ingestion of diethyltoluamide-containing insect repellents. *JAMA* 1987;258:1509.

Thompson DF. Pralidoxime chloride continuous infusion [Letter]. *Ann Emerg Med* 1987;16:831.

Wadia RS, et al. Neurological manifestations of organophosphorus insecticide poisoning. *J Neurol Neurosurg Psychiatry* 1974;37:841.

Emergency Toxicology, Second Edition,
edited by Peter Viccellio.
Lippincott–Raven Publishers, Philadelphia © 1998.

26

Herbicides and Fungicides

Sandra A. Craig

Department of Emergency Medicine, Carolinas Medical Center,
Charlotte, North Carolina 28232-2861

Modern advances in agriculture and industry have presented us with a bewildering array of products that are designed to inhibit undesired growth of weeds and fungi. Many of these agents produce toxic effects in humans when not used according to specific guidelines. This chapter outlines the toxic effects and recommended therapy for the most commonly encountered herbicides, including bipyridyliums, chlorophenoxyacid derivatives, chlorophenols, glyphosate, sodium chlorate, and substituted urea compounds. The final section discusses four commonly used fungicidal agents: ethylenebis dithiocarbamates, dithiocarbamates, thiuram disulfate, and hexachlorobenzene. For further information on these or other compounds, the reader is referred to Micromedex's *Poisindex* or regional poison control centers.

HERBICIDES

I. **Bipyridyliums**

    A. **Properties of agents.** The bipyridylium compounds paraquat and diquat are nonselective contact type herbicides well known for their toxic effects in humans. These diquaternary nitrogen compounds are highly soluble divalent cations, stable to light and heat, but inactivated on contact with soil. Human toxicity therefore results from ingestion or dermal contact with the agents prior to their application to weeds and soil. Bipyridyliums are poorly absorbed by inhalation owing to the large size of the suspended droplets, and significant toxicity has not been reported by this route.

        1. The **mechanism of toxicity** is incompletely understood. These agents are reduced in biological tissues to free radicals, which react with oxygen to form superoxide and hydrogen peroxide, which are thought to induce tissue damage either by lipid peroxidation of cell membranes or by alteration of cellular redox states with consequent depletion of NADPH.

        2. The **toxicity profiles** of paraquat and diquat are generally similar but differ in one important aspect. Paraquat actively accumulates in the lung by an energy-dependent, specific uptake process within 10 h of ingestion, resulting in severe acute or delayed pulmonary effects that are not seen after diquat ingestion.

    B. **Clinical presentation.** Exposure to bipyridylium herbicides by brief dermal contact or inhalation of spray mist produces mild symptoms consisting of local skin irritation, reversible irregularities in nail morphology, keratoconjunctivitis, and occasional epistaxis. It should be noted that death has resulted from prolonged dermal contact with paraquat when it was used to kill body lice or scabies.

1. Symptoms of **paraquat** ingestion are somewhat dose dependent.
   a. Doses of **less than 20 mg/kg** generally produce transient vomiting and diarrhea, which resolve within days without further sequelae.
   b. Patients who ingest **20 to 50 mg/kg** present with oropharyngeal burns, pseudomembranes, vomiting, and abdominal pain, followed by diarrhea and acute renal and hepatic insufficiency due to acute tubular necrosis and centrilobular necrosis of the liver. Elevations in BUN, creatinine, liver enzymes, and active urine sediment typically resolve within days. This initial symptomatic improvement is followed within 2 to 10 weeks by a progressive pulmonary fibrosis and death.
   c. Ingestions of **more than 50 mg/kg** of paraquat (approximately one mouthful of a standard 20% commercial solution) kill within 72 h owing to multiple organ failure consisting of renal tubular necrosis, myocarditis, liver necrosis, and pulmonary hemorrhage. Pneumothorax, pneumomediastinum, pneumopericardium, and subcutaneous emphysema may accompany severe ingestion.
2. Oral ingestion of **diquat** likewise produces symptoms in a dose-dependent manner, although specific dose correlations are not known.
   a. **Small ingestions** may be followed by an asymptomatic period of 24 to 48 h and then transient gastrointestinal (GI) upset, vomiting, and diarrhea.
   b. **Moderate ingestions** lead to ulcerations of the GI mucosa, diarrhea, and acute renal failure similar to those seen with diquat, but without delayed pulmonary fibrosis. GI fluid sequestration is more pronounced and may lead to shock.
   c. **Massive ingestions** of diquat, like paraquat, cause death within hours owing to multi-organ failure.

C. **Diagnosis.** Acute bipyridylium poisoning is diagnosed by **history** of exposure along with typical **clinical findings.** Accidental ingestion may occur when these solutions are placed in household drinking bottles for storage, therefore emetics and stenching agents have been added to the formulations as a deterrent to accidental ingestion. Many of these cases represent intentional self poisoning as part of a suicide attempt. The diagnosis can be rapidly confirmed using the **dithionite urine test** in which 10 mL of urine is added to 2 mL of 1% sodium thionite in 1 N sodium hydroxide. A blue coloration of the solution indicates the presence of bipyridyliums.

D. **Laboratory evaluation**
1. Quantitative analysis of blood or urine for paraquat or diquat can be done by radioimmunoassay, colorimetry, or gas-liquid chromatography, with results in approximately 1 h. In cases of paraquat ingestion, serum levels are helpful for predicting outcome. Proudfoot et al. (1) showed that patients with serum levels of less than 2.0, 0.6, 0.3, 0.16, and 0.10 mg/L at 4, 6, 10, 16, and 24 h were more likely to survive. Plasma levels of both paraquat and diquat peak within 1 to 2 h after ingestion and decline rapidly during the first 48 h due to glomerular filtration and active secretion by the renal tubules, assuming good renal function.
2. **Prognostic factors** with paraquat poisoning include the following: plasma levels within the first 24 h; amount ingested; concentration of ingested solution (20% solution most toxic); time between ingestion and last meal (food absorbs paraquat

and neutralizes its toxic effects); presence of gastric lesions as seen by early endoscopy; and presence of renal tubular necrosis.

E. **Treatment** is identical for both paraquat and diquat ingestion and must begin as soon as the diagnosis is suspected, focusing on prevention of further GI absorption and maintenance of renal clearance of the toxin.

1. There is no specific antidote.

2. All patients should receive activated charcoal with sorbitol. Fuller's earth and bentonite, previously recommended as adsorbents for bipyridyliums, are rarely available and less effective than charcoal. Gastric lavage is of uncertain benefit and best reserved for patients who present within 1 to 2 h of ingestion.

3. Once absorbed, these toxins are most efficiently eliminated via renal filtration and active secretion. Early and aggressive use of i.v. fluids to maintain glomerular filtration is important. Furosemide and mannitol are thought to be useful adjuncts.

4. Treatment is difficult in patients who develop renal failure, as only relatively small amounts of toxin are removed by hemoperfusion. Continuous hemoperfusion techniques (8 h daily for 2 to 3 weeks) have been used with success in some cases, but must begin within a few hours of ingestion in order to prevent significant tissue uptake.

5. **Antioxidant therapy** including administration of deferoxamine (100 mg/kg over 24 h) and continuous infusion of acetylcysteine (300 mg/kg/d) has been effective in animal studies and anecdotally in cases of human ingestions of up to 160 mg/kg of paraquat.

6. Oxygen therapy is to be avoided in patients who ingest paraquat as it appears to enhance the pulmonary fibrotic reaction. PEEP should be used as needed to maintain oxygenation.

II. **Chlorinated phenoxyacids**

A. The chlorinated phenoxyacid derivatives are plant growth hormone type compounds which are thought to produce toxic effects through uncoupling of oxidative phosphorylation. This group includes 2,4-dichlorophenoxyacetic acid (2,4-D), 2,4,5-trichlorophenoxyacetic acid (2,4,5-T), and 4-chloro-2-methylphenoxypropionic acid (mecoprop). Systemic toxicity in humans has been reported following ingestion, inhalation of vapors, and skin contact with these compounds. The chlorinated phenoxyacids are widely used herbicides and were used extensively during the Vietnam conflict as an exfoliant known as Agent Orange.

B. **Clinical features** of acute phenoxyacid toxicity occur within 6 h in cases of ingestion.

1. Depressed level of consciousness occurs early in **severe cases,** followed by fibrillary twitching of the muscles, hypertonia, and areflexia. Tachycardia, diaphoresis, flushing and hyperpyrexia with hypoxia, metabolic acidosis, and elevations in creatine phosphokinase (CPK) and aldolase are well documented.

2. Patients who ingest **small quantities** or are exposed by **dermal contact** may undergo a more benign course consisting of nausea, vomiting, diarrhea, headache, myalgias, and muscular weakness. These symptoms may persist for several weeks and may be followed by development of peripheral neuropathies as long as 6 weeks after exposure and persisting up to 2 years.

C. **Diagnosis** is made by eliciting a history of exposure to a phenoxyacid herbicide. Most cases involve occupational exposure during manufacturing or agricultural use, or intentional ingestion as part of a suicidal attempt. Such a history, along with clinical signs of hypermetabolism due to oxidative uncoupling, strongly supports a diagnosis of phenoxyacid herbicide poisoning.

D. **Laboratory Evaluation** may reveal transient mild elevations in the WBC and liver enzymes. Patients with hypertonia may have laboratory evidence of rhabdomyolysis with increases in serum CPK, aldolase, lactic dehydrogenase (LDH), and myoglobinuria. Severe cases may demonstrate arterial hypoxia with metabolic acidosis and respiratory alkalosis. Elevations in BUN are occasionally seen but do not seem to reflect a significant degree of renal insufficiency. Phenoxyacid derivatives can be quantitated in serum and urine by gas chromatography, high-performance liquid chromatography, or ultraviolet spectrophotometry.

1. Human data relating levels with clinical symptoms is scant. There is one report of fatality after ingestion of 2,4-D to a serum level of 80 mg/kg, with other reports of survival despite levels of 2,4-D as high as 400 mg/L.

2. The oral LD_{50} is thought to be approximately 400 mg/kg.

E. **Management** of patients with acute phenoxyacid herbicide poisoning is primarily supportive. Hair and skin should be cleansed in cases of dermal exposure in order to prevent ongoing skin absorption. Activated charcoal is recommended in cases of ingestion. Patients with severe hypertonia may be unable to utilize intercostal muscles for ventilation and often exhibit diaphragmatic breathing. These patients would benefit from a period of positive pressure mechanical ventilation. Hyperpyrexia should be treated with tepid baths and fans. Phenoxyacids are rapidly and completely absorbed and excreted unchanged in the urine. Alkaline diuresis therefore would theoretically increase the rate of clearance of the toxin from the body; several cases of rapid clinical improvement after institution of alkaline diuresis have been reported.

F. **Long term occupational exposure** to phenoxyacid herbicides has been associated with chloracne, lymphoma, and soft tissue sarcoma in several retrospective series. Many of the cited cases were exposed to several compounds created in the manufacturing process, including chlorinated phenols and dioxins; the specific agent responsible for these effects has not been delineated.

III. **Chlorophenols**

A. **Properties of agents.** The chlorophenols comprise a group of polychlorinated aromatic compounds that, like phenoxyacid herbicides, produce toxic effects by uncoupling of oxidative phosphorylation and induction of a hypermetabolic state. These compounds are used as fungicides, herbicides, pesticides, and insecticides; and they are usually encountered as liquid solutions that are applied as preservatives to wood, paint, and rubber products. Human toxicity typically occurs after cutaneous absorption or inhalation of vapors when these preservative solutions are applied without protective garments or in poorly ventilated areas. Pentachlorophenol is the most widely used agent in this class and is consequently responsible for most cases of human chlorophenol toxicity.

B. **Clinical features** of acute pentachlorophenol toxicity reflect the generalized hypermetabolic state.

1. **Symptoms** may develop within 2 h if the absorbed dose is large, or may arise after days to weeks of repeated low-grade exposure. Initial features include lethargy, hyperpyrexia, diaphoresis, weight loss, tachypnea, nausea, and vomiting. Anorexia and polydipsia are common. Larger exposures lead to pulmonary edema, coma, and death followed by immediate onset of intense rigor mortis. There is one case report of profound intravascular hemolysis after using pentachlorophenol to clean wooden furniture without use of protective gloves or clothing.

2. Up to 4 years after contact, repeat, low level exposure to pentachlorophenol has been associated with aplastic anemia or pure RBC aplasia that is almost uniformly fatal. Patients who develop aplastic anemia or RBC aplasia are at high risk for subsequent or concomitant malignancies, especially Hodgkins and non-Hodgkins lymphoma, leukemia, and soft tissue sarcoma. Other, less serious effects of chronic low-grade pentachlorophenol toxicity include dermatitis, chronic urticaria, pemphigus vulgaris, chronic sinusitis, conjunctivitis, and recurrent headache.

C. **Diagnosis** of chlorophenol toxicity is by history of exposure to the agent and recognition of the clinical hypermetabolic state. It is often made retrospectively or after several patients develop symptoms from a common source, usually in a workplace where protective measures are not enforced.

D. **Laboratory confirmation** of the diagnosis is by gas chromatography of serum or urine. Serum levels correlate with severity of the symptoms, as there is little storage of chlorophenols in human tissue. Other findings include an increase in the measured basal metabolic rate, mild elevation in WBC count, and, in patients who develop renal tubular degeneration, transient increases in BUN and creatinine. Progressive anemia with decreased haptoglobin and elevations in serum LDH and bilirubin are seen in patients who develop intravascular hemolysis.

E. **Management** of chlorophenol poisoning is entirely supportive. Skin and hair should be washed with soap and water in cases of dermal exposure. Activated charcoal with sorbitol is recommended in cases of ingestion; because chlorophenol herbicides are usually dissolved in petroleum distillates, induced emesis carries the risk of aspiration pneumonia. Pentachlorophenol is 80% excreted in the urine; careful attention to hydration and maintenance of glomerular filtration is thus important, with liberal use of i.v. fluids. Hyperpyrexia is treated with tepid baths and fans. Antipyretics are of no value. Packed RBCs may be required in patients with significant hemolysis. Exchange transfusion is helpful in symptomatic infants but impractical in adults.

F. Cases which arise after exposure in the workplace should be **reported** to public health officials so that work conditions, ventilation, and use of protective clothing can be reviewed and further toxicity prevented.

IV. **Glyphosate**

A. Glyphosate is the active ingredient in herbicidal formulations such as Roundup, Rodeo, Bronco, and Weedoff. Glyphosate inhibits the enzyme 5-enolpyryl-shikimate-3-phosphate which promotes the synthesis of aromatic amino acids in plants. Animals, however, do not utilize such an enzyme and it is now thought that human toxicity is attributable to the surfactant component polyoxyethyleneamine (POEA) in these formulations. The toxicity profile is similar to that of other surfactant substances and is limited to cases of exposure by ingestion.

B. **Clinical findings** in acute glyphosate-surfactant toxicity include sore throat, abdominal pain, and vomiting with GI bleeding and ileus in severe cases. Hematemesis and melena may last several days. Endoscopy reveals erosion of the pharynx, esophagus, and stomach. Pneumonia and pulmonary edema have been observed with severe ingestions and generally develop within 12 h of presentation. Hypotension and oliguria are common in cases of massive intentional ingestion.

C. **Diagnosis** is by clinical history. Adults usually ingest glyphosate herbicides in a suicidal attempt while pediatric ingestions are usually accidental. Laboratory confirmation of glyphosate ingestion can be accomplished using high performance liquid chromatography or in less than 1 h using ion exchange chromatography. Serum LDH, amylase, and white cell count are often elevated. Electrolytes may reveal metabolic acidosis.

D. **Treatment** for glyphosate herbicide ingestion is entirely supportive; there is no specific antidote.

1. Large amounts of i.v. fluids may be required to maintain blood pressure and urine output. Patients should be observed for GI bleeding although antacids and H_2 blockers are of unknown benefit.

2. Activated charcoal is of theoretical benefit since it adsorbs surfactant in vitro, but no clinical studies have proven its efficacy. There are no data to support or refute the benefit of interventions such as hemodialysis, hemoperfusion, or forced diuresis.

3. Ingestions of less than 100 mL and accidental ingestions are generally nonfatal, but intentional ingestion of as little as 200 mL can cause death. Suicidal patients tend to ingest alcohol or other depressive substances in combination with these formulations, which may contribute to the CNS clouding and pneumonia seen in these patients.

V. **Sodium chlorate**

A. **Properties of agent.** Sodium chlorate is a powerful oxidizing agent which is widely available for use as a herbicide.

1. It is a white crystalline substance similar in appearance to table sugar, accounting for some cases of accidental ingestion. The compound is dissolved in water before application to plants and poisoning has been reported after inhalation of atomized droplets of the solution.

2. Initial **toxic effects** are due to the irritant effect of chloride ion on the GI mucosa. Following absorption, the chlorate ion reacts with thiol groups on the RBC and may cause it to lyse. Within the RBC, chlorate oxidizes hemoglobin to methemoglobin, resulting in methemoglobinemia. Sodium chlorate is also a potent nephrotoxin and acute tubular necrosis is common.

B. **Initial clinical features** of acute sodium chlorate poisoning include nausea, vomiting, abdominal pain, and diarrhea. Fifty percent of patients are cyanotic and 20% experience dyspnea. With severe ingestions, the patient may present in frank coma. Early deaths are due to hyperkalemia from massive hemolysis or tissue hypoxia secondary to methemoglobinemia which can be more than 70%. Survivors often become anuric during the first 48 h.

C. **Diagnosis** is generally made when there is a history of ingestion of the substance or exposure to droplets of the prepared solution. Mortality is quoted at 64% in one small series, and is higher is cases of accidental ingestion due to delay in diagnosis and initiation of specific therapy. The fatal dose is 20 to 30 g, but survival has occurred after ingestion up to 100 g in patients who received early specific antidotal therapy and early dialysis. Supportive therapy alone is of little benefit, and deaths have occurred after ingestion of as little as 2 to 3 g.

D. Laboratory Findings. Electrolyte abnormalities include hyperkalemia and azotemia. Methemoglobinemia is usually present and imparts a chocolate brown tint to the blood when it is exposed to air. Increases in serum lactic dehydrogenase (LDH) and urine free hemoglobin are due to intravascular hemolysis, which may be massive.

E. Treatment of sodium chlorate poisoning must be prompt and specific.

   1. Patients who present early should undergo gastric lavage and administration of activated charcoal.

   2. Sodium thiosulfate given as 2 to 5 g in 200 mL of 5% sodium bicarbonate may inactivate the chlorate ion and can be given orally or by i.v. infusion.

   3. Although methemoglobinemia is usually treated by infusion of methylene blue, efficacy of this treatment in cases of chlorate poisoning may be limited due to lack of NADPH available for reduction of methemoglobin (2).

   4. Patients with acute renal failure should undergo early hemodialysis or peritoneal dialysis, which aids in removal of sodium chlorate.

   5. Potassium and hemoglobin should be closely monitored; transfusions may be required in cases of massive hemolysis.

VI. Substituted ureas

A. Properties of agents. The substituted urea herbicides include agents such as mono-linuron, monuron, chlortoluron, diuron, and fenuron which are effective against annual grasses and broad leafed weeds. Human toxicity has been reported following ingestion of these agents, either alone or in combination products such as Gramonol, which contains a mixture of urea herbicide plus paraquat. The substituted urea herbicides are metabolized to hydroxychloroaniline derivatives which are potent oxidants of heme iron in erythrocytes. Human toxicity is manifested primarily by development of methemoglobinemia.

B. Clinical features of urea herbicide toxicity are determined by the degree of methemoglobinemia. Normal blood contains approximately 1% methemoglobin, and concentrations of 5% may be tolerated without adverse effects. Concentrations of 10% to 20% usually manifest as asymptomatic central cyanosis, while levels of 20% to 50% are associated with dyspnea, fatigue, weakness, dizziness, headache and tachycardia. Concentrations above 50% may lead to seizures, coma, cardiac dysrhythmias, and death. Human ingestions of less than 28 mg/kg of monolinuron have been associated with methemoglobin levels of 18% to 36%, while ingestions of 40 mg/kg have resulted in methemoglobin concentrations of 52%.

C. Diagnosis is by clinical history, often that of intentional ingestion in a suicidal attempt. While patients may present with ashen gray skin and lips characteristic of central cyanosis and elevated methemoglobin concentrations, it should be remembered that methemoglobinemia is caused by metabolites of the urea herbicides rather than the parent compound. Symptoms may not manifest for 12 to 14 h after ingestion and patients should be observed for signs of methemoglobinemia during this time. Methemoglobin levels should be measured in patients with central cyanosis or other symptoms consistent with methemoglobinemia.

D. Treatment of substituted urea herbicide ingestion focuses on GI decontamination, adequate period of observation, and reversal of symptomatic methemoglobinemia.

1. Activated charcoal is of theoretic benefit, though no clinical studies have examined its efficacy in cases of urea herbicide ingestion.

2. Patients with suspected urea herbicide ingestion should be observed for a minimum of 12 to 14 h since onset of methemoglobinemia may be delayed.

3. Methylene blue is a relatively safe and specific treatment for methemoglobinemia. Its use is generally reserved for patients with concentrations of more than 30% or those with pregnancy or comorbid pulmonary or cardiac disease. Intravenous administration of 1 to 2 mg/kg of 1% methylene blue over 5 min effectively reverses signs of methemoglobinemia in these patients.

FUNGICIDES

The fungicides are a diverse group of chemical compounds used primarily in the agricultural industry to control fungal disease of cereals, fruits, plantations, and other crops. Commonly used agents include ethylenebis (dithiocarbamates) such as maneb, zineb, nabam, mancozeb, propineb, metiram; dithiocarbamates, including ferbam and ziram; thiuram disulfate, or thiram, and its derivative ethylene thiourea (ETU); and hexachlorobenzene. These compounds are present in small amounts throughout the food chain and are supplied in large quantities to agriculture for use on crops.

I. **Ethylenebis (dithiocarbamates)** are regarded as relatively harmless due to low mammalian toxicity and biological instability to light, heat, and moisture. Human toxicity after acute exposure is rare, although contact dermatitis is well documented. Two cases of acute renal failure have been reported in humans exposed to maneb in an agricultural setting. There are no reported cases of chronic toxicologic or carcinogenic effects from concentrations commonly found in the environment.

II. The **dithiocarbamates** have been studied extensively in rats and dogs, produce no chronic toxic or carcinogenic effects in usual environmental concentrations. No cases of significant acute human toxicity have been reported.

III. **Thiuram disulfate** can cause ocular symptoms, including lacrimation, photophobia, conjunctivitis, decreased visual acuity, and delayed dark adaptation in patients with prolonged occupational contact. Dermatitis is well documented in humans, and is treated with topical or systemic steroids and avoidance. Thiuram can also cause an alcohol sensitization reaction similar to that of disulfiram (antabuse) in topically exposed individuals.

IV. **Ethylene thiourea (ETU)** is a degradation product of the ethylenebis (dithiocarbamates) and has not been linked to significant acute or chronic human toxicity.

V. **Hexachlorobenzene (HCB)** is a fungicide used on seed grains including rye, barley, oats, and wheat. It also occurs as an industrial waste product in the manufacture of some chlorinated solvents and pesticides. Long term low level ingestion has been shown, in human subjects, to cause **porphyria cutanea tarda**, a systemic illness due to disturbed porphyrin metabolism.

A. It has a predilection for children ages 4 to 14 years but is found in infants and adults as well.

B. Symptoms include weakness, anorexia, growth delay, photosensitive skin with hyperpigmentation and hypertrichosis, and porphyrinuria. Skin lesions consist in vesicles and bullae, which may advance to comedo and milium type lesions, ulcers, or scars. Hepatomegaly and rheumatoid arthritic changes are common.

C. An infantile form of PCT known as **pembre yara** or **pink sore** is seen in children ages 2 months to 5 years. Findings include fever, diarrhea, vomiting, and red plaques over the hands, legs, and feet.

D. **Diagnosis** of PCT is made by demonstrating elevated coproporphyrins and uroporphyrins in a 24-h urine specimen. The urine typically exhibits a port-wine color that turns dark on exposure to light. Urine and teeth may exhibit red fluorescence on exposure to ultraviolet radiation.

E. **Treatment** is limited to removal of HCB from the environment. No cases of PCT or other human toxicity have been noted during routine handling of HCB by vegetable spraymen, transporters of wastes containing HCB, or in the general public via the food chain.

Reference

1. Proudfoot A, et al. Paraquat poisoning: significance of plasma paraquat concentrations. *Lancet* 1979;2:330.
2. Singlemann E, Wetzel E, Adler G, et al. Erythrocyte membrane alterations as the basis of chlorate toxicity. *Toxicology* 1984;30:135.

Selected Readings

Bergner H, Constantinidis P, Martin J. Industrial pentachlophenol poisoning in Winnipeg. *Can Med Assoc J* 1965;92:448.

Berwick P. 2,4-Dichlorophenoxyacetic acid poisoning in man. *JAMA* 1970;214:1114.

Bismuth C, et al. Prognosis and treatment of paraquat poisoning: a review of 28 cases. *J Toxicol Clin Toxicol* 1982;19:461.

Casey PB, et al. Methemoglobinemia following ingestion of a monolinuron/paraquat herbicide (Gramonol). *Clin Toxicol* 1994;32:185.

Courtney K. Hexachlorobenzene: a review. *Environ Res* 1979;20:225.

Crome P. Paraquat poisoning 1986. *Lancet* 1986;1:333.

Flanagan RJ, et al. Alkaline diuresis for acute poisoning with chlorophenoxy herbicides and ioxynil. *Lancet* 1990;335:454.

Gaudreault P, Friedman P, Lovejoy F. Efficacy of activated charcoal and magnesium citrate in the treatment of oral paraquat intoxication. *Ann Emerg Med* 1985;14:123.

Hardell L, Johansson B, Alexson O. Epidemiological study of nasal and nasopharyngeal cancer and their relation to phenoxy acid or chlorophenol exposure. *Am J Ind Med* 1982;3:248.

Hassan A, Seligmann H, Bassan H. Intravascular hemolysis induced by pentachlorophenol. *BMJ* 1985;291:21.

Helliwell M, Nunn J. Mortality in sodium chlorate poisoning. *BMJ* 1979;1:1119.

Koizumi A, et al. Acute renal failure and maneb (manganous ethylenebis [dithiocarbamate]) exposure. *JAMA* 1979;242:2583.

Lambert J, et al. Skin lesions as a sign of subacute pentachlorophenol intoxication. *Acta Dermatol Venereol (Stockh)* 1986;66:170.

Lheureux P, et al. Survival in a case of massive paraquat ingestion. *Chest* 1995;107:285.

Okonek S, et al. Activated charcoal is as effective as Fuller's earth or bentonite in paraquat poisoning. *Klin Wochenschr* 1982;0:270.

Okonek S, et al. Two survivors of severe paraquat intoxication by "continuous hemperfusion." *Klin Wochenschr* 1979; 57:957.

Onyeama H, Oehme F. A literature review of paraquat toxicity. *Vet Hum Toxicol* 1984;6:494.

Park J, Darrien I, Prescott L. Pharmacokinetic studies in severe intoxication with 2,4-D and mecoprop. *Clin Toxicol* 1976;417:154

Parrot F, Bedry R, Favarel-Garrigues J. Glyphosate herbicide poisoning: use of a routine amino acid analyzer appears to be a rapid method for determining glyphosate and its metabolite in biological fluids. *Clin Toxicol* 1995;33:695.

Prescott L, Park J, Darrien I. Treatment of severe 2,4-D and mecoprop intoxication with alkaline diuresis. *Br J Clin Pharmacol* 1979;7:111.

Roberts H. Aplastic anemia and red cell aplasia due to pentachlorophenol. *South Med J* 1983;76:45.

Sawada Y, et al. Probable toxicity of surface-active agent in commercial herbicide containing glyphosate. *Lancet* 1988; 1:229.

Shelley W. Golf course dermatitis due to thirma fungicide. *JAMA* 1964;188:415.

Suskind R, Hertzberg V. Human health effects of 2,4,5-T and its toxic contaminants. *JAMA* 1984;251:2372.

Vanholder R, et al. Diquat intoxication—report of two cases and review of the literature. *Am J Med* 1980;70:1267.

Emergency Toxicology, Second Edition,
edited by Peter Viccellio.
Lippincott–Raven Publishers, Philadelphia © 1998.

27

Rodenticides

Scott M. Sasser

*Department of Emergency Medicine, Carolinas Medical Center,
Charlotte, North Carolina 28232-2861*

Rodenticides represent the modern human attempt to control an ever-burgeoning rodent population. Although early Chinese, Mediterranean, and Near Eastern literature contains references to rat and mouse overpopulation, the practice of using chemical rodenticides other than strychnine did not develop until the beginning of the 20th century. Still occasionally employed by professional exterminators, many of the early agents, such as arsenic oxide and zinc phosphide, have been abandoned due to serious human toxicity. The anticoagulant preparations, currently the most commonly used rodenticides, have proven safer. However, consequential human poisonings can and do occur with these preparations. The search for a rodenticide nontoxic to humans continues. Whereas rodenticide consumption in adults tends to be deliberate, most pediatric intoxications occur accidentally. Representing the vast majority of rodenticide ingestions, pediatric cases are often due to inappropriate storage of these agents in easily accessible areas. Rodenticides are less popular for suicide attempts but are occasionally used (1–3,29–31). The Federal Insecticide, Fungicide, and Rodenticide Act classifies rodenticides as high toxicity, moderate toxicity, or low toxicity, depending upon the LD_{50} of the agent (26) (see Table 27-1 below).

I. **Anticoagulants.** Initially discovered in the first half of the 20th century during the search for the cause of "Sweet Clover Disease" in cattle, the anticoagulant class contains the coumadin derivatives and the indanediones (19,21).

  A. **Properties**

    1. **Sources and forms: 4-hydroxycoumarin derivatives** include warfarin, difenacoum, bromadiolone, and brodifacoum. **Indanedione derivatives** include diphacinone, pindone, and chlorphacinone. Warfarin may be obtained in 0.025% and 0.5% concentrations. The long-acting anticoagulants **(LAAs),** which include the superwarfarin compounds brodifacoum and difenacoum and the indanedione derivative chlorphacinone, are marketed in 0.005% to 2% concentrations. Prolin consists of warfarin (0.025%) plus sulfaquinoxaline (0.025%), an antibiotic that eradicates vitamin K–producing organisms in the gut.

    2. **Physical and chemical properties.** Warfarin is a tasteless, odorless, colorless compound. Diphacinone forms yellow, odorless crystals, and pindone emits a moldy, acrid odor. All compounds are available in one or more of the following forms: bait packs, powders, concentrates, pellets, tablets, or capsules.

    3. **Mechanism of action/pathophysiology.** All compounds induce a coagulopathic state by inhibiting activation of the vitamin K–dependent clotting factors II, VII, IX,

and X (4,5). Specifically, they block two enzymes (2,3-epoxide reductase and quinone reductase) in the vitamin K–epoxide cycle, decreasing available reduced vitamin K necessary for gamma-carboxylation activation of these factors (Fig. 27-1) (4,5). Experimental evidence indicates that warfarin may also produce direct capillary damage via its benzalacetone moiety (6).

   a.   **Warfarin** rodenticides must be ingested repeatedly over a period of days to induce bleeding in both humans and rodents; thus, a one-time accidental ingestion usually poses no clinical problem. The need for repeated ingestion has made warfarin somewhat ineffective as a rodenticide. This combined with the emergence (via a single autosomal dominant gene) of warfarin-resistant rats, led to the development of more potent rodenticides, the long-acting anticoagulants (LAAS) or superwarfarins (21,26).

   b.   **Long-acting anticoagulants,** which have no medicinal use, can produce a prolonged coagulopathy in humans after a single ingestion. They are thought to bind more avidly than warfarin to a lipophilic site in the liver, thus exerting a prolonged effect. Extended coagulopathies have been reported with difenacoum, chlorphacine, and brodifacoum (1–3,7–10,).

4. **Pharmacology and pharmacokinetics.** Warfarin and LAAs are well absorbed from the gastrointestinal (GI) tract over a 2- to 3-h period. Case reports exist documenting percutaneous absorption as well (32). The elimination half-life of warfarin ranges from 37 to 42 h in humans, and that of brodifacoum has been measured at 156 h in rats and 120 days in dogs. The terminal half-life of brodifacoum has been reported to be anywhere from 20.3 to 62 days (24). Case reports of LAA poisonings in humans indicate effects may persist for up to 76 days (23), with two cases reporting prolonged anticoagulation (for 120 and 300 days, respectively).

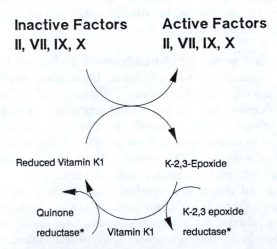

Inactive Factors
II, VII, IX, X

Active Factors
II, VII, IX, X

Reduced Vitamin K1

K-2,3-Epoxide

Quinone
reductase*

Vitamin K1

K-2,3 epoxide
reductase*

FIG. 27-1. Anticoagulant rodenticide–vitamin K interaction.
* = warfarin and long-acting anticoagulant sensitive.

Warfarin must either be consumed in massive quantities or eaten over 3 to 7 days to produce effects, whereas a single brodifacoum dose of 0.12 mg/kg has been sufficient to induce prolonged anticoagulation. On a molecular basis, brodifacoum is approximately 100 times more potent than warfarin. The volume of distribution (V_d) of warfarin is 0.1 to 0.17 L/kg, whereas that of brodifacoum has been estimated at 1.0 L/kg. High lipid solubility, resulting in hepatic concentration, a prolonged elimination half-life, a large V_d, and an enterohepatic recirculation contribute to this protracted effect. Both warfarin and the LAAs undergo hepatic conversion to inactive metabolites that are excreted in the urine.

B. Clinical presentation

1. **History.** Patients are typically asymptomatic unless their presentation is delayed. A history of ingesting rodenticides or consuming pellets found on the floor should alert the physician to a possible anticoagulant ingestion. Taking the time to examine any containers brought in by the patient, parents, or emergency medical service personnel can aid in substance identification. Quantify the amount and time of ingestion.

2. **Physical examination.** The physical exam may initially be normal. Over a period of several days, as the anticoagulant effects take place, patients may experience **spontaneous bleeding** from numerous sites. This includes gingival bleeding, spontaneous ecchymoses, gross hematuria, epistaxis, and GI hemorrhage. During the clinical examination, one should search for signs of occult hemorrhage, including guaiac testing and urinalysis for occult blood in the stool and urine. Often rodenticide baits contain a blue or green **dye** to facilitate detection of contamination of commercial food sources. Children who ingest these compounds may present with dye in and around the mouth. However, this finding has not proven to be predictive of a significant ingestion (11).

3. **Clinical course.**

    a. **Warfarin** rodenticides lengthen the prothrombin time initially by 24 h, with peak effects experienced at 36 to 72 h, after ingestion. Effects subside approximately 4 to 5 days after the final dose and are further diminished by vitamin K therapy (see **I.E.2.a**).

    b. The peak effects of the **LAA compounds** are not well documented in humans. In a comparative study of brodifacoum and warfarin in warfarin-sensitive rats, the two compounds produced an equal rate of deregulation of prothrombin complex activity (PCA), which is a concentrate of the vitamin K–dependent clotting factors (12). Human case reports indicate that patients poisoned with LAAs typically seek help 4 days or more after consumption and have marked coagulopathies at that time (1,7,9,23,24). Patients frequently bleed from numerous sites, requiring fresh frozen plasma and packed RBCs. Anticoagulation may persist for months, and it necessitates prolonged vitamin K_1 therapy and often hospitalization.

C. Differential diagnosis (Table 27-2)

D. Laboratory analysis

1. **General tests.** Check a baseline prothrombin time (PT), partial prothrombin time

(*Text continues on page 430*)

TABLE 27-1. *Management of specific rodenticide ingestions*

Name of rodenticide (LD$_{50}$ <50 mg/kg)	Physical characteristics	Toxic mechanism	Estimated fatal dose	Diagnostic presenting signs and symptoms	Onset	Antidote
Highly toxic (LD$_{50}$ <50 mg/kg)						
Thallium	White, crystalline, odorless, tasteless	Binds Na$^+$K$^+$ ATPase pump, causing membrane depolarization. Combines with mitochondrial sulf-hydryl groups interfering with oxidative phosphorylation. Riboflavin deficiency.	14 mg/kg	Anorexia, abdominal pain, diarrhea, paresthesias, myalgias, neuropathy, delirium, coma, convulsions, Delayed alopecia.	Delay of 12–24 h	Potassium chloride Prussian blue Activated charcoal (even with delayed presentation)
Sodium monofluoroacetate (Compound 1080), sodium fluoroacetate (SMFA), and fluoroacetamide (Compound 1081)	White, crystalline, odorless, tasteless, water-soluble	Converts fluoroacetate to fluorocitrate and interferes with the Krebs cycles especially in cardiac and CNS cells.	3–7 mg/kg (Compound 1080) 13–14 mg/kg (Compound 1081)	Seizures, coma, ST-T changes, tachycardia, PVCs, VT, VF	2–20 h	Experimental regimens: ? glycerol monoacetate; ? ethanol loading regimen Calcium for hypocalcemia
Strychnine	Bitter taste	Competitively inhibits spinal cord motoneuron postsynaptic glycine receptors	Children: 15 mg Adults: variable	Restlessness, anxiety, twitching, multiple "spinal convulsions" with extensor muscle contraction, intense pain, trismus, or facial grimacing known as "risus sardonicus," inability to swallow, skeletal fractures secondary to muscle contractions. Patient is conscious and muscles are relaxed between seizures.	10–20 min; 40 min to death	Quiet room, diazepam and/or phenobarbital i.v. ? Paralysis with nondepolarizing neuromuscular blocker Activated charcoal
Zinc phosphide	Heavy, gray crystalline powder; water-insoluble; "rotten fish," "phosphorus" odor. Normally used as 1% concentration	Releases phosphine on contact with water or in GI tract.	40 mg/kg	Phosphorus or fishy breath; black vomitus; GI and cardiovascular toxicity; pulmonary edema; agitation, coma, convulsions; hepatic/renal toxicity	Within hours; onset may be delayed with inhalation	Gastric lavage or emesis Calcium for hypocalcemia H2 antagonists (e.g., cimitidine, ranitidine)

Agent	Physical description	Mechanism	Toxic dose	Signs and symptoms	Onset	Treatment
Elemental phosphorus (yellow phosphorus)	Yellow, waxy paste; fat-soluble (water insoluble)	Causes local irritation and burns; later GI, liver, renal damage; interferes with clotting.	1 mg/kg (more toxic if dissolved in alcohol, fats, oils)	Skin burns, luminescent vomitus and stools with garlicky odor; hypocalcemia; jaundice; cardiac arrhythmias; coma; cardiac arrest	1–2 h	Lavage, activated charcoal, catharsis; Diazepam or barbiturates for seizures; Calcium for hypocalcemia
Arsenic	White crystalline powder	Combines with sulfhydryl groups and interferes with a variety of enzymatic reactions.	? 120 mg	Dysphagia, nausea and vomiting, bloody diarrhea with mucous shreds; seizures; cardiovascular collapse; garlic odor; altered mental status, late sensory/motor neuropathy	Symptoms 1 h; Death 1–24 h	Gastric lavage or emesis, charcoal; Dimercaprol or penicillamine until urine arsenic level is <50 µg/24 hr; Hemodialysis to remove chelated compound if renal failure
Vacor, N-3 pyridylmethyl-N-p-nitrophenyl urea	Yellow and resembles corn meal or yellow-green powder (House Mouse Tracking Powder) Odor peanuts	Interferes with nicotinamide metabolism in pancreas (destroying pancreatic beta cells), central and peripheral nervous systems, and heart.	Toxic dose: 5 mg/kg	Nausea and vomiting, severe abdominal pain; severe orthostatic hypotension; hyperglycemia with or without ketoacidosis; GI perforations; pneumonia; neuropathy	4–48 h	Emesis or lavage followed by activated charcoal; Nicotinamide (niacinamide) 500 mg i.v. or i.m. followed by 200 mg i.v. or i.m. q 2 h to total of 3 g in 24 h, 100 mg p.o. 3 times day for 2 weeks; Manage diabetic ketoacidosis with insulin
Moderately toxic (LD$_{50}$ 50–500 mg/kg) Alpha-naphthyl-thiourea (ANTU)	Odorless, slightly bitter, fine blue gray powder, water insoluble	Tracheobronchial hypersecretions, pulmonary edema.	>4 g/kg	Dyspnea; rales; cyanosis; hypothermia	?	Emesis or lavage followed by charcoal and catharsis
Chloralose, alpha-chloralose, chloralosane, glucochoral	Crystalline powder, soluble in glacial acetic acid and ether, soluble in water and petroleum ether	Metabolized to trichloroacetic acid and trichloroethanol.	?	Hypersecretion of respiratory tract; vomiting; vertigo; trembling; sense of inebriation; bilateral myoclonic disturbances resembling seizures; hyperthermia	1 h or more, but may appear in minutes	Airway management; Quiet room; Diazepam

(PTT), and CBC in all patients who ingest a superwarfarin compound. Type and cross-match blood for all patients requiring hospitalization. Further laboratory evaluations are dictated by other considered diagnoses (Table 27-1).

2. **Toxin-specific tests**

   a.   Hoffman et al. (7) recommended monitoring factor **VII-X complex levels** as sensitive indicators of toxicity. Because factor VII has a half-life of 4 to 6 h, declines in factor VII-X complex activity would be detected earlier than alterations in the PT and would thus permit earlier diagnosis. Also, following serial factor levels might assist in decisions regarding dosage and continuation of vitamin K therapy. In the case of a deliberate **brodifacoum overdose,** the authors noted significant depressions of factor VII-X complex activity (levels of approximately 20% to 30% activity) occurring simultaneously with normal PTs. Thus, monitoring PT levels alone might erroneously result in inadequate vitamin K treatment.

   b.   **Warfarin** may be detected at blood levels of 0.6 to 3.1 µg/m by gas chromatography in patients on long-term therapy. High-performance liquid chromatography (HPLC) combined with ultraviolet and fluorescent detection can quantitate serum concentrations down to 3 to 12 ng/m (fluorescence) and 20 to 75 ng/mL (ultraviolet) for some superwarfarin rodenticides, including chlorophacinone, brodifacuom, and difenacoum (33). Hollinger et al. (24) suggest that if plasma brodifacuom levels are found to correlate between individuals, they may prove of benefit in planning duration of therapy.

   c.   **Range of toxicity**

      (1)   Human consumption of **warfarin** rodenticide 1 to 2 mg/kg/day for 6 days has produced a significant coagulopathy (13). Accordingly, a 70-kg person would need to consume 0.6 to 1.2 lb of a 0.025% warfarin bait per day for 6 days to achieve these amounts.

      (2)   Data from human consumption of **LAA compounds** varies. Significant toxicities have been reported with ingestions of 250 and 625 mg of chlorphacinone, 7.5 mg of brodifacoum (0.12 mg/kg), and 500 mg of difenacoum. Bachmann and Sullivan (14) induced prolonged bleeding in rats with brodifacoum 0.2 mg/kg, whereas no effect was obtained with 0.1 mg/kg.

E. **Management**

   1. **General measures.** GI decontamination procedures should be initiated in all patients with a history of LAA ingestion or with a recent (within 3 h) ingestion of warfarin. Basic treatment includes activated charcoal and a cathartic. Multiple-dose activated charcoal (MAC) is indicated for significant LAA ingestions. Ipecac or gastric lavage may be indicated for recent (within 2 to 3 h) ingestions of any LAA compounds or for consumption of more than 1.5 lb of 0.025% warfarin bait (corresponds to warfarin of more than 0.025 mg/kg). A baseline PT should be obtained in all patients seen in a hospital setting. It should be noted that at least one group of authors are recommending that there be no decontamination procedures for one time ingestions of plain warfarin-related or superwarfarin-related rodenti-

cides in the absence of clinical symptoms. This view is based upon AAPCC and literature data which shows few serious illnesses and infrequent deaths, despite a large number of ingestions (19).

2. **Toxin-specific measures**
   a. **Vitamin K**
      (1) **Vitamin K₁** (phylloquinone, or Aquamephyton) should be administered only to those patients who have a demonstrably prolonged PT. Administering a one-time dose to patients prior to emergency department discharge only delays the onset of coagulopathy in seriously poisoned patients and lengthens the follow-up period.
      (2) **Vitamins K₂, K₃, and K₄ cannot be used.** Vitamin K₂ is not commercially available. Vitamins K₃ and K₄ are provitamins that are converted slowly to their active forms. The use of K₃ has been associated with skin and respiratory tract irritation and hemolytic anemia.
      (3) Initial doses for an adult are 5 to 10 mg s.q. and for children 1 to 5 mg s.q. Large doses of 40 mg/kg/day in 3 to 5 divided doses may be required for weeks to months to treat superwarfarin poisonings.
         (a) Intravenous vitamin K₁ has produced anaphylactoid reactions and should be used only in cases of life-threatening hemorrhage where absorption by other routes may be erratic (15).
         (b) Final dosages should be titrated to achieve normal coagulation parameters. Depressed coagulation factors begin to normalize after 4 to 6 h.
   b. **Prothrombin complex** (PCA) has been used in one reported case, but the PT began to lengthen within 9 h after the last dose. Given the infectious risk, this treatment should be reserved for severe bleeding complications, such as severe GI hemorrhage and intracranial bleeding. Because the effect of vitamin K₁ does not begin for 4 to 6 h and may not peak for 24 to 36 h, fresh frozen plasma (initial dose 10 to 20 mL/kg) should be given initially for bleeding control, with packed RBCs administered as needed. Monitor the PT to determine the amount of fresh frozen plasma needed.
3. **Complicating factors and controversies.** One animal study and several case reports have suggested that daily phenobarbital administration may induce hepatic microsomal activity and thus hasten the metabolism of the long-acting anticoagulant compounds (9,10,14). No human studies exist to support this treatment, and others speculate that sedating an anticoagulated patient may be dangerous.

F. **Indications for hospitalization**
   1. Clinical or laboratory evidence of coagulopathy
   2. Suicidal ideations
G. **Disposition and follow-up.** In cases of accidental ingestion of any of the above LAA compounds, patients should have repeat PTs at 24 and 48 h after exposure and should be given strict instructions to return to the emergency department sooner if they develop any signs of bleeding. For significant accidental or intentional overdose, patients should be hospitalized for close monitoring of the PT or measured clotting factors for a minimum

of 48 h. Once the coagulopathy is controlled with vitamin K_1, patients can be managed with outpatient oral K_1 therapy unless psychiatric considerations or patient noncompliance mandate continued admission.

II. **Other rodenticides.** There exists a number of other compounds, restricted for use by professional exterminators, that are now infrequently used and seldom implicated in human poisonings.

   A. **Thallium.** Although prohibited since 1965 for pesticide use in the United States, this toxic heavy metal is still used in many industrial processes, homeopathic remedies, and as a rodenticide in many developing countries (20).

      1. **Toxic mechanisms of action**

         a. Substitution for potassium, with higher affinity, for the sodium-potassium ATPase pump, resulting in membrane depolarization.

         b. Via binding to sulfhydryl groups and interfering with sulfhydryl-containing enzymes. This involves the mitochondrial respiratory chain, thus interfering with oxidative phosphorylation.

         c. Thallium binds with riboflavin and riboflavin cofactors, leading to riboflavin deficiency.

         d. Interfering with protein synthesis, and causing increased intracellular calcium (20).

      2. **Initial symptoms** include gastroenteritis, peripheral neuropathy, paresis of the extremities, respiratory depression, coma, psychosis and death. Alopecia is characteristically seen 2 to 3 weeks after ingestion. **Mee's lines,** single white lines across the nails secondary to nail dystrophy, are a late finding (3 to 4 weeks postintoxication).

      3. **Levels** can be measured in the hair, urine, and blood.

      4. **Treatment** includes activated charcoal (even in cases of delayed presentation), slow intravenous potassium chloride infusions, and oral Prussian blue (potassium ferric cyanoferrate II); the latter absorbs thallium, interrupting enterohepatic circulation and leading to fecal elimination. When used by themselves, chelating agents have not proven helpful; however, initial trials with chelator-Prussian blue combinations have proven encouraging (20,26).

   B. **Sodium monofluoroacetate** (compound 1080) and **fluoroacetamide** (compound 1081) are potent rodenticides that have found new uses as coyote, rabbit, and opossum poisons (34).

      1. **Toxic mechanism of action.** Transformation of fluoroacetate to fluorocitrate. This action results in the substitution for citrate in the Krebs cycle, thus blocking cellular energy production.

      2. **Initial symptoms** are predominantly neurological and cardiovascular and include dysrhythmias, seizures, and death (26). Symptoms usually occur within 1 to 2 h of ingestion. Hypocalcemia may occur.

      3. **Levels** are detectable with gas chromatography (34).

      4. **Treatment** is supportive with vigorous gastric decontamination and MDC. The efficacies of two controversial therapies, glycerol monoacetate and ethanol, remain unproven in humans (16,17).

C. Strychnine. Initially introduced as a rodenticide in 16th century Germany, strychnine continues to be used commercially today.

1. **Toxic mechanism of action.** Strychnine competitively blocks ventral horn motoneuron postsynaptic receptor sites for glycine, the major inhibitory neurotransmitter in the spinal cord.

2. **Initial symptoms** typically appear within 30 min following exposure and include nausea and vomiting, diaphoresis, blurred vision, and "spinal convulsions"— severe symmetric extensor muscle spasms during which **patients are conscious.** Diaphragmatic, thoracic, and abdominal muscle contractions can compromise respiration, and the generalized muscle activity may cause hyperthermia, lactic acidosis, rhabdomyolysis, and acute renal failure. The disease closely resembles tetanus, but the latter develops more slowly.

3. **Levels** may be obtained (to as low as 0.01 ppm) by thin-layer chromatography and HPLC using urine and gastric aspirates (25).

4. **Treatment.** Emesis is contraindicated in the patient with potential for development of seizures. Gastric decontamination is recommended; however, the possibility of inducing seizure activity remains. Airway and seizure control may need to be instituted prior to decontamination procedures. Other treatment measures include supportive care, intravenous diazepam, phenobarbital, and potentially nondepolarizing paralytic agents to control the muscular contractions (25,26).

D. Zinc phosphide. A potent rodenticide with a disagreeable, often described as "fishy" odor, may be absorbed by inhalation, via broken skin, and by oral ingestion.

1. **Toxic mechanism of action.** On contact with water or weak acids, phosphine gas and free radicals are released.

2. **Symptoms.** Some patients succumb to pulmonary edema within a few hours in some patients; however, most patients die within 30 h of exposure secondary to cardiovascular collapse due to a direct myocardial toxic effect.

3. **Treatment.** GI decontamination should be performed with aspiration of gastric contents followed by installation of milk, starch or lavage with 3% to 5% sodium bicarbonate (to neutralize gastric acid) (18). Calcium disodium ethylenediaminetetraacetate (EDTA) has been utilized by some investigators (26). The role of zinc in the compound's toxicity remains unclear.

E. Arsenic is present in the inorganic form in several rodenticides.

1. **Toxic mechanism of action.** By binding to sulfhydryl groups, arsenic interferes with a number of enzymatic reactions.

2. **Symptoms.** With **acute exposures,** initial GI symptoms are followed by cardiovascular collapse, cerebral edema, seizures, and possibly death due to circulatory failure. Delayed sequelae include peripheral neuropathy, jaundice, and renal failure. **Chronic poisoning** may be more difficult to diagnose. Abdominal pain, diarrhea, skin hyperpigmentation and hyperkeratosis, and a symmetric sensory neuropathy are often seen.

3. **Treatment** includes the usual decontamination measures and chelation therapy with **dimercaprol** (British anti-Lewisite, or BAL), preferably, or D-penicillamine until the 24-h urinary excretion of arsenic does not exceed 50 µg/L. Hemodialysis to remove the chelated compound may be necessary if renal failure ensues.

TABLE 27-2. *Differential diagnosis of anticoagulant rodenticide ingestion*

Inherited disorders
  Hemophilia A and B
  Von Willebrand's disease
  Factor deficiencies: II, VII, X, fibrinogen
Acquired disorders
  Medicinal coumadin overdose
  Heparin use
  Vitamin K deficiency: malnutrition, malabsorption
  Hepatic insufficiency
  Disseminated intravascular coagulation
  Circulating anticoagulants, e.g., lupus anticoagulant, inhibitors of clotting factors

F. **Vacor,** a compound that interferes with nicotinamide metabolism, produced severe human toxicity by destroying pancreatic beta cells and was withdrawn from the U.S. market in 1978. Storage of old compound may still result in toxic cases, the latest being reported in 1986. **Treatment** includes supportive therapy and niacinamide (initial dose for adults is 500 mg i.v. or i.m.; for small children, it is one-half the adult dose).

G. **Red squill** contains several compounds with chemical and pharmacologic properties similar to those of the digitalis glycosides. Because of its emetic properties, poor GI absorption, and decreased potency (compared to that of digitalis), red squill has seldom been associated with human toxicity.

H. Newer compounds include **bromethalin** and **cholecalciferol,** which to date have not been implicated in human poisonings.

  1. In rodents, bromethalin uncouples oxidative phosphorylation and reduces nerve impulse transmission, leading to decreased cellular energy production, tremor, cerebral edema, convulsions, coma, and death. Dogs and cats intoxicated with bromethalin have developed CNS excitation, seizures, and death. Bromethalin may be detected in tissues using gas chromatography with electron capture (27,28).

  2. Initially made available in 1985, cholecalciferol (vitamin D_3) potentially poses the threat of vitamin D intoxication if ingested. Measurement of serum 25-hydroxy cholecalciferol may be helpful. Treatment is aimed at the resulting hypercalcemia (35,36). Each pellet contains 2,308 units of vitamin D_3. The estimated LD_{50} for a 10-kg child is 338 pellets.

I. Details about these rodenticides and other compounds less frequently used are listed in Table 27-1.

References

1. Chong L, Chau W, Ho C. A case of "superwarfarin" rodenticide poisoning. *Scand J Hematol* 1986;35:314–315.
2. Barlow AM, Gay AL, Park BK. Difenacoum (neosorexa) poisoning. *BMJ* 1982;285:341, 541.
3. Murdoch DA. Prolonged anticoagulation in chlorphacinone poisoning [Letter]. *Lancet* 1983;1:355–356.
4. Olson R. Vitamin K. In: Colman RW, et al., eds. *Hemostasis and thrombosis.* Philadelphia: Lippincott, 1972.
5. Fasco MJ, Hildebrandt EF, Suttie JW. Evidence that warfarin anticoagulant action involves two distinct reductase activities. *J Biol Chem* 1982;257:11210–11212.
6. Ellenhorn MJ, Barceloux DG. *Medical toxicology: diagnosis and treatment of human poisoning.* New York: Elsevier Science, 1988.

7. Hoffman RS, Smilkstein MJ, Goldfrank LR. Evaluation of coagulation factor abnormalities in long-acting anticoagulant overdose. *J Toxicol Clin Toxicol* 1988;26:233–248.

8. Jones EC, Gershon GH, Sheldon NC. Prolonged anticoagulation in rat poisoning. *JAMA* 1984;252:3005–3007.

9. Lipton RA, Klass EM. Human ingestion of a "superwarfarin" rodenticide resulting in a prolonged anticoagulant effect. *JAMA* 1984;252:3004–3005.

10. Burucoa C, et al. Chlorophacinone intoxication: a biological and toxicological study. *J Toxicol Clin Toxicol* 1989; 27:1–2, 79–89.

11. Smolinske SC, et al. Superwarfarin poisoning in children: a prospective study. *Pediatrics* 1989;84:490–494.

12. Leck JB, Park BK. A comparative study of the effects of warfarin and brodifacoum on the relationship between vitamin K_1 metabolism and clotting factor activity in warfarin-susceptible and warfarin-resistant rats. *Biochem Pharmacol* 1981;30:123–128.

13. Holmes RW, Love J. Suicide attempt with warfarin, a bishydroxycoumarin-like rodenticide. *JAMA* 1952;148:935.

14. Bachmann KA, Sullivan TJ. Dispositional and pharmacodynamic characteristics of brodifacoum in warfarin-sensitive rats. *Pharmacology* 1983;27:281–288.

15. Barash P, Kitahata LM, Mandel S. Acute cardiovascular collapse after intravenous phytonadione. *Anesth Analg Curr Res* 1976;55:304–306.

16. Egekeze JO, Oehme FW. Sodium monofluoroacetate (SMFA, Compound 1080): a literature review. *Vet Hum Toxicol* 1979;21:411–416.

17. Hutchens JO, et al. The effect of ethanol and various metabolites on fluoroacetate poisoning. *J Pharmacol Ther* 1949;95:62.

18. Flomenbaum NE, et al. Rodenticides. In: Goldfrank LR, et al., eds. *Goldfrank's toxicologic emergencies.* Norwalk, CT: Appleton & Lange, 1990:702.

19. Burgess JL, Robertson WO. Washington's experience and recommendations RE: anticoagulant rodenticides. *Vet Hum Toxicol* 1995;3(4)7:362.

20. Mulkey JP, Oehme FW. A review of thallium toxicity. *Vet Hum Toxicol* 1993;35:445–453.

21. Mack RB. Not all rats have four legs: superwarfarin poisoning. *NC Med J* 1994;55:554–556.

22. Travis SF, et al. Spontaneous hemorrhage associated with accidental brodifacuom poisoning in a child. *J Pediatr* 1993;122:982–984.

23. Kruse JA, Carlson RW. Fatal rodenticide poisoning with brodifacuom. *Ann Emerg Med* 1992;21:331–336.

24. Hollinger BR, Pastoor TP. Case management and plasma half-life in a case of brodifacuom poisoning. *Arch Intern Med* 1993;153:1925–1928.

25. Smith BA. Stychnine poisoning. *J Emerg Med* 1990;8:321–325.

26. Flomenbaum NE. Rodenticides. In: Goldfrank LR, et al., eds. *Goldfrank's toxicologic emergencies.* 5th ed. Norwalk, CT: Appleton & Lange, 1994:1127.

27. Dorman DC, et al. Diagnosis of bromethalin toxicosis in the dog. *J Vet Diagn Invest* 1990;2:123–128.

28. Dorman DC, et al. Neuropathologic findings of bromethalin toxicosis in the cat. *Vet Pathol* 1992;29:139–144.

29. Litovitz TL, et al. 1995 annual report of the American Association of Poison Control Centers toxic exposure surveillance system. *Am J Emerg Med* 1996;14:487–537.

30. Litovitz TL, et al. 1994 annual report of the American Association of Poison Control Centers toxic exposure sureveillance system. *Am J Emerg Med* 1995;13:551–597.

31. Litovitz TL, et al. 1993 annual report of the American Association of Poison Control Centers toxic exposure sureveillance system. *Am J Emerg Med* 1994:12:546–584.

32. Abell TL, et al. Cutaneous exposure to warfarin-like anticoagulant causing an intracerebral hemorrhage: a case report. *Clin Toxicol* 1994;32:69–73.

33. Kuijpers EA, et al. A method for the simultaneous identification and quantification of five superwarfarin rodenticides in human serum. *J Anal Toxicol* 1995;19:557–562.

34. Allender WJ. Determination of sodium "fluoroacetate" (compound 1080) in biological tissues. *J Anal Toxicol* 1990; 14:45–49.

35. Scheftel J, et al. Elevated 25-hydroxy and normal 1,25-dihydroxy chleocalciferol serum concentrations in a successfully treated case of vitamin D3 toxicosis in a dog. *Vet Hum Toxicol* 1991;33:345.

36. Talcott PA, et al. Accidental ingestion of a chleocalciferol-containing rodent bait in a dog. *Vet Hum Toxicol* 1991; 33:252–256.

Selected Readings

Boyd RE, et al. Strychnine poisoning: recovery from profound lactic acidosis, hyperthermia, and rhabdomyolysis. *Am J Med* 1983;74:507.

Gehring PJ, Hammond PB. The interrelationship between thallium and potassium in animals. *J Pharmacol Exp Ther* 1967;155:187–201.

Gordon AM, Richards DW. Strychnine intoxication. *JACEP* 1979;8:520–522.

Hadler MR, Shadbolt RS. Novel 4-hydroxycoumarin anticoagulants active against resistant rats. *Nature* 1975;253:275–277.

Heath A, et al. Thallium poisoning—toxin elimination and therapy in three cases. *J Toxicol Clin Toxicol* 1983;20:451–463.

Kumer K, Nwangwu PU. Clinical toxicology of warfarin from commercial rodenticides: symptoms, diagnosis and management. *Clin Toxicol Consult* 1981;3:23.

Lisella FS, Long KR, Scott HG. Toxicology of rodenticides and their relation to human health. *J Environ Health* 1970; 33:137.

Morgan B, Tomaszewski C, Rotker I. Spontaneous hemopentoneum from brodifacoum overdose. *Am J Emerg Med* 1996; 14:656–659.

Peters R, Wakelin RW. Biochemistry of fluoroacetate poisoning: the isolation and some properties of the fluorotricarboxylic acid inhibitor of citrate metabolism. *Proc R Soc Lond (Biol)* 1953;140:497.

Saddique A. Thallium poisoning: a review. *Vet Hum Toxicol* 1983;25:16–22.

Emergency Toxicology, Second Edition,
edited by Peter Viccellio.
Lippincott–Raven Publishers, Philadelphia © 1998.

28

Toxicity of Household Products

Howard C. Mofenson and Thomas R. Caraccio

Department of Emergency Medicine, Long Island Regional Poison Control Center, Winthrop University Hospital, Mineola, New York 11501

INTRODUCTION

I. Household product toxicity most often involves childhood ingestions. The ingestion of a household product by a child is the most common pediatric medical emergency (1–3). A poison control center (PCC) plays an important role in household poisonings. Most household products are of relatively low toxicity, with the exception of products that contain ethanol or other alcohols in high concentrations, drain and oven cleaners, phenol disinfectants, toilet bowl cleaners, and some hair cosmetics and artificial-fingernail products (2,3). The management of household product ingestions consists of calling the regional PCC for proper identification of the product ingredients and offering first aid advice. Emesis induction and emergency department (ED) visits and hospitalization are often unnecessary unless there are mitigating circumstances.

II. It has been estimated that **over a million children a year** will be exposed to potentially poisonous substances. About 60% will be under the age of 6 years. In 1961, 450 children age 1 to 5 years died of poisoning annually; in the 1990s, these deaths were reduced approximately to 50 a year (2,3).

III. During the past few decades, PCCs have reduced the number of **ED visits and served as medical cost containment.** For example, the Long Island Regional PCC has reduced ED visits from 12% of our calls involving children under 6 years of age in 1969 to approximately 8% in 1995, despite a 50% increase in exposures in this age group of aprroximately 13,000 exposures. Our center managed over 18,000 patients at home in 1995. These patients were spared unnecessary expenses of visits to emergency facilities. The total cost savings of our center last year was estimated at almost $3,600,000 based on an average emergency room (ER) fee of $200. This is accomplished by offering telephone information and first aid advice with follow-up.

IV. Other regional poisoning control centers report similar experiences. **In Massachusetts**, an estimated 6,500 unnecessary visits to EDs secondary to ingestions occur annually. **In Louisiana**, where a PCC closed, self-referral to health care facilities increased fourfold with annual cost attributable to unnecessary outpatient visits estimated to be $1.4 million (4). In addition, there are the human health complications and the financial expense of unnecessary delays in seeking early medical care for poisonings when a PCC is not readily available. For example, a liver transplant for patient with a delay in seeking medical care for acetaminophen poisoning resulted in $250,000 initial medical costs, whereas appropriate hospital antidotal treatment would have cost $2,500.

INCIDENCE

I. Hundreds of new household products are introduced to the marketplace annually. Most household products are associated with fastidiousness and hygiene. Table 28-1 contains a list of the **10 most common categories** of substances responsible for household exposures. These 10 categories of agents accounted for 40% of the exposures reported to the American Association of Poison Control Centers National Database in 1994 (6). Table 28-2 lists the names of common dangerous household products. Pharmaceuticals are the leading substances ingested in overdose. They will be discussed individually.

II. **Data collected by the American Association of Poison Control Centers (AAPCC) Toxic Exposure Surveillance System (Tess) in 1994** (4) is used in the introduction of many of the household products to offer the reader the national experience. In certain instances, the statistics of our PCC experience has been added to show correlation or discrepancy of local statistics from the national.

A. The **total number of exposures 1,926,438** documented by the AAPCC represents an estimated 83% of the human exposures reported to PCCs.

B. **Ages.** Approximately 1,036,967 (62%) exposure were under 6 years (64.3% were nontoxic), 121,512 (6.3%) between 6 to 12 years, 137,450 (7.1%) between 13 to 19 years, 424,512 (22.1%) between 20 to 59 years, 94,473 (3.9%) between 60 to 89 years, and 1,871 (0.1%) more than 90 years. Children younger than 3 years were involved in 40% of reported exposures.

C. **Site of care.** The majority (2.1% of the exposures reported were managed in a non-health care facility (usually at the home site); treatment in a health care facility occurred in 23.8%. Of the exposures managed in a health care facility, 55.4% were treated and released, 12.4% were admitted for critical care, and 7.2% were admitted for noncritical care.

D. **Fatalities.** There were 766 deaths reported; 75 were in the pediatric age category (under 19 years of age). Young children younger than 6 years of age accounted for 28 of fatalities due to poisonings.

E. The **terms** "minor," "moderate," and "major" outcomes are used in the AAPCC statistics.

TABLE 28-1. *Top 10 categories of household exposures*

Category	Number	Most common substance
Cleaners	196,921	Bleaches
Cosmetics and personal products	162,807	Perfumes, cologne, after shave
Plants	103,616	GI irritants
Hydrocarbons	64,634	Gasoline
Foreign bodies: toys/miscellaneous	70,891	Desiccants
Insecticides and pesticides	61,882	Organophosphates and carbamates
Arts and crafts supplies	36,107	Magic Markers, ink
Paints/lacquers/varnishes, strippers	24,872	Latex paint
Deodorizers	17,902	Air fresheners
Rodenticides	16,478	Anticoagulants (includes long-acting types)

Data from ref. 4: 1,926,438 human cases reported by 65 poison centers during 1994.

TABLE 28-2. *Potentially common dangerous household products*

Product	Potentially hazardous agent
Disinfectants	Cresol, phenol, hexachlorophene
Cleaning agents and solvents	
Bleaches	Sodium hypochlorite, oxalic acid, perborates, and boric acid
Window cleaner	Ammonia
Carpet cleaner	Ammonia, turpentine, naphthalene, 1,1,1 trichloroethane
Oven cleaner	Potassium and sodium hydroxide
Dry cleaning fluids and spot removers	1,1,1 trichloroethane, petroleum distillates, perchloroethylene
Paints and varnishes	Turpentine, xylene, toluene, methanol, methylene chloride, acetone
Emissions from heating or cooling devices	Nitrogen oxide
Gas stove pilot light	Carbon monoxide
Indoor-use charcoal grill	Freon
Leak from refrigerator or air conditioner	

Modified from ref. 381.

1. **Minor** outcome means mild effects (skin or mucous membrane irritation, GI symptoms, drowsiness, first degree burn, tachycardia without hypotension, transient cough) that resolved rapidly without treatment.

2. **Moderate** outcome indicates more prolonged, more systemic effects (corneal abrasion, acid-base disturbance, high fever, disorientation, hypotension) that resolved rapidly to treatment.

3. **Major** outcome indicates life-threatening effects or residual disability or disfigurement (repeated seizures, required intubation, ventricular tachycardia with hypotension, cardiac or respiratory arrest, esophageal stricture, and disseminated intravascular coagulation).

4. **Death** indicates the patient died as a direct result of exposure or as a direct complication of the exposure.

III. **Over 900,000 patients are treated in EDs annually.** Studies suggest that 30% of poisoning between 1 to 6 years are **repeated poisonings** (5,6,7). Single-agent poisonings are most common in early childhood, whereas intentional ingestions in adolescents and adults often involve several drugs. Children's ingestions of household products are often nontoxic, whereas adolescent and adult ingestion often require intensive care.

IV. The concept of a **"hazard factor"** was recently introduced for childhood ingestions. It consists of assigning a score to each substance based on the frequency the substance was involved and the severity of toxicity (6). The three most commonly implicated **categories** (30.4%) were **cosmetics or personal care products, cleaning agents, and plants.** Of the 10 substances commonly ingested, only two—hydrocarbons and insecticides—have high hazard factors (6).

V. The **most dangerous areas in the home** for the ingestion of household products are the kitchen (50%), bathroom (20%), and bedroom (10%). Studies conducted during the late 1970s indicate that household product ingestions made up over 70% of calls reported by PCCs (1).

VI. The **formulations of many household products** change; therefore, the date of the product or the date of purchase is important when establishing the identity of the toxic agent. Household products often contain more than one ingredient in a single product, and the first aid for one ingredient may be contraindicated with the other; therefore, the experienced judgment of a regional PCC or toxicologist is often necessary (7).

VII. Suspicion of poison in a child. Children should be suspected of being poisoned under the following circumstances (7).

   A. There is a history of ingestion of an inedible substance.

   B. The child is in the at-risk age group (1 to 5 years).

   C. The child has an abrupt onset of an illness, particularly nonfebrile or complex febrile convulsion or coma without any explanation.

   D. The illness involves multiple systems without an apparent explanation.

   E. There is an unusual odor from the mouth, or there are stains on the clothing or stains or burns on the skin around the mouth or the oral mucosa.

   F. Unexplained hematemesis is present.

VIII. Unlabeled container. Ingestion of a product from an unlabeled container or one on which the label is illegible is a frustrating experience. In most cases, immediate induction of emesis, use of activated charcoal, or both should be considered when significant quantities are ingested unless they are contraindicated. Contraindications to these include the following.

   A. Ingestion of a **caustic or corrosive.** This event can be determined by the symptoms of dysphagia, drooling, or burns on the skin or in the mouth. The caretaker may also apply the material to a small area of his/her skin; if the material produces irritation, one may assume it may have the properties to produce esophageal mucosal damage.

   B. Ingestion of **petroleum distillates,** as indicated by the odor, usually does not require GI decontamination procedures.

   C. **Risk of aspiration** by loss of the protective reflexes of the upper airway, as in coma, convulsions, or necrologic disorders that impair the protective reflexes, should not have GI decontamination.

   D. In all other circumstances, it is safe to carry out GI decontamination, although it may be unnecessary.

IX. "Accidental" ingestions

   A. A survey of PCCs suggested that "accidental" ingestions in children more than 5 years of age are often not "accidental" but intentional, and they deserve investigation as to the motivation for the act (7). This type of event may actually be a "cry for help," indicating an intolerable home situation. Psychological factors may also play a role in some ingestions by children even younger than 5 years (8,9).

   B. **"Accidental" ingestions** in children under 1 year of age should undergo adequate investigation, as it is unlikely that the developmental skills under 1 year of age would be sufficient to accomplish many "accidental" ingestions. In 1994, there were over 3 million reports of child abuse or neglect in the United States, of which 1 million were substantiated. That year 1,300 victims died. The **"chemical" maltreatment** of young children appears to be much more prevalent than was once believed.

      1. **"Munchausen by proxy" syndrome,** or the administration of chemicals and drugs to children to produce iatrogenic disease by caretakers, has been reported with increasing frequency in the literature (10). **"Munchausen by proxy" syndrome** has **four features.**

      a. Illness simulated by parent or caretaker

      b. Repeated presentation of child for medical care that results in multiple procedures

      c. Denial by parent or caretaker of knowledge about cause of illness

      d. Abatement of symptoms when the child is separated from parent or caretaker

  C. "Accidental" ingestions should be **investigated** under the following circumstances:

    1. Age more than 5 years may be a "cry for help"

    2. More than one episode of "accidental" ingestion

    3. Bizarre clinical manifestations that suggest "Munchausen by proxy" syndrome

    4. "Accidental" ingestions by a child less than 1 year of age

  D. Necropsy child abuse cases should include toxicologic analysis.

X. **Signal words** on containers of insecticides, fungicides, and rodenticide are mandatory. They alert the consumer and health care professionals to potential toxicity of products. Table 28-3 indicates the suggested use of signal words for household products (11–13).

XI. **Prevention of children household ingestions.** The ultimate goal is prevention of ingestions and poisonings by educating consumers and caretakers (parents, grandparents, babysitters) about childproofing the child's environment and the proper handling of toxic products. Poison control information specialists should educate callers. ED and hospital personnel should educate parents and patients upon discharge about poison prevention. A list of poison prevention instructions appears in Table 28-4.

XII. **Nontoxic ingestion** (11–13) (see Chapter 4 and Table 28-5). The criteria for nontoxic ingestion include the following.

  A. Absolute identification of the product.

  B. Absolute assurance that a single product was ingested.

  C. Assurance that there is no signal word on the container.

  D. A good approximation of the amount ingested.

  E. The ability to call back at frequent intervals to determine if symptoms have developed.

HOUSEHOLD PRODUCTS

  I. **Cleaning agents**

    A. **Bleaches.** Household bleach commonly contains sodium hypochlorite in concentrations less than 8% (often 5.25%). Industrial and commercial products contain hypochlorite in concentrations more than 10%. Other substances used as bleach in the home include hydrogen peroxide, borate, and oxalic acid and have different concentrations and pH, and may produce toxicity (3). In 1994, the AAPCC reported 47,306 exposures to household bleach, with 2,148 moderate outcomes, 41 major outcomes, and two deaths (4).

TABLE 28-3. *Suggested use of signal words for household products*

Category (Gosselin)	Signal words on label	LD_{50} (mg/kg)	Household measures
1–2	None	5,000	≥1 pint
3	Caution	500–5,000	1 oz to 1 pint
4	Warning	50–500	1 tsp to 1 oz
5–6	Danger	<50	1 tsp to taste

Based on the Federal Insecticide and Fungicide Act of 1960.

TABLE 28-4. *List of suggestions to caretakers for prevention of childhood poisoning*

Advocating child-resistant containers and refastening immediately after use.
Keeping products in their original containers and storing food, chemicals, and medications separately.
Using safety catches on all storage areas.
Purchasing the least toxic product to do the job and in the smallest amount possible.
Never taking or giving medicine in front of children who are not the patients; never referring to medicine as "candy."
Purchasing a bottle of ipecac syrup.
Keeping medication and chemicals out of sight and out of reach.

1. **Hypochlorite** is a common household bleach which usually contains 3% to 8% sodium hypochlorite and has a pH of about 10.5 to 11. **Calcium hypochlorite** (48% in Minute Mildew Remover, Tilex Instant Mildew Remover sodium hypochlorite 5% with sodium hydroxide 1%), household mildew remover is more caustic than ordinary household bleach. **Swimming pool disinfectants** may contain up to 20% hypochlorite and are more caustic. There were 45,311 exposures reported to AAPCC in 1994, with 2,080 moderate outcomes, 39 major outcomes, and two deaths (4).

   a. **Toxicity:** The local effect of hypochlorites is due to the oxidizing caustic action of available chlorine. They have the potential to injure the oropharynx, esophagus, stomach and eyes, producing clinical states that vary from mild irritation to corrosion depending on amount ingested, the physical form, the duration of exposure, the pH and the concentration of the product. In the stomach it forms hydrochlorous acid.

   b. **Sodium hypochlorite** (Carrel-Dakin solution, hydrochlorous acid, NaOCl) is a green-yellow solution with characteristic "swimming pool" odor.

      (1) Sodium hypochlorite solutions are manufactured by adding chlorine gas to 12% to 15% sodium hydroxide until the solution is neutral. **Household laundry bleach** (Clorox, Dazzle) is usually 5.25% sodium hypochlorite, pH 10.5 to 11, free sodium hydroxide 0.005% to 0.015% with 5% free chlorine. Most household hypochlorite bleaches contain less than 8% and rarely produce serious damage.

      (2) **Medically significant** are caustics in concentrations over 10%, but even 20% concentrations rarely produce strictures (16). Granular bleaches are potentially more toxic because they are more concentrated.

      (3) **Ingestion** of general household strength hypochlorite bleach rarely produces esophageal burns (14,15,16). The signs of possible esophageal damage include difficulty in swallowing, drooling, burns in the mouth or oropharynx, pain in mouth, throat, chest, or abdomen. Stricture or perforation is unlikely although 2 cases of strictures were reported with high concentrations (14). Sodium hypochlorite in high concentrations may cause hypotension, bradycardia, and cardiac arrest. Massive ingestions may produce hyperchloremic metabolic acidosis (18,19).

TABLE 28-5. *Usually nontoxic ingestion, unless ingested in very large quantity.*
(LI Regional Poison Center 1996)

A&D ointment	Glitter glues and pastes
Abrasives	Glowstick/jewelry
Adhesives	Golf ball core (may cause mechanical injury)
Air fresheners	Grease
Ajax Cleaner	Gypsum
Aluminum foil	Hair products (conditioner, shampoos, not Lin-
Antacids	dane)
Antibiotic ointments	Hand lotions and creams
Antiperspirants	Hydrogen peroxide 3%
Ashes (wood, fireplace)	Indelible markers
Baby products (cosmetics)	Ink (blue, black)
Baby wipes	Iodophor disinfectant
Ballpoint pen inks	Kaolin
Bathtub floating toys	Kitty litter
Bath oil (castor oil and perfume)	Lanolin
Battery (convention if bitten)	Latex paint
Bleach (<5%)	Laxatives
Body conditioners	Lipstick
Bubble bath (detergents)	Lotrimin cream
Calamine lotion	Lubricants
Candles	Lysol Disinfectant Spray (70% ethanol)
Caps (for toy pistols)	Magic Marker
Cat food	Makeup (eye, liquid facial)
Caulk	Mascara (domestic)
Chalk (calcium carbonate)	Massengil Disposable Douches
Charcoal and charcoal briquettes	Matches (book type, three books)
Cigarette ashes	Mineral oil
Cigarettes (less than one)	Mineral Gro Plant Food
Clay (modelling)	Newspaper
Cold packs (a swallow)	Nutrasweet
Colognes[a]	PAAS Easter egg dyes (after 1980)
Comet Cleaner	Paints (indoor latex acrylic)
Contraceptive pills (without iron)	Pencil lead (graphite)
Corticosteroids and their ointments	Perfumes[a]
Crayola Markers	Petroleum jelly (Vaseline)
Crayons (marked AP, CP, CS-140)	Photographs
Crazy Glue (cyanoacrylate)	Plastics
Cyclamate	Plaster (non–lead-containing)
Dehumidifying packets (silica or charcoal)	Play-Doh
Deodorants (spray and refrigerator)	Polaroid picture coating
Detergents (phosphate type, anionic)	Porous tip ink marking pens
Dishwashing liquid soap (not automatic	Preparation H suppository/ointment
electric dishwasher) (Mr Clean, Dawn,	Prussian blue (ferricyanide)
Joy, Tide, Wisk)	Putty
Disposable diapers—not aspirated	Rouge
Erasers	Rubber cements
Etch-A-Sketch	Rust
Eye makeup	Rug cleaners/shampoos
Fabric softener	(most: Glory, Resolve, Woolite)
Felt-tip markers and pens	Saccharin
Fertilizer (nitrogen, phosphoric acid, and potash)	Sachets (essential oils)
Fingernail polish	Shampoo (liquid)
Fish bowl additives	Shaving creams
Fluoride—caries preventive	Shoe polish
Glade Plug In	Silica gel

(continued)

TABLE 28-5. *Continued*

Silly putty	Toothpaste (even fluoride)
Soaps and soap products	Vaseline
Soil Shackles	Vitamins (even fluoride), excluding iron
Starch	Warfarin (single dose)
Sunscreen and tan preparations	Water color paint
Sweetening agents	Windex Glass Cleaner With Ammonia D
Teething rings (fluid may have bacteria)	Zinc oxide
Thermometers (mercury, phthalate alcohol)	Zirconium oxide
Toilet water[a]	

[a]Depends on the alcohol content.

(4) **Inhalation** of gases produced by **mixing chlorine bleach** with acids (bisulfide in toilet bowl cleaner, vinegar and rust removers) result in liberation of chlorine gas or when mixed with household ammonia liberates chloramine gas. There were 2,852 chloramine cases reported in 1994 to the AAPCC, with 382 moderate outcomes, three major outcomes, and no deaths. There were 749 chlorine gas cases reported, with 130 moderate outcomes, one major outcome, and no deaths.

(a) **Chlorine gas** is a greenish yellow gas, heavier than air with a pungent odor. It has high water solubility, an oxidizing action due to nascent oxygen, free oxygen radicals and the caustic effect of hydrochloric acid producing an irritating effect on the mucous membranes, eyes, and upper respiratory tract. Low levels of 1 to 2 part per million (ppm) can be tolerated for 8 h. Odor is detected at 3 to 5 ppm. At 15 to 30 ppm moderate symptoms and 40 to 60 ppm are life-threatening. Exposure to 1,000 ppm (0.1%) is fatal in a few minutes. If severe and prolonged exposure, pulmonary toxicity can occur producing cough, stridor, wheezing, bronchospasm, pneumonitis and rarely noncardiac pulmonary edema.

(b) **Chloramine gas** is produced by mixing sodium hypochlorite with ammonia which produces monoamine, dichloramine and nitrogen trichloride. Another source is the addition of bleach to ammonia such as toilets with standing urine or sewage tanks. Chloramine decomposes in the mucous membrane to form hydrochlorous acid and ammonia. Hydrochlorous acid liberates hydrochloric acid and nascent oxygen to cause respiratory irritation. These gases are less water-soluble and may produce more delayed onset of irritation than chlorine gas. Severe cases have occurred following prolonged exposure over several hours or days in a poorly ventilated area (20,21).

(5) **Ocular injuries.** An immediate burning sensation follows ocular exposure, followed by erythema, lacrimation, edema and photophobias but

these injuries are unlikely to cause permanent damage, and lesions heal within 3 weeks. More serious injury may occur from commercial hypochlorite bleach or undiluted swimming pool hypochlorite.

(6) **Dermal exposure** of high concentrations may produce erythema, blistering, and onycholysis.

(7) **Intravenous injection** has been described inadvertently or intentionally by patients with acquired immune deficiency syndrome (AIDS). Small amounts such as 0.3 mL of 5.6% sodium hypochlorite from a 1-mL U 100 insulin syringe have not been reported to cause serious consequences. Intravenous injection produces high osmolar gap (16,23,24).

(8) **Management**

(a) **Ingestion: Avoid** gastrointestinal (GI) decontamination procedures (emesis, gastric lavage, activated charcoal). Rinse mouth and dilute with water or milk by mouth if the patient can swallow. The dilution amount should be small to avoid inducing vomiting. **Esophagoscopy** is considered only if unusually large amounts have been ingested and the patient is symptomatic with persistent vomiting, unable to swallow, hematemesis, drooling, has persistent retrosternal pain, or stridor, or if the product is much stronger (more than 10%) than the average hypochlorite household bleach concentration (14,15,17).

(b) **Inhalation of gases produced by mixing bleach with ammonia or acids.** Remove from the contaminated area. If a household inhalation exposure occurs with coughing and respiratory distress and fails to respond to fresh air within a few minutes to an hour, the patient should be evaluated by a physician for respiratory therapy (oxygen, humidification, bronchodilators, intubation and positive end expiratory pressure therapy). Pulmonary edema rarely occurs. Chloramine may have a delayed onset (20,21). Pulmonary function can be monitored short-term with continuous pulse oximetry, chest radiograph and arterial blood gases. Nebulized sodium bicarbonate 4 mL of 3.75% may provide relief, but has not been scientifically investigated to recommend for routine use (20,21).

(c) **Ocular and dermal exposure** requires removal of contaminated clothes and immediate gentle irrigation with water of the skin and eyes for at least 15 min.

(d) **Intravenous injections** need observation and supportive care. Small amounts of 5.6% solution are usually not of serious nature (16,23,24).

2. **Oxalic acid** is the simplest dicarboxylic acid. Commercially it is used as a bleach, cleanser, ink eradicator, metal polisher, rust remover, and leather tanner. It is naturally present as a salt in many **plants** (4,25,26). It may cause caustic damage and later renal damage and hypocalcemia (precipitation of insoluble calcium oxalate salt).

a. **The oxalate forms in plants** (27)
   (1) **Soluble** salts contain sodium, potassium, lithium and iron. Soluble oxalates rarely give systemic toxicity, convulsions and tetany due to hypocalcemia, and renal damage.
   (2) **Insoluble** salts contain calcium and magnesium. High oxalate foods bind calcium and render it unavailable for absorption.

b. **Toxicity. The ingestion of plants** (e.g., dieffenbachia and others) with high oxalate concentrations usually causes only mild irritation and burning in the mouth and esophageal mucosa. **Deaths** have been reported from eating boiled rhubarb leaves and stems. The deaths were attributed to anthraquinone glycoside in these plants which may cause cardiac failure and death (24,25) not the oxalates. The **lethal amount** of ingested oxalic acid ranges from 15 to 30 g (27). An adult human injected 20 mg/kg i.v., which produced cardiac failure secondary to profound hypocalcemia and death (27). **Oxalic acid** less than 10% is a strong irritant and more than 10% is corrosive.

c. **Kinetics:** In normal adults, 2% to 5% of the ingested dose is absorbed (27). **Endogenous intermediatory metabolism** in humans produces oxalates as an end product of glyoxylate, glycine, and ascorbic acid metabolism (27). About 40% of urinary oxalate is derived from the oxidative deamination of glycine to glyoxylate which is catalyzed by the liver enzyme glycine oxidase. Patients with **hereditary primary oxaluria** have a defect in enzyme transaminating glyoxylate to glycine. Pyridoxine deficiency which inhibits the transamination process results in increased urinary oxalate in the rat (25). Ethylene glycol is metabolized to oxalates which deposit in the tissues. Urinary excretion peaks in about 4 h and persists up to 24 h.

d. **Manifestations.**
   (1) **Acute ingestion of oxalic acid** results in metallic taste, burning of the **GI tract,** hemorrhagic vomiting, diarrhea, and melena. The QT interval may be prolonged and conduction defects may occur. There may be a rapid onset of shock, hypocalcemic tetany, cardiovascular collapse, oliguric renal failure and seizures which leads quickly to death. Oxalate crystals may block the **renal** tubules and cause oliguria, anuria, hematuria,453 and renal failure. **Hypocalcemia** may develop due to oxalates combining with the calcium to form unionized insoluble calcium oxalate which can result in tetany, muscle fasciculations, and convulsions (27).
   (2) **Dermal contact with oxalic acid** causes burning, itching, yellow colored nails and acrocyanosis in persons working with oxalic acid without gloves (28). Hypocalcemia can occur from extensive dermal burns (28).
   (3) **The ingestion of oxalate containing plants.** In most instances of plant oxalate ingestion, the patients remain asymptomatic (25,26). There were 14,548 exposures reported to the AAPCC in 1994, with 72 moderate outcomes, three major outcomes, and no deaths (4).

(a) **Insoluble oxalate** concentrations (*Caladium, Dieffenbachia sequine* [dumbcane], *Colocasia antiquorum* [elephant's ear], *Arisaema triphyllium* [Jack-in-the-pulpit], *Philodendron scandus* (philodendron), *Narcissus*, or daffodil) usually cause only mild irritation and burning in the mouth and esophageal mucosa. Individuals who ingest parts of these plants may develop facial swelling, rash, oropharyngeal edema, and allergic type symptoms from the oxalate crystals.

(b) **Soluble oxalates** may rarely give systemic toxicity which are convulsions and tetany due to hypocalcemia, and renal damage. Examples include *Rheum rhaponticum* (rhubarb), *Oxalis spp* (shamrock, sorrel, soursob), Parthenocissus (American Ivy), and *Parthenocissus creeper* (Virginia creeper).

(c) **Chronic ingested oxalates** may have adverse effects on the kidneys, and bladder (nephrocalcinosis), nervous system and metabolic system (tetany and seizures). It has been estimated 66% of renal calculi and 75% of bladder **calculi** in the United States are composed of calcium oxalates (12). The manifestations of chronic ingestions may be those of **renal calculi** including **renal colic** and urinary tract calculi (28).

(d) **Management. Ocular or dermal contact** irrigation and dilution for at least 15 min. Chemical burns have been caused by oxalic acid and should be treated similar to any burn and if extensive, consider systemic hypocalcemia (28).

(e) **Ingestion of oxalates and oxalic acid**

  (i) For **Plant ingestions,** the administration of milk may be recommended. Plant parts may require evaluation for obstruction of the airway.

  (ii) **Oxalic acid ingestions less than 10%** may be managed by gastric lavage with calcium gluconate of 1 to 2 g or calcium carbonate (Tums) orally or via lavage tube or milk. However, lavage may not be advisable when the concentration is more than 10% (27).

  (iii) **Oxalic acid more than 10% may be caustic.** Immediate first aid treatment consists of dilution with milk. Emesis, gastric lavage and activated charcoal are not recommended. Endoscopy may be required for evaluation.

  (iv) **Control seizures** with calcium if hypocalcemia exists and diazepam.

  (v) **Chronic exposure** producing renal calculi are managed by analgesia and brisk **diuresis.** Surgical removal or lithotripsy may be required for large calculi (29).

(f) **Laboratory.** Urinary findings of crystals of oxalate exist both in envelope shaped and needle-like forms. An abdominal scout film may be helpful in localizing calculi. **Monitor** serum calcium bound and unbound, serum electrolytes, BUN, creatinine, and urinalysis. The upper limit of the **normal serum oxalate** is 1.4 mg/L. Fatal amount is more than 18 mg/L (27).

3. **Boric acid** was used as an antiseptic, disinfectant, astringent, and fundiostatic agent in baby talcum powder, and is used as a food preservative, water softener, astringent and antiseptic, mild antiseptic eyewash (5%, 10%), optic solution (5%), ant and roach pesticide (40% tablet, 99% powder or crystals), and in topical skin products (5%). Borax cleaners contain 21.5% boron by dry weight. One teaspoonful of 100% boric acid powder equals 2.9 to 4.4 g of boric acid (9,34). In 1994, the AAPCC reported 3,477 exposures to boric acid chemicals and 922 cleaners. Most cases were asymptomatic, with 63 moderate outcomes, three major outcomes, and one death (4).

   a. **Toxicity:** Most accidental ingestions are minimally toxic. Serious poisoning occurs with ingestion of 1 to 3 g in neonates, 5 g in infants and 20 g in adults. The potentially fatal dose is believed to be much higher than the quoted values of 20 g in adults and 5 g in children (30–32).

   b. **Kinetics:** Boric acid is well absorbed from the GI tract, open wounds, inflamed and denuded skin (32), and serous cavities. **Volume distribution** (V_d) is 0.17 to 0.50 L/kg. The **elimination route** is renal, with 50% of the dose excreted in the urine within 12 h and 80% to 100% in 5 to 7 days. **Elimination half-life** ($t_{1/2}$) is 12 to 27 h. Normal blood levels are less than 5 µg/mL (30,32,34).

   c. **Manifestations** (31,32,35)

      (1) **Acute boric acid ingestion** include acute gastroenteritis with **blue-green vomitus** and diarrhea. Sometimes the stools are black. CNS stimulation is produced. In severe cases, seizures and coma can occur. Renal failure may develop. An erythematous rash may develop as early as 6 h (usually 2 to 3 days) after ingestion. The rash desquamates in 3 to 5 days, giving the "boiled lobster" appearance (30–35).

      (2) **Chronic** application of boric acid to the diaper area produces a rash. Ingestion of formula with boric acid contamination for several days produces very serious poisoning with seizures, renal failure, and extensive desquamation of the skin similar to staphylococcal scaled skin syndromes (Ritter's disease) (31–33).

   d. **Management** (for initial management, see Table 28-6).

TABLE 28-6. *Initial management of boric acid ingestion*

Body weight	Amount ingested	Management
<30 kg	<200 mg/kg	Observe at home.
	>400 mg/kg	Emergency department for evaluation.
>30 kg	<6 g ingested	Observe at home.
	>12 g	Emergency department for evaluation.

Modified from refs. 29, 30, and 33.

(1) **Decontamination. Ingestion:** Syrup of ipecac is contraindicated due to the potential of seizures. Activated charcoal does not absorb boric acid (31,32). **Dermal exposure**: Remove from skin with soap and water (31,32).

(2) Treat the seizures with diazepam or lorazepam.

(3) Exchange transfusion or hemodialysis may be used in serious poisoning. Hemodialysis may be required for renal failure (30,31,35).

B. Caustics and corrosives (alkali or acid) are some of the most dangerous substances in the home. Approximately 30,000 caustic exposures occur annually in the United States. There were 21,533 **alkali cleaner exposures** reported to AAPCC in 1994, with 1,660 moderate outcomes, 100 major outcomes, and four deaths (4). There were 8,541 **acid cleaner exposures** reported in 1994, with 803 moderate outcomes, 11 major outcomes, and three deaths (4). Caustic exposures make up about 5% of human exposures to toxins and account for about 10 deaths per year. Approximately 5,000 esophageal burns occur each year and 10% result in strictures. Approximately 99% are in children less than 7 years and about 56% are under the age of 2 years (3,4,5,6). The **Federal Hazardous Substance Act** and the Poison Prevention Packaging Act of 1970 requires that corrosive agents that have concentrations of active ingredients greater than 2% be sold in child resistant containers. Acid and alkali are grouped together as caustics and corrosives but their pathophysiology differs (see Chapter 20).

1. Alkaline products that produce injury are drain cleaners (sodium hydroxide in Crystal Drano 50%, Liquid Drano 2% to 10%, Drano Professional (liquid) 34%, Liquid Plumber 2% to 10% with 5% to 10% hypochlorite, Red Devil Drain Opener 96% to 100%), oven cleaners (Dow Oven Cleaner 4%), cuticle removers, denture liquid cleaner (Efferdent potassium monoperborate, Polident sodium tripolyphosphate less than 15%), disk batteries (sodium or potassium hydroxide 40%), and Clinitest tablets (sodium hydroxide 50%). An alkaline caustic are those with pH more than 12, the level which produces ulceration of the esophagus. There were 3,117 alkali drain cleaner exposures reported in 1994 to AAPCC, with 460 moderate outcomes, 28 major outcomes, and four deaths (4).

a. Ammonia is a highly volatile alkali that is highly water-soluble. In 1994 there were 3,850 chemical exposures reported to AAPCC, with 24 moderate outcomes, one major outcome, and one death. There were also 3,850 ammonia cleaner exposures, with 191 moderate outcomes, one major outcome, and no deaths (4).

(1) **Anhydrous ammonia (NH_3)** is a water-soluble, colorless, irritating, noxious gas used as fertilizer; in manufacture of plastics, explosives, nylon and as a commercial refrigerant gas. Anhydrous ammonia reacts with water to form ammonium hydroxide which is used as household cleaning agent (household ammonia).

(2) **Aqueous household ammonias are 5% to 10% solutions. These** are alkaline and causes irritation, rarely burns and no strictures. Greater than 10% is corrosive (36,37). **Ingestion of industrial strength** 30% or greater can produce effects similar to other caustics including strictures.

Aqueous ammonia plus chlorine bleach produces chloramine gas which may cause pulmonary injury. Systemic systems may occur after 7% ammonia, but it is unlikely to produce strictures (36,37).

(3) **Aromatic spirits of ammonia** contains 0.33 to 0.44 mL 18% ammonia in 36% alcohol-water solution with lemon, nutmeg, and lavender oils. This can cause local irritation, but no strictures have been reported (36).

(4) **Management** of ingestions with dilution is similar to other caustics. Ocular exposure may produce severe damage and requires copious immediate and prolonged irrigation with water or saline for at least 15 min and continue until there is no pain. A detailed eye examination including fluorescein dye and slit-lamp examination is recommended for any exposure (36,37) (see Chapter 20).

b. **Disc batteries** are salts of zinc, cadmium, nickel, and lithium in concentrated sodium or potassium hydroxide 40%. Cylindrical batteries also contain sodium and potassium hydroxide (pH 12 to 13) which can leak out and produce burns. Disc batteries are in 8- to 25-mm casings. It is estimated that there are 2,100 button battery ingestions per year (38). There were 1,904 disc battery ingestions reported to AAPCC in 1994, with 85 minor outcomes, 23 moderate outcomes, four major outcomes, and no deaths (4).

(1) Older (introduced in the early 1980s), larger batteries (more than 23 mm) lodged in the esophagus and caused pressure necrosis, electrical injury and/or alkaline damage including perforation and tracheoesophageal fistula (40). Leaking mercury from batteries did raise the urine mercury level but did not produce toxicity except in one patient (39,40).

(2) The smaller batteries with stronger casing make disc battery ingestion less of a problem (38).

(3) An initial radiograph for localization is advised to make sure the battery is not lodged in the esophagus. Stool confirmation of passage of the battery is recommended, although 97% negotiate the passage without problems (38,39). For algorithm on the management of disc battery ingestions, see Fig. 28-1.

c. **Clinitest tablets** contain sodium hydroxide 50% and have copper sulfate, sodium carbonate and citric acid. The sodium hydroxide 50% (alkaline corrosive) reacts with citric acid to generate heat (thermal burns) in the presence of copper sulfate as a catalyst and sodium bicarbonate. Attractive to children (colored speckles) and mistaken by visually impaired, they adhere to the mucosa and usually produce esophagitis, alkaline burns, and strictures in upper esophagus (41). Fortunately these tablets are rarely used since simpler methods of testing the urine are available and blood glucose monitoring has come into vogue. There was only one patient reported in 1994.

d. **Common alkali and specific toxicity.** For a list of common caustic materials found around the home, see Table 28-7.

(1) **Ammonium hydroxide** (NH_3OH) 5% to 10% is irritant, more than 10% is corrosive. Household ammonia is usually 5% to 10%. Ammoniated products are only a small percent of ammonia.

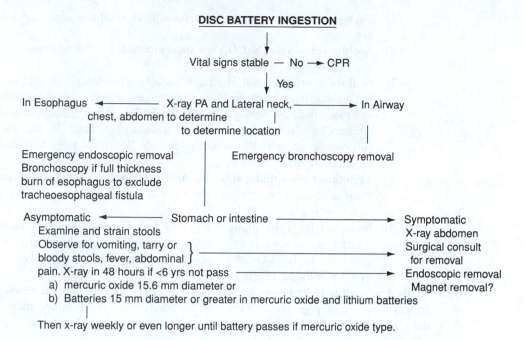

DISC BATTERY INGESTION

Vital signs stable — No → CPR

Yes

In Esophagus ← X-ray PA and Lateral neck, → In Airway
chest, abdomen to determine
to determine location

Emergency endoscopic removal
Bronchoscopy if full thickness
burn of esophagus to exclude
tracheoesophageal fistula

Emergency bronchoscopy removal

Asymptomatic ← Stomach or intestine → Symptomatic
Examine and strain stools
Observe for vomiting, tarry or
bloody stools, fever, abdominal
pain. X-ray in 48 hours if <6 yrs not pass
a) mercuric oxide 15.6 mm diameter or
b) Batteries 15 mm diameter or greater in mercuric oxide and lithium batteries

X-ray abdomen
Surgical consult
for removal
Endoscopic removal
Magnet removal?

Then x-ray weekly or even longer until battery passes if mercuric oxide type.

FIG. 28-1. Algorithm on the management of disc battery ingestions.

(2) **Calcium oxide** (lime) when mixed with water forms calcium hydroxide. Dry calcium hydroxide is corrosive. Calcium hydroxide ($CaOH_2$) pH 11 to 13 is used in making Portland cement and is listed as a strong irritant.

(3) **Metasilicate** is in nonphosphate detergents with pH 12.0. It is listed as a corrosive but in clinical experience appears to be a strong irritant.

(4) **Potassium hydroxide** (KOH, caustic potash, lye) less than 1% is weak irritant, more than 1% is a corrosive.

TABLE 28-7. *Common caustic and corrosive materials found around the home*

Acids	Alkali
Ammonia	Lime (calcium oxide)
Cement and cement cleaners	Lye (K^+ and Na^+ hydroxide)
Clinitest tablets	Metal cleaners
Coffee pot cleaners	Mildew removers
Denture cleaners	Oven cleaners
Drain cleaners	Pipe smokers' cleaners
Electric dishwasher detergents	Rust removers
Formaldehyde	Toilet bowl cleaners
Hair bleaches, permanents, straighteners	Wart removers
Hydrofluoric acid	

(5) **Potassium permanganate** ($KMNO_4$) is an oxidizer with corrosive properties.

(6) **Sodium carbonate** ($NaCO_3$) is a strong irritant. It is found in nonphosphate detergents.

(7) **Sodium hydroxide** (NaOH, caustic soda, lye) less than 0.5% (pH 12.8) is a weak irritant, less than 1% is a irritant, more than 1% is a corrosive, and more than 2% strong corrosive (pH 13.6). Most household drain cleaners have reduced their NaOH content to less than 2%, but some still contain up to 100% sodium hydroxide. The most toxic household products are drain cleaners.

(8) **Trisodium phosphate, silicates, and carbonates** (laundry and automatic dishwasher detergents) are listed as caustic but are irritants (see Detergents).

(9) **Sodium tripolyphosphate** is a caustic found in automatic dishwasher detergents and some laundry detergents (Electrosol Dishwasher Detergent 20% to 40%, Oxydol Laundry Detergent 25% to 49%, Polident Powder less than 15%).

2. **Acids** are found in toilet bowl cleaners, metal cleaners, swimming pool cleaners, battery acids, and phenolic compounds. In addition to local injury there is the potential for systemic absorption and acidosis, electrolyte disturbances, and hemolysis.

  a. **Common acids and specific toxicity**

   (1) **Acetic acid** used as disinfectant and hair wave neutralizer; less than 5% is vinegar, 5% to 10% is weak irritant, and more than 50% is corrosive.

   (2) **Carbolic acid** (Phenol) is used as disinfectant and dye and can produce seizures, coma, and respiratory arrest.

   (3) **Chromic acid** is used in photography, plating, tanning, and can produce renal and hepatic toxicity.

   (4) **Hydrochloric acid** (HCl) less than 5% is a weak irritant, 5% to 10% is strong irritant, and more than 10% is corrosive. Toilet bowl cleaners may contain up to 10% to 25% and can produce dermal damage and esophageal and gastric injury. There were 2,772 exposures to HCL, with 1,172 minor outcome, 370 moderate outcomes, 15 major outcomes, and four deaths (4).

   (5) **Hydrofluoric acid (HFA)** is a weak acid (produces less free hydrogen ions in solution) and has poor dissociation which allows greater penetration of tissues (see Chapter 20).

  b. In 1994, there were 1,370 cases of **exposure** to hydrofluoric acid, with 543 minor outcomes, 342 moderate, 22 major, and no deaths (4). HFA is contained in rust removers and used in metal and glass etching, and masonry cleaners.

  c. The fluoride binds avidly with calcium and magnesium demineralizing the bone and interrupting calcium and magnesium functions. Locally HFA produces intensive pain, extensive dermal damage, and extensive ocular damage.

Inhalation causes extensive pulmonary injury and extensive systemic manifestions of acidosis, hypocalcemia, hypomagnesemia, and hyperkalemia. Large areas of local dermal injury can result in systemic toxicity (50–52).

d. Dilute 5% to 15% HFA produces asymptomatic injury for 12 to 24 h, 20% to 40% delayed symptoms for few hours and concentrated more than 50% immediate symptoms and risk of morbidity and mortality.

e. Most of the cases of significant HFA exposure require medical evaluation and management in an ED and consultation with a plastic surgeon (50–52).

    (1) **Management** is immediate decontamination of skin and eyes with water or saline. Local management consists of topical calcium gluconate gel (3.5 g/5 oz KY Jelly) in a surgical glove. If it fails to relieve the pain, use subcutaneous infiltration of calcium gluconate (0.5 mL/cm$_2$). Removal of fingernails may be necessary if pain persists. Some toxicologists use intra-arterial 10% calcium gluconate (10 mL in 50 mL D5W) over 4 h or a tourniquet-limited (Bier block) calcium gluconate. Systemically administer calcium and magnesium as needed (50–52).

    (2) **Nitric acid 5%** is used in engraving and in some gun barrel cleaners, more than 5% is a corrosive.

    (3) **Phosphoric acid** is used in metal cleaning and disinfectants; 15% to 35% is weak irritant, 35% to 60% is strong irritant, and more than 60% is corrosive.

    (4) **Oxalic acid** is used in rust remover, tanning and cleaning, and bleach; less than 10% is strong irritant, and more than 10% is corrosive and can produce hypocalcemia and renal failure (see oxalates and oxalic acid under Bleach).

    (5) **Selenious acid 2%** is used in gun bluing solution. It has corrosive effects similar to other acids. However multisystem failure with shock (decreased inotrophy, vasodilation), adult respiratory distress syndrome, hepatic, and renal failure may occur. Deaths have occurred in a few hours after ingestion of as little as 15 to 20 mL of 2% in children (40,41) (see gun bluing under Sport Equipment).

    (6) **Sulfuric acid** (H_2SO_4)-(battery acid or oil of vitriol) is used as toilet cleaner, drain cleaner, and metal cleaner. Dilution of less than 5% is an irritant, less than 10% is strong irritant, more than 10% is corrosive, and more than 15% strong corrosive. Sulfuric acid also acts as a desiccant and turns the skin black.

    (7) **Toilet bowl and drain cleaners** (Cost Cutter Bowl Cleaner HCl 9.55%, Lysol Toilet Bowl Liquid HCl 8.5%, Mr Plumber Liquid H_2SO_4 99%, Saniflush Toilet Bowl Cleaner sodium bisulfide 75%, SnoBol HCl 15%, and Vanish Toilet Bowl Cleaner granular sodium bisulfide 75%).

3. **Location of the damage.** The squamous epithelium of the esophagus is somewhat believed to be resistant to acid burns but susceptible to alkali burns. The columnar epithelium of the stomach is effected by acids. Nevertheless both acids and alkali can damage either the esophagus or the stomach or both (42–44).

4. **Manifestations.** It is possible to have serious gastric or esophageal injury without external physical evidence of injury in the oropharynx, but it is unlikely to have such injury without some combination of GI or respiratory symptoms. Vomiting, drooling, and stridor are among the best predictors (42–44).

5. **Management of alkali and acid ingestions** (Fig. 28-2).

    a. **Dilution.** Copious irrigation of the eyes and skin. Hold eyelids open. Dilution with water or milk after ingestion. Do not give excess fluid that may cause vomiting—about 15 mL/kg is adequate. Neutralization produces in vitro exothermic reaction and is not recommended.

    b. No emesis, or gastric lavage is recommended except in large acid ingestion with a flexible small bore tube and the possibility of dangerous systemic effects (48).

    c. **Endoscopy** is valuable to predict early hemorrhage or perforation and late risk

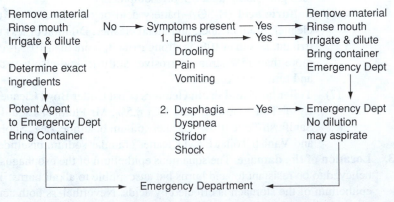

Basic Therapy

<u>Immediately</u> dilute and irrigate with milk or water.
  1. If spilled or splashed
     Irrigate the exposed skin and eyes
     Remove clothes and continue irrigation
  2. If ingested
     * Remove any residual material and rinse mouth.
     * If can swallow and vital signs stable
     a) Swallow small amounts milk and water.
         Maximum 30 ml child, 150 mL adult
     b) Avoid making vomit
        NO EMETIC, LAVAGE, ACTIVATED CHARCOAL.

History: 1. Type of substance
          2. Examine container
          3. Time exposed
          4. Presence of vomiting and hematemesis
          5. Presence of pain and location
          6. Presence of drooling, dyspnea, stridor

Remove material   No ⟶ Symptoms present ⟶ Yes ⟶ Remove material
Rinse mouth   1. Burns ⟶ Yes ⟶   Rinse mouth
Irrigate & dilute   Drooling   Irrigate & dilute
                                  Pain   Bring container
Determine exact   Vomiting   Emergency Dept
ingredients

Potent Agent   2. Dysphagia ⟶ Yes ⟶   Emergency Dept
to Emergency Dept   Dyspnea   No dilution
Bring Container   Stridor   may aspirate
                                  Shock

                        Emergency Department

FIG. 28-2a. Algorithm for management of caustics.

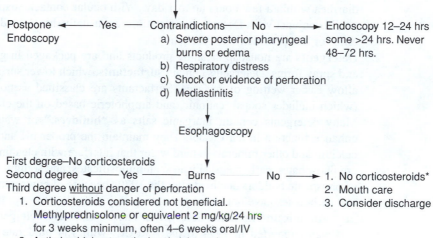

Emergency Department Procedures
1. Establish airway
2. Establish vital functions
3. Remove foreign materials, rinse mouth
Irrigate eye and skin and dilute by swallowing.
4. Establish vascular access
5. Examine oropharnyx–describe findings
6. Order "nothing by mouth"
7. Obtain hemoglobin, hematocrit, urinalysis
serum electrolytes, glucose, BUN, creatinine
8. If hematemesis or perforation, cross match blood
9. Chest and abdominal x-ray
10. Obtain consent for endoscopy

Postpone ◄──── Yes ──── Contraindictions──── No ────► Endoscopy 12–24 hrs
Endoscopy   a) Severe posterior pharyngeal   some >24 hrs. Never
                       burns or edema   48–72 hrs.
              b) Respiratory distress
              c) Shock or evidence of perforation
              d) Mediastinitis

Esophagoscopy

First degree–No corticosteroids
Second degree ◄──── Yes ──── Burns ──── No ────► 1. No corticosteroids*
Third degree <u>without</u> danger of perforation   2. Mouth care
1. Corticosteroids considered not beneficial.   3. Consider discharge
    Methylprednisolone or equivalent 2 mg/kg/24 hrs
    for 3 weeks minimum, often 4–6 weeks oral/IV
2. Antimicrobial not routinely administered
3. Intravenous therapy until can swallow saliva
    (usually in 48 hrs) then advance to soft diet
4. Cinefluoroscopy in 3 weeks include stomach and duodenum.
5. If stenosis develops, stop corticosterods and consider
    bougienage and dilation in several weeks.
Third degree <u>with</u> danger of preforation–No Corticosteroids

Follow-up–1. Monthly for first year
           2. Consult physician if dysphagia occurs at anytime
               and inform physician of history of esophageal burns.

*Corticosteroids are not recommended as therapy for any
degree burn of the esophagus. However, some clinicians still
administer corticosteroids in second degree burn. It is a
clinical judgment that is left up to the physician.

FIG. 28-2b. *Continued*

of stricture. The indications for endoscopy are controversial. Some authorities recommend all patients, regardless of symptoms, who ingest caustics undergo endoscopy (42,44) but other authorities are selective using vomiting, stridor and drooling, visual lesions as criteria (43,46,47).

d. **Corticosteroids** after ingestions are controversial. A prospective small series showed no benefit (44,45) but a meta-analysis flawed by lack of controlled studies suggested benefit (49). If steroids are used they should be used for several weeks, with antibiotics initially (49).

C. Soap and detergents

1. **Soaps are salts** of fatty acids and are of low toxicity. If bar soaps or liquid hand soaps are ingested, they may produce nausea, vomiting within a few minutes, and diarrhea within a few hours up to 1 day. With ocular contact, soaps may produce a mild conjunctivitis. Dermal manifestations are usually due to mild irritative properties or a hypersensitivity reaction.

2. **Detergents** are nonsoap cleaning products and are packaged in granular, liquid, and spray forms. Detergents contain **surfactants,** which lower surface tension and allow easier wetting of surfaces. Surfactants are classified as nonionic, anionic (which includes soaps), cationic, and amphoteric based on the electrical charge. Many detergents contain inorganic salts as **"builders,"** or water softeners to enhance function in hard water. They maintain the proper pH and combine with calcium and other minerals in hard water that interfere with cleaning. The builders are phosphates, carbonates, silicates, aluminosilicates, and sodium citrate. The use of phosphate builders declined after the 1970s because of environmental concerns, and carbonates have not been used extensively since 1970.

   a. **Anionic and nonionic detergents.** There were 8,292 detergent cleaner exposures reported in 1994 to the AAPCC, with 154 moderate outcomes, one major outcome, and no deaths (4).

   (1) **Anionic are the most common form of commercial detergents.** They are negatively charged ions. Examples are sodium alkyl benzene sulfonate in Ajax Cleaner, dodecyl benzene sulfonate in Comet Cleaner. The detergent cleaners that fit into this category are Bold Granular Laundry Detergent, Cheer Laundry detergent, Dash Laundry Detergent, FAB Granular Laundry Detergent, Glory Concentrated Rug Shampoo, Oxydol, Tide (sodium silicate 15%), Top Job, Wisk, and Woolite Rug Cleaner. These are laundry soaps, low suds soaps for automatic washers and hand soaps (55–57). These are toxicologically irritants.

   (2) **Nonionic detergents** are electrically neutral. Nonionic detergents contain ethoxylated alcohols or alkoxylated alcohols or sulfonates with a pH near neutral. They are less irritating than anionic detergents and usually do not cause serious damage. They are found in heavy laundry liquids, nonphosphate granular products and low suds laundry products. Examples are ERA Laundry Detergent, Ivory Snow liquid, Joy Dish Detergent, Mr Clean Liquid Household Cleaner, and Mop & Glow Wax (55–57).

   (3) The **toxicology of anionic and nonionic detergents**—GI absorption is minimal. Neither anionic or nonionic detergents have significant systemic toxicity. Locally, they may produce mucosal and skin irritation and superficial mucosal erosion if in contact for an extended period of time. Theoretically they could produce hypocalcemia but this has rarely occurred (55–57,59).

(4) **Most nonphosphate detergents** contain carbonates or silicates. In 1972 significant corrosive injury to the esophagus and stomach of cats was demonstrated if the detergent contained more than 30% to 35% carbonates, more than 10% silicates, or had a pH of 11.5 or more (58). However, the most saturated solutions of nonphosphate detergents usually have pH values of 11.0 to 11.5 or less and ulceration of the esophagus occurs at pH 12 (58).

b. **Laundry detergents** are mainly anionic and nonionic detergents with builders. There were 13,878 exposures reported in 1994 to AAPCC for laundry detergents, with 282 moderate outcomes, seven major outcomes, and one death with a liquid laundry detergent (4).

(1) **Serious respiratory consequences** have been reported from ingestion and **inhalation of powdered laundry detergent powder** (Arm and Hammer). Between 1979 and 1987, eight patients, ages 1.5 to 2.0 years, required hospital admission (60). The most frequent symptoms were drooling and stridor. Four required endotracheal intubation. All patients were extubated within 48 h and asymptomatic at 72 h. Three children had objective evidence of minimal esophageal damage. One patient was reported to develop symptoms of mucosal injury 5 h after ingestion (60).

(2) **Liquid laundry detergents** containing alkyl ethoxylates, when ingested in estimated amounts of more than 10 ml/kg, may produce ataxia and CNS depression (61). The AAPCC in 1994 reported 3,599 exposures, with 70 moderate outcomes, one major, and one death (4).

c. **Automatic dishwashing machine detergents** (ADMD) (e.g., Electrosol is tripolyphosphate, Cascade 25% to 50% phosphates, Calgonite sodium phosphate less than 50%) are reported to have the potential to produce caustic injuries. They are available in both liquid and granular forms. Even in the absence of oral irritation they may produce gastroesophageal damage (59,61,62). The AAPCC in 1994 reported 4,980 granular exposures, with 27 moderate outcomes, one major outcome, and no deaths. There were also 1,998 liquid exposures, with 15 moderate outcomes, one major outcome, and no deaths (4).

(1) Exposure to small amounts of **liquid ADMD,** despite a pH of 11.8 to 12.7, usually does not appear to result in serious esophageal injury. An analysis of liquid automatic dishwasher detergent exposure showed that more than 91% of exposed patients did not have adverse reactions, and 8% had only oral irritation. However, ocular exposure may produce eye irritation and corneal abrasions (61).

(2) The residual sludge remaining in the **powder** dispenser at the end of the wash cycle is highly concentrated and especially hazardous for producing damage (61,62).

d. **Cationic detergents** are quaternary ammonium compounds in such disinfectants as hexachlorophene (PhisoHex 2%), benzalkonium (Zephiran 1:1,000 to 1:10,000), and cetylpyridium (Creepryn 1:1,000 to 1:10,000). Cationic detergents are also in fabric softeners, such as "Downey" and "Purex," but they are at a much lower concentration than in disinfectants. The AAPCC in 1994 reported 3,426 exposures, with 143 moderate outcomes, nine major outcomes, and no deaths. Industrial cationic detergent exposures were 700, with 94 moderate outcomes and two deaths (4)

(1) The estimated **toxic dose** of cationic detergents is 30 mg/kg, and the potentially fatal dose is 1 to 3 g. Most of these substances are in concentrations of 2% or less and are not toxic unless large quantities are ingested (57,59).

(2) **Manifestations of cationic detergents** (mild irritants) in very low concentrations (e.g., fabric softener). Strong irritant in most 0.1% to 0.5% concentrations (disinfectants). In concentrations of less than 2% rarely cause systemic toxicity and convulsions. In high concentrations of 7.5% to 15% industrial/institutional products or algicide can be caustic.

(3) **Management of cationic detergent exposure.** If a fabric softener is ingested, the recommendation is dilution with milk or water and home observation. If less than 7.5% cationic detergent is ingested, manage by observation only; if more than 7.5%, manage by dilution with milk or water, skin and ocular exposure is decontaminated with copious irrigation with water, and medical evaluation. Avoid emesis (57,59).

3. **Hard surface cleaners.** They contain small amounts (4% to 10%) of isopropyl alcohol and glycols. Liquid products require no dilution, such as the "spray on/wipe off" types, and are generally nontoxic.

4. **Scouring powders and liquids.** Except for products that are metal cleaners with oxalic acid, or sulfuric acid with a pH about 1.5, most of these agents are alkaline (pH 9.5 to 12.3) and do not represent a significant toxicologic problem.

5. **General management for detergent ingestion** (Fig. 28-3)

a. Spontaneous vomiting is frequent. However, persistent vomiting, dysphagia, stridor, severe abdominal pain, bloody vomitus, or an extraordinarily large ingestion warrants immediate medical attention (57). Most detergent ingestions do not produce damage.

b. If detergent **with caustic properties is ingested** remove any residual material from the mouth and rinse. If the patient can swallow and vital signs stable, immediately dilute with small amounts milk and water. The amount of diluting fluid should be limited to 60 ml in a child and 150 ml in an adult in order to avoid distention of the stomach. **Determine if there is skin or eye exposure,** if so, these areas should be immediately irrigated with water for at least 15 min.

c. **Gastric emptying** is *not* indicated because it is both unnecessary and may result in further damage. **Activated charcoal** is not administered because it is ineffective and may obscure burns from the endoscopist. **Cathartics** are not recommended.

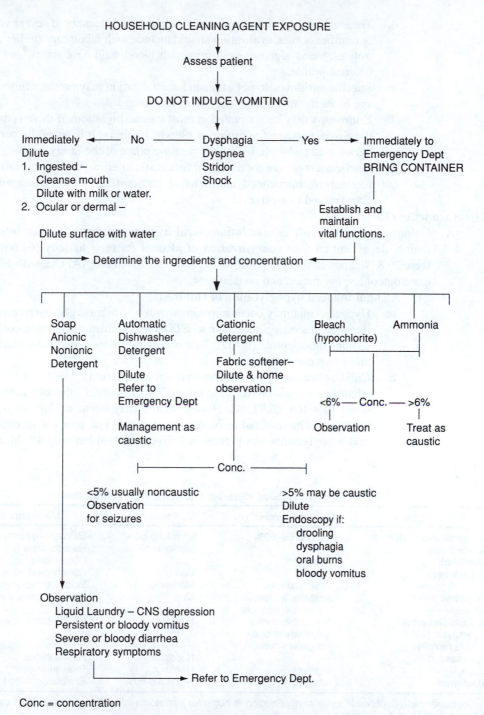

FIG. 28-3. Household cleaning agent exposure.

    d. There are no toxicologic "screens" for household cleaners. If severe vomiting or diarrhea occurs, **evaluation** should include such laboratory studies as electrolytes, blood glucose, stool for occult blood, acid-base status, and a renal function profile.

    e. **Specific antidotes** do not exist, and neutralization may produce further damage by its thermal action and is not recommended.

    f. **Endoscopy** may be warranted in most caustic ingestions if there is drooling, dysphasia, persistent vomiting or bloody vomiting. It is generally performed between 12 and 48 h, before the necrotic phase of the injury begins.

    g. **Corticosteroids** are controversial for caustic injuries. **Antimicrobials** are not routinely recommended unless using corticosteroids (see Management of Caustics and Corrosives).

II. Cosmetics (Table 28-8)

    A. Colognes, perfumes, aftershave lotions, oral hygiene products, suntan lotions are mainly dependent on their **concentration of alcohol** for their toxicity (64,66). There were 29,847 exposure to these products in 1994 reported to the AAPCC, with 139 moderate outcomes, five major, and no deaths (4).

    1. Alcohol-induced hypoglycemia in children.

      a. Hypoglycemia may occur in patients with low hepatic glycogen reserve and impaired gluconeogenesis due to ETOH metabolism depleting nicotinamide adenine dinucleotide (NAD). This occurs in children, the malnourished and those on weight reduction diets.

      b. Children are highly susceptible to develop profound hypoglycemia at blood ethanol concentration (BEC) as low as 20 to 50 mg/dL. Ethanol inhibits gluconeogenesis (64–66,73,74). Hypoglycemia may occur as late as 6 h after ingestions with minimal alcoholic symptoms. In one series of alcohol ingestion hypoglycemia was present in 24% of children but only 4% of adults at

TABLE 28-8. *Cosmetics ingredient, toxicity, and management*

Product type	Major toxic ingredient	Toxicity	Management
Colognes and perfumes	Ethanol 50–90%	>1 mL/kg 50%	Evaluation; blood glucose
Conditioners	—	Nontoxic	Reassurance
Deodorants	Aluminum	Low	Observation
Depilatories	Sulfides	Low	Observation
	Thioglycolates	Moderate	Induce emesis; evaluation
Fingernail polish remover	Acetone, toluene, aliphatic acetates	Mild	Induce emesis if >2 mL/kg
Artificial fingernail remover	Acetonitrile forms cyanide in body	High	Induce emesis; evaluation
Cuticle remover	Potassium hydroxide	—	Evaluation
Eye makeup	—	Nontoxic	Reassurance
Lipstick	Pigments	Nontoxic	Reassurance
Mouthwash	Ethanol	>1 mL/kg 50%	Evaluation; blood glucose

Reassurance in nontoxic ingestions; observation at home for symptoms in low toxicity; evaluation by medical personnel for toxic ingredients.

blood ethanol concentrations less than 67 mg/dL and only 1% of adults at levels less than 50 mg/d.

2. One study involving 119 children reported all but one who ingested less than 60 ml of **colognes, perfumes, or aftershave lotions** and remained asymptomatic (67,68). Of four children who ingested 60 to 105 ml of these products by history, only two developed slurred speech and ataxia (68).

3. **Indications for referral and evaluation** include if more than 1 ml/kg of 50% (100 proof) ethanol is ingested which will produce a blood ethanol concentration of 50 mg/dL or if there are any symptoms. If hypoglycemia is not detected by 4 h after ingestion and if no symptoms the patient can be discharged (64). If symptoms, treat as alcoholic intoxication and treat hypoglycemia with glucose i.v. if present.

B. **Deodorants (personal)** are composed of aluminum and zinc and are considered to have low toxicity (3). In 1994 there were 10,759 exposures to deodorants, with 67 moderate outcomes, one major outcome, and no deaths (4).

C. **Depilatory preparations** act through combination of an alkali and acid salt (usually ammonium). They may have corrosive action. Some preparations are sulfides or thioglycolates and are often irritants to the skin and GI tract. Large doses of thioglycolates may produce hypoglycemia and convulsions (3).

In 1994 there were 10,750 exposure depilitory preparations, with 67 moderate outcomes, one major outcome, and no deaths.

D. **Fingernail and toenail cosmetics** are the fad of 1990s.

1. **Fingernail polish/remover** ingested in large amounts may cause CNS depression due to the acetates, acetone, toluene, and aromatic hydrocarbons. Nail polish comes in less volume and is very viscous, therefore little toxicity would be expected (3). The ingestion of 2 to 3 mL/kg of **acetone** in children or 200 mL in adults has caused CNS depression. Acetone exhibits low toxicity. There were 8,434 exposures to nail polish reported to the AAPCC, with 68 moderate outcomes, two major, and no deaths. In addition, there were 3,282 exposures to acetone nail polish removers, with 23 moderate outcomes, one major outcome, and no deaths. In industry, there were 1,226 exposures to acetone reported, with 64 moderate outcomes, one major outcome, and no deaths.

2. **Artificial-fingernail remover** may contain **acetonitrile** (vinyl cyanide), which breaks down in vivo to form cyanide or **nitroethane** which may form methemoglobinemia.

    a. **Acetonitrile** (cyanomethane, methyl cyanide, vinyl cyanide). Acetonitrile is a highly polar solvent used in artificial nail removal. Commercial products available that have contained acetonitrile include Nailene Salon Quality Glue Remover, Ardell Instant Glue Remover, Artificial Nail Tip and Glue Remover, Super Nail Wrap-Off Instant Glue Dissolver, Super Nail Tip-Off, and Super Nail Glue-Off, and Originals (75,76).

        (1) **Toxicity.** Acetonitrile median oral lethal dose in pigs ranges from 177 mg/kg to 1.7 to 8.5 g in adult male rats. A 16 month old child had a blood cyanide concentration of 6 µg/mL 12 h after exposure to acetonitrile. Serum cyanide levels greater than 3.0 µg/mL are potentially lethal (75,76).

The oxidative metabolism of acetonitrile in vivo via the cytochrome P-450-dependent hepatic microsomal enzyme system slowly release hydrogen cyanide. The metabolism accounts for the latent period of 3 to 12 h. The half-life of acetonitrile is 32 h (cyanide is 15 h) (75).

(2) **Manifestations** may not occur for 3 to 12 h. They include irritability, vomiting, tachypnea, tachycardia, coma, convulsions, apnea, and severe metabolic lactic acidosis, and cardiovascular collapse. The difference between oxygen saturation of the pulse oximeter versus the arterial blood gases provide a diagnostic clue in the presence of patients with altered consciousness and respiratory insufficiency. The calculated oxygen saturation is normal but the measured oxygen saturation via the pulse oximeter is lower because some of the hemoglobin is not carrying oxygen. When the oxygen saturation difference from the arterial blood is greater than 5, a dysfunctional hemoglobin is suspected (76–80).

(3) **Management**

(a) **GI decontamination**—Avoid the induction of emesis because of rapid neurologic symptoms. Gastric lavage and activated charcoal/cathartic are recommended although there is no data on the efficiency of charcoal in this setting.

(b) In the management of cyanide intoxication due to acetonitrile, **sodium thiosulfate alone** may be preferred because of the prolonged release of cyanide from organic nitriles. The sodium nitrite is for acute inorganic cyanide intoxication. This topic is controversial and there is no data (76–80). Hydroxycobalamin (vitamin B_{12a}) has been utilized successfully (77).

(c) Hemodialysis and charcoal hemoperfusion have also been used (76–79).

(d) Ingestion of acetonitrile warrants close medical observation for 24 h (76–80).

b. **Nitroethane** ($CH_3CH_2NO_2$) is a colorless liquid with a fruity odor. It has been used as rocket propellant and an industrial solvent. It is now commercially available in an artificial fingernail glue remover with name "Remove" Brand of artificial nail remover (Gena Laboratories, Duncanville, Texas).

(1) **Toxicity.** A case of life-threatening methemoglobinemia (methb) occurred in a child who ingested 100% nitroethane artificial nail remover. Initially it was mistaken as acetone nail polish remover. The methemoglobinemia may be delayed 7 to 10 h and be recurrent. It is metabolized to aldehyde and nitrite with the end product as nitrite. Complete clearance has been reported to occur in rats in 30 h.

(2) **Manifestations.** There is a report of a delay in methb. Abrupt onset of cyanosis unresponsive to oxygen, in a previously well child is the hallmark of methb. Methb levels of 10% to 15% produce visible cyanosis, levels of 30% to 50% produces headache, dysphoria, lethargy, and vomiting, and a level of 70% is potentially fatal.

(3) Management.

(a) Establish and maintain vital functions.

(b) GI decontamination with emesis, gastric lavage, and activated charcoal although there is no data on their effectiveness.

(c) The antidote for methhb is **methylene blue (MB)** i.v. for blood concentration over 20% to 30%. The dose is 1 to 2 mg/kg (0.1 to 0.2 mL/kg) 1% sterile saline solution. It should be administered **slowly over 5 min** and may be repeated only once in 1 to 2 h, if necessary. The maximum total dose should not exceed 7 mg/kg. Flush the vein out immediately after administration with 10 to 20 mL saline to minimize local pain. Improvement should be seen within 15 min with a maximum response within 30 min. Methb blood concentrations should be obtained 1 h after administration. Patients with glucose-6-phosphate dehydrogenase deficiency do not respond to MB because it utilizes reduced nicotinamide adenine dinucleotide phosphate derived from the hexose monophosphate shunt pathway.

(d) Patients who ingest nitroethane should be observed for 24 h because of delayed and recurrent methemoglobinemia (81,82).

c. **Nailprimer or artificial nail extender. Methacrylic acid** (2-methypropanenoic acid, MA) is a liquid with a disagreeable odor. It is combustible and emits toxic gases. It has caustic action. It is used in bone cements and as an artificial nail extender.

(1) **Toxicity and manifestations.** It is described as a skin irritant and sensitizer capable of causing skin burns on prolonged contact, however once polmerized becomes inert and nontoxic. It has produced severe burns of eyes. Vasodilation and transient hypotension have been reported after its use as a bone cement. Its vapor is irritating to the eyes and respiratory tract. Direct cardiotoxicity has been noted. The permissible exposure level (PEL) is 20 ppm and immediately dangerous to life and health (IDLH) 3 ppm. Based on structural analogues, compounds containing the acrylate moiety may be carcinogens. Occupational asthma has been associated with various methyl methacrylates (83).

(2) A 21-month-old boy ingested an unknown amount of methacrylic acid. Vomiting developed followed immediately by respiratory distress. Esophagoscopy revealed 1st and 2nd degree burns of the entire esophagus with a deep burn along the lesser curvature of the stomach. Bronchoscopy showed marked edema of epiglottic, aryepiglottic folds and both main stem bronchi. The patient required a total of 28 days hospitalization including 6 days of positive pressure ventilation and 15 days of parenteral nutrition (81).

(3) **Kinetics.** Possibly metabolized in the liver and hydroxylated to an alcohol then oxidized to aldehyde and to pyruvate, where it enters the Krebs cycle (83).

(4) **Management** consists of decontamination with charcoal/oathartic although there are no studies; supportive care including parenteral nutrition if severe GI ulceration (83).

d. **Acrylic fingernails** containing *N,N*-dimethyl-*p*-toluidine solution, a component used in the fabrication of artificial fingernails have been reported to produce a severely delayed and recurrent methemoglobinemia. Exposure warrants 24 h close observation (84). A 16 month old girl became symptomatic after ingesting 15 ml (6 mg/kg) of an artificial fingernail preparation containing this chemical. She developed a **methemoglobin level** of 43%. She was treated with methylene blue and completely recovered (84). Management is GI decontamination and treatment of methemoglobinemia with methylene blue.

E. **Hair products.** The AAPCC in 1994 reported 21,511 exposures to hair products, with 567 moderate outcomes, 21 major outcomes, and no deaths (4).

1. **Dyes and bleaches.** Permanent color requires oxidizers such as **hydrogen peroxide** 3% to 6%, which is usually of low toxicity (see Hydrogen Peroxide). Metallic hair dyes usually contain small amounts of toxic metals, and only large ingestions require treatment. **Hair sprays** that are chronically inhaled may cause hilar adenopathy and pulmonary infiltrates (thesaurosis) (3).

2. **Hair-straightening** and **hair-waving preparations** may contain 1% to 3% sodium hydroxide or ammonium hydroxide plus potassium carbonate or bicarbonate, and may cause corrosive injury. Management is the same as a potential caustic material (3).

3. **Permanents** are usually composed of 1% to 3% sodium hydroxide. They are highly alkaline with a pH of 13. The ingestions should be treated as a caustic ingestion. Ocular exposures require immediate irrigation of the eye and a thorough eye examination.

   a. **"Cold" permanent waves** introduced in the 1940s are usually produced by the use of two solutions: the waving fluid, which is alkaline thioglycolate solution (ammonium thioglycolate, thioglycerol), and the reducing agent and the fixation-neutralization solution, which is an acid hydrogen peroxide. No teratogenicity has been implicated with these chemicals.

      (1) The **thioglycollate** can cause irritation and immediate type hypersensitivity reaction and in large amounts cause hypoglycemia and cyanosis.

      (2) The **fixation solution** is an irritant but is rapidly degraded to oxygen and water (see Hydrogen Peroxide).

   b. **"Hot" permanent waves** introduced in the 1970s uses glyceryl monothioglycerate in solutions having a pH 2.0 to 2.5 and has resulted in second degree scalp burns.

   c. **Permanent wave neutralizers** may contain **perborates** (see Boric Acid) or nephrotoxic **bromates** (85–93). Hairwave neutralizers that contain bromates are listed in Table 28-9.

      (1) **Bromates** are used to improve and preserve the textures of bread. Sodium (10%) and potassium (2%) bromate are oxidizing agents in

TABLE 28-9. *Hair neutralizers that contain bromates*

Product	Manufacturer	Bromate content
Biowave	Redken	10–25%
Curl & Condition	Redken	10–25%
RK Trichoperm Style	Redken	15–18%
Revlon	Revlon	10%
Trichoperm	Redken	15–18%
California Curl	Morrow	7%

certain permanent hair wave neutralizers. Bromates have been removed from most products, but certain commercial products still contain the dangerous nephrotoxin: Biowave (10% to 25%), Curl & Condition (10% to 25%), RK Trichoperm Style (15% to 18%), Revlon (10%), Trichoperm (15% to 18%), and California Curl (7%). A total of 17 cases of bromate intoxication have been reported up to 1989 (90).

(a) **Toxicity:** The **toxic amount** in children is estimated at 250 to 500 mg/kg (90). The potentially **fatal amount** is about 5 g. Serious poisonings have occurred after 2 to 4 oz of a 2% solution of potassium bromate in children. There are 10 deaths reported (85–93).

(b) **Kinetics** has not been well defined. Bromates may be converted into hydrobromatic acid in the stomach causing gastritis. Bromates are converted into bromides in the body. The route of elimination is renal. Volume of distribution is 0.24 L/kg. The mechanism of toxicity is unclear although bromates may produce damage as an oxidizing agent or have an irritating effect on renal tubule (88).

(c) **Manifestations.** GI symptoms occur within 1.5 to 2 h postingestion due to the caustic action of hydrobromic acid. Irreversible neurosensory **hearing loss** and tinnitus develops within 6 to 24 h (90–92). **Renal impairment** develops within 24 to 48 h and improves in the majority of cases by the fourth day postingestion. Some renal impairment can persist for days to weeks and may be permanent (87,90,92). **Death** from bromate intoxication is usually due to renal failure. CNS depression and seizures may develop with uremia. Methemoglobinemia, hemolysis (87) and thrombocytopenias have been reported. Bromate intoxication may **mimic hemolytic uremic syndrome (HUS)** in infants and small children (90,93).

(d) **Management.** GI decontamination is to administer sodium bicarbonate orally 5 g in 8 oz of water (may prevent the formation of hydrobromic acid). **Do not administer oral sodium thiosulfate** because in the presence of gastric hydrochloric acid, it may form irritating and toxic hydrogen sulfide. Activated charcoal may be administered although there are no studies of effectiveness (88,93). **Sodium thiosulfate i.v.** 100 to 500 mL 1% solution is advised as an infusion or 0.2 to 1 mL/kg up to 10 to 50 mL of 10% solution over 30 to 60 min. Thiosulfate theoretically acts to reduce absorbed bromate to a relatively innocuous bromide ion. There is controversy about its use although it is fairly innocous (90,93). Correct dehydration, shock, electrolyte, and acid-base disturbances (91). **Transfusions** of packed red blood cells may be necessary if hemolysis develops. Do not use **methylene blue** for methemoglobinuria since it enhances the toxicity of bromates (87,89–93). **Hemodialysis** does not enhance the elimination of bromates but may be necessary for renal failure that does not improve within 48 h. Administer oxygen and consider exchange transfusion (88,91).

(e) **Laboratory.** Be sure to specify **bromates** if desired blood concentration or bromides will be determined. **Monitor** renal function (BUN, creatinine, urine specific gravity, electrolytes, and urinary output). Monitor hemoglobin, hematocrit, and serum electrolytes. Check for neurosensory deafness (91).

4. **Shampoos.** Plain shampoos are nontoxic. Dry shampoos can be dangerous and contain methanol or isopropyl alcohol. Bubble baths and shampoos in the bath water are not toxic but have caused irritation cystitis, urethritis, and vaginitis. **Selenium shampoos** contain 2% selenium sulfide, a nonabsorbable salt, which is less toxic than the soluble selenites (1 to 5 mg/kg caused moderate toxicity in adults), selenates and selenium compounds. Ten mL of typical shampoo is 100 to 250 mg of poorly absorbed sulfate. It is of low level toxicity, produces vomiting and usually requires over 1 to 2 oz to produce toxicity. Most of the symptoms are GI with burning sensation in the mouth and a garlic taste and smell to the breath. There are no reports of deaths. Management consists of avoiding emesis and administering supportive care and monitoring electrolytes (94) (see Soluble Selenious Acid of High Toxicity).

5. **Lightening agents** typically contain oxidizers (including ammonia), metasilicates (alkalinizers) and detergents. The pH varies from 9.5 to 11.5. They are considered moderately toxic. Management should be the same as a caustic.

F. **Ointments, creams, and plain soaps** are usually nontoxic.

G. **Dental care products**
  1. **Mouthwash.** The Consumer Product Safety Commission had received 2,000 reports of poisoning by **mouthwash with alcohol** over a 5-year period and three deaths in the last 10 years. All these incidents involved children under 5 years. In 1994 there were 6,948 exposures to ethanol containing mouthwash reported to AAPCC, with 154 moderate outcomes, 17 major outcomes, and two deaths. There were also 1,220 exposures to **fluoride mouthwash**, with three moderate outcomes, no major outcomes, and no deaths (4).
      a. Mouthwash preparations may contain as much as 26% **ethanol** (Listerine 26.9% or 53.8 proof). It is recommended that children under 6 years not use

mouthwash and mouthwash should be in safety packaging if it contains more than 5% ethanol. Treatment is for alcohol intoxication and treat hypoglycemia if present (69–74).

    b. **Fluoride** in mouth rinses contain between 0.05% to 2% sodium fluoride. One gram of sodium fluoride equals 452 mg of elemental fluoride. The toxic dose of fluoride is more than 5 mg/kg and the lethal dose is about 16 mg/kg (95–97).

  2. **Toothpaste with flouride.** In 1994 there were 3,339 exposures reported to AAPCC, with 19 moderate outcomes, one major outcome, and no deaths (4). The maximum amount of sodium fluoride in a tube of **toothpaste** is usually less than 264 mg. Pediatric exposures rarely result in intoxications. The immediate treatment of fluoride ingestion is milk followed by gastric lavage with 10% calcium gluconate. Do not induce emesis. Activated charcoal is ineffective. Further treatment is i.v. 10% calcium gluconate and hemodialysis (95–97).

  3. **Denture cleaner** liquids may be alkalies and could damage esophageal tissue. Treat as a caustic. There were 1,087 exposures in 1994 reported to AAPCC, with five moderate outcomes, no major outcomes, and no deaths (4).

H. **Skin lighteners** contain hydroquinones, which in large amounts can produce cyanosis and convulsions. Management is supportive. Activated charcoal has been recommended although there are no studies of its effectiveness (3).

I. **Talc, talcum powder**

  1. Talc is a naturally occurring hydrous magnesium silicate similar in chemical composition, but not morphologically, to various asbestos minerals.

  2. In 1994, the AAPCC reported 3,008 exposures to talcum powder, with 51 moderate outcomes, one major outcome, and no deaths (4). Moss indicated approximately 50 exposures/year were reported to the New York City PCC in 1969 (99). The Long Island PCC reported 211 exposures in 1981 (two of which were hospitalized and one required assisted ventilation) (100); 85 exposures were reported in 1985 (106) and 52 in 1989. There has been a decline in our area since the publicity about the possible health effects.

    (1) **A survey of 100 parents** of infants (2 weeks to 6 months) revealed 46 used talcum powder, 68% routinely (101). Another study showed that majority of parents who used baby power were unaware of the aspiration hazard (99). Powdering of a baby is not essential to good infant skin care (101,102). If parents decide to use a powder they should be advised to sprinkle the powder on their own hands and apply it to the infant rather than creating a cloud of powder by shaking the can directly onto the baby (110).

    (2) **Massive aspiration** of talcum powder is likely to occur **during the diaper-changing period** 73% of episodes occurred during this time (104). Some of the powder containers **resemble infant formula bottles** (100,106,109).

    (3) A review of over 25 cases of **talcum powder aspiration reports** in infants revealed a mortality of 20% (107). These cases however represent only the most severe episodes.

(4)   Parents should be aware of the controversy regarding long-term health risks of talc. The composition of the talc depends on the geographic location of the mines. **The American Conference of Governmental Industrial Hygienists** currently have two threshold limits values (TLVs) for talc; one for respirable dust containing no asbestos fibers at 2 mg/m^3 or, one for fibrous talc which follows the asbestos limit of two fibers per milliliter for fibers greater than 5 μm in length (114) There is controversy about **talc's relationship to asbestos and cancer** (111,112,115).

(5)   **Condoms, ovarian cancer and fertility.** There is circumstantial evidence that talcum powder applied to the perineal area in females over several years may be associated with increased risk of cancer of the ovary. Studies have shown that particles of powder make their way up the fallopian tube and talc has been found imbedded in ovarian cancer specimens (116). Talc placed on the surface of condoms and diaphragms also reached the ovaries via the fallopian tubes (117). Talc is found in the majority of condoms manufactured in the United States (117).

(6)   Talc is **harmless if ingested** but can be hazardous when inhaled.

(7)   **Inhalation.** Infants may die within hours from pulmonary edema or aspiration pneumonia. Baby powder has caused adult respiratory distress syndrome (109,119). There are reports of **chronic exposure** to talc resulting in pulmonary fibrosis (talcosis), usually in industrial workers (105,112), and in chronic cosmetic overuse (102). **Inhalation talcosis** has been reported in a child following massive inhalation of talc (107).

(8)   **Prevention** The powder containers should not look like a formula bottle and it should be kept out of the infant's reach when diapering. The container type should deliver only a limited amount of powder when inverted. The routine of giving a free sample of powder on discharge from the hospital nursery should be abandoned. Parents should be instructed regarding the proper method to powder an infant. There is controversy about the long-term exposure to talcum powder. Talcum powder should be removed from condoms and diaphragms.

(9)   **Management** of talc aspiration consists of procedures to establish and maintain the vital functions. Respiratory support is the main treatment. Bronchopulmonary lavage is not effective because talc is insoluble in water.

III.   **Disinfectants**

A.   **Disinfectants in over-the-counter (OTC) preparations** are of low concentration, but the highly concentrated substances found in **herbicides** and **germicides** may produce toxicity. Most of the disinfectants are acids, alkali, pine oil, phenol, hypochlorite, and cationic detergents. Disinfectant exposures reported to the AAPCC in 1994 were 21,795, with 816 moderate outcome, 25 major outcomes, and two deaths (4).

B.   **Pine oil**. Pine Sol, one of the widely used pine oil preparations, was a 25% to 35% pine oil. Since 1985, it has contained only 19.9% pine oil and 80% inert ingredients, which includes 10.9% isopropyl alcohol and soap. Additional ingredients are added to pine oil to increase the viscosity and reduce the danger of aspiration and pulmonary toxicity.

1. **Incidence.** In 1994, there were 10,656 pine oil exposures (the largest number of disinfectant exposures) reported to the AAPCC, with 240 moderate outcomes, 17 major outcomes, and one death (4).
2. **Pine-scented formulations** have a small percentage of pine oil and are of minimal toxicity.
3. **Pine oil** is a mixture of highly lipophilic, volatile oil that is an unsaturated hydrocarbon of low viscosity called "cyclic terpenes." It is related to turpentine. It not a petroleum distillate and is not as toxic to the lungs as petroleum distillate products.
4. **Toxicity.** Pine oil is estimated to have **one-fifth the toxicity of turpentine** in animals. Turpentine ingestions of 15 to 60 mL cause GI symptoms, and 120 to 180 mL is a potentially lethal dose (114,115) (see Art Materials). Systemic absorption of pine oil produces the pulmonary toxicity, but **aspiration is not necessary to produce pneumonitis** (120–123). Death occurred in a child who ingested 15 cc of 100% solution. The adult fatal amount is estimated to be 60 to 120 mL of 100%, although survival has been reported after a 400-mL ingestion (122). The authors of a retrospective study of 22 cases over a 10-year period (1977 to 1986) concluded that with volumes over 1 oz of Pine Sol 20% or 5 mL of 100% or if the patient is symptomatic, the patient should have gastric lavage and activated charcoal with a cathartic and be observed (121). An abstract of a prospective study of 66 patients presented in 1986 led the authors to conclude that patients ingesting less than 20% pine oil did not become ill (123).
5. **Kinetics.** Pine oil is readily absorbed from the GI tract. It is also absorbed from the vagina and uterus (used in abortion attempts). The **onset of toxic action** following ingestion is 90 min. It is metabolized in the liver to a triol metabolite that is excreted in the urine and the lungs. The terminal half-life ($t_{1/2}$) is 1.5 days (122).
6. **Manifestations**. A clue is the odor of pine oil on the breath. Spontaneous vomiting, lethargy, and ataxia develop within 90 min postingestion in children. An intentional ingestion of as much as 9 to 10 oz of pine oil in adults has produced emesis, lethargy, tachycardia and tachypnea, hypertension, pneumonitis, and transient coma. There are no long-term sequelae or deaths that have been reported. CNS depression was present in 50% of patients. This may develop rapidly but is quickly reversible. Pulmonary toxicity may be due to systemic absorption as well as aspiration, but most recover within 24 h. Pulmonary complications occurred in one series in 27%. Renal failure may occur (120–123,125).
7. **Management.** Referral to a medical facility for several hours observation and GI decontamination is recommended if children ingest 1 oz or more of a 20% solution or are symptomatic (120,121). Others recommend gastric emptying of the stomach only if over 2 mL/kg of 20% is ingested (123). More concentrated solutions should be referred for proportionately less amounts and any amount of 100% solution warrants medical evaluation and consideration of GI decontamination. **Induced emesis is avoided** because of the rapid onset of CNS depression and gastric lavage is withheld in minor ingestions or if the presentation is delayed. Activated charcoal and cathartic is recommended within the first few hours postingestion. However, there is no data available on charcoal or gastric lavage effectiveness. Supportive care of the **complications** is all that is available.

C. **Boric acid** (see boric acid under Bleach).

D. **Hydrogen peroxide (H_2O_2)** is a clear colorless, odorless, liquid oxidizing agent found in many households at low concentrations (3% to 9%) for various medicinal applications (3%) (antiseptic/ disinfectant, loosening secretions, cerumen removal, gargle, douche enemas) and as a clothes (6%) and hair bleach (6%). Higher concentrations more than 10% often 35% are used as strong oxidizing agents in industry (126–128). "Food grade hydrogen peroxide" (35%) from health-food stores or by mail is used illegally to lengthen the shelf life of milk and refrigerated perishables.

1. **Incidence and outcomes.** The 1994 AAPCC report listed 13,449 peroxide exposures, with 126 moderate outcomes, two major, and one death. Under topical agents, there were 7,797 exposures, with 66 moderate outcomes, one major outcome, and no deaths (4). The percentage of the H_2O_2 in products and their relationship to outcomes was not listed.

   a. A retrospective study of 670 patients from LI with 3% hydrogen peroxide ingestions over a 3 year period revealed 85% had no symptoms, 14% had minor symptoms, and one patient had major symptoms with multiple gastric ulcers and erosions (129).

   b. Another study of 325 patients exposed to different concentrations by different routes indicated that 41 exposures involved H_2O_2 concentrations less than 10%. Of these, 58% had no symptoms, 38% had minor symptoms, and two (4%) had major symptoms. In this study, 284 exposures involved more than 10% concentration of H_2O_2. Of these, 29% developed no symptoms, 53% had minor symptoms, and three (17.6%) had major symptoms and one died (130).

2. **Mechanism of toxicity** of H_2O_2 results from its interaction with catalase in the tissue which produces the liberation of water and oxygen as it decomposes. One milliliter of 3% H_2O_2 liberates 10 mL of oxygen. When the amount of oxygen evolved exceeds its maximum blood solubility, then venous embolism occurs. **Higher strength** preparations more than 10% are caustic (127,129,131) to the skin and mucosa and systemically are more likely to produce fatal air embolism (126,127,132–141).

3. **Toxicity:** Most cases of household strength 3% to 10% H_2O_2 ingestion, or dermal and ocular exposure are benign (129,130).

   a. **Ingestion of 3%** concentration may produce a mild GI irritation, rarely significant mucosal erosions (128,129), rarely portal vein embolization (128) and in large amounts death (130,135). There is a single report of a 2-year-old child who developed portal vein embolization after ingesting 3% H_2O_2 (128). One of the reported pediatric ingestion fatalities involved up to 8 oz of 3% H_2O_2 in a 16 month old; all others were 30% to 35% or greater (130,132). Ingestions of more than 10% are more likely to produce mucosal ulcerations and fatal air embolism (126,127,131–137).

   b. Hydrogen peroxide should not be administered where the evolved oxygen gas cannot dissipate freely.

   c. There are many reports of **oxygen embolization** after irrigation of tissues **during surgery** (126–127,132–137). Gas embolism and intestinal gangrene was noted from colonic irrigation with 1% H_2O_2 in the treatment of meconium ileus (136). An 81-year-old man developed cerebral embolism immediately after ingestion of 30 mL of 35% hydrogen peroxide (140).

4. **Manifestations**
   a. Ingestion of H_2O_2 in concentrations of **3% to 10%** may produce white foam from the mouth, mild gastric irritation, gastric distention and emesis, rarely GI erosions or embolism; **10% to 20%** in addition to the above can result in burns to exposed tissues; **20% to 40%** in addition to the above can produce rapid loss of consciousness followed by respiratory arrest.
   b. **Oxygen embolization** to the portal vein and heart may restrict blood flow resulting in ischemia and ECG changes and electromechanical dissociation asystole (132,140).
   c. **Radiographic findings** of gas in mesenteric, gastric, splenic or portal vein, inferior vena cava and right ventricle has been reported (135,140).

5. **Management**
   a. **GI decontamination is not indicated.** Vomiting should not be induced. Asymptomatic patients who have ingested small amounts of 3% hydrogen peroxide may be observed at home but symptomatic patients with persistent vomiting, hematemesis, abdominal distention or discomfort should be medically evaluated. Patients ingesting higher concentrations especially more than 10% should be medically evaluated. Administration of milk to dilute may be useful.
   b. **Endoscopy** may be needed if symptoms, especially hematemsis, are present, high concentrations more than 10% are ingested, or hematemesis is present (129).
   c. **Gastric distention** may require decompression via nasogastric tube. A careful examination should be performed to detect any gas formation. The use of antiulcer regimes such as antihistamine H-2 blockers has not been evaluated.
   d. **Trendelenburg positioning** should be avoided and may trap air in the apex of the right ventricle and cause obstruction of blood flow.
   e. A **Radiograph** of the abdomen and chest is advised if there are symptoms or if a high concentration is ingested to detect intravascular oxygen embolization. Embolization is most commonly seen in the portal venous system (140).
   f. **Hyperbaric oxygen** has been used in severe embolization cases but there are no controlled studies.
   g. **Laboratory.** A screening test for the presence of hydrogen peroxide involves adding 1 drop of 15% titanium chloride to an acidified mixture of equal parts of gastric contents and ethyl ether. A yellow to deep orange coloration of the aqueous layer occurs due to the formation of H_2TiO_4 which is an indication of ingested peroxide (141).

E. **Iodine and iodofores.** Iodine is used as a local dermal disinfectant, and in the treatment of hyperthyroidism. There were 1,757 exposures to iodine and iodide antiseptics reported in 1994 to the AAPCC, with 46 moderate outcomes, four major outcomes, and no deaths (4).

1. Iodine is poorly soluble in water so liquid preparations are in 50% or higher ethanol. USP Tincture (2% iodine, 2.4% sodium iodide) are in 15-mL bottles (720 iodine mg/15 mL), "strong" iodine tincture (7% iodine and 5% potassium iodide or 350 mg of iodine/5 mL). Lugol's solution (5% iodine and 10% potassium iodide) is used preoperatively to reduce vascularity of the thyroid and to prevent absorption of iodine in the treatment of hyperthyroidism. **Organic bound iodides** (iodophor) includes povidone iodine (0.2% to 1% available iodine) diluted to 7.5% for surgical scrubs or antiseptic solutions so the dilute solutions are 0.15 to 7.5 mg/mL. **Betadine** is 1% iodine. Iodine **ointment** is 4% iodine.

2. **Toxicity:** The potentially fatal dose is 2 to 4 g of free iodine. Food in the GI tract inactivates iodine to harmless iodide salts. **Organic bound iodides** have 1/5 toxicity of their iodine base. **Mechanism of toxicity** is similar to an acid because of its oxidizing properties. Iodine in the body tissues forms complexes with amino groups to form an iodophor which liberate iodine slowly in small amounts causing sustained action, is nontoxic and not caustic. Dermal absorption of iodine has been reported in burn patients (142,143) in treatment of other wounds topically (144,145) and in newborns (146).

3. **Manifestations of iodine toxicity:** If ingested may cause corrosive gastroenteritis, blue vomitus if starch is present, and hematemesis, renal failure, metabolic acidosis, increased osmolarity, shock and hypersensitivity reactions. One case of pyloric stenosis is reported. Enlargement of the parotid glands was reported with chronic use. Strong iodine solution may cause dermal burns and systemic absorption. Severe hypersensitivity reactions have been reported.

4. **Management:** Maintain airway because of edema from sensitivity reactions. Iodines and iodofors are not usually of sufficient concentration or amount to produce toxicity (147).

   a. Milk is given immediately and may be followed by 15 g of cornstarch or flour in 500 mL of water or 1% to 5% sodium thiosulfate (produce purple color). Milk may be repeated every 15 min to relieve gastric irritation. Avoid other GI decontamination procedures. Most household ingestions of tincture of iodine or providine iodine only require milk and observation.

   b. If signs of esophageal or gastric damage occur then endoscopy is recommended.

   c. If anaphylactoid reaction occurs, treat with epinephrine.

   d. Monitor urinary output and renal profile if the patient becomes toxic.

   e. Elimination can be enhanced by osmotic diuresis or salt loading.

F. **Phenol and its derivatives** (see Chapter 21). Phenol (carbolic acid) is an aromatic alcohol derived from coal tar which is used in explosives, fertilizers, paints, resins, and disinfectants. Chlorinated phenol derivatives are much less toxic than pure phenol (148). Phenols have local caustic properties as well as systemic toxicity (148–150). The AAPCC reported 3,387 exposures in 1994, with 109 moderate outcomes, three major outcomes, and one death (4).

   1. **Hexachlorophene** (Phisohex) is a chlorinated biphenol used as a local antiseptic. There were 154 exposures reported to AAPCC in 1994, with 39 moderate outcomes, three major outcomes, and no deaths.

a. It produced neurotoxicity from chronic dermal application to premature infants (151,152) and pediatric burn patients. The acute ingestion of large amounts at high concentrations more than 3% or in doses more than 0.5 mg/kg can produce toxic effects including dermal (erythema and desquamation), GI (vomiting and diarrhea), and neurological effects (lethargy, coma, seizures) with fatalities after both acute and chronic exposure.

2. **Chlorhexidene** (Hibiclens) has little system absorption and is an irritant at low concentrations and caustic at high concentrations. Anaphylaxis has been reported.

3. **Pentachlorophenol (herbicides)** used a diaper rinse produced transdermal intoxication in neonates associated with profuse diaphoresis (153,154). In the newborn skin absorption of phenols disinfectants has also produced hyperbilirubinemia (155).

4. **Other phenol and phenol related compounds** include Chloraseptic (1.4% phenol), creosol (antiseptic), creosote (wood preservative), eugenol (see Eugenol and Clove Cigarettes), guaiacol (antiseptic), hydroquinone, mouth washes gargles contain 0.5% to 1.5%, resorcinol (antiseptic), tetrachlorophenol (fungicide), thymol (fungicide), and phenol eardrops 5.4% to 7.5%.

5. **Toxicity**
   a. **Mechanism of toxicity.** Phenol is a general protoplasmic poison (denatures protein) with corrosive local effects. Systemically it is a CNS stimulant. Phenol derivatives are less toxic than pure phenol.
   b. **The oral toxic and lethal amounts** are not well documented. In adults they have been reported in single ancedotal reports as low as 1.0 g, or 50 to 500 mg in infants, but documentation is not provided. Other sources quote an estimated lethal dose as between 3 to 6, or 10 to 30 g with references not well documented. Ingestions of 45, 56, and 65 g have been associated with coma and cardiovascular collapse but survival (148–150,152,157). **Inhalation PEL** is 5 ppm. **IDLH** is 100 ppm.
   c. **A 10% solution** produces local skin necrosis. Infant death occurred after 2% application to umbilicus for 11 h (148,149).

6. **Kinetics:** Phenol is well absorbed by inhalation, dermal application, and ingestion. The route of elimination is by biotransformation in the liver to ethereal or phenylglucuronide or phenylsulfate metabolites and small amounts are oxidized to catechol and quinol which are conjugated.

7. **Manifestations**
   a. **Systemic**—Symptoms develop in 5 to 30 min postingestion and may produce early convulsions, coma, acidosis, and shock. Initially phenols may produce a transient excitement phase followed by coma. Convulsions may occur as long as 18 h postingestion. Hemolysis and methemoglobinemia (especially with dinitrophenol, a herbicide) have been noted (148–150). Brown-black urine on standing may be found due to oxidation of phenol metabolites.
   b. **Local**—produces **dermal** lesions which are initially painless white patches and later turns erythematous and finally stain brown. Phenols produce mucosal burns with a coagulum. They produce eye irritation and corneal damage.

    c. When phenols are **ingested** they cause extensive local corrosion with pain, nausea, vomiting, sweating, and diarrhea. Phenols have not been reported as producing esophageal strictures.

    d. **Inhalation** produces respiratory tract irritation and chemical pneumonia.

8. Management

    a. Immediate medical evaluation, if significant ingestion (phenol more than 1 g or 50 mg in infants; hexachlorophene more than 0.5 mg/kg) or if symptomatic. Establish and maintain vital functions. Establish vascular access. Treat shock (fluids), dysrhythmia (lidocaine) and convulsions (diazepam). Protect personnel with gowns and rubber gloves. If inhalation administer 100% oxygen, intubate and give assisted ventilation as needed.

    b. **If ingested.** Avoid emesis, alcohol and oral mineral oil and dilution and which may increase absorption. **Gastric lavage** is usually not recommended. Immediately give **activated charcoal** by small bore nasogastric tube, if necessary. In vitro studies indicate activated charcoal adsorbs phenol (158). However activated charcoal may interfere with endoscopic visualization. Castor oil has been reported to delay absorption but this is not supported by clinical studies. **Over 1 g phenol is of concern in a small child.**

    c. **Immediately decontaminate the skin** with copious amounts of water followed by undiluted **polyethylene glycol** (GoLytely or from Sigma Chemical Co.). Repeatedly sponge the area with sponges soaked in propylene glycol. **Wash the area thoroughly with soap and water after treatment** (159). Isopropyl alcohol has been effective in burns less than 5% in animals. Further studies are needed to determine degree of absorption of isopropyl alcohol in larger burns (159).

    d. Immediately **decontaminate the eyes** with copious amounts of tepid water for at least 15 min. Follow up with examination and fluorescein stain of eyes for corneal abrasion. If pain persists obtain ophthalmologic consultation.

    e. **Control convulsions** with diazepam.

    f. Treat **methemoglobinemia** if greater than 30%, or if respiratory distress, with methylene blue 1 to 2 mg/kg of 1% solution slowly i.v.

    g. Manage the **metabolic acidosis** with 1 to 2 mEq/kg of sodium bicarbonate if necessary.

    h. In vitro studies suggest **charcoal hemoperfusion** removes free phenol (160).

G. Laboratory

    1. **Nontoxic amounts in the blood** are free phenol 0 to 4 mg/dL, conjugated phenols 0.1 to 2.0 mg/dL, and total phenol 0.15 to 7.96 mg/dL. Phenol is found in the urine normally and is naturally present in foods, a byproduct of salicylate metabolism. The maximum **permissible phenol in urine of exposed workers is 80 mg/L**, which is also the level used to monitor workers exposed to benzene.

    2. **In potentially toxic exposures**, monitor arterial blood gases (if dyspnea or pulmonary symptoms), blood electrolytes, glucose, renal and liver function, ECG, and urinalysis. Monitor for hemolysis with CBC and other tests if indicated. If cyanotic, obtain methemoglobin level. Phenol 1.5 g in 50% solution resulted in blood levels of 6.8 μg/mL. A fatal postmortem blood level from 30% dermal absorption was 2.7 mg/dL (157).

3. **A 10% ferric chloride test** on acidified urine may show a violet or blue color if phenol metabolites are present. A positive ferric chloride test is also seen with salicylates and phenothiazines.

IV. **Pesticides** (see Chapter 25). **Pesticides** that are highly toxic include arsenic, cyanide, fluoride, sodium monofluoroacetate (Compound 1080), phosphorus (white), strychnine and thallium. These pesticides should not be in the home. Their management is described under separate sections.

A. **Arsenic. Roach pellets containing lead arsenate** 16.2% and boric acid are still sold in certain states but they have been being phased out by the EPA since 1989. Inorganic arsenic is a rodenticide. Arsenic binds sulfhydryl groups and interferes with ezymatic reactions. The fatal dose of arsenic is about 120 mg. There were 430 exposures reported in 1994 to the AAPCC, with three moderate outcomes, no major outcomes, and no deaths (4).

1. **Terro Ant Killer** (2.28% sodium arsenate, 0.91% inorganic arsenic). Recommendations: if less than 5 mL are ingested advise observation, if greater than 5 mL are ingested, administer ipecac syrup to induce emesis and observe at home. If any symptoms other than a brief mild GI effect, refer for medical evaluation. These suggestions are based on 149 cases (155,156) and an incidence of 1593 case reports with 96.1% nontoxic or minor effect and 0.8% major effect (163). A prior study of 57 patients advocated GI decontamination and BAL chelation for all cases of sodium arsenate ant killer ingestion (163), however this is no longer the current standard for this type of ingestion (161).

2. **Indications** to start dimercaprol (BAL) therapy after arsenic exposure include

a. **Toxic exposure** to a potentially fatal dose of arsenic, such as arsenic trioxide 120 mg, or 1 to 2 mg/kg. If the patient's condition has stabilized or the symptoms are resolved an oral chelator such as D-penicillamine or succimer may be given until the urinary arsenic concentration is less than 50 μg/24 h.

b. **Symptoms of arsenic poisoning,** such as gastroenteritis or cardiac abnormalities can occur within 1 to 3 h after exposure.

c. If excessive absorption has occurred over an extended period or ingestion occurred 48 h prior to treatment and the patient can take oral medication, penicillamine may be the treatment of choice (see Chapter 23).

B. **Rodenticides** (see Table 28-10 and Chapter 25)

1. **Sodium monofluoroacetate** (SMFA, Compound 1080) is a clear odorless, tasteless compound that is metabolized to fluorocitrate that inhibits the Krebs cycle and oxidative phosphorylation which produces acute hypoxia. The potential lethal dose is 5 mg/kg. In 1994 there were eight exposures reported to the AAPCC, with no symptomatic outcomes or deaths (4). Management is GI decontamination, and the possible antidote is glycol monacetate (166).

2. **Thallium** was banned as depilatory in 1965, as an insecticide in traps, and a rodenticides in 1975, although it is still used in other countries. Thallium acts similar to arsenic and produces gastroenteritis, delayed neurologic signs and alopecia. Poten-

tial lethal dose is 12 mg/kg. Administer oral activated charcoal or Prussion blue (not available in United States). Forced saline diuresis and hemoperfusion is recommended (167,168).

3. **Yellow phosphorous paste** which had the appearance of butter was available for application to food as a rodenticide. Potential lethal dose is 1 mg/kg. Phosphorous compounds produce a very malodorous fluorescent stool ("the smoking stool syndrome") hepatorenal and multisystem failure (168–169). Phosphorous analogs are **aluminum, calcium phosphide** and zinc phosphide are gray, yellow or brown powder that liberate phosphine gas (170,171). Zinc phosphide has gray color with rotten egg odor. They are absorbed orally, dermally and by inhalation (171). They may produce cardiac, delayed pulmonary edema, multisystem failure, and death (171).

   a. **Management**

      (1) **Ingested phosphorous** is GI decontamination with milk by gastric lavage (not water) and activated charcoal. Emesis is not recommended. Supportive care of multiple organ failure. Hemodialysis and hemoperfusion are not useful.

      (2) **Phosphides** is removal from exposure, and administer respiratory and general supportive care.

4. **Strychnine** is a white powder with a bitter taste that causes refractory spinal seizures with clear mentation. There were 186 reports to AAPCC in 1994, with 21 moderate outcomes, five major outcomes, and no deaths (4). It interferes with the neuroinhibitor glycine at the postsynaptic glycine receptors (172). The potential lethal dose is 1.5 mg/kg.

   a. **Management.** Do not induce emesis. Gastric lavage can be done after controling hyperactivity and convulsions. Administer activated charcoal, but repeated doses have not been documented to be effective. Control convulsions with benzodiazepies and consider neuromuscular blockers (172–176). Rhabdomyolysis and myoglobinuria are managed with fluid diuresis, diuretics and alkalinization. Hyperthermia is treated by cooling, and antipyretics are ineffective (183).

5. **Anticoagulant rodenticides** produce cumulative toxicity. Anticoagulants are often blue-green pellets (superwarfarin Talon), odorless and tasteless. Single doses of the **warfarin** (coumarin) **or superwarfarins** (brodifacoum) are not usually toxic unless extraordinary amounts have been ingested (177,178). There were 12,868 exposures of superwarfarin long acting type in 1994 reported to AAPCC, with 54 moderate outcomes, 16 major outcomes, and one death. There were also 1,333 standard anticoagulant exposures, with six moderate outcomes, two major outcomes, and one death (4). Hypoprothrombinemia may occur without symptoms in some cases. From January 1993 to November 1995, the LIRPCC received 215 calls involving anticoagulant pesticides exposures. The majority of cases involved superwarfarins (189 cases) versus 26 containing regular acting warfarin. The majority (71%) were accidental ingestions in children less than 6 years of age. There were 12 patients that were symptomatic with vomiting, the most common

TABLE 28-10. *Rodenticides*

Agent	Mechanism of action	Manifestations	Onset	Management
Highly toxic LD$_{50}$ <50 mg/kg				
Thallium PFD 12 mg/kg Gizmo Rat Killer	Combines with —SH groups, interferes oxidative phosphorylation	GI upset, alopecia, neuropathy, delirium, convulsions	12–24 h, delayed	Oral prussian blue, AC, hemoperfusion
Appearance: white, crystalline, odorless, tasteless				
Na monofluoro-acetate (1080), Na fluoroacetate (SMFA) PFD 5 mg/kg, fluor-acetamide (1081) PFD 10 mg/kg	Interferes with Krebs cycle	Convulsions, cardiac dysrhythmias	30 min to 20 h	Glycol monoacetate?, clinical benefit, ethanol loading?, calcium if hypocalcemia
Appearance: white crystalline, odorless, tasteless, water-soluble				
Strychnine PFD 1.5 mg/kg EL ROY Mouse Bait	Interferes with glycine inhibition of spinal cord	Convulsions (spinal type), trismus, conscious	10–20 min	Anticonvulsants, neuromuscular nonpolarizing blockers
A bitter-tasting colorless, odorless, white powder				
Zinc Phosphide 1% PFD 40 mg/kg Field Rat Powder	Releases phosphine gas	"Fish breath" odor, black vomitus, CV collapse, pulmonary edema, hepatore-nal damage, multi-ple organ failure	2–3 h	Milk, avoid water lavage, supportive
Appearance: heavy, gray, cystalline powder, water-insoluble				
Elemental (yellow), phosphorous PFD 1 mg/kg Blue Death Rat Killer	Local burns, hepa-torenal damage	Garlic odor, lumines-cent vomitus and stools, cardiac toxicity, coma, "smoking stool syndrome"	1–2 h	GI decontamination, anticonvulsants
Appearance: yellow, waxy, paste, fat-soluble, water-insoluble				
Arsenic PFD 120 mg Rose Rat Killer	Combines with —SH groups, interferes enzymes	Garlic breath, bloody diarrhea, convulsions	1 h	GI decontamination, BAL or penicillamine
Appearance: white, crystalline, powder				
N-3 pyridylmethyl-*N*-p-nitrophenyl urea PFD 5 mg/kg Bann 1979 Vacor House Mouse Tracking Powder	Interferes with nico-tinamide metabo-lism in pancreas, Related to alloxan and streptozocin, neuropathic	GI upset, diabetes mellitus, autonomic dysfunction (blad-der, bowel dysfunc-tion, hypotension, motor and sensory neuropathy)	4–48 h	GI decontamination, nicotinamide 500 mg i.v./i.m. 200 mg g 2 h up to 3 g a day, then 100 mg oral 3 × a week for 2 wk

(continued)

TABLE 28-10. *Continued*

Agent	Mechanism of action	Manifestations	Onset	Management
Vacor yellow-green powder looks like corn meal or cereal, smells like peanuts				
Moderate toxicity LD$_{50}$ 50–500 mg/kg				
Alpha-naphthyl-thiourea PFD >4 g/kg Antu	Damages pulmonary capillaries, gives pulmonary edema	Pulmonary edema (rare in humans)	?	GI decontamination, supportive
Appearance: bitter-tasting, fine blue-gray powder, water-insoluble				
Chloralose alpha-chlorase chloralosane, glucohol PLD unknown	Metabolized trichloroacetic and trichlorethanol	Hypersecretion respiratory tract, myoclonic-like seizures	Min to 1 h	Airway care, diazepam
Appearance: crystalline powder, soluble in glacial acetric acid				
Cholecalciferol 0.75% baits LD$_{50}$ 336 pellets in 10-kg child (V-D 2308 units/pellet) Quintox, Rampage, Ortho Mouse B Gone, Ortho Rat, B Gone	Vitamin D intoxication	Hypercalcemia, hypertension, dysrhythmias	—	Emesis, lavage, AC, treat hypercalcemia
Appearance: Packets 1-10 oz				
Mild toxicity LD$_{50}$ 500–5,000 mg/kg				
Red Squill, PLD?	Cardiac glycoside	GI upset, cardiac toxicity, dysrhythmias	—	GI decontamination, treat dysrhythmia, digoxin FAB
Appearance: bitter taste				
Norbormide PLD >300 mg?	Vasoconstriction	Hypothermia in rat (not humans)	—	GI decontamination hypotension

PFD = potential fatal dose; CV = cardiovascular collapse; AC = activated charcoal.
Modified from refs. 164–190.

effect (3.7%). The amounts ingested were usually limited to a few pellets in these cases but exact amounts were unknown. Activated charcoal/cathartics was administered in 17 cases. The outcome in 11 out of 12 cases was minor. None of the ingestions had developed abnormal coagulation times. In one case with a moderate outcome, a 13-year-old girl ingested an unknown amount of brodifacoum with a toxic amount of aspirin (574 mg/kg). The patient developed salicylate intoxication. She completely recovered after a few days of treatment and did not have evidence of prolonged bleeding.

   a.   **Toxicity. Warfarin** is usually found in concentrations of 0.025% to 0.050%, and persons ingesting the agent usually remain asymptomatic unless over 20 mg are ingested. **Superwarfarins** (4-hydroxycoumarin derivatives) are

40 to 100 times more potent than warfarin and in massive overdose may produce a prolonged anticoagulant effect that lasts weeks to months if over 1 mg is ingested. However the majority of overdoses from superwarfarins remain asymptomatic (177,178).

b. We do not feel, based on our experience, that GI decontamination, hospital visits, or prothrombin determinations are necessary for single accidental ingestions of regular warfarin or superwarfarin rodenticides in children under 6 years of age involving small amounts such as a few pellets. The **management** of **intentional or repeated ingestions** require medical evaluation and management if the amount of a single ingestion is exceeded based on the chart in Fig. 28-4.

   (1) GI decontamination with emesis can be done immediately at the site, activated charcoal should be used in the ED.

   (2) The antidote is **vitamin K_1** as phytonadione (Mephyton Oral or Aqua-Mephyton) which is specific therapy if clinical bleeding occurs. There is controversy concerning its administration for only laboratory abnormalities in the prothrombin time. Larger doses of vitamin K_1 and fresh frozen plasma may be needed for clinical bleeding. Prophylactic vitamin K_1 is not recommended.

c. **Laboratory.** Initial and followup prothrombin times are not recommended unless there is clinical evidence of bleeding (177,178) (see Chapters 30 and 39).

6. **Vacor** (nitrophenylurea compound, PNU) is a phenyl urea rodenticide that looks like cereal and smells like peanuts. Potential lethal dose is 5 mg/kg. It was banned in 1979. There was only one exposure report to AAPCC in 1994. PNU intoxication results in autonomic and peripheral neuropathy (by interfering with nicotinamide adenine dinucleotide [NAD-NADP] necessary for energy transfer reactions) and produces irreversible diabetes mellitus (destroys the beta cells of the pancreas).

   a. **Management** is GI decontamination with emesis at the site, gastric lavage, and activated charcoal. The specific antidote is nicotinamide (niacinamide, vitamin B_3) 500 mg i.v./i.m. initially then 200 mg every 2 h up to 3 g a day for 48 h. Nicotinic acid (niacin) is not a substitute for nictinamide in treatment of PNU (179–183) (see Chapter 30).

7. **Antu** (alpha-naphthathiourea) is a blue gray powder that is rarely toxic in humans but causes increased pulmonary capillary permeability and pulmonary edema in rats. The potentially lethal dose is more than 4 g/kg. There were only 14 reports of exposures to AAPCC in 1994, and no toxicity occurred (4).

8. **Arsenic** is a white powder with garlic odor. Potential lethal dose is 120 mg in adults (see Chapter 23).

9. **Norbromide** causes vasoconstriction and ischemia in rats but not in humans.

10. **Red squill** is of low toxicity and acts like digitalis intoxications.

D. **Organophosphate (OPI) and carbamate insecticides** (see Chapter 28)

E. **Organochlorine pesticides** (see Chapter 28 and Lindane)

F. **Insect repellents.** Insect repellents are primarily for mosquitos, fleas, chiggers, and some biting flies, but hymenoptera are not deterred by available chemical repellents. These

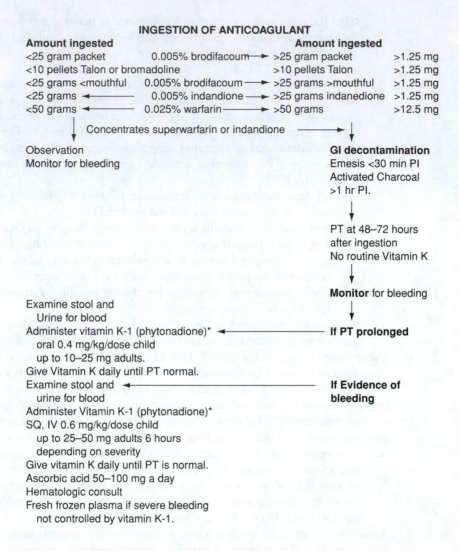

INGESTION OF ANTICOAGULANT

Amount ingested

		Amount ingested	
<25 gram packet	0.005% brodifacoum ⟶	>25 gram packet	>1.25 mg
<10 pellets Talon or bromadoline		>10 pellets Talon	>1.25 mg
<25 grams <mouthful	0.005% brodifacoum ⟶	>25 grams >mouthful	>1.25 mg
<25 grams ⟵	0.005% indandione ⟶	>25 grams indanedione	>1.25 mg
<50 grams ⟵	0.025% warfarin ⟶	>50 grams	>12.5 mg

Concentrates superwarfarin or indandione ⟶

Observation
Monitor for bleeding

GI decontamination
Emesis <30 min PI
Activated Charcoal
>1 hr PI.

PT at 48–72 hours
after ingestion
No routine Vitamin K

Monitor for bleeding

Examine stool and
   Urine for blood
Administer vitamin K-1 (phytonadione)* ⟵ **If PT prolonged**
   oral 0.4 mg/kg/dose child
   up to 10–25 mg adults.
Give Vitamin K daily until PT normal.
Examine stool and ⟵ **If Evidence of**
   urine for blood **bleeding**
Administer Vitamin K-1 (phytonadione)*
SQ, IV 0.6 mg/kg/dose child
   up to 25–50 mg adults 6 hours
   depending on severity
Give vitamin K daily until PT is normal.
Ascorbic acid 50–100 mg a day
Hematologic consult
Fresh frozen plasma if severe bleeding
   not controlled by vitamin K-1.

* Note: **Administer** Vitamin K-1 (phytonadione or (Mephyton oral or Aquamephyton).
DO NOT USE K-3 (menadione) or K-4 (menadiol).
PI = postingestion
PT = Prothrombin time
FFP = fresh frozen plasma.
Note: **Reversal of anticoagulation** may be dangerous for patients who require anti-coagulation, i.e. prosthetic heart valve patients, deep vein thrombosis. They may require heparin anticoagulation in these circumstances. Heparin may be used in pregnant patients for bleeding emergencies.

FIG. 28-4. Ingestion of anticoagulant.

chemicals are not harmful to wool or cotton but should be used with caution on other natural fibers or synthetics and may damage watch crystals and eye lens (181–184). There were 6,216 exposures to insect repellents in 1994 reported to AAPCC, with 119 moderate outcomes, 11 major outcomes, and one death (4).

1. **N,N-diethyl-M-toluamide** (**DEBT,** synonyms benzamide, diethylamide, M-det, M-delphene, M-toluic acid diethylamide) was produced in 1953 and marketed initially in 1956. It is a colorless to amber liquid found in aerosols, pump sprays, lotions/creams, roll-on sticks, and impregnated towelettes.

   a. Products containing DEET include "Muskol" (spray 25%, lotion 100%), "Deep Woods Off" (liquid 100%, aerosol 40%), "Jungle Plus" (100%), "Jungle Formula" (75%), "Repel" (20%), "Off" (aerosol 15%, towelettes 32.31%), Cutter (spray 17.9%), and "6–12 Plus" (5%). The preparation with the lowest concentration was "Skedaddle Insect Protection for Children" 9.5% DEET. DEET will dissolve certain plastics including watch faces and eye lenses.

   b. DEET is usually in an **ethyl or isopropyl alcohol vehicle.** The application of 30% DEET will prevent 90% of attachments of ticks (191–194), but the maximum suggested safe application to the skin is unknown for duration, frequency, and concentration.

   c. **Toxicity:** (195–198) DEET is lipophilic and structurally related to doxapram, an analeptic CNS stimulant. Toxicity has occurred following both dermal and oral exposure. There is no documented safe amount for children since the studies on safety were done on adults.

      (1) Since **Gryboski's report in 1961** (200) there have been 5 additional patients with encephalitis (201–204) reported following prolonged and extensive use and two died. In the two decades of DEET (1975 to 1995) use, there have been associated 13 deaths (205), seizures, encephalopathies, and other illness associated with DEET exposure. Most of the cases of toxicity involved the use of DEET from 10% to 50% and were related to overdose and misuse (205).

      (2) **Severe toxicity** has occurred after **ingestion** of 25 mL of 50% solution in a 1-year-old. Severe toxicity and death has occurred after ingestion of 50 mL 100% solution in adults. Extensive dermal application of 105 to 15% solutions for 2 days to 3 months have been linked to encephalopathy in children (200–204). **Neurotoxic effects** have been observed in adults exposed to more than 2 g by ingestion. **The mechanism of CNS toxicity** is undefined but it is postulated to be type I hypersensitivity reaction (206), direct CNS stimulation or interference with ammonia metabolism (207,208).

      (3) Patients heterozygous for sex-linked **ornithine transcarbamylase deficiency** (a urea cycle enzyme defect with overall prevalence of 1:30,000) may be at increased risk of toxicity. One such patient died of topical application (207,208). A 29-year-old man experienced seizures with fewer than 3 dermal applications (207,208).

    (4) **A retrospective analysis** of 9,086 human exposures between 1985 to 1989 reported to AAPCC revealed five patients experienced serious or potentially life-threatening effects and one death occurred in a patient who ingested 8 oz (205).

    (5) At present **the safe concentration of DEET is not known** especially for children. It is recommended it not be applied to children's hands and face and to wash the DEET off thoroughly when the patient returns indoors. Do not apply DEET near the eyes, or mouth or on damaged skin (cuts, blisters, sunburn or rashes). Do not apply in enclosed areas and avoid breathing in the repellent.

  d. **Kinetics.** DEET is absorbed by the oral and dermal routes. About 9% to 56% of the topically applied dose is absorbed within 6 h. **Onset of action after toxic ingestion** is rapid with coma and seizures occurring within 30 to 60 min. **Peak** plasma concentrations from GI absorption are usually within 1 h after ingestion and 6 h after dermal application. The **volume distribution** is 2.1 L/kg. The plasma **half-life** ($t_{1/2}$) is 2.5 h. The skin and fatty tissue retain DEET and its metabolites for 1 to 2 months after topical application and may act as reservoirs for DEET. DEET is eliminated by **hepatic oxidative metabolism** through the P450 enzyme system. About 10% to 15% is excreted in the urine unchanged. Elimination half-life ($t_{1/2}$) is 4 h. DEET and its metabolites may be detected in the urine for 2 weeks after ingestion and from 1 to 3 months after dermal application. DEET and metabolites have an **enterohepatic recirculation** (196–198).

  e. **Manifestations:** Although DEET is generally of low toxicity, in high concentrations or sprayed repeatedly on children, it has been associated with encephalopathy (200–204), seizures (209), coma, cerebral edema (200–203) and death (195). The encephalopathy can last up to 6 weeks after exposure. Hypotension and bradycardia have been noted (210). There are 5 known cases of hepatitis reported in Russia following DEET ingestion (181). Dermal and anaphylactoid reactions have been reported (206,211,212) DEET is teratogenic in chickens (213).

  f. **Management**

    (1) **Establish and maintain** the vital functions.

      Treat **convulsions** with i.v. diazepam or lorazepam and phenobarbital if recurrent seizures.

    (2) If DEET is **ingested** perform gastric lavage and administer activated charcoal initially with a cathartic. Emesis is not advised because of rapid onset of seizures. Repetitive doses of activated charcoal are advised because of the enterohepatic recirculation.

    (3) If **dermal exposure** remove clothes and wash the skin thoroughly with tepid water and soap. **Ocular** decontamination is by copious irrigation with water for at least 15 min. If irritation, pain, swelling, lacrimation and photophobia persist medical consultation should be sought.

(4) **Cerebral edema** is treated with hyperventilation, fluid restriction, head elevation, mannitol, and consideration of intracranial pressure monitoring. Monitor for inappropriate secretion of the antidiuretic hormone.

g. **Laboratory:** DEET serum level 8 h after topical application is 0.3 mg/dL (0.016 mmol/L) in asymptomatic patients. The DEET **blood concentration in a fatal case** was 16.8 to 24 mg/dL (168 to 240 µg/mL). Monitor blood glucose, electrolytes, and renal and hepatic parameters. A blood ammonia is recommended. With chronic oral and dermal exposures consider cranial tomography and cerebrospinal fluid (CSF) examination to exclude other causes for neurologic effects. A sterile CSF pleocytosis usually lymphocytic predominance has been associated with DEET exposure.

2. **Permethrin** is an alternative repellent for protection against mosquitoes, ticks, and fleas. Permethrin 1%, introduced in 1989, is a synthetic pyrethoid chemical insecticide structurally similar to a natural compound found in *Chrysanthemum cinerareaefolium*. Permethrin 0.5% provided 100% protection against the ticks that produce Lyme disease, compared with 86% protection for 20% DEET and 92% protection for 30% DEET, respectively. Permethrin 5% has been used safely in children as young as 2 months old (192). There were 11,030 exposures in 1994 to pyrethrins reported to AAPCC, with 596 moderate outcomes, 23 major outcomes, and 0 deaths (4). Permanone Tick Repellent is an aerosol spray to be applied **only on the outer surface of the clothes.** Do not saturate clothes. **Hang the treated** clothing outdoors to dry for several hours before wearing. Keep away from face and eyes because it may cause ocular irritation and corneal damage. Immediately wash off any skin accidently exposed to the product.

   a. **Toxicity:** Permethrin is toxic to the nervous system of insects but in mammals is poorly absorbed. In the absence of skin lesions, only 2% is absorbed. It may cause **allergic reactions**, but adverse systemic effects have not been reported (215,216). It is suspected of carcinogenic potential. The **toxic dose** in adults is more than 200 mL of 1% solution. The estimated **fatal dose** is 1 to 2 g/kg (217). It should not be used in infants under 2 months. Permethrin may cause ocular irritation and corneal abrasions (214,215). The mechanism of action in parasites is by disruption of the sodium transport in the nerve cell membranes. **Piperonyl butoxide** or similar compounds of low toxicity are usually added to enhance insecticide action, although they are not insecticides by themselves.

   b. **Kinetics.** In mammals it is poorly absorbed through the skin (less than 2%), but readily absorbed orally. It has low bioavailability due to high first pass metabolism. **Onset** of symptoms occurs in about 30 min. Pyrethrins are rapidly inactivated by ester hydrolysis, or hydrolyzed to chrysanthemumic acid and an alcohol which is oxidized to the aldehyde and acid or conjugated with glucuronide. They are slowly excreted as inactive metabolites in the urine and bile and may remain detectible in the tissues for up to 3 weeks. Duration of action is 14 days (216,218,219).

    c. **Manifestations: Overdose** produces nausea, vomiting, dizziness, weakness and coma, fasciculation, and seizures in doses over 200 mL in adults. Inhalation may cause bronchospasm. Paresthesia and peripheral neuropathy may occur after prolonged dermal application (216,218). Most complications are hypersensitivity reactions, which occur in 50% of those sensitive to ragweed. Ingestion of massive quantities may cause CNS stimulation, tremors, ataxia, and cardiopulmonary arrest. Corneal abrasions may occur with eye exposure. A death has been associated inhalation of a shampoo (217).

    d. **Management:** Establish and maintain vital functions.

       (1) **Decontamination procedures: Dermal:** Wash skin thoroughly with water. **GI:** Avoid emesis because of seizures. Gastric lavage with activated charcoal if substantial ingestion of more than 1 g/kg. Avoid fats and oils, which increase intestinal absorption. **Ocular:** Copious irrigation of the eyes with water or 0.89% saline for at least 15 min followed with fluorescein dye evaluation for corneal abrasion. If pain presists, obtain an ophthalmologic consultation.

       (2) **Treat allergic reactions** with supportive care, bronchodilators for bronchospasm, epinephrine, and diphenhydramine for anaphylactoid-allergic reactions.

       (3) **Seizures:** Diazepam or lorazepam.

   3. **Avon "Skin So Soft,"** a concentrated bath oil, is used as a "folk medicine" insect repellent and may offer short-lived (30 min) protection. It has not been scientifically investigated. There are no reports of toxicity.

   4. **R-11** 2,3,4,5-Bis(2-butylene tetrahydro-2-furaldehyde). There is a warning from EPA of animal studies showing reproductive problems and tumors in mice and rats. It was found in "Deep Woods Off" (and has been removed from it) and in "Cutter's Insect Repellent." It is listed in products as R-11.

  G. **Products for the treatment of lice and scabies**

   1. **Lindane (a gamma isomer of hexachlorocyclohexane).** It comes as Kwell in 1% cream, lotion, and shampoo. Lindane is an organochlorine insecticide used for the treatment of lice and scabies.

    a. **Toxicity:** Ingestions of less than 5 mL in a child or less than 15 mL in adult has not been associated with seizures. However, too frequent or prolonged and improper topical application has also caused seizures (two whole-body applications on two successive days has caused seizures). Ingestion of **1 g can produce seizures in a child and 10 to 30 g may be lethal in adults** (222–224) Deaths in infants and children have been reported from the improper topical application of lindane. It is an animal carcinogen. There are some reports of aplastic anemia, including a 21-year-old man who applied it for 3 weeks as a scabicide. Although not labelled a teratogen, caution is advised with its use in pregnancy (225,226). **The mechanism of action** is to increase the synaptic activity by increasing the neurotransmitter release from the presynaptic terminals.

    b. **Kinetics:** GI absorption occurs within 30 min and peak effects are in 2 h. It achieves brain levels three times greater than the blood. Lindane is metabolized by the liver into chlorophenol derivatives. Lindane is an enzyme inducer and has an enterohepatic recirculation. Following dermal application the half-life is 18 to 21 h (230).

    c. **Manifestations** (220–230). Onset of the signs of toxicity are within 15 min to 6 h following acute exoposure. Initially nausea and vomiting may occur. CNS stimulation including hyperirritability, restlessness, muscle spasms, loss of equilibrium, tonic-clonic seizures may develop within 15 min. Death may occur secondary to respiratory depression. Rhabdomyolysis and myoglobinuria secondary to seizures may result in renal failure. Hepatic damage has been reported in animals. Postapplication side effect of lindane is pruritic, dermatitis which occurs in 18% of the patients when lindane is applied in the treatment of scabies. The rash gradually disappears in about 2 weeks. Pruritis is a side effect of lindane not a sign of reinfestation. The duration of the toxic manifestations is short, subsiding within 12 h.

    d. **Management:** Establish and maintain the vital functions.

        (1) **If ingested** avoid emesis because of the rapid onset of seizures (within 15 min). Activated charcoal, initially with a cathartic, should be administered and repeated every 4 h because of the enterohepatic recirculation. No fats or oils should be administered because thery will enhance absorption. **Dermal decontamination** is accomplished with soap and water. Avoid oil-based solvents.

        (2) **Control seizures** with diazepam. Phenytoin has appeared to enhance the convulsive toxicity in rats and many clinicians avoid its use (216).

  2. **Permethrin (Pyrethrum, Pyrethrin, Pyrethroid)** [Ambush Fog, Elimite, Mustrol, Permit, Picket, Allergan Herbert, A-200, Pyrinate (OTC), Alfadex RID (OTC), Tisit (OTC) CAS 8003-34-7]. It is used in the treatment of lice and scabies, and as an insect repellent in the prevention of tick infestation (229,221) (see Permethrin).

H. **Moth repellents.** Mothballs, cakes, and nuggets were available as three types: camphor (discontinued), naphthalene, and paradichlorobenzene. According to the AAPCC in 1994, there were 4,919 mothball exposures (3,865 in children under 6 years). Naphthalene was involved in 1,877, with 15 moderate outcomes, one major outcome, and no deaths; paradichlorobenzene was involved in 207, with one moderate outcome, no major outcomes, and no deaths. In 2,811, the chemical demothing agents was not identified; there were 27 moderate outcomes, three major outcomes, and no deaths (4). Mothballs weigh between 0.5 to 3.6 g. For rapid differentiation test, see Table 28–11.

  1. **Camphor** is now banned in mothballs (233,234,235) and camphorated oil (20% camphor in cotton seed oil) in the United States (233). In accordance with FDA regulations, OTC drug products may not contain concentrations of camphor that exceeed 11% (233). One gram of camphor, which is toxic to children, is in over 30 common topical products (237) (Table 28-12).

TABLE 28-11. *Mothing agents differentiation*

Mothballs	Paradichlorobenzene	Naphthalene	Camphor
Form	Crystals, nuggets	Balls, flakes	—
Appearance	Wet and oily	Dry	—
Water test			
Plain water	Sinks	Sinks	Floats
Salt water[a]	Sinks	Floats	Floats
Melting pt	Yes 3 min 53°C	None at 80°C	—
Soluble			
Water	None	None	—
Alcohols	Yes	Yes	—

[a]Three tablespoonsful (45 g) of table salt in half glass (100 mL) of water stirred vigorously. This test may be done at home.

a. Toxicity. Camphor poisoning was first reported in 1925 (236). Camphor is a rapidly acting neurotoxin with both excitatory and depressant properties. The ingestion of more than **60 mg/kg or a single dose of 1 g** in a child has resulted in syncope, cyanosis, hypotension, dysrhythmias, mental state changes, and convulsions, which may be recurrent and rarely caused death (237–247). The mean **fatal dose is more than 5 g in adults and more than 1 g in children.** In Phelan's review of 748 patients, 42% had seizures following ingestion of 700 to 6,000 mg of camphor (238).

b. Kinetics. Camphor is a colorless, transparent white crystals with a penetrating aromatic odor and a pungent taste. It is highly lipid-soluble. It is readily and rapidly **absorbed** through the skin, mucous membranes, and GI tract, and

TABLE 28-12. *Amount of products that contain >1 g of camphor*

Amount	Product (percentage camphor)
20 mL	Ben-Gay vaporizing rub (5%)
5 mL	Camphorated oil (20% in cotton seed oil), banned in the United States
9.2 mL	Campho-Phenique first Aid Gel (10.80%, 4.66% phenol)
9.2 mL	Campho-Phenique Liquid (10.85%)
11 mL	Mentholatum (9%, 1.35% menthol, 1.96% eucalyptus oil, 1.4% turpentine spirits)
10 mL	Camphorated spirits (10% camphor in isopropyl alcohol)
17.5 mL	Musterole (5.7%)
27 mL	Heet Spray (3.6%)
33 mL	Heet Lotion (3%)
28 mL	Minit-Rub (3.5%)
29 mL	Sloan's Liniment (3.4%)
21 mL	Vicks Vaporub (4.8%, 2.6% menthol, 1.2% eucalyptus oil, 4.5% turpentine spirits)
23 mL	Vick's Vaposteam (4.2%)
20 mL	Children's Ben Gay Vaporizng Rub (5%)
26 mL	Soltice's Quick Rub (Children's) (3.75%)
29 mL	Sloans's Liniment (3.35%)
25 mL	Musterole Regular (4%)
16 mL	Save the Baby (6%)
26 mL	Camphorated tincture of opium (paregoric) (0.38%)

because of its nonpolar structure it crosses the placenta. **Protein binding** is 61% and **volume distribution** (V_d) is 2 to 4 L/kg. Camphor's absorption from the GI tract is enhanced by fatty substances and alcohol (238–241). The route of elimination is by hepatic hydroxylation and metabolism to the active form **campherol,** then oxidation to ketones and carbonic acid. Carbonic acid conjugates with glucuronide prior to renal excretion of inactive glucuronide compounds. Half-life is 93 to 167 min (237,238,240,241).

    c. **Manifestations.** The clinical syndrome begins with a feeling of warmth, followed by oral and epigastric burning, nausea, and vomiting. The **onset** of CNS simulation convulsions may be within 5 (usually 15 to 30) min, with **peak action** in 90 min after ingestion. A clue is the distinctive odor of camphor on the breath or in the urine (234–241). Elevation of the liver enzymes may occur and mimic Reye's syndrome (241,242). Other disturbances are anxiety, confusion, dizziness, and facial fasciculations, which may precede the seizures. Renal impairment has been described (225,234).

    d. **Management**

      (1) Indication for referal to ED: Children ingest more than 30 mg/kg or adults who ingest more than 3,000 mg of camphor need medical evaluation and monitoring for 6 h in an emergency facility (239,245). Establish seizure precautions.

      (2) Treat seizures with diazepam or lorazepam and if refractory administer phentobarbital. Maintence anticonvulsant therapy is unwarrented.

      (3) GI decontamination including gastric lavage and activated charcoal are of doubtful efficacy. **Avoid the induction of emesis** because of early onset of seizures (245). **Avoid** giving fats, oils, alcohol or milk which increase absorption and increase risk of aspiration (241).

      (4) **Charcoal hemoperfusion** is used in cases unresponsive to conventional therapy and with refractory seizures. Less than 1% of the ingested dose is removed by this method and it is **rarely** used (230,231). Amberlite XAD-4 resin hemoperfusion or lipid dialysis are no longer available or recommended (45,246). There are no specific antidotes but **N-acetylcysteine** may be effective in preventing liver damage in chronic poisoning (242,245).

      (5) **Deposition.** Patients who are asymptomatic or who have only mild GI symptoms during 6 h after ingestion are at low risk for serious intoxication (234,239).

    e. **Laboratory** Camphor plasma concentration are not readily available and do not correlate with symptoms. However, patients are asymptomatic at 1.5 µg/mL and have seizures at about 19.5 µg/mL (241).

2. **Naphthalene** is found in moth repellents and toilet bowl deodorizers.

    a. **Mechanism of toxicity.** Naphthalene must be metabolized to its toxic metabolites (especially **alpha-naphthol**) which act as toxic oxidants. This explains the typical delay of several days before hemolysis occurs. The toxic metabolites in the presence of decreased levels of reduced glutathione, combine with hemoglobin and cell wall structures to produce hemolysis. Naphthalene is also a CNS stimulant (248–250).

    (1) The ingestion of **250 to 500 mg** of pure naphthalene (one mothball weighing 0.5 to 3.6 g) may cause hemolysis in patients with **glucose-6-phosphate dehydrogenase (G6PD)** deficiency. The amount necessary to produce **seizures** may be as little as 1 to 2 g (248–250).

    (2) **G6PD deficiency** is X-linked and occurs in 13% of the black males and 2% (heterozygous and homozygous) of the black females (248). It is also found in Italians, Greeks, Sephardic Jews, Filipinos, Asians, and Africans. Acute hemolysis due to naphthalene was reported in 21 Greek infants (nine did not have G-6-PD) (252,253,254). Neonates and young infants are susceptible to hemolysis because they may have a physiologic deficiency in G6PD and glucuronidation is immature (252).

    (3) **Persons without G6PD deficiency** require several grams (more than one mothball) to produce toxicity. The lowest fatal dose is 50 mg/kg.

  b. **Kinetics:** Naphthalene is absorbed erratically from GI tract depending on the diet. It is also absorbed dermally and by inhalation.

    (1) Any oil or fat (milk) enhances GI and dermal absorption. **Skin absorption** may occur from clothes stored in naphthalene particularly if baby oil is applied (248,249).

    (2) **Inhalation** exposure has resulted in intoxications and has caused cataracts in animals (253).

    (3) Elimination is by hepatic **oxidative metabolism** into its toxic metabolites alpha and beta naphthols and alpha and beta naphthoquinones, which are responsible for the hemolysis. **Alpha naphthol** has the greatest hemolytic activity. The metabolites are detoxified by glucuronide conjugation. Small amounts are excreted through the lungs, GI tract and kidneys(248,250,253).

  c. **Manifestations:** Significant acute symptoms are often absent. The major toxic effect is the occurrence of hemolytic anemia within 3 days in children of susceptible ethnic groups more likely to have G-6-PD deficiency.

    (1) **Hemolysis** usually starts on day 1 to 3 postexposure. Hemoglobinuria and methemoglobinemia may occur. The urine may be brown or black, due to elimination of naphthalene or a metabolite, prior to the onset of hemolysis (248,250,253).

    (2) **Other findings** may include nausea, vomiting, diarrhea, fever, jaundice, dark urine, flank pain and renal failure which may last up to 2 weeks. Coma and convulsions may occur in severe cases. Rarely hepatocellular damage may occur 3 to 5 days postexposure.

    (3) **Chronic ingestion** has resulted in toxicity.

  d. **Drugs and chemicals that may precipitate hemolytic anemia in G6PD deficiency patients are** (i) analgesics and antipyretics (254)—acetaminophen (242), acetanilid, acetophenetidin (phenacetin), aminopyrine (Pyramidon), aniline, antipyrine, *p*-aminosalicylic acid (255), acetylsalicylic acid (258);

(ii) antimalarials—chloroquine, pentaquine, plasmaquine, quinacrine, quinine, quinicide; (iii) nitrofurans; (iv) sulfonamides; (v) sulfonylureas; (vi) miscellaneous—ascorbic acid, chloramphenicol, dimercaprol (BAL), fava beans, methylene blue, nalidixic acid, *p*-aminobenzoic acid, penicillamine, phenylhydrazine, probenecid, procainamide, quinidine, sodium nitrite, tripelennamine, vitamin K (water-soluble type) (252).

e. **Management** (Fig. 28-5): Attempt to identify the type of mothball from the container, if available or from the salt water test.

(1) Decontamination: If ingested, syrup of ipecac–induced emesis is most effective if induced within 30 min postingestion in the alert asymptomatic patient. Mothballs may be too large for the lavage tube. Activated charcoal and cathartic should be administered although its effectiveness has not been confirmed. Do not administer milk, fatty meals, or oil, which enhance absorption, for 6 h postingestion. Decontaminate the skin and discard contaminated clothing. Washing does not completely remove naphthalene.

(2) If the patient is of an **ethnic or racial background prone to G6PD deficiency** ingests half a mothball of naphthalene, emesis and medical evaluation are indicated. If the patient is asymptomatic and the blood smear, hemoglobin, hematocrit and reticulocyte count, and urinalysis are normal, home observation for vomiting, diarrhea, abdominal pain, dark urine, and yellow color to eyes or skin may be permitted. However, the patient and these tests should be monitored for the next 5 days. A rapid test for G6PD deficiency test is available (251).

(3) If the patient is **not of an ethnic background prone to G6PD deficiency,** ingests more than one mothball emesis, medical evaluation and followup as above are indicated.

(4) **If hemolysis develops.** If transfusion is needed in G6PD deficiency patients use blood from a donor with normal G6PD. Transfuse to 80% of normal G6PD value. If methemoglobinemia is greater than 30% and respiratory distress consider methylene blue. During hemolysis the patient's G6PD deficiency red blood cells are destroyed but parents blood could be checked for G6PD deficiency.

(5) **Renal status.** If hemolysis is present monitor urinary output and BUN and creatinine. Establish good hydration, alkalinize with sodium bicarbonate and create a brisk diuresis with furosemide 1 mg/kg/dose to avoid precipitation of hemoglobin in the renal tubules. Attempt to keep the urinary pH 7 to 8. If renal shutdown, dialysis is indicated until the hemolytic process is completed.

(6) **Corticosteroids** have been reported as helpful in limiting the hemolysis and might be considered in patients showing hemolysis or evidence of impending hemolysis. However, there is no scientific data to support this therapy.

(7) If **methemoglobinemia** develops treat with 1% methylene blue 1 to 2 mg/kg if symptomatic or methemoglobin more than 30%.

Exposure to demothing agent —— No ——▶ Other etiologies
Obtain sample of agent
|
Aroma test presumptive
Naphthalene ◄—— Floats ◄—— Salt water Test ——▶ Sinks ——▶ Paradichlorobenzene
| |
Italians, Greeks, Sephardic Jews   500-5000 mg/kg
Filipinos, Asians, Africans: or
G6PD deficiency: 250 mg naphthalene   20 grams tolerated
        or   If large amount
No G6PD deficiency: 5 gms naphthalene (>1 mothball)   (over 1 mothball or
| several bites of
GI decontamination if ingested toxic amount   deodorant cake)
    Emesis preferred |
    Activated charcoal   GI decontamination
    Cathartic   if ingested
No oils, milk, fatty meals   Emesis preferred
Dermal decontamination and discard clothing   Activated charcoal
Remove from environment and remove demothing agent   Cathartic
| No oils, milk
▼

1. Test G-6-PD deficiency —— (+) ——▶ observe for hemolysis
2. CBC on patient
a) Heinz bodies —— (+) ——▶ impending hemolysis
b) "Eccentrocytes —— (+)——▶ hemolysis
3. If hemolysis present in the patient, test parents for A+
   variant G-6-PD deficiency
4. Reticulocyte count >7% will yield normal G-6-PD values
   even if deficiency exists
5. Coomb's test, osmotic fragility, heptoglobin
6. Sickle cell hemoglobin electrophoresis
7. Liver and renal function
8. Cyanotic -- monitor methemoglobin
9. Cultures if infection suspected
|

Manifestations   Manifestations
1. Hemolysis starts 1–3 days postexposure   1. Only 1 fatal case
2. Recovery begins 7–10 days   2. Tremors, hemolysis
3. No cholylithiasis   3. Renal and liver failure
| |
Management   Management
1. Transfusion from donor with normal G-6-PD blood. 1. Symptomatic
2. Good hydration, urinary diuresis, alkalinization.
3. Monitor urinary output. If renal shutdown, dialysis.
4. Consider corticosteroids if show Heinz bodies.
5. Methemoglobin >30% with dyspnea.

FIG. 28-5. Hemolysis or exposure to demothing agent.

(8) If patient has deficiency, instruct parents as to the avoidance of chemicals and drugs that may precipitate hemolysis.

f. **Laboratory. Heinz bodies** on the peripheral smear are due to denatured protein in the erythrocytes, signify impending hemolysis and **eccentrocytes** (a dense asymmetrical distribution of hemoglobin in the red blood cell) are found in active hemolysis. Reticulocyte counts greater than 7% will yield normal G-6-PD even if deficiency exists.

3. **Paradichlorobenzene** (PDB) is most commonly used and has a high lethal amount and rarely produces death even in large overdoses. PDB produces only GI upset (256). PDB products are consistently **radiopaque**, whereas naphthalene products are radiolucent (232).

a. **Toxicity.** The toxic amount is estimated as 500 to 5,000 mg/kg or an LD_{50} of 2.5 to 3.2 g/kg. There is one report of a 3-year-old boy who developed methemoglobinemia and hemolysis (256). Up to 20 g has been tolerated in adults (256).

b. **Management**

(1) GI decontamination is recommended only if large amounts are ingested such as several mothballs or the entire cake deodorant. Avoid milk and oily foods for at least 6 h postingestion because they increase absorption. Treat hemolysis or methemoglobinemia if they occur (256).

V. **Art hazards.** Health hazards are associated with the six major art processes: art painting, sculpture, printmaking, photography, glasswork, and ceramics. Artists may have excessive exposure to toxic chemicals because of poor ventilation and inadequate protective equipment and lack of regulation. Often art work is done in the home which may expose the entire family to the hazard (257,258). Children come in contact with art materials and equipment at home, in the school, in day-care centers, and during summer camp, church and synagogue activities, work shops after school activities and by hospital patients in art therapy programs. There were 36,107 exposures to arts, crafts and office supplies (27,347 under 6 years of age) reported to AAPCC in 1994, with 179 moderate outcomes, eight major outcome, and no deaths (4).

A. **Safety in the art materials and regulations**

1. The **Center for Safety in the Arts** was established in 1972. It is a national clearinghouse that provide information, education and a newsletter to interested parties (1-212-227-6220) (258).

2. Prior to the passage of the **Labeling of Art Materials Act (LHAMA)** of 1988 (259), the **Federal Hazardous Substance Act (FHSA)** required safe and adequate labels and regulated only the acute hazards of art materials as determined by a single-dose animal test(260). The distinction between toxic and nontoxic was defined only by the LD_{50} and if less than half of the animals died the product was labelled "nontoxic." These tests were designed for adults, not for children since adult animals were used. Obviously there were many instances where children's art products were labelled inappropriately "nontoxic." Long-term or chronic hazards, carcinogenic properties and sensitivity were not addressed (257,260,261).

3. In 1992 the **Consumer Product Safety Commission** (CPSC) voted to issue guidelines required by LHAMA for evaluating art materials and other household prod-

ucts as to whether they represent a chronic hazard to supplement existing definitions of acute toxicity and flammability (262). The CPSC recommends parents buy only crayons that conform to **ASTM D-4236** safety standards which means that a toxicologist has reviewed the formula of the art material for chronic hazards.

4. In addition, the **Arts and Crafts Material Institute** (ACMI, formerly called the Crayon, Watercolor, and Craft Institute), has developed and instituted a voluntary certification program that attempts to provide standards for the safety of children's art products. Products bearing labels **AP** (approved product) or **CP** (certified product) were certified by an authority in toxicology to contain no materials in sufficient quantities to be toxic or injurious to the body if ingested. This is tested for immediate toxicity, not long-term. This validity of the program depends on the skill of the toxicologist and checks and balances of the program. The **CP seal** additionally, approves the product standard of worksmanship (261).

5. **The State of California Department of Health** has developed a list of approved art materials suitable for children which is the gold standard of safety. Unfortunately smaller manufacturers may not have participated in the ACMI program (257).

B. **Children** are particularly at risk. They have a faster metabolic rate, larger surface area, developing nervous system, and those under 5 years put everything in their mouth. **Children between the ages of 2 to 12 years** routinely use rubber cement, felt tip markers (aromatic hydrocarbon), water-based glues (polyvinyl acetate emulsions), pottery glazes (lead), enamels spray fixatives, wheat wall paper paste, modeling clay (toxic preservatives), and paper mache (flour and water but colored sections of newspaper sections may contain toxic materials such as lead) (257,263).

1. **Art materials recommended for children under 12 years** include water colors (but some may contain small amounts of ammonia, formaldehyde), crayons and school pastels if they have ACMI certified (CP) or approved (AP) label indicating they are nontoxic. Professional pastels, however may be toxic because of their organic and inorganic constituents. Indoor latex acrylic water-based paints are nontoxic unless they contain dangerous fungicides. Art materials safe for children should certify the product is safe by the **Art & Craft Material Institute, Inc. (AMCI),** a nonprofit trade association of manufacturers who produce art and craft materials. If the product bears the seal **"CP Nontoxic"** (certified product) or **"AP Nontoxic"** (approved product) it is a safety guarantee. The ACMI recommends that children under Grade 6 use only AP and CP labeled products. Children should use art materials labeled as nontoxic and carry a statement "conforms to ASTMD-4236" or similar wording. If an adult material contains a **potentially hazardous material,** the label of a ACMI-certified product will identify the specific chemical. Art activities of children under age of 12 years should be supervised by an adult. Guidelines for choosing and safely using children's art materials materials are given in Tables 28-13 and 28-14.

   a. Specific hazards for children include **lead and solvents.**

      (1) Although **lead** is banned from households paints, artists paints (especially oil paints), automobile spray paints, ceramic glazes and copper enamels band related materials are exempt. Lead fumes may be inhaled

TABLE 28-13. *Guidelines for choosing and safely using children's art materials*

1. No dusts or powders that can be inhaled or get into eyes.
2. No organic solvents or solvent-containing products.
3. No aerosol spray or air brushes, etc.
4. Nothing that stains skin or clothing (or cannot be washed out of clothing).
5. No acids, alkali, bleaches, or other irritant or corrosive chemicals.
6. No donated or found materials unless the ingredients are known
7. No old materials. Do not allow children to use grandmother's old art supplies. In the past, art materials were more toxic and had less labelling. Rubber cement contained carbon tetrachloride, chloroform, and benzene, and old instant papier mâché contained asbestos.
8. Choose only government-approved supplies (State of California) or those carefully investigated.
9. Adult supervision of all art activities is recommended for children under the age of 12 years.
10. Encourage cleanliness and a thorough clean-up. Materials should be carefully stored when not in use. Do not eat or drink while using art materials.
11. Open cuts or sores should be well protected when working with art materials.
12. If child is having an adverse reaction, note the child's name and product and how it was used and route of entry—inhaled, ingested, on the skin.

during soldering of stained glass, firing of lead-containig ceramic glazes, and casting of toy soldiers.

(2) **Solvents** are hazardous by ingestion, inhalation and absorbed through the skin. Methyl alcohol which can cause blindness is found in paint strippers, duplicating fluids, shellacs and some dyes.

(3) **Other toxic art materials** may include asbestos (paper maches, modeling compounds, soapstone), silica, "strong sensitizers" as formaldehyde (particle board), nickel (ceramic glazes), dichromates (metal dye mordants) and many tropical woods.

C. **Specific Art Material Hazards include**

1. **Ceramic glazes** are made of leaded or nonleaded silicate complexes.

   a. The AAPCC in 1994 reported 269 ceramic glaze exposures, with five moderate outcomes and no major outcomes or deaths (4). More than 10 cases of

TABLE 28-14. *Arts and Crafts Materials Institute guidelines for acceptable levels of contaminants in art materials*

Contaminant	Acceptable level (ppm)
In pigments	
Polychlorinated biphenyls	50
Cadmium (weak acid leachable)	1000
In products	
Formaldehyde	400
Cobalt (weak acid leachable)	100
Nickel (weak acid leachable)	500
Asbestos (fibers of >5 μm)	0.1%
Nitroaromatic amines	10

lead poisoning in 1992 resulted in nursing homes where residents ingested lead from liquid ceramic glazes given accidently in in small medicine cups (261). All ingestions of lead glaze should be considered having the potential for lead poisoning. Although lead is no longer used in pottery glazes in the United States, pottery in Third World countries still contains lead glazes. Drinking or eating acid foods will solubilize lead from the glaze and make it available for absorption (261,264).

    b. **The pigments used in glazes** are heat stable, insoluble, and do not represent a hazard (263).

    c. **Heavy metals** used in glazes in the United States include **arsenic, antimony, barium, cadmium, chromium, lead, and uranium** (252).

2. **Clays:** Binders in some clay used in modeling may produce allergic manifestations. There were 1,672 exposures reported in 1994 to the AAPCC, with 12 moderate outcomes and no major outcomes or deaths (4).

    a. Certain clays contain up to 32% **free silica.** Grinding or sanding dry clays create a potential hazard from inhalation of poisonious materials and should be done either outdoors or in a ventilated hood (262).

    b. Clay dust should be routinely vaccumed from the studio. Clays also contain alumina and experimental studies indicate when the two silica and alumina are combined silicosis is prevented (250,252).

    c. Sulfur dioxide emitted from the initial firing of clay can produce pulmonary disease (261).

3. **Crayons and chalk**

    a. Childrens' crayons are waxed or pressed and are **nontoxic,** but **industrial crayons** contain lead chromate and are **highly toxic.** The average crayon weight is 14 g and contains about 70 µg of lead/crayon. There were 2,999 exposures reported in 1994 to the AAPCC, with four moderate outcomes, no major outcomes, and no deaths, There were 2,079 exposures to chalk reported, with three moderate outcomes, no major outcomes, and no deaths (4).

    b. A variety of crayon products from China have recently been reported as containing 4,000 µg/g of lead and had the safety label ASRM D-4236 illegally. These products have been confiscated (267).

4. **Glass and stoneware etching**

    a. **Hydrofluoric acid for etching** requires protective equipment to prevent severe damage to the skin, fingernails, and bones. Flouride binds the body calcium causing systemic hypocalcemia and dysrhythmias (42). It is important to use impermeable protective gloves of sufficient length to cover the forearm, full face shield, plastic apron overalls, respirators or self contained breathing apparatus when exposed to vapor (see Hydrofluoric Acid) (261).

    b. **Glassworking** includes hot glass blown and casted, neon art (glass tubes filled with neon) and stained glass (cutting and joining pigmented glass. Hot glass art is produced from bags of **silica** ("batch") in powdered form. Silica exposure can result in silicosis. Prolonged thermal exposure can result in catarcts. Toxicity may occur from inhaling elemental mercury or from the arc producing ozone. **Elemental mercury** is poorly absorbed from the GI tract when volatized and may produce "erethism" (bizarre insidious behavior changes), neuropathy and tremors (261). **Stained glass** has the hazard of lead exposure and zinc chloride fumes from the soldering (265).

5. **Glues** may be water-based with polyvinyl acetate emulsions, organic glues have solvents and superglues have cyanoacylate which can cause adhesions of skin and conjunctiva. There were 22,077 exposures to glues reported in 1994 to AAPCC, with moderate outcomes of 977, major outcomes of 9, and one death (4).

   a. **Cyanoacrylate variety** "instant glues." The chemical composition indicate these glues belong to a family of polymers whose monomer is formed from formaldehyde with a cyanoacrylate ester: ethyl cyanoacrylate (90.6%), hydroquinone (0.4%), polymethylmethacrylate (9.0%), and organic sulfonic acid (trace). There were 12,245 exposures reported in 1994 to APCC, with 640 moderate outcomes, four major outcomes, and no deaths (4). The vapors of cyanoacrylate ahesives may be irritating. Cyanide gas is not released unless combustion occurs.

   (1) **Toxicity** is related to mechanical irritation. Cyanoacrylates produce **rapid adhesion** to adjacent surfaces when exposed to air. Exposure is unlikely to cause toxicity other than adhesion of mucous membranes, skin, eyelids and other areas of contract (268–270). They have been used in clinical ophthalmology to seal corneal perforations.

   (2) Phargneal or esophageal adhesion is unlikely since cyanoacrylates polymerize so rapidly that little if any of the monomer will pass beyond the oropharynx without polymerization (268). Respiratory and eye irritation may occur from inhalation when cyanoacrylate glue is heated.

   (3) The **first aid management of cyanoacrylate** (268)

   (a) Do not attempt to separate bound surfaces forcibly because several layers of skin may become detached. The application of prolonged soaking in warm water may result in sufficient softening of the bond to separate tissue surfaces. This may take several hours to accomplish. Do not burn skin with hot water, and do not use acetone or alcohol on or near the eyes.

   (b) Mineral oil, vegetable oil, or petroleum jelly (vaseline) aids in the removal of glue from tender dermal areas and about the eyes (268,270). Eyelid or eyeball adhesions are managed by copious irrigation with warm water. The adhesion usually resolves within 48 h. Irrigation and flouroscein stain of the eye should follow the separation. Secondary keratoconjunctivitis, corneal abrasion and traumatic iritis are treated with topical ophthalmic antibiotics drops, ocular lubricants, cycloplegic agents and patching as required (270–271).

   b. **Library paste** ASTM D-4236 (e.g., Elmer's Glue) has a nontoxic rating.

   c. **Toluene/xylene model glues** are aromatic hydrocarbons. There were 2,092 exposure in 1994 reported to AAPCC, with 53 moderate outcomes, two major outcomes, and no deaths (4). An infant or child biting into a tube rarely causes toxicity (see Hydrocarbons in Chapter 18).

  d.   All other glues such as rubber, contact and water proof are slightly toxic.

6.   **Kilns** (both electric and gas-fired) need ventilation perferably a canopy hood. **Many toxic gases** are emitted by kilns during firing including formaldehyde, cadium, carbon dioxide, carbon monoxide (gas fired kilns), flouride, nitrogen, ozone, sulfur dioxide (from sulfur clays), chlorine, fluorine, carbon monoxide (from gas-fired kilns). Lead, selenium, cadmium and antimony from glazes may vaporize during the firing (258,261,263).

7.   **Metal casting:** When casting metals, the artist must wear protective clothing and provide exhaust ventilation to eliminate toxic fumes including metal fumes, sand (silica) from olding, bindings of phenol, formaldehyde or urea formaldehyde (261).

8.   **Paints** are solvents or pigment agents. They can be **water-based mediums** (water color, acrylic, gouache) or **solvent-based mediums** (oil, alkyd, and lacquer). Professional paints can be toxic because they contain a considerable amount of metal pigment. There were 986 exposures to artists paint reported in 1994 to AAPCC, with 12 moderate outcomes, one major outcome, and no deaths (4).

  a.   **Pigments.** Powdered pigments are added to organic media such as linseed oil to make paints and the paints are thinned with solvents (acetone, benzene, turpentine, methanol, and methylene chloride). Acrylic paints are water-based instead of oil-based but have similar pigments and may release ammonia when they dry (261,263).

  (1)   **Inorganic pigments** are potentially hazardous because they may contain excess levels of soluble toxic heavy metal compounds such as lead, mercury and arsenic. The following have been tested and had negative carcinogenic results by at least one route cadmium sulfide, chrome oxide green (valence III is insoluble and unlikely to cause poisoning, whereas chrome valence VI is soluble and toxic), cobalt black, titanium dioxide, molybdate. The insolubility and stability of most of the pigments may account for their low toxic potential. Heavy metals are used to produce **whites** (barium, magnesium, titanium and lead), **ultramarine blue** (cobalt); **blues, purples and greens** (managanese, copper, arsenic "Paris Green or emerald green"); **reds, orange and yellows** (zinc, cadmium, chrome), and **violets** (arsenic). The Potentially toxic pigments are:

  (a)   **Cadmium** (yellow and orange) in acute massive ingestions has stomatitis, profound gastroenteritis and pulmonary edema developing in 1 to 4 days and a mortality of 15% (272). Acute respiratory exposure begins like metal fume fever with decreased smell, edema of the face and larynx, yellow discoloration of the teeth (yellow rings) cough, and dyspnea. It is potentially carcinogenic. Chronic exposure produces respiratory (pneumonitis, emphysema), gastroenteritis, testicular necrosis, calciuria, and renal stones, and beta-2 microproteinuria, hypochromic anemia, osteoporosis ("Itai Itai" or the Japanese "Ouch ouch" disease), vertigo, headache, and shivering (272,273).

(b) **Arsenic** (violet and Paris or emerald green) acutely produces severe gastroenteritis ("rice water stools"), hypotension, shock and seizures. By prolonged low level exposure peripheral sensorimotor neuropathy, encephalopathy, dermatitis, gastroenteritis, hematologic abnormalities and renal failure can occur. Arsenic is teratogenic and carcinogenic (275).

(c) **Lead** in white, **copper** in green, **zinc** in yellow have the potential of heavy metal toxicity (261,263).

(d) **Cobalt** (blue) and barium are cardiotoxins (263).

(2) **Organic pigments** tested have not been found to have carcinogenic potential (263) except for pigment orange 5 which produced liver tumors in rats and mice. This pigment is formed by a nitro aromatic amine with mutagenic properties (263). **Driers** are metal soaps added to oil-based paints and etching inks to levels of 0.4% of zinc zirconium, cerium, cobalt, and manganese. None of these driers in these amounts have appreciable toxicity (263).

(3) Some painters who prefer to **grind their own pigments** might inhale the toxic dust. Those mixing large amounts should use exhaust ventilation or respiratory protective equipment. The concern with water-based paints is with the toxic pigments. **Most metallic pigments are only slightly soluble in the stomach and thus unlikely to cause acute poisoning.** However there is concern over chronic exposure (263,266).

(4) The use of toxic pigments requires **strict cleaniness** practices. The painter should always clean his hands and fingernails after painting and keep contaminated hands away from his face. Absorption can occur from "pointing" or licking or molding brush tips with lips to obtain a fine point is dangerous (261,263).

(5) **Acrylic paints** are water-based. They can be hazardous if they contain the same pigments found in oil paints in toxic amounts, including toxic cadmium colors, manganese colors, chrome yellow, and zinc yellow. In addition, they may contain **mercury** perservatives, small amounts of **ammonia** (0.2%, which gives ammonia odor but no toxicity) and **formaldehyde** (0.5% or 1 ppm) which should not cause respiratory symptoms. Some people however are very sensitized to formaldehyde and small amounts can cause eye nose and throat irritation and an allergic response, especially if heated (261,263). There were 3,105 exposure reports in 1994 to AAPCC, with three moderate outcomes and no major outcomes or deaths (4).

(6) **Aerosols:** Spray coatings, fixitives, and adhesives may be irritating to the eyes and the skin, may be toxic in varying degrees, and are fire hazards. Care is necessary in using these materials. They should be used outdoors or with appropriate window or wall ventilation units. When using **air brushing with water-based paints,** a respirator with a paint sprayfilter should be used (261).

9. **Photography.** There were 470 exposures of phographic developers, stops, and fixes reported in 1994 to AAPCC, with 28 moderate exposure outcomes, one major outcome, and no deaths (4). Photographic developers are the most toxic chemical used in the process, e.g., hydroquinones (a phenolic compound) and metals (261). The stop baths are usually weak solutions of acetic acid, stop hardener is potassium chrome alum (chromium), fixing baths contain sodium thiosulfate, acetic acid and preservatives. None of these produce serious disease from short term effects (261).

10. **Plastics.** Plastics when heated releases monomers (polyvinyl chloride), methylmetharylate, acrylic glues, polyurethane (toluene 2-4 diisocyanate a potent sensitizer), polystyrene (methyl chloride release), fiberglass and polyester of eposy resins.

11. **Printmaking** is the process of the application of liquid or semiliquid pigment media to a prepared surface which is transferred to paper in a pressing device. **Lithographing** uses fine-grained lime stone instead of metal plates. **Intaglio** utilizes the surface of copper, aluminium or zinc plates which are etched by exposure to inorganic acids. In **photoetching** a copper or zinc plate is coated with a light sensitive emulsion and a photographic transparency is placed on top of it. The plate is exposed to a carbon arc and later the plate is bitten with organic solvent and acid (261). Printmakers are exposed to organic and inorganic acids, alkali, hydrofluoric acid, nitric acid and hydrochloric acid. Inks are complex mixtures of pigment, oil, stabilizers, and various organic solvents. Eugenol, an antiskinning agent, is a strong respiratory and dermal irritant. CNS toxicity can be caused by organic solvent exposure in lithography and photoetching (261).

12. **Rubber cement and rubber paint thinner** may contain large amounts of flammable and highly toxic hexane. Hexane can cause dermatitis, narcosis from the inhalation of large amounts and peripheral neuropathy from chronic inhalation (266,276,277).

13. **Silk Screen painting** involves pigments (lead, cadmium, manganese, solvents (mineral spirits, toluene and xylene) and photoemulsions (ammonium dichromate) and can produce peripheral neuropathy (266,276,277).

14. **Soldering and brazing:** The fumes from the solders containing cadmium are poisonous. Some fluxes may irritate the upper respiratory system. Proper ventilation is manditory when utilizing these metal joining methods. In addition, acid fluxes can burn the skin on contact (261).

15. **Solvents** are the greatest potential threat to the health of amateur painters. Inhalation of toxic solvent vapors is the most serious. Solvents are also flammable (261).

   a. **Carbon tetrachloride** and **benzene** are among the most toxic solvents and they should not be used.

   b. Among the **most common solvents** used are the **aromatic hydrocarbons** (Tables 28–15, 28–16, and 28–17), toluene (renal tubular acidosis, death) and xylene and halogenated hydrocarbons (1,1,1 trichloroethane produces liver and renal damage, and death). Excessive absorption of *n*-**hexane** solvent produces peripheral neuropathy (276–278).

   c. Mineral spirits and other **petroleum distillates** are dangerous acutely if aspirated (unlikely because of the high viscoity of paints).

d. Turpentine (gum spirits, spirits of turpentine). Turpentine, an oleoresin distillate, is a mixture of terpenes in various proportions. **Gum turpentine** in oil-based paints is not toxic to the kidneys, but can produce skin allergies. Steam distilled turpentine is toxic to the kidneys (261). It is a common paint remover and used for mixing paints. There were 1,282 exposure reported in 1994 to AAPCC, with 60 moderate outcomes, three major outcomes, and no deaths (4).

(1) **Toxicity** is associated with local tissue irritation and central nervous sytem (CNS) depression. Systemic toxicity may occur after a single dose of 30 to 45 mL in adults, although other adults have tolerated larger amounts. The literature on turpentine reports as little as 15 mL has been reported to be fatal in children and 120 to 180 mL in adults. In general **in excess of 2 mL/kg** should be considered potentially toxic (279,280,283,380).

(2) **Kinetics:** Turpentine has high volatility, low viscosity, and high fat solubility. Absorption occurs rapidly through the GI tract. Inhaled turpentine is absorbed and is widely distributed in the body. Turpentine persists in adipose tissue. It is metabolized in the liver and eliminated

TABLE 28-15. *Common examples of aliphatic halogenated hydrocarbons*

	Estimated toxic dose (ingested 100%)[a]	TLV-TWA ppm ACGIH	Synonyms
1,2-dichloromethane[b]	0.3 mL/kg,[a] one swallow adult, lethal >0.5 mL/kg	1	Methylene chloride
1,2-dichloroethylene	150–200 mL toxic, in adults or large intentional ingestion	200	Acetylene dichloride
1,2 dichloropropane	0.3 mL/kg toxic, one swallow	75	Propylene dichloride
Tetrabromoethane	1 mL/kg toxic, several swallows	—	Acetylene tetrabromide
Tetrachloroethane	0.3 mL/kg toxic, one swallow	1	Acetylene tetrachloride
Tetrachloroethylene	1 mL/kg toxic, several swallows	50	Perchloroethylene
Tetrachloromethane	0.3 mL/kg toxic, one swallow	5	—
1,1, 1-Trichloroethane	5.0 mL/kg fatal, 150–200 mL toxic in adults or large intentional ingestion	350	Methyl chloroform, Triethane, Glamorene Spot Remover, Scotchgard, typewriter correction fluid
Trichlorethylene	0.3 mL/kg toxic, more than one swallow	50	Vapor degreaser, typewriter correction fluid, fire retardant
Trichloromethane	0.3 mL/kg toxic, one swallow	10	Cleaning agent, fumigant, insecticide
1,1,2 trichloro— 1,2,2-fluoroethane	>200mL? toxic adult	—	
Trichloroethane 1,1,2	0.5 mL/kg toxic, lethal >2.0 mL/kg	10	Vinyl trichloride
Carbon tetrachloride	3–5 mL total amount, lethal 4 mL total	2	—

[a] Estimated fatal dose assumes pure 100% of the halogenated hydrocarbon in the ingested product. At this dose, it is recommended that medical evaluation is needed. A swallow in a 2-year-old is ~5 mL (0.3 mL/kg), in an adult 15–20 mL. Large intentional amount is 120–150 mL in adults. The decision for medical evaluation should be based on the most toxic substance present at concentrations exceeding 10–20%.

[b] Amount methylene chloride in a single Christmas Tree bubbling fluid light (0.5 mL) is nontoxic if ingested in small children.

TABLE 28-16. *Initial management of hydrocarbon ingestions*

Symptoms	Contents	Amount	Initial management
None	Petroleum distillate only	<5 ml/kq	None
None	Heavy hydrocarbon	Any amount	None[a]
	Mineral seal oil	—	None
None	Petroleum distillate with dangerous additive (heavy metals pesticide)	Depends on additives' toxicity: >15 mL/kg or 150–200 mL	Gastric lavage with small bore tube
	Aromatic hydrocarbons	>1 mL/kg	—
	Halogenated hydrocarbons[b]		
	A. Very toxic compounds	>0.3 mL/kg	Gastric lavage
	B. Moderate toxic compounds	>0.5 mL/kg	Gastric Lavage
	C. Low-toxicity compounds	>1.0 mL/kg	Gastric lavage
	D. Xmas bubbling light	0.5 mL	None
Loss of protective airway reflexes, comatose, seizures	Petroleum distillate with dangerous additive, aromatic, or halogenated hydrocarbons		Gastric lavage, ET tube prior to gastric lavage

[a] Emesis may be necessary if machine oil contains triorthocresyl phosphate (TOCP), which causes weakness, sensory impairment, and "partially reversible damage to the spinal cord."

[b] Amounts of halogenated hydrocarbons ingested assume 100% of product. (A) More than one swallow in adult or 0.3 mL/kg in a child of 100% 1,2-dichloromethane (methylene chloride), 1,2-dichloropropane (propylene dichloride), tetrachloroethane (acetylene tetrachloride), tetrachloromethane, trichloroethylene, tetrachloroethylene, trichloromethane, tetrabromoethane (acetylene tetrabromide). (B) Several swallows in an adult or 0.5 mL/kg in a child of 100% of 1,2 dichloroethane (ethylene dichloride), 1,2-dichloroethylene (acetylene dichloride), 1,1,2-trichloroethane (vinyl chloride), tetrabromoethane and tetrachloroethylene (perchloroethylene), 1,1,2,2-tettra-chloro-ethylene. (C) A large intentional ingestion in an adult (150–200 mL) or >1 mL/kg in a child of 100% of 1,2 dichloroethylene or tetrachloromethane, 1,1,1 trichloroethane (methyl chloroform), 1,1,2-trichloro 1,2,2-fluoroethane. (D) The amount dichloromethane (methylene chloride) in a single Christmas Tree bubbling fluid light (0.5 mL) is nontoxic if ingested in small children.

through the kidneys and lungs. Excretion of turpentine or metabolites in the **urine gives the odor of violets.**

(3) **Manifestations**

(a) **GI effects.** Burning sensation in throat and GI tract following ingestion.

(b) **Respiratory** symptoms develop in about 20% of ingestions cough, dyspnea, bronchospam, and pulmonary edema have been reported. Inhalation produces tachypnea. Pneumonitis occurs with systemic absorption not only with aspiration. Pulmonary function abnormalities may exist for years after turpentine pneumonitis (281).

(c) **CNS** depression is common. Convulsions are rare.

(d) **Urinary tract.** Hemorrhagic cystitis (282) but not nephritis may develop. Dysuria and hematuria occurred 12 h to 3 days postingestion. Abnormalities on urinalysis are found which may last 5 to 10 days.

(e) **Hematologic abnormalities** include one case of thrombocytopenic purpura (283)

TABLE 28-17. *Types of hydrocarbons*

Petroleum distillates (aliphatic hydrocarbons, straight chain)

Product	Synonym	Use	Systemic	Pulmonary
Kerosene	Coal oil	Fuel	1+	4+
Gasoline	Petro spirit	Fuel	1+	4+
Mineral spirits	Stoddard, mineral turpentine, varasol, white spirit	Solvent	3+	3+
Petroleum naphtha	Legroin	Lacquer, lighter fluid, solvent	3+	3+
V.M. and P naphtha	Varnish naphtha, painter's naphtha	Thinner	3+	3+
Petroleum ether	Benzine	Rubber solvent	4+	0
Fuel or diesel	Light gas oil	Fuel	1+	0
Mineral seal oil	Signal oil	Furniture polish	0	4+
Lubricating oil	Motor oil, cutting oil, transmission fluid	Lubrication	0	0
Mineral oil	Liquid petrolatum	—	0	0
Turpentine	Paint thinner	—	3+	3+
Pine oil	—		2+	2+

Aromatic hydrocarbons (cyclic with benzene ring)

Product	CNS	Pulmonary
Xylene	4+	0
Toluene	4+	0
Benzene	4+	0

Aliphatic halogenated hydrocarbons (mostly solvents, spot removers, and stain protectors)

	Estimated toxic dose (ingested 100%)[a]	TLV-TWA ppm ACGIH	Synonyms
1,2 dichloromethane	0.3 ml/kg, one swallow adult, lethal >0.5 mL/kg	1	Methylene chloride
1,2-dichloroethylene	150–200 mL toxic in adults or large intentional ingestion	200	Acetylene dichloride
1,2 dichloropropane	0.3 mL/kg toxic, one swallow	75	Propylene dichloride
Tetrabromoethane	1 mL/kg toxic, several swallows	—	Acetylene tetrabromide
Tetrachloroethane	0.3 mL/kg toxic, one swallow	1	Acetylene tetrachloride
Tetrachloroethylene	1 mL/kg toxic, several swallows	50	Perchloroethylene
Tetrachloromethane	0.3 mL/kg toxic, one swallow	5	
1,1,1-Trichloroethane	5.0 mL/kg fatal, 150–200 mL toxic in adults or large intentional ingestion	350	Methyl chloroform, Triethane, Glamorene Spot Remover, Scotchgard, typewriter correction fluid
Trichlorethylene	0.3 mL/kg toxic, more than one swallow	50	Vapor degreaser, typewriter correction fluid, fire retardant
Trichloromethane	0.3 mL/kg toxic, one swallow	10	Cleaning agent, fumigant, insecticide

(continued)

TABLE 28-17. *Continued*

	Estimated toxic dose (ingested 100%)[a]	TLV-TWA ppm ACGIH	Synonyms
1,1,2 trichloro- 1,2,2-fluoroethane	>200 mL? toxic adult	—	
Trichloroethane 1,1,2	0.5 mL/kg toxic, lethal >2.0 mL/kg	10	Vinyl trichloride
Carbon tetrachloride	3–5 ml total amount, lethal 4 mL total	2	—

Dangerous additive (see text)

Heavy hydrocarbons: Asphalt, motor oil (lubricating oil, engine oil), diesel oil (fuel oil, home heating oil), petroleum liquid (mineral oil, suntan oils), petroleum jelly (Vaseline), paraffin wax, transmission oil, cutting oil, greases.

Special products: mineral seal oil

[a] Estimated fatal dose assumes pure 100% of the halogenated hydrocarbon in the ingested product.

(4)   **Management**

  (a)   **Decontamination**

    (i)   If **inhaled**, remove the patient from the environment. If **ingested**, there is controversy about the measures to use for gastric emptying. Emesis is indicated only for large ingestions within the first 30 min after ingestion.

    (ii)   If **over 2 mL/kg is ingested,** removal by induced emesis **under medical supervision** has been recomended if the patient has not vomited spontaneously (279,283). In 255 patients ingesting hydrocarbons with 35% to 37% ingesting turpentine, pulmonary complications developed less frequently (27%) in those with syrup of ipecac-induced emesis than those receiving gastric lavage (56%) without cuffed endotracheal tube (279). However, **a small nasogastric tube aspiration** has been advocated by some toxicologists. These methods have not been scientifically compared. It is not anticipated that activated charcoal will be useful and may precipitate vomiting (280).

    (iii)   **Dermal** decontamination should be carried out by removal of contaminated garments and a thorough washing although there is no evidence of dermal absorption.

  (b)   **Monitor** for CNS depression, pulmonary symptoms, and evidence of urinary irritation. If pulmonary symptoms obtain a chest radiograph. Examine the urine for abnormalities and if present obtain renal function tests. Urinary output should be monitored. Pulmonary function tests should be followed if respiratory symptoms.

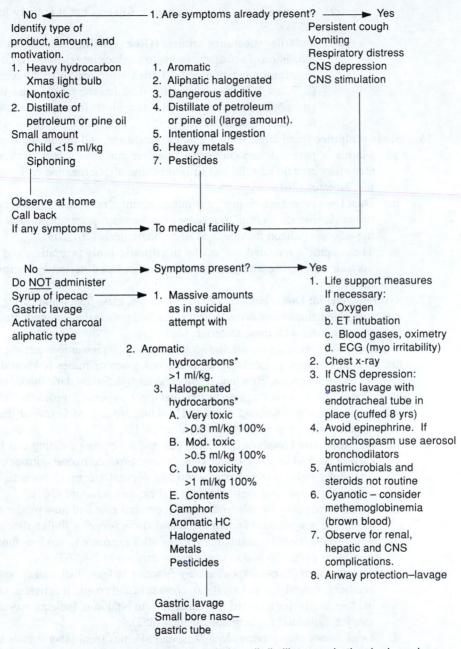

No ◀——————— 1. Are symptoms already present? ——————▶ Yes

Identify type of
product, amount, and
motivation.

1. Heavy hydrocarbon
   Xmas light bulb
   Nontoxic
2. Distillate of
   petroleum or pine oil
Small amount
   Child <15 ml/kg
   Siphoning

1. Aromatic
2. Aliphatic halogenated
3. Dangerous additive
4. Distillate of petroleum
   or pine oil (large amount).
5. Intentional ingestion
6. Heavy metals
7. Pesticides

Persistent cough
Vomiting
Respiratory distress
CNS depression
CNS stimulation

Observe at home
Call back
If any symptoms ——————▶ To medical facility ◀——

No ——————————▶ Symptoms present? ——▶ Yes

Do NOT administer
Syrup of ipecac ——————▶ 1. Massive amounts
Gastric lavage   as in suicidal
Activated charcoal   attempt with
aliphatic type

2. Aromatic
   hydrocarbons*
   >1 ml/kg.
3. Halogenated
   hydrocarbons*
   A. Very toxic
      >0.3 ml/kg 100%
   B. Mod. toxic
      >0.5 ml/kg 100%
   C. Low toxicity
      >1 ml/kg 100%
   E. Contents
   Camphor
   Aromatic HC
   Halogenated
   Metals
   Pesticides

1. Life support measures
   If necessary:
   a. Oxygen
   b. ET intubation
   c. Blood gases, oximetry
   d. ECG (myo irritability)
2. Chest x-ray
3. If CNS depression:
   gastric lavage with
   endotracheal tube in
   place (cuffed 8 yrs)
4. Avoid epinephrine. If
   bronchospasm use aerosol
   bronchodilators
5. Antimicrobials and
   steroids not routine
6. Cyanotic – consider
   methemoglobinemia
   (brown blood)
7. Observe for renal,
   hepatic and CNS
   complications.
8. Airway protection–lavage

Gastric lavage
Small bore naso–
gastric tube

FIG. 28-6. Ingestion of petroleum and pine oil distillates and other hydrocarbons.

    (c) **Acetone** is one of the least toxic solvents but it is higly flamable (257).

    (d) **Volatile substance abuse (Glue sniffing)** is the intentional inhalation of volatile solvents to produce intoxication (285). Fatalities from inhalation of 1,1,1-trichloroethane or trichloroethylene (277,284,285), polyneuropathy from hexane rubber cement (277), encephalopathy and renal tubular acidosis from toluene (286,287) has been reported.

16. **Stone sculpture** (marble, scapstone, granite, sandstone, and pneumatic tools)
    a. Marble is pure calcium carbonate, however common stones such as field stone may contain harmful and irritating minerals. Serpentine rock may contain asbestos (261).
    b. **Dust** from prolonged chipping, grinding, slicing, and polishing in stone scupturing (soapstone, granite, sandstone) can produce pneumoconiiosis including silicosis (silicon dioxide) and silicotuberculosis (261,263).
    c. The scuptor's repeated use of the **pneumatic tools** (vibration and noise) may affect hearing and produce vibration-induced peripheral neuropathy (261).

17. **Synthetic media:** Direct contact with certain resins, glass fibers, and curing agents can cause skin irritations. Adequate ventilation and personal cleanliness are important when working with these materials (261).

18. **Welding:** When welding metals, the sculptor must take precautions against serious fire hazards, eye injury, inhalation of poisonous gases or fumes (carbon dioxide, carbon monoxide, ozone, phosgene if solvents nearby). Safety dark shades of green glass goggles and masks against ultraviolet light exposure, protective clothing should be worn when welding. Forms of welding are arc, MIG (metal inert gas) welding and TIG (tungsten inert gas) welding (261).
    a. **Oxyacetylene** (combination of oxygen and acetylene) welding can liberate carbon monoxide and the arc welding may produce ozone, nitrogen oxide, ultraviolet light, infrared irradiation and present electrical hazards. It also represents a potential thermal injury and explosive hazard (261).
    b. **Metal fumes** may be released from copper and zinc and may produce pneumonitis or a syndrome known as "**metal fume fever**" a flulike illness often with metallic taste in mouth, the evening after exposure to noxious fumes and resolution within 36 h after cessation of exposure (258,263).
    c. **Molybdenum fumes** exposure may produce fatigue, listlessness, anorexia, headache, arthralgias and myalgias, chest pain and cough. It activates xanthine oxidase, a cofactor required for transferases to bind iron. Patients may develop gouty arthritis and hypochromic anemia (252).
    d. **Lead fumes** may produce lead poisoning. Fumes from other metals such as nickel and cadmium may also produce intoxication (258,263).
    e. **MIG and arc welders** emit **ozone (O_3)** a pungent odor, water-soluble upper respiratory irritant that may produce respiratory distress, dyspnea, cyanosis and pulmonary edema. Other symptoms are increase RBC fragility, altered

visual response, and a decrease in RBC cholinesterase. Symptoms subside in 1 to 2 weeks (261).

    f. **TIG welders** in addition to flux flumes of the arc and MIG produce intense ultraviolet radiation which may produce second degree burns on uncovered skin, keratopathy, and damage to the retina (261).

19. **Wood working:** Contact with some exotic woods (e.g., Western Red Cedar) used for carving contain caustic oils that may cause contact dermatitis or other allergic reactions in the respiratory tract.

    a. Wood working from **machining produces** dust, noise and fire. Glues used in wood working contain epoxy resins, solvents (toluene), and formaldehyde which may produce reactions and respiratory irritation (261).

    b. **Paint strippers** contain methylene chloride (which is metabolized in the body to carbon monoxide) (288), toluene, methanol and other solvents are potential hazards (261).

    c. **Paints and finishes** (lacquers, varnishes, shellac) contain mineral spirits, toluene, and turpentine.

    d. **Preservatives** in wood are chromated copper arsenate, pentachlorphenol, and creosote and, if exposed chronically, may produce intoxications (261,263).

20. **Hazards to artists** (261)

    a. Neurotoxins: carbon disulfate, manganese, mercury, organophosphate plasticizers, organic solvents (toluene, xylene).

    b. Peripheral neuropathies: methyl ethyl ketone, *n*-hexane.

    c. Cardiotoxicity: heavy metals (barium, cobalt), organic solvents (methylene chloride, toluene)

    d. Pulmonary fibrosis: silica, talc, scrapstone, asbestos

    e. Asthma: wood and stone dust, fibers, reactive dyes, formaldehyde, turpentine, polyurethane, isocyanate.

    f. Hypersensitivity pneumonitis: wood dust and heavy metals.

    g. Irritation of upper respiratory tract: highly water-soluble nitrogen dioxide (welding, carbon arc, etching and enameling), chromium gas (etching acid), hydrogen chromide (heating, plastics, and polyvinyl chloride), caustic dusts (lime, dichromate, soda ash, and potassium).

    h. Antiskinning agents: eugenol, clove oil

    i. Pneumoconiosis: iron oxides, aluminium, and barium sulfate.

    j. Hepatitis: chlorinated hydrocarbons, phenol, ethyl alcohol, nitrobenzene, cadmium, styrene, arsenic, toluene, lead, and xylene. Manganese involves the liver but hepatitis has not been reported.

    k. Renal toxis: oxalic acid, turpentine, ethylene glycol, mercury. Chronic renal disease with B-2 microglobulin and proteinuria.

    l. Severe dermatitis: grinding fiberglass, photograhic developers, exotic woods, soaps, drying agents, and solvents.

    m. Hematologic: cyanosis (hydroxyamine a color developer), polyvinyl chloride, nitrates, cobalt.
Anemia: lead, cadmium, benzene, and naphthalene.

    n. Teratogens and carcinogens: cadmium, chromium, zinc, arsenic.

        Additional sources of information are: For more information: Center for Safety in the Arts, 5 Beekman Street, Suite 820, New York, NY 212-227-6220 Dr. Michael McCann. To receive a list of ACMI products that are ABMI-certified for children, contact ACMI, 100 Boylston St., Ste. 1050, Boylston, MA 02116.

        Another important source is the manufacturer's **material safety data sheet** (MSDS). These sheets are required by the Occupational Health and Safety Administration (OSHA) for hazardous material. They provide information on ingredients, industrial standards, health hazards and reactive chemicals.

VI. **Miscellaneous**

  A. **Swimming pools/aquarium.** There were 6,700 exposures reported in 1994 to the AAPCC, with 366 moderate outcomes, with seven major outcomes, and no deaths (4). With the exception of copper sulfate and some pH kits that contain sodium hydroxide, these products are of low toxicity because if they were toxic to humans they would also be toxic to marine animals (297).

    1. **Home aquarium products** (294–297)

      a. **Antimicrobials,** used to control algae, fungi bacteria and parasites. Antibiotics are given in trace amounts except for penicillin and tetracycline which may be given in therapeutic doses for man. Idiosyncratic and hypersensitivity reactions are possible.

      b. **Antichlorine** products such as sodium thiosulfate, potassium permanganate, and silver salts are in dropper bottles, low concentrations and have low toxicity.

      c. **pH indicators** such as bromothymol blue. Bromothymol blue is the most commonly used pH indicator and is in low concentration and size container and low toxicity. Some kits contain sodium hydroxide, a caustic with potential toxicity.

      d. **Miscellaneous substances** include vitamins, aquarium salts, and copper sulfate. Aquarium salts contain sodium chloride. Quinine 1% is in small amounts but has caused severe allergic reactions. Methylene blue when present is of low toxicity (294–297).

      e. **Management** includes determining the ingredients of the product. The liquid products are of low potential hazard. Dropper bottles are more concentrated but have less volume than nondropper bottles. Treat sodium hydroxide and copper sulfate if in toxic range. Majority of other products are nontoxic (294–297).

    2. **Swimming poolside toxicology** (294–297). Chemicals adequately diluted in a swimming pool pose no threat to swimmers. Its before adding to the pool, in undiluted form that they can produce damage through direct contact with the skin, eyes, inhalation of the powder or gas and even ingestion.

      a. **Swimming pool disinfectants and purifiers**

        (1) These compounds are used as germicide, algicide and deodorants. They are available in tablet and powder form (e.g., Pittchlor, Pittabs, HTH) and have **over 70% calcium hypochlorite** (70% available chlorine) is in their formulation, whereas the household preparations as bleaches are less than 8%. Sodium hypochlorite is a common substitute. **Cyanuric acid** is a less popular pool sanitizer and when mixed with water is nonirritating.

(2) **Hypochlorite** is a **strong oxidant** which should be stored in a dry cool place. Contact with organic matter (kerosene, turpentine, greases, beverages, rags), acids, or high temperature may cause decomposition with the release of heat, free chlorine and oxygen creating a **fire hazard.** **Metals** such as iron and manganese oxide in contact with calcium hypochlorite can result in a reaction that releases oxygen and pressure and cause containers to explode. Scoops should be enamel, glass or porcelain (see hypochlorite under Bleach).

(3) **Skin and ocular contact** even properly diluted in a pool can produce dermatitis and conjunctivitis in susceptible individuals. Undiluted it can produce skin burns and corneal abrasions.

(4) **Ingestion** can cause severe gastritis drooling, pain on swallowing (dysphagia), ulcers, perforation, strictures, chest and abdominal pain,

(5) **Inhalation** of fumes can cause irritation of upper respiratory tract with dyspnea, cough, wheezing, or frank noncardiac pulmonary edema.

(6) **Management.** Maintain adequate airway, oxygenation and assisted ventilation if necessary (see hypochlorite under Bleach).

  (a) **Decontamination** consists of moving the victim into fresh air, irrigation of skin and eyes immediately if exposed. If a skin burn is present evaluation by a professional is necessary.

  (b) **Inhalation** requires immediate removal from the contaminated environment and evaluation by a health professional if symptoms persist. Oxygen is required to correct hypoxia, bronchodilator for bronchospasm, and positive end expiratory pressure (PEEP) for noncardiac pulmonary edema. The nebulized use of sodium bicarbonate is controversial. Chest and abdominal radiographs may be helpful to confirm the presence of perforation (295–297).

  (c) **Ingestions** may produce esophageal damage. Immediately dilute with milk or water. Do not use any of the common measures of GI decontamination (emesis, gastric lavage or activated charcoal. Endoscopy may be needed later to exclude esophageal damage (295–297).

b. **Swimming pool testing.** The desirable pH is 7.4 to 7.8 and records should be kept. The standard phenol red indicator has a range of 6.8 to 8.2. If the reading is 6.8 the pool should be corrected to 7.2 or above with **sodium bicarbonate.** If the pH is more than 7.8, lower the pH with 100% **sodium bisulfide** (fine granular powder) which forms sulfuric acid on contact with water. This acid can be harmful if it contacts skin, eyes or is ingested in undiluted form (297).

  (1) **Phenol red** and **orthotolidine** are harmless in the concentrations used to check the chlorine concentrations of the pool. If the orthotolidine preparation contains hydrochloric acid in concentrations of more than 10% it can cause significant burns (296,297).

   c. **Algicides**

      (1) **Quaternary ammonia compounds** (*n*-alkyl dimethyl benzyl ammonium chloride 42 and *n*-dialkyl methyl benzyl ammonium chloride) (295–297)

         (a) Most of the products have concentrations of 10% but even at concentrations of 0.5% can cause conjunctival and mucosal irritation. Solutions of 20% are caustic. Ingestions of 100 to 400 mg/kg have been reported as being fatal because of systemic effects (coma, convulsions, and respiratory paralysis). In higher concentrations they can produce corrosion. Treat as a caustic and provide supportive therapy.

         (b) **Copper sulfate anhydrous** 6.5% is a permanent algicide that can be toxic if swallowed in undiluted form.

   d. **Pool clarifiers are flocculents** that attract tiny suspected particles and then settle to the bottom. They may be nontoxic polymers or a few contain highly toxic ethylene glycol.

   e. **Iron remover** is a concentrate of sodium salts of amino carboxylic acids.

B. **Deodorants.** There were 10,750 exposures reported in 1994 to the AAPCC, with 67 moderate outcomes, one major outcome, and no deaths (4). They are much less toxic now that they contain paradichlorobenzene than in past years when they contained naphthalene.

   1. **Room deodorizers usually** contain **paradichlorobenzene (PDB).**

         (a) **A small bite** into a cake of this type of deodorant is not an indication for emesis; however, more than this amount or the swallow of a mothball would warrant emesis. PDB is radiopaque and an alternative in toilet bowl deodorizers, cetrimonitum bromide is also radiopaque (256).

         (b) In massive amounts **PBD** may result in tremors and hepatic or renal dysfunction. Paradichlorobenzene is classified as Gosselin category 3 toxicity (500 to 5,000 mg/kg is the LD_{50} (256). No serious intoxications have been reported from its ingestion except for a 3-year-old who developed a hemolytic anemia (256) (see Demothing Agents).

         (c) Older cake products were **naphthalene** which could produce methemoglobinemia and hemolysis. People with glucose-6-phosphate dehydrogenase (G6PD) deficiency are at greater risk of hemolysis. Many liquid products are perfumed alcohol and cationic detergents (see Demothing Agents).

   2. **Personal deodorants** (see Cosmetics)

C. **Matches** (298,299) There were 1,532 exposures in 1994 reported to the AAPCC, with four moderate outcomes and one major outcome (4).

   a. In the past, matches contained lead thiosulfate 2% to 3% and antimony trisulfide 10% to 15%, and these have mostly been eliminated.

    b. Since most strikers are insolubilized it is not likely a child would ingest any of the constituents unless he chewed up the paper and all.

    c. The two potentially toxic chemicals in match heads are a trace of **potassium chlorate** (2.5 mg) and **potassium dichromate** (180 to 270 mg). The percentage of potassium dichromate is so small it can be ignored. A match head contains potassium chlorate 10 to 12 mg/head or 220 mg in 20-light book matches. The estimated lethal dose for chlorates is 30 g for a 70 kg man or 428 mg/kg. **The ingestion of two books of 20 match heads is considered nontoxic.** Long before the child could ingest so many matches they would develop gastric irritation and vomiting from the paper. The ingestion of 2 entire books of matches requires no intervention (298,299).

    d. **Red phosphorous sesquisulfide** used in "strike on rough surface match tips" are nonabsorbable, nonsoluble and nontoxic (298).

D. **Fireworks.** There were 516 exposure reported in 1994 to the AAPCC, 15 moderate outcomes, no major outcomes, and no deaths (4). The 1976 regulations of the U.S. Consumer Product Safety Commission mandates that those sold or distributed for consumer use be limited to 50 mg powder (300,301).

    1. **Sparklers.** Gold sparklers contain barium nitrate plus gums, paste and chalk dextrin, iron, and aluminum. Green sparklers contain potassium perchlorate in addition to the ingredients in the gold and red sparklers contain stronium carbonate and nitrite in addition to the other ingredients.

        a. Soluble barium salts are very toxic. The toxic dose is 0.2 g, lethal dose 1 to 15 g or 100 mg/kg. Barium stimulates the smooth and cardiac muscle. It results in vomiting, abdominal pain blood stools, shallow respirations, coma, convulsions and death from cardiac or respiratory failure.

        b. Stronium bromide: adult dose is 1 mg, which is in excess of the amount in a sparkler.

        c. Nitrates are vasodilators and may produce vomiting, abdominal pain, bloody stools, and methemoglobinemia. The amount in a sparkler is not sufficient to produce toxicity. The potentially fatal dose in adults is 10 g.

        d. Perchlorates may produce effects similar to nitrates.

        e. The management of an ingested sparkler should consist of emesis or gastric lavage with sodium thiosulfate. Treat methemoglobin with methylene blue.

    2. The formulation of **Caps** is usually potassium chloride, antimony sulfide, amorphous (red) phosphorous, and gum. Antimony is an insoluble salt, red phosphorous has low toxicity, and chlorates are in too small a quantity to produce methemoglobinemia. A roll of 50 caps contains a total of 200 mg of these ingredients. GI decontamination is not indicated and it is unlikely toxicity will occur.

E. **Tobacco products.** There were 8,758 exposures reported in 1994 to the AAPCC, with 154 moderate outcomes, five major outcomes, and no deaths. Children under 6 years were involved in the majority of exposures (more than 90%). Over 60% of these exposures resulted in no toxicity, and 1.8% resulted in moderate to major toxicity. There were 285 exposures from plants, with 17 moderate outcomes, four major outcomes, and no deaths. There were 23 exposures to nicotine insecticides with no toxicity listed (4).

(1) **Tobacco use, through smoking** is linked more than 430,000 deaths per year in the United States. About 114,000 of these deaths are caused by lung cancer. On the basis of 30 epidemiologic studies the EPA has concluded that environmental tobacco smoke is a **human carcinogen.** Research on the hazards of smoking tobacco has recently shown an association between exposure to tobacco smoke by **passive smoking** and adverse health effects including lung cancer, respiratory diseases, brain tumors, asthma, asthmatic exacerbations, and sudden infant death syndrome (302–309).

(2) **Nicotine** is highly toxic alkaloid found in the plant *Nicotiana tobacum* which contains 1% to 6% nicotine alkaloid in leaves and stem and in tobacco products. Nicotine is used as an **insecticide,** usually 1% to 14%, although "Black Leaf" insecticide contains 40%. Deaths have been associated with using tobacco leaves as salads (1% to 6% nicotine/leaf by weight), tobacco enemas for intestinal parasites, ingestion of concentrated pesticides, and dermal exposure to nicotinic solutions, from saliva expectorated into spittoons (314).

(3) **Smoking tobacco.** A **cigarette** of 1 g contains about 1.5% nicotine malate or 13 to 19 mg/cigarette, a **cigar** is 15 to 40 mg, **a cigarette butt** 5 to 7 mg/butt, **snuff** containers are about 30 g, of which 1.5% is nicotine or a total of 45 mg, **chewing tobacco** is 2.5% to 8% nicotine, **cigarette butts** contain 25% of original nicotine content or 5 to 7 mg per butt (Table 28-14).

(4) **Smokeless tobacco** (Table 28-18)

   (a) **Snuff** 1.5% nicotine. Dry snuff is inhaled. Wet snuff is more alkaline and absorbed more readily reaching plasma levels of cigarette smoking in 10 min (314). GI symptoms and unresponsiveness have occurred after 7.5 to 15 g. In general **greater than a pinch is a toxic ingestion in a child** (314). Eight to 10 dips of snuff is equivalent to smoking 30 to 40 cigarettes a day (303).

TABLE 28-18. *Nicotine content of tobacco products*

Source	Nicotine content (mg)	Dose (mq) nicotine
Cigarette whole	13–19	1
Cigarette butt	5–7	4.5–6.3 mg
Clove cigarette	Twice tobacco as regular cigarette	
Cigar	15–40	0.2–1
Snuff	12–15 mg/g dry, 5–50 mg/wet	2–3.5
Chewing tobacco	6–8 mg/g	2–4
Nicorette gum	2–4 mg/piece	1–2
Tobacco leaf	1–6%	
Nicotine patch	8.3–11.4	1–2
Insecticides	Up to 40%	1–2

Modified from refs. 314 and 315.

(b) **Chewing tobacco** 2.5% to 8% nicotine is sweeter in taste than smoking tobacco. **Any amount is considered toxic in a child** (314). Nicotine content of a "chaw" is 7.8 mg/g of tobacco and 8 to 10 "chaws" is equivalent to smoking 30 to 40 cigarettes.

(c) **Nicotine gum** (nicotine polyacrolex, Nicorette) contains 2 mg/piece (in US) or 4 mg/piece in Canada and Europe of nicotine. It is buffered to a pH of 8.5 for enhanced absorption. Nicotine is rapidly and completely absorbed through the oral mucosa. About 30 min of chewing releases 90% of the nicotine, 1 h of chewing a 2-mg piece produced 11.8 ng/mL, and a 4-mg piece 23.2 ng/mL nicotine plasma concentrations, respectively. The gum must be chewed to release nicotine. **Any amount of chewed gum is considered a toxic ingestion in a child.** If intact gum is swallowed little absorption occurs (316,318,319).

(d) **Nicotine transdermal systems** are usually in three doses and provide 21, 14, and 7 mg of nicotine over 16 to 24 h. These provide average plasma nicotine concentrations of 17, 12, and 6 ng/mL, respectively (smoking provides 20 to 50 ng/mL) (321,324,325). A 21 mg/24 h is equivalent to smoking for 15 h (314) The elimination half-life of transdermal absorbed nicotine is 3 to 6 h. The amount of nicotine remaining in a transdermal patch after use is 27% to 73%. Although there is limited experience with dermal patch ingestion, in accidental dermal application, the toxicity appears to be minimal. **Patients should be cautioned about smoking and using the patches** (321,322,324) (Table 28-19).

(5) **Insecticides.** Nicotine was widely used as an insecticide. It is still available as a dust for leaf-eating insects (0.05% to 4.0%) and as a concentrated solution (40%). Dermal intoxication can occur with the 40% solution. A 5-g solution ingested by a 17-year-old produced cardiac arrest in 2 min and later death (314). **Any amount of 40% insecticide is considered toxic by ingestion in a child.**

(6) In **adults** the absorption of 2 to 5 mg of the alkaloid rapidly can produce centrally mediated nausea and vomiting which usually empties the stom-

TABLE 28-19. *Nicotine content of dermal patches*

Product	Patch doses, total nicotine, (mg/patch)	Manufacturer	Amount of nicotine undelivered in 24 h		
			mg	Percentage	mg
Nicoderm	7 (35), 14 (78), 21 (114)	Marion Merrell Dow	15.5	74	from 21
Prostep	11, 22 (15–30)	Lederle	5.9	27	from 22
Nicotrol	15 (24.9), 10 (16), 5(8.3)	Warner-Lambert	10	40	from 16
Habitrol	7 (17.5), 14 (35), 21 (52.5)	Ciba-Geigy	8.4	40	from 21

In parenthesis is the amount that could be absorbed (mg).
Data from refs. 314, 382, and 383.

ach and is protective. **The fatal dose** of nicotine in adults is reported to be about 40 to 60 mg (0.6 to 0.85 mg/kg) or the amount in 2 g of tobacco (two cigarettes) (314). However this dose spread out throughout the day in a smoking adult does not result in obvious clinical manifestations. Survival has been reported following ingestions of 1 to 4 g.

(7) **Mechanism of toxic action** (314,316). Nicotine stimulates the peripheral autonomic ganglia at lower doses with predominately sympathetic effects (tachycardia, hypertension), and at higher doses cholinergic effects (salivation and bronchial secretion). It binds to the CNS dopaminergic receptors (alertness, mood, reward, appetite depression) and in overdose directly effects CNS vomiting center and may produce seizures and respiratory arrest. Nicotine produces ganglionic and neuromuscular junction blockage (fasciculations and depolarizing paralysis of skeletal muscle).

(8) **Kinetics:** Nicotine is a tertiary amine similar to acetylcholine. **Absorption** occurs by all routes. **GI** absorption is slow and incomplete, and nicotine is poorly absorbed from tobacco in GI tract (314,327). Bioavailability is only 30% to 40%. **The onset of action by inhalation** occurs within minutes. Nicotine intoxication has not been reported by passive inhalation. The **ingestion onset** is within 15 to 30 min. **Mucosal absorption** is more rapid than ingestion and produces a higher serum concentration and lasts longer (315,327). The duration is 1 to 2 h with mild exposure and 48 to 72 h after severe exposure (314). Death may occur within 5 min. The route of elimination is 90% by hepatic cytochrome P-450 enzymes **metabolism** (80% to 90%) to low or inactive major metabolites cotinine and nicotine-1′N′-oxide. Both are rapidly excreted by the kidneys. Protein binding is less than 5%. It is metabolized more rapidly by a smoker. The **half-life** of nicotine in smokers is 0.8 h, in nonsmokers is 1.3 h and for cotinine is 15 to 20 h (314,327). The half-life of nicotine with **gum/cigarette** is 1 to 2 h and with **transdermal** patches more than 4 h (321–325). An alkaline urine reduces the nicotine excretion to 2% to 10% from an acid urine excretion of 23% to 30% (314). The volume of distribution (V_d) is 1 to 3 L/kg and is higher in nonsmokers. Nicotine **crosses the placenta** surpassing the maternal serum. Nicotine is found in the breast milk in small quantities (91 ppb) (328). The recommended plasma level of nicotine to avoid physiologic withdrawal is 5 to 35 ng/mL.

(a) **Cotinine** is an indicator of smoke absorption (307,309, 314). It has been found in the urine of 60% of 433 infants of mothers who smoked in their infants' presence (306,307)

(9) **Manifestations: The onset** with small doses is within 15 min after exposure. Delayed onset and prolonged duration may occur with nicotine gum and transdermal patches. Black Leaf Insecticide (40) nicotine may cause pallor, hypotension, retching, and death, often within 1 h.

(a) **Phase I adrenergic and cholinergic effects** (314,327) (Tables 28-20 and 28-21). Amounts of 1 mg/kg may cause nausea, and induce emesis. Initially pallor, tachycardia, hypertension (ganglionic sympathetic stimulation) followed in severe cases by hypotension and bradycardia (ganglionic blockade), profuse salivation, abdominal pain and diarrhea, and diaphoresis (cold sweats). Weakness, headache, ataxia, confusion can occur. Early excitation, fasciculations, tremors and seizures may occur within 30 min. **Miosis** occurs with small doses.

(b) **Phase II ganglionic and neuromuscular junction blockade effects** (314,327) tachycardia and hypertension occurs initially followed by bradycardia and hypotension, **mydriasis** with large doses, hyperpyrexia, later paralysis including respiratory muscle paralysis, seizures, dysrhythmia, and coma. Ileus and urinary retention may occur. Duration in mild cases is 1 to 2 h and 24 to 48 h in severe intoxications. A catecholamine release may cause polymorphonuclear leucocytosis and glycosuria. Death occurs from cardiovascular collapse and respiratory arrest (Table 28-20).

(c) Differential diagnosis. The sudden onset of an **atraumatic afebrile seizure** in a nonepileptic child should suggest **intoxicants** such as nicotine (319). Camphor, cocaine, cyanide, lidocaine, phencyclidine, and strychnine may also cause seizures. Nicotine ingestion should be considered in a child with **unexplained vomiting. Other cholinergic intoxicants** do not produce the biphasic course of nicotine toxicity and **other agents that cause paralysis** do not have cholinergic manifestations.

(10) There is a great deal of **controversy about the toxicity and management of cigarette ingestions by children.**

(a) A retrospective review of 223 consecutive children under 6 years with cigarette ingestions by the Long Island Regional Poison Control (LIRPCC) 1993 to 1995, 17.9% exhibited manifestations (mild GI symptoms in 39, diaphoresis and lethargy in one, 26 (11.7%) were managed in an ED setting by observation for an average of 6 h. None required admission to a hospital. No moderate, major, or fatal outcomes occurred in our series.

TABLE 28-20. *Nicotine intoxication: changes that occur between phases I and II*

	Phase I	Phase II
Pupils	Miosis	Mydriasis
Heart rate	Tachycardia	Bradycardia
CNS	Stimulation	Depression
Blood pressure	Hypertension	Hypotension

TABLE 28-21. *Nicotine intoxication*

Ingestion (mg)	Manifestations
<40	Headache resolves in 1–2 h
50–80	Loss of consciousness, nausea, diaphoresis, hypotension, headache resolves in 24 h
80	Chest pain and tightness
150	Decreased respiration, tachycardia, nausea, vomiting, headache, diaphoresis, numbness for 10 d

Modified from ref. 384.

(b) National data indicate 15,235 exposures in children under 6 years were reported to the AAPCC 1993 to 1994. Of these, 23% were treated in a hospital, 97% were asymptomatic or had minor toxicity, and there were no deaths (4).

(c) In 1985, Smolinske et al. (318) investigated 51 cases of tobacco exposure in children under 6 years, 23 had GI symptoms, but no other toxicity. They estimated that 1.4 to 1.9 mg/kg tobacco would produce severe toxicity, 0.2 to 1.8 mg/kg mild toxicity and 0.3 to 1 mg/kg no toxicity. Nakamura, et at (333) in Japan reported 1,000 cases of tobacco ingestions in children, none required hospitalization. A study by Malizzia et al. (334) in 1983 described ingestions of cigarettes (nicotine and marijuana) in 10 children in Rome, Italy and reported that four patients ingesting two cigarettes developed salivation, vomiting, diarrhea, tachypnea, tachycardia, and hypertension. Respiratory depression, dysrrhythmias and convulsions developed within 60 min and four patients required artificial ventilation. A letter by Petridou et al. (335) described 15 Greek children exposed to chewing or swallowing cigarettes. All required admission to a hospital for at least 24 to 48 h. The predominant symptoms were tachycardia and vomiting which peaked at 16 h after exposure despite ingestions of less than 2 cigarettes. Bonadio reported that 1 in 20 children reviewed in Wisconsin with tobacco ingestion became moderately ill and required 24 h hospitalization after ingesting cigarettes (336). McGee et al. (337) in a 2-year retrospective review of 341 tobacco ingestions in children under 6 years in 1989 indicated 62 were symptomatic. Vomiting occurred in the majority, two patients experienced irritability and 1 had lethargy. Children who ingested more than six butts or two whole cigarettes were referred to a medical care facility. Eight such patients were and remained asymptomatic (337). In a second study McGee and colleagues reviewed the data for 4 years on 700 exposures, 143 children vomited usually in less than 20 min and symptoms resolved, 557 were asymptomatic. Children who ingested more than 2 cigarettes or 6 butts were referred to the ED; 20 had symptoms; however, 24 remained asymptomatic (338).

(11) Management: Establish and maintain vital functions.

(a) **Conclusions on ingestion of tobacco products by children.** The minimal toxic amount of nicotine appears to be 1 mg/kg or about the amount in 1 fresh cigarette. Children who ingest more than one fresh cigarette, three cigarette butts, one cigar butt, a pinch of snuff, chew any amount of chewing tobacco, chew nicotine gum (330–338), suck for over 30 min on a transdermal nicotine patch, or are exposed to any amount of 40% nicotine insecticide should be considered as potentially toxic and require medical evaluation and observation. In other circumstances of small ingestions (less than the above previous stated amounts) gastric emptying is not necessary (332–335). If there are signs of early nicotine toxicity such as persistent vomiting, sympathetic or cholinergic intoxication such as pallor, diaphoresis, salivation and wheezing the patient should be medically evaluated in a medical facility.

(b) **GI decontamination: Avoid emesis** because of the rapid onset of convulsions, coma and persistent vomiting may be a sign of intoxication. **Gastric lavage** (avoid alkaline lavage solutions which enhance absorption and decrease excretion of nicotine) if recent ingestion. **Activated charcoal/initial cathartic** may be administered. Although activated charcoal binds nicotine, its value in acute poisoning has not been documented. Pharmacokinetic studies have indicated nicotine appears to have a enterohepatic recirculation therefore **repeated doses of activated charcoal** may theoretically be of value in serious exposures (314).

(c) **Dermal decontamination** may be needed if exposed to nicotine liquids and dermal patches. Wash the area thoroughly with cool water and dry. Alkaline soaps, may increase absorption. Nicotine may continue to be absorbed for several hours after removal because of deposit in the skin.

(d) Seizure precautions and **control convulsions** with diazepam or lorazepam.

(e) **Atropine** should be used for cholinergic excess.

(f) **Phentolamine or beta and alpha blockers (labetalol** for sympathetic overstimulation and severe hypertension.

(g) **Hypotension** may be treated with positioning, fluids and vasopressors like dopamine or norepinephrine if necessary.

(h) **Acid diuresis** theoretically may decrease reabsorption and enhance elimination but has not been investigated. **It is not recommended.**

(i) **Mecamylamine** (Inversine) is an oral specific antagonist to CNS nicotine effects, however it is **not useful** for treating nicotine toxicity which includes vomiting, seizures and hypotension.

        (j)   Measures to enhance elimination such as hemodialysis and hemo-perfusion are not useful (314).

    (12) Disposition. Observe the asymptomatic patient in the ED for 6 h. For the ingestion of intact gum tablets or transdermal patches, observe for 12 to 24 h.

    (13) Laboratory

        (a)   **Monitor:** CBC (leucocytosis occurs with intoxications), electrolytes, blood glucose (hyperglycemia with intoxications), BUN, creatinine, arterial blood gases, liver function tests, serum nicotine, ECG, blood pressure, and urinalysis.

        (b)   The **biologic markers of tobacco** are cotinine, thiocyanate and carbon monoxide in blood, urine and saliva. **Carbon monoxide** can be inexpensively measured via expiration. It is a good marker of short-term use. **Thiocyanate** is a metabolite of hydrogen cyanide commonly found in cigarettes. It takes up to 6 weeks to reach presmoker's thiocyanate level after discontinuing tobacco use. Smoking induces elevation in thiocyanate levels which may be useful for determining measures of passive exposure. Plasma concentrations of **cotinine** in children living with smokers is four times (0.004 µg/ml) higher than those in children from nonsmoking environments (0.001 µg/mL) (290,291). Active smokers have cotinine blood concentrations more than 13.7 ng/mL, passive inhalation have 1.0 to 13.7 ng/mL, and nonsmokers have less than 1.0 ng/mL, which is the minimal concentration detectable (324,325).

        (c)   **Nicotine** in the blood is the most specific test and should be measured with radioimmunoassay or gas chromatography but these are expensive. Nicotine is unstable over time so tests measure only short-term use. Plasma levels of nicotine from pipe smoking is 4 to 6 ng/ml (0.004 mg/L) (321), cigarette smoking 18.3 ng/mL 5–30 ng/mL (321), chewing 2 mg of nicotine gum is 29.5 ng/mL, chewing 4 mg of nicotine gum is 40.7 ng/mL (309,314,323), transdermal 21 mg = 17 ng/mL, 14 mg = 12 ng/ml, and 7 mg = 6 ng/mL (310). The **toxic serum level** is more than 50 ng/mL, and the **fatal serum concentration** in the literature is more than 200 ng/mL.

F. Azide, sodium (NaN2) Sodium azide is used as antimicrobial preservatives of laboratory reagents, in the explosive industry for shell detonators and in pharmaceuticals. It was used until 1950 as a direct vasodilator to treat hypertension. Azide is used as a gas generant (350 to 600 g sodium azide) with copper and iron oxides in **automobile safety airbags.** Its explosive decomposition to nitrogen gas produces rapid inflation of the airbag. There have been 16 reported poisonings in the English literature, including seven deaths (342–349).

1. **Automobile airbags** are rubberized nylon bags that inflate on spark ignition of sodium azide and yield nitrogen gas, ash, and a small amount of sodium hydroxide (342).
   a. Automotive airbags may produce **"slap-like" thermal burns** (all reported cases were mild) by the conversion of the ignition canister containing sodium azide to release "hot" nitrogen in 1/20th of a second (350).
   b. Sodium azide undergoes complete combustion in ignition and should not represent a hazard (342,348). Small amounts of sodium hydroxide released is quickly converted to sodium carbonate and bicarbonate which is dispersed as a white powder (344,346). Two cases of "**airbag keratitis**" have been reported when the airbag broke (351).

2. **Toxicity:** Sodium azide toxicity is similar to cyanide and hydrogen sulfide. It has been shown to be mutagenic in rodents.
   a. Inhibits the iron containing **respiratory enzyme** cytochrome oxidase producing cellular asphyxiation, inhibiting mitochondrial oxidative phosphorylation and other oxidative systems stopping aerobic metabolism and change the production from pyruvate to lactate (342).
   b. Converted into **nitric acid** in vivo which has an effect similar to the endothelium relaxing factor and causes vasodilation (342).
   c. **Ingestion** of 150 mg produced breathlessness, tachycardia, nausea, vomiting and diarrhea within 1 min and later polydipsia, T wave changes on the ECG, leukocytosis and numbness for 10 days (343). It is reported that 700 mg produced myocardial failure in 72 h (349). The human hypotensive dose was 0.2 to 4 µg/kg. Ingestion of 1 to 2 g quickly produce GI symptoms, hypotension, seizures and multiple organ failure and death in 1 to 2 h. The fatal ingested dose is estimated to be 10 to 20 g although deaths have been reported with amounts greater than 13 mg/kg (342,352) (Table 28–9).
   d. **Inhalation.** Sodium azide is stable in neutral solutions but is hydrolyzed in aqueous solutions to hydrazoic acid, a toxic gas with a pungent odor. The pungent odor does not give adequate warning. An elevated cyanide blood concentration was reported in one patient. Inhalation of 1,024 ppm of hydrazoic acid (HN_3) for 60 min is anticipated to be **fatal. The TLV** is 0.1 ppm, and PEL is 0.3 ppm. American Conference of Governmental Industrial Hygienists ceiling limit (ACGIH TLC-C) is 0.29 mg/m^3 for sodium azide and 0.11 ppm for hydrazoic acid. Air concentrations as low as 0.3 ppm may result in mucosal irritation, hypotension and headache.

3. **Kinetics:** Sodium azide is a stable, neutral, white crystalline solid. Azide in contact with water or acidified is hydrolyzed to hydrazoic acid (HN_2)a toxic and explosive gas. Acute toxicity of HN_2 is compared to hydrogen sulfide and hydrogen cyanide. It is rapidly absorbed from the GI tract, skin contact, and the respiratory tract.

4. **Manifestations**
   a. Large ingestions produce rapid onset within 1 to 2 h of GI and neurological manifestations but with smaller ingestions symptoms may be delayed for several hours.

    b. The severity of the manifestations are dose related. Several grams may produce death in 1 to 2 h or as late as 24 h after exposure (342–344,351).

    c. Ingestion and inhalation produces neurological symptoms of faintness, muscle weakness, convulsions, coma and respiratory failure.

    d. Cardiovascular—hypertension or hypotension, tachycardia, and cardiac dysrhythmias. Myocardial ischemia and cardiomyopathy has been reported and may delayed several days (349,352).

    e. Respiratory—bronchitis, hyperpnea, apnea and pulmonary edema.

    f. Neurological—muscle weakness and flaccidity, coma, convulsions.

    g. Metabolic—acidosis (352)

    h. Keratitis has been reported from automobile airbags that broke when they inflated (351).

5. Management. Caution: In the acid environment of the stomach, azide salts are converted into the toxic gas hydrazoic acid that may represent a danger to health care providers. Keep the patient in well ventilated areas, quickly isolate vomitus and gastric washing and avoid exposure to hydrazoic acid, wear appropriate respiratory protective equipment including self contained breathing apparatus and chemical protective clothing. **Explosive hazard:** Contact with heavy metals, including copper or lead in water pipes may form metal azides that may explode.

    a. Establish and maintain the vital functions. Intensive support of respiratory and cardiovascular system is essential. Monitor the ECG and establish vascular access.

    b. If ingested. Gastric lavage may produce hydrazoic acid and a toxic gas although it is recommended (342). Avoid emesis because of rapid onset of manifestations. Activated charcoal is probably ineffective but there are no studies. Caution vomitus and gastric washings should be quickly isolated.

    c. Inhalation. Remove victim from exposure and administer supplemental oxygen.

    d. Dermal contact. Provide skin decontamination with removal of the contaminated clothing and use copious washing of affected areas.

    e. The cyanide antidote kit (sodium nitrite and sodium thiosulfate) and dicobalt edetate has been used but reported to be ineffective (342), although there are some animal reports of some protection by sodium nitrite and *p*-aminopropriophenone (PAPP) (352).

    f. There is role for dialysis or hemoperfusion.

    g. Examine the eyes thoroughly for evidence of injury in cases of automobile airbag rupture (fluorescein stain and slit-lens examination) (351).

    h. Reports of delayed cardiac toxicity suggest admission and monitoring for cardiac injury for 3 to 5 days with ECG and cardiac enzymes, if significant exposure.

6. Laboratory. Azide produces a positive ferric chloride test of the gastric aspirate giving a red precipitate. Monitored studies may include arterial blood gas studies with oxygen saturation, electrolytes, blood lactate, creatine kinase, methemoglobin, and co-oximeter.

VII. Sport equipment

    A. Gun bluing solution includes selenious acid which interferes with the sulfhydryl-containing enzymes and is a caustic. There were 52 exposures reported in 1994 to AAPCC, with nine moderate outcomes and no major outcomes or deaths (4). However there are **four fatalities in children** under 6 years reported to the AAPCC from 1983 to 1990, from selenious acid-containing gun bluing that warrants discussion. The normal recommended selenium in diet is 50 to 200 µg/day and 10 to 100 times that amount may be toxic (353,354,355).

        1. Toxicity

            a. **As little as 20 mL of gun bluing (2% selenious acid) has been fatal** (353–355).

            b. It produces hypersalivation, vomiting, seizures, dermal burns and garlic odor to the breath.

            c. Chronic toxicity will be caused by doses of 3.2 to 6.7 mg daily. About 31 mg/day for 11 days produced toxicity.

            d. Normal blood selenium is 0.1 µg/ml.

        2. Management

            a. **Management** is GI decontamination with cautious lavage (although it has been unsuccessful in 2 cases) and activated charcoal/cathartic and supportive therapy. In vitro experiments suggest that oral **vitamin C** can reduce selenium salts to elemental selenium which is poorly absorbed. It seems reasonable to administer several grams although results in animals are equivocal. **The shampoo** contains selenium sulfate salt which is poorly absorbed and will cause vomiting on its own therefore small amounts are not toxic (94) (see Selenium Shampoo).

            b. **Dye decontamination:** Flush eyes with copious amounts of water for at least 15 min. Consider an ophthalmological consult if irritation, lacrimation, or photophobia persist for more than 15 min.

            c. **Dermal decontamination:** Wash the exposed area thoroughly with soap and water.

            d. **Monitor** the serum electrolytes if vomiting or diarrhea is protracted. Replace fluids as appropriate. Monitor liver transaminases.

            e. **Chelation** with BAL and CaNa$_2$EDTA has been studied in animal and are equivocal and not recommended. *N*-acetylcysteine may have therapeutic value but further studies are needed. Bromobenzene is dangerous and should not be used. Vitamin C i.v. may be helpful but has not been clinically investigated.

            f. **After selenious acid ingestion** consider endoscopic examination to exclude gastroesophageal damage.

            g. **Deposition.** The patient should be medically observed for at least 6 to 12 h postingestion.

VIII. Environmental household toxicity

    A. Formaldehyde (HCHO, formalin, methylaldehyde, methylene glycol). There were 123 exposures to urea formaldehyde reported to the AAPCC, with 11 moderate outcomes and no major outcomes or deaths (4).

1. Formaldehyde is a colorless, flammable gas with a pungent, irritating odor. It is usually found as a 37% clear solution in water with 12% to 15% methanol **(formalin)** (36).

2. NIOSH has listed 29 **product uses** for formaldehyde. The most common in mobile homes is particle board (357), plywood, adhesives, permanent press fabrics or clothes treated with crease-resistant resins, embalming fluid, and cosmetics. Cigarette smoke contains about 30 ppm of formaldehyde by volume. The potentially highly exposed population is approximately 400,000 persons (pathologists, funeral service workers, medical, dental and nursing students) (357,358).

3. **Urea formaldehyde** was used as insulation foam until 1982 and releases formaldehyde. Cured polyurethane does NOT release free formaldehyde (356).

4. **Toxicity:** Formaldehyde is toxic by inhalation and ingestion.

   a. **Mechanism of toxicity:** Formaldehyde causes coagulation necrosis by covalently binding with protein and causes cell necrosis, mucous membrane irritation and severe system acidosis.

   b. **Direct contact** with skin produces contact dermatitis and with eyes conjunctivitis.

   c. **Inhalation acts** on humans principally as an irritant of the eyes and upper respiratory tract, and impairs the mucociliary mechanism. The low threshold of response and the disagreeable, irritating odor prevents one from breathing intolerable amounts.

      (1) The **College of American Pathologists** and **OSHA** recommends no higher than 1 ppm time-weighted average per 8-h workday (TLV-TWA), PEL-weighted average is 3 ppm, and IDLH is 100 ppm, If the formaldehyde levels are greater than 0.05 ppm, it is recommended to remove the source or use barrier paints.

      (2) Formaldehyde causes hypersensitivity reactions. The gas produces irritation of mucous membranes, cough, wheezing (359) and pulmonary edema (356,358).

   d. **Ingestion** of as little as 30 mL of 37% formaldehyde has caused death in an adult (359), although 60 to 90 mL of 100% formaldehyde is the usual potentially fatal amount. Ingestion can produce coagulation necrosis of the esophagus like any mineral acid (360). Systemically it can produce formic acid acidosis in 8 to 12 h with anion gap, shock, and hepatorenal syndrome. There have been **no reports of systemic formaldehyde producing blindness** or retinal eye damage (358).

   e. Certain regulatory agencies regard formaldehyde as a **possible human carcinogen.** It has mutagenic and carcinogenic properties (362). Formaldehyde and hydrogen chloride form a potent **carcinogen bischloromethyl ether.** Formaldehyde is known to cause nasal tumors in some rodents (360,363). The **Environmental Protection Agency (EPA) assessment of cancer risk** over a 70-year lifetime at "ambient exposure levels" is 1.3 cases per 100,000.

5. **Manifestations** (Table 28-22) of the concentration of formaldehyde and effects.

6. **Kinetics:** Well absorbed through GI tract and by inhalation, less absorption der-

mally. Metabolized within 15 min to formic acid and then to carbon dioxide and water. Half-life of formate is 1.5 h.

7. **Prevention of exposure**
   a. If formaldehyde levels in a home are greater than 0.05 ppm, reduce exposure by removal, and provide ventilation and vapor barrier painting.
   b. Engineering controls of the work environment consist of using hoods and local exhaust ventilation. Monitor the work environment.

8. **Management**
   a. Remove from environment, establish and maintain vital functions and administer supplemental warm humidified oxygen.
   b. Protective measures for levels of formaldehyde up to 30 ppm: use specific chemical cartridge respirator with full facepiece. For unknown or levels up to 100 ppm use air-supplied respirator operated in a positive pressure mode.
   c. **Dermal exposure** requires removal of contaminated clothing, immediate irrigation of exposed areas with copious amounts of tepid water.
   d. **Ocular exposure** requires immediate irrigation with copious amounts of water with eyelids retracted for at least 15 min.
   e. **If ingested** immediate therapy is to administer 8 to 12 oz of milk. Activated charcoal absorbs formalin and may be useful although there is no scientific data. **Do not** induce emesis because of risk of corrosive injury. **Do not** use activated charcoal if plan endoscopy.
   f. **Consider endoscopy** to exclude gastroesophageal damage if concentrated solution is ingested.
   g. **Treat formic acid metabolic acidosis** with sodium bicarbonate if present. Alkalinization helps promote excretion of formate.
   h. **Administer folic acid or sodium folate** 1 mg/kg/dose every 4 h up to 50 mg total dose i.v. in acute formaldehyde ingestions.
   i. **Treat bronchospasm** with aerosol beta-2 agonists bronchodilators or theophylline.
   j. **If spill occurs** cleanup management is with absorbent material NOT sodium bisulfate or isopropyl alcohol.
   k. **Hemodialysis** is effective and is indicated if severe acidosis or if the methanol level is elevated.

TABLE 28-22. *Concentration of formaldehyde and effects*

ppm	Effects
0.05–1.0	Odor threshold
0.40–0.80	Coughing and wheezing
1–5	Irritation of eyes, nose, and throat
	Lacrimation, laryngitis, bronchitis
10–20	Dyspnea, palpitations
>50	Lung damage, pneumonitis, noncardiogenic pulmonary edema, death
100	Immediately dangerous to life and health (IDLH)
15 ppm for 6 h for 16 months	In rats, squamous cell carcinoma of nasal turbinates

9. **Laboratory:** Formate levels may indicate the severity of the intoxication. More than 12 mg/dL is extremely toxic. Monitor CBC, electrolytes, BUN, creatinine, and liver function tests. Plasma formaldehyde levels are not useful, but formate levels may indicate the degree of toxicity.

B. **Radon.** In 1988, the International Agency for Research on Cancer (IARC) concluded there was enough evidence to classify radon as a carcinogen in human beings (364–366). According to the EPA, there are several thousand (5,000 to 20,000) with lung cancer deaths per year attributable to radon (364). A Swedish study found the number of cancer related radon deaths depend greatly on the rate of cigarette smoking (370)

1. In October 1988 the EPA and the Office of the Surgeon General jointly **recommended that all homes in the United States below the third floor be tested for the presence of radon.** The indoor **Radon Abatement Act** was passed in October 1988 and in 1990, Congress appropriated grants to states to develop and enhance programs to reduce radon risks in the homes and schools. It is now the standard of practice to measure radon in the homes at the time of real estate transactions (366).

2. Approximately 5% to 10% of single family homes (about 8 million homes) in United States exceed the **EPA guideline of less than 4 picocurie/L of air** (366–369). The highest concentrations of radon are found along the "Reading Prong or Fault" which involves areas in Pennsylvania, New York and New Jersey. However other areas also exist (364–366).

   a. **Radium,** an ubiquitous element obtained from uranium, produces radon. Uranium is found in some granite and shale deposits and in phosphate-containing soils and rocks.

   b. **Radon** is a naturally occurring colorless, odorless "gas" (not truly a gas but particulate matter) that is the decay product of radium found in some areas where there are faults in the Earth's crust. Radon is in the air we breath, however outdoors it is diluted to low concentrations and poses no problem. Indoors in a closed space radon can accumulate to significant levels. The magnitude of the radon buildup depends on the type of construction and concentration of radon in the soil (366).

   c. **The decay progeny "daughters" of radon** may attach to particulate matter such as cigarette smoke and be inhaled. During subsequent decay the progeny of radon emit **alpha particles of radiation** that can injure adjacent bronchial cells and lung tissue and increase risk of lung cancer (366).

   d. **Radon can be detected only by testing. Short-term testing** usually for 3 to 7 days but as long as 90 days is done with charcoal canisters ($10 to $25), charcoal liquid scintillation detectors, electrode ion detectors, and alpha tract detectors. **Long-term testing** of more than 90 days and lasting up to 1 year will give better evaluation if performed with alpha track ($20 to $50) and electrode ion detector most commonly. These devices measure radon "gas" and report in pCi/L. **Wintertime testing** is best because of negative pressure (364–369).

   e. The EPA urged that all detached and row homes, schools, day care facilities, as well as all apartments below the third floor, should be inspected for radon and if levels are elevated, remedial action be taken. **Other factors found to predispose homes to elevated levels of radon** include soil porosity, foundation type, location, building materials used, entry points for soil gas, building ventilation rates, and source water supply (366).

    f.   **Cigarette smokers** are at greater risk for lung cancers than nonsmokers similarly exposed to radon. Radon and cigarette smoking are synergistic carcinogens. Smoking creates more particulate matter to be inhaled and enhances the exposure. The risk of lung cancer from radon exposure in a smoker of a pack of cigarettes a day is 15% risk and a nonsmoker has a 1% risk of developing lung cancer (366,367,369). However there are reports confirming exposure to radon daughters in the absence of smoking which is still a potent carcinogen (371,376).

3.   **Management**

    a.   Remedial action consists of **abatement** (sealing basement cracks), discouraging smoking, increased ventilation and not placing bedrooms or playrooms in basement areas where radon concentrations are typically highest.

    b.   **Effective reduction** of exposure may sometimes be as simple as increasing the ventilation in a basement or other areas. Balanced heat exchangers properly installed can be useful.

    c.   **Exposure levels of radon.** If the level is above 200 pCI/L evacuate until levels are reduced, if the levels are 20 to 200 pCi/L, reduce these over several months, and if the levels are 4 to 20 pCI/L, these should be reduced over years to months. The State Radon offices can recommend qualified contractors for radon abatement contractors (364–368).

C.   **Asbestos.** Asbestos refers to a group of naturally occurring silicate minerals with a fibrous structure amosite, crocidolite, chrysotile and the asbestiform types tremolite, actinolite and anthophylite.

    1.   Asbestos was widely used from 1950 to 1970s in areas requiring sound proofing, thermal proofing or durability including floor and ceiling coverings, heating and water pipe insulation and brake linings. It was often applied as spray on material. **The rise in mesothelioma,** a malignancy of the pleura and the peritoneum, was the **"sentinel disease" for asbestos.**

    2.   Asbestos Hazard Emergency Response Act is administered by the EPA (372,373). In 1986 EPA estimated that friable asbestos may be present in as many as **35,000 schools** in United States built between 1946 to 1973, potentially exposing 15 million children and 1.4 million adults (374). Children may be at greater risk because of long life expectancy, high activity rates, higher breathing rates and more time spent near the floor (374,375).

    3.   **Smoking cigarettes** in addition to asbestos exposure increases the risk of cancer of the lung more than exposure to either one alone.

    4.   **Toxicity.** The **mechanism of toxicity** is unknown but appears to be related to the time of clearance of asbestos from the lungs.

        a.   Inhalation of thin fiber longer than 5 μm produces processes that are associated with pulmonary fibrosis and lung cancer. Shorter fibers are phagocytosed and removed from the lungs.

    b. Amosite and crocidolite are cleared more slowly from the lungs and are associated with the development of mesothelioma than is chrysolite. About 90% of the asbestos used in United States was chrysolite. Crocidolite is more strongly associated with cancer of the lung than chrysotile (375,376).

    c. The **safety guidelines** indicate that the levels of contamination range is greater than 0.2 fibers per cubic centermeter of air longer than 5 μm down to 0.05 fibers. The Occupational Safety and Health Administration PEL action standard for 8 h time-weighted average is 0.2 fibers/cc (375,377,378).

5. The **manifestations of pulmonary malignancy** is the gradual development of cough and dyspnea weight loss and chest pain. In advanced disease, restriction of expansion of the chest develops and inspiratory crackles are heard, clubbing and cyanosis of the fingers. Chest radiograph shows fibrosis especially of the lower lobes. Lung cancer is increased in cigarette smokers.

6. The type of disease is **asbestosis,** a slowly progressing fibrosing disease of the lungs. **Pleural plaques** which are usually asymptomatic involve the parietal pleura. **Pleural effusions** may occur as early as 5 to 10 years after exposure. **Mesothelioma** is not associated with cigarette smoking (376). The latent period for these diseases to develop are 30 to 40 years (376–378).

7. **Biopsies of the lung** include discrete foci of fibrosis in bronchiolar walls with presence of asbestos bodies (ferruginous bodies) which are fibers coated with hemosiderin and glycoproteins or both.

8. **Asbestos that is in good condition and not respirable is not a health risk.** However frayed or friable (easily crumbled) asbestos can release fibers into the air and exposure to fibers can be associated with lung cancer, asbestosis, benign pleural disease, and mesothelioma. The occurrence is influenced by the type of asbestos material inhaled, concentration, dimension of fibers and exposure duration (377–378).

    a. The **management** for friable asbestos is to encapsulate, removal may increase ambient air asbestos fibers (376–378). There is no specific treatment.

        (1) Prevention is the most important measure and all exposed should be encouraged to stop smoking and observe workplace control measures.

        (2) If renovation is planned in areas that had asbestos it should be done by certified contractors.

        (3) Those assisting acute exposure victims should wear respirators, protective equipment, and disposable gown and caps. Water down dried material should be used to prevent dispersion.

        (4) Acute dermal exposure and ingestion is not known to be harmful.

IX. **Microwave radiation. Nonionizing radiation** or longer wavelength radiation does not dislodge orbital electrons or destroy physical integrity of impacted atom. The longer **wavelengths** of the electromagnetic spectrum include radio waves, microwaves, infrared waves, and visible and ultraviolet radiation, which have relatively low energies and are nonionizing. Microwaves are at the opposite end of the spectrum from gamma waves, and their hazard to biologic systems is from the **heat of production.**

SUMMARY

I. Most household products are of relatively low toxicity, with the exceptions of products that contain ethanol or other alcohols in high concentrations, drain and oven cleaners, artificial-nail removers, phenol disinfectants, toilet bowl cleaners, some hair cosmetics, and organophosphate and carbamate insecticides.

II. Most ingestions of household products do not result in intoxications; however, they may be markers of inadequate supervision, behavioral problems, and chemical maltreatment.

III. Childhood poisoning may mimic many diseases, and specific presentations should make the physician suspicious of an intoxication.

IV. Significant reductions in childhood morbidity and mortality due to poisoning have occurred by using proved preventative measures, proper first aid, and the regionalization of PCCs.

References

1. Anonymous. Unintentional poisoning among young children—United States 1979-1978. *MWWR* 1983;32:117.
2. Done AK. Toxicity of household products. *Pediatr Clin North Am* 1970;17:579.
3. Litovitz TL, Felberg L, Soloway R, et al. 1994 Annual Report of American Association of Poison Control Centers Exposure Surveillance System. *Am J Emerg Med* 1995;13:551–597.
4. King W, Palmissano P. Poison control centers: can their value be measured? *South Med J* 1991;84:722–726.
5. Litovitz TL, et al. Recurrent poisonings among pediatric poisoning victims. *Med Toxicol Adv Drug Exp* 1989;4:381–386.
6. Litovitz TL, Manoguerra A. Comparison of pediatric poisoning hazards: an analysis of 3.8 million exposure incidents. *Pediatrics* 1992;89:999–1006.
7. Waldman JM, Mofenson HC, Greensher J. Evaluating the functioning of a poison control center. *Clin Pediatr* 1976;14:75.
8. McIntire MS, Angle CR. The taxonomy of suicide as seen in poison control centers. *Pediatr Clin North Am* 1970;17:697.
9. Sobel R. Psychiatric implications of accidental childhood poisoning. *Pediatrics* 1970;17:653.
10. Shnaps Y, et al. The chemically abused child. *Pediatrics* 1981;68:119.
11. Mofenson HC, Greensher J. The non-toxic ingestion. *Pediatr Clin North Am* 1970;17:584.
12. Mofenson HC, Greensher J, Caraccio TR. Ingestions considered non-toxic. *Emerg Clin North Am* 1984;2:159.
13. Gosselin RE. How toxic is it? *JAMA* 1957;163:1333.
14. French RJ, et al. Esophageal stenosis produced by the ingestion of bleach: report of two cases. *South Med J* 1970;63:1140.
15. Landau GD, Saunders WH. Effect of chlorine bleach on the esophagus. *Arch Otolaryngol* 1964;80:174–176.
16. Froner GA, Rutherford GW, Roeach M. Injection of sodium hypochlorite in by intravenous drug abusers [Letter]. *JAMA* 1987;258:325.
17. Pike DG, Peabody JW, Davis EW, et al. Re-evaluation of the dangers of Clorox ingestion. *J Pediatr* 1963;63:303–305.
18. Ward MJ, Routledge PA. Hypernatremia and hyperchloremic acidosis after bleach ingestion. *Hum Toxicol* 1988;7:37–38.
19. Spiller HA, Ross MP, Nickols GR. Fatal caustic ingestion of sodium hypochlorite associated hypernatremic-hyperchloremic acidosis. *Vet Hum Toxicol* 1994;36:373.
20. Gapary-Gapanavicius M. Chloramine-induced pneumonitis from mixing household cleaning agents. *BMJ* 1982;285:1086.
21. Faigel HC. Mixtures of household cleaning agents. *N Engl J Med* 1964;271:618.
22. Recommendations for preventing transmission of human T-lymphotrophic virus type III lymphadenopathy associated virus in the workplace. *MMWR* 19856;34:685–694.
23. Hoy RH. Accidental systemic exposure to sodium hypochloride (chlorox) during dialysis. *Am J Hosp Pharm* 1981;38:1512–1514.
24. Morgan DL. Intravenous injection of household bleach. *Ann Emerg Med* 1992;21:1394–1395.
25. McIntire MS, Guest JR, Porterfield JR. Philodendron: an infant death. *Clin Toxicol* 1990;28:177.
26. Fassett DW. *Oxalates in toxicants occurring naturally in foods.* 2nd ed. Washington, DC, National Academy of Science, 1973.

27. Woolf A. Oxalates. *Clin Toxicol Rev* 1993;16:24.
28. Saydjara R, Abston S, Desai MH. Chemical burns. *Burn Care Rehabil* 1986;7:404–408.
29. Menon M, Mahle CJ. Oxalate metabolism and renal calculi. *J Urol* 1982;127:148–151.
30. Aronow R, ed., for the Committee on Accident and Poison Prevention, AAP. *Handbook of common poisoning in childhood*. 2nd ed. Evanston, IL: AAP, 1983:107–114.
31. Litovitz TL, et al. Clinical manifestations of toxicity in a series of 784 boric acid ingestions. *Am J Emerg Med* 1988;6:209–213.
32. Linden CH, Hall AH, Kulig KW, et al. Acute ingestions of boric acid. *Clin Toxicol* 1986;24:269–279.
33. Rubinstein AD, Musher DM. Epidemic boric acid poisoning simulating staphylococcal toxic epidermolysis in a newborn Ritter's disease. *J Pediatr* 1970;77:884.
34. Baker MD, Bogema SC. Ingestion of boric acid by infants. *Am J Emerg Med* 1986;4:358–361.
35. Goldbloom RB, et al. Boric acid poisoning: a report of four cases and a review of 109 cases from the world literature. *J Pediatr* 1953;43:631–643.
36. Klein J, Olsen KR, McKinney HE. Caustic injury from household ammonia. *Am J Emerg Med* 1985;3:320.
37. Wason S, Stephan M, Briede C. Ingestion of aromatic ammonia smelling salts capsules. *Am J Dis Child* 1990;144:139–140.
38. Litovitz T, Schmitz B. Ingestion of cylindrical button batteries: an analysis of 2382 cases. *Pediatrics* 1992;89:747–757.
39. Mofenson HC, Greensher J, Caraccio TR. Ingestion of flat disc batteries. *Ann Emerg Med* 1983;12:88.
40. Kulig K, et al. Disc battery ingestion: elevated urine mercury levels and enema removal of battery fragments. *JAMA* 1983;249:25–32.
41. Burlington JD. Clinitest burns of the esophagus. *Ann Thorac Surg* 1975;20:400.
42. Gaudrealt P, Parent M, McGuigan M, et al. Predictability of esophageal injury from signs and symptoms: a study of caustic ingestions in 378 children. *Pediatrics* 1983;71:767–770.
43. Crain EF, Gershel JC, Meezey AP. Caustic ingestions as predictors of esophageal injury. *Am J Dis Child* 1984;138:163–165.
44. Anderson KD, Rouse TM, Randolph JG. A controlled trial of corticosteroids in children with corrosive injury of the esophagus. *N Engl J Med* 1990;323:637–640.
45. Lovejoy FH Jr. Are steroids necessary in caustic burns of the esophagus? [Editorial]. *N Engl J Med* 1990;323:668.
46. Previtera C, Guisti F, Gugleilimi. Predictive value of visible lesions (cheeks, lips, oropharynx) in suspected caustic ingestions: may endoscopy reasonably be omitted in completely negative pediatric patients? *Pediatr Emerg Care* 1990;6:176–178.
47. Gorman RL, Khin-Maung-Gyi MT, Klein-Schwartz W. Initial symptoms as predictors of esophageal injury in alkaline corrosive ingestions. *Am J Emerg Med* 1992;10:189–194.
48. Penner CE. Acid ingestion: toxicology and treatment. *Ann Emerg Med* 1980;7:374.
49. Ferguson MK, Miglione M, Staszak VM, et al. Early evaluation and therapy for caustic esophageal injury. *Am J Surg* 1989;157:116–120.
50. Cox RD, Osgood KA. Hydrofluoric acid. *Clin Toxicol* 1994;32:123–136.
51. Berolini JC. Hydrofluoric acid burns. *J Emerg Med* 1992;10:163–168.
52. Burkhart KK. Hydrofluoric acid burns. *Ann Emerg Med* 1994;24:9–13.
53. Carter RF. Acute selenium poisoning. *Med J Aust* 1966;1:525–562.
54. Pentel P, Fletcher D, Jensen J. Fatal acute selenium toxicity. *J Forensic Sci* 1985;30:556–562.
55. Cann HW, et al. Toxicity of household detergents and treatment of their ingestion. *Am J Dis Child* 1960;100:290.
56. Lawrence RA, Haggerty RJ. Household agents and their potential toxicity. *Mod Treat* 1971;8:511.
57. Temple AR, Veltri JC. Outcome of accidental ingestion of soaps, detergents and related household products. *Vet Hum Toxicol* 1979;21:9.
58. Lee JF, et al. Corrosive injury of the stomach and esophagus by nonphosphate detergents. *Am J Surg* 1972;123:652–656.
59. Temple AR, Spoerke DG, eds. *Cleaning products and their accidental exposure*. New York: Soap and Detergent Association, 1989.
60. Einhorn A, et al. Serious respiratory consequences of detergent ingestions in children. *Pediatrics* 1989;84:P472–P474.
61. Krenzelok EP. Liquid automatic dishwashing detergents: a profile of toxicity. *Ann Emerg Med* 1989;18:60–63.
62. Kynaston JA, et al. The hazards of automatic dishwasher detergents. *Med J Aust* 1989;151:5–7.
63. Haddad LM. Phenol, dinitrophenol, and pentachlorophenol. In: Haddad LM, Winchester JF, eds. *Clinical management of poisoning and drug overdose*. Philadelphia: WB Saunders, 1983:810.
64. Vogel C, Carraccio TR, Mofenson HC, et al. Alcohol intoxication in young children. *Clin Toxicol* 1995;33:25–33.
65. Leung AK. Ethyl alcohol ingestion in children: as fifteen year review. *Clin Pediatr* 1986;25:617–619.
66. Committee on Drugs, AAP. Ethanol in liquid preparations intended for children. *Pediatrics* 1984;73:405.
67. Scherger DL, et al. Ethyl alcohol (ethanol) containing cologne, perfume, and after shave ingestions in children. *Am J Dis Child* 1988;142:630–632.

68. Hornfelt CS. A report of acute ethanol poisoning in a child: mouthwash versus cologne, perfume and aftershave. *Clin Toxicol* 1992;30:115–121.
69. Selbst DSM, DeMaio JG, Boenning D. Mouthwash poisoning: report of a fatal case. *Pediatrics* 1985:24:162–163.
70. Henretig F, Vuignier B. Mouthwash ingestions in young children [Abstract]. *Vet Hum Toxicol* 1989;31:338.
71. Leung AK. Acute alcohol toxicity following mouthwash ingestion. *Clin Pediatr* 1985;24:470.
72. Leung AK. Ethanol-induced hypoglycemia from mouthwash. *Drug Intell Clin Pharm* 1985;19:480–481.
73. Simon HK, Cox JM, Sucov A, et al. Serum Alcohol clearance in intoxicated children and adolescents presenting to the ED. *Acad Emerg Med* 1994;1:520.
74. Ricci LR, Hoffman SA. Ethanol-induced hypoglycemic coma in a child. *Ann Emerg Med* 1982;11:202–204.
75. Freeman JJ, Hayes EP. Microsomal metabolism of acetonitrile to cyanide. *Biochem Pharmacol* 1988;37:1153–1159.
76. Caravati EM, Litovitz TL. Pediatric cyanide intoxication and death from acetonitrile-containing cosmetic. *JAMA* 1988;260:3470–3473.
77. Bismuth C, Baud FJ, Djeghout H, et al. Cyanide poisoning from propionitrile exposure. *J Emerg Med* 1987;5:191–195.
78. Geller RJ, Elkins BR, Ikonian RC. Cyanide toxicity from acetonitrile containing false nail remover. *Am J Emerg Med* 1991;9:288–270.
79. Kurt TL, Day LC, Reed WG, et al. Cyanide poisoning from glue on nail remover. *Am J Emerg Med* 1991;9:271–272.
80. Losek JD, Reock AL, Boldt RR. Cyanide poisoning from a cosmetic nail remover. *Pediatrics* 1991;88:337–340.
81. Osterhoudt FC, Wiley CC, Dudley R, et al. Artificial nail remover (nitroethane) poisoning. *J Pediatr* 1995;126:819–821.
82. Hornfeldt CS, Rabe WH. Nitroethane poisoning from an artificial fingernail remover. *J Toxicol Clin Toxicol* 1994;32:321–324.
83. Dowett R, Woolf A. Gastrointestinal corrosive injury due to ingestion of methacrylic acid [Abstract 138]. *Vet Hum Toxicol* 1994;36:373.
84. Potter JL, Krill EC, Neal E, et al. Methemoglobinemia due to ingestion of *N,N*-dimethyl-*P*-toluidine, a component used in the fabrication of artificial fingernails. *Ann Emerg Med* 1988;17:1098–1100.
85. Anonymous. Neutralizers in home permanent waving kits. *JAMA* 1950;144:397.
86. Dunsky I. Potassium bromate poisoning. *Am J Dis Child* 1947;74:719–730.
87. Gradus D, et al. Acute bromate poisoning associated with renal failure and deafness presenting as hemolytic anemia. *Am J Nephrol* 1984;4:188–191.
88. Warshaw BL, et al. Bromate poisoning from permanent wave preparations. *Pediatrics* 1985;76:975–978.
89. Lue JN, Jognson CE, Edwards DC. Bromate poisoning from ingestion of professional hair care neutralizer. *Clin Pharm* 1988;7:66–70.
90. Lichtenberg R, Zeller WP, Gatson R, et al. Clinical and laboratory observations: bromate poisoning. *J Pediatr* 1989;144:891–894.
91. McElwee NE, et al. Bromate poisoning. *Clin Pharm* 1988;7:570–572.
92. Malsumolo I, Morizono T, Paparella MM. Hearing loss following potassium bromate. Two case reports. *Otolaryngol Head Neck Surg* 1980;88:625–629.
93. McElwee NE, Kearney TE. Sodium sulfate unproven as bromate antidote. *Clin Pharm* 1988;7:570–572.
94. Cummins LM, Kimura ET. Safety evaluation of selenium sulfide anti-dandruff shampoos. *Toxicol Appl Pharmacol* 1971;20:89–96.
95. Heifetz SB, et al. The amounts of fluorine in self-administered dental products. *Pediatrics* 1986;77:876.
96. Eichler HG, Lenz KI, Fuhrmann M, et al. Accidental ingestion of NaF by children: report of a poison control center and one case. *Int J Clin Pharmacol Ther Toxicol* 1982;20:334–338.
97. Augustein WL, Spoerke DG, Kulig RW, et al. Fluoride ingestion in children: a review of 87 cases. *Pediatrics* 1991;88:907–912.
98. Rodgers GA, ed. *AAP handbook pediatric poisoning.* Elk Grove Village, IL: AAP, 1994.
99. Moss MH. Dangers from talcum powder. *Pediatrics* 1969;43:1058.
100. Mofenson HC, Greensher J, DiTomasso A, et al. Baby powder—a hazard. *Pediatrics* 1981;68:265–266.
101. Hayden CF, Sproul GT. Baby powder use in infant skin care: parental knowledge and determinants of powder usage. *Clin Pediatr* 1984;23:163–165.
102. Cetta F, Lambert GH, Ros SP. Newborn chemical exposure from over-the-counter skin care products. *Clin Pediatr* 1991;30:286–289.
103. Cotton WH, Davidson PJ. Aspiration of baby powder. *N Engl J Med* 1985;313:1662.
104. Cruthirds TP, Cole FH, Paul RN. Massive aspiration of baby powder causing pulmonary talcosis. *South Med J* 1977;70:626.
105. McCormick MA, Lecouture PG, Gaudrealt P, et al. Hazards associated with diaper changing. *JAMA* 1982:2159–2160.
106. Mofenson HC, Caraccio TR, Okun S, et al. Hazards of baby powder [Letter]. *Pediatrics* 1986;78:546–547.
107. Brouillete P, Weber ML. Massive aspiration of talcum powder by an infant. *CMAJ* 1978;119:354–355.
108. Molnar JJ, Nathenson Edberg S. Fatal aspiration of talcum powder by a child: report of a case. *N Engl J Med* 1962;266:36–37.

109. Gould SR, Barnardo DE. Respiratory distress after talc inhalation. *Br J Dis Chest* 1972;66:230.
110. Wells IP, Dubbin PA, Whimster WF. Pulmonary disease caused by the inhalation of cosmetic talcum powder. *Br J Radiol* 1979;52:586–588.
111. Wehner AP, Zwicker GM, Cannon, et al. Inhalation of talc baby powder by hamsters. *Ed Cosmet Toxicol* 1977;15:121–129.
112. Kleinfeld M, Messite J, Kooyman O, et al. Mortality among talc miners and millers in New York State. *Arch Environ Health* 1967;14:663–667.
113. Griffiths K. Asbestos, silicates and particulate materials in tissue. *Clin Chem* 1977;22:1141.
114. Threshold limit values for chemical substances and physical agents in the work environment with intended changes for 1983–1984. Presented at the American Conference of Governmental Industrial Hygienists, Cincinnati, 1983.
115. Ng TK. Talc and mesothelioma. *Med J Aust* 1984;Apr 14:452–453.
116. Cramer DW. Ovarian cancer and talc. *Cancer* 1982;50:372–376.
117. Kasper CS, Chandler PJ. Possible morbidity in women from talc on condoms. *JAMA* 1995;273:846–847.
118. Fanconi S, et al. Long-term sequelae in children surviving adult respiratory syndrome. *J Pediatr* 1985;216–222.
119. De LaRocha SR, et al. Normal pulmonary function after baby powder inhalation causing adult respiratory distress syndrome. *Pediatr Emerg Care* 1989;5:43–48.
120. Brook MP, et al. Pine oil cleaner ingestion. *Ann Emerg Med* 1989;18:391–395.
121. Conrad F, Wruk KM, Spoerke DG, et al. Pine oil cleaner ingestions. A prospective study [Abstract]. *Vet Hum Toxicol* 1988;28:484.
122. Ellenhorn MJ. Ellenhorn's *Med Toxicol*. Baltimore: Williams & Wilkins, 2nd ed., chap 54. 1997; 1081–1082.
123. Wruk CF, et al. Pine oil cleaner ingestions [Abstract 64]. Presented at the AAPCC/AACT/ABMT/CAPCC Meeting, Sante Fe, September 25–30, 1986.
124. Rosseaux CC, et al. Acute Pine Sol toxicity in a cat. *Vet Hum Toxicol* 1986;28:316–317.
125. Hill RM, et al. An investigation of recurrent pine oil poisoning in an infant by the use of gas chromatographic mass spectrometric methods. *J Pediatr* 1975;87:115–118.
126. Giberson TP, Ken JD, Pettigrew DW, et al. Near fatal hydrogen peroxide ingestion. *Ann Emerg Med* 1989;18:778–779.
127. Sleigh JW, Litter JP. Hazards of hydrogen peroxide. *BMJ* 1985;291:1786.
128. Rackoff WR, Menton DF. Gas embolism after the ingestion of hydrogen peroxide. *Pediatrics* 1990;85:593–594.
129. Mofenson HC, Caraccio TR, Wheeler T. Toxicity of 3% hydrogen peroxide (H_2O_2) OTC [Abstract 4]. *Clin Toxicol* 1995;33:488.
130. Dickenson KF, Caravati EM. Hydrogen peroxide exposure—325 exposures reported to a regional poison control center. *Clin Toxicol* 1994;32:705–714.
131. Davis RK, Brodeur AE, Shields J. The danger of hydrogen peroxide as a colonic irrigating solution. *J Pediatr Surg* 1967;2:131–133.
132. Christensen DW, Fraught WE, Black RE. Fatal oxygen embolization after hydrogen peroxide ingestion. *Crit Care Med* 1992;20:543–544.
133. Gervish SP. Gas embolism due to hydrogen peroxide. *Anesthesia* 1985;40:1244.
134. Tsai SK, Lee TY, Mok MS. Gas embolism produced by hydrogen peroxide irrigation of fistula during anesthesia. *Anesthesiology* 1985;63:316–317.
135. Cina SJ, Downs JCU, Conradi SE. Hydrogen peroxide: a source of lethal oxygen embolism. *Am J Forensic Med Pathol* 1994;15:44–30.
136. Shaw A, Cooperman A, Fusco J. Gas embolism produced by hydrogen peroxide. *N Engl J Med* 1967;277:238–241.
137. Bassan MM, Daudai M, Shalev O. Near fatal systemic oxygen embolism due to wound irrigation with hydrogen peroxide. *Postgrad Med J* 1982;58:448–450.
138. Humberston CL, Dean BS, Krenzelok EP. Ingestion of 35% hydrogen peroxide. *Clin Toxicol* 1990;28:95–100.
139. Luu TA, Kelley MT, Strauch JA, et al. Portal vein gas embolism from hydrogen peroxide ingestion. *Ann Emerg Med* 1992;21:1391–1393.
140. Sherman SJ, Boyer LV, Sibley WA. Cerebral infarction immediately after ingestion of hydrogen peroxide solution. *Stroke* 1994;25:1065.
141. Gonzolas TA, Vance M, Helpern M, et al. *Legal medicine, pathology and toxicology*. New York: Appleton-Century-Crofts, 1954.
142. Lavelle KJ, Doedens DJ, Kleit SA, Forney RB. Iodine absorption in burn patients treated topically with povidone iodine. *Clin Pharm Ther* 17:355;1975.
143. Peitsch J, Meakins JL. Complications of povidone iodine absorption in topically treated burn patients. *Lancet* 1:280;1976.
144. D'Auria J, Lipson S, Garfield JM. Fatal iodine toxicity following surgical debridement of a hip wound: case report. *J Trauma* 1990;30:353–355.
145. Aronoff GR, Friedman SJ, Doedens DJ, Lavelle RJ. Case report: increased serum iodide concentration from iodine absorption through wounds treated topically with povidone iodine. *Am J Med Sci* 279:173;1980.

146. L'Allemard D, Gruters A, Heidemann P, Schurnbrand P. Iodine-induced alterations of thyroid function in newborn infants after prenatal and perinatal exposure to povidone-iodide. *J Pediatr* 102:935;1983.

147. Mofenson HC, Caraccio TR, Greensher J. Iodine. In: Haddad LM, Winchester JF, eds. *Clinical management of poisoning and drug overdose*. Philadelphia: WB Saunders, 1983:697.

148. Haddad LH, et al. Phenol poisoning. *JACEP* 1979;8:267.

149. Liao JTP, Ohme FV. Phenol poisoning. *Vet Hum Toxicol* 1980;22:160–163.

150. Spiller HA, Qusadrani-Kushner HA, Cleveland P. A five year evaluation of acute exposures to phenol disinfectant (26%). *Clin Toxicol* 1993;31:307–313.

151. Halling H. Suspected link between exposure to hexachlorophene and malformed infants. *Ann NY Acad Med* 1979; 320:426–435.

152. Lockhart AD. How toxic is hexachlorophene? *Pediatrics* 1972;50:229–235.

153. Robson AM, Kissane JM, Elvick NH, et al. Pentachlorophenol poisoning in a nursery for newborn infants. I. Clinical features and treatment. *J Pediatr* 1969;75:309–316.

154. Armstrong RW, Eichner ER, Klein DE, et al. Pentochlorophenol poisoning in a nursery for newborn infants. II. Epidemiology and toxicologic studies. *J Pediatr* 1969;75:317–325.

155. Wysocki D, Flynt J, Golfield M, et al. Epidemic neonatal hyperbilirubinemia and the use of phenol disinfectant detergent. *Pediatrics* 1987;61:165–170.

156. Warner MA, et al. Cardiac dysrhythmia associated with chemical peeling with phenol. *Anesthiology* 1985;62:366–367.

157. Soares ER, Tift JP. Phenol poisoning: three fatal cases. *J Forensic Sci* 1982;27:729.

158. Neuvonen PJ. Clinical pharmacokinetics of oral activated charcoal in acute intoxications. *Clin Pharmacokinet* 1982;7:465–489.

159. Hunter DM, Timerding BL, Leonard RB, et al. Effects of isopropyl alcohol, ethanol and polyethylene glycol/industrial methylated spirits in the treatment of acute phenol burns. *Ann Emerg Med* 1992;21:1303–1307.

160. Kazliuka EN, Chang TMS. In vitro assessment of the removal of phenols by activated charcoal hemoperfusion. *Int J Artif Organs* 1972;2:215–221.

161. Kingston RL, Hall S, Sioris L. Clinical observations and medical outcome in 149 consecutive cases of ingestion of arsenate-containing ant killer. *Clin Toxicol* 1993;31:581–591.

162. Scalzo AJ, et al. Asymptomatic presentation of pediatric arsenic ingestion from sodium arsenate ant killer [Abstract 41]. Presented at the Meeting of the AACT/AAPCC/ABMT/CAPCC, Atlanta, October 1989.

163. Kerjes MP, Maurer JR, Trestrail JH, et al. An analysis of arsenic exposures reported to Blodgett Regional Poison Control Center. *Vet Hum Toxicol* 1987;29:75–78.

164. Flomenbaum NK, et al. Rodenticides. In: Goldfrank LR, et al, eds. *Goldfrank's toxicologic emergencies*. Norwalk, CT: Appleton & Lange, 1990.

165. DiPalma J. Human toxicity from rat poisons. *Am Fam Physician* 1981;24:186–189.

166. Egekeze JD, et al. Sodium monofluoroacetate (SMFA compound 1080). A literature review. *Vet Hum Toxicol* 1979;21:411–416.

167. Lehrmann F, et al. Parameters for the absorption of thallium ions by activated charcoal and Prussian blue. *Clin Toxicol* 1984;22:331.

168. Simon F, Pickering LK. Acute yellow phosphorous poisoning: the smoking stool syndrome. *JAMA* 1976;235:1343–1344.

169. McCarron M, Gladdis GP, Trotter AT. Acute yellow phosphorous poisoning from pesticide. *Clin Toxicol* 1981; 18:693–711.

170. Wilson R, Lovejoy FH Jr, Jaeger RJ. Acute phosphine poisoning abroad a grain frighter—epidemiologic, chemical and pathologic findings. *JAMA* 1980;244:148.

171. Gupta S, Ahlawat SK. Aluminum phosphide poisoning—a review. *Clin Toxicol* 1995:33:19–24.

172. Lambert JR, et al. Management of acute strychnine poisoning. *CMAJ* 1981; 124:1268–1270.

173. Edmunds M, et al. Strychnine poisoning: clinical and toxicological observations on a non-fatal case. *Clin Toxicol* 1986;24:245–255.

174. Smith BA. Strychnine poisoning. *J Emerg Med* 1990;8:321–325.

175. O'Callaghan WG, et al. Unusual strychnine poisoning and its treatment; report of eight cases. *BMJ* 1982;285:478.

176. Boyd RE, Brenan PT, Deng U. Strychnine poisoning, Recovery from profound lactic acidosis, hyperthermia, and rhabdomyolysis. *Am J Med* 1983;74:507–511.

177. Smolinske SC, Scharger DI, Kearns PS, et al. Superwarfarin poisoning in children: a prospective study. *Pediatrics* 1989;84:490–494.

178. Katona B, Wason S. Superwarfarin poisoning. *J Emerg Med* 1989;7:627–631.

179. Miller LV, et al. Diabetes mellitus and autonomic dysfunction after vacor rodenticide ingestion. *Diabetes Care* 1976;1:73.

180. Gallanosa AG, et al. Diabetes mellitus associated with autonomic and peripheral neuropathy after vacor rodenticides: a review. *Clin Toxicol* 1981;18:441–449.

181. Johnson D, et al. Accidental ingestion of vacor rodenticide: the symptoms and sequele in a 25 month old child. *Am J Dis Child* 1980;134:161.

182. LeWitt P. The neurotoxicity of the rat poison vacor. *N Engl J Med* 1980;392:73–77.

183. Presser PR, et al. Diabetes mellitus following rodenticide ingestion (Vacor) in man. *JAMA* 1978;239:1148.

184. Morgan DP. *Recognition and management of pesticide poisonings.* 3rd ed. Washington, DC: U.S. EPA, 1982.

185. Moore FM, Kudisch M, Richter K, et al. Hypercalcemia associated with rodenticide poisoning in three cats. *JAVMA* 1988;193:1099–1100.

186. Gunther R, Felice LJ, Nelson RK, et al. Toxicity of a vitamin D_3 rodenticide to dogs. *JAVMA* 1988;193:211.

187. Talcott PA, Mather GC, Kowitz. Accidental ingestion of a calciferol-containing rodent bait in dog. *Vet Hum Toxicol* 1991;33:252–256.

188. Chew DJ, Meuteen DJ. Disorders of the calcium and phosphorus metabolism. *Vet Clin North Am* 1982;12:1099–1100.

189. Forshee SK, Forester SD. Hypercalcemia secondary to cholecalciferol rodenticide toxicosis in two dogs. *JAVMA* 1990;195:1265–1268.

190. Dougherty S, Center SA, Dzanis. Salmon calcitonin as adjunct treatment for vitamin D toxicosis in a dog. *JACMA* 1990;196:1269–1272.

191. Anonymous. Insect repellents. *Med Lett* 1989;31:45–47,111.

192. Schreck CE, Shoddy EL, Spellman A. Pressured sprays of permethrin or DEET on military clothing for personal protection against Ixodes dammini (Acar ixodes). *J Med Entomol* 1986;23:396–399.

193. Evans SR, Korch GW, Lawson MA. Comparative field evaluation of permethrin and DEET military uniforms for personal protection against ticks (Acari). *J Med Entomol* 1990;27:829–834.

194. Wheater RH. Insect repellents. *JAMA* 1985;253:1458.

195. Tenenbein M. Severe toxic reactions and death following the ingestion of diethyltoluamide-containing insect repellents. *JAMA* 1987;68:1509–1511.

196. de Garbino J, Laborde A. Toxicity of an insect repellent: *N,N*-diethyltoluamide. *Vet Hum Toxicol* 1983;25:422–423.

197. Lurie AA, et al. Pharmacokinetics of insect repellent, *N,N*-diethyltoluamide. *Med Parasitol* 1979;47:72.

198. Davies MH, et al. Toxicity of diethyltoluamide-containing insect repellents. *JAMA* 1988;259:2239.

199. Anderson A. *N,N*-Diethyl-*M*-toluamide (DEET). *Clin Toxicol Rev* 1989;11:1.

200. Gryboski J, Weinstein D, Ordway NK. Toxic encephalopathy apparently related to the use of an insect repellent. *N Engl J Med* 1961;264:289–291.

201. Zadikoff CM. Toxic encephalopathy associated with the use of insect repellent. *J Pediatr* 1979;95:140–142.

202. Roland EH, Jan JE, Rigg JM. Toxic encephalopathy in a child after brief exposure to insect repellents. *Can Med Assoc J* 1985;132:155–156.

203. Edwards DL, Johnson CE. Insect repellent–induced toxic encephalopathy in a child. *Clin Pharm* 1987;6:496–498.

204. Oransky S, Roseman D, Fish T, et al. Seizures temporally associated with use of DEET insect repellent, New York–Conn. *MMWR* 1989;38:678–680.

205. Veltri JC, Osimitz TG, Bradford DC. Retrospective analysis of calls to poison control centers resulting from exposure to the insect repellent *N,N*-diethyl-*M*-toluamide (DEET) 1985–1989. *Clin Toxicol* 1994;32:1–16.

206. Miller JD. Anaphylaxis associated with insect repellent. *N Engl J Med* 1982;307:1341–1342.

207. Heick HMC, Shipman BY, Norman MG, et al. Insect repellent, *N,N*-diethyltoluamide effect on ammonia metabolism. *Pediatrics* 1988;82:373–376.

208. Heich HMC, Shipman RT, Norman MG, et al. Reye Syndrome associated with insect repellent in a presumed heterozygote for ornithine carbamyl transferase deficiency. *J Pediatr* 1980;97:471.

209. Lipscomb JW, Kramer JE, Leikin JB. Seizure following brief exposure to the insect repellent *N,N*-diethyl-*m*-toluamide. *Ann Emerg Med* 1992:21:315–317.

210. Clem JR, Haverman DF, Raebel MA. Insect repellent (*N,N*-diethyl-*m*-toluamide) cardiotoxicity in an adult. *Ann Pharmacother* 1993;27:289–293.

211. Malbach HI, Johnson HL. Contact urticaria syndrome: contact urticaria to diethyl-toluamide (immediate type hypersensitivity). *Arch Dermatol* 1975;111:726.

212. Mayenburg JV, Radkowski. Contact urticaria to diethyltoluamide contact. *Dermatitis* 1983;9:171.

213. Kuhlmann RS, et al. *N,N*-Diethyl-meta-toluamide: embryonic sensitivity. *Teratog Teratol* 1981;23:48A.

214. Anonymous. Permethrin 1% aerosol for ticks. *Med Lett* 1989;31:45.

215. Taplin D, Meinking TL. Pyrethrin and pyrethrin and pyrethoids in dermatology. *Arch Dermatol* 1990;126:213–221.

216. Dorman DC, Beasley VR. Neurotoxicity of pyrethrin and pyrethoid insecticides. *Vet Hum Toxicol* 1991;33:238–243.

217. Wax PM, Hoffman RS. Fatality associated with inhalation of pyrethrin shampoo. *J Toxicol Clin Toxicol* 1994;32:457–460.

218. He F, Wang S, Lui L, et al. Clinical manifestations and diagnosis of acute pyrethoid poisoning. *Arch Toxicol* 1989;63:54–58.

219. Culver CA, Malina JJ, Talbert RL. Probable anaphylactoid reaction to pyrethrin pediculicide shampoo. *Clin Pharmacol* 1988;7:846–849.

220. Anonymous. Permethrin 1% for head lice. *Med Lett* 1989;31:45.

221. Schultz MW, et al. Comparative study of 5% permethrin cream and 1% lindane lotion for the treatment of scabies. *Arch Dermatol* 1990;126:167–170.
222. Davies JE, et al. Lindane poisonings. *Arch Dermatol* 1983;119:142–144.
223. Kurt TL, Bost R, Gilliland M, et al. Accidental lindane (Kwell) ingestions. *Vet Hum Toxicol* 1986;28:569–571.
224. Jaeger U, Podczeck A, Haubenstock A, et al. Acute oral poisoning with lindane solvent mixtures. *Vet Hum Toxicol* 1984;26:11–14.
225. Rauch AF, Kowalsky SF, Lesar TS, et al. Lindane (Kwell)–induced aplastic anemia. *Arch Intern Med* 1990;150: 2393–2395.
226. Rugman FP, Cosstick R. Aplastic anemia with organochlorine pesticide. Case reports and review of evidence. *J Clin Pathol* 1990;43:98–103.
227. Ginsburg CM, Lowry W, Reisch JS. Absorption of lindane (gamma benzene hexachloride) in infants and children. *J Pediatr* 1977;91:998–1000.
228. Telch J, Jarvis DA. Acute intoxication with lindane (gamma benzene hexachloride). *CMAJ* 1982;126;662–663.
229. Lee B, Groth P. Scabies: transcutaneous poisoning during treatment. *Pediatrics* 1977;59:643.
230. Tilson HA, Hong JS, Mactutus CF. Effects of 5,5-diphenylhydantoin (phenytoin) on neurobehavioral toxicity of organochlorine insecticides and permethrin. *J Pharmacol Exp Ther* 1985;233:285–289.
231. Koyama K, et al. Test for differentiating mothballs. *Vet Hum Toxicol* 1991;33:425–427.
232. Woolf AD, Saperstein A, Zawin J, et al. Radiopaqucity of household air refresheners and moth repellents. *Clin Toxicol* 1993;31:415–428.
233. Varano C. Hazards of camphorated oil. *Pharm Int* 1980;1:5.
234. Committee on Drugs, AAP. Camphor revisited: focus on toxicity. *Pediatrics* 1994;94:127–128.
235. Committee on Drugs, AAP. Camphor. Who needs it? *Pediatrics* 1978;62:404–406.
236. Hall HH. Camphor liniment poisoning. *JAMA* 1925;84:1571.
237. Geller RJ, Spyker DA, Garretson LK, et al. Camphor toxicity: development of a triage strategy. *Vet Hum Toxicol* 1984;26:8–10.
238. Phelan WJ III. Camphor poisoning: the over-the-counter dangers. *Pediatrics* 1976;57:428–430.
239. Siegel E, Wason S. Camphor toxicity. *Pediatr Clin North Am* 1986;33:375–379.
240. Dean BS, Burdick JD, Goetz PD. In vivo evaluation of the adsorptive capacity of activated charcoal for camphor. *Vet Hum Toxicol* 1992;34:297–299.
241. Kresel JJ. Camphor. *Clin Toxicol Rev* 1982;4:1–2.
242. Enez JF, Brown AL, Arnold WC, et al. Chronic camphor poisoning mimicking Reyes' syndrome. *Gastroenterology* 1983;84:394–398.
243. Gibson DE, Moore CP, Pfaff JA. Camphor Ingestion. *Am J Emerg Med* 1989;7:41–43.
244. Aronow R. Camphor poisoning [Editorial]. *JAMA* 1976;235:1200.
245. Koppel C, Martens F, Schirop T, et al. Hemoperfusion in acute camphor poisoning. *Intensive Care Med* 1988:14: 431–433.
246. Wascie-Taylor BH, Widdop B, Davidson AM. Camphor intoxication treated by charcoal hemoperfusion. *Postgrad Med J* 1981;57:725–726.
247. Winter ML, Rice BS, Snodgrass WR. Seizures and serum camphor concentrations in man. *Vet Hum Toxicol* 1991; 33:375.
248. Shannon K, et al. Severe hemolytic anemia in black children with glucose-6-phosphate dehydrogenase deficiency. *Pediatrics* 1982;70:364.
249. Metzer-Lange M, et al. Naphthalene-induced hemolysis in a black female toddler deficient in glucose-6-phosphate deficiency. *Pediatr Emerg Care* 1989;5:24–26.
250. Todisco V, Lamour J, Finberg L. Hemolysis from exposure to naphthalene mothballs. *N Engl J Med* 1991;325: 1660–1661.
251. Kucharski E, Gorman R, Klein-Schwartz W. A prospective evaluation of naphthalene moth ball repellent toxicity. *Vet Human Toxicol* 1991;33:425–427.
252. Beutler E. Glucose-6-phosphate dehydrogenase deficiency. *N Engl J Med* 1991;324:169–173.
253. Valcs T, Doxidis SA, Pessas T. Acute hemolysis due to naphthalene inhalation. *J Pediatr* 1963;63:904–915.
254. Heintz B, Bock TA, Rierdorf H, et al. Hemolytic crisis after acetaminophen in glucose-6-phosphate dehydrogenase deficiency. *Klin Wochenschr* 1989;67:1068.
255. Meloni T, Forteleoni G, Ogana A, et al. Aspirin-induced acute hemolytic anemia in glucose-6-phosphate dehydrogenase deficiency children with systemic arthritis. *Acta Haematol* 1989;81:208–209.
256. Halowell M. Acute hemolytic anemia following ingestion of paradichlorobenzene. *Arch Dis Child* 1959;34:74.
257. Siedlicki JT. Amateur artists: heed health hazards. *JAMA* 1968;204:86.
258. McCann MF. *Artists beware New York*. New York: Lyons and Burford Publishers, 1982.
259. Regulations [16 CAR 1500,14(b)(8),11500.135] *Fed Reg* 1992;46626-45674. Public Law 100-695. 100th Congress to amend the Federal Hazardous Substance Act to require labeling of chronically hazardous art materials and for other purposes. Nov 18, 1988.

260. Federal Hazardous Substance Act Regulation (16 C. 1500). *Fed Reg* 1973;38:20712–27038.
261. Lesser SH, Weiss SJ. Art hazards. *Am J Emerg Med* 1995;13:451.
262. Consumer Product Safety Commission Part II (16 CFR Part 1500). *Fed Reg* 1992;57:46527–46671.
263. Arena JM, Drew RH. *Poisoning: toxicology symptoms and treatments*. Springfield, IL: Charles C. Thomas Publisher, 1989.
264. Lead ingestion and ceramic glazes. *MMWR* 1992;41:1.
265. Sartrelli E, Lori F, Gori R. Lead silicate toxicity: a comparison among different compounds. *Anvil Res* 1985;35: 420–425.
266. Rutter HA, Copeland C. *Biological availability of cadmium from cadmium pigments: final report*. Hazelton Laboratories America, 1977.
267. News from CPSC. Release 94–021. Jan. 3, 1994.
268. Bock GW. Skin exposure to cyanoacrylate adhesive. *Ann Emerg Med* 1984;34:846.
269. Osterhout DE, Gludieux GV, Wade CWR, et al. Digestive tract absorption of alkyl alpha cyanoacrylate beta 14. *Oral Surg* 1969:27:410.
270. DeRespinis PA, et al. Instant glue mistaken for eyedrops. *JAMA* 1990;263:2301.
271. Striet S, et al. Cyanoacrylate. *Ann Ophthalmol* 1981;13:315.
272. Grum EE, Besnitz EA. Case studies in environmental medicine. 10 cadmium toxicity. U.S. Dept. HHS PHS ATSDR, June 1990.
273. Lucas PA, et al. Fatal cadmium fume inhalation. *Lancet* 1980;2:205.
274. Emerson BY. "Ouch, ouch" disease: the osteomalacia of cadmium nephropathy. *Ann Intern Med* 1970;73:854.
275. Kosett M. *Case studies in environmental medicine: arsenic toxicity*. USDHH, Public Health Service. Agency for Toxic Substances and Disease Registry, June 1990.
276. Paulson GW. Polyneuropathy due to *n*-hexane. *Arch Intern Med* 1976;136:880.
277. Anonymous. Toxic occupational neuropathy. *MMWR* 1980;29:529.
278. Garroit J, Petty CS. Death from inhalation abuse: toxicologic and pathologic evaluation of 34 cases. *Clin Toxicol* 1980;16:305–315.
279. Ng R, Darwish H, Stewart DA. Emergency treatment of petroleum distillate and turpentine ingestion. *Can Med Assoc J* 1974;111:537–538.
280. McGuigan MA. Turpentine. *Clin Toxicol Rev* 1985;8:1–2.
281. Wedin GP. The risk of pneumonitis following turpentine ingestion. *Clin Toxicol* 1984;22:485–492.
282. Klein FA, Hacker RH. Hemorrhagic cystitis associated with turpentine ingestion. *Urology* 1980;16:1980.
283. Wahlberg P, Nyman D. Turpentine and thrombocytopenia [Letter]. *Lancet* 1969;2:215.
284. Wise MG. Trichloroethane (TCE) and central sleep apnea: a case study. *J Toxicol Environ Health* 1983;11:101.
285. Bass. Sudden sniffing death. *JAMA* 1970;212:2075.
286. Patel R. Renal damage associated with toluene inhalation. *Clin Toxicol* 1986;24:213–223.
287. Taber SM. Renal tubular acidosis associated with toluene "sniffing." *N Engl J Med* 1974;290:765–768.
288. Sturman K, Mofenson HC, Caraccio TR, et al. Methylene chloride inhalation. An unusual form of drug abuse. *Ann Emerg Med* 1985;14:903.
289. Clark DG, Tinston DJ. Acute inhalation toxicity of some halogenated and nonhalogenated hydrocarbons. *Hum Toxicol* 1982;1:239.
290. Hall FB, Hine CH. Trichloroethane intoxication: report of two cases. *J Forensic Sci* 1966;11:404.
291. Stewart RD. Acute tetrachloroethylene intoxication. *JAMA* 1969;208:1471.
292. Rosenburg N. Nervous system effects of toluene and other organic solvents. *West J Med* 1989;150:571–575.
293. Filey CM, Heston RK, Rosenberg NL. White matter dementia in chronic toluene abuse. *Neurology* 1990;40:532–534.
294. Wood BR, Colombo JL, Benson BE. Chlorine inhalation toxicity from vapors generated by swimming pool chlorinator tablet. *Pediatrics* 187;79:429–430.
295. Howland MA. Poolside toxic hazards. *Emerg Med* 1986;89–93.
296. *Clearinghouse for Poison Control Centers Bulletin: swimming pool and aquarium hazards*. U.S. Department of Health Education and Welfare National, Food and Drug Administration, Bureau of Drugs. January–February 1976.
297. Arena JM, Drew RH. *Poisoning: toxicology symptoms and treatments*. Springfield, IL: Charles C. Thomas Publisher, 1989.
298. Siedlechi JT. Toxicology of matches. *JAMA* 1966;197:200.
299. Steffen C, Seitz R. Severe chlorate poisoning. Report of a case. *Arch Toxicol* 1981:48:282.
300. Arena JM, Drew RH. *Poisoning: toxicology symptoms and treatments*. Springfield, IL: Charles C. Thomas Publisher, 1989.
301. Anom. *Fourth of July poisoning hazard*. National Clearinghouse for Poison Control Centers, U.S. Department of Health Education and Welfare, Public Heath Service. June 1959.
302. Committee on Environmental Hazards, AAP. Effects of cigarette smoking on the fetus and child. *Pediatrics* 1969;44:757–759.
303. Committee on Environmental Hazards, AAP. Smokeless tobacco—a carcinogen hazard to children. *Pediatrics* 1985;76:1009–1011.

304. Chilmonczyk BA, Salmun AM, Megathlin RN, et al. Association between exposure to environmental tobacco smoke and exacerbations of asthma in children. *N Engl J Med* 1993;328:1663–1669.
305. Smoking attributable mortality and years of potential life lost—United States 1988. *MMWR* 1991;40:62–63,69–71.
306. Klonoff-Cohen HS, et al. The role of passive smoking in sudden infant death syndrome. *JAMA* 1995;273:795–798.
307. Bergman AB, Wieser BA. Relationship of passive smoking to sudden infant death syndrome. *Pediatrics* 1976;58:665–668.
308. Greenberg RA, et al. Ecology of passive smoking by young infants. *J Pediatr* 1989;114:774–780.
309. Pattishall EM, Strope GL, Etzel RA, et al. Serum cotinine as a measure of tobacco smoke exposure in children. *Am J Dis Child* 1985;139:1101–1104.
310. Committee on Environmental Health, AAP. Tobacco-free environment: an imperative for the health of children and adolescents. *Pediatrics* 1994;93:866–868.
311. Etzel RA, Pattishall EN, Haley NJ, et al. Passive smoking and middle ear effusion among children in day care. *Pediatrics* 1992;90:228–232.
312. Murray AB, Morrison BJ. The decrease in severity of asthma in children of parents who smoke since the parents have been exposing them to less cigarette smoke. *J Allergy Clin Immunol* 1993;91:102–110.
313. Martinez FD, Cline M, Burrows B. Increased incidence of asthma in children of smoking mothers. *Pediatrics* 1992;89:21–26.
314. Blanehead J. Nicotine. *Clin Toxicol Rev* Part I—1993;11:1. Part II—1993;12:15.
315. Salmon M. Nicotine. In: Goldfrank LR, et al., eds. *Toxicologic emergencies.* 5th ed. Norwalk, CT: Appleton & Lange, 1994:997–1008.
316. Mensch AR, Holden M. Nicotine overdose after a single piece of nicotine gum. *Chest* 1984;86:801–802.
317. McNabb ME, Ebert RV, McCuster K. Plasma nicotine levels produced by chewing nicotine gum. *JAMA* 1982;248:865–868.
318. Smolinske SC, Spoeke DDG, Spiller SK, et al. Cigarette and nicotine chewing gum toxicity in children. *Hum Toxicol* 1988;7:27–31S.
319. Ebert RV, McKendree E, McNabb MD, et al. Effect of nicotine gum on plasma nicotine levels of cigarette smokers. *Clin Pharmacol Ther* 1984;35:495–498.
320. Benowitz NL, Savanapridi JP III. Determinants of nicotine intake while chewing nicotine polacrilex gum. *Clin Pharmacol Ther* 1987;41:467–473.
321. Anom. Nicotine patches. ;itMed Lett *1991;34:37–38.*
322. Benowitz NL, Jacob P, Olsson P, et al. Intravenous nicotine retards transdermal absorption of nicotine: evidence of blood flow-limited percutaneous absorption. *Clin Pharmacol Ther* 1992;52:223–230.
323. Jacob P, Benowitz NL, Shulgin AT. Recent studies of nicotine metabolism in humans. *Pharmacol Biochem Behav* 1988;30:249.
324. Transdermal nicotine study group. Transdermal nicotine for smoking cessation. *JAMA* 1991;266:3133–3138.
325. Mulligan SC, Masterson JG, Devane JG, et al. Clinical and pharmacokinetic properties of a transdermal nicotine patch. *Clin Pharm Ther* 1990;47:332–337.
326. Miller NS, Cocores JA. Nicotine dependence: Diagnosis, chemistry, pharmacologic treatments. *Pediatr Rev* 1993;14:275–279.
327. Goodman AG, Rall TW, Niels AS, et al. *Goodman and Gilman's. The pharmacologic basis of clinical therapeutics.* 8th ed. New York: Pergamon Press, 1990:545–549.
328. Luck W, Nau H. Nicotine and cotinine concentrations in serum and urine of infants exposed to passive smoking or milk from smoking mothers. *J Pediatr* 1985;107:816–820.
329. Sisselman SG, Mofenson HC, Caraccio TR. Childhood Poisoning from ingestion of cigarettes. *Lancet* 1996;347:200–201.
330. Singer J, Janz T. Apnea and seizures caused by nicotine ingestion. *Pediatr Emerg Care* 1990;6:135.
331. Litovitz TL, Felberg L, Soloway R, et al. 1993 annual report of American Association of Poison Control Centers Exposure Surveillance System. *Am J Emerg Med* 1994;12:546–584.
332. Smolinske SC, Spoeke DDG, Spiller SK, et al. Pediatric nicotine overdose. *Vet Hum Toxicol* 1985;28:308.
333. Nakamura NH, Mituzani T, Yamashita M. 1000 cases of tobacco ingestions in children. Presented at the meeting of the AAPCC/AACT/ABMT/CAAPC, Boston, August 6–17, 1983.
334. Malizia G, Andreucci G, Alfani F, et al. Acute intoxication with nicotine alkaloids and cannabinoids from in children from ingestion of cigarettes. *Hum Toxicol* 1983;2:315–316.
335. Petridou E, Polychronopoulou A, Kouri N, et al. Childhood poisoning from ingestion of cigarettes. *Lancet* 1995;346:1296.
336. Bonadio WA, Anderson Y. Tobacco ingestions in children [Letter]. *Clin Pediatr* 1989;28:592–593.
337. McGee D, Picciotti M, Spevack T. Two-year review of tobacco ingestions [Abstract]. *Vet Hum Toxicol* 1991;33:370.
338. McGee D, Brabson T, McCarthy J. Four-year review of cigarette ingestions in children. *Pediatr Emerg Care* 1995;11:13–16.
339. Borys DJ, Tetzer SC. CNS depression in an infant after ingestions of tobacco. *Vet Hum Toxicol* 1988;30:20–22.

340. Jarvus MJ, Tunstall-Peedoe H, Feyerabend C, et al. Comparison of tests used to distinguish smokers from nonsmokers. *Am J Public Health* 1987;77:1435–1438.
341. McKusher K, McNabb E, Bone R. Plasma nicotine levels in pipe smokers. *JAMA* 1982;248:577–578.
342. Klein-Schwatz W, Gorman RL, Odera GM, et al. Three fatal sodium azide poisonings. *Med Toxicol* 1989;4:219–227.
343. Richardson SC, Giles C, Swan CH. Two cases of sodium azide poisoning by accidental ingestion of Isoton. *Clin Pathol* 1975;28:350.
344. Albertson TE, Reed S, Siefkin A. A case of fatal sodium azide ingestion. *J Toxicol Clin Toxicol* 1986;24:339–351.
345. Howard JD, Skogerboe KJ, Case GA, et al. Death following accidental sodium azide ingestion. *J Forensic Sci* 1990;35:193–196.
346. Abrams J, El-Mallalh RS, Meyer R. Suicidal sodium azide ingestion. *Ann Emerg Med* 1987;16:1378–1380.
347. Emmett EA, Ricking JA. Fatal self-administration of sodium azide. *Ann Intern Med* 1975;83:224.
348. Edmonds EA, Bourne MS. Sodium aside poisoning of 5 laboratory technicians. *Br J Indust Med* 1982;39:308–307.
349. Judge KW, Wart NE. Fatal azide-induced cardiomyopathy presenting as acute myocardial infarction. *Am J Cardiol* 1989;64:830–831.
350. Conover R. Chemical burn from automotive air bag [Letter]. *Ann Emerg Med* 1992;21:770.
351. Ingraham HJ, Perry HD, Donnenfeld ED. "Airbag keratitis." *N Engl J Med* 1991;324:1599–1600.
352. Lawson RS. Sodium azide. *Clin Toxicol Rev* 1993;15.
353. Koppel C, Baudish H, Beyer KH. Fatal poisoning with selenious dioxide. *J Toxicol Clin Toxicol* 1986;24:35.
354. Nantel AJ, Brown M, Dery P, et al. Acute poisoning by selenious acid. *Vet Hum Toxicol* 1985;27:531–533.
355. Pentel P, Fletcher D, Jensen J. Fatal acute selenium toxicity. *J Forsenic Sci* 1985;30:556–562.
356. Harris JC, et al. Toxicology of urea formaldehyde and polyurethane foam insulation. *JAMA* 1981;245:243.
357. Richie IM, et al. Formaldehyde-related health complaints of residents living in mobile and conventional homes. *Am J Public Health* 1987;77:323–328.
358. Warfew GA. The health hazards of formaldehyde. *J Appl Toxicol* 1983;3:121–126.
359. Frigas E, et al. Bronchial challenge with formaldehyde gas: Lack of bronchoconstriction in 13 patients suspected of having formaldehyde-induced asthma. *Mayo Clin Proc* 1984;59:295–299.
360. Kochhar R, et al. Formaldehyde-induced corrosive gastric cicatrization. Case report. *Hum Toxicol* 1986;5:381.
361. Council on Scientific Affairs. Formaldehyde. *JAMA* 1989;2261:1183–1187.
362. Halperin WE, et al. Nasal cancer in a worker exposed to formaldehyde. *JAMA* 1983;249:510–512.
363. Albert RE, et al. Nasal cancer in rat induced by gaseous formaldehyde and hydrogen chloride. *J Natl Cancer Inst* 1982;68:597–503; and 1987;77:323.
364. Council on Scientific Affairs, AMA. Radon in the home. *JAMA* 1987:258:668–672.
365. International Agency for Research on Cancer (IARC). *Monograph on evaluation of carcinogenic risks to humans. Vol. 43. Man-made mineral fibers and radon.* Lyon: IARC, 1988.
366. Upfai M, et al. *Radon toxicity. ATSDR case studies in Environmental Medicine.* USDHHS, USPHS, ATSDR, September 1992.
367. Committee on Environmental Hazards, AAP. Radon exposure: a hazard to children. *Pediatrics* 1989;83:799–802.
368. Samet JM, Nero. Sounding board: indoor radon and lung cancer. *N Engl J Med* 1989;320:591–594.
369. Sun M. Radon's health risks. *Science* 1988;239:250.
370. Radford EP, Renard KG. Lung cancer in Swedish iron miners exposed to low doses of radon daughters. *N Engl J Med* 1984;310:1385.
371. Ames BN, Magraw R, Gold LS. Ranking possible carcinogenic hazards. *Science* 19987;236:271–280.
372. Council on Scientific Affairs. A physicians' guide to asbestos-related disease. *JAMA* 1984;252:2593–2597.
373. Brody AR, Mossman BY, et al. Controversy over asbestos significance. *Science* 1990;248:797–802.
374. Spooner CM. Asbestos in schools: a public health problem. *N Engl J Med* 1979;301:782–783.
375. Craighead JE, Mossman BY. The pathogenesis of asbestos associated disease. *N Engl J Med* 1982;306:1446.
376. Committee on Environmental Hazards, AAP. Asbestos exposure in the schools. *Pediatrics* 1987;79:301.
377. Mossman BY, Gee JB. Asbestos-related diseases. *N Engl J Med* 1989;320:1721–1730.
378. Council on Scientific Affairs, AMA. Asbestos removal, health hazards, and the EPA. *JAMA* 1991;266:696–697.
379. Rogers G, ed., for the Committee on Injury and Poison Prevention, AAP. *Handbook of common poisonings in children.* Elk Grove, IL: AAP, 1994.
380. Olsen KR, ed. *Poisoning and drug overdose.* 2nd ed. Norwalk, CT: Appleton & Lange, 1994.
381. Goldman RH, Peters JM. The occupational and environmental history. *JAMA* 1981;246:2831.
382. *Facts and Comparisons,* Nicotine Transdermal Nicotine Patch Monograph April 1992.
383. Lawson KS. Nicotine Toxicity. *Clin Toxicol Rev* 1993;15:4.

Emergency Toxicology, Second Edition,
edited by Peter Viccellio.
Published by Lippincott–Raven Publishers, Philadelphia.

29

Industrial Exposure to Toxins

†Clark S. Homan and °James V. Writer

†*Department of Emergency Medicine, State University of New York at Stony Brook,
Stony Brook, New York 11794-7400;* °*Walter Reed Army Institute of Research,
Washington, D.C. 20307-5100*

For many people, the workplace is the site of greatest potential exposure to toxic agents. The recognition of occupation as a threat to health can be traced back to the ancient Greeks, who reported occupational lead poisoning. New chemicals are approved for use in the work environment before the complete impact upon industrial toxicology is completely recognized (1). Today, workers are exposed to more than 50,000 chemicals, with hundreds of new ones added to the inventory each year. Most have not been evaluated for human health effects, and no standards exist suggesting safe or permissible levels of exposure for most chemicals. Private and government agencies try to evaluate toxins and to recommend standards for exposures or worker protection. The number of chemicals and the paucity of human epidemiologic and animal experiment data hamper these efforts. The American Conference of Governmental Industrial Hygienists, in their *Threshold Limit Values and Biological Exposure for 1993–94,* listed just over 600 chemicals and their recommended allowable exposures. In 1994, excluding illness due to physical agents and repeated trauma, there were 160,900 reported workplace illnesses (U.S. Bureau of Labor Statistics, *personal communication, 1996*). Skin disorders and diseases, many of which are the result of the local or systemic effects of toxins, accounted for 40.8% of the total. Dust diseases of the lung and other respiratory conditions due to toxic agents were responsible for 17.4% of the total number of these reported occupational diseases and illnesses. Another 4.5% were attributed to a poisoning without further elaboration. The American Association of Poison Control Centers Toxic Exposure Surveillance System reports that occupational exposures are more subacute or chronic, demonstrated greater morbidity and mortality and was associated with an increased use of health care resources when compared to other poisonings (2). Despite laws requiring employers to maintain records of occupational injuries and illness, these numbers are likely to be an underestimate of occupational poisoning. One study of compliance with Occupational Safety and Health Administration (OSHA) record-keeping requirements showed that only 75% of the companies surveyed kept records (3). Furthermore, many chronic illnesses and cancers that are due to workplace exposures may not be associated with specific industrial processes or toxins. This chapter provides the reader with an overview of occupational exposure to toxins and directs the reader to appropriate sources of information. Other chapters in this book discuss in detail the toxicology of the most common occupational exposures, including heavy metals, pesticides, toxic gases, irritants, and solvents. The reader should keep in mind that workers in many industries, professions, and work environments, including high technology and white collar workers, are at

---

The views of the authors do not purport to reflect the position of the Department of the Army or the Department of Defense.

risk of illness or disability due to workplace exposures. The "clean rooms" of "silicon valley" are among the most hazardous places in modern industry because of exposure to solvents and fixing solutions. Occupational disease is not limited to workers in heavy industry. Specific questions about the patient's occupation, workplace, and job duties with potential exposure to hazardous materials should be included in all histories.

I. **Occupational history.** The work- and job-related history may reveal an association between the patient's signs and symptoms and exposure to a toxic agent. The essentials of an occupational history include the present employment and past job experience.

   A. **Present employment history.** Ask the patient to elaborate his or her job characteristics. This information includes data about the workplace, employer, type of job hazards, relation of symptoms to job exposure, and implementation of control measures.

      1. **Employment-related data**

         a. **Name of employment firm and nature of business** often provides insight as to what type of exposure is present in the workplace. General types of industrial hazards may be identified by simply asking for the title or name of the firm or corporation.

         b. **Length of employment** gives the clinician an idea of the total overall exposure the patient may have encountered. Changes in the specific job performed and types of control measures must be taken into account when assessing the patient's total extent of exposure.

         c. **Specific job performed** and overall factory process. The information obtained here is important for determining what job hazards may be directly encountered by the patient, including:

            (1) The specific job process

            (2) General process description of the workplace as a whole

            (3) Processes in nearby areas

            (4) Chemicals with which they worked. For example, a worker in a clothing factory may perform the job of treating clothing material with flame retardants. The chemical exposure of the worker to the flame retardant is obvious, but a more thorough history about the overall process performed at the plant would have revealed that the clothing material was freshly dyed and treated with stain resistors in neighboring rooms. Hence, this patient is directly exposed to not one but three chemical hazards on a continued basis.

         d. **Symptoms in relation to work.** The onset of symptoms while in the workplace helps to establish a cause-and-effect relation between the toxic exposure and the clinical disease process. Specific events such as the following are noted.

            (1) Time of onset of symptoms

            (2) Type of symptoms experienced

            (3) Location in the physical plant at onset of symptoms

            (4) Specific job being performed at onset of symptoms

            (5) Specific chemical names or processes that may represent potential or known hazards present in the immediate and nearby areas of the workplace

(6) If removal of the patient from the workplace area results in an improvement of the patient's symptoms

(7) Coworkers who work nearby in the physical plant with similar signs, symptoms, and previous diagnosis as a result of toxic exposure in the same work environment

e. **Control measures** include protective work gear, monitoring of toxins present in the work environment, periodic medical evaluations, engineering protection, administrative policies, and worker education. The presence of control measures shows that the employer has recognized a potential hazard and has implemented a plan that attempts to minimize the chance of exposure. Existing control measures must be evaluated for their efficacy. Hazards for which effective control measures are not in place must be addressed immediately to ensure effective preventive management of the worker.

B. **Prior employment history.** Present employment history may not reveal any source of occupational hazard. However, prior employment may disclose singular or multiple sources of hazardous exposure and therefore must be actively sought. Many disease processes have a long latency from time of exposure to the time of onset of signs and symptoms, e.g., mesothelioma due to asbestos exposure.

II. **Approach to gathering data on industrial toxins.** One of the most significant changes and advances in data gathering since the last edition of this book is the accessibility of the internet by almost anyone with a computer. There are a number of sources of general information on using the internet in nearly every bookstore. A good review of internet resources of interest to physicians and other health care providers is also available (4).

A. The number of toxic substances to which a worker may be exposed is so voluminous that one cannot be expected to be familiar with every presentation, diagnosis, and management. Attempts must initially be made to **identify the specific toxin** to which the patient has been exposed. The practitioner is referred to Table 29-1 for sources to assist in the identification of the toxin in those cases where the name of the specific agent in not known. Regional poison control centers may be utilized as resources of toxin identification and specific therapy.

B. The **employer** may be contacted with the patient's permission. Employers are mandated by state and federal legislation to assist the physician in the care of patients who have medical problems secondary to work-related causes. A supervisor or safety officer may provide the name of the specific agent and additional history regarding the mechanism of exposure. Employee health departments may provide the results of prior testing performed on the patient.

C. **Material safety data sheet** (MSDS) can supply the physician with important information on routes of exposure, toxicity, composition of mixtures, emergency treatment, and further sources of information. Under the OSHA Hazard Communication Act, manufacturers must prepare MSDSs for their products, and users must have MSDSs on file for all products used. The MSDS is particularly helpful when evaluating patients exposed to products with brand or trade names because the MSDS describes the composition of the product. When a recipe is incomplete because of trade secret protection, the manufacturer can be contacted directly for more complete information.

TABLE 29-1. *Resources for identification of toxic materials*

Clayton, G. D., and Clayton, F. E. *Patty's Industrial Hygiene and Toxicology* (3rd ed.). New York: Wiley, 1985.

National Institute for Occupational Safety and Health. *NIOSH Pocket Guide to Chemical Hazards.* Washington, DC: NIOSH, 1985.

Plunket, E. R. *Occupational Diseases: A Syllabus of Signs and Symptoms.* Stamford, CT: Bartlett Book Co., 1977.

Rumack, B. H. *Poisindex Information System.* Denver: Micromedex, 1990.

Proctor, N. H., Hughes, J. P., and Fischman, M. L. *Chemical Hazards of the Workplace,* 2nd ed. Philadelphia: Lippincott, 1988.

Sax, N. I., and Lewis, R. J. *Hazardous Chemicals Desk Reference.* New York: Van Nostrand Reinhold, 1987.

Sax, N. I., and Lewis, R. J. *Dangerous Properties of Industrial Materials,* 7th ed. New York: Van Nostrand Reinhold, 1989.

MEDLINE
MEDLARS   Call National Library of Medicine (301) 496-4000 for
TOXLINE   information on these on-line databases.

CHEMTREC (for transportation emergencies, i.e., rail car derailments, call [800] 424-9300).

American Chemical Society
1155 16th Street, NW
Washington, DC 20036

American Industrial Hygiene Association
475 Wolf Ledges Parkway
Akron, OH 44311

American Conference of Governmental Industrial Hygienists
6500 Glenway Ave, Bldg D-5
Cincinnati, OH 45211

Local U.S. and state EPA and OSHA offices

Local poison control centers

D. If more information than is provided on the MSDS or by the manufacturer is needed, the physician can obtain it from various internet sites or from one of the **on-line database services** of the National Library of Medicine (Table 29-1).

E. Another important resource for industrial toxin identification and management is the **Chemical Transportation Emergency Center** (CHEMTREC). This organization is sponsored by the Chemical Manufacturers Association. Practitioners may obtain data on chemical toxins in the workplace by calling the toll free number (800) 424-9300.

F. **Unions** are another source of information that should not be overlooked. Committees on health and safety or shop stewards may give information as the MSDS and track history of the manufacturer. The American Federation of Labor and Congress of Industrial Organizations (AFL-CIO) located in Washington, D.C., can give information on which of the member chapters may be most helpful for the particular case at hand.

III. **Routes of exposure.** Inhalation and skin contact are the two most common routes of exposure in the workplace. Ingestion, intentional or accidental, is an important but less common route of exposure.

A. **Inhalation** is often considered the most significant route of entry. Almost anything that is airborne can be inhaled. Inhaled toxins gain direct entry to the circulation and can quickly produce systemic toxicity. If the substance is a primary irritant or asphyxiant, it may present an immediate threat. The initial respiratory or systemic reaction may range from asymptomatic (i.e., cancer induction) to rapidly fatal. All unprotected workers in a contaminated environment are at risk.

B. The **skin** is the largest organ in the body and forms the most important protective barrier. It is especially prone to local irritation and sensitizing reactions. Some substances, such as organic solvents, are absorbed through the skin in significant quantities, resulting in systemic toxicity. It is important to remember that abraded skin allows certain substances to enter the systemic circulation that would not be able to penetrate normal skin.

C. **Ingestion** is not a significant route of entry for industrial toxins. Occupational ingestions are usually accidental and may be associated with smoking, eating, or drinking in a contaminated workplace. Workers who violate good industrial hygiene and eat, drink, or smoke around hazardous chemicals are at risk of increasing their body burden of some toxins, especially heavy metals, such as lead and mercury.

IV. Range of disease

A. Pulmonary disease. Occupational lung diseases result from the inhalation of irritants or toxins in the work area. The particular disorder may be caused entirely by the exposure (e.g., pneumoconiosis) or may precipitate clinical episodes of preexisting diseases (e.g., asthma). Occupational lung disease is common. Prompt and accurate recognition is important to ensure therapeutic discontinuance of exposure. Prevention of the disease among other exposed workers may be facilitated by appropriate recognition.

1. Pneumoconiosis is the condition that results from prolonged inhalation exposure to dusts, usually over months or years. Silicosis, coal worker's pneumoconiosis, and asbestosis are the most common forms. Pneumoconiosis may be caused by numerous other substances such as kaolin, talc, fibrous glass, and metal dusts from antimony, barium, and tin. Autopsies have shown large deposits of these dusts present in the lung parenchyma years after cessation of exposure.

a. Silicosis lung disease is the most common form of pneumoconiosis. Mine workers and sandblasters are at highest risk. Silica deposition in the lung parenchyma results in a local inflammatory reaction characterized by leukocyte infiltration and subsequent granuloma formation. Silicotic nodules ranging from 1 mm to 1 cm in diameter may initially appear in the upper lobes, seen on chest roentgenogram, but become distributed over the entire lung fields over time. Pulmonary function ranges from mild decreases in expiratory flow rates and volumes to severe obstructive and restrictive spirometric patterns.

b. Coal worker's pneumoconiosis is secondary to inhalation of coal dust composed primarily of carbon. Macules are histologic aggregations of macrophages and coal dust that usually measure 1 to 2 mm in diameter; they may be detectable during the earlier forms of the disease on chest films. Mild forms of the disease present with cough and sputum production and may progress to frank emphysema with the characteristic obstructive spirometric flow patterns.

c. Asbestosis is an interstitial lung disease that results from the inhalation of asbestos fibers. Asbestos is a known human carcinogen. Latency ranges between 5 and 40 years depending on the concentration of exposure. OSHA has established permissible occupational exposure as less than 0.2 fibers/cc of air averaged over an 8-h work day. Asbestos bodies present in the pulmonary tissue are the only histologic finding specific to this disease. Interstitial fibrosis is the predominating but nonspecific characteristic. The chest film is not as helpful diagnostically. Early disease shows linear-shaped densities at the bases, and progression results in gradual increase in size and number of these densities. Early clinical disease is characterized by a decrease in the diffusing capacity for carbon monoxide and a reduced forced vital capacity. Progression leads to a restrictive pattern on lung spirometry.

d. Control over the work environment is essential for the **prevention** of all forms of pneumoconiosis. Dust sources must be enclosed. Exhaust and dust collection systems should be provided. If engineering or administration controls are not feasible, personal protective equipment should be provided. The effectiveness of these measures must be tested by continual measurement of the airborne agent. Persons with prior pulmonary disorders must be screened and not permitted to partake in high risk employment. Annual medical examinations should include chest roentgenograms and spirometric testing for early detection of occupational lung disease.

2. Other types of pulmonary pathology secondary to industrial toxins include **irritant lung reactions** due to inhaled agents that produce local toxic effects. Examples of these agents are chlorine, ammonia, hydrogen chloride, and hydrogen fluoride. Irritation of the eyes, nasopharynx, and upper airways is usually mild so long as the patient is removed from the source. Sawmill and wood dust exposures are associated with allergic alveolitis (5). More severe and chronic forms of lung disease develop if exposure is repeated and prolonged.

3. **Lung cancer** has long been recognized as an industrial occupational hazard. Recent reports in the literature indicate that the incidence is higher than in previous observations (6,7). Occupational lung cancer has been observed in women as well as men (8).

4. **Occupational asthma** is defined as airway narrowing caused by exposure to airborne substances in the working environment. The diagnosis must be made by confirming variations in lung spirometry. Occupational asthma has been recognized in many industries including welders (9,10), potato processing (11), and timber/woodworking (12). A common factor among occupational asthma is exposure to airborne particulate matter which is subsequently inhaled by the worker. A causal relation either by history or skin testing must then be established between these variations of lung function and exposure to the workplace. Transfer of the employee to an area without exposure is necessary once this diagnosis is made.

B. **Carcinogens**

1. Since World War II, the occupational exposure to chemical carcinogens has been increasingly recognized as an important cause of cancer. Four percent to 5% of all cancers are believed to be secondary to an occupational etiology (13,14).

2. Chromates have been linked to gastrointestinal cancer (15,16) as well as lung cancer (17). Estimates of occupationally induced lung cancer range from 3% to 17%

(18). The semiconductor industry employs agents that include arsenic, gallium and inium which have been shown to cause cancer in animals and have been strongly implicated in human carcinogenesis (19). The recognition of exposure to agents such as vinyl chloride (causing hepatic hemangiosarcoma) and asbestos (causing pleural and peritoneal mesothelioma) has helped focus public attention on the field of occupational cancer research and prevention.

3. At present, hundreds of chemicals have been shown to cause cancer in animals. The International Agency for Research on Cancer (IARC) has identified 25 agents and industrial processes which are carcinogenic to humans (20). There is an increasing employer and public realization that exposed workers are at an increased risk of cancer. However, personal habits such as smoking and diet contribute more to the personal risk than occupational exposure.

4. Chemicals known to produce cancer in humans are listed in Table 29-2. Chemicals that are not proved to cause cancer but carry a reasonable suspicion that they do are listed in Table 29-3.

C. **Reproductive disorders** secondary to occupational exposure (Table 29-4) fall generally within the two categories of disorders of fertility and teratogenic pre- and postnatal maldevelopment. These disorders affect both males and females of reproductive age. Such patients present to the physician with great fear and concern, often due to extensive media coverage about a specific agent or because they have had contact with a friend or relative who has experienced adverse effects from an exposure. An appropriate response by the physician must be based on factual information from the literature. The actual and possible exposure as well as specific safety systems present in the workplace in question must also be evaluated to provide appropriate patient counseling.

D. **Skin disorders** account for almost half of all reported occupational disorders.

1. **Contact dermatitis** accounts for at least 90% of all occupational skin diseases. Other forms of occupational skin diseases include urticaria, acne, eczematous dermatitis, granulomas, ulcerations, skin tumors, and pigment changes. Irritant reactions due to repeated contact with such chemicals as petroleum distillates are usually mild. Usually local irrigation, removal from exposure, and prevention of additional exposures is all that is required.

TABLE 29-2. *Substances and technologic or manufacturing processes known to be carcinogenic*

4-Aminobiphenyl	Coke oven emissions
Arsenic and certain arsenic compounds	Cyclophosphamide
Asbestos	Diethylstilbestrol (DES)
Auramine manufacture	Hematite underground mining
Benzene	Isopropyl alcohol manufacture (strong-acid process)
Benzidine	Melphalan
N, N-Bis(2-chloroethyl)-2-naphthylamine (chlornaphazine)	Mustard gas
	2-Naphthylamine
Bis(chloromethyl) ether (BCME) and technical grade chloromethyl methyl ether (CMME)	Nickel refining
	Soots, tars, and mineral oils
Chlorambucil	Thorium dioxide
Chromium and certain chromium compounds	Vinyl chloride

TABLE 29-3. *Substances that may reasonably be anticipated to be carcinogens*

2-Acetylaminofluorene	7*H*-Dibenzo(*c,g*) carbazole
Acrylonitrile	Dibenzo(*a,h*)pyrene
Aflatoxins	Dibenzo(*a,i*)pyrene
Aminoanthraquinone	1,2-Dibromo-3-chloropropane (DBCP)
1-Amino-2-methylanthraquinone	1,2-Dobromoethane (EDB)
Amitrole	3,3′-Dichlorobenzidine
o-Anisidine and *o*-abisidine hydrochloride	1,2-Dichloroethane (EDC)
Aramite	Diepoxybutane
Benzi(a)anthracene	Di(2-ethylhexyl) phthalate
Benzo(b)fluoranthene	4-Dimethylaminoazobenzene
Benzo(a)pyrene	3,3′-Dimethylbenzidine
Beryllium and certain beryllium	Dimethylcarbamoyl chloride
compounds	Dimethyl sulfate
Cadmium and certain cadmium	1,4-Dioxane
compounds	Direct Black 38
Carbon tetrachloride	Direct Blue 6
Chloroform	Ethylene thiourea
p-Cresidine	Formaldehyde
Cupferron	Hexachlorobenzene
Cycasin	Hydrazine and hydrazine sulfate
2,4-Diaminoanisole sulfate	Hydrazobenzene
2,4-Diaminotoluene	Indeno(*1,2,3c-d*)pyrene
Dibenz(a,h)acridine	Iron dextran complex
Dibenz(a,j)acridine	Kepone (chlordecone)
Dibenz(a,h)anthracene	

2. **Direct mechanical injury** may result in nail dystrophy, blisters, calluses, lichenification of skin, and abrasions. Vibration may induce a vasoconstrictive disorder, similar to Raynaud's disease, known as vibration white finger syndrome (VWFS). Abrasions and contusions should be cleaned with a disinfectant after all visible foreign bodies are removed. Proper dressings are then applied to protect the wound from any additional exposure encountered in the workplace.

3. **Hot water scald burns** are usually more superficial than chemical burns unless there is prolonged hot water-to-skin contact. Cool compresses are used to cool down the burn and stop the progression of the thermal injury. Chemical burns, particularly those caused by acids and alkalies, produce deep, penetrating injuries (21). Immediate and copious lavage with water must be implemented for these injuries (22).

TABLE 29-4. *Agents/conditions causing reproductive disorders*

Heavy metals: methyl mercury, phenyl mercuric acetate, inorganic mercury salts, lead, thallium, strontium, selenium, chelating agents (EDTA)
Azo dyes: trypan blue, Evans blue, Niagara sky blue 6B
Fungicides
Herbicides
Insecticides
Physical agents or conditions: radiation, hypo- and hyperthermia, carbon monoxide, carbon dioxide, hypoxia
Infections: rubella and cytomegalovirus, syphilis, gonorrhea

V. **Worker protection**
   A. **Federal level**
       1. The Occupational Safety and Health Act of 1970 created the Occupational Safety and Health Administration (**OSHA**) within the U.S. Department of Labor. This agency was created "to assure as far as possible every working man and woman in the Nation safe and healthful working conditions and to preserve our human resources." Specifically, OSHA is a regulatory agency that promulgates legally enforceable standards, oversees their implementation, and enforces the standards. Employees who believe that a health hazard exists at their workplace should contact the local OSHA area office and request an inspection. The OSHA standards are known as permissible exposure levels, or PELs. The PELs are enforceable standards.

       2. The National Institute of Occupational Safety and Health (**NIOSH**) exists within the U.S. Public Health Service. Its primary function is to conduct research into occupational health issues. Unlike OSHA, NIOSH has no legal authority to enforce its recommendations. Created under the Occupational Safety and Health Act of 1970, the agency is responsible for conducting research and developing and recommending health and safety standards such as limiting exposure to potentially hazardous materials or conditions in the workplace.

          a. NIOSH is mandated to evaluate all known and available medical, biologic, chemical, engineering, trade, and other information relevant to potential hazards. These reviews are used by OSHA and the Mine Safety and Health Administration in promulgating enforceable standards.

          b. NIOSH produces a series of publications that are of interest to the health care professional.

             (1) **Criteria documents** define and support recommended workplace exposure limits and preventive measures.

             (2) **Current intelligence bulletins** are based on evaluations of new data on a particular hazard.

             (3) **Special hazard reviews, occupational hazard assessment,** and **technical guidelines** support and complement NIOSH's other publications and recommended standards.

             (4) **The Registry of toxic effects of chemical substances (RTECS)** is an example of a N.I.O.S.H. document which provides valuable information to health care personnel (23).

       3. **Right-to-know** (R-T-K) is the collective name for federal, state, and local laws designed to increase workers' awareness of hazards in the workplace. The OSHA Hazard Communication Standard Act of 1983 is the oldest of the R-T-K laws. Originally it covered only chemical manufacturers, importers, and distributors, but in May 1985 coverage was extended to all manufacturers. Then in August 1988 the standard was expanded to include all workplaces where hazardous materials may be handled. The Standard Act has three goals.

          a. It helps to force manufacturers and end-users determine the hazardous properties of substances used.

b. It mandates the education of employees and employers in the safe handling of hazardous materials and the recognition of possible adverse health effects.

c. It forces employers to disclose the hazardous properties of materials handled in a facility.

4. In addition to workers, the **community** in which an industry is located may be at risk of exposure through accidental release of hazardous materials. This problem has been addressed in SARA Title III Emergency Response and Community Right-To-Know legislation designed to protect emergency responders and the community. In brief, the legislation requires users to notify local agencies of the hazards that may be encountered during an emergency. It is also hoped that community awareness of hazardous materials will cause communities to encourage businesses to practice good environmental hygiene and thereby reduce the risk of exposure. Under SARA, chemical releases must be reported to the appropriate state, local, and federal agencies.

5. Other legislation of interest is the Toxic Substance Control Act (**TOSCA**), which requires premarket testing of all chemicals. As a result, the physical properties and some toxicologic data are available for all chemicals in use.

6. **Other federal agencies** with a peripheral interest in workplace health and safety are the U.S. Environmental Protection Agency, the Centers for Disease Control, and the Department of Transportation, which regulates the transport of toxic material.

B. **State/local level.** At the state level, worker health and safety may be protected by agencies similar to OSHA. These state OSHAs may promulgate rules, conduct inspections, and enforce state standards. Local, county, or city agencies may investigate workplace health hazards, especially those that may have effect on the general community. As of April 1988 there were 44 states that had R-T-K laws in place. The local or state department of health should be informed of all toxin exposure cases that are work-related.

C. **Nongovernmental agencies.** A wide array of nongovernmental agencies participate in controlling occupational exposure to toxins. Unions, nonprofit organizations, and professional organizations collect data, conduct research, provide education, promote health and safety at work, and suggest exposure limits and hazard abatement. The National Safety Council (Chicago), American Conference of Governmental Industrial Hygienists (ACGIH, Cincinnati), and the American Industrial Hygiene Association (AIHA, Fairfax, VA) are excellent sources of information on workplace health and safety. The ACGIH annually publishes a handbook, *Threshold Limit Values and Biological Indices,* that contains recommended levels of exposure for more than 600 chemical and physical agents.

VI. **Industrial hygiene**

A. The **industrial hygienist** is a professional trained to recognize, evaluate, and control hazardous occupational exposures. Many large manufacturers employ their own industrial hygienists, and small operations may depend on consulting industrial hygienists. Unfortunately, for some workplaces industrial hygiene surveys are conducted by OSHA or NIOSH only when a problem or the threat of a problem exists.

1. The industrial hygienist may be an excellent source of data when a physician suspects an occupational etiology of the patient's disease or symptoms.

2. The hygienist should be familiar with the hazards in a workplace as well as the degree of exposure and the controls that have been implemented to reduce the hazard.

3. Illnesses traced back to the workplace should prompt a review of the site by the company's own industrial hygienist, a contract hygienist, or by OSHA.

B. **Exposure limits** in the occupational environment may be set using one of two criteria or a combination of both.

1. **Threshold limit values** (TLVs) are exposure limits set by the American Conference of Governmental Industrial Hygienists. They are suggested levels for 8-h time-weighted average exposures, short-term exposures (less than 15 min), and ceiling levels for more than 600 hazards.

2. **Permissible exposure levels** (PELs) are promulgated by OSHA and are legally enforceable exposure limits. The original set was based on the then current TLVs. Today, there may be some differences between the suggested and legal limits.

3. TLVs and PELs set limits on contamination in the **ambient environment.** Direct measurement of exposure through **biological samples** may be preferable to environmental sampling when available. Some hazards, such as lead, arsenic, PCBs, some organic solvents, and their metabolites, can be measured in blood, urine, tissue, or expired air. Appropriate biologic sampling should be ordered when evaluating a patient for an occupational disease. Because biologic sampling controls for individual differences in uptake, distribution, metabolism, storage, and excretion of toxic substances, it gives a more accurate picture of exposure.

VII. **Determination of exposure limits.** Human epidemiology, animal experimentation, and chemical analogy are the three general methods for determining workplace exposure limits. Each has its advantages and disadvantages.

A. **Human epidemiology** is the preferred source of data when determining human workplace exposure limits. Data are scarce, however, and when available they are often complicated by low exposures, short or irregular exposure periods, poor data on dose, changes in dose over time, and exposure to a mixture of toxins in and out of the workplace.

B. **Animal experimentation** provides the bulk of toxicity data. However, some large assumptions must be made about toxic responses. Researchers and regulators must assume that animal and human systems behave similarly when exposed to proportionate doses of toxins. Animals are often dosed at levels above those found in the workplace. The results of such studies are then incorporated into models to obtain a human dose that produces little or no effect, i.e., one case of cancer in one million exposed people. Thalidomide is an example of animal model failure to predict human response. This medication did not cause birth defects in the animals in which it was tested. Much of the available animal data have not been verified by human epidemiology.

C. **Chemical analogy.** Animal experiments are expensive and time-consuming. Therefore exposure levels for a given substance may be established based on the behavior of similar or analogous chemicals. Similar chemicals, however, may have a wide range of toxic effects. Benzene, toluene, and xylene have similar chemical structures and properties, for example, but benzene is a potent human carcinogen whereas toluene and xylene are not.

VIII. **Obligations of the health care provider.** Once a work-related illness is diagnosed, the physician has several responsibilities to both the patient and coworkers. The goal of future management is prevention of the progression of illness in the patient and prevention of subsequent illness in the coworkers.

    A. The **patient** should be informed that the illness may be job-related and educated regarding short-term and long-term health implications.

        1. Patient counseling includes methods and avenues of consultation that minimize exposure and subsequent risk. These measures may include protective clothing and change of such habits as hand washing, showering, and eating in relation to the source of exposure. Ideally, a change in the work environment, such as transfer to another area of the plant, is sought from the employer.

        2. Patients should be advised to inform their employer of their illness in writing. This step is necessary particularly if the patient is suffering from a disability and seeks benefits from Social Security or medical insurance.

        3. Legal consultation should be advised if the illness results in disability, wage loss, medical expenses, or damages due to pain and suffering.

        4. All patients diagnosed as having a work-related illness must have health care monitoring established on a regular basis to follow their illness.

    B. The patient's **co-workers** may develop similar job-related illnesses if exposed in the same manner as the patient. The employer should be notified of the physician's concerns, which is best done through the medical department. Unions are helpful in educating and warning coworkers. Many unions have specific programs that assist and promote investigation and corrective action to be taken by the employer. Appropriate union contacts may be obtained from the patient.

    C. **Committees on occupational safety and health** (COSH) are union-based groups that are often helpful for investigating and correcting work-related health hazards. These committees have many locations nationwide. Health effects of industrial toxins, implementation of control measures, legal rights of workers, and access to governmental agencies are some of the services provided by COSH groups.

    D. **The local U.S. Occupational Health and Safety Administration** office should be contacted if the employer resists implementing control measures and corrective action. Health departments on a state or local level should be notified if a significant health hazard is determined to be present.

References

1. Liebowitz AJ. The industrial hygiene impact of new materials and technology. *Am Ind Hyg Assoc J* 1990;51: A350–A353.
2. Litovitz TL, Oderda G, White D, Sheridan MJ. Occupational and environmental exposures reported to poison centers. *Am J Public Health* 1993;83:739–743.
3. Seligman PJ, et al. Compliance with OSHA record keeping requirements. *Am J Public Health* 1988;78:1218.
4. Glowniak JV. Medical resources on the internet. *Ann Intern Med* 1995;123:123–131.
5. Enarson DA, Chan-Yeung M. Characterization of health effects of wood dust exposures. *Am J Ind Med* 1990;17:33–38.
6. Simonato L, Fletcher AC, Anderson AA, Anderson K, Becker N, Chang CJ. An historical prospective study of European stainless steel, mild steel, and shipyard welders. *Br J Ind Med* 1991;48:145–154.

7. Langard S. Role of chemical species and exposure characteristics in cancer among persons occupationally exposed to chromium compounds. *Scand J Environ Health* 1993;19:81–89.
8. Brownson RC, Alavanja MCR, Chang JC. Occupational risk factors for lung cancer among nonsmoking women: a case control study in Missouri (United States). *Cancer Causes Control* 1993;4:449–454.
9. Donoghue, AM, Glass WI, Herbison GP. Transient changes in the pulmonary function of welders: a cross-sectional study of Monday peak flow. *Occup Environ Med* 1994;51:553–556.
10. Sjogren B, Plato N, Alexandersson MD, Eklund A, Falkenberg C. Pulmonary reactions caused by welding-induced decomposed trichloroethylene. *Chest* 1991;99:237–238.
11. Hollander A, Heederick D, Kauffman H. Acute respiratory effects in the potato processing industry due to bioaerosol exposure. *Occcup Environ Med* 1994;51:73–78.
12. Halpin DMG, Graneek BJ, Turner-Warwick M, Newman-Taylor AJ. Extrinsic allergic alveolitis and asthma in a sawmill worker: case report and review of the literature. *Occup Environ Med* 1994;51:160–164.
13. Doll R, Petro R. *The causes of cancer: quantitative estimates of avodable risks of cancer in the United States today.* New York: Oxford University Press, 1981.
14. Higginson J. Proportion of cancers due to occupation. *Prev Med* 1980;9:180–188.
15. Royle H. Toxicity of chromic acid in the chromium plating industry. *Environ Res* 1975;10:39–53.
16. Sorahan T, Burges DCL, Waterhouse JAH. A mortality study of nickle/chromium platers. *Br J Ind Med* 1987;44: 250–258.
17. Davies JM. Lung cancer among workers making lead chromate and zinc chromate pigments at three English factories. *Br J Ind Med* 1984;41:158–169.
18. Vineis P, Thomas T, Hayes R, et al. Proportions of lung cancer in males, due to occupation, in different areas of the USA. *Int J Cancer* 1988;42:851–856.
19. Fowler BA, Yamauchi H, Conner EA, Akkerman M. Cancer risks for humans from exposure to the semiconductor metals. *Scand J Environ Health* 1993;19 suppl 1:101–103.
20. Vainio H, Hemminki K, Wilbourn J. Data on the carcinogenicity of chemicals in the IARC Monographs programme. *Carcinogenesis* 1985;6:1653–1655.
21. Homan CS, Maitra SR, Lane BP, Thode HC, Sable M. Therapeutic effects of water and milk for acute alkali injury of the esophagus. *Ann Emerg Med* 1994;24:14–20.
22. Homan CS, Maitra SR, Lane BP, Thode HC, Davidson L. Histopathologic evaluation of the therapeutic efficacy of water and milk dilution for esophageal acid injury. *Acad Emerg Med* 1995;2:587–591.
23. National Institute of Occupational Safety and Health (NIOSH). *Registry of toxic effects of chemical substances (RTECS).* Cincinatti: NIOSH, 1990.

Selected Readings

Klassen CD, Amdur MO, Doull J, eds. *Casarett and Doull's toxicology: the basic science of poisons.* 5th ed. New York: McGraw-Hill, 1996.
American Conference of Industrial Hygienists. *Threshold limit value and biological exposure indices for 1995–96.* Cincinnati: American Conference of Industrial Hygienists, 1995.
Barlow SM. *Reproductive hazards of industrial chemicals: an evaluation of animal and human data.* London: Academic Press, 1982.
Encyclopedia of occupational health and safety. Vols. I and II. 3rd ed. Washington, DC: International Labor Office, 1983.
Hamilton A, Hardy J, Finkel AJ. *Hamilton and Hardy's industrial toxicology.* 4th ed. Littleton, MA: J. Wright, 1983.
Kusnetz S, Hutchinson MK, eds. *A guide to the work-relatedness of disease.* DHEW (NIOSH) Publ. No. 79-116. Washington, DC: U.S. Government Printing Office, 1979.
Lauwerys PR, Hoet P. *Industrial chemical exposure guidelines for biologic monitoring.* (1st ed.). Boca Raton, FL: Lewis Publishers, 1993.
Levy BS. *Occupational health: recognizing and preventing work-related disease.* 2nd ed. Boston: Little, Brown and Company, 1988.
Lewis RS, Sweet D, eds. *Registry of toxic effects of chemical substances 1983–1984, cumulative supplement to the 1981–1982 edition (Vols. 1 and 2).* Cincinnati: USGPO (Department of Health and Human Services), 1985.
Lippman M, ed. *Environmental toxicants: human exposures and their health effects.* (1st ed.). New York: Van Nostrand Reinhold, 1992.
Mackison FW, Stircott RS, Partridge LJ, eds. *Occupational health guidelines for chemical hazards.* DHHS Publ. No. (NIOSH) 81-123. Washington, DC: U.S. Department of Health and Human Services and Department of Labor, 1985.
McCunney RJ. *Handbook of occupational medicine.* 2nd ed. Boston: Little, Brown and Company, 1994.
Plog BA. *Fundamentals of industrial hygiene.* 3rd ed. Chicago: National Safety Council, 1988.

Reproductive health hazards in the workplace. Washington, DC: Congress of the United States, Office of Technology Assessment, 1985.

Rom WN. *Environmental and occupational medicine.* 2nd ed. Boston: Little, Brown and Company, 1992.

Rosenstock L, Cullen MR. *Textbook of clinical occupational and environmental medicine.* Philadelphia: WB Saunders, 1994.

United States Superintendent of Documents, U.S. Department of Labor. *Code of Federal Regulations, title 29, parts 1900 through 1910.* Washington, DC: U.S. Government Printing Office, 1988.

Wexler P. *Information resources in toxicology.* 2nd ed. New York: Elsevier Science, 1988.

Zenz C, ed. *Occupational medicine: principles and practical applications.* 2nd ed. Chicago: Year Book Medical Publishers, 1988.

PART IV

Medical Toxicology

Emergency Toxicology, Second Edition,
edited by Peter Viccellio.
Lippincott–Raven Publishers, Philadelphia © 1998.

30
Salicylates

Gregory L. Almond

*Department of Emergency Medicine, New York Medical College/Metropolitan Hospital Center,
New York, New York 10029*

I. **Introduction.** Salicylate poisoning is a potentially life-threatening ingestion. Most households have enough aspirin in the medicine cabinet to produce a life-threatening ingestion. This ease of availability of salicylate, along with the lack of a discrete toxidrome, mandates the clinician to always consider this condition in the differential diagnosis of any patient with any condition that is not obvious. There are four groups of patients who are considered at risk for salicylate poisoning. The incidence of accidental acute pediatric ingestions is declining due to the use of childproof caps as well as the limited number of tablets per bottle. Public awareness of the association of Reye's syndrome with salicylate ingestion has contributed to the downward trend in accidental pediatric poisonings from salicylates. Occasionally, a child may be overzealously treated with salicylates by an anxious parent during the first few days of the child's illness resulting in chronic toxicity. Acute toxicity may result from a single large ingestion taken as an attempted suicide. The elderly patient may suffer chronic toxicity following a gradual alteration in the patient's metabolic elimination processes, or due to the simultaneous ingestion of medications, such as acetazolamide, that enhance the toxicity of salicylate.

II. **Available preparations.** Salicylates are common in many over-the-counter (OTC) oral preparations, including PeptoBismol, various cold preparations, and antacids. Topical preparations such as methylsalicylate (oil of wintergreen) may contain as much as 1,400 mg of salicylate per cc (16). Small children may accidentally ingest these rubifacients. Fatalities have occurred with doses as small as 1 tsp. The topical preparations are a potential source of systemic toxicity, as dermal absorption may occur with exercise or exposure to heat.

III. **Pharmacology and properties**

A. **Mechanism of action.** Therapeutic salicylate levels result in antiinflammatory, analgesic, and antipyretic effects primarily through inhibition of prostaglandin biosynthesis. In toxicity, salicylates cause a variety of metabolic derangements. Salicylates uncouple oxidative phosphorylation to result in hyperthermia, an increased metabolic rate, and hyperpnea. This hyperactive state leads to increased insensible fluid losses. The increased energy demand promotes tissue glycolysis and gluconeogenesis. Hyperglycemia may result. However, hypoglycemia and neuroglycopenia are common in chronic intoxication or late in the course of acute toxicity. Salicylates directly inhibit certain enzymes in the Kreb's cycle, possibly as a result of magnesium chelation (10). This inhibition results in increased amounts of organic acids (e.g., pyruvate and lactate) which contribute to metabolic acidosis. Stimulation of lipid metabolism and altered levels of serum glucose leads to elevated levels of ketones and organic acids (e.g., B-hydroxybutyric acid, aceto-acetic acid, and acetone). An inhibition of aminotransferases results in increased levels of circulating amino acids and an aminoaciduria (10). These mechanisms also contribute to the metabolic acidosis. Organic aciduria occurs and results in an increased renal excretion of sodium, potassium and water. The increased excretion of bicarbonate secondary to compensation for the respiratory alkalosis results in renal potassium losses. Renal tubular damage may ultimately result in proteinuria with sodium chloride and water retention (10). Metabolic alkalosis may result from vomiting and volume contraction (10).

B. **Absorption and distribution.** Acetylsalicylic acid, a weak acid with a pK_a of 3.5, is predominantly nonionized in the low pH environment of the stomach. Once dissolved, it is absorbed rapidly from the stomach and intestines by passive diffusion. Absorption is usually complete within 2 to 4 h depending upon the formulation. Concretions may form, especially with large ingestions, resulting in a delayed peak serum level and prolonged toxicity. The major factor determining the absorption rate of salicylic acid is the formulation (17). Enteric-coated preparations are absorbed slowly with a delayed peak serum level of 4 to 6 h (22). Buffered preparations are absorbed rapidly. These preparations form salts upon disintegration which enhances absorption (20). Effervescent tablets dissolved prior to ingestion are absorbed most rapidly (27). Other factors that affect salicylate absorption include the rate of gastric emptying, the volume of food in the stomach, the pH of stomach contents, concurrent ingestions, exercise, posture, and disease states associated with altered gastrointestinal (GI) transit time (21). Salicylates are classified as acetylated (acetylsalicylic acid and diflunisal) and nonacetylated (salicylsalicylic acid, sodium salicylate, choline salicylate, magnesium salicylate, and trilisate which are metabolized to salicylic acid derivatives). Aspirin and salicylic acid have pK_a's of 3.5 and 3.0, respectively. This allows the compound to be highly ionized at the pH of normal blood. Any process resulting in a lower serum pH will allow the salicylate to exist in the nonionized state. This allows easy entry of these compounds into various tissues of the body, including the central nervous system (CNS).

C. **Metabolism and elimination.** Salicylate metabolism occurs through hepatic conversion to salicyluric acid, a phenolic glucuronide, an acyl glucuronide, and gentisitic acid. Salicylic acid may be excreted unchanged in the urine. Hepatic enzymes are saturated at upper therapeutic as well as toxic levels of salicylate which results in zero-order elimination kinetics. At toxic levels, renal excretion becomes significant. Aciduria promotes the resorption of nonionized salicylate in the renal tubules that can prolong toxicity. The volume of distribution of salicylates in adults (11) is 9.6 to 12.7 L/kg and in children (28) is 0.12 to 0.14 L/kg. The volume of distribution is pH dependent and increases with acidemia. Salicylates are excreted in breast milk and may represent a hazard for the infants of nursing mothers (8).

IV. **Clinical presentation.** A patient who is suffering from salicylate toxicity may present with a wide range of signs and symptoms, depending upon the circumstances, time since ingestion, co-ingestions, state of health of the patient and many other factors. Patients with lethal ingestions may have only minimal symptoms if they present soon after their exposure. The clinician must be suspicious of salicylate toxicity in any patient who presents with an altered consciousness, hyperventilation, hyperpyrexia, vomiting, an abnormal serum glucose, anion gap metabolic acidosis, acid-base disturbances, tinnitus, noncardiogenic pulmonary edema (NCPE) (12), or coma. The conscious patient whose intent was to commit suicide may not voluntarily give the history of an ingestion. The examiner must question the presence of diminished auditory acuity or deafness, vertigo, hallucinations, dyspnea, nausea or vomiting, convulsions, fever, diaphoresis, hematemesis, abnormal bleeding, bruising, or melena as possible manifestations of salicylism. The progression of signs and symptoms is dependent upon the amount of salicylate ingested and pH of the serum. For the same level of salicylate, increased symptomatology will be present at a lower pH. A complete medication history, including all OTC medications, must be carefully reviewed. Simultaneous drug ingestions which may enhance toxicity include furosemide (1) by inhibiting salicylate excretion; acetazolamide (5,14,24) by enhancing the ability of nonionized salicylate to penetrate into the CNS tissue; and any drug that produces hypercarbia through blunting of the respiratory drive. The resulting acidemia will promote salicylate distribution throughout the body.

A. **Acute salicylate intoxication**

   1. **General.** A single ingestion of less than 150mg/kg of salicylates will generally result in negligible clinical toxicity. A single ingestion of 150 to 300 mg/kg may result in mild to moderate toxicity. An ingestion of greater than 300 mg/kg will result in prolonged and more severe effects including marked hyperpnea and prominent neurological disturbances. Ingestions of greater than 500 mg/kg are considered potentially lethal. Toxicity can occur with chronic administration of greater than 100 mg/kg/24 h for 2 or more days (26). Tachypnea and nausea may be the only physical findings in the mildly intoxicated patient. Tinnitus and Kussmaul respiration may be present as well. Disorientation, coma, and seizures are manifestations of severe toxicity. These findings can represent underlying cerebral edema. Renal failure and cardiovascular collapse are also possible.

   2. **Respiratory.** Tachypnea occurs early in a pure salicylate intoxication, due to a direct effect on the CNS respiratory center. The depth and rate of respiration is increased, leading to a respiratory alkalosis. A compensatory increase in bicarbonate excretion by the kidneys occurs. Respiratory acidosis secondary to CNS depression may occur with either severe salicylate intoxication, the simultaneous ingestion of sedative hypnotic agents (9) or pulmonary edema (10). Pulmonary edema will be evident by the presence of rales or cyanosis and may occur in moderate to severe toxicity. The physician must be careful not to miss a significant salicylate intoxication in an elderly patient assumed to have cardiogenic pulmonary edema which is actually salicylate-induced noncardiogenic pulmonary edema. Heffner (13) noted that certain patients including smokers and the elderly are at an increased risk of salicylate-induced pulmonary edema. Diagnosis of this disorder is essential because it demands immediate removal of the salicylate by hemodialysis. Coingestion of a sedative hypnotic agent will blunt the initial respiratory alkalosis. As tachypnea is a classical sign of salicylate intoxication, the absence of this sign may allow the intoxication to be misdiagnosed. In addition, the sedative hypnotic agent will blunt the ventilatory response to metabolic acidosis resulting in acidemia and worsening toxicity.

3. **Metabolic.** Respiratory alkalosis is the predominant early acid-base disturbance and is followed quickly by a combined respiratory alkalosis and metabolic acidosis. In children, systemic metabolic acidosis predominates, as they have a higher metabolic rate, an increased respiratory quotient and less ability to increase their tidal volume. As toxicity evolves, a combined respiratory and metabolic acidosis develops. This is significant for severe illness and high mortality.

4. **GI.** Nausea and vomiting occur secondary to direct irritative effects of the GI tract and through a centrally mediated mechanism. Decreased GI motility and pylorospasm occurs with larger ingestions of salicylate. GI bleeding can occur secondary to gastritis and exacerbation of peptic ulcer disease. GI bleeding is excluded by rectal exam. Concretions of salicylate may form resulting in delayed and prolonged toxicity.

5. **Hepatic.** Hepatitis may occur with any salicylate ingestion. DIC may be expected with moderate to severe toxicity. The effect of platelet inhibition alone will not cause bleeding.

B. **Differences between acute versus chronic salicylate intoxication.** The patient with an acute ingestion of salicylate is likely to be younger than the patient presenting with a chronic ingestion. Chronic exposure of salicylate is defined as an increased dose or frequency of salicylate with a duration of exposure greater than 8 h. The diagnosis of chronic salicylate ingestion is less obvious than acute. The acutely intoxicated patient will more likely have ingested the salicylate intentionally, while the chronic ingestion is more often accidental or iatrogenic. The predominate clinical scenario of an acute ingestion will be GI and metabolic versus the chronic ingestion with mostly CNS disorders, renal insufficiency, and pulmonary edema. Serum levels are more often significantly elevated and predictive of outcome in the acute ingestions than in the chronic ingestions. Mortality rates approach 25% with chronic ingestions while there are only rare mortalities (less than 1%) in patients with acute ingestions. The clinician must be aware of the lack of correlation of salicylate levels with clinical toxicity in patients with chronic or cumulative ingestions and must remain conservative in their evaluation and treatment of these patients.

C. **Differential Diagnosis.** The differential diagnosis of salicylate intoxication includes all causes of an increased anion gap metabolic acidosis including ketoacidosis (diabetic, alcoholic, starvation), renal failure, sepsis and hepatic cirrhosis. CNS trauma or infection and toxicity from carbon monoxide, cyanide, methanol, ethylene glycol, theophylline, isoniazid, metformin, and iron poisoning must also be considered. Reye's syndrome should be considered in children. In the elderly, the combination of increased temperature, rales, tachypnea and altered mental status may be easily mistaken for severe CHF or pneumonia with sepsis.

V. **Laboratory evaluation**

A. **General.** Necessary laboratory studies in patients with signs and symptoms consistent with salicylate toxicity include electrolytes, BUN and creatinine, glucose, calcium, arterial blood gas, acetaminophen level, complete blood count, platelets, prothrombin time, partial thromboplastin time, and urinalysis. The salicylate-induced platelet abnormality is not reflected in the PT, PTT, or platelet count. It is a functional disorder that is reflected as a prolongation of the bleeding time. Creatinine phosphokinase may be included to assess for the presence of rhabdomyolysis. Urine is noted for the pH, the presence of ketones, and hemoglobin. If hemoglobin is present, a microscopic examination of the urine is performed to exclude the presence of RBCs. If no RBCs are present, the presence of myoglobin must be considered and a urinary myoglobin requested. An electrocardiogram is obtained for all patients as a screening test for potentially life threatening electrolyte abnormalities secondary to dehydration, hypokalemia, hyperkalemia, or hypocalcemia. A chest x-ray is necessary to exclude pulmonary edema. A noncardiogenic source of the pulmonary edema is supported by the presence of a normal sized heart. If the patient has an abnormal mental status, a lumbar puncture may be necessary to exclude a diagnosis of meningitis in the febrile salicylate-intoxicated patient. Spinal fluid is analyzed for evidence of CNS infection and hemorrhage. Obtain a CT scan prior to performing the LP if head trauma or bleeding is suspected. Coagulation factors should be replaced prior to LP if coagulopathy is present.

B. **Salicylate levels.** A quick qualitative test for the presence of salicylates may be done by adding several drops of 10% ferric chloride to 1 mL of urine (5). A purple color change indicates the possible presence of salicylates. A formal serum quantification assay is then necessary. False positives are common and result from acetoacetic acid or phenylpyruvic acid (3), but a false negative ferric chloride test is rare. If no Ferric chloride is available, the Ames Phenistix may be utilized. However, it must be interpreted cautiously because this reagent strip will turn brown in the presence of salicylates as well as phenothiazines. The addition of one drop of 20N H_2SO_4 to the strip will bleach out the color if caused by phenothiazines, but not salicylate (5). Monitoring serum salicylate levels are important in acute ingestions. Levels are repeated every 2 h in significant ingestions until the peak value has been determined. The salicylate level can then be repeated every 4 to 6 h until it is less than 30 mg/dL. This is necessary because salicylate levels can rebound unexpectedly, necessitating a more aggressive therapy. Factors responsible for these rises are erratic gut absorption and redistribution effect. The Done nomogram (6) is no longer recommended for use because of several limitations. The nomogram was based on pediatric patients with acute nonenteric coated ingestions and normal blood pH. Thus, the application of this graph to other clinical settings would be inappropriate. The nomogram also could result in delayed therapy since the first level is obtained at 6 h postingestion. Toxicity should be determined and therapy initiated much earlier than 6 h postingestion. Additionally, Done's criteria for distinguishing between mild, moderate and severe toxicity are not consistent with today's standard and may misguide the clinician. For patients with chronic ingestions (26), salicylate levels do not correlate well with the patient's clinical status. Management is reliant upon clinical manifestations.

VI. **Management**

A. **General.** In the more severely intoxicated patient, standard Advanced Cardiac Life Support measures must be instituted. A rectal temperature should be obtained because the oral route may be falsely low from tachypnea and mouth breathing. Severe hyperpyrexia (i.e., greater than 105°F) must be aggressively treated by either ice water immersion or covering the patient with a wet sheet and having a fan blow over the patient. The treatment of salicylate-induced noncardiogenic pulmonary edema is similar to other types of noncardiogenic pulmonary edema (with the addition of hemodialysis), and includes intubation for ventilation, oxygenation, and the use of positive end expiratory pressure (PEEP). A patient who has recently ingested a potentially lethal amount of salicylate may initially be asymptomatic, particularly if the ingestion was an enteric coated preparation. These patients must not be discharged prematurely. Glucose administration is necessary to all salicylate intoxicated patients with altered mental status for the treatment of presumptive neuroglycopenia (15). Hydration must be maintained as salicylate intoxication results in dehydration through insensible and GI fluid losses. Patients in pulmonary edema will not be able to tolerate the fluid load and must be considered for hemodialysis. Respiratory and metabolic acidosis must be prevented or corrected to prevent salicylate from becoming nonionized and diffusing across tissue boundaries. Intubation or the administration of sodium bicarbonate may be indicated.

   B. Gastric decontamination. Gastric Lavage with a 40-French lavage tube in the adult patient or emesis with syrup of Ipecac may be indicated for the asymptomatic patient who presents within 1 to 2 h following the ingestion of a large amount of salicylate. Even later presentations may benefit from gastric lavage because of delayed gastric emptying and bezoar formation. Critically ill patients or those with rising salicylate levels require gastric lavage regardless of their time of presentation. The airway should be secured prior to this procedure. Any patient with suspected salicylate exposure requires an oral dose of activated charcoal (1 g/kg) with a cathartic such as sorbitol. Repetitive activated charcoal is indicated for all moderately to severely intoxicated patients. Whole bowel irrigation may be useful in toxic patients whose salicylate levels are not declining. Concretions and enteric coated preparations can be removed by this procedure. Polyethylene glycol electrolyte lavage solution is administered (PO/NGT) at a rate of 1 to 2 L/h (adult) or 500 mL/h (child). Bicarbonate lavage is not recommended because salicylate absorption can be enhanced. A drug level that remains elevated despite the above therapy requires an upper GI endoscopy to identify and break up large concretions.

   C. Alkalinization of urine. Alkalinization of the urine with sodium bicarbonate is indicated in any patients with other than mild salicylate poisoning. Raising the pH of the urine favors the ionized form of salicylate that is poorly diffusible back across membranes which results in the salicylate becoming trapped in the urine (5). Alkalinizing agents such as trimethamine should not be used, as salicylate may become "trapped" in the tissues (5) as these agents alkalinize intracellularly as well as extracellularly. Acetazolamide is not used because it will alkalinize the urine at the expense of acidifying the serum. This will result in higher levels of nonionized salicylate and worsening toxicity (14). A bolus of 1 to 2 mEq/kg of sodium bicarbonate over 5 min is followed by a bicarbonate infusion at 0.2 to 0.4 mEq/Kg/h. This solution may be prepared by adding 2 to 3 ampules of sodium bicarbonate (88 to 132 mEq/L) to 1 L of D5W. Potassium chloride is added to the solution as 20 to 40 mEq/L to compensate for alkalemia-induced hypokalemia. The bicarbonate infusion is to be titrated to a serum pH greater than 7.40 and a urine pH of 7 to 8 (10). Hypokalemia and dehydration must be corrected to assure successful alkalinization of the urine (26). Frequent monitoring of urine pH is necessary.

If the urinary pH remains less than 7.0 after the initial alkalinization, rebolus with bicarbonate and increase the maintenance rate of bicarbonate infusion. Monitor the arterial pH to prevent rises above 7.55. This shifts the oxyhemoglobin dissociation curve leftward, and interferes with the release of oxygen to tissues. In severe poisoning, larger amounts of bicarbonate will be required and should be used as long as the serum pH is followed (10). The alkalinization of children may be difficult because the excess inorganic acid production and accompanying aciduria may not be compensated for with bicarbonate administration. Alkalinization can be stopped in the patient with acute ingestion of salicylate when the salicylate level is less than 25 mg/dL.

D. Hemodialysis. Hemodialysis is the preferred method of extracorporeal removal. While charcoal hemoperfusion is effective for clearing salicylates from the serum compartment, electrolyte abnormalities can not be corrected. Given the significant mortality rate from salicylism in spite of treatment, hemodialysis is indicated if any of the following is present.
1. Renal insufficiency
2. Serum salicylate level greater than 100 mg/dL in an acute exposure and 60 mg/dL in a chronic exposure.
3. Metabolic acidosis refractory to bicarbonate and volume therapy
4. Altered mental status or seizures
5. Pulmonary edema
6. Hepatic insufficiency affecting coagulation
7. Progressive rise in salicylate level despite attempts at urinary alkalinization

VII. Disposition. All infants with any sign of salicylism should be admitted. Patients with acute salicylate ingestions resulting in mild to moderate symptoms should be admitted to a medical ward after appropriate stabilization. Close monitoring for clinical deterioration is necessary. Patients requiring intensive care are those with altered mental status, pulmonary edema, renal insufficiency, requirement for aggressive monitoring of fluid and electrolytes, and anticipation for hemodialysis. Swan-Ganz monitoring should be considered for any patient with hemodynamic instability, pulmonary edema, renal failure or evidence of congestive heart failure. Patients that may be medically cleared after an exposure are those demonstrating the following: serial salicylate levels that have decreased to less than 25 mg/dL while off alkalinization therapy; no acid base disturbance; and no CNS, cardiovascular or pulmonary symptoms. If this can not be accomplished in the Emergency Department, then the patient should be admitted. Psychiatric evaluation is mandatory for any intentional overdose.

References

1. Berg KJ, Loew D. Inhibition of furosemide-induced natriuresis by acetylsalicylic acid in dogs. *Scand J Clin Lab Invest* 1977;37:125–131.
2. Brady CE, Dipalma JA, Morawaski SG, et al. Urinary excretion of polyethylene glycol 3350 and sulfate after gut lavage with a polyethylene glycol electrolyte lavage solution. *Gastroenterology* 1986;90:1914–1918.
3. DiPiro JT, Michael KA, Clark BA, et al. Absorption of polyethylene glycol after administration of a PEG electrolyte lavage solution. *Clin Pharm* 1986;5:153–155.
4. Danon A, Ben-Shimon S, Ben-Zvi Z. Effect of exercise and heat exposure on percutaneous absorption of methyl salicylate. *Eur J Clin Pharmacol* 198631:49–52.
5. Done AK. Aspirin overdosage: incidence, diagnosis, and managment. *Pediatrics* 1978;62:8903–8897.

6. Done AK. Salicylate intoxication: significance of measurements of salicylate in blood in cases of acute ingestion. *Pediatrics* 1960;26:800.
7. Done AK, Temple AR. Treatment of salicylate poisoning. *Mod Treat* 1971;8:528–551.
8. Findlay WA, De Angelis RL, Kearney MF, et al. Analgesic drugs in breast milk and plasma. *Clin Pharmacol Ther* 1981;29:625–633.
9. Gabow P, Anderson RJ, Potts DE, et al. Acid-base disturbances in the salicylate-intoxicated adult. *Arch Intern Med* 1978;128:1481–1484.
10. Goldfrank LR, Bresnitz EA, Hartnett L. Salicylates. In: Goldfrank LR, ed. *Goldfrank's toxicologic emergencies.* 3rd ed. New York: Appleton-Century-Crofts, 1986.
11. Grahm GG, Champion GD, Day RO, et al. Patterns of plasma concentrations and urinary excretion of salicylate in rheumatoid arthritis. *Clin Pharmacol Ther* 1977;22:410.
12. Heffner J, Starkey T, Anthony P. Salicylate-induced noncardiogenic pulmonary edema. *West J Med* 1979;130:263–266.
13. Heffner JE, Sahn SA. Salicylate-induced pulmonary edema. *Ann Intern Med* 1981;95:405–409.
14. Hill JB. Salicylate intoxication. *N Engl J Med* 1973;286:1110.
15. Hill JB. Experimental salicylate poisoning: observations on the effects of altering blood pH on tissue and plasma salicylate concentrations. *Pediatrics* 1971;47:658.
16. Johnson PN, Welch DW. Methyl salicylate/aspirin (salicylate) equivalence: who do you trust? *Vet Hum Toxicol* 1984; 26:317.
17. Klinenberg JR, Miller F. Effect of corticosteroids in blood salicylate concentration. *JAMA* 1965;194:601–604.
18. Leventhal LJ. Salicylate-induced rhabdomyolysis. *Am J Emerg Med* 1988;7:409–410.
19. Levy G. Pharmacokinetics of salicylate elimination in man. *J Pharm Sci* 1965;54:959.
20. Levy G, Hayes BA. Physiochemical basis of the buffered acetylsalicylic acid controversy. *N Engl J Med* 1960; 262:1053.
21. Needs CJ, Brooks PM. Clinical pharmacokinetics of the salicylates. *Clin Pharmacokinet* 1985;10:164–177.
22. Ross-Lee LM, et al. Aspirin pharmacokinetics in migraine. The effect of metrochlopropamide. *Eur J Clin Pharmacol* 1982;24:777–785.
23. Spahn H, et al. Pharmacokinetics of salicylates administered with metoprolol. *Arzneimittelforschung* 1986;36: 1697–1699.
24. Sweeney KR, Chapron DJ, Brandt JL, et al. Toxic interaction between acetazolamide and salicylate: case reports and a pharmacokinetic explanation. *Clin Pharmacol Ther* 1986;40:518–524.
25. Temple AR. Pathophysiology of aspirin overdosage toxicity, with implications for management. *Pediatrics* 1978;62: 873–876.
26. Temple AR. Acute and chronic effects of aspirin toxicity and their treatment. *Arch Intern Med* 1981;141:364–369.
27. Volans GN. Effects of food and exercise on the absorption of effervescent aspirin. *Br J Clin Pharmacol* 1974;1: 137–141.
28. Wilson JT, et al. Efficacy, disposition and pharmacodynamics of aspirin, acetaminophen, and choline salicylate in young febrile children. *Ther Drug Monitor* 1982;4:147–180.

Emergency Toxicology, Second Edition,
edited by Peter Viccellio.
Lippincott–Raven Publishers, Philadelphia © 1998.

31

Acetaminophen

Howard C. Mofenson and Thomas R. Caraccio

*Department of Emergency Medicine, Long Island Regional Poison Control Center, Winthrop
University Hospital, Mineola, New York 11501*

I. **Properties of the agent.** Acetaminophen (paracetamol) APAP), *N*-acetyl-*p*-aminophenol, one of the coal tar analgesics, is a major active metabolite of phenacetin and acetanilid. Phenacetin was produced in 1887 from the more toxic aniline dye derived, acetanilid. Acetanilid and phenacetin have produced methemoglobinemia in humans, but acetaminophen has rarely been reported to do so, although it does produce methemoglobinemia in dogs. Analgesics accounted for 10.5% of all exposures. Acetaminophen overdose producing hepatotoxicity was first reported in the United Kingdom in 1966 (1,2). In 1994, there were 102,619 exposures of APAP reported (about one-third in combination with other products): 903 of those patients had major medical problems, and 100 died (0.0009%) (3). No children have been reported to have died from an acute overdose, but there are reports of liver failure and death in children from overdoses (4–9). APAP has been implicated in about 7% of the annual reported poison exposures and about 35% of emergency department visits and hospital admissions (3). In the United Kingdom, 150 people die annually after APAP overdose.

A. **Sources.** APAP is available as tablets and capsules: regular strength 325 mg, extra strength 500 mg. It is also supplied as suppositories: 120, 325, 650 mg. For children's preparations, see Table 31-1. A sustained release acetaminophen was introduced in August, 1994 in 650 mg (325 mg regular acting and 325 mg extended release) APAP/caplet.

B. **Mechanism of action and pathophysiology**

   1. **Mechanism of action** of APAP is mediated by interference with prostaglandin synthesis through inhibition of prostaglandin synthetase in the arachidonic acid cascade in the CNS. APAP has very little activity as an inhibitor of the peripheral prostaglandin synthetase enzyme, which explains its weak antiinflammatory action. Its antipyretic action is directly on the hypothalamus.

   2. **Therapeutic dose** is 10 to 15 mg/kg up to 2.6 g/24 h. (9). **The minimal toxic amount** is approximately 3 g or more or 140 mg/kg (some say 200 mg/kg) (4–9, 38,39) in a child and 7.5 g or more in an adult (Table 31-1). Liver toxicity usually follows ingestion of more than 15 g in adults. Those who have liver disease, or depleted glutathione stores or deficiency in glutathione synthetase may experience toxicity after taking as small an amount as 7.5 g (10–15).

   3. **Mechanism of toxicity.** Mitchell and others (11–14) showed during the 1970s that a portion of the ingested dose undergoes metabolism by the P450 mixed function oxidase to a reactive, arylating, intermediate metabolite, ***N*-acetyl-*p*-benzoqui-**

TABLE 31-1. *Amount of preparations equals the toxic amount of 140 mg/kg*

Age	Weight (kg)	Drops (15 mL) 100 mg/mL)	Elixir (60 and 120 mL 160 mg/5 mL)	Chewable Tablets (80 mg)	Tablets (160 mg)	Tablets (325 mg)	Caplets (500 mg)
<1 mo	3.5	4.9 mL	15.4 mL	6 tabs	3 tabs	1.5 tabs	1 cap
1 mo	4.0	5.6 mL	17.6 mL	7 tabs	3.5 tabs	1.72 tabs	1.12 cap
6 mo	7.0	9.8 mL	30.8 mL	12.8 tabs	6.4 tabs	3.0 tabs	1.96 cap
1 yr	10.0	14.0 mL	44.0 mL	17.5 tabs	8.8 tabs	4.3 tabs	2.8 cap
2 yr	12.0	16.8 mL	52.8 mL	21 tabs	10.5 tabs	5.16 tabs	3.36 cap
3 yr	14.0	19.6 mL	61.6 mL	24.5 tabs	12.3 tabs	6.02 tabs	3.92 cap
5 yr	18.0	25.2 mL	79.2 mL	31.5 tabs	15.8 tabs	7.74 tabs	5.04 cap
6 yr	20.0	26.2 mL	88.0 mL	35 tabs	17.5 tabs	8.6 tabs	5.60 cap
9 yr	28.0	39.2 mL	123.2 mL	49 tabs	24.5 tabs	12.1 tabs	7.84 cap
10 yr	32.0	44.8 mL	140.8 mL	56 tabs	28 tabs	13.8 tabs	8.96 cap
12 yr	34.0	47.6 mL	149.6 mL	59.5 tabs	30 tabs	14.6 tabs	9.52 cap
14 yr	40.0	56.0 mL	176.0 mL	70.0 tabs	35 tabs	17.2 tabs	11.20 cap
15 yr	50.0	70.0 mL	220.0 mL	87.5 tabs	44 tabs	21.5 tabs	14.00 cap
Adult	60.0	84.0 mL	264.0 mL	105.0 tabs	52.5 tabs	25.8 tabs	16.80 cap
Adult	70.0	98.0 mL	308.0 mL	122.0 tabs	61 tabs	30.1 tabs	19.60 cap

noneimine (**NAPQI**) (less than 5%), a strong oxidizing agent, that is subsequently reduced by the sulfhydryl groups of glutathione to a nontoxic form. The glutathione conjugate is ultimately converted to cysteine and mercapturic acid conjugate. When there is not sufficient glutathione available, NAPQI forms covalent bonds with cellular proteins which are believed to produce hepatocellular centrilobular necrosis and renal injury.

4. **Overdose** of APAP saturates the conjugation pathways and produces an increase in the toxic metabolite that overwhelms the glutathione detoxification mechanism (the natural protective stores of cellular glutathione). When the glutathione is less than 30%, NAPQI causes cell death (10–12,16,17) (Fig. 31-1).

5. **Chronic intoxication** producing hepatotoxicity may occur in adults ingesting 10 to 15 g/day and in chronic alcoholics ingesting 3 to 4 g/day for a few days (16). Simultaneous acute ethanol probably protects the liver by enzyme inhibition. Chronic alcohol use is reported to increase the hepatotoxicity of APAP through enzyme induction (17–26). Chronic intoxication may occur in children receiving 150 mg/kg/day for 2 to 4 days. Two of these children were given several doses of 650-mg suppositories (5). Clinically, it may resemble Reye's syndrome. Pathologically, it shows centrilobular necrosis of the liver (characteristic of APAP pathology), rather than the diffuse pathology of Reye's syndrome (4–9).

6. **Chronic alcoholism** has also been reported to enhance APAP toxicity (17–26). In these circumstances, the acetaminophen plasma concentration may not be in the toxic range, although lethal hepatotoxicity has been reported. It has been advised that this subgroup be treated at plasma concentrations 50% below threshold levels by the British Formulary (25). Six alcoholic patients with severe acetaminophen hepatotoxicity were reported in a 2-year period. The patients had a marked elevation of transaminases and sometimes the prothrombin time. The authors emphasize

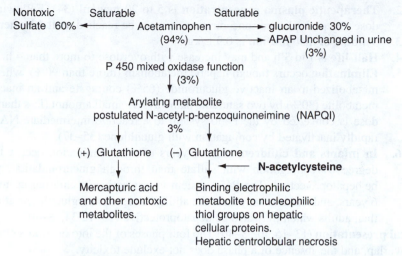

FIG. 31-1. Metabolism of acetaminophen in adults.

that reliance on APAP plasma levels (which do not appear hepatotoxic) and insufficient history regarding use of alcohol and acetaminophen may cause a misdiagnosis (21). See differential diagnosis. Five patients developed severe hepatic injury after 6.4 g of APAP in less than 20 h (27). Lauterberg (20) found glutathione deficiency in alcoholic patients.

7. **Eating disorders** such as anorexia nervosa or starvation may deplete glutathione and increase the risk for severe liver damage at single modest overdose or after multiple high therapeutic doses doses. Chronic alcoholism, acetaminophen, and malnutrition or fasting are synergic because all three deplete the level of reduced glutathione from the liver mitochondria (19,28).

8. **Chronic use of phenytoin, phenobarbital** (25–29), and other drugs that induce the cytochrome P450 may produce an increase in APAP's toxic metabolite, **NAPQI**. In these circumstances, the APAP plasma concentration may not be in the toxic range, although lethal hepatotoxicity has been reported. It has been advised that this subgroup be treated at plasma concentrations below threshold levels (25–29). Hepatotoxicity associated with multiple drug therapy for **tuberculosis** has been reported especially with isoniazid (30). Although there are no specific reports of APAP administration, reduction of glutathione in AIDS may be detrimental in acquired human immunodeficiency virus infection (AIDS) (31–33).

9. Table 31-1 calculates the amount of the commonly used preparations that would be expected to produce toxicity.

C. **Pharmacokinetics** (34)
1. **GI absorption time** is 0.5 to 1.0 h. Although the time may be delayed by the presence of other drugs, the extent of absorption is not affected. The peak plasma concentration following an oral therapeutic dose occurs at 20 to 90 min.

2. **Therapeutic plasma concentration** is 5 to 20 mcg/ml (34). Following an overdose, the peak plasma concentration may not be reached until 4 h after ingestion.
3. **Volume of distribution** is 0.9 L/kg.
4. **Half-life** is 1 to 3 h and may increase with overdose to more than 4 h.
5. **Elimination** occurs though hepatic metabolism (more than 90%), where APAP is metabolized to an inactive glucuronide (65%) conjugate and an inactive sulfate metabolite (30%) by two saturable pathways. A small amount (less than 5%) of the dose is converted by the P450 system to a reactive intermediate NAPQI that is rapidly inactivated by conjugation with glutathione (35–37).
6. **In infants and children** under 6 years of age, elimination occurs to a greater degree by conjugation with sulfate than through glucuronidation, which may be hepatoprotective. The P450 system is less active in children up to the age of 6 years, and children may have the ability to regenerate glutathione at a faster rate than adults which may also be hepatoprotective (10–12,34,38–40).

II. **Clinical presentation** (13–15,36,38–40) The four phases of the intoxication's clinical course may overlap, and the absence of a phase does not exclude toxicity.
   A. **Phase I** occurs within the first few hours after ingestion and consists of malaise, diaphoresis, nausea, vomiting, and drowsiness. Vomiting is more frequent in children, and diaphoresis does not occur. In adults symptoms may be delayed for 12 to 24 h. Loss of consciousness is **not** a feature; and if it is present either another cause or another drug has been taken concomitantly or in place of APAP. In extremely large acetaminophen overdoses producing blood levels greater than 800 µg/ml at 15 h after ingestion, central nervous system (CNS) effects including coma, apnea, hypotension, hypothermia and metabolic acidosis have been reported in young children (41,42).
   B. **Phase II** is a period of diminished symptoms.
   C. **Phase III** occurs 72 to 96 h after ingestion with peak liver function abnormalities. Although the degree of elevation of the hepatic enzymes does not correlate with outcome, values greater than 1000 IU/L indicate hepatotoxicity. SGOT values up to 30,000 IU/L have been reported. Fewer than 1% of patients in stage III develop fulminant hepatotoxicity. If the hepatic damage is extensive, hepatic failure develops about the fourth to fifth day. Signs and symptoms include altered consciousness, hypoglycemia, and coagulation abnormalities. Jaundice does not usually become obvious before the fourth or fifth day.
      a. **Acute fulminant liver failure (AFHF)** is a clinical syndrome resulting from massive necrosis of liver cell leading to encephalopathy and severe impairment of hepatic function. The encephalopathy is usually present and prior liver disease is usually absent. The condition is potentially reversible (65).
      b. **Encephalopathy classification** (65)
         (1) **Grade I**—Confused or altered mood
         (2) **Grade II**—Inappropriate behavior or drowsiness (mild obtundation)
         (3) **Grade III**—Stuporous but arrestable, markedly confused behavior
         (4) **Grade IV**—Coma with or without decerebrate posturing unresponsive to painful stimuli.
   D. **Phase IV** occurs at 7 to 10 days, with hepatic enzyme abnormalities reaching resolution. Complete hepatic recovery can occur within 3 to 6 months. If extensive liver damage has

occurred, sepsis and disseminated vascular coagulation may ensue. Death may occur at 7 to 10 days.

1. **Transient renal failure** may develop at 5 to 7 days after ingestion. The renal damage occurs in some patients without evidence of hepatic damage (44,45). Acetaminophen's metabolite, para-aminophenol is nephrotoxic and concentrates in the renal papillae and APAP inhibits prostaglandin synthesis which causes vasoconstriction of the renal vasculature and medullary ischemia. Chronic daily use of APAP has been estimated as doubling the risk of end-stage nephropathy compared to those who took it twice a week (44–52). **Back pain, proteinuria,** and **hematuria** may occur at 36 to 48 h and are reported to herald renal failure.

2. **Other complications. Myocardial necrosis** (53), hemolytic anemia (54), methemoglobinemia (54), skin rashes, and pancreatitis (55,56) have been reported but are quite rare.

III. **Differential diagnosis.** As APAP is widely available and often a co-ingestant with other overdoses, it is important to screen for it in every patient who presents in a coma or who has taken an intentional ingestion. Other hepatotoxins to be considered if plasma levels fail to reveal APAP include *Amanita phalloides* mushroom and halogenated hydrocarbons. Most other hepatotoxins, however, produce symptoms early, which serves to differentiate them. Medically, infectious hepatitis, "shock liver, and Reye's syndrome should be excluded."

IV. **Laboratory analysis.** Early symptoms of toxicity may be minimally absent. Despite reports questioning the routine screening for APAP (57), it is recommended that all comatose patients and all those with intentional drug overdoses be screened. It is important that an appropriately timed plasma specimen be obtained for diagnostic evaluation and effective management of the overdosed patient because of the unreliability of historical information.

A. **Methods:** Nonspecific rapid colorimetric methods may underestimate APAP level. **Appropriate reliable methods** are radioimmunoassay, high pressure liquid chromatography (HPLC) and gas chromatography (GC). **Spectroscopic assays often give false elevated values** (61,62).

B. **Cross reactions.** Salicylate, salicylamide, diflunisal, and methyldopa increase the APAP level. Each mg/dl increase in creatinine increases the APAP plasma level 30 mcg/ml (61,62).

C. **Use of the level.** The plasma APAP value should be determined no sooner than 4 h after ingestion (after the distribution phase) and should be plotted on the **modified Rumack-Matthew (RM) nomogram** (28,63) to assess potential toxicity (Fig. 31-2).

D. The Rumack-Matthew nomogram used in the United States (Fig. 31-2) has a "probable hepatic toxicity risk line" and a lower "possible hepatic toxicity line." It is recommended that the antidote NAC (Mucomyst) be administered if the intersecting concentrations and time coordinates are above the lower line and that the course of therapy be completed **even if the subsequent values fall below the toxic zone** (40,63). However, English toxicologists using i.v. NAC therapy and "treatment line" recommend discontinuing NAC if the plasma APAP falls below "the treatment line" (28,60). Woo et al. using oral NAC recommend NAC therapy be discontinued if plasma APAP is undetectable and liver enzymes are not elevated (59). A multicenter study is planned to investigate the different protocols.

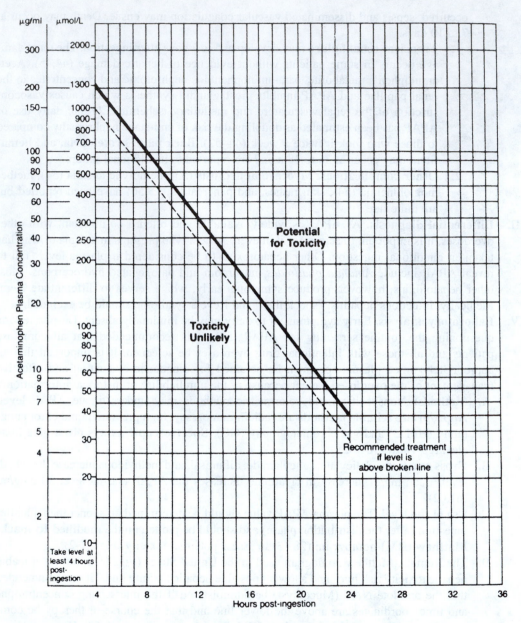

FIG. 31-2. Nomogram

E. Limitations of the nomogram. The nomogram is based on the plasma APAP concentrations after a **single** ingestion. The applicability of the "treatment lines" for children has never been proven and its validity beyond 15 h is uncertain (60). However, 417 children with potentially serious amounts were analyzed on the protocol and there were no deaths or hepatic abnormalities on discharges. Hepatotoxic effects were shown to be less in this pediatric population due to differences in metabolism (14). **Concomitantly ingested drugs** (i.e., opioid-acetaminophen combination, anticholinergic agents) **or carbohydrate-rich foods** may change the gastric emptying time and the peak time. Additional concentrations may be needed to determine the peak (40,64). We recommend repeat plasma APAP concentrations be obtained, 2 to 4 h after the initial 4-h level if this level is 20 μg/ml or greater or if the patient has a history of ingesting a toxic amount (more than 140 mg/kg). Delayed toxic plasma APAP concentrations, after 4-h nontoxic APAP concentrations have been reported and are more common than the single report in the literature would indicate (64).

F. If the plasma APAP concentrations cannot be determined and a significant overdose is suspected, **oral therapy** should be started within the first 8 to 10 h (58). If it is unclear how long since ingestion, err on the longest-duration side. If the time of ingestion is unknown but is between 4 to 24 h, a patient with a serum APAP level of more than 5 mcg/ml requires treatment with **N-acetylcysteine (NAC)** for the full prescribed course (59,60) (Fig. 31-2).

G. Liver enzyme elevation. We found the liver enzymes may increase as early as 4 h after ingestion and as late as 36 h (64). The pattern of liver test profiles typically seen in the different types of hepatitis may be helpful in differentiating the etiologies (Table 31-2).

H. Monitor **liver and renal profiles** including bilirubin, prothrombin time, serum amylase (55,56), coagulation tests, and blood glucose. CBC, platelet count, phosphate (66), electrolytes, HCO3, ECG (53), and urinalysis should be obtained in toxic cases.

TABLE 31-2. *Clinical features differentiating hepatotoxicity*

	Alcoholic with APAP hepatotoxic	Suicide ingestion of acetaminophen	Alcoholic hepatitis	Viral hepatitis
AST/SGOT (IU/L)	Markedly increased more than ALT	Normal initially, later may be marked increased	Usually <300	Hundreds to thousands
ALT/SGPT (IU/L)	Increased but less AST	Normal initially, later may be marked increased	Normal or slight increase	Variable, less than AST
AST/ALT ratio	>2	<2	>2	>1
Prothrombin time	Increased to markedly increased	Normal initially, later may be increased	Increased but usually under 30 sec	Increased
Acetaminophen	Normal or slight increase	Increased	Normal	Normal
Acute viral studies[a]	Negative (−)	Negative (−)	Negative (−)	+/(−)[b]

[a] Hepatitis B surface antigen, hepatitis B core IgM, Hepatitis A IgM.
[b] May be negative with nonA, nonB viral hepatitis.
APAP, acetaminophen; AST, aminotransferase (SGOT); ALT, alanine aminotransferase (SGPT).
Adapted from ref. 21.

I. **Prognostic laboratory values.** The following factors have been demonstrated to be of significance in predicting mortality in patients with fulminant hepatic failure. (HHF) due to acetaminophen toxicity (65). [See also Section IIc].

      (1) Absolute blood pH below 7.3. This has a 95% positive predictive value (PPV) for mortality (65).

      (2) In nonacidemic patients, the combination of grade III coma, creatinine greater than 3.3 mg/dL and PT greater than 100 s (PPV 57%). The creatinine as an independent predictor was of the least value (PPV 35%).

      (3) Factor V less than 10% activity and grade III coma. (PPV 91%). Factor VIII/V greater than 30%. (PPV 95%) (120).

      (4) Persistent rise in PT from day 3 to 4. PPV 93% (60). Some authorities start prophylaxis against hepatic encephalopathy if the IN PT ratio rises to more than 3.0 (11–14,36,38).

      (5) The total bilirubin has been identified as a marker for survival. The higher the value the more likely the patient was to live (65). This is contrary to earlier reports.

V. **Management** (Fig. 31-3)

  A. **GI decontamination.** If patient presents within 1 h of a substantial ingestion, it would seem reasonable to **administer activated charcoal** (AC) and a **cathartic** to adult patients. This would probably be unnecessary in young children most of whom will have taken on minor overdoses (28,67–69).

    1. **Studies on GI decontamination of APAP.** Studies on gastric lavage within 6 h produced a mean of 39% fall in APAP plasma concentration (70). Syrup of ipecac-induced emesis lowered the APAP plasma level by 41% (67). A volunteer study of ipecac-induced emesis at 60 min after ingestion reduced the area under the curve (AUC) by 21% (68). In 20 patients 50 g of AC 1 h after ingestion produced a mean fall of 52% in the plasma APAP. **Emesis is best avoided** in the emergency department because it may interfere with the retention of AC and NAC (51). The use of **gastric lavage has been questioned** because it is labor-intensive and may contribute to delayed AC administration. Studies have indicated that AC effectively absorbs significant amounts of APAP when given in an 8:1 ratio (69–80).

    2. **Charcoal controversy** (69–80). In vivo studies demonstrated a decrease in serum NAC, about 30%, when the antidote N-acetylcysteine (NAC), was administered 30 min after the activated charcoal (76). It had been suggested AC not be used with NAC, that increasing the dose of NAC, gastric lavage of charcoal and separation of the AC and NAC may result in sufficient hepatoprotection (77,78). However further studies indicated that not even this separation was not necessary (79,80). **Therefore, the administration of activated charcoal does not interfere with NAC** sufficiently to warrant separation of AC from NAC or increasing the dose of NAC (79,80). However the separation of the AC and NAC is still recommended on the basis that the combination is more likely produce vomiting of NAC.

    3. **Multiple doses of AC** has been shown to decrease the circulating APAP by "gastrointestinal dialysis" however the clinical significance as far as lowering the

ACETAMINOPHEN (APAP) INGESTION

Caution. An Acetaminophen Extended Release (Tylenol ER is embossed on the caplet side) was introduced in August, 1994 containing 650 mg APAP/caplet. The blood levels of this product have not been extensively studied in overdose. See addendum at end of algorithm for suggested management of extended release preparation overdose.

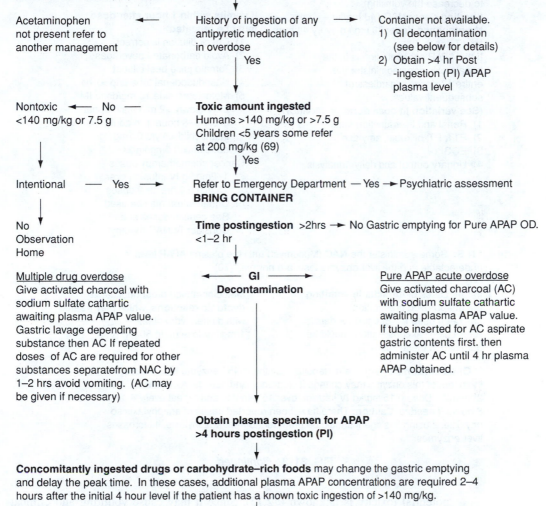

Acetaminophen not present refer to another management ← History of ingestion of any antipyretic medication in overdose → Container not available.
1) GI decontamination (see below for details)
2) Obtain >4 hr Post -ingestion (PI) APAP plasma level

↓ Yes

Nontoxic ← No — **Toxic amount ingested**
<140 mg/kg or 7.5 g Humans >140 mg/kg or >7.5 g
Children <5 years some refer at 200 mg/kg (69)

↓ Yes

Intentional — Yes → Refer to Emergency Department — Yes → Psychiatric assessment
BRING CONTAINER

No
Observation
Home **Time postingestion** >2hrs → No Gastric emptying for Pure APAP OD.
<1–2 hr

Multiple drug overdose
Give activated charcoal with sodium sulfate cathartic awaiting plasma APAP value. Gastric lavage depending substance then AC If repeated doses of AC are required for other substances separatefrom NAC by 1–2 hrs avoid vomiting. (AC may be given if necessary) ← **GI Decontamination** → **Pure APAP acute overdose**
Give activated charcoal (AC) with sodium sulfate cathartic awaiting plasma APAP value. If tube inserted for AC aspirate gastric contents first. then administer AC until 4 hr plasma APAP obtained.

**Obtain plasma specimen for APAP
>4 hours postingestion (PI)**

Concomitantly ingested drugs or carbohydrate–rich foods may change the gastric emptying and delay the peak time. In these cases, additional plasma APAP concentrations are required 2–4 hours after the initial 4 hour level if the patient has a known toxic ingestion of >140 mg/kg.

APAP blood level hepatoxic or enzyme inducer (Alcoholism or anticonvulsants) Lower nomogram values 50% (controversial) → Specimens obtained after 24 hr PI may be useful in management but can not be used on nomogram. → APAP blood levels can not be obtained for 8 hrs. Start NAC therapy.

FIG. 31-3. Acetaminophen (APAP) ingestion.

(continued)

↓

**Administer N–acetylcysteine
(NAC)** Do not double loading dose
because AC was or is given
(separate the two if possible
to decrease the vomiting)
Loading dose: NAC 140 mg/kg — Vomits ⟶
Maintenance dose: 70 mg/kg every 4 hours
for 17 doses. *
If the APAP concentration is in the
hepatotoxic zone administer the
entire 17 doses regardless of
subsequent values.
(See variation in dose duration Monitor)
1) Renal and liver function tests
2) PTT, PT, bilirubin, amylase
3) ECG
4) Urinary output and daily urinalysis

**If vomits within 1 hour after dose
must be repeated**
1) Check dilution is correct
2) Avoid carbonated beverages
3) Tomato juice best diluent
4) Nasodueodenal tube drip >1 hr
5) Metoclopramide 10 mg/dose IM
   or IV slowly >2 min may repeat
   every 6–8 hours prn adults. In
   infant/child <6 yrs 0.1mg/kg/
   dose max 0.5mg/kg/24h.
Cancer chemotherapy doses
   1–2mg/kg IV infusion over
   15 min q 2 hrs for 2 doses
6) Ondansetron may be used
   See caution doses at end **
7) Consider IV NAC therapy

* N.B. Some administer the **NAC** (Mucomyst) until the plasma APAP level is
undetectable and the liver enzyme tests are normal. (70)

In rare cases of **intractable vomiting**
the unapproved preparation
has been used IV. See text for details.
A toxicological consultation should be
obtained in these cases.

Metoclopramide/droperidol cause
dystonic reactions, which may treated
with diphenhydramine.
1 mg/kg/dose up to 50 mg IV

** Ondansetron (Zofran) is a metabolized by the P-450 enzyme thus inducers or
inhibitors of this enzyme may change it clearance and half-life. Available as
2 mg/mL. Dose 0.15 mg/kg IV infusion over 15 minutes and repeat every 4 and
8 hours if needed. **Caution:** There have been reported cases of anaphylaxis so
physicians using this agent should be prepared to treat anaphylaxis. It increases
liver enzymes.

FIG. 31-3. *Continued*

potential toxicity is unknown (72,73). Since it may cause vomiting and clinical
effect is uncertain MDAC is not recommended unless co-ingestants warrant it.

4. **Saline sulfate cathartics** are preferred because they may enhance the activity of
the sulfate metabolic pathway and provide hepatic protection. Saline cathartic
should be avoided in the presence of renal failure (12–14,81).

B. *N*-Acetylcysteine (NAC) is used for hepatotoxic overdose on the basis of nonrandomized
trials carried in UK using a "200 treatment line" (82,83) and in North America using a
"150 treatment line" (28,38,58). Patients were treated only if presented within 24 h.

Addendum

Deviations from conventional therapy of APAP
1. Variations in the duration of NAC therapy

   a. Short Course of NAC Therapy. Some experts recommend **variable duration** of NAC therapy. Woo et al. are discontinuing the NAC therapy if the APAP blood levels become nondetectable, **and** the liver function tests remain normal after 24 hours [59]. If the plasma acetaminophen (APAP) level is not detectable and there is no elevation of the aspartase aminotransferase (AST), there is little benefit from further NAC therapy. Similarly when the dose is unknown or appears to be excessive (>140–200 mg/kg) the same logic applies for dicontinuing therapy [114]. However, in some patients it has been noted that the aspartase aminotransferase (AST) does not start to rise until after 36 hours post-ingestion and we recommended therapy be discontinued **after the aspartase aminotransferase** has remained normal after 36 hrs [115].

   b. Late treatment with N-acetylcysteine has been shown to decrease the morbidity and mortality in patients with **fulminant hepatic failure** caused by acetaminophen and other hepatotoxins. The mean time of therapy was reported as late as 53 hours after ingestion of acetaminophen. This benefit requires that the treatment be continued indefinitely until the encephalopathy resolves or the patient dies [115–118].

2. Extended Release Acetaminophen overdose

In August of 1994 **Extended Relief (ER) Caplets** were introduced. Each caplet contains 325 mg of immediate release acetaminophen, and 325 mg of extended release acetaminophen. Using **a single 4-hour plasma APAP level may under-estimate the peak concentration** of APAP because of a possible delayed peak and lead to failure to treat patients with potentially toxic APAP levels [119]. In a report of 8 patients with **extended release overdose,** there were 4 patients whose elimination phase was not apparent until 5–12 hours after ingestion, suggesting continued absorption beyond the usual 2–4 hours. The mean elimination half-lives for 8 patients was 3.3 +/– 0.7 (range 2.1–4.9 hours) [119]. **It is recommended** that **at least 1** additional APAP levels be drawn **4-8 hours after the first level,** with initiation of NAC therapy if either level is above the nomogram line but not if both levels fall below the line. Additional levels are useful in the presence of co-ingestants [119].

FIG. 31-3. *Continued*

1. **Mechanism of action.** NAC is an *N*-acetyl derivative of the amino acid cysteine, which constitutes the central portion of the glutathione molecule. Presumably NAC is metabolized by the hepatocyte to a glutathione precursor (cysteine) that provides protective levels of a glutathione surrogate to detoxify the hepatotoxic reactive metabolite NAPQI by providing sulfhydryl groups (10–13,37,38,82–88). It may also enhance sulfation conjugation (11,58,89). Although the treatment has never been evaluated in a controlled trial, there is substantial evidence for its beneficial effect (60).

2. **Controversy** exists over the route of administration (82–92). Theoretically, oral administration results in more availability of the antidote at the site of injury (liver) via the portal circulation and avoids anaphylactoid reactions. However, the i.v. route avoids the risk of treatment failure by vomiting and the Prescott et al. (83,84) protocol is much shorter, 20 h versus 72 h. Prescott (83) estimated 15% of patients continue to vomit after admission. Adverse reactions using the i.v. route are reported to be about 15% and most are minor, however anaphylactoid reactions have occurred with i.v. administration (60,83–93).

   a. **Oral NAC**—The **dose** of oral NAC for the treatment of APAP intoxication is a **loading dose of 140 mg/kg** (10% NAC: 1.4 ml/kg; 20% NAC: 0.7 ml/kg) followed by 70 mg/kg q4h for 17 additional maintenance doses (1/2 of the loading dose), giving a total of 1,330 mg/kg over 72 h. An additional dose is administered if the patient vomits the dose within 1 h after administration. The original solution is administered as a 5% solution diluted in fruit juice or a noncarbonated soft drink (11–13,36,50,66). This is the basis of our present day therapy in the United States. There were no deaths among the treatment group that presented within 10 h with levels in the toxic range defined as a "150 treatment line." NAC was protective regardless of initial plasma APAP concentration (47). NAC treated patients within 16 h had no deaths, however there were 11 deaths among 2,540 patients with elevated liver enzymes before treatment with NAC was started. Of 1,630 patients who did not complete the full course only 33 had hepatotoxicity (58). Table 31-3 calculates the amount (rounded off) of the **loading dose** of 20% NAC (0.7 ml/kg) and the diluent required for a 20% solution to make a less irritating 5% solution for oral administration. **The maintenance dose** is one-half the loading dose. If only 10% NAC is available, the loading dose (in milliliters of 10% NAC) is double the amount of the 20% solution and the diluent is the same as this amount added to the 10% solution to make 5%, i.e., a 70-kg person requires 100 ml 10% NAC and 100 ml diluent. The maintenance dose is one-half the loading dose of 10% NAC.

b. **Intravenous (i.v.) NAC.** An i.v. preparation has been used in Europe and Canada for about 20 years but is not approved in the United States. **Anaphyl-**

TABLE 31-3. *Table of NAC dilutions for loading dose*

Body Weight (kg)	Mycomyst mL 20%	Grams NAC	Diluent mL add to 20%	5% solution total mL
140–149	100–105	20–21	300–315	400–420
130–139	90–95	18–19	230–285	320–380
120–129	85–90	17–18	255–270	340–360
110–119	75–80	15–16	225–240	300–320
100–109	70–75	14–15	210–225	280–300
90–99	65–70	13–14	195–210	260–280
80–89	55–65	11–13	165–195	220–260
70–79	50–55	10–11	150–165	200–220
60–69	40–50	8–10	120–150	160–200
50–59	35–40	7–8	105–120	140–160
40–49	30–35	6–7	90–105	120–140
30–39	20–30	4–6	60–90	80–120
20–29	15–20	3–4	45–60	60–80
10–19	7.5–15	1.5–3	23–45	30–60

Calculation equation for determining the loading dose dilution:

Equation: 140 mg × 70 kg (pt wt kg) = 9,800 mg NAC

$$20\% = \frac{20\,g}{100\,mL} = \frac{9.8\,g\ NAC}{X\,mL} = X = 49\ mL\ of\ 20\%\ NAC;\ dilute\ to\ 5\%\ by\ adding\ volume\ of\ diluent\ equal\ to\ three\ times\ the\ volume\ of\ 20\%\ NAC\ dose$$

The maintenance is half the loading dose.

actoid response to i.v. NAC has been described. They usually begin within 20 min after starting therapy and subsides when stopped. There have been 38 cases compiled. The frequency was estimated at 0.3% to 3% of courses of correctly administered NAC and 11 of 15 overdose or ten times more frequent. The reactions consisted of bronchospasm, angioedema, rash, pruritus and hypotension (94). **The duration of the i.v. regime is 48 h.** The loading dose is 140 mg/kg of 0.2 g/mL NAC (**diluted to 3% solution** made by adding one part of NAC to five parts of D5W. This is infused slowly through a 22-micropore filter over 1 h followed by the **12 maintenance doses of 70 mg/kg** diluted in a similar manner of 1:5 in DSW and administered over 1 h every 4 h over 48 h (60). In circumstances when i.v. administration of the oral preparation is **absolutely** necessary, a 20- to 30-μm filter is required. The 48-h i.v. regime is comparable when compared with patients with the 72-h (3 day) oral and the 20-h i.v. regimen when started within 10 h. The 48-h i.v. regime when started within 10 to 24 h is as effective as the 72-h oral NAC and superior to the 20-h i.v. regime when more than 16 h has occurred after ingestion. The optimum treatment after 16 h postingestion is unclear.

3. **Variations in the duration of NAC therapy.** Some experts recommend **variable durations** of NAC therapy. Woo et al. are stopping the NAC therapy if the blood levels fall to nondetectable and the liver function tests remain normal at 24 h (59). If there is neither a detectable acetaminophen level nor any elevation of the aspartase aminotransferase there is little benefit of NAC and the patient does not require therapy. Similar logic should be applied when the dose is unknown or appears to be excessive or toxic (114). However some liver function tests do not start to rise until after 24 h so it is best to be sure the liver enzymes do not rise after 36 h (115). **Late treatment** with *N*-acetylcysteine has been shown to decrease the morbidity and mortality in patients with fulminant liver failure caused by acetaminophen when the mean time of therapy was 53 h after ingestion. This benefit requires that the treatment be continued indefinitely until the encephalopathy resolves or the patient dies (115–118).

    a. **Intravenous NAC protocol for 20 h:** Prescott et al. (83,84,90) have used a 20-h regimen of 300 mg/kg administered as 150 mg/kg i.v. in 200 mL D5W over 15 min followed by 50 mg/kg in 500 mL D5W over 4 h followed by 50 mg/kg in 500 mL of D5W over 4 h, then 100 mg/kg in 1,000 mL D5W over 16 h. In 60 patients, they reported a 3% incidence of hepatic toxicity if therapy was started within 12 h of exposures, but a 67% incidence of toxicity if it was started between 10 to 16 h of exposure.

    b. **Intravenous NAC protocol for 48 h:** Smilkstein et al. (89) reported on 179 patients with acute overdose who received NAC for potential toxic plasma APAP levels on the Rumack-Matthew nomogram. Multiple and chronic overdoses were excluded. **Hepatotoxicity** defined as AST or ALT of more than 1,000 IU/L was uncommon in all groups treated within 10 h (4.3%). Hepatotoxicity was found in 5 of 50 (10%) of "probable risk" when started within 10 h and in 23 of 85 (27.1%) of those who were started within 10 to

24 h. Among the "high risk" patients started at 16 to 24 h, hepatotoxicity occurred in 11 of 19 (57.9%) patients. Two of 179 (1.1%) patients died. **Adverse reactions** occurred in 32 of 223 patients (14.3%) consisting of a transient (resolved within 1 h) skin rash or mild urticaria in 29 (91%) of patients. Adverse reactions did not require discontinuation of i.v. NAC (89).

4. **For acetaminophen overdoses: administer and complete an entire course of NAC** if a toxic dose has been ingested or if the initial plasma concentration (specimen obtained 4 h after ingestion) is above the toxic line (more than 150 mcg/ml at 4 h or more than 40 mcg/ml at 12 h) on the nomogram shown in Fig. 31-2 (35). However some experts discontinue NAC when the plasma APAP concentration is undetectable if the liver enzymes are not elevated at 24 h (59,60) or 36 h (59,121). Since this is controversial we recommend consulting with a Regional Poison Control Center and Medical toxicologist for further advice.

5. **NAC is most effective when administered during the first 8 to 10 h after ingestion** (28,38,58,60,64). The loss of efficacy 16 h after ingestion is not complete (58,60). There is no advantage to giving the NAC earlier than 4 to 6 h after ingestion. The benefits of late NAC therapy (i.e., beyond 10 h from the time of ingestion) from both prospective (107,114) and retrospective studies (95,96) show improved survival (95,96,107,114), improved cardiovascular response (107) and fewer incidences of cerebral edema (114).

6. **Procedure for oral administration.** NAC should be offered orally in a covered "takeout beverage container" through a straw. It is preferably diluted with slightly acidic tomato juice or a "flat" soft drink. If emesis occurs within 1 h of administration, the dose should be repeated. If vomiting occurs, check the dilution: If the correct dilution is vomited, it may be necessary to place a radiopaque tube past the stomach into the duodenum and administer the antidote by a slow drip over 1 h.

   a. If these measures are unsuccessful, give an antiemetic drug such as **metoclopramide** (Reglan) 10 mg/dose i.v. over 1 to 2 min every 30 min (maximum 1 to 2 mg/kg/24 h). In children, give metoclopramide 0.1 mg/kg up to a maximum of 0.5 mg/kg/day. (The manufacturer states that metoclopramide may increase APAP absorption, but this point is probably clinically unimportant.)

   b. **Ondansetron** (Zofran) is used as a last resort, if metoclopramide fails. It is metabolized by the P-450 enzyme, thus inducers or inhibitors of this enzyme may change its clearance and half-life. It is available in a concentration of 2 mg/mL. Dose 0.15 mg/kg i.v. infusion over 15 min and repeat every 4 and 8 h if needed. There have been reported cases of anaphylaxis so physicians using this agent should be prepared to treat anaphylaxis. It increases liver enzymes (97).

7. **Extended release (ER) acetaminophen overdose.** In August 1994, ER tablets were introduced. Tylenol ER is embossed on the caplet side. Each tablet contains 325 mg of immediate relief acetaminophen and 325 mg of ER per tablet. Using a single 4-h serum acetaminophen may underestimate the peak concentration of APAP ER because of a possible delayed second peak (119). In a report of eight

patients with ER overdoses, there were four patients in whom the elimination phase was not apparent until 5 to 12 h after ingestion, suggesting continued absorption beyond the usual 2 to 4 h. The mean elimination half-lives for eight patients was 3.3 ± 0.7 (range 2.1 to 4.9 h) (119). A single 4-h level may lead to failure to treat patients with potentially toxic levels. It is recommended to draw at least one additional level at 4 to 6 h after the first with initiation of NAC therapy if either level is above the nomogram line but not if both levels fall below the nomogram line. Additional levels may be useful in the presence of coingestants (119).

8. **Chronic acetaminophen intoxication**. Repeated chronic overdose can produce toxic levels and hepatotoxicity. NAC administration appears justified in the presence of hepatotoxicity caused by APAP no matter what the time since the last dose(122). Indications for therapy with NAC are:

   (1) history of more than recommended dose for several days or repeated APAP overdosing at risk of hepatotoxicity

   (2) Elevated liver function tests

   (3) Serum acetaminophen level inconsistent with therapuetic dose

   (4) Persistent vomiting

   (5) Chronic administration of 4 to 6 g daily for 3 to 4 days especially in chronic alcoholics is considered an indication for NAC if the liver function tests are abnormal.

C. **Avoid** administering the agents listed in Table 31-4 as they may compete with APAP for the conjugation pathway or stimulate enzyme induction and increase the toxic metabolite (40). It has been reported that the APAP plasma concentration may not be in the toxic range when the patient is chronically using enzyme inducers (16–29,40), but the toxicity due to the metabolite may be present. Some experts recommend that NAC be started at 50% below the range of toxicity. A Regional Poison Control Center and

TABLE 31-4. *Agents to avoid in acetaminophen overdose.*
AVOID the following agents which may compete with acetaminophen for the conjugation pathway or stimulate enzyme induction with chronic use and increase the formation of the toxic metabolite.

Agents that decrease conjugation	Enzyme Inducers
Phenolphthalein	Barbiturates
Dicoumarol	Chronic alcohol abuse
Testosterone	Phenytoin
Hydroxyzine	Imipramine
Morphine	Chloral hydrate
Chloramphenicol	Ethchlorvynol
Prednisolone	Glutethimide
Tetracycline	Haloperidol
Estrogens	Meprobamate
Salicylamide	Phenylbutazone
Vitamin C	Tolbutamide
Salicylate	

Medical Toxicologist should be consulted for further guidance since this is controversial. The medications that decrease conjugation should be avoided in patients with potential **APAP** toxicity.

D. **Pregnancy.** The available data appear to indicate no teratogenicity for APAP or NAC. Animal data indicate that the fetal liver cells are capable of oxidizing drugs during early pregnancy and can form toxic metabolites. **It is recommended that pregnant patients with a toxic blood concentration of APAP be treated with NAC to prevent hepatotoxicity in both fetus and mother.** Animal data seems to indicate that the transplacental NAC is clinically insignificant. In a series of 609 patients in pregnancy with an overdose of APAP, 24 had APAP considered toxic and were treated with NAC. Of 10 treated within 10 h, eight delivered normal infants and two had elective abortions. Of 10 patients treated within 10 to 16 h, three delivered normal infants and two had elective abortions and three spontaneous abortions. In four patients treated at 16 to 24 h postingestion, one patient died and had a stillborn, one spontaneous abortion, 12 elective abortion, and one a normal infant (52,103,104,106). **Currently, there are no recommendations for either the early termination or delivery of a fetus in the setting of APAP toxicity.** The treatment of hepatic and renal failure in this setting differs from that of any other etiology.

E. **Fulminant hepatic failure** (FHF)—Obtain expert consultation and consider liver transplantation.

   1. **Administer a course of NAC** (if not previously administered) and continue until recovery. A retrospective study of i.v. NAC administered 10 to 36 h postingestion in 100 patients who developed acetaminophen-induced and other types of fulminant liver failure, reported progression to severe coma significantly less and a lower mortality. It is postulated that NAC replenishes the sulfhydryl groups, restores full activity to endothelial-derived releasing factor and may enhance the endogenous production of nitric oxide which dilates hepatic vessels and improves microcirculatory hepatic blood flow leading to improved tissue oxygenation. (60,96,107)

   2. A randomized study involving 50 patients with **APAP-induced liver failure** who presented at 33 to 96 h after ingestion, 25 patients received NAC 150 mg/kg i.v. followed by 50 mg/kg over 4 h and 100 mg/kg over an additional 16 h. The final infusion was continued until the patients recovered from encephalopathy or died. Survival was significantly more common in the NAC treated patients 48% vs 20% among controls. (96)

   3. **Liver transplant.** Liver transplant has a definite but limited role in acute APAP overdose (96). Some investigators have considered an SGOT transaminase level above 10,000 IU/L as indication for considering evaluation for a liver transplant.

      a. **Indicators.** See prognostic factors in Section III.J for guidance in addition to contacting a Regional Poison Control Center, Medical Toxicologist and Liver Transplant Unit.

      b. **The contraindications for liver transplantation are** acceptable alternative therapy; suboptimal quality of outcome; impairment of other organ systems; major systemic infection; and the disease is expected to recur (110).

      c. Of six liver transplants for APAP poisoning, four survived for 1 year and two died. Of eight who did not get transplants, one survived. In another group of 17 patients recommended for liver transplant, 10 actually had surgery, six of seven not transplanted died, and seven out of 10 transplanted survived. The authors recommend transfer to a liver unit for PT (in seconds) greater than the interval from ingestion in h; PT more than 50 s; metabolic acidosis on presentation; and an established encephalopathy. There were no deaths in patients who were not encephalic at transfer (111). Two additional patients successfully received liver transplants in whom the authors considered this an option because of rapidly progressive encephalopathy, hemolysis, and hepatorenal failure (112). The liver transplants reported

F. Dialysis is recommended if renal failure persists more than 48 h. Hemodialysis reduces the half-life of APAP, but there is no evidence it alters the clinical course (44–52). Hemoperfusion in three patients with grade 3 encephalopathy produced no benefit (104). Dialysis was usually performed from 4 to 19 days after ingestion (113).

G. Other antidotes. No other effective antidotes in the US. Some authorities in England and Finland prefer methionine as an antidote (60). Cimetidine, a cytochrome P450 enzyme antagonist, has been suggested as an antidote, but the results are equivocal and it needs time to produce enzyme inhibition (98–103).

VI. Disposition

A. Patients asymptomatic with nontoxic plasma APAP levels obtained at least 4 h after ingestion and an additional APAP done 4 h after the first level, when indicated, may be transferred or discharged after psychiatric evaluation.

B. Patients with a potential hepatotoxic concentration of APAP should be admitted and receive a full course of NAC therapy.

C. Early antidotal therapy is beneficial. Patients who ingest over 140 mg/kg or 7.5g, should receive therapy within the first 8 h until a plasma APAP level is obtained.

D. NAC has been shown to be beneficial even after 24 h if the liver enzymes are elevated or there are other laboratory signs of liver impairment.

E. The Regional Poison Center should be consulted in situations where the role of NAC therapy is unclear.

VII. Deviations from conventional therapy of APAP

A. **Variations in the duration of NAC therapy**

1. **Short course of NAC therapy.** Some experts recommend **variable duration** of NAC therapy. Woo et al. are discontinuing the NAC therapy if the APAP blood levels becomes nondetectable, **and** the liver function tests remain normal after 24 h (59). If the plasma acetaminophen (APAP) level is not detectable and there is no elevation of the aspartase aminotransferase (AST), there is little benefit from further NAC therapy. Similarly when the dose is unknown or appears to be excessive (140 to 200 mg/kg) the same logic applies for discontinuing therapy (114). However, in some patients it has been noted that the aspartase aminotransferase (AST) does not start to rise until after 36 h postingestion and we recommended therapy be discontinued **after the aspartase aminotransferase** has remained normal after 36 h (115).

2. **Late treatment** with *N*-acetylcysteine has been shown to decrease the morbidity

and mortality in patients with **fulminant hepatic failure** caused by acetaminophen and other hepatotoxins. The mean time of therapy was reported as late as 53 h after ingestion of acetaminophen. This benefit requires that the treatment be continued indefinitely until the encephalopathy resolves or the patient dies (115–118).

B. **ER acetaminophen overdose.** In August of 1994, **ER caplets** were introduced. Each caplet contains 325 mg of immediate release acetaminophen, and 325 mg of ER acetaminophen. Using **a single 4-h plasma APAP level may under-estimate the peak concentration** of APAP because of a possible delayed peak and lead to failure to treat patients with potentially toxic APAP levels (119). In a report of eight patients with **ER overdose,** there were four patients whose elimination phase was not apparent until 5 to 12 h after ingestion, suggesting continued absorption beyond the usual 2 to 4 h. The mean elimination half-lives for eight patients was 3.3 ± 0.7 (range 2.1 to 4.9 h) (119). **It is recommended** that **at least one additional** APAP levels be drawn **4 to 8 h after the first level,** with initiation of NAC therapy if either level is above the nomogram line but not if both levels fall below the line. Additional levels are useful in the presence of co-ingestants (119).

References

1. Davidson DGD, Eastham WN. Acute liver necrosis following overdose of paracetamol. *BMJ* 1966;2:497–499.
2. Thomson JS, Prescott LF. Liver damage and impaired glucose tolerance after paracetamol overdose. *BMJ* 1966;2: 506–507.
3. Litovitz TL, Felberg L, Soloway RA. 1994 annual report of the American Association of Poison Control Centers Toxic Exposure Surveillance System. *Am J Emerg Med* 1995;13:551.
4. Henretig FM, Selbst SM, Forrest C. Repeated acetaminophen overdose. *Clin Pediatr* 1989;28:525.
5. Agran PF, Zenk KE, Romansky SG. Acute liver failure and encephalopathy in a 15 month old infant on repeated doses of acetaminophen. *Am J Dis Child* 1983;137:1107.
6. Swetnam SM, Florman AL. Probable acetaminophen toxicity in an 18 month old infant due to repeated overdosing. *Clin Pediatr* 1984;23:104.
7. Nogen AG, Bremner JF. Fatal acetaminophen in a young child. *J Pediatr* 1978;92:832.
8. Blake KV, et al. Death of a child associated with multiple overdoses of acetaminophen. *Am J Dis Child* 1988;7:391.
9. Nobota MC, et al. Acetaminophen accumulation in pediatric patients after repeated therapeutic doses. *Eur J Clin Pharmacol* 1984;27:57.
10. Mitchell JR, et al. Acetaminophen-induced hepatic necrosis. I. Role of drug metabolism. *J Pharmacol Exp Ther* 1973; 187:185.
11. Mitchell JR, Thorgeirsson SS, Potter WZ. Acetaminophen-induced hepatic injury: protective role of glutathione in man and rational for therapy. *Clin Pharmacol Ther* 1974;16:676.
12. Rumack BH, Peterson RC, et al. Acetaminophen overdose: 662 cases with evaluation of oral acetylcysteine treatment. *Arch Intern Med* 1981;141:380.
13. Rumack BH. Acetaminophen overdose: incidence, diagnosis, and management in 416 patients. *Pediatrics* 1978; 62:898.
14. Rumack BH. Acetaminophen overdose in young children: treatment and effects of alcohol and additional ingestants in 416 cases. *Am J Dis Child* 1984;138:428–433.
15. Mathis RD, et al. Subacute acetaminophen overdose after incremental dosing. *J Emerg Med* 1987;6:37.
16. Goldfinger R, et al. Concomitant alcohol and drug use enhancing acetaminophen toxicity. *Am J Gastroenterol* 1978; 70:385.
17. Leser PB, Vietti MM, Clark WD. Lethal enhancement of therapeutic doses of acetaminophen by alcohol. *Dig Dis Sci* 1986;31:103.
18. Seeff L, et al. Acetaminophen hepatotoxicity in alcoholics. *Ann Intern Med* 1986;104:399.
19. Lieber CS. Medical disorders of alcoholism. *N Engl J Med* 1995;333:1058–1064.
20. Lauterberg BH, Velez ME. Glutathione deficiency as a risk factor for paracetamol hepatotoxicity. *Gut* 1988;29: 1153–1157.

21. Kumar S, Rex DK. Failure of physicians to recognize acetaminophen hepatotoxicity in chronic alcoholics. *Arch Intern Med* 1991;151:118.
22. Cheung L, Potts RG, Meyer KC. Acetaminophen treatment nomogram. *N Engl J Med* 1994;330:1907–1908.
23. Davies A. Acetaminophen poisoning and liver function. *N Engl J Med* 1994;331:1311.
24. Whitcomb DC. Acetaminophen poisoning and liver function. *N Engl J Med* 1994;331:1311–1312.
25. British National Formulary, no. 27. London: British Medical Association, 1990.
26. McClements BM, Hyland M, Callender ME. Management of paracetamol poisoning complicated by enzyme induction due to alcohol or drugs. *Lancet* 1990;1:1526.
27. Minton NA, Henry JA, Frankel RJ. Fatal paracetamol poisoning in an epileptic. *Hum Toxicol* 1988;7:33.
28. Vale JA, Proudfoot AT. Paracetamol (acetaminophen) poisoning. *Lancet* 1995;346:547–552.
29. Bray GP, Harrison PM, O'Grady JG. Long-term anticonvulsant therapy worsens outcome in paracetamol-induced fulminant hepatic failure. *Hum Exp Toxicol* 1992;11:265–270.
30. Nolan CM, et al. Hepatotoxicity associated with acetaminophen usage in patients receiving multiple drug therapy for tuberculosis. *Chest* 1994;105:408.
31. Staal FJT, Ela SW, Roederer MM, et al. Glutathione deficiency and human immunodeficiency virus infection. *Lancet* 1992;339:909–912.
32. Buhl R, Holroyd KJ, Mastrangeli A. Systemic glutathione deficiency in symptom-free HIV-seropositive individuals. *Lancet* 1989;11:1294–1297.
33. Kaalebi T, Kinter A, Poli G, et al. Suppression of human immunodeficiency virus expression in chronically infected monocytic cells by glutathione, glutathione ester, and *N*-acetylcysteine. *Proc Natl Acad Sci USA* 1991;88:986–990.
34. Miller RP, Roberts RJ, Fisher LM. Acetaminophen elimination kinetics in neonates, children, and adults. *Clin Pharmacol Ther* 1976;19:284.
35. Peterson RG, Rumack BH. Age as a variable in acetaminophen overdose. *Arch Intern Med* 1981;141:390.
36. Rumack BH. Acetaminophen overdose in children and adolescents. *Pediatr Clin North Am* 1986;33:691.
37. Mitchell JR, et al. Acetaminophen-induced hepatic injury: protective role of glutathione in man and rationale for therapy. *Clin Pharmacol Ther* 1974;18:676.
38. Yerman B, Tseng J, Caraviti E. Pediatric Acetaminphen ingestion: a prospective study of referral criteria [Abstract 115]. *Clin Toxicol* 1995;33:530.
39. Gorman S, Klein-Schwartz W, Oderda G. Pediatric Acetaminophen ingestion—when is health care referral necessary? [Abstract 16]. Presented at the AACT/AAPCC/ABMT/CAPCC 23rd Annual Meeting, Toronto, Oct. 1–4, 1991.
40. Linden CH, Rumack BH. Acetaminophen overdose. *Emerg Clin North Am* 1984;2:103.
41. Lieh-Lai M, Sarnaik A, Newton J, et al. Metabolism and pharmacokinetics in a severly poisoned young child. *J Pediatr* 1984;105:125–128.
42. Flanagan RJ, Mani TK. Coma and metabolic acidosis in severe acute paracetamol poisoning. *Hum Toxicol* 1986;5:179–182.
43. Singer A, Caraccio TR, Mofenson HC. The temporal profile of increased transaminase levels in patients with acetaminophen-induced liver dysfunction. *Ann Emerg Med* 1995;26:49–53.
44. Wilkerson SP, et al. Frequency of renal impairment in paracetamol overdose compared with other causes of liver disease. *J Clin Pathol* 1977;30:141.
45. Habersang RW. Severe hepatotoxicity, renal failure and panocytopenia in a young child after repeated acetaminophen overdose. *Clin Pediatr* 1994;33:42.
46. Ronco PM, Flahault A. Drug-induced end-stage renal disease. *N Engl J Med* 1994;321:1711–1712.
47. Curry RW, Robinson D, Sughrue MJ. Acute renal failure after acetaminophen ingestion. *JAMA* 1982;247:1012.
48. Coden I, et al. Paracetamol-induced acute renal failure in the absence of fulminant liver damage. *BMJ* 1982;28:21.
49. Prescott LP, Proudfoot AJ, Cregren RJ. Paracetamol-induced acute renal failure in the absence of fulminant liver disease. *BMJ* 1982;28:421.
50. Jeffrey WH, Lafferty WE. Acute renal failure after acetaminophen overdose: report of 2 cases. *Am J Hosp Pharm* 1981;38:1355.
51. Phillans P, Hall C. Paracetamol-induced renal failure in the absence of severe liver damage. *S Afr Med J* 1985;67:791.
52. Kaysen GA, et al. Combined hepatic and renal injury in alcoholics during therapeutic use of acetaminophen. *Arch Intern Med* 1985;145:2019.
53. Sanerkin NG. Acute myocardial necrosis in paracetamol poisoning [Letter]. *BMJ* 1971;3:478.
54. McClean D, et al. Paracetamol and methemoglobinemia. *BMJ* 1968;1:390.
55. Gilmore IT, Tourase E. Paracetamol-induced pancreatitis. *BMJ* 1977;2:753.
56. Mofenson HC, Caraccio TR, Naraz H, Steckler G. Acetaminophen-induced pancreatitis. *J Toxicol Clin Toxicol* 1991;29:223–230.
57. Ashbourne JF, Olsen KR, Khayam-Bashi H. Value of rapid screening for acetaminophen in all patients with intentional drug overdose. *Ann Emerg Med* 1989;18:1036.

58. Smilkstein MJ, Knapp GL, Kulig KW, et al. Efficacy of oral *N*-acetylcysteine in the treatment of acetaminophen overdose. *N Engl J Med* 1988;319:1557.

59. Woo OF, Anderson IB, Kim SY, et al. A shorter duration of *N*-acetylcysteine for acute acetaminophen poisoning [Abstract 57]. *Clin Toxicol* 1995:33:508.

60. Harrison PM, Keays R, Bray GP, et al. Serial prothrombin time as a prognostic indicator in paracetamol-induced fulminant liver failure. *BMJ* 1990;301:964–966.

61. Bridges R, Kinneburgh D, Keehn B, et al. An evaluation of the common methods for acetaminophen quantitation for small hospitals. *Clin Toxicol* 1983;20:1.

62. Osterloh J. Limitations of acetaminophen assays. *J Toxicol Clin Toxicol* 1983;20:19.

63. Rumack BH, Matthew H. Acetaminophen poisoning and toxicity. *Pediatrics* 1975:55:871–876.

64. Tighe TV, Walter FG. Delayed toxic acetaminophen level after initial four hour nontoxic level. *Clin Toxicol* 1994;32:431–434.

65. O'Grady JG, Alexander GJM, Hayllar KM, et al. Early indicators of prognosis in fulminant liver failure. *Gastroenterology* 1989;97:439–445.

66. Jones AF, Harvey JM, Vale JA. Hypophoshataemia and phosphaturia in paracetamol poisoning. *Lancet* 1989;2: 608–609.

67. Underhill TJ, Greene MK, Dove AF. A comparison of the efficacy of gastric lavage, ipecacuahana and activated charcoal in the emergency management of paracetamol overdose. *Arch Emerg Med* 1990;7:148–154.

68. Amitai Y, Mitchell AA, McGuigan MA. Ipecac-induced emesis and reduction of the plasma concentrations of drugs following accidental overdose in children. *Pediatrics* 1987;80:364–367.

69. McNamara RM, et al. Efficacy of activated charcoal: cathartic versus ipecac in reducing serum acetaminophen in simulated overdose. *Ann Emerg Med* 1989;18:934.

70. Dordon B, et al. Reduction in the absorption of paracetamol by activated charcoal and cholestyramine: a possible therapeutic measure. *BMJ* 1973;1:86.

71. Levy G. Effect of activated charcoal on acetaminophen absorption. *Pediatrics* 1976;58:432.

72. Bainbridge CA, et al. In vitro absorption of acetaminophen onto activated charcoal. *J Pharm Sci* 1977;66:480.

73. Klein-Schwartz W, et al. Absorption of oral antidotes for acetaminophen poisoning (methionine and *N*-acetylcysteine) by activated charcoal. *Clin Toxicol* 1981;18:283.

74. Chinmouth RW, et al. *N*-Acetylcysteine absorption by activated charcoal. *Vet Hum Toxicol* 1980;22:392.

75. North DS, et al. Effect of activated charcoal administration on acetylcysteine levels in humans. *Am J Hosp Pharm* 1981;38:1022.

76. Renzi F, et al. Concomitant use of activated charcoal and *N*-acetylcysteine. *Ann Emerg Med* 1985;14:568.

77. Elkins BHR, et al. The effect of activated charcoal on *N*-acetylcysteine in absorption in normal subjects. *Am J Emerg Med* 1987;5:483.

78. Chamberlain J, Gorman R, Oderda GM, et al. Use of activated charcoal in a simulated poisoning with acetaminophen: a new loading dose for *N*-acetylcysteine. *Ann Emerg Med* 1993;22:1398–1402.

79. Brent J. Are activated charcoal-*N*-acetylcysteine interactions of clinical significance? [Editorial]. *Ann Emerg Med* 1993;22:1900–1903.

80. Spiller HA, Krenzelok EP, Grande GA, et al. A prospective evaluation of the effect of activated charcoal before oral *N*-acetylcysteine in acetaminophen overdose. *Ann Emerg Med* 1994;23:519.

81. Slattery JT, Levy G. Reduction in acetaminophen by sodium sulfate in mice. *Res Commun Chem Pathol Pharmacol* 1977;18:167.

82. Prescott LF, et al. Treatment of severe paracetamol poisoning with intravenous *N*-acetylcysteine. *Arch Intern Med* 1981;141:386–389.

83. Prescott FF, Illingworth RN, Critchley JAHH, et al. Intravenous treatment is the treatment of choice for paracetamol poisoning. *BMJ* 1979;2:1097.

84. Prescott L. Paracetamol overdose: pharmacologic considerations and clinical management. *Drugs* 1983;25:290.

85. Lauterberg BH, et al. The effects of age and glutathione depletion on hepatic glutathione turner in vivo determined by acetaminophen probe analysis. *J Pharmacol Exp Ther* 1980;213:54.

86. Jollow DJ, et al. Acetaminophen-induced hepatic necrosis. II. Role of covalent binding in vivo. *J Exp Pharmacol Ther* 1973;187:195.

87. Potter WZ, et al. Acetaminophen-induced hepatic necrosis. III. Cytochrome oxidase P-450-mediated covalent binding in vitro. *J Exp Pharmacol Ther* 1973;187:203.

88. Slattery JT, et al. Dose-dependent pharmacokinetics of acetaminophen: evidence of glutathione depletion in humans. *Clin Pharmacol Ther* 1987;41:413.

89. Smilkstein MJ, Bronstein AC, Linden C, et al. Acetaminophen overdose 48 hours intravenous *N*-acetylcysteine treatment protocol. *Ann Emerg Med* 1991;20:1058–1063.

90. Prescott LF, et al. Treatment of severe paracetamol poisoning with intravenous *N*-acetylcysteine. *Arch Intern Med* 1981;141:386–389.

91. Mant TGK, et al. Adverse reactions to acetylcysteine and effects of overdose. *BMJ* 1984;2:217.
92. Batemann DN, et al. Adverse reactions to intravenous *N*-acetylcysteine. *Hum Toxicol* 1984;3:393.
93. Vale JA, Wheeler DC. Anaphylactoid reactions to IV NAC. *Lancet* 1982;2:988.
94. Sunman W, Hughes AD, Sever PS. Anaphylactoid response to intravenous acetylcysteine [Letter]. *Lancet* 1992;339:1231–1232.
95. Flanagan R. The role of acetylcysteine in clinical toxicology. *Med Toxicol* 1987;2:93.
96. Harrison PM, Keays R, Bray GP, et al. Improved outcome of paracetamol-induced hepatic failure by late administration of acetylcysteine. *Lancet* 1990;335:1572.
97. Comparison dexamethasone and ondansetron in prophylaxis of emesis induced in moderately emetogenic chemotherapy. *Lancet* 1991;338:483–487.
98. Kadri AZ, Fisher R, Winterton MC. Cimetidine and paracetamol hepatotoxicity. *Hum Toxicol* 1988;7:205.
99. Speeg KV Jr, Mitchell MC, Maldonaldo AL. Additive protection of cimetidine and *N*-acetylcysteine treatment against acetaminophen-induced hepatic necrosis in the rat. *J Pharmacol* 1985;234:550.
100. Critchley JAJH, et al. Is there a place for cimetidine or ethanol in the treatment of paracetamol? *Lancet* 1983;2:1375.
101. Vendemiale G, et al. Effect of acute and chronic cimetidine administration on acetaminophen metabolism in humans. *Am J Gastroenterol* 1987;82:1031.
102. Slattery JT, et al. Lack of effect of cimetidine on acetaminophen disposition in humans. *Clin Pharmacol Ther* 1989;46:591.
103. Burkhart K, et al. Cimetidine as adjunct treatment for acetaminophen overdose. *Vet Hum Toxicol* 1989;31:337.
104. O'Grady JG, et al. Controlled trials of charcoal hemoperfusion and prognostic factors in fulminant hepatic failure. *Gastroenterology* 1988;94:1186.
105. Riggs BS, et al. Acute acetaminophen overdose during pregnancy. *Obstet Gynecol* 1989;74:247.
106. Selden SS, Curry SC, Clark RF. Transplacental transport of *N*-acetylcysteine in a ovine model. *Ann Emerg Med* 1991;20:1069–1071.
107. Harrison PM, Wenon JA, Gimson AES, et al. Improvement by acetylcysteine in hemodynamics and oxygen transport in fulminant hepatic failure. *N Engl J Med* 1991;324:1852–1857.
108. O'Grady JG, Alexander GJM, Halylar KM, et al. Early indicators of prognosis in fulminant liver failure. *Gastroenterology* 1989;97:439–445.
109. Harrison PM, Keays R, Bray GP, et al. Serial prothrombin time as a prognostic indicator in paracetamol induced fulminant liver failure. *BMJ* 1990a;301:964–966.
110. Whitington PF, Ballisteri WF. Liver transplantation in pediatrics: indications, contraindications, pretransplant management. *J Pediatr* 1991;118:169–177.
111. Mutimer DJ, Ayres RCS, Neuberger JM, et al. Serious paracetaminol poisoning and the results of liver transplantation. *Gut* 1994;35:809–814.
112. O'Grady JG, Wendon J, Tan KC, et al. Liver transplantation after acetaminophen overdose. *BMJ* 1991;303:221–223.
113. Mrvos R, Schneider SM, Dean BS, et al. Orthoptic liver transplants necessitated by acetaminophen-induced hepatotoxicity. *Vet Hum Toxicol* 1992;34:425–427.
114. Keays R, Harrison PM, Wendon JA, et al. IV acetylcysteine in paracetamol induced fulminant hepatic failure: a prospective controlled treatment. *BMJ* 1991;303:1026–1029.
115. De Roos FJ, Hoffman RS. Drug-induced hepatoloxicity. *N Engl J Med* 1996;334:863.
116. McNamara RM, et al. Efficacy of activated charcoal cathartic versus ipecac in reducing serum acetaminophen in simulated overdose. *Ann Emerg Med* 1989;18:934–938.
117. Harrison PM, Keays R, Bray GP, et al. Improved outcome of paracetamol-induced hepatic failure by late administration of acetylcysteine. *Lancet* 1990;335:1572–1573.
118. Harrison PM, Wendon JA, Gimson AES, et al. Improvement by acetylcysteine of hemodynamics and oxygen transport in fulminant hepatic failure. *N Engl J Med* 1991:324:1852–1957.
119. Cetaruk EW, Dart RC, Horowitz RS, et al Extended-release Acetaminophen overdose [Letter]. *JAMA* 1996:275:688.
120. Pereira LMMB, Langley PG, Hayllar KM, et al. Coagulation Factor V and VIII/V Ratio as predictors of outcome in paracetaminol induced fulminant hepatic failure: relation to other prognostic indicators. *Gut* 1992;33:98–102.
121. Bizovi K, Keyes N, Rivas J, et al. Tylenol ER, late rise in APAP level after overdose. *Clin Toxicol* 1996;33:510.
122. Habersang RW. Severe hepatotoxicity, renal failure and panocytopenia in a young child after repeated acetaminophen overdose. *Clin Pediatr* 1994;33:42.
123. De Roos FJ, Hoffman RS. Drug-induced hepatotoxicity. *N Engl J Med* 1996;334:863.

Emergency Toxicology, Second Edition,
edited by Peter Viccellio.
Lippincott–Raven Publishers, Philadelphia © 1998.

32

Nonsteroidal Antiinflammatories

†Richard Y. Wang, °Bonnie Simmons, and *Diane Sauter

†*Department of Emergency Medicine, Brown University, Rhode Island Hospital, Providence, Rhode Island 02903; °Department of Emergency Medicine, North General Hospital, Mt. Sinai Affiliate, New York, New York 10035; *Metropolitan Hospital, New York, New York 10029*

Nonsteroidal antiinflammatory drugs (NSAIDs) have become the mainstay of therapy for arthritis and are widely prescribed for common strains and sprains. The introduction of over-the-counter (OTC) NSAIDs has led to a greater availability of these agents and thus an increase in accidental and nonaccidental poisonings. In general, patients who ingest toxic quantities of NSAIDs manifest gastrointestinal (GI) and central nervous system (CNS) disturbances that are usually self-limiting. There are, however, an increasing number of serious and even fatal outcomes resulting from acute renal and hepatic failure, respiratory depression, coma, convulsions, cardiovascular collapse, and cardiac arrest (1).

I. **Properties of the agent**
   A. **Sources and forms.** The NSAIDs comprise a large group of drugs with similar therapeutic actions and side effects. A variety of formulations exists. Ketorolac (Toradol) can be administered parenterally. Diclofenac, ketorolac, flurbiprofen, and suprofen can be found as **ophthalmic solutions. Sustained release** preparations are available with diclofenac, naproxen, and indomethocin.
   B. **Mechanism of action and toxicity.** These compounds inhibit cyclooxygenase, the enzyme that mediates the initial step of the synthesis of prostaglandins. It is this inhibition that accounts for the antiinflammatory and analgesic properties of these nonsteroidal agents. The **side effects** common to all the NSAIDs are also the result of prostaglandin inhibition. They occur even at therapeutic levels (2).
      1. **GI:** nausea, vomiting, abdominal pain, GI hemorrhage from local irritation.
      2. **Hematologic:** blood dyscrasias and hemorrhage, which results from impaired platelet aggregation. Reversible prolongation in bleeding time occurs with NSAID use.
      3. **Renal:** sodium, potassium, and water retention and renal failure secondary to volume depletion, acute interstitial nephritis nephrotic syndrome, and papillary necrosis.
      4. **Cardiac:** worsening of congestive heart failure secondary to sodium and water retention.
      5. **Obstetric:** delay in the onset of labor, prolonged labor, and an increased risk of hemorrhage for the mother and fetus. NSAID use may cause closure of the ductus arteriosus by inhibition of prostaglandin synthesis.
      6. **Gynecologic:** dysfunctional uterine bleeding.

7. **Neurologic:** minor CNS disturbances, including drowsiness, blurred vision, and cognitive dysfunction in the elderly.

8. **Hypersensitivity reactions:** acute exacerbations of asthma in 8% to 20% of adult asthmatics with nasal polyps, occurring within minutes to hours after ingestion of an NSAID (2).

C. **Drug interactions.** The NSAIDs, through effects on renal prostaglandins, may cause increased toxicity when given in conjunction with certain other drugs, including other NSAIDs, oral anticoagulants, oral hypoglycemics, sulfonamides, phenytoin, methotrexate, digitoxin, and lithium.

D. **Physical and chemical properties.** For the purpose of systematic evaluation of this wide range of compounds, it is helpful to subdivide the NSAIDs into six groups based on their chemical structure (2).

1. **Salicylates.** Salicylate toxicity is discussed elsewhere (see Chapter 30).

2. **Pyrazolones.** This group includes phenylbutazone and oxyphenbutazone (withdrawn from the market). **Phenylbutazone** is available for veterinary use and can be found in some herbal preparations.

   a. **Pharmacokinetics.** Phenylbutazone is rapidly and completely absorbed from the GI tract, with peak plasma levels reached in 2 h. More than 98% is protein-bound. It is extensively **metabolized** by oxidation and conjugation with glucuronic acid. Its elimination **half-life** is unusually long, approximately 75 h. It is a more effective antiinflammatory agent than many of the other NSAIDs, but serious, even life-threatening side effects limited its use (1,3).

   b. **Clinical presentation.** Toxicity may be classified as mild, early-onset severe, and delayed-onset severe (1).

      (1) **Mild toxicity** is characterized by drowsiness, abdominal pain, and nausea.

      (2) **Early-onset severe:** Symptoms include vomiting and diarrhea, GI hemorrhage, hyperventilation, dizziness, **seizures** (especially in children), metabolic acidosis, respiratory alkalosis and electrolyte disturbances, hematuria, sodium and water retention, hypotension, pulmonary edema, coma, and respiratory or cardiac arrest. In addition, hypoprothrombinemia, thrombocytopenia, agranulocytosis, and aplastic anemia have been described (1,3).

      (3) **Delayed-onset severe:** Renal failure and hepatic necrosis have been described as long as 1 week after ingestion (3–5). Severe toxicity has been reported following the ingestion of 4 g in an adult.

   c. **Laboratory evaluation.** As the toxicity of the individual agents is evaluated in the same manner, the following statements may apply to all NSAIDs. In general, serum levels of NSAIDs are not widely available and are of little use. Although plasma ibuprofen levels have been measured in the past and a nomogram exists (6), neither is considered by most toxicologists to be clinically useful and is not recommended by these authors. A baseline urinalysis, BUN, and serum creatinine should be obtained initially. More consequential medical illnesses and ingestions should be evaluated.

    d. Management and disposition

       (1) The toxicity of phenylbutazone may be associated with life-threatening symptoms. **Aggressive treatment** is indicated in all settings in which reasonable suspicion of an ingestion exists even when the patient is asymptomatic, especially children.

       (2) **Gastric lavage** followed by repeated doses of oral activated **charcoal** and one dose of a **cathartic** is indicated initially. Patients who have already vomited usually do not require lavage because they have emptied their own stomachs. Similarly, patients with diarrhea do not need cathartics. Management from this point is symptomatic and supportive. Respiratory and cardiac parameters must be closely monitored. Renal function must be observed for signs of insufficiency. Forced diuresis is of no value, as the drug is largely protein-bound. Hemoperfusion may be attempted in extreme cases, although there is, as yet, no clear evidence that it is beneficial (2).

3. Indoleacetic acids (pyroles). This group includes the drugs **diclofenac,** etodolac, **ketorolac,** indomethacin, sulindac, tolmetin, and zomepirac (taken off the market).

    a. Pharmacokinetics. Indomethacin is rapidly and nearly completely absorbed from the GI tract. It is 90% protein-bound and has an elimination **half-life** of 2 to 11 h (7). Indomethacin undergoes **enterophepatic recirculation.**

    b. Clinical presentation. Indomethacin is generally considered to have less toxicity than phenylbutazone. Following the ingestion of indomethacin, patients may complain of nausea, vomiting, abdominal pain, and tinnitus; and they may exhibit drowsiness, lethargy, confusion, disorientation, and restlessness. The usual course is self-limiting. Vascular headaches commonly occur even with therapeutic serum levels. They are often described as frontal in location and often occur after the morning dose.

    c. Management and disposition. Gastric lavage should be performed in cases of serious overdosage. Activated charcoal should be given and repeated every 4 h for symptomatic ingestions of sustained/delayed (e.g., diclofenac) formulations or NSAIDs that undergo enterohepatic recirculation. The remainder of the treatment is supportive and symptomatic.

    d. Other indoleacetic acids. No serious side effects have yet been described in the few reported cases of sulindac or tolmetin overdose. **Sulindac** is metabolized into a sulfone that is responsible for the severe characteristic diarrhea often observed. **Tolmetin** is often prescribed for the pediatric population because it has fewer CNS side effects than indomethacin. **Zomepirac** was taken off the market because of reported cases of severe anaphylactic reactions at therapeutic doses.

4. Phenylpropionic acids. The agents in this group include fenoprofen, flurbiprofen, **ibuprofen,** ketoprofen, naproxen, oxaprozin, and benoxaprofen (taken off the market). In general, overdoses with propionic acids do not result in significant morbidity or mortality, although deaths after overdoses with ibuprofen and fenoprofen have occurred (1). Ibuprofen, the most widely used of the group, is also, to date, the most extensively studied. It is an analgesic antiinflammatory with moderate antipyretic action.

a. **Pharmacokinetics.** Ibuprofen is rapidly **absorbed** from the GI tract and is approximately 99% protein-bound. Its elimination **half-life** is 2.0 to 2.5 h. Neither the rate of absorption nor elimination seems to be altered by overdose. Symptoms therefore usually appear within 4 h and have a short duration. A single dose of ibuprofen is **metabolized** by the liver and is completely **excreted** in the urine within 24 h.

b. **Clinical presentation**

(1) Poisoning with **ibuprofen** is usually manifested by mild GI symptomatology. Toxicity, in general, is without major consequences if managed appropriately. In the presence of normal renal function, patients usually recover fully within 24 h. However, there have been a number of reports of severe, sometimes fatal outcomes following the onset of acute renal or hepatic failure, hypotension, and coma (6,9–12).

(2) In general, the amount of ibuprofen ingested does not correlate well with symptomatology in adults. One patient remained asymptomatic after the ingestion of 24 g of ibuprofen (6).

(a) **Therapeutic dose range** in adults is 400 to 2,400 mg/kg/day and 20 to 50 mg/kg/day in children. More than 400 mg/kg is associated with serious toxicity in children.

(b) Common **symptoms** of poisoning with ibuprofen include nausea, anorexia, vomiting, abdominal pain. Rarely, GI hemorrhage occurs, especially in the elderly (13). CNS depression, drowsiness, lethargy, nystagmus, tinnitus, hyperventilation, headache, diplopia, and seizures have been reported (6). Other symptoms include rash, hypotension, bradycardia, apnea, hypoprothrombinemia, and hypothermia.

(c) Renal insufficiency and renal failure secondary to papillary necrosis are reversible after supportive therapy (14). Also described are hematuria, proteinuria, metabolic acidosis with increased anion gap in adults and children, respiratory depression, and cardiac arrest (15).

c. **Management and disposition**

(1) **Ingestion of less than 100 mg/kg:** Dilute with milk or water to decrease GI toxicity.

(2) **Ingestion of more than 100 mg/kg:** Emesis with syrup of ipecac or gastric lavage should be performed. Emesis is contraindicated in patients with any CNS depression, including an absent or depressed gag reflex, and in children who have ingested in excess of 400 mg/kg or whose medical history is significant for a seizure disorder.

(3) After gastric emptying is accomplished, activated **charcoal** and a saline **cathartic** should be administered. The activated charcoal dose should be repeated every 4 h for symptomatic ingestions of delayed release

formulations (e.g., ibuprofen). The remainder of treatment is symptomatic and supportive.

(4) **Hypotension** is best treated initially with i.v. fluids. If it persists, dopamine or norepinephrine may be required.

(5) Seizures are best controlled initially with i.v. diazapam followed by barbiturates.

(6) Symptomatic bradycardia, when it occurs, may respond to atropine.

(7) Severe **metabolic acidosis** (pH less than 7.10) may require the administration of sodium bicarbonate. Ibuprofen is an acidic compound, and although urine alkalinization has been recommended in the past to enhance urinary excretion, the drug's short half-life and extensive protein binding make it an ineffective intervention.

(8) In general, other than GI decontamination, there are no effective methods to enhance drug elimination. Dialysis has no role in the treatment of ibuprofen ingestions.

(9) As the amount of drug ingested is not a predictor of subsequent toxicity, all symptomatic adults and those who have attempted suicide must be observed for 24 h. Asymptomatic adults must be observed for 4 h. At that time, unless there is the need for psychiatric evaluation, discharge may be considered.

(10) As a general guide for **children,** an ingestion of less than 100 mg/kg is unlikely to result in toxicity. Under these circumstances and when the history is clear, observation at home with instruction about potential dangers may be appropriate. Ingestions of 100 to 200 mg/kg may be treated with emesis and observation at the hospital, or in a reliable home setting, for 4 h following the ingestion of 200 to 400 mg/kg. Children should be treated in a hospital setting with gastric decontamination and the administration of activated charcoal and a cathartic. A period of observation of not less than 4 h is appropriate with admission of patients who develop symptoms. Ingestion of more than 400 mg/kg in a child warrants concern. Gastric lavage should be performed immediately. Patients must be observed carefully for the development of seizure activity (16).

d. **Other propionic acids**

(1) The elimination half-life of **fenoprofen** is 2 h. It is extensively metabolized; only 5% is excreted unchanged in urine. One clinical study documented drowsiness as the only reported symptom in a pediatric population following the ingestion of excessive fenoprofen (1). Approximately half of the adults studied remained asymptomatic, and the other half developed drowsiness, ataxia, tinnitus, nausea, hypotension, tachycardia, and panting respirations. One woman developed hypothermia and coma after an isolated massive ingestive of fenoprofen. Within 5 h, she developed respiratory depression and cardiac arrest from which she could not be resuscitated. One British study documented the occurrence of hematuria and acute renal failure following the ingestion of large quantities of fenoprofen.

(2) **Naproxen** has been reported to induce GI symptoms as well as pulmonary infiltrates with associated eosinophilia and resolution following discontinuation of the drug (2). **Benoxaprofen** was taken off the market after many cases of severe toxicity manifested by vomiting, severe dizziness, lethargy, irritability, and hepatic failure. The elderly (less than 70 years) were particularly sensitive to toxic effects, and several hundred deaths apparently resulted from the toxicity of this agent. Treatment considerations are similar to those of the other phenyl propionic acids.

5. **Anthranilic acids.** Two members in this group are mefenamic acid and **meclofenamate.** Overdoses of the two may be treated in a similar manner. To date, there are no reported cases of overdose with meclofenamate. There is, however, one reported case of meclofenamate-included colitis (17).

   a. **Pharmacokinetics.** Mefenamic acid is well absorbed following oral dosing, and it has a **half-life** of 3 h. More than 50% is excreted unchanged in the urine, the remainder being excreted as the 3-hydroxymethyl conjugate.

   b. **Clinical presentation.** Toxicity with **mefenamic acid** may produce no symptoms. Muscle twitching, either focal or generalized, has been reported. It may begin within a few hours of ingestion and last several minutes (18). **Seizures** are a common occurrence following overdose. They may not begin until 4 h after ingestion and are not necessarily dose-related. Other symptoms may include severe diarrhea, rash, and an elevated BUN. These symptoms generally have their onset following at least 1 week of use, and they usually subside within 24 h after the last dose. Coma has been reported.

   c. **Management and disposition.** Treatment consists in basic poison management including gastric lavage and the administration of oral activated charcoal. Patients require close observation for the development of seizure activity, which may have an onset several hours after ingestion. As the drug has a relatively short half-life, recovery is generally is rapid.

6. **Oxicams**

   a. **Pharmacokinetics.** Piroxicam is structurally distinct from the other NSAIDs (19). It is extensively protein-bound and has a long elimination **half-life** of 45 h, resulting in moderately severe clinical toxicity.

   b. **Clinical presentation. Piroxicam** can cause a **photosensitivity** reaction. Patients must be instructed to use sunscreen when outside. Most patients who ingest excessive amounts of piroxicam usually do not develop symptoms, although severe symptoms have been reported, including GI hemorrhage, dizziness, excitability, hyperventilation, hematuria, proteinuria, renal and hepatic dysfunction, and hypoprothrombinemia (20).

   c. **Management and disposition**. Gastric lavage is performed, followed by repeated doses of oral activated charcoal for symptomatic ingestions. Piroxicam undergoes **enterohepatic circulation** (21).

II. To date, there is limited knowledge about many of the drugs in the NSAID family. Early, aggressive management is indicated for the pyrazolones (phenylbutazone and oxyphenbutazone) and anthranilic acids (mefenamic acid and meclofenamate), as these two groups are potentially the most toxic. Significant ingestions of the phenylpropionic acids, especially fenoprofen, may also result in life-threatening symptoms. The other NSAIDs appear thus far to be less problematic, although in each subgroup cases of severe toxicity have been reported. GI distress, electrolyte imbalance, and dehydration are common presenting disorders which can be effectively managed within a 24-h time period.

References

1. Court H, Volans GN. Poisoning after overdose with nonsteroidal anti-inflammatory drugs. *Adverse Drug React Acute Poisoning Rev.* 1984;3:1.
2. Howland MA, Weisman RS, Goldfrank LR. Nonsteroidal antiinflammatory agents. In: Goldfrank LR, et al., eds. *Goldfrank's toxicologic emergencies.* 4th ed. Norwalk, CT: Appleton-Century-Crofts, 1990:243–248.
3. Strong JE, et al. Phenylbutazone self-poisoning treated by charcoal haemoperfusion. *Anaesthesia* 1979;34:1038.
4. Prescott LF, Critchley JAJH, Balali-Mood M. Phenylbutazone overdosage: abnormal metabolism associated with hepatic and renal damage. *BMJ* 1980;281:1106.
5. Berlinger WG, et al. Hemoperfusion for phenylbutazone poisoning. *Ann Intern Med* 1982;96:334.
6. Hall AH, et al. Ibuprofen overdose; 126 cases. *Ann Emerg Med* 1986;15:1308.
7. Alvan G, et al. Pharmacokinetics of indomethacin. *Clin Pharmacol Ther* 1975;18:364.
8. Duggan DE, et al. The metabolism of indomethacin in man. *Pharmacol Exp Ther* 1972;181:563.
9. Barry WS, Meinzinger MM, Howse CR. Ibuprofen overdose and exposure in utero: results from a postmarketing voluntary reporting system. *Am J Med* 1984;77:35.
10. Hunt DP, Leigh RJ. Overdose with ibuprofen causing unconsciousness and hypotension. *BMJ* 1980;281:1458.
11. Court H, Streete P, Volans GN. Acute poisoning with ibuprofen. *Hum Toxicol* 1983;2:381.
12. Bennet RR, Dunkelburg JC, Marks ES. Acute oliguric renal failure due to ibuprofen overdose. *South Med J* 1985;78:490.
13. Beard K, et al. Nonsteroidal anti-inflammatory drugs and hospitalization of gastroesophageal bleeding in the elderly. *Arch Intern Med* 1987;147:1621.
14. Lee CY, Finkler A. Acute intoxication due to ibuprofen overdose. *Arch Pathol Lab Med* 1986;110:747.
15. Linden CH, Townsend PL. Metabolic acidosis after acute ibuprofen overdose. *J Pediatr* 1987;3:922.
16. Hall AH, et al. Ibuprofen overdose—a prospective study. *West J Med* 1988;148:653.
17. Doman DB, Goldberg HJ. A case of meclofenamate sodium-induced colitis. *Am J Gastroenterol* 1986;81:1220.
18. Prescott LF. Clinical features and management of analgesic poisoning. *Hum Toxicol* 1984;3:75.
19. Nuki G. Nonsteroidal analgesic anti-inflammatory agents. *BMJ* 1983;1:39.
20. Vale JA, and Meredith TJ. Acute poisoning due to nonsteroidal anti-inflammatory drugs. *Med Toxicol* 1986;1:12.
21. Ferry DG, et al. Enhanced elimination of piroxicam by administration of activated charcoal or cholestyramine. *Eur J Clin Pharmacol* 1990;39:599.

Emergency Toxicology, Second Edition,
edited by Peter Viccellio.
Lippincott–Raven Publishers, Philadelphia © 1998.

33

Antiinfective Agents

Joseph J. Sachter

Bronx, New York 10471-1804

Most of the more commonly used antibiotics are relatively nontoxic in overdose. Data demonstrate that, of more than 50,000 exposures involving antimicrobials, only five resulted in fatalities: three were complicated by other, more toxic substances, whereas the other two involved chloroquine (1). Although exposure to most antibiotic agents tends to be benign, this is in fact a common overdose. A recent study showed that one of eight drug-related emergency department (ED) visits involved antibiotics, the third most common drug class (ahead of respiratory drugs and pain medications) (2). This introduction contains a brief discussion of five commonly used antibiotics. The four drugs discussed in detail afterward have all caused fatalities in acute overdose. The toxicity of drugs utilized only via parenteral routes (e.g., aminoglycosides) is beyond the scope of this chapter. The reader is referred to a more comprehensive text (see Selected Readings) or the regional poison control center. Antiinfective agents discussed in separate chapters include quinine (see Chapter 51) and isoniazid (see Chapter 48).

I. **Commonly used antibiotics**

   A. **Cephalosporins.** This group of antibiotics, which currently includes nine oral and more than 16 parenteral preparations in three generations, appears to be relatively free of severe, acute toxicity. GI side effects (diarrhea, nausea, and vomiting) are the most common. Approximately 5% to 15% of parents who display allergy to penicillin have similar hypersensitivity reactions to the cephalosporins. Adverse reactions may include renal dysfunction (especially when used with other nephrotoxic drugs) and coagulopathies (especially with moxalactam) (3).

   B. **Erythromycin and other macrolide antibiotics.** Generally considered among the safest of the antibiotics, erythromycin's ability to enhance the effects of theophylline and digoxin are important in the setting of multiple-drug ingestions. Although rare, it has been linked with pseudomembranous colitis and Torsade de pointes (4). In the early 1990s, reports began to surface about **potential adverse interactions between erythromycin and two nonsedating antihistamines, terfenadine (Seldane) and astemizole (Hismanal).** These second generation H1 blockers were noted to cause prolonged QT intervals, Torsade de pointes, and, occasionally, sudden death in overdose situations. These agents are metabolized via P-450 metabolic pathways, and agents that inhibit these pathways, such as erythromycin, can—when taken in conjunction with these antihistamines—cause serious side effects even at recommended doses (5). The effect can be exacerbated in patients with liver dysfunction (especially cirrhosis) or patients taking antifungal agents such as ketoconazole or fluconazole. A recent study showed no similar effects with recommended doses of loratidine (Claritin), another nonsedating antihistamine and erythromycin (6). Two new antibiotics, azithromycin (Zithromax) and clarithromycin (Biaxin), share structural similarities to erythromycin. Their extended half-lives (once and twice daily dosing, respectively) and broad spectrum of coverage have made them popular choices in the outpatient setting. Although there are no case reports detailing interactions between these newer macrolide antibiotics and either terfenadine or astemizole, the structural similarities have caused many authorities to include such warnings. In the multiple overdose setting, the physician should also be aware that erythromycin may cause more rapid delivery of alcohol from the stomach to the small intestine and consequent reduced absorption by the gastric mucosa. It also appears to slow small bowel transit time, increasing overall alcohol absorption (7).

C. **Metronidazole.** Severe reactions from single large overdoses are rare. The largest acute overdose, almost 20 g, in a 27-year-old woman, resolved without sequelae (8). Chronic ingestions have reportedly resulted in both central (seizures, ataxia, and mental status changes) and peripheral (peripheral neuropathies) nervous system toxicity. The former are usually single episodes with recovery over a period of hours to days; the latter are paresthesias of the lower extremities that resolve over a period of months. Most of these case reports involved patients with severe underlying illnesses. Because metronidazole **inhibits alcohol dehydrogenase,** its most significant interaction is with alcohol, resulting in a disulfiram-like reaction (see Chapter 43). Reports have also appeared regarding the deliberate use of a combination of metronidazole and alcohol among teenagers to achieve a sense of giddiness.

D. **Penicillin.** Again, even large oral overdoses of penicillin are judged to be safe, usually resulting only in GI side effects. Physicians should be aware that this class of antibiotics is frequently involved in all types of hypersensitivity reactions. Although deaths are uncommon (more than 0.1%), the widespread use of these drugs is believed to result in approximately 500 fatalities per year from anaphylaxis, far more than for any other type of drug. Large, usually repetitive parenteral dosing has resulted in CNS toxicity, ranging from abnormalities of the mental status to frank seizures, often unresponsive to anticonvulsants. This may be a manifestation of the "caine reaction," resulting from the inadvertent i.v. administration of procaine penicillin preparations intended for intramuscular use.

E. **Quinolones.** Ciprofloxacin and norfloxacin are the two antibiotics available in this class of antibiotics. Overdoses have not been reported. The physician should be aware that these medications are absolutely contraindicated in children and pregnant women. Relatively small doses (100 mg/kg/day) have caused erosion of cartilage in immature animals, leading to permanent disability (9).

F. **Tetracycline.** Severe toxicity following an acute ingestion is rare. Reported complications of the chronic ingestion of increased dosages include benign intracranial hypertension and a Fanconi-like syndrome (polyuria, polydipsia, glycosuria, and hypokalemia) (10).

G. **A final word.** The reader is reminded to exercise caution when caring for patients who have ingested any of the above substances. Antibiotic ingestion frequently occurs as part of a multiple-substance overdose, often in combination with over-the-counter (OTC) medications. Many of these substances, including aspirin, acetaminophen, antihistamines, and decongestants, can cause significant morbidity. The physician must maintain a high index of suspicion for concurrent ingestion of these and other substances.

II. **Drugs causing fatalities in overdose**
  A. **Chloramphenicol**
    1. **Properties of the agent**
        a. Sources and forms. Chloramphenicol is available in a wide variety of preparations, including 250- and 500-mg capsules, a suspension (150 mg/5 mL), topical applications (creams, ointments, and a 0.5% or 1.0% solution), and parenteral forms.
        b. Physical and chemical properties. Chloramphenicol was originally discovered as a naturally occurring product of *Streptomyces venezuelae,* an actinomycete. It is currently synthesized from dichloroacetic acid.
        c. Mechanism of action. Chloramphenicol binds to the 50 S subunit of the 70 S ribosome, inhibiting protein synthesis. It is a broad-spectrum, bacteriostatic antibiotic.
        d. Pharmacokinetics. Chloramphenicol is rapidly and almost completely (75% to 90%) absorbed via the GI tract following oral administration. A dose of 15 mg/kg results in a serum level of 10 µg/mL (oral) to 20 µg/mL (i.v.). Peak levels occur 2 to 3 h after oral ingestion. The half-life is slightly less than 3 h in adults, twice that in children, and as long as 24 h in neonates. The apparent volume of distribution is approximately 1 L/kg; protein binding is roughly 50%.
    2. **Clinical presentation**
        a. **History.** Recent antibiotic use or availability is the most obvious and important element of the initial history. Chloramphenicol is prescribed infrequently in the United States, although its broad spectrum of coverage and relatively low cost make it a popular alternative in Third World countries, especially Africa and Asia. Thus recent travel or emigration from these regions increases the possibility of chloramphenicol involvement.
        b. **Physical examination**
            (1) The most serious form of chloramphenicol toxicity is the **"gray baby syndrome."** The syndrome begins with GI disturbances, including vomiting, anorexia, abdominal distention, and diarrhea, followed by hypothermia, progressive hypotension and pallor, and cyanosis. Further deterioration is marked by respiratory depression, hypotension, arrhythmias, and finally circulatory collapse. Virtually all deaths reported occurred in infants (age less than 3 months) receiving large dosages (more than 100 mg/kg). The syndrome has been reported in older children—a 14-year-old girl who responded to charcoal hemoperfusion (11)—as well as in adults (12).
            (2) **Hematologic toxicity** remains the most important toxic side effect associated with chloramphenicol usage. Two types of abnormality have been reported.

(a) **Aplastic anemia** has been termed "idiosyncratic" because it is not related to the route of administration and is rare. The occurrence rate has been estimated at less than one in 25,000 (13). Contrary to popular belief, aplastic anemia has been associated with both parenteral and oral routes of administration. The anemia is usually irreversible and thus carries an extremely poor prognosis.

(b) **Bone marrow depression** is a more common side effect. The effect is dose-related (serum levels are invariably more than 25 µg/L), progressive, and reversible upon discontinuation of the medication. It is marked by anemia and reticulocytopenia. Leukopenia and thrombocytopenia may also occur. Both serum iron and total iron-binding capacity are elevated. It has been postulated that the depression is secondary to the inhibition of mitrochondrial protein synthesis.

c. **Differential diagnosis.** Although chloramphenicol is used less frequently than in the past, anyone, especially infants, presenting with vomiting, anorexia, lethargy, and hypotension—especially without fever and leukocytosis—should be questioned about antibiotic usage. A history of chloramphenicol administration in this setting should prompt consideration of rapid diagnostic and therapeutic intervention (see below). However, because chloramphenicol is usually reserved for severe illnesses, the presence of concomitant infection makes many of the above criteria problematic. Changes in skin color (as well as hemodynamic instability) may result from cyanosis secondary to hypoxemia, shock, or both. In addition, the blue-gray color associated with methemoglobinemia/sulfhemoglobinemia may be mistaken for the gray baby syndrome described above.

d. **Laboratory studies.** Initial studies should include a CBC (with reticulocytes) and liver function tests. Although there is a correlation between peak chloramphenicol levels and subsequent toxicity, its use is complicated by a relatively short half-life (in adults) as well as lack of routine availability. Because the possibility of a multiple-substance overdose often cannot be excluded, other drug levels (e.g., acetaminophen) are usually indicated.

e. **Management and disposition**

(1) **Gut decontamination** is indicated. The relatively rapid absorption of chloramphenicol from the GI tract makes ipecac-induced emesis relatively less effective unless the ingestion was a recent one (0.5 to 1.0 h). Lethargy, obtundation, seizure activity, and an absent gag reflex are contraindications to the use of ipecac. The reader is cautioned that emesis may also complicate or delay the administration of activated charcoal.

(2) **Supportive care** remains the mainstay of treatment for the more serious hematologic consequences of chloramphenicol overdose. Respiratory support, administration of fluids or pressors, and monitoring and treatment of electrolyte disturbances may be indicated.

- **(3)** The bone marrow depression sometimes seen with chronic chloramphenicol use may be treated with the administration of blood products.
- **(4)** Hemodialysis has not been shown to be efficacious in this setting. Case reports do, however, indicate that charcoal hemoperfusion is beneficial (14).

B. Chloroquine. From a toxicologic viewpoint, chloroquine is without question **the most dangerous antimicrobial agent available today.** The proper adult loading dose (two tablets) has caused the death of a 3-year-old child (15). The documented ingestion of more than 600 mg chloroquine (1 g chloroquine phosphate) by a child or more than 1,500 mg by an adult is an absolute medical emergency requiring rapid and vigorous intervention regardless of the initial clinical presentation. In 1989, of more than 1.5 million exposures reported to poison control centers, only 140 involved antimalarials. However, it should also be noted that the only two deaths directly associated with antimicrobial use were chloroquine ingestions (1). Although chloroquine overdose is relatively rare in the United States, its use as an effective agent for suicide has been promoted in Europe (especially France), Africa, and the Middle East.

1. **Properties of the agent**
   a. **Sources and forms**
      - **(1)** Chloroquine is considered the treatment of choice for susceptible strains of malaria.
      - **(2)** The drug is usually dispensed as chloroquine phosphate, with 500 mg of the latter equivalent to 300 mg of chloroquine.
      - **(3)** It is available in 250- and 500-mg tablets (containing 150 and 300 mg of chloroquine, respectively).
      - **(4)** Recommended dosage for the chemoprophylaxis of malaria (as well as treatment of amebiasis) is two 500-mg tablets daily for 2 days, followed by one tablet weekly.
      - **(5)** Chloroquine hydrochloride is primarily used for intramuscular injection.
   b. **Physical and chemical properties.** Chloroquine is a 4-aminoquinolone derivative. It is a white powder that is water-soluble and discolors with exposure to sunlight.
   c. **Mechanism of action.** Chloroquine is considered a schizonticidal agent; that is, it attacks the asexual form of the malarial parasite. It is believed that the drug inhibits both DNA and RNA polymerases. With acute toxic ingestions, chloroquine is believed to **act directly on the myocardium,** depressing myocardial contractility and causing conduction disturbances. Its cardiotoxic effect has been likened to that of **quinidine,** and occasionally classic ECG changes such as widened QRS complex and a prolonged QT interval are noted.
   d. **Pharmacokinetics.** Chloroquine is rapidly and completely absorbed from the GI tract. Approximately half the drug is protein-bound. The apparent volume of distribution is high, probably more than 100 L/kg.
2. **Clinical presentation.** Significant chloroquine ingestions result in rapid deterioration. Headache, visual disturbances, dysphagia, and vomiting have been reported

as the initial symptoms. Although not a universal finding, movement disorders and seizures are frequently reported. Hypotension, respiratory depression, circulatory collapse, and cardiac arrest may soon follow.

a. **History.** A history of travel to countries where malaria is endemic is important. Parents must be questioned regarding the possibility of accidental ingestions among symptomatic children. A history of dysphagia or diplopia suggest the diagnosis.

b. **Physical examination.** Unfortunately, no signs are pathognomonic for chloroquine ingestion. The combination of neurologic and cardiologic abnormalities suggest the etiology.

c. **Differential diagnosis.** Given the wide range and possible severity of initial symptomatology, the differential diagnosis is vast. The combination of severe neurologic and cardiologic abnormalities in the setting of acute overdose may suggest tricyclic antidepressants, digitalis, class IA antiarrhythmics, phenothiazines, theophylline, or even carbamazepine.

d. **Laboratory studies.** Initial studies should include arterial blood gases and an ECG. Chloroquine levels are often difficult to obtain, but may have significant prognostic value (see **e.(3),** below).

e. **Management and disposition**

(1) The need for **rapid and vigorous intervention,** especially in the pediatric setting, cannot be overemphasized. Chloroquine is absorbed so rapidly and clinical deterioration can be so precipitous that the induction of emesis in the face of a documented supratherapeutic ingestion is probably contraindicated. When there is reasonable suspicion of a significant chloroquine ingestion, **sedation (with a benzodiazepam), intubation, and vigorous lavage using an orogastric tube are indicated.** Activated charcoal should then be given.

(2) Traditional management focuses on supportive care, using dopamine as the initial pressor of choice for hypotension. However, a 1988 French study (16), though small, yielded such impressive results that it bears review. The authors first retrospectively studied 51 chloroquine ingestions over a two year period. Ten of the eleven patients (91%) who ingested more than 5 grams of chloroquine died, whereas all 40 who ingested less than 5 g survived. The authors then used a multiple-drug regimen to treat the next 11 patients who presented with large (more than 5 g) ingestions and compared the results with those of the original 11 patients. The therapy consisted of rapid intubation (using thiopental; now contraindicated, see **e.(4),** below), gastric lavage, diazepam 2 mg/kg administered over 30 min, and epinephrine in boluses of 0.25 µg/kg/min until a systolic pressure of 100 mm Hg was achieved. Only one of the 11 patients who received the regimen died (p = 0.0003).

(3) It should be noted that the above regimen was started on the scene and that the patients were conscious at the initiation of the study. Animal studies (17) also suggest that diazepam may have a protective effect after acute chloroquine ingestion. Given the above, diazepam (in the intubated patient) appears to be a reasonable and proper intervention. The use of epinephrine (rather than dopamine or norepinephrine) is controversial but is not unreasonable in the setting of a documented, symptomatic chloroquine overdose.

(4) A just published retrospective study (18) from France gives valuable additional information about management and prognosis in acute chloroquine ingestions. The study reviewed 167 documented ingestions admitted to a special toxicology centered ICU over a five-year period, by far the largest such study ever published. The authors report an overall mortality of approximately 10%, with no correlation to amount ingested by history. They did however find a strong correlation with peak blood chloroquine levels; In patients with levels of more than 25 mmol/L, mortality was 21%, versus 1.6% in those with levels between 12 and 25 mmol/L (a single case where epinephrine was accidentally discontinued) and no fatalities among patients with levels of less than 12 mmol/L. The retrospective nature of the study did not allow the others to comment on the relative importance of the regimen advocated by Riou (see **e.(2),** above), although 87% of the patients received at least one arm of this combination therapy. The overall mortality rate here supports the use of aggressive interventions discussed earlier. The authors do however caution against the use of thiopental. Of nine patients who experienced cardiac arrest after care had begun, seven (77%) succumbed immediately after injection of thiopental. It is unclear whether other barbiturates, such as etomidate, would have similar adverse effects, but given the evidence available to date, the use of benzodiazepines as the primary agent for both induction and sedation appears warranted.

C. Dapsone

   1. Properties of the agent

      a. Sources and forms

         (1) Dapsone is a synthetic sulfone that is considered the drug of choice for the treatment of leprosy and dermatitis herpetiformis. Current recommendations for the treatment of leprosy include the concurrent administration of dapsone with clofazimine and rifampin. It has also been used for chemoprophylaxis of chloroquine-resistant malaria and treatment of the bite of the brown recluse spider.

         (2) It is available in 25- and 100-mg tablets.

         (3) Dosage is typically 1 mg/kg in children and 100 mg/day in adults.

      b. Physical and chemical properties. Dapsone is 4,4′-diaminodiphenylsulfone. It shares an S-benzene amino ring group with other sulfonamide-type antibiotics.

      c. Mechanism of action. Like other sulfonamides, dapsone interferes with folic acid synthesis by **competition with paraaminobenzoic acid (PABA).** The toxic effect of the drug is largely due to its interaction with hemoglobin to produce both **methemoglobin and sulfhemoglobin.** In addition, dapsone can interact directly with erythrocytes to produce a hemolytic anemia.

    d. **Pharmacokinetics**

      (1) Dapsone is slowly but completely absorbed from the GI tract, with peak levels occurring 3 to 4 h after ingestion.

      (2) The apparent volume of distribution is 1 L/kg.

      (3) Between 50% and 75% of the drug is bound to plasma proteins. Dapsone is acetylated in the liver to monoacetyldapsone (MADDS), which is 100% protein-bound.

      (4) Plasma half-life is variable, ranging between 12 and 48 h; the half-life appears to be extended with higher (i.e., toxic) plasma concentrations.

      (5) The drug is believed to undergo significant enterohepatic recirculation, making activated charcoal one of the mainstays of treatment (see below).

2. **Clinical presentation**

    a. **History.** Use of dapsone or a history of the diseases mentioned above are the critical elements. Although leprosy is often thought a rare or exotic illness, more than 20 million people worldwide suffer from it. Depending on the type and severity, dapsone may be prescribed for periods of 10 years and longer.

    b. **Physical examination**

      (1) Methemoglobinemia resulting from the ingestion of dapsone has been described as **cyanosis without respiratory distress.** In actuality, the clinical presentation is much more varied (19). Cyanosis unresponsive to oxygen administration and chocolate brown blood (especially arterial) are reliable clues to methemoglobinemia, which frequently accompanies dapsone toxicity. The cyanosis may be subtle (confined to the nails and buccal mucosa) or dramatic. Dyspnea may also be present.

      (2) **Neurologic disturbances** are the other frequent consequence of dapsone overdose. Changes in mental status usually begin with restlessness and agitation and often progress to lethargy and eventual unresponsiveness. Ataxia, dyskinesia, and even tonic-clonic seizures may occur.

      (3) **Chronic dapsone toxicity** (variously known as the dapsone, sulfone (20), or diaminodiphenylsulfone syndrome) appears weeks into therapy and is characterized by **exfoliative dermatitis, fever, and lymphadenopathy.** Hepatic involvement characterized by jaundice and abdominal pain may also occur.

    c. **Differential diagnosis**

      (1) Cyanosis responsive to oxygen or respiratory support is likely due to cardiopulmonary pathology.

      (2) There are many other compound that can cause methemoglobinemia with one review (21) citing more than 80 such substances. Methemoglobinemia can be caused by either direct (e.g., nitrates and nitrites) or indirect (e.g., sulfonamide) oxidation. Cyanosis that appears to be methemoglobin-related but that does not respond to methylene blue therapy (see below) may be due to sulfhemoglobinemia. Sulfhemoglobinemia is usually a late component of acute dapsone toxicity.

(3) Other causes of methemoglobinemia unresponsive to methylene blue include hemoglobin M disease, NADPH methemoglobin reductase deficiency, and G6PD deficiency.

d. Laboratory studies

(1) Initial laboratory studies should include arterial blood gases (normal after dapsone ingestion). CBC and an ECG (to help rule out a cardiac etiology for the patient's cyanosis).

(2) **Methemoglobin level** is useful to confirm the diagnosis, but not as important as the patient's clinical status for determining early treatment. Because a multiple-substance ingestion often cannot be excluded, other drug assays (e.g., acetaminophen) are usually indicated.

(3) The availability of more sophisticated laboratory tests (lactic acid dehydrogenase, dapsone and monoacetyl dapsone (MADDS) levels, serum haptoglobin, and NADPH methemoglobin reductase levels) are more useful during the later stages of management (see below).

e. Management and disposition

(1) Unlike many of the other antibiotics discussed above, a dapsone overdose is often dangerous and potentially lethal. Toxicity resulting from the ingestion of 20 to 25 mg/kg has been reported (22). The situation is further complicated by the fact that patients receiving vigorous intervention (methylene blue, exchange transfusion) have died (23), whereas some receiving only supportive care have survived.

(2) Any patient who is symptomatic following a dapsone ingestion— including those who are "asymptomatic" but cyanotic—should be admitted to hospital. Because the **development of hemolytic anemia secondary to a dapsone overdose may take 1 week to develop,** physicians at small hospitals may want to consider transferring a stable patient to a large center, especially if the small facility is unable to perform the sophisticated laboratory studies mentioned above.

(3) Initial evaluation includes the tests discussed above.

(4) Management of the cyanotic patient begins by ruling out other, more common (and treatable) causes of cyanosis.

(5) The relatively **slow absorption of dapsone from the GI tract** (see **II.C.1.d**) increases the importance of gastric emptying procedures. However, the fact that the drug undergoes enterohepatic recirculation and clearly **responds to multiple-dose activated charcoal** (23) lessens the value of any substance (e.g., ipecac) that limits or delays the administration of this effective and otherwise benign intervention.

(6) Induction of emesis is of course contraindicated in any patient with impaired mental status.

(7) Critically ill patients should be intubated and undergo lavage with a 30- to 40-French orogastric tube.

(8) **Activated charcoal** is a mainstay of treatment. In one study (23) four times a day dosing resulted in a four- to fivefold diminution of the plasma half-life of both dapsone and its principal metabolite MADDS. Other methods of elimination, including hemodialysis, peritoneal dialysis, and charcoal hemoperfusion do not have proved efficacy in this setting.

(9)   Methylene blue therapy in this setting is reserved for patients who have symptoms of methemoglobinemia in addition to cyanosis (e.g., confusion, diaphoresis, shortness of breath, angina, or tachycardia) or methemoglobin levels in excess of 30% to 35%. The reader is reminded that the cyanosis associated with dapsone overdose may be due in part to **sulfhemoglobinemia,** which **does not respond to treatment with methylene blue.** The usual initial dose of methylene blue is 1 mg/kg i.v. given over 10 min. Consultation with the regional poison control center is strongly recommended before its use. Further information on this treatment can be found in Chapter 11.

D.   Rifampin

1.   Properties of the agent

a.   Sources and forms. Rifampin is a semi-synthetic antibiotic derived from Streptomyces mediterranei. It is available in 150- and 300-mg capsules. Its two primary clinical uses are for treatment of tuberculosis and as prophylaxis for individuals exposed to *Neisseria meningitidis.* It is also used with dapsone to treat Hansen's disease (leprosy).

b.   Physical and chemical properties. Rifampin is a macrocyclic antibiotic. Its most striking physical property (shared by its primary metabolite desacetyl-rifampicin) is its deep red color, which is responsible for the characteristic deep orange staining of tissues and urine associated with rifampin ingestion.

c.   Mechanism of action. The drug inhibits the action of the enzyme RNA polymerase, and induces certain hepatic microsomal enzymes, thereby increasing the metabolism (and decreasing the effectiveness) of a broad range of medications, including anticoagulants, steroids, beta-blockers, quinidine, and methadone.

d.   Pharmacokinetics. Rifampin is well absorbed from the GI tract, with peak levels occurring within approximately 3 h. Plasma half-life is 1.5 to 5.0 h. The apparent volume of distribution has been calculated at 1.6 L/kg. Approximately three-fourths of the drug is protein-bound.

2.   Clinical presentation. There are three reported cases of death secondary to acute rifampin toxicity (24–26); all three involved alcohol, and one (24) involved co-ingestion of large doses of ethambutol. Serum rifampin levels (when measured) were 5 to 20 times therapeutic levels. Death occurred relatively quickly and was preceded by seizures in one case.

a.   History. Patients with tuberculosis taking **rifampin** invariably use **isoniazid** as well. Therefore the physician encountering an acute overdose should be familiar with the presentation of this substance (see Chapter 48). Concurrent alcohol use is an important element of the history (see **II.D.2.c–e**).

b.   Physical examination

(1)   The classic presentation of acute rifampin toxicity has been described as **"red man syndrome"**—with deep, orange-red staining of skin, mucous membranes, and urine (27). Note that the latter is not specific for toxicity, as even a single 300-mg capsule can change the color of the patient's urine. The skin is discolored (at least with an acute overdose) by the patient's sweat; thus, the color can be "washed off," a characteristic not found with other causes of discoloration.

(2) The patient often has many episodes of **vomiting** and may complain of severe **pruritus** as well.

(3) Intermittent dosing of rifampin can lead to a **flu-like syndrome,** sometimes accompanied by wheezing, dyspnea, and skin lesions.

(4) **Leukopenia and thrombocytopenia** are sometimes found. The reaction is believed to be immune-mediated.

(5) **Nephrotoxicity** via a similar mechanism, though rare, has been reported.

c. **Differential diagnosis.** The orange-red tinge of the skin and sclera may of course be seen with frank jaundice. Jaundice (secondary to liver dysfunction) has been seen with rifampin use as well. It is much more common when isoniazid is taken as well, especially in patients with prior hepatic pathology (alcoholic or infectious hepatitis). More benign causes of the skin and scleral discoloration include carotenemia (from ingesting large amounts of carrots and sweet potatoes) as well as lycopenemia (tomatoes are the culprit here).

d. **Laboratory studies.** Baseline tests include CBC, liver function tests (including bilirubin), and an alcohol level. Rifampin levels may be useful if readily available.

e. **Management and disposition**

(1) Patients with documented or suspected large ingestions (more than 5 g in adults or 1 g in children), especially in conjunction with alcohol ingestion, are potentially in danger and should be admitted for observation.

(2) Because rifampin undergoes enterohepatic recirculation, multiple-dose activated charcoal is probably beneficial.

(3) The use of any substance (e.g., ipecac) that limits or delays the administration of this effective and otherwise benign intervention is problematic. Ipecac is best reserved for the relatively rare overdose characterized by recent (more than 1 h) ingestion of a known substance that is unlikely to produce rapid clinical deterioration.

(4) Induction of emesis of course is contraindicated in patients with diminished mental status. Critically ill patients should be intubated (to protect their airway) and undergo lavage with a 30- to 40-French orogastric tube.

References

1. Litovitz TL, et al. 1989 annual report of the American Association of Poison Control Centers. *Am J Emerg Med* 1990; 8:398.
2. Prince BS, et al. Drug-related emergency department visits and hospital admissions. *Am J Hosp Pharm* 1992;49: 1696–1700.
3. Lee S, et al. Coagulopathy associated with moxalactam. *JAMA* 1982;248:1100.

4. Nattel S, et al. Erythromycin-induced long QT syndrome: concordance w/quinidine and underlying cellular electro-physiologic mechanism. *Am J Med* 1990;89:235.

5. Honig PK, et al. Erythromycin changes terfenadine pharmacokinetics and electrocardiographic pharmacodynamics. *Clin Pharm Ther* 1992;51:156.

6. Brannan MD, et al. Loratidine administered concomitantly with erythromycin: pharmacokinetic and electrocardio-graphic evaluations. *Clin Pharm Ther* 1995;58:269–278.

7. Edelbroek MA, Horowitz M, Wishart JM, Akkermans LM. Effects of erythromycin on gastric emptying, alcohol absorption, and small intestinal transit in normal subjects. *J Nucl Med* 1993;34:582–588.

8. Siegel JA. Analysis of metronidazole in human serum: an unusual overdose case. *J Forensic Sci* 1984;29:639.

9. *Physician's desk reference*. Oradell, NJ: Medical Economics, 1995:1496–1498.

10. Fox SA. Tetracycline toxicity presenting as a multisystem disease. *Mt Sinai J Med* 1976;43:129.

11. Schaible DH, et al. Chloramphenicol induced "gray adolescent syndrome." *Vet Hum Toxicol* 1985;28:316.

12. Thompson WI. Overdoses of chloramphenicol. *JAMA* 1975;234:149.

13. Wallerstein RO, et al. Statewide study of chloramphenicol therapy and fatal aplastic anemia. *JAMA* 1969;208:2045.

14. Mauer SM, et al. Treatment of an infant with severe chloramphenicol intoxication using charcoal column hemoperfu-sion. *J Pediatr* 1980;96:136.

15. Cann HM, et al. Fatal acute chloroquine poisoning in children. *Pediatrics* 1961;27:95.

16. Riou B, et al. Treatment of severe chloroquine poisoning. *N Engl J Med* 1988;318:1.

17. Crouzette J, et al. Experimental assessment of the protective activity of diazepam on the acute toxicity of chloroquine. *J Toxicol Clin Toxicol* 1983;20:271.

18. Clemessy JL, Taboulet P, Hoffman JR, et al. Treatment of acute chloroquine poisoning: a 5-year experience. *Crit Care Med* 1996;24:1189–1195.

19. Woodhouse KW, et al. Acute dapsone poisoning: clinical features and pharmacokinetic studies. *Hum Toxicol* 1983;3:507.

20. Tomecki KJ, Catatlano CJ. Dapsone hypersensitivity: sulfone syndrome revisited. *Arch Dermatol* 1981;117:38.

21. Curry S. Methemoglobinemia. *Ann Emerg Med* 1982;11:214.

22. Elonen E, et al. Acute dapsone intoxication: a case with prolonged symptoms. *Clin Toxicol* 1979;14:79.

23. Reigert JR, et al. Repetitive doses of activated charcoal in dapsone poisoning in a child. *J Toxicol Clin Toxicol* 1982/83;19:1061.

24. Jach DB, et al. Fatal rifampicin-ethambutol overdosage. *Lancet* 1978;2:1107.

25. Broadwell RO, et al. Suicide by rifampin overdose. *JAMA* 1978;240:2283.

26. Plomp TA, et al. A case of fatal poisoning by rifampin. *Arch Toxicol* 1981;48:245.

27. Newton RW, Forest A. Rifampin overdosage—"the red man syndrome." *Scott Med J* 1975;20:55.

Selected Readings

AMA Division of Drugs. *AMA drug evaluations*. Chicago: American Medical Association, 1983.

Dreisbach RH. *Handbook of poisoning*. Los Altos, CA: Lange Medical Publications, 1987.

Ellenhorn MJ, Barceloux DG. *Medical toxicology*. New York: Elsevier Science, 1988.

Goldfrank LR, et al., eds. *Goldfrank's toxicologic emergencies*. 4th ed. Norwalk, CT: Appleton & Lange, 1990.

Meyers BR. *Antimicrobial prescribing*. Princeton: Antimicrobial Prescribing, 1985.

Emergency Toxicology, Second Edition,
edited by Peter Viccellio.
Lippincott–Raven Publishers, Philadelphia © 1998.

34

Laxative Abuse

Thomas G. Lemke

Department of Emergency Medicine, Brown University, Rhode Island Hospital,
Providence, Rhode Island 02903

I. **Introduction.** Toxicity from laxative ingestion is rare in that most (e.g., bulk forms, emollients, and saline) remain unabsorbed within the gastrointestinal (GI) tract. During 1994, the American Association of Poison Control Centers reported 13,172 contacts regarding laxative exposure. Of this number, only eight patients were hospitalized, with resulting death in three (1). Minor or no symptoms were found in the vast majority. Exceptions to this usual benign course are the following:

   A. **Magnesium**-containing agents may cause hypermagnesemia.

   B. **Lactulose**-containing agents may induce lactic acidosis.

   C. **Profound diarrhea from any of these agents** may cause fluid and electrolyte abnormalities.

II. **Available preparations.** These agents are best grouped by mechanism.

   A. Irritant/stimulant (e.g., castor oil, bisacodyl, phenolphthalein)

   B. Bulk-producing (e.g., Metamucil, psyllium)

   C. Osmotic agents (lactulose, magnesium salts)

   D. Hyperosmotic agents (glycerin)

   E. Lubricant (mineral oil)

   F. Of the many different types of laxatives, there are only three that can cause significant toxicity.

      1. Magnesium-containing agents, such as Milk of Magnesia, magnesium citrate, and Epsom salts (magnesium sulfate)

      2. Lactulose-containing agents like Cephulac and Chronulac

      3. Phenolphthalein (Ex-Lax)

III. **Pharmacology and properties**

   A. Mechanism

      1. Lactulose. Lactulose is poorly absorbed from the GI tract; therefore, both the lactulose and its bacterial breakdown products (e.g., lactic acid, acetic acid, formic acid) form an osmotic load drawing water into the intestine. The increase in stool water results in catharsis. Its toxic effects result primarily from excessive loss of fluid and electrolytes leading to hypovolemia, hypokalemia, and hypernatremia. One report of lactic acidosis resulting from administration of lactulose to a patient suffering from hepatic encephalopathy exists (2). It was postulated that in this case

an adynamic ileus prevented the patient from rapidly excreting the lactic acid. Serum lactate rapidly accumulated and led to the patient's death.

2. Magnesium. When taken orally, magnesium causes excretion of cholycystokinin, which increases both intestinal secretion and motility. In large amounts, systemic absorption of magnesium can cause hypermagnesemia with resultant neuromuscular paralysis. Conversely, therapeutic amounts of magnesium given to patients with marginal renal function (and therefore unable to excrete a magnesium load) may also result in hyermagnesemia. While the precise mechanism is unclear, magnesium exerts its toxic effects via impairment of neuromuscular transmission creating a curare-like effect. Layzer speculates that as calcium ions couple the electrical impulse with acetylcholine release, displacement of calcium ions by magnesium ions negate this effect (3).

3. Phenolphthalein. Effective as a cathartic because of a direct stimulant effect upon the intestinal tract, increasing peristalsis and GI motor activity. While toxicity is rare, it appears that phenolphthalein is capable of exerting a direct toxic effect upon liver, kidney, and pancreas. In at least two instances, the unabsorbed portion of an oral phenolphthalein load was felt to be the cause of GI bleeding. While red stools are common in phenolphthalein ingestions, actual bleeding is not. A local irritant effect from the acidic breakdown products is felt to be the likely cause (4).

B. Pharmacokinetics

1. Lactulose. In that lactulose is poorly absorbed across the intestinal mucosa, it usually remains confined to the intestinal tract. Excretion of lactulose itself is almost entirely fecal with less than 2% excreted by the kidney (5). The breakdown products, particularly lactic acid, may be absorbed and require further metabolism prior to excretion.

2. Magnesium. Approximately 30% to 40% of magnesium is normally absorbed. Increasing oral loads result in decreased absorption rates, often below 10% (6). Once absorbed, magnesium becomes the second most common cation in the body. Almost half of the body's magnesium resides in bone with a majority of the remainder divided between liver and striated muscle (7). Only about 1% is found in extracellular fluid. Magnesium is excreted primarily by the kidney with up to 97% excreted during magnesium overload (8). Excretion, however, mirrors creatinine clearance, and therefore the ability to excrete a magnesium load decreases in patients with renal failure (9).

3. Phenolphthalein. A majority of an oral phenolphthalein load remains unabsorbed with only 15% crossing the intestinal mucosal barrier. After absorption, the drug is excreted by the kidney. An enterohepatic circulation path exists that may prolong the cathartic effect.

IV. Clinical presentations

A. Lactulose. GI symptoms tend to predominate, usually in the form of vomiting, diarrhea, abdominal cramping, and flatulence. If fluid and electrolyte losses have been profound, dehydration and weakness may dominate the clinical picture.

B. Magnesium. Evidence of magnesium toxicity usually occurs in one of two settings: renal failure and therapeutic misadventures by both physician and patient. The success of multiple dose charcoal treatment has, unfortunately, been accompanied by the inappropriate use of multiple dose cathartics (10).

1. The **neuromuscular system** effects are usually most apparent beginning with muscle weakness, twitching, and tremor, then proceeding to delirium, hyperreflexia, and convulsions. Unchecked, the final result of rising magnesium levels is coma (11).

2. The effects of hypermagnesemia on the **heart** are equally profound, if not as immediately apparent. Early findings may only consist of QT prolongation, some T wave flattening, and PVCs. If untreated, PR, QRS, and QT intervals may all become prolonged. If still untreated, atrial fibrillation and Torsade de Pointes may ensue (8). Loss of deep tendon reflexes precedes all cardiac manifestations.

3. Problems in both of the above listed organ systems may be exacerbated by metabolic changes including hypocalcemia and refractory hypokalemia. In the setting of a cathartic overdose, these symptoms are likely due to hypermagnesemia but the possibility of endocrinopathies (hypothyroidism, hypoadrenalism, and hyperparathyroidism) must also be considered. All of the above symptoms tend to correlate with the level of serum magnesium (Table 34-1) (12).

C. **Phenolphthalein.** Like other stimulant laxatives, diarrhea and occasionally vomiting dominate the clinical picture. In the rare, life-threatening case, hematochezia, oliguria, and evidence of a consumptive coagulopathy may complicate the patient's course.

D. **Chronic laxative poisoning.** The above listed effects are all the result of acute toxicity. When abused over time, however, laxatives are capable of producing a syndrome known as **"cathartic colon."** The patient has chronic constipation, with diminished haustrations of the colon. The finding of melanosis coli on sigmoidoscopy is specific for chronic anthraquinone abuse. Abuse over more that 15 years is usually necessary for the complete syndrome to manifest itself. No firm cause of this syndrome has been identified but some have speculated that it is due to chronic sodium and potassium loss. In that a similar clinical picture could result from other diseases of the colon (both intrinsic large bowel diseases and hypersecretory states) the work-up of these patients should include parameters outside of toxicology.

E. **Differential diagnosis.** Alternate causes of acute diarrhea are best considered by mechanism (13).

1. Secretory (e.g., cholera, islet cell tumors)
2. Exudative (e.g., ulcerative colitis, shigella, amebiasis)

TABLE 34-1. *Relation of serum magnesium levels to physical findings*

Magnesium level (mEq/L)	Physical findings
4	Depression of deep tendon reflexes
4–7	Somnolence, bradycardia, hypotension, nausea, vomiting, diarrhea, urinary retention, cutaneous vasodilation
10	Paralysis, respiratory depression
15	Asystole

Data from ref. 10.

   3. Decreased absorption
      a. Osmotic (e.g., lactase deficiency)
      b. Anatomic derangement (e.g., subtotal colectomy, gastrocolic fistula)
      c. Motility disorders (e.g., hyperthyroidism, irritable bowel syndrome)

V. **Laboratory evaluations.** Regardless of the type of laxative ingested, many of the laboratory abnormalities are the result of fluid and electrolyte losses. **Hypokalemia** and **hypernatremia** are frequent findings regardless of the agent ingested. In lactulose ingestions, the possibility of **lactic acidosis** must be considered (occurring within 24 h in the one reported case). If a magnesium-containing laxative is ingested, **hypophosphatemia** may occur (14). In that most laxatives never reach the blood stream, obtaining serum levels of these compounds is of no value. **Magnesium levels,** on the other hand, are valuable because of the correlation between clinical effects and serum levels. As expected, magnesium salts will be found in the **stools** of these patients. If the stool turns red when combined with **sodium hydroxide,** phenolphthalein ingestion can be inferred.

VI. **Management**
   A. General. As with any overdose, the **ABCs** should take precedence over any attempt to ascertain the specific effects of the toxin. Once these are assured, GI decontamination should be considered. Clearly, use of cathartics is inappropriate. **Emesis and/or gastric lavage** may be indicated, particularly if the ingestion has been large and recent. **Activated charcoal,** while effectively binding most laxatives, has little effect on magnesium. As with all overdoses, the possibility of coexisting poisons and associated medical illnesses must be considered.
   B. Magnesium (Fig. 34-1)
      1. In that the kidney is capable of excreting large quantities of magnesium, patients without immediate life threatening symptoms may be treated with **saline loading and furosemide-induced diuresis,** assuming the patient's renal function is adequate (15). An appropriate initial dose of furosemide would be 40 mg i.v.
      2. **Calcium** (0.2 to 0.5 mL/kg of 10% calcium gluconate up to 10 mL over 10 min) may successfully ameliorate both cardiac and respiratory depression by displacing magnesium from its binding sites. While not all patients will require calcium, those manifesting respiratory or cardiac signs/symptoms should receive it. If symptoms recur, this dose may be repeated and serum calcium levels followed.
      3. In patients unable to tolerate a fluid load (either due to cardiac or renal disease), in patients in which diuresis has failed, or in those with resistant cardioxicity, **hemodialysis** is indicated.
   C. Lactulose. If lactic acidosis develops in patients receiving lactulose, every attempt to **purge the lactulose** from the patient's intestinal tract should be pursued. Whole bowel irrigation with polyethylene glycol-electrolyte lavage solution (e.g., GoLytely) may be used if no contraindications exist. **Intravenous bicarbonate** may be administered for refractory acidemia, but this has not been shown to alter the course of the disease.
   D. Phenolphthalein. All children ingesting more than one gram of phenolphthalein should be referred to a treatment center and receive activated charcoal and possibly emesis/lavage. Profound diarrhea may mandate rehydration either i.v. or via balanced oral replacement solutions (e.g., Pedialyte).

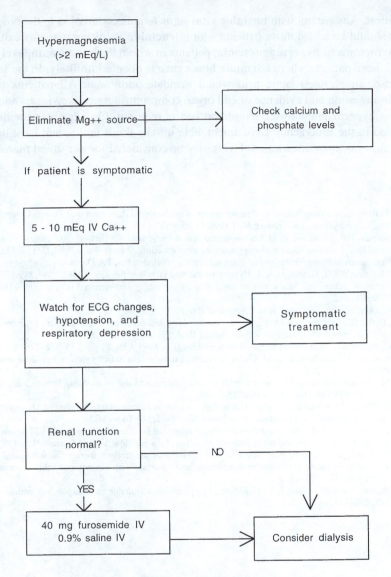

FIG. 34-1. Management of hypermagnesemia.

VII. Disposition. Any patient with **unstable vital signs** requires admission to the hospital. To this number should be added those patients with **intractable vomiting,** patients exhibiting signs and/or symptoms of **hypermagnesemia,** patients in whom the **magnesium level may be rising,** and those patients where **adequate home care is deemed unlikely.** In the setting of lactulose use, an elevated lactic acid would mandate admission. All patients with phenolphthalein ingestion and evidence of end organ compromise must likewise be admitted. If the patient is hypermagnesemic, a monitored bed is required. Conversely, patients adequately rehydrated in the Emergency Department, able to take fluids orally, and have no electrolyte abnormalities or toxic magnesium levels may be considered for outpatient management.

References

1. Litovitz TL, Felberg L, Soloway RA, et al. Annual report of the National Association of Poison Control Centers Toxic Exposure Surveillance System. *Am J Emerg Med* 1994;13:551–557.
2. Mann NS, Russman HB, Mann SK, et al. Lactulose and severe lactic acidosis [Letter]. *Ann Intern Med* 1985;103:637.
3. Weiss BD, Wood GA. Laxative abuse causing gastrointestinal bleeding. *J Fam Pract* 1982;15:177–181.
4. Layzer RB. *Neuromuscular manifestations of systemic disease.* Philadelphia: FA Davis Co, 1985.
5. Nelson DC, McGrew WRG, Hoyumpa AM. Hypernatremia and lactulose therapy. *JAMA* 1983;249:1295–1298.
6. Morris ME, Leroy S, Sutton SC. Absorption of magnesium from orally administered magnesium sulfate in man. *Clin Toxicol* 1987;25:371–382.
7. Mordes JP, Wacker W. Excess magnesium. *Pharmacol Rev* 1978;29:273–299.
8. Sutton RAL, Dirks JH. Calcium and Magnesium: renal handling and disorders of metabolism In: Brenner BM, Rector FC, eds. *The kidney.* 3rd ed. Philadelphia: WB Saunders, 1986:551–617.
9. Wacker WEC, Parish AF. Magnesium metabolism (concluded). *N Engl J Med* 1968;278:772–776.
10. Jones J, Heiselman D, Dougherty J, et al. Cathartic-induced magnesium toxicity during overdose management. *Ann Emerg Med* 1986;15:1214–1218.
11. Reinhert R. Magnesium metabolism: a review with special reference to the relationship between intracellular content and serum levels. *Arch Intern Med* 1988;148:2415–2420.
12. Fassler CA, Rodriguez M, Badesch DB, et al. Magnesium toxicity as a cause of hypotension and hypoventilation: occurrence in patients with normal renal function. *Arch Intern Med* 1985;145:1604–1606.
13. Goldfinger SE. Constipation, diarrhea, and disturbances of anorectal function. In: Braunwald E, Isselbacher KJ, Petersdorf RG, et al., eds. *Harrison's principles of internal medicine.* 11th ed. New York: McGraw-Hill, 1987:177.
14. Rasmussen HS, Cintin C, Aurup P, et al. The effect of intravenous magnesium therapy on serum and urine levels of potassium, calcium, and sodium in patients with ischemic heart disease, with ans without acute myocardial infarction. *Arch Intern Med* 1988;148:1801–1805.
15. Smilkstein MJ, Smolinske SC, Kulig KW, et al. Severe Hypermagnesernia due to multiple-dose cathartic therapy. *West J Med* 1988;148:208–211.

Emergency Toxicology, Second Edition,
edited by Peter Viccellio.
Lippincott–Raven Publishers, Philadelphia © 1998.

35

Hypervitaminosis

*Cameron Cushing and †Angela C. Anderson

*Department of Emergency Medicine, †Department of Pediatrics, Brown University,
Rhode Island Hospital, Providence, Rhode Island 02903*

A vitamin is defined as "a substance that is essential for the maintenance of normal metabolic functions, but is not synthesized in the body and therefore, must be furnished from an exogenous source" (1). Because of the largely unsubstantiated beliefs that megadoses of vitamins can prevent or ameliorate the effects of aging and cancer, vitamins portend a large potential for misuse and toxicity. This is compounded by the fact that vitamins are neither perceived nor regulated as drugs by the Food and Drug Administration (FDA). **Water-soluble** vitamins, including the B and C complexes, do not have a large spectrum of toxicity. They rarely accumulate in the body because they are readily excreted by the kidneys. However, these complexes may produce significant toxicity, particularly if they are consumed chronically, and in large quantities. **Fat-soluble** vitamins, including vitamins A, D, E, and K, are generally more toxic and represent the greater of well described toxidromes. Scientific committees throughout the world periodically survey the established literature to generate a recommended dietary allowance (RDA) as a daily goal for intake of vitamins. Failure to consume a vitamins' RDA for prolonged periods will be manifested as the clinical syndromes of vitamin deficiency; conversely, chronic consumption of vitamins in quantities that exceed the RDA become manifested as the clinical toxidrome known as hypervitaminosis (Table 35-1).

I. **Vitamin A.** Night blindness, a currently known consequence of vitamin A deficiency, was first described in Egypt around 1500 B.C. Vitamin A was later discovered through the observation that animals with xerophthalmia (dryness and thickening of the conjunctiva) could be cured by adding vitamin A–rich substances (e.g., butter, egg yolk, and cod liver oil) to their diets (2,3). Dietary sources of vitamin A include the following: liver (mammalian, polar bear and shark), dairy products (butter, cheese, whole milk and egg yolk), yellow or green fruits and vegetables (corn, spinach, broccoli, etc.), and fish oils. The RDA for vitamin A is 5,000 IU/day. Signs and symptoms of acute toxicity have occurred following the ingestion of 1.5 million IU of vitamin A. Chronic toxicity can occur following the ingestion of 10 times the RDA over a period of several weeks to months. Although vitamin A overdose is rare, toxicity has been observed in individuals whose diets consisted of large quantities of animal liver, and in patients taking commercially available preparations used for the treatment of dermatologic diseases.

A. **Available preparations.** Vitamin A is available in capsules (10,000, 25,000, and 50,000 IU), oral solution (50,000 IU/mL), and tablets (10,000 IU). A parenteral form is also available (50,000 IU/mL).

TABLE 35-1. *Toxidromes observed with vitamins*

Vitamin	Toxidrome	Treatment
A	Increased ICP	Supplement withdrawal
	Skin desquammation	ICP management
	Liver abnormalities	Hypercalcemic management
	Hyperostosis	
	Arthritis and myopathy	
	Retinoic dysmorphic syndrome	
B_1	Anaphylaxis (i.v.)	Supplement withdrawal
		Supportive care
B_2	Yellow urine and perspiration	Supplement withdrawal
B_3	Anaphylaxis (niacin flush)	Supplement withdrawal
	Liver abnormalities	Supportive care
	Dermatologic abnormalities	
	Myopathy	
B_6	Peripheral neuropathy (sensory)	Supplement withdrawal
B_{12}	Allergic reaction	Supplement withdrawal
	Dermatitis	Supportive care
C	Diarrhea	Supplement withdrawal
	Nephrolithiasis	Hydration
	Hyperoxaluria	Supportive care
	Red cell hemolysis	
D	Hypercalcemia and related signs and symptoms	Supplement withdrawal
		Low calcium diet
		Prednisone
		Calcitonin
		Diuretics
		Hydration
E	Increased bleeding	Supplement withdrawal
		Vitamin K
K	Anaphylaxis (i.v.)	Supplement withdrawal
	Hemolysis and hyperbilirubinemia in preterm newborns	Supportive care

B. **Pharmacology and properties**

1. **Mechanism of action and toxicity.** Naturally occurring vitamin A (retinal) is the prosthetic group for the photosensitive pigment in rods and cones of the retina. Retinal also serves a function in the maintenance of epithelial cell structure; basal epithelial cells in the presence of retinal are stimulated to produce mucous and inhibit keratinization. Synthetic analogs, termed "retinoids," have been in wide use since 1982 for the treatment of severe acne and keratinization disorders, such as eczema. These analogs do not maintain vitamin A's actions on vision and reproduction, but have retained the roles of epithelial differentiation and mucous production.

2. The presence of large quantities of vitamin A will exceed the capacity of retinol binding protein. Free vitamin A then nonspecifically binds to plasma proteins and is delivered to peripheral tissues where it enacts tissue damage by producing unstable cellular membranes through the generation of free radicals.

3. **Pharmacokinetics.** Vitamin A and its congeners are absorbed in the small intestine and esterified within epithelial cells in preparation for transport and deposi-

tion. The esterified form is then transported in chylomicrons, via the lymphatic system, to the liver where it is unesterified. Ninety percent of vitamin A exists as the unesterified free alcohol retinol, which is stored in the liver. A percentage of retinol is conjugated in the liver with glucuronic acid and then oxidized to the active metabolites retinal and retinoic acid. These metabolites are excreted via the feces and urine; only in cases of renal failure is retinol excreted unchanged in the urine. Retinol is mobilized from the liver by the carrier protein retinol binding protein, which normally binds 95% of free retinol and protects tissues from the surface active properties of vitamin A.

C. **Clinical manifestations**

   1. **Acute vitamin A toxicity** has been reported in fishermen who ingested large quantities of polar bear, shark, or seal liver (4). A single dose of 1.5 million units of vitamin A produces acute toxicity in adults (5). Adult symptoms may mimic those observed in patients with elevated intracranial pressures and include headache, nausea, lethargy, irritability, and vomiting. Vitamin A toxicity has been also observed in children following ingestions of 150,000 IU. Patients present with the symptoms mentioned above and may also have bulging fontanels.

   2. **Chronic vitamin A toxicity** has been reported in individuals using over-the-counter (OTC) commercial vitamin preparations. Chronic toxicity may result from the ingestion of 3,000 IU/kg/day over a period of weeks to months (6). The clinical presentation may include dermatologic, central nervous system (CNS), hepatic, bone, and rheumatologic abnormalities.

      a. **Dermatologic and CNS manifestations.** Initial manifestations usually involve dermatologic changes such as red desquamation (especially over the hands and feet), as well as cheilosis, pruritus, alopecia, and a seborrhea-like skin eruption (4). CNS abnormalities include pseudotumor cerebri, papilledema, diplopia, vision loss, and symptoms associated with increased intracranial pressure.

      b. **Hepatic manifestations.** Hepatic enlargement, ascites, and portal hypertension have also been described in patients with hypervitaminosis A (7). Hepatocellular injury with associated elevations in serum hepatic enzymes is rare but has been reported (8).

      c. **Bone abnormalities.** Hyperostosis may occur in more than 80% of patients taking high doses of synthetic retinoids for a few years or more (9). It usually involves the cervical and thoracic spines and may cause a decreased range of motion that mimics seronegative spondyloarthropathy or diffuse idiopathic skeletal hyperostosis (10). Polydypsia, polyuria, and hypercalcuria can occur secondary to elevated serum calcium levels generated from bone resorption (11). Boney changes may be asymptomatic and found adventitiously on x-ray or scintigraphic examination (12).

      d. **Rheumatologic manifestations.** Arthritis, vasculitis and myopthy are rheumatologic manifestations of chronic vitamin A toxicity. Symptoms include muscle pain and stiffness, and edema of the lower extremities. Three cases of Wegner's granulomatosis have been described (9).

3. **Side effects observed with therapeutic doses.** Synthetic retinoids, taken in therapeutic doses, may cause acute and chronic abnormalities. Both oral and topical forms have been shown to induce toxicity. Early side effects are seen often within 48 h (13). These include acne flare, erythema, and xerosis of the face or scalp, and drying of mucous membranes which can cause rectal, vaginal, and nasal bleeding. Late side effects arise after 48 h and include musculoskeletal symptoms, fatigue, depression, insomnia, depressed libido, menstrual irregularities, visual complaints, hair loss, hepatic dysfunction, and bone resorption. Pseudotumor cerebri was described in a 14-year-old boy following 3 weeks of treatment with a synthetic retinoid and tetracycline (14).

4. **Teratogenic effects.** In pregnancy, the risk of retinoid-induced infant malformations experienced in the first trimester approaches 25% to 30% and is termed the "retinoic acid dysmorphic syndrome" (15). It results from the toxic effects of vitamin A on cephalic neural crest cells. CNS defects, optic atrophy, small or absent ears, micrognathia, cleft palate, and thymic and congenital heart defects have been described (15).

5. **Differential diagnosis** (adapted from Haddad and Winchester, 1990) (Table 35-2) (11)
   a. Elevated intracranial pressure
      (1) Benign increased intracranial pressure
      (2) CNS tumor
      (3) Intracranial hemorrhage
      (4) Hydrocephalus
      (5) Corticosteroid- or tetracycline-induced
      (6) Addison's or hypoparathyroidism
   b. Papuloerythematous dermatitis
      (1) Eczematous dermatitis
      (2) Drug eruptions
      (3) Exanthematous diseases
   c. Corticohyperostosis and hypercalcemia
      (1) Caffey disease
      (2) Hypervitaminosis D
   d. Hepatomegaly and abnormal liver function tests
      (1) Hepatitis
      (2) Obstructive liver disease
      (3) Genetic-metabolic disorders
      (4) Infiltrative-vascular diseases of the liver

D. **Laboratory evaluation.** Definitive diagnosis of hypervitaminosis A is made by measuring serum retinol levels. Vitamin A toxicity generally occurs when serum retinol values exceed 100 µg/dL. However, these values can only be reliable when serum protein levels are normal. Decreases in retinol binding protein may allow for vitamin A toxicity at serum retinol levels as low as 60 µg/dL (16). Conversely, renal disease may cause elevated retinol binding proteins which protect the body from vitamin A poisoning, even at serum retinol levels greater than 100 µg/dL. Supportive findings include elevations in serum calcium, alkaline phosphatase, bilirubin, prothrombin time, and sedimentation rate. Anemia and hypoalbuminemia may also be present. Elevation of hepatic transaminases is rare but has been reported following the chronic ingestion of 25,000 IU/day (8). Peak transaminase elevations have been observed as late as two months following *discontinuation* of retinoid therapy (17). Toxicity from synthetic retinals may also cause elevated triglycerides and cholesterol (both HDL and LDL fractions).

E. **Management.** The majority of toxic ingestions of vitamin A may be managed with supplement withdrawal. Symptom regression usually occurs within several weeks. Acute vitamin A ingestions of more than one million IU in adults, or 100,000 IU in children, should be treated with gastric decontamination and administration of activated charcoal. Patients who present with symptoms of elevated intracranial pressure may require CT scan imaging of the head and lumbar puncture to dismiss the possibility of other intracranial abnormalities. Mannitol diuresis, dexamethasone, and hyperventilation can be instituted for significant intracranial pressure elevations. Hypercalcemia can be treated with fluid hydration and diuretics. Occasionally, there may be permanent liver disease or skeletal deformities with chronic ingestions of vitamin A.

F. **Disposition.** Hypercalcemia and significant elevations in intracranial pressures require immediate recognition and hospital admission. Abnormal liver function tests require close follow-up.

II. **Vitamin B_1.** The Neiching, a Chinese medical book written in 2697 B.C., first described beriberi as a disease entity. It subsequently became widespread in East Asia. In 1926, Jansen and Donath isolated "antiberiberi," later named "thiamine" (vitamin B_1), from rice bran extract. The RDA of thiamine is 1.5 mg/day. Thiamine deficiency may result from poor dietary intake, however, in the United States, excess alcohol intake is the most common cause of vitamin B_1 deficiency (18). Ethanol interferes with intestinal transport of thiamine and inhibits the conversion of inactive thiamine to active thiamine. Significant thiamine deficiency causes abnormalities in the cardiovascular system ("wet beriberi"), or the CNS and peripheral nervous system ("dry beriberi"). Cardiomegaly, peripheral edema, sinus tachycardia, and high output failure dominate the presentation of wet beriberi. Dry beriberi is characterized by Wernicke-Korsakoff encephalopathy, and peripheral motor and sensory deficits. Though largely nontoxic, intravenous administration of thiamine has resulted in some cases of anaphylaxis. Individuals who may require immediate intravenous administration include those with wet and dry beriberi, Alzheimer's disease, Maple syrup urine disease, and those with acute coma or hypothermia.

A. **Available preparations.** Tablet preparations are available in the following doses: 5, 10, 25, 50, 100, 250, and 500 mg. Parental forms are available in 100 and 200 mg/mL concentrations.

B. **Pharmacology and properties**

1. **Mechanism of action and toxicity.** Thiamine is an essential cofactor in a number of enzymatic reactions, and is ultimately necessary for ATP and DNA synthesis, carbohydrate metabolism, and nerve conduction. In the absence of thiamine, pyruvic acid is not converted to acetyl-CoA, and is thus not able to enter the aerobic oxidative pathway. Accumulations of pyruvic acid then promote a lactic acidosis. In addition, decreased thiamine levels cause a deficiency of serum transketolase

which has been linked with Wernicke's encephalopathy. Anaphylactic reactions have been described in hypersensitive individuals receiving intravenous thiamine. Transient vasodilatation and hypotension have resulted in vascular collapse, and even death (19). Pain on injection and contact dermatitis may also result from immediate sensitivity mechanisms.

2. **Pharmacokinetics.** Absorption of thiamine occurs in the small intestine via both active transport and passive diffusion through a Na^+-dependent channel. Thiamine is then bound to serum proteins, largely albumin. Gastric absorption of thiamine is decreased in alcoholics, and in patients with malabsorption or cirrhosis. Approximately 1 mg/day is degraded by the tissues, accounting for the RDA of 1 mg/day. When excess thiamine is administered, tissue stores are first saturated, and the excess is renally excreted as intact thiamine or its metabolites. The pathways for degradation and excretion of thiamine are not well identified.

C. **Clinical presentation.** Pain at the injection site and contact dermatitis may occur in approximately 1% of individuals who receive thiamine. In rare instances, anaphylactic reactions have been known to occur with rapid thiamine injection resulting in hypotension, angioedema, and weakness. No adverse effects have been noted in patients using thiamine during pregnancy.

D. **Management.** Treatment of thiamine-induced anaphylaxis is similar to that of other histamine mediated processes; it involves rapid infusion of crystalloids, and administration of epinephrine and histamine blocking agents. Pressor agents may be necessary in extreme cases.

E. **Disposition.** Anaphylaxis resulting in vascular collapse would necessitate hospital admission for cardiovascular support. Contact dermatitis may be managed on an OUTpatient basis.

III. **Vitamin B_2.** Riboflavin is a water-soluble fluorescent yellow compound discovered by Blyth in 1879 and noted to have vitaminic properties in 1933. Common food sources include milk, meat, eggs, nuts, enriched flour, and green vegetables. Deficient states arise from inadequate dietary intake and malabsorption. Patients predisposed to ribflavin malabsorption include those with tropical sprue, celiac disease, malignancy, resection of the small bowel, and GI or biliary obstruction. The RDA for riboflavin is 1.7 mg/day.

A. **Available preparations.** Riboflavin is available in 10-, 25-, 50-, and 100-mg tablets.

B. **Pharmacology and properties**

1. **Mechanism of action and toxicity.** As a bound coenzyme, riboflavin functions in numerous oxidation-reduction reactions, and in energy production via the respiratory chain. Riboflavin carries OUT its functions as one of two coenzymes, flavin mononucleotide (FMN) and flavin adenine dinucleotide (FAD). No substantiated toxicologic effects have been attributed to the use of riboflavin.

2. **Pharmacokinetics.** Riboflavin is absorbed in the proximal small intestine by a transport system which becomes saturated when serum levels of ribflavin exceed 25 mg/dL. Bile salts facilitate the uptake of riboflavin. Within plasma, riboflavin circulates bound to albumin, as well as to other plasma proteins, including immunoglobulins. Riboflavin circulates via the enterohepatic system. Greater than 90% of riboflavin is excreted unchanged in the feces; a smaller amount is

excreted, unchanged, in the urine. The elimination half-life of riboflavin is approximately 1 h.

C. **Clinical manifestations.** Riboflavin is essential in tissue respiration. Deficient states are characterized by cheilosis, stomatitis, keratitis, seborrhea, and ocular changes which include corneal vascularization. In chronic deficiency, a normocytic, normochromic anemia may develop. No toxicologic effects have been noted with the use of riboflavin. Toxicity from ingestion of excess riboflavin is doubtful. There has been one report of EEG abnormalities in two patients undergoing long-term treatment with riboflavin and niacin (20). In large doses, riboflavin will enhance the yellow color of urine and may produce yellow perspiration.

D. **Laboratory findings.** Riboflavin is measured by urinary or erythrocyte concentrations. Daily urinary concentrations should be greater than 50 mcg; erythrocyte concentrations should be greater than 10 mcg/dL.

E. **Management.** There is a paucity of information in the literature regarding riboflavin toxicity. Primary management includes cessation of excessive intake. In the deficient state, supplementation of 5 to 30 mg/day is prescribed.

F. **Disposition.** The clinical manifestations of riboflavin toxicity require, at most, withdrawal of supplementation and outpatient management.

IV. **Vitamin B$_3$.** Pellagra, characterized by "the three D's" of diarrhea, dermatitis, and dementia, was first recognized by the Spanish physician Casals who noted that the disease was most prevalent among maize eating populations (2,3). In 1937, Elvehjem discovered that nicotinic acid (niacin) was effective in treating this disease (2,3). In 1955, large doses of niacin were noted to be effective in reducing serum cholesterol, and consequently, mortality from heart disease (2,3). Tryptophan is the amino acid precursor for niacin. Therefore, pellagra can be observed in patients who malabsorb tryptophan (Hartnups disease), or in patients suffering from the carcinoid syndrome in which stores of tryptophan are depleted during the synthesis of serotonin. Toxic effects from niacin have been reported in patients taking the vitamin in both therapeutic and excessive doses. These effects primarily include niacin-induced hepatitis, anaphylaxis, and dermatologic abnormalities. The RDA of niacin is 20 mg/day.

A. **Available preparations.** Niacin (nicotinic acid) is available in three forms: 25- to 500-mg capsules; 250- to 750-mg extended release capsules; and 50 or 100 mg/mL solutions for intravenous injection. Niacinamide tablets are available in doses of 50 to 500 mg.

B. **Pharmacology and properties**

1. **Mechanism of action and toxicity.** Nicotinic acid and niacinamide are converted to their active forms, nicotinamide adenine dinucleotide (NAD) and nicotinamide adenine dinucleotide phosphate (NADP) respectively, in the process described below. Theses active forms function as oxidants in a wide variety of essential reactions. Niacin promotes histamine release which can result in severe skin flushing, pruritus, and gastrointestinal disturbances. This reaction is termed "The Niacin Flush" and routinely lasts for 2 to 3 h. Liver damage is a potentially significant complication of niacin use. It is most commonly seen in patients undergoing treatment for hyperlipidemia. Niacin (or its metabolites) appears to be directly hepatotoxic; centrilobular cholestasis and parenchymal necrosis can be seen on liver biopsy in

most patients (21). The hepatotoxic reactions observed following niacin use are usually reversible, however fulminant hepatic failure has been described. The spectrum of niacin-induced hepatotoxicity is preparation dependent and dose related. Slow release preparations were developed to reduce the histamine-associated side effects of niacin. However, hepatic damage is more severe in patients taking these sustained release preparations than in those prescribed crystalline niacin (21–23). Hepatitis resulting from slow-release preparations has been observed in patients taking as little as 3 gram/day for 2 days (23). Rechallenge with crystalline preparations has been performed successfully without recurrence of transaminase elevations (21).

2. **Pharmacokinetics.** Niacin and its amide forms are readily absorbed from all portions of the gastrointestinal tract by both facilitated and passive diffusion processes. Niacin is concentrated in the liver and erythrocytes where it is converted to NAD and NADP. Excess quantities are metabolized in the liver and further excreted in the urine. Niacin levels may be measured through the urinary excretion of its metabolites, *N*-methylnicotinamide (NMN) and 2-pyridone.

3. **Drug-drug interactions.** Niacin deficiency can result from the use of isoniazid. Isoniazid depletes pyridoxine—a necessary coenzyme in the tryptophan to niacin pathway. Niacin also potentiates the effects of ganglionic blocking agents (e.g., tryptophan) and may result in orthostatic hypotension.

C. **Clinical manifestations.** Niacin-induced histamine mediated reactions cause skin flushing, pruritus, hypotension, and tachycardia. Hepatocellular and cholestatic hepatotoxicity can present as malaise, nausea, vomiting, jaundice, or reversible maculopathy of the retina. Myopathies, manifested by leg myalgias and cramps, have been observed with chronic overdoses. Dermatologic abnormalities, including acanthosis nigrans, have been associated with nicotinic acid use (24). Niacin may also aggravate asthma and peptic ulcer disease.

D. **Laboratory findings.** Niacin-induced hepatitis may cause elevations in aspartate aminotransferase, alanine transferase, bilirubin, and lactate dehydrogenase levels, and a prolongation of prothrombin time. Other laboratory abnormalities include hypoalbuminemia, impaired glucose tolerance, hyperuricemia, and phosphaturia.

E. **Management.** As with most adverse reactions associated with vitamin ingestions, discontinuation of the vitamin is the most important therapy in patients with niacin toxicity. Anaphylaxis may require fluids, antihistamines, steroids, pressors and careful cardiovascular monitoring. Pre-treatment with aspirin may ameliorate the immediate effects of the niacin flush. Hepatotoxicity requires supportive therapy and close follow-up of liver function studies.

F. **Disposition.** Elevated liver function tests may necessitate hospital admission—especially if bleeding times are prolonged. Patients who have had severe histamine reactions should be monitored until they are asymptomatic for at least 4 to 6 h.

V. **Vitamin B$_6$.** Vitamin B$_6$ (pyridoxine) is a water-soluble B complex vitamin found in many foods including cereals, legumes, vegetables, liver, meat, and eggs. Signs of deficiency in adults include stomatitis, cheilosis, glossitis, irritability, depression, and confusion. Conditions in which plasma pyridoxine concentrations have been found to be decreased include asthma, renal disease, alcoholism, coronary artery disease, breast cancer, Hodgkin's disease, sickle cell anemia, diabetes, and smoking. Also, vitamin B_6 deficiency can be inherited as an autosomal recessive disorder which presents in infancy as intractable seizures and abnormal EEG patterns. Pyridoxine has been promoted in the treatment of psychiatric disorders including schizophrenia, autism, and hyperkinesis. It has also been used in the treatment of vomiting in pregnancy, carpal tunnel syndrome, and isoniazid overdose. Toxic effects, though rare, can be related to overzealous administration of the vitamin in supplement forms. The RDA of vitamin B_6 is 2 mg/day.

A. **Available preparations.** Pyridoxine hydrochloride is available in tablets of 5 to 500 mg, and as an injection of 100 mg/mL.

B. **Pharmacology and properties**

1. **Mechanism of action and toxicity.** Pyridoxine has multiple functions because of its complex interactions with amino acids and other nitrogenous compounds. Therefore, it is involved in a number of metabolic activities which include (but are not limited to) the following: transaminase reactions in gluconeogenesis; the conversion of tryptophan to niacin; lipid and cholesterol metabolism; modulation of endocrine functions via competitive binding of steroid receptor sites; and the synthesis of neurotransmitters. Sensory neuropathies have been associated with long-term use of greater than 2 mg/day of pyridoxine. Although the mechanism of this effect is unknown, it has been suggested that megadosing may affect the function of the dorsal root ganglia (25).

2. **Pharmacokinetics.** The primary forms of vitamin B_6 are absorbed by a non-saturable passive process in the jejunum. Phosphorylated forms are retained; nonphosphorylated forms pass through the intestine. The coenzyme form is bound to albumin in plasma, and to hemoglobin within the red blood cell. Removal of the phosphoryl group occurs in the liver by the action of aldehyde oxidase. The product is then excreted as 4-pyridoxic acid. Approximately 1000 micromoles of pyridoxine are stored in the body; the largest depot resides in the muscle. The turnover rate of pyridoxine is 25 to 33 days.

3. **Drug-drug interactions.** Several common drugs interfere with vitamin B_6 metabolism or promote pyridoxine catabolism. Ethinyl estradiol and mestranol cause increased retention of pyridoxine in tissues. Ethanol, conversely, causes increased vitamin B_6 breakdown. Some drugs interfere with the *activity* of pyridoxine. These include theophylline and caffeine which inhibit pyridoxal kinase. Finally, pyridoxine antagonizes the actions of levodopa, barbiturates, and phenytoin (5).

C. **Clinical manifestations.** Pyridoxine elicits low toxicity after either oral or intravenous administration. The use of 2 to 5 mg of pyridoxine per day for several months to treat disorders such as premenstrual syndrome and neurologic diseases, has resulted in a small number of cases of chronic neurotoxicity (25). Observed symptoms include paresthesias, ataxia, perioral numbness, loss of position and vibration sense, sensory neuropathies, and photosensitivity. These peripheral neuropathies result from both central and peripheral neuronal degeneration. Similar doses given to laboratory rats induced convulsions and death. Although the neuropathy associated with pyridoxine toxicity is described most typically as sensory in nature, a mild motor neuropathy was reported in a patient who chronically ingested large doses of the vitamin (10 g/day for 5 years) (26).

D. **Laboratory evaluation.** Direct methods for assessing vitamin B_6 status include measurement of the plasma coenzyme form pyridoxal phosphate, and total vitamin B_6 levels. Additionally, the major metabolic product of vitamin B_6, 4 pyridoxic acid, can be measured in the urine. Indirect methods include the measurement of tryptophan and methionine urinary metabolites, and erythrocyte transaminase activity.

E. **Management.** Complete, albeit slow, recovery usually occurs with cessation of pyridoxine therapy.

F. **Disposition.** Pyridoxine dependent seizures usually warrant hospital admission and neurologic evaluation. Neuropathies may be managed on an outpatient basis with immediate withdrawal of megadosing.

VI. **Vitamin B_{12}.** Vitamin B_{12} (cobalamin) was isolated in 1948 and was initially termed the "antipernicious anemia principle" (2,3). The natural source of cobalamin is synthesis by microorganisms in soil or sewage. Primary food sources can be found in meat, liver, fish eggs, and milk. Deficiency is most always the result of inadequate ingestion or absorption. The vitamin is essentially nontoxic, though rare cases of anaphylaxis have been reported. The RDA for adolescents and normal adults is 2 mcg/day, which should be increased in pregnancy.

A. **Available preparations.** Oral preparations are available in 25- to 1,000-mcg tablets. Parenteral injection forms come in concentrations of 30 to 1,000 mcg/mL.

B. **Pharmacology and properties**

1. **Mechanism of action and toxicity.** The primary roles of vitamin B_{12} are in the synthesis of thymidine and in DNA synthesis. Ineffective DNA synthesis results in ineffective hematopoiesis which causes megaloblastosis and pancytopenia. Vitamin B_{12} is also necessary in myelin synthesis; neurologic damage occurs in deficient states. Other vitamin B_{12} activities include methionine synthesis, fat and carbohydrate metabolism, and maintenance of sulfhydryl groups in the reduced form. There have been rare reports of transient diarrhea, itching, urticaria, and anaphylaxis associated with vitamin B_{12} use. These effects are believed to result from a sensitivity to impurities in the preparation of cyanocobalamin.

2. **Pharmacokinetics.** Vitamin B_{12}, normally bound to animal protein, is freed from its polypeptide linkages by gastric acid. It then attaches to gastric intrinsic factor (secreted by parietal cells) to form a complex which binds to receptors on the brush border of the ileal mucosa. The transport protein, transcobalamin II, then picks up cobalamin, transports it through the portal vein, and promotes endocytosis of cobalamin into the tissues. Vitamin B_{12}, largely in its coenzyme form, is stored in the liver. Total body stores average from 2 to 5 mg, and whole-body turnover is between 0.1% and 0.2% daily. Excretion occurs via the enterohepatic circulation and the kidneys.

C. **Clinical Manifestations.** Vitamin B_{12} is nontoxic in quantities up to 10,000 times the RDA. Rare instances of allergic reactions, characterized by pruritis, urticaria, and anaphylaxis, have been described (3). Reported dermatologic abnormalities associated with vitamin B_{12} use include contact dermatitis from occupational exposure and an acneiform eruption from high-dose ingestion (27,28).

D. Laboratory findings. Normal plasma values of vitamin B_{12} range from 200 to 900 pcg/mL and are measured by microbiological assays or radioimmunoassays.

E. Management. Dermatologic and allergic reactions resolve with discontinuation of vitamin exposure or ingestion. Allergic reactions can be treated with routine supportive therapy.

F. Disposition. Frank anaphylaxis resulting in hemodynamic or vascular compromise may necessitate hospital admission. Less severe anaphylactic reactions may be managed on an observation or outpatient basis.

VII. Vitamin C. Scurvy was first described as far back as the Roman civilizations and the Crusades (2). Sea explorers of the 16th century were described as having the physical symptoms of scurvy which include bleeding and rotting gums, swollen and inflamed joints, dark blotches of the skin, and muscle weakness. It was later discovered that species which lack the enzyme which converts L-gulonolactone to L-ascorbic acid, cannot synthesize vitamin C. These species include man, monkeys, and guinea pigs. Vitamin C has a purported role as a reductant and scavenger of free radicals useful in the prevention of cancer. Toxicity of vitamin C has been reported in rare cases, and occurs most commonly in individuals who, encouraged by these reports, ingest large quantities. The RDA for ascorbic acid is 60 mg/day.

A. Available preparations. Vitamin C (ascorbic acid) supplements are available in 1- to 500-mg tablets. Concentrations of the parenteral injection form range from 100 to 500 mg/mL. Ascorbic acid is also found in high concentrations in green tea which is popular in Japan (29).

B. Pharmacology and properties

1. **Mechanism of action and toxicity.** The functions of ascorbic acid are related to its role as a reductant; it is especially critical in reactions which require a reduced cofactor. The vitamin also acts as a scavenger of superoxide and hydroxyl radicals. The role of ascorbic acid as a reductant and scavenger of free radicals portends its utility in the detoxification of carcinogens. Ascorbic acid is also essential in the formation of collagen and glycosaminoglycans, and as a cofactor in the production of carnitine, necessary in the transport of long chain fatty acids across the mitochondrial membrane. Decreased resistance to infectious agents has been noted in ascorbic acid deficiency, prompting some to promote using megadoses of vitamin C in the treatment of the common cold. Much of the toxicity of ascorbic acid is related to osmotic effects in the intestine. Homeostatic mechanisms attempt to eliminate unnecessary quantities, resulting in nausea and diarrhea. Patients with intestinal malabsorption syndromes may be at increased risk for ascorbate-induced hyperoxaluria and nephrolithiasis (30–32). This is because intestinal malabsorption of ascorbate allows for a significant amount of oxalate to be formed from the unabsorbed ascorbate. The excess oxalate is absorbed and then excreted by the kidney. The conversion of ascorbate to oxalate appears to occur at the level of the gut since intravenous administration of ascorbate does not increase urinary oxalate excretion (31).

2. **Pharmacokinetics.** Ascorbic acid is absorbed in the small intestine in an energy dependent process which is saturable at elevated concentrations. Ascorbic acid is oxidized to dehydroascorbic acid and diketogulonic acid, which are metabolized subsequently to oxalic acid, threonic acid, xylose, and ascorbate-2-sulfate. In large

doses (or elevated blood concentrations of vitamin C), unabsorbed forms pass through the intestine and provide an osmotic load which can precipitate diarrhea or intestinal discomfort. At threshold blood levels of approximately 1.2 mg/dL, ascorbic acid is excreted unchanged via the kidneys.

3. **Drug-drug interactions.** Studies have also shown that **vitamin C deficiency** disrupts the cytochrome P450 system and therefore causes disorders in drug metabolism (33). Oral contraceptives have been shown to lower ascorbic acid levels (34).

Vitamin C excess may contribute to elevated iron absorption, especially in elderly men, and hence may be dangerous in patients with hemochromatosis, thalassemia, or sideroblastic anemia (31). Large doses of vitamin C may also interfere with heparin or coumadin anticoagulation (32).

C. **Clinical manifestations.** Studies which investigate the toxicity of high-dose vitamin C (1 to 15 g/day) are inconclusive (3). Many investigators have suggested that vitamin C can be taken in quantities of up to 10,000 mg/day for 3 years without adverse effect (35). The primary side effects, nausea and diarrhea, are ascribed to the osmotic load of excess vitamin in the intestine and resolve when excess supplementation is stopped. As described earlier, some patients may be predisposed to ascorbate-induced urolithiasis. These patients include those with ileal resection, small intestinal disease, jejuno-ileal bypass, or those with known hyperoxaluria or recurrent calcium-stone formation (30,31). Acute red cell hemolysis has been described in patients with glucose 6 phosphate dehydrogenase (G6PD) deficiency and paroxysmal nocturnal hemoglobinuria exposed to large quantities of vitamin C (see laboratory evaluation) (29,36). These patients presented with anemia, jaundice, dyspnea, and hemoglobinuria.

D. **Laboratory evaluation**

1. **Oxaluria.** When serum ascorbic acid levels exceed 2 mg/dL, urinary oxalic acid levels may elevate and precipitate oxalic acid renal stones (30,37).

2. **Red cell hemolysis.** Although low doses of ascorbic acid are known to protect against hemolysis of G6PD deficient red cells, excess vitamin C can promote red cell destruction. In fact, acute hemolysis was attributed to high-dose ascorbic acid treatment in a 32-year-old man with G6PD deficiency (36). The mechanism of ascorbic acid–induced hemolysis in G6PD deficiency is unknown; it is postulated that the production of hydrogen peroxide and other substances that deplete glutathione may be involved (36). Ascorbic acid has also induced hemolysis in patients with paroxysmal nocturnal hemoglobinuria (29).

3. **Redox chemistry interference.** Laboratory studies which rely on redox chemistry (serum cholesterol, glucose, and cerruloplasmin) are biased by high levels of vitamin C (3).

E. **Management.** Cessation of vitamin C supplementation usually results in resolution of symptoms and laboratory abnormalities. However, abrupt withdrawal is not recommended. This is because a rebound deficiency state after excess vitamin C supplementation has been reported (35). Chronic megadosing of ascorbic acid may induce metabolic elimination pathways and cause a precipitous drop in plasma ascorbic acid levels following abrupt discontinuation. Although further studies are needed, a gradual withdrawal is recommended in individuals taking high levels of the vitamin.

F. Disposition. Significant nephrolithiasis may necessitate intravenous pyelography and hospital admission.

VIII. Vitamin D. Cholecalciferol, or vitamin D, was first recognized during the seventeenth century for its use in the prevention of a bone deforming disease. This disease, later termed rickets, was characterized by enlargement of long bone epiphyses, bowing of the legs, bending of the spine, and weak or atonic muscles. Later, the physiologic function of vitamin D was deemed essential in maintaining extra and intracellular concentrations of calcium and phosphorus. Patients who routinely require vitamin D supplementation include those with renal osteodystrophy, hypoparathyroidism, rickets, osteoporosis, and defective absorption of vitamin D. In addition, patients receiving phenytoin and phenobarbital over prolonged periods metabolize vitamin D at accelerated rates. The RDA of vitamin D is 400 mg/day.

A. Available preparations. Ergocalciferol (calciferol) is vitamin D_2. It is derived from plants and is found in irradiated bread and milk. Commercially it is available in 1.25-mg tablets and capsules, and as an oral solution (0.25 mg/mL). Dihydrotachysterol (DHT) is the reduced crystalline form of vitamin D_2 and is available in tablets (0.125 to 0.4 mg), capsules (0.125 mg), and oral solutions (0.2 and 0.25 mg/mL). Vitamin D_3 (cholecalciferol) is the natural form of vitamin D that is produced when 7-dehydrocholesterol in the skin is exposed to sunlight. The section below describes its in vivo conversion to calcifediol and calcifitriol. Calcifediol is commercially available in 20 to 50 µg capsules. Calcifitriol is marketed in 0.25- to 0.5-g tablets and in an injectable form (1 or 2 µg/mL). There is no practical physiologic difference between vitamins D_2 and D_3.

B. Pharmacology and properties

1. **Mechanism of action and toxicity.** Vitamin D, in concert with parathyroid hormone and calcitonin, acts to maintain serum concentrations of calcium and phosphorus. Overall, vitamin D increases serum calcium levels through its action on bone resorption, intestinal calcium absorption, and renal calcium excretion. It stimulates bone resorption and thereby provides calcium and phosphorous for bone mineralization, thus preventing rickets and osteomalacia. Vitamin D also enhances intestinal absorption of calcium. Finally, vitamin D promotes reabsorption of calcium in the proximal tubules of the kidney. The manifestations of vitamin D toxicity are related to the effects of hypercalcemia. Toxicity related to the symptoms of hypercalcemia may be noted among individuals exceeding daily doses of 60,000 IU over prolonged periods (2).

2. **Pharmacokinetics.** Dietary and intrinsically synthesized vitamin D are prohormones that require activation before they can carry out their biological effects on target tissues. These prohormones are readily absorbed from the small intestine in a process which is dependent on bile salts. They travel to the liver where the first step of activation occurs: this involves the hydroxylation of vitamin D to form 25-hydroxyvitamin D (25-$[OH]_2D_3$ or calcifediol). This metabolite undergoes further hydroxylation in the proximal tubules of the kidney to form 1,25-dihydroxyvitamin D (1,25-$[OH]_2D_3$ or calcifitriol). Calcifitriol is the active metabolite of vitamin D. Both calcifediol and calcifitriol are

available for clinical use. Vitamin D and its metabolites circulate in the plasma bound to the carrier protein alpha-globulin. Excess vitamin D is stored in fatty tissue. The majority of vitamin D excretion occurs in bile; a small amount may be found in urine. Vitamin D absorbed from the intestine has an elimination half-life of 19 to 25 h. The plasma half life of calcifediol is approximately 19 days, while that of calcifitriol is between 3 and 5 days.

3. **Drug-drug interactions.** Phenytoin and phenobarbital have been shown to decrease serum levels of vitamin D, presumably through accelerated metabolism.

C. **Clinical manifestations.** Vitamin D doses of approximately 1,000 to 3,000 IU/kg are potentially dangerous. Massive doses of vitamin D can acutely cause symptoms within 2 to 8 days—these effects are related to hypercalcemia. Symptoms related to hypercalcemia include polydipsia, polyuria, vomiting, diarrhea, weakness, fatigue, anorexia, and headache. The differential diagnosis is listed in Table 35-2. Prolonged ingestions of greater than 60,000 IU/day of vitamin D may result in excessive calcium deposition in the vasculature, heart, bone, lungs, and kidneys. Prolonged insults to these organs may result in anemia, hypertension, renal failure, and death. Cardiac arrhythmias may arise secondary to hypercalcemia and may be potentiated in patients using digitalis. Vitamin D toxicity has caused toxic effects in children when taken in doses of 10,000 IU/day for 4 months (11). Prolonged feeding with premature formulas may lead to hypervitaminosis D because of the high concentrations of vitamin D and calcium found in those formulas (38). Childhood manifestations of vitamin D toxicity include growth arrest and developmental delay in addition to the symptoms described above (2,39). Hypervitaminosis D and hypercalcemia in pregnant women may suppress parathyroid function in the newborn. This suppressed parathyroid activity may lead to neonatal hypocalcemia, tetany, and seizures.

D. **Laboratory findings.** Circulating calcifediol levels reflect vitamin D intake and body pool size; the normal range is 10 to 50 pg/mL, while vitamin D intoxication is often accompanied by levels above 200 pg/mL. Other laboratory abnormalities associated with vitamin D excess include hypercalcemia, hypercalcuria, and hyperphosphatemia. Hypochromic anemia, azotemia, and a decreased alkaline phosphatase are also commonly found. Potential roentgenographic findings include metastatic calcifications or osteoporosis.

E. **Management.** The management of hypervitaminosis D involves discontinuation of vitamin D therapy and administration of a low calcium diet. Refractory cases and patients with associated cardiotoxicity of hypercalcemia may be treated with saline hydration, furosemide, and prednisone at 1 mg/kg/day. Prednisone decreases calcium absorption from the gut and calcium mobilization from the bone. Patients with calcium levels exceeding 14 mg/dL may benefit from treatment with calcitonin 4 to 8 IU/kg intramuscularly every 6 to 12 h.

F. **Disposition.** Patients with acute ingestions of 100 times the RDA or more may require decontamination and administration of activated charcoal and cathartics in the emergency department. Cardiac effects related to hypercalcemia necessitate hospitalization. The effects of chronic exposure may require a low calcium diet, though may be managed on an outpatient basis, if no cardiotoxic effects are present.

IX. Vitamin E. The discovery of alpha-tocopherol in 1922 by Evans and Bishop can be traced to early observations that rats fed diets deficient in this vitamin often suffered fetal demise (3). The term "tocopherol" is derived from the Greek "*tos*" (childbirth), "*phero*" (to bring forth), and "*ol*" (pertaining to the alcohol portion of the molecule). Vitamin E supplementation has been recommended in disease states such as ischemic heart disease and intermittent claudication for its role as an antioxidant. It has also been used to prevent or ameliorate axonal dystrophy and retrolental fibroplasia. The RDA of vitamin E is 400 mg/day. Due to the large belief that megadoses may be beneficial, many take supplements in the range of 100 to 800 mg/day and may be susceptible to toxic effects.

A. Available preparations. Vitamin E is found in tablets and capsules ranging form 50 to 1,000 IU. Oral drops are available in concentrations of 50 mg/mL. An injectable form for intramuscular use is available from the manufacturer.

B. Pharmacologic properties

   1. Mechanism of action and toxicity. There is widespread agreement and at least in vitro evidence that vitamin E functions as a biologic antioxidant to protect cellular membranes from oxidative destruction (3,40). As a lipid-soluble cofactor, vitamin E functions as a free radical scavenger in biologic membranes, halting fatty acid peroxidation. Theories that aging processes and carcinogenesis are mitigated by the effects of free radicals suggest that vitamin E may ameliorate both processes. It has been proposed that vitamin E functions as a "sparing agent" of protein sulfhydryl groups during periods of oxidative stress, as found in ischemic injury and drug-induced injury. Proposed functions include regulation of nucleic acid synthesis and gene expression. Isolated toxidromes have occurred through unknown mechanisms. These include gastrointestinal disturbances, weakness, headache, gonadal dysfunction, and blurred vision (40).

   2. Pharmacokinetics. Tocopherols are intestinally absorbed in a saturable process which is dependent on lipid digestion. Bile salts and pancreatic enzymes are important in the absorptive process. Tocopherols are transported, in association with lipoproteins, by lymphatic vessels to the venous system. They are absorbed by most tissues but are primarily sequestered in adipose tissues. Vitamin E is enzymatically metabolized, and excreted in the feces, perhaps in association with bile salts.

C. Clinical manifestations. Reported toxic effects include an increased bleeding tendency, impaired immune function, decreased levels of vitamin K–dependent clotting factors, and impaired leukocyte function (3). Intravenous vitamin E (E-Ferol) was formerly used in premature infants as prophylaxis against retinopathy of prematurity and hemolytic anemia. This resulted in several deaths secondary to the development of ascites, epatosplenomegaly, cholestatic jaundice, azotemia, and thrombocytopenia (41). The exact mechanism of this syndrome is unknown. Toxicity was thought to be related to the cumulative effects of one of the additives of the injectable form; consequently E-Ferol production was discontinued (41). Subsequent studies suggest that the toxicity results from the vitamin itself (42).

D. Laboratory findings. Toxicity can occur when serum tocopherol levels exceed 3 to 4 mg/dL. An elevated prothrombin time may occur secondary to vitamin E's anti–vitamin K effect. Serum elevations of the following substances have been noted during vitamin E use: creatinine kinase, cholesterol, triglycerides, thyroxine, triiodothyronine, and urinary estrogens and androgens. These elevations have resolved with discontinuation of vitamin E (40). It is recommended that plasma levels be monitored during the use of pharmacologic doses of vitamin E for the treatment of retrolental fibroplasia. These patients should also be observed for evidence of hemolysis and thrombocytopenia.

    E. **Management.** Treatment of hypervitaminosis E involves discontinuation of the drug and supportive therapy. Coagulation deficits should be managed with administration of intramuscular vitamin K.

    F. **Disposition.** Coagulation abnormalities may necessitate hospitalization. In most cases, however, vitamin E toxidromes can be managed on an outpatient basis.

X. **Vitamin K.** Phytonadione (vitamin K) was discovered by Henrik Dam in 1929, in studies of chicks fed fat free diets which developed hemorrhages and coagulopathy (2). It was later discovered that vitamin K activates the clotting factors prothrombin (factor 2), proconvertin (factor 7), Christmas factor (factor 9), and Stuart factor (factor 10) which each undergo hepatic synthesis. Deficient states can be seen in patients with poor nutrition, malabsorption, or defective hepatic synthesis. Vitamin K is useful in the treatment of hypoprothrombinemia, oral anticoagulant overdoses, hemorrhagic diseases of the newborn, and hemorrhage associated with vitamin K deficiency. The recommended daily allowance for vitamin K is 1 μg/kg; the average diet usually satisfies the daily requirement. Some vitamin K is synthesized endogenously by bacteria in the gut. Hypersensitivity reactions have been described, following intravenous vitamin K administration, and represent this vitamin's spectrum of toxicity. The major effect has been acute cardiovascular collapse (36).

    A. **Available preparations.** Vitamin K_1 (phytonadione), synthesized in plants, is the only naturally occurring vitamin K that has therapeutic uses. Phytonadione is present in green tea, beef liver, and green leafy vegetables such as broccoli. It is commercially available as an oral preparation in 5-mg tablets, and as intravenous or intramuscular solutions in concentrations of 2 or 10 mg/mL. Vitamin K_3 (menadione) is the precursor of vitamin K_2 (menaquinone-4) which is synthesized in animals by gram-positive bacteria. Menadione is available in 5-mg tablets.

    B. **Pharmacology and properties**

        1. **Mechanism of action and toxicity.** The clotting factors 2,7,9, and 10 are biologically inactive proteins in the liver that remain inactive in the absence of vitamin K. Vitamin K acts as an essential cofactor in their activation which involves post-translational carboxylation of these proteins as well as the anticoagulant, protein C. In adequate doses, vitamin K reverses the inhibitory effects of coumadin on these coagulation factors. Severe anaphylactic reactions from rapid infusion of intravenous vitamin K have occurred; the mechanism of this hypersensitivity reaction or anaphylaxis is unknown, though may be related to the injection vehicle (36). The injectable form of phytonadione is preserved in benzyl alcohol which has known toxic effects when given in higher than recommended concentrations in newborns (43). These effects include gasping respirations, metabolic acidosis, renal failure, hematologic abnormalities, cardiovascular collapse, and death, and has occurred following administration of 99 to 234 mg/kg/day of benzyl alcohol (39).

        2. **Pharmacokinetics.** Phytonadione is absorbed from the gastrointestinal tract only in the presence of bile salts. After absorption, vitamin K_1 is transported by the lymphatic system and then concentrated in the liver. Vitamin K_1 is then rapidly metabolized to polar metabolites which are excreted in the bile and urine. Mena-

dione absorption is not dependent upon the presence of bile salts. It travels directly to the blood stream and is excreted as glucuronide and sulfate conjugates.

3. **Drug-drug interactions.** Coumadin anticoagulants antagonize the action of vitamin K. This results in an initial inhibition of protein C resulting in a paradoxical hypercoagulable state. Later, a reduction of factors 2, 7, 9, and 10 result in the hypocoagulable state.

C. **Clinical manifestations.** Intravenous administration of phytonadione has caused anaphylactic reactions characterized by flushing, dyspnea, chest pain, cardiovascular collapse, and even death (36,39). Erythematous, pruritic, indurated lesions have resulted from chronic injection of the intramuscular form. Parenteral vitamin K administration has caused hemolysis and hyperbilirubinemia in newborn infants, particularly those born prematurely (43).

D. **Laboratory findings.** Vitamin K administration will decrease prothrombin times within 12 to 48 h following an oral dose and within 3 to 8 h following a parenteral injection. Hemolysis and hyperbilirubinemia following vitamin K administration in a newborn may suggest the diagnosis of vitamin K overdose.

E. **Management.** Anaphylactic reactions may require treatment with intravenous fluid resuscitation and administration of epinephrine and histamine blockers.

F. **Disposition.** Anaphylactic reactions resulting in cardiovascular compromise warrant hospital admission. Mild hypersensitivity reactions resulting in cutaneous effects can be managed on an outpatient basis.

XI. **Differential diagnosis of hypervitaminosis D** (11). Symptoms are consistent with those found in hypercalcemia; these include:

A. Hyperparathyroidism
B. Paget's disease
C. Neoplasm
D. Nonparathyroid endocrinopathies
   1. Hyperthyroidism
   2. Adrenal insufficiency
   3. Pheochromocytoma
   4. Acromegaly
E. Other pharmacologic agents
   1. Milk-alkali syndrome
   2. Thiazide diuretics
   3. Vitamin A
   4. Calcium or lithium
F. Hypersensitivity to vitamin A
   1. Granulomatous disease, e.g., sarcoidosis
   2. Idiopathic infantile hypercalcemia
G. Miscellaneous
   1. Newborn physiologic hypercalcemia
   2. Immobilization
   3. Phosphate depletion in uremia
   4. Hypophophatasia

References

1. Krenzelok E. Vitamin toxicity. Selected aspects of acute and chronic overdosage. *Clin Toxicol Forum* 1993;2:1–5.
2. Gilman A, Rall T, Nies A, Taylor P. *Goodman and Gilman's—The pharmacologic basis of therapeutics.* 8th ed. New York: McGraw-Hill, 1993.
3. Shils M, Olson J, Shike M, ed. *Modern nutrition in health and disease.* 8th ed. Philadelphia: Lea & Febiger, 1994.
4. Inkeles S, Conor W, Lingworth D. Hepatic and dermatologic manifestations of chronic hypervitaminosis in adults. *Am J Med* 1986;80:491.
5. Ellenhorn M, Barceloux D, ed. *Medical toxicology.* 1st ed. New York: Elsevier Science, 1988.
6. Amine E, Corey J, Hegsted D, Hayes K. Comparative hematology during deficiencies of iron and vitamin A in the rat. *Journal of Nutrition* 1970;100(9): 1033–1040, September.
7. Robbins S, Cotran R, Kumar V, ed. *Pathologic basis of disease.* 3rd ed. Philadelphia: WB Saunders, 1984.
8. Kowalski T, Falestiny M, Furth E, Malet P. Vitamin A hepatotoxicity: a cautionary note regarding 25,000 IU supplements. *Am J Med* 1994;97:523–528.
9. Kaplan G, Haettich B. Rheumatological symptoms due to retinoids. *Baillieres Clin Rheumatol* 1991;5:77–97.
10. Nesher G, Zuckner J. Rheumatologic complications of vitamin A and retinoids. *Semin Arthritis Rheum* 1995;24: 291–296.
11. Haddad L, Winchester J. *Clinical management of poisoning and drug overdose.* 2nd ed. Philadelphia: WB Saunders, 1990.
12. Vahlquist A. Long-term safety of retinoid therapy. *J Am Acad Dermatol* 1992;27:829–833.
13. Bruno N, Beacham B, Burnett J. Adverse effects of isotretoin therapy. *Cutis* 1984;33:484.
14. Lee A. Pseudotumor cerebri after treatment with tetracycline and isotretinoin for acne. *Cutis* 1995;55:165–168.
15. Lammer E, Chen D, Hoar R, Agnish D, et al. Retenoic acid embryopathy. *N Engl J Med* 1985;313:837.
16. Mahoney C. Vitamins A and D and their analogues. In: Haddad L, Winchester J, ed. *Clinical management of poisoning and drug overdose.* Philadelphia: WB Saunders, 1990:1440–1446.
17. Sanchez M, Ross B, Rotterdam H, Salik J, Brodie R, Freeberg I. Retinoid hepatitis. *J Am Acad Dermatol* 1993;28: 853–858.
18. Rivlin R. Disorders of vitamin metabolism: deficiencies, metabolic abnormalities, and excesses. In: Wyngaarden J, Smith L, ed. *Textbook of internal medicine.* Philadelphia: WB Saunders, 1988:1228–1240.
19. Stephen J, Grant R, Yeh C. Anaphylaxis from administration of intravenous thiamine. *Am J Emerg Med* 1992;1:61–63.
20. Santanelli S, Gobbi G, Albani F, Gastaut H. Appearance of EEG abnormalities in two patients during long-term treatment with vitamin B vitamins. *Neurophysiol Clin* 1988;18:549–553.
21. Henkin Y, Johnson K, Segrest J. Rechallenge with crystalline niacin after drug-induced hepatits from sustained-release niacin. *JAMA* 1990;264:241–243.
22. Rader J, Calvert R, Hathcock J. Hepatic toxicity of unmodified and time-release preparations of niacin. *Am J Med* 1992;92:77–81.
23. Etchason J, Miller T, Squires R, et al. Niacin-induced hepatitis: a potential side effect with low-dose time-release niacin. *Mayo Clin Proc* 1991;66:23–28.
24. Stals H, Vercammen C, Peeters C, Morren M. Acanthosis nigrans caused by nicotinic acid: case report and review of the literature. *Dermatology* 1994;189:203–206.
25. Schaumberg J, Kaplan J, Windenabk A, et al. Sensory neuropathy from pyridoxine abuse. A new megavitamin syndrome. *N Engl J Med* 1983;309:445–448.
26. Morra M, Philipszoon M, D'Andrea G, Cananzi A, L'Erario R, Milone F. Sensory and motor neuropathy caused by excessive ingestion of vitamin B_6: a case report. *Funct Neurol* 1993;8:429–432.
27. Rodriguez A, Echechipia S, Alvarez M, Muro M. Ocupational contact dermatitis from vitamin B_{12}. *Contact Dermatitis* 1994;31:271.
28. Sherertz E. Acneiform eruption due to "megadose" vitamins B_6 and B_{12}. *Cutis* 1991;48:119–120.
29. Dam H, Schonheyder F. The antihaemorrhagic vitamin of the chick. *Nature* 1935;135:652–653.
30. Urivetzky M, Kessaris D, Smith A. Ascorbic acid overdosing: a risk factor for calcium oxalate nephrolothiasis. *J Urol* 1992;147:1215–1218.
31. Cook J, Monsen E. Vitamin C, the common cold and iron absorption. *Am J Clin Nutr* 1977;30:235–241.
32. Rosenthal G. Interaction of ascorbic acid and warfarin. JAMA3 1971;215:1671.
33. Basu T, Schorah C. *Vitamin C in health and disease.* Westport: AUI Publishing, 1982.
34. Briggs M. Megadose vitamin C and metabolic effects of the pill. *BMJ* 1981;283:1547.
35. Anderson T. Large-scale studies with vitamin C. *Acta Vitaminol Enzymol* 1977;31:43–50.
36. Barash P, Kitahata L, Mandel S. Acute cardiovascular collapse after intravenous phytonakione. *Anesth Analg Curr Res* 1976;55:304–306.

37. Lawton J, Conway L, Crosson J, Smith C, Abraham P. Acute oxalate nephropathy after massive ascorbic acid administration. *Arch Intern Med* 1985, 145(5).
38. Nako Y, Fukushima N, Tomomasa T, Nagashima K. Hypervitaminosis D after prolonged feeding with a premature infant formula. *Pediatrics* 1993;92:862–863.
39. Ellenhorn M, Schonwald S, Ordog G, Wasserberger J. *Ellenhorn's medical toxicology—diagnosis and treatment of human poisoning.* 2nd ed. Baltimore: Williams & Wilkins, 1997.
40. *American hosptial formulary service drug information.* AHFS, 1996.
41. Bove K, Kosmetatos N, Wedig K, et al. Vasculopathic hepatotoxicity associated with E-Ferol syndrome in low birth weight infants. *JAMA* 1985;254:2422–2430.
42. Hale T, Rais-Bashrami K, Montgomery D, Harkey C, Habersang R. Vitamin E toxicity in neonatal piglet. *J Toxicol Clin Toxicol* 1995;33:123–130.
43. *Physicians' desk reference.* 49th ed. Montvale, NJ: Medical Economics, 1995.

Emergency Toxicology, Second Edition,
edited by Peter Viccellio.
Lippincott–Raven Publishers, Philadelphia © 1998.

36

Anticoagulants

Mara J. Stankovich and Daniel L. Savitt

*Department of Emergency Medicine, Brown University, Rhode Island Hospital,
Providence, Rhode Island 02903*

I. Hemorrhage observed in cattle fed spoiled sweet clover silage led to the eventual isolation of 4-hydroxycoumarin (1). A compound structurally similar to vitamin K, acting as a vitamin K antagonist, it induces a coagulopathy. Derivatives of this compound have been used as oral anticoagulants since the early 1940s and include ethyl bicoumacetate, sodium warfarin, acenocoumarin, and bishydroxycoumarin. Less commonly used are the indanedione derivatives (phenindione, diphenadione, and anisodione) which are associated with more adverse effects.

II. **Available preparations**

   A. Pharmaceutical preparations of warfarin, the most commonly available oral anticoagulant, are available in 1-, 2-, 2.5-, 5-, 7.5-, and 10-mg tablets. In the United States, approximately 95% of rodenticides contain an anticoagulant (2). To counteract warfarin-resistance in rats, more potent coumarin compounds have been synthesized and are readily available in garden and hardware stores. These long-acting anticoagulant compounds are collectively termed the "superwarfarins." They are divided into two classes: the indanedione derivatives (Diphacinone, Pindone, Chlorphacinone) and the 4-hydroxycoumarin derivatives (Difenacoum, Bromadione, Brodifacoum) (3). Brodifacoum is the most commonly available superwarfarin for rodenticidal use. The concentration of these agents varies from 0.005% to 2% (4).

   B. At therapeutic doses, oral anticoagulants are used to treat or prevent intravascular thrombosis. They have no in vitro activity and are not used when extracorporeal anticoagulation is needed. Larger doses contained in rodenticides are used to induce fatal hemorrhage in rodents. The minimum toxic dose of oral anticoagulants ranges from 6 to 15 mg/kg. The toxic dose of the rodenticidal anticoagulant compounds is difficult to quantify on a milligram per kilogram basis. Clinical bleeding may occur from as little as 1 mg of a superwarfarin agent. In children, a dose of 0.15 mg/kg (or 30 g of a 0.005% bait) will cause a coagulopathy (5). One should rely on clinical signs and degree of hypoprothrombinemia rather than the estimated amount ingested to determine toxicity.

III. **Pharmacology and properties**

   A. **Mechanism of action.** The oral anticoagulants exert their effect by inhibiting the enzyme, epoxide reductase, in generating active vitamin K_1 (6). Active vitamin K_1 functions to carboxylate and thereby activate coagulation Factors II, VII, IX, and X; the so-

627

TABLE 36-1. *Drugs that potentiate anticoagulant action*

Allopurinol	Metronidazole
Amiodarone	NSAIDS
Anabolic steroids	Penicillin
Cephalosporins	Phenothiazines
Chloramphenicol	Quinine
Cimetidine	Sulfonamides
Clofibrate	Sulfonylureas
Disulfiram	Tetracycline
Ethanol	Thyroxine
Heparin	Tricyclic antidepressants
Laxatives	

called "vitamin K–dependent factors." Vitamin K also activates Proteins C and S, both of which have anticoagulation properties. The effect of anticoagulant agents on hemostasis is delayed until the normal clotting factors are cleared from the circulation. The half-lives of the vitamin K–dependent factors are as follows: Factor VII, 4 to 7 h; Protein C, 8 h; Factor IX, 24 h; Protein S, 30 h; Factor X, 36 to 48 h; and Factor II, 50 h. The prothrombin time (PT) is used clinically to monitor the degree of anticoagulation.

B. Pharmacokinetics

1. The pharmacokinetics of warfarin have been well-studied while that of the super-warfarins are less clearly defined. The **absorption** of warfarin and the super-warfarins from the gastrointestinal (GI) tract is rapid and nearly complete. Coagulopathy has also been reported from industrial exposure via inhalation and dermal contact (7). Approximately 99% of warfarin is bound to serum albumin. Onset of action occurs within 12 h but activity does not peak until 96 h because of the longer half-lives of Factors II and X (8).

2. The oral anticoagulants are completely **metabolized** by hepatocytes and byproducts are excreted in the stool and urine. It is presumed that the superwarfarins undergo biotransformation by the same mechanism. The **plasma half-life** of warfarin is 35 to 40 h. The half-life of brodifacoum from case reports varies between 20 to 62 days (9). The half-lives for other superwarfarins are unknown, but are at least three times that of warfarin based on studies in laboratory rodents (10).

3. Duration of action. Warfarin can induce anticoagulation for 3 to 5 days. In the case of superwarfarin ingestion, coagulopathy can persist for 45 days to 8 months because these compounds are more lipophilic and bind with approximately 100-fold greater affinity to hepatic epoxide reductase (11). Numerous drug interactions exist (Table 36-1).

4. The warfarin-like anticoagulants **cross the placenta** and are contraindicated in pregnancy, especially during the third trimester because of teratogenicity.

IV. Clinical manifestations

A. Accidental overdose is the **leading cause** of warfarin toxicity. Exposures of this nature are less likely to produce symptoms because the amount ingested is usually insufficient to interfere with coagulation. Superwarfarin ingestions account for the majority of anticoagulant overdoses reported to poison control centers. In 1994, there were 12,868 exposures to a superwarfarin compound and 2,312 to standard warfarin preparations (12). The majority of accidental poisonings occur in children secondary to ingestion of the agents themselves or rat feces which contain undigested rodenticide. Intentional ingestions have been used to malinger, commit murder, attempt suicide, induce abortion, and for Munchausen-by-proxy.

B. **Minor bleeding** may occur in 2% to 10% of patients on anticoagulant therapy. Back or flank pain, hematuria, and ecchymosis are the most common presenting complaints. Headache, chest or abdominal pain, difficulty breathing or swallowing, and shock with overt bleeding may also be seen.

C. **Ecchymosis** is the most frequent sign of anticoagulant overdose. Also seen are hematuria, GI bleeding, epistaxis, spontaneous hematoma formation, compartment syndrome, vaginal bleeding, gingival bleeding, and hemoptysis (in order of decreasing frequency) (13). Petechiae and hemarthroses are seen less commonly. Rodenticide bait pellets often contain a nontoxic dye so that the presence of a blue or green-stained oral mucosa or hands may suggest rodenticide ingestion.

D. **Fatalities** occur with intracerebral hemorrhage, retroperitoneal hemorrhage, and bleeding into the submandibular space leading to upper airway obstruction (14). In nonoverdose situations, bleeding is more likely to occur in patients with ischemic cerebrovascular disease, hypertension, underlying malignancies, ulcer disease, and trauma (15). Fatalities average two to three per year and are caused by both standard warfarin and superwarfarins in near-equal proportions (12).

E. Nonhemorrhagic adverse reactions to warfarin include skin necrosis, urticaria, nausea, diarrhea, and dermatitis. Skin necrosis is more prevalent in those with Protein C deficiency and usually occurs within 3 to 10 days from treatment onset. Initiation of coumadin therapy may also cause release of atheromatous microemboli resulting in "purple toes syndrome" which is managed by discontinuation of the drug and observation for gangrenous extension. The indenadione derivatives can produce polyuria, polydipsia, and tachycardia when given in large doses. Less commonly, they are associated with granulocytopenia and increased liver transaminases.

F. The differential diagnosis of a coagulopathy accompanied by a prolonged PT includes vitamin K deficiency, hepatic failure, inherited coagulation disorders, DIC, and amyloidosis.

V. **Laboratory evaluation.** Initial laboratory studies should include a measurement of the PT, aPTT, a complete blood count, urinalysis, liver function tests, and stool hemoccult test. Vitamin K–dependent factor deficiency can be confirmed with a plasma mixing study which involves combining equal volumes of the patients plasma and normal plasma resulting in correction of the PT. However, this is not usually done in an emergency department setting. Although rarely used, assays for clotting factor activity can be performed. These are considered the most precise way of measuring the effect of the oral anticoagulants because a normal PT may exist despite markedly decreased factor activities. The serum Factor VII–X complex will decrease 12 h postingestion and precedes a change in the PT so that quantification of this complex may be useful in detecting patients at risk for the development of a coagulopathy (16). When more widely available, this test could be used as an early sensitive screening tool in acute ingestions. Moreover, it could serve as a useful adjunct in determining the need for further treatment when vitamin K therapy has been discontinued. Serum warfarin levels can be determined by radioimmunoassays although they are not routinely performed in the acute setting.

VI. Management

A. An algorithmic management of anticoagulant toxicity. Initial management should include assessment of the ABC's and stabilization of the patient. Ipecac-induced emesis may be performed early in cases of acute ingestion, especially in children. It is not recommended for repeated ingestions or patients on chronic therapy because of the risk of inducing hemorrhage. To enhance elimination and excretion of the drugs the use of activated charcoal, cholestyramine, and a cathartic has been advocated. Charcoal should be repeated at least once unless contraindicated. Cholestyramine may interrupt enterohepatic recirculation of warfarin, thereby increasing clearance (17). The duration of cholestyramine therapy will depend on the PT Identification of the ingested agent is cru-

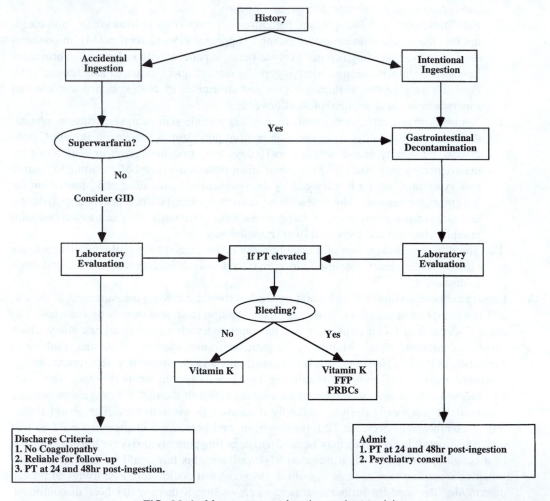

FIG. 36-1. Management of anticoagulant toxicity.

cial to proper management because the superwarfarins are more refractory to therapy and are associated with a relapse if therapy is withdrawn prematurely.

B. Marked hypoprothrombinemia (greater than three to four times control) without evidence of bleeding can be managed by discontinuing use of the drug and administering low-dose vitamin K (10 mg in adults, 1 to 5 mg in children). An effect on the PT will not be seen for 6 to 12 h following vitamin K administration. If bleeding is present despite a therapeutic PT an occult lesion must be sought. A larger dose of vitamin K should be administered if there is evidence of bleeding and an abnormal PT (10 to 50 mg in adults, 0.6 mg/kg in children). This should be repeated every 4 h if bleeding persists and/or the PT is prolonged more than 19 seconds (or an INR of 1.5). Superwarfarin ingestion may require large and prolonged administration of vitamin K in doses that need to be individualized. Up to 125 mg/day have been used in cases of superwarfarin ingestion, although the oral route must be employed in addition to the i.v. route in order to deliver such a large amount. This can be tapered as the coagulation parameters normalize. In the case of severe hemorrhage or intracranial bleeding, immediate reversal of coagulopathy is required. Fresh frozen plasma (FFP), in a dose of 10 to 20 mL. FFP/kg for a child or 4 to 6 U in adults, is then the initial treatment of choice. Alternatively, prothrombin complex/Factor IX concentrate can be infused, although this is associated with many adverse effects such as transmission of hepatitis, HIV, and embolic phenomenon. Volume loss is treated with crystalloid infusion and blood transfusion as needed. The PT should be checked every 12 h until stable and vitamin K administered until the value is within the normal range. Cases of superwarfarin overdoses may require extended therapy lasting several weeks.

C. Antidotes.

1. Vitamin K is synthesized by bacteria in the intestinal tract or can be obtained from dietary sources such as green vegetables and vegetable oils. It exists in three forms: phytonadione (vitamin K_1), menaquinone (vitamin K_2), and menadione (vitamin K_3). The daily requirement of vitamin K is 1 µg/kg in the adult and 10 µg/kg in the neonate. Phytonadione is the indicated form of vitamin K for the treatment of oral anticoagulant-induced coagulopathy. Trade names include Aquamephyton, Konakion, Mephyton. It is available in 5 mg tablets and in 2 or 10 mg/mL solutions. Menadione (Synkavite) is available in 5 mg tablets and is useful in cases of vitamin K deficiency but is ineffective in reversing anticoagulation because it requires hepatic metabolism to vitamin K_1 (18). **Adverse effects**: i.v. infusion of phytonadione has been associated with flushing, chest pain, dyspnea, and anaphylactoid shock (19). Physicians should be prepared for this eventuality. Dilution of 10 to 20 mg of phytonadione in 125 mL of D5W and infusion at a rate of 1 mg/min is recommended, though adverse reactions have been reported even despite these measures. Therefore, the i.v. route should be reserved for serious toxicity (20). Subcutaneous and i.m. injections of phytonadione have not been associated with life-threatening adverse reactions, however, the onset of action using these routes of administration is variable and should not be relied on in cases of anticoagulant-induced hemorrhage. If the risk of bleeding is low, the intramuscular route is preferred. Oral administration may be used once hemorrhage has ceased and the PT is normal.

2. **Fresh frozen plasma (FFP)** should be used in cases of severe bleeding or airway compromise. In an adult, 4 to 6 U of plasma infused i.v. will restore circulating clotting factors to near normal, although without concomitant administration of vitamin K, the factors will be degraded rapidly and repeated transfusions will be necessary. Patients should be monitored for signs of volume overload.

3. **Phenobarbital** is of no proven benefit in humans. It has been reported anecdotally to decrease the duration of anticoagulant effect in cases of overdose via the stimulation of hepatic microsomes (10).

VII. **Disposition considerations**

A. Intentional overdose warrants close observation because larger amounts and more toxic substances are likely to have been ingested. Psychiatric evaluation and admission are also indicated.

B. Asymptomatic patients with a normal PT and reliable follow-up can be discharged with instructions to return for PT measurement in 24 and 48 h or with the onset of any symptoms.

C. **Admission criteria.** Any patient with PT prolongation, bleeding, or those having attempted suicide should be admitted for evaluation and serial PT measurements. These should be followed until coagulation tests are normal. The patient can then be safely discharged on oral vitamin K with follow-up laboratory tests to ensure efficacy of outpatient treatment. Suicidal patients should be referred for psychiatric care when medically stable.

VIII. **Heparin.** Heparin, so named because of its abundance in the liver, was discovered in 1922. It is a negatively charged glycosaminoglycan found in many mammalian tissues. Commercial forms of heparin are derived from bovine lung tissue and porcine intestinal mucosa and exist as sodium and calcium salts. These are used both therapeutically and prophylactically for intravascular thrombosis. Low molecular weight heparins include enoxaprin and fragmin. These have different pharmacokinetic properties and are most commonly used for prophylaxis.

IX. **Available preparations.** Heparin is available in a variety of concentrations ranging from 1,000 to 20,000 USP U/mL. Enoxaprin is available in a premixed solution at a concentration of 3,000 USP U/0.3 mL. Fragmin is also available for clinical use in the United States and is distributed in a solution of 2,500 USP U/0.2 mL. The recommended dose of standard heparin varies and is considered adequate when the aPTT is in the therapeutic range. The low molecular weight heparin compounds, when used at recommended doses, will not affect clotting parameters, thereby obviating the need for routine coagulation tests. Three thousand units of enoxaprin or 5,000 U of fragmin is usually given twice daily for DVT prophylaxis.

X. **Pharmacology and properties**

A. **Mechanism of action**—Heparin induces anticoagulation by accelerating the action of antithrombin, a natural plasma anticoagulant (21). Antithrombin neutralizes thrombin (Factor Xa) to prevent clot formation. It also inactivates factors IX, XI, XII, and kallikrein which are part of the intrinsic and common pathways of the coagulation cascade. Thus, the activated partial thromboplastin time (aPTT), which reflects the integrity of the intrinsic pathway, is used to monitor heparin therapy. At higher concentrations heparin accelerates the action of heparin co-Factor II, which is similar in action to antithrombin. Heparin can both promote and inhibit platelet aggregation and may prolong the bleeding time (8). At supratherapeutic levels heparin may affect the PT.

B. **Pharmacokinetics**

1. Heparin is only available for parenteral use because its large size and negative charge prevent GI absorption. Intramuscular injection may result in hematoma formation so i.v. or subcutaneous administration is preferred. Onset of action is immediate when given i.v. A delay of 20 to 60 min may result from subcutaneous administration. Approximately 95% of heparin is bound to plasma proteins.

2. **Plasma half-life** is dose-dependent. The half-life of standard doses (100 to 800 U/kg) varies between 1 and 5 h. The duration of heparin's action is 1 to 3 h. This may be shortened in the presence of an intravascular thrombus and prolonged in patients with renal and hepatic disease. Heparin is also potentiated by concomitant administration of antiplatelet drugs, nonsteroidal anti-inflammatory agents, and thrombolytics. Plasma half-lives of the low molecular weight heparin compounds range from 3 to 5 h.

3. Heparin is primarily **metabolized** by the enzyme heparinase in the liver. Inactive metabolites and a small amount of unmetabolized drug may be found in the urine.

4. Heparin **does not cross the placenta** and may be used subcutaneously when anticoagulation is needed in pregnancy (22).

XI. **Clinical manifestations**

A. Most cases of heparin toxicity are iatrogenic and occur in neonates because it is frequently used to flush arterial catheters. These patients are more sensitive to an excess of heparin because of their small body size and immature livers. Toxicity is dose-dependent and correlates with the degree of aPTT prolongation (15). Patients with bleeding may have an underlying cause such as recent invasive procedure, intramuscular injection, occult malignancy, or ulcer disease. Women, especially over the age of 60, are at an increased risk of bleeding from heparin for unknown reasons (23). Also at an increased risk are those with renal failure, ethanol abuse, and hepatic failure.

B. At therapeutic levels (aPTT 60 to 90) complications of heparin therapy are few. During the first few days of therapy, a mild transient thrombocytopenia (platelet count more than 100,000/μL) may occur in 2% to 5% of patients. A more severe thrombocytopenia may develop in 7 to 14 days which would necessitate the discontinuation of the drug. Although rare, heparin can induce a paradoxical thrombosis, despite thrombocytopenia, leading to limb ischemia, myocardial infarction, and stroke. This may be seen 5 to 10 days after the initiation of therapy. Hemorrhagic manifestations of heparin toxicity are similar to those seen with overdose of the oral anticoagulants. Low molecular weight heparins are thought to have less bleeding complications though these can induce a thrombocytopenia as well. There are no data regarding overdoses of the low molecular weight heparin because these compounds have only recently been introduced for clinical use.

    C. Nonhemorrhagic adverse reactions seen with chronic heparin use are osteoporosis, aldosterone suppression with hyperkalemia, alopecia, and anaphylaxis.

    D. The differential diagnosis of coagulopathy with an abnormal aPTT includes heparinoid use, liver failure, inherited coagulation disorder, and DIC.

XII.   **Laboratory evaluation.** Heparin therapy is most commonly monitored by measuring the aPTT and platelet count. Ideally, the aPTT should be maintained at 1.5 to two times the control or the patient's baseline for the treatment of thrombosis. The risk of hemorrhagic complications increases greatly at levels higher than this. Prophylactic therapy with low dose heparin usually does not affect coagulation parameters. The reptilase time test or protamine sulfate titration may be used to determine the presence of heparin when the cause of a prolonged aPTT is unclear. Although not widely used, heparin levels can be measured and should be maintained higher than 0.3 to 0.5 U/mL. A toxic level has not been clearly defined.

XIII.   **Management**

    A. Initial management of heparin overdose should always include assessment of the airway, breathing, and circulation. Laboratory studies should include PT, aPTT, CBC, and, if indicated, a type and crossmatch.

    B. If the aPTT is significantly prolonged but no bleeding has resulted, discontinuation of the drug for one to two half-lives will be adequate therapy. If external hemorrhage occurs, control of bleeding should be attempted using compression. If this fails or if bleeding is internal, immediate reversal of heparin-induced coagulopathy should be instituted using protamine sulfate, a positively-charged molecule derived from fish sperm which binds tightly to heparin and prevents interaction with antithrombin. The dose of protamine sulfate required is based on the amount of heparin expected to be remaining in circulation (1 mg protamine per 100 U heparin). For example, assuming a half-life of 1 h, 500 U heparin will be remaining in circulation 1 h after infusion of 1,000 U heparin. The necessary dose of protamine needed to counteract this would be 5 mg. Protamine can itself be an anticoagulant by binding to platelets and fibrinogen when given in excess. Infusion should be slow (not to exceed 50 mg over 10 min) to avoid adverse reactions. Intravascular fluid volume should be replaced with crystalloid and/or blood transfusion. Exchange transfusion is an acceptable alternative in neonates for the removal of heparin (24).

    C. **Antidote toxicity.** Systemic hypotension may occur with rapid infusion of protamine. This is an anaphylactic response seen in patients with prior exposure to protamine, those with fish allergies, and less commonly in diabetics on NPH insulin. Pulmonary vasoconstriction may occur without previous exposure. Hypotension may be prevented by rapid fluid administration after protamine (25).

XIV.   **Disposition considerations.** The majority of patients with heparin toxicity are already hospitalized which allows for close observation of hemodynamic status and serial evaluation of laboratory studies. In cases of intentional overdose, suicidal intent must be assessed and psychiatric consult obtained if warranted.

References

1. Allen EV, Barker MW, Waugh JM. A preparation from spoiled sweet clover. *JAMA* 1942;110:1009 to 1015.
2. Fitzgerald KT. Poisoning in companion animals by anticoagulant rodenticides. *Rocky Mountain Poison Center Bull* 1986;5.
3. Katona B, Wason S. Superwarfarin poisoning. *J Emerg Med* 1989;7:627–631.
4. Katona B, Wason S. Anticoagulant rodenticides. *Clin Toxicol Rev* 1986;8:1–2.
5. Smolinske SC, Scherger DL, Kearns PS, Wruk KM, Kulig KW, Rumack BH. Superwarfarin poisoning in children: a prospective study. *Pediatrics* 1989;84:490–494.
6. Whitlon DS, Sadowski JA, Suttie JW. Mechanism of coumarin action: significance of vitamin K–epoxide reductase inhibition. *Biochemistry* 1978;17:1371–1377.
7. Baselt RC, Cravey RH. *Disposition of toxic drugs in man.* 3rd ed. Chicago: Year Book Publishers, 1989:851–854.
8. Hirsh J. Mechanism of action and monitoring of anticoagulants. *Semin Thromb Hemostasis* 1986;12:1–11.
9. Van der Meer FJM, Rosendaal FR, Vandenbroucke JP, Briet E. Bleeding complications in oral anticoagulant therapy. *Arch Intern Med* 1993;153:1557–1562.
10. Watts RG, Castleberry RP, Sadowski JA. Accidental poisoning with a superwarfarin compound (Brodifacoum) in a child. *Pediatrics* 1990;86:883–887.
11. Lipton RA, Klass EM. Human ingestion of a superwarfarin rodenticide resulting in a prolonged anticoagulation effect. *JAMA* 1984;252:3004.
12. Routh CR, Triplett DA, Murphy MJ, Felice LJ, Sadowski JA, Bovill EGT. Superwarfarin ingestion and detection. *Am J Hematol* 1991;36:50–54.
13. O'Reilly RA, Aggeler PM. Covert anticoagulant ingestion: study of 25 patients and review of world literature. *Medicine* 1976;55:389–399.
14. Boster SR, Bergin JJ. Upper airway obstruction complicating warfarin therapy with a note on reversal of warfarin toxicity. *Ann Emerg Med* 1983;12:711–715.
15. Levine MN, Hirsh J. Hemorrhagic complications of anticoagulant therapy. *Semin Thromb Hemostasis* 1986;12:39–57.
16. Hoffman RS, Smilkstein MJ, Goldfrank LR. Evaluation of coagulation factor abnormalities in long-acting anticoagulant overdose. *Clin Toxicol* 1988;26:233–248.
17. Renowden S, Westmoreland D, White JP, Routledge PA. Oral cholestyramine increases elimination of warfarin after overdose. *BMJ* 1985;291:513–514.
18. Murdoch DA. Prolonged anticoagulation in chlorphacinone poisoning. *Lancet* 1983;1:355–356.
19. de la Rubia J, Grau E, Montserrat I, Zuazu I, Paya A. Anaphylactic shock and Vitamin K_1. *Ann Intern Med* 1989;110:943.
20. O'Mara K, Mavichak V. Trauma and oral anticoagulant. *Ann Emerg Med* 1983;12:700–703.
21. Rosenberg RD. Actions and interactions of antithrombin and heparin. *N Engl J Med* 1975;292:146–151.
22. Stevenson RE, Burton OM, Ferlauto GJ, Taylor HA. Hazards of oral anticoagulants during pregnancy. *JAMA* 1980;243:1549–1551.
23. Jick H, Slone D, Borda IT, Shapiro S. Efficacy and toxicity of heparin in relation to age and sex. *N Engl J Med* 1968;279:284–286.
24. Schreiner RL, Wynn RJ, McNulty C. Accidental heparin toxicity in the newborn intensive care unit. *J Pediatr* 1978;92:115–1166.
25. Horrow JC. Protamine: a review of its toxicity. *Anesth Analg* 1985;64:348–361.

Emergency Toxicology, Second Edition,
edited by Peter Viccellio.
Lippincott–Raven Publishers, Philadelphia © 1998.

37

Poisoning by Antidysrhythmic Drugs

Howard C. Mofenson, Thomas R. Caraccio, and William Heino

Department of Emergency Medicine, Long Island Regional Poison Control Center,
Winthrop University Hospital, Mineola, New York 11501

Antidysrhythmic agents that exert their primary therapeutic effect on the cardiovascular system and might be accidentally ingested by young children or taken orally for attempted suicide by adolescents and adults are covered in this chapter. Most of the drugs have been studied in patients with cardiac disorders, so it is difficult to extrapolate their effects to the hearts of healthy victims. Although many dysrhythmias have serious consequences for children and adults with significant cardiac and metabolic disorders, they appear to be relatively benign in healthy patients. Beta-blockers, calcium channel blockers, and digitalis glycosides and phenytoin are not discussed in this chapter, as they are covered in other chapters.

I. **Incidence.** A study conducted between 1970 and 1986 indicated that the number of prescriptions written for antidysrhythmic agents increased by 300% during that period, from 3.8 million to 11.4 million (1). Antidysrhythmic drugs accounted for 1,015 cases (3.5%) of all cardiac drug exposures reported to the American Association of Poison Control Centers' national database in 1994: 51.3% of exposures resulted in minimal or no toxicity; 45.4% moderate toxicity; 2.2% caused life-threatening manifestations; and 1.1% resulted in death (2).

II. **Normal sinus rhythm**

   A. The normal cardiac conduction in the heart begins within the pacemaker cells at the sinoatrial (SA) node, the "electrical generator." The spread of electrical activity leads to depolarization over, first, the right atrium then the left atrium—by three tracts rapidly or more slowly through the atrial myocardium to the atrioventricular (AV) node. The AV node then presents the impulses to the bundle of His, which conducts them between the atria and the ventricles. At the point where the membranous septum becomes the muscular septum, the His bundle divides into the right and left bundles with two divisions (anterior and posterior) and finally terminates in the His-Purkinje system. The ECG depicts the depolarization of the atrial and ventricular muscle. This depolarization leads to synchronous contraction of the atria and ventricles.

   B. Although all myocardial tissues are capable of automatic depolarization, it occurs most rapidly at the SA node, the normal pacemaker of the heart. If the SA node is slowed sufficiently by reflexes or disease, other cardiac tissues may assume the pacemaker function.

   C. Most dysrhythmias are the consequences of abnormal impulse formation (automaticity), where an ectopic focus depolarizes faster than the intrinsic pacemaker; abnormal impulse conduction and reentry due to ischemia, acidosis, hypoxia, and stretching; or a combination of the above. The drugs of choice for common dysrhythmics are listed in Table 37-1.

TABLE 37-1. *Drugs of choice for common arrhythmias*

Dysrhythmia	Choice	Alternative	Remarks
Atrial fibrillation and flutter	Diltiazem, verapamil, digoxin, esmolol	Class IA	Digoxin, beta-blocker, verapamil may be dangerous in WPW
Supraventricular tachycardia	Adenosine	Esmolol, digoxin, calcium channel blocker	Cardioversion or atrial pacing in some patients
Ventricular premature contractions due to encainide/flecainide	Asymptomatic—no therapy	Symptomatic—beta-blocker	Post myocardial infarction beta-blocker decrease mortality
Sustained VT	Lidocaine if stable	Procainamide, bretylium	Cardioversion if unstable/ refractory to medication
Ventricular fibrillation	Lidocaine	Procainamide, bretylium, amiodarone	Defibrillation
Cardiac glycoside VT	FAB	Phenytoin, procainamide	Self-limited if stopped FAB; caution with cardioversion can produce VF; use as last resort
Torsades de pointes	Magnesium	Cardiac pacing, isoproterenol	Mg may be effective even if serun magnesemia is normal

VT, ventricular tachycardia; VF, ventricular fibrillation; K, potassium; WPW, Wolf Parkinson White syndrome; FAB, fragment of digoxin antibodies; Mg, magnesium.

III. Classification of antidysrhythmic drugs

A. Antidysrhythmic drugs are used for the prevention and treatment of disorders of cardiac rhythm. The tachydysrhythmias represent a major concern, whereas the bradydysrhythmias may be readily treated with atropine, isoproterenol, or cardiac pacing. Antidysrhythmic agents act on the cardiac conduction tissues by affecting the properties of the membrane so that ionic exchanges occurring during transmission of the action potential are altered, with automaticity or excitability being either increased or decreased; interfering with the responsiveness of specialized tissues so conduction of the impulse is altered, resulting in circuit or reentry rhythms; and altering the duration of the action potential and refractoriness of the tissue, interfering with or causing cessation of the mechanism of the abnormal rhythm.

B. Ideally, the classification would be linked to the key electrophysiologic abnormalities that underlie the various dysrhythmias. However, current knowledge does not permit classification on this basis. As a framework for toxicologic discussion, we have chosen the classification of Vaughan-Williams (3), which defines five groups and is based on the electrophysiologic properties of the drug (Table 37-2).

C. Figure 37-1 depicts the normal electrophysiologic action potential as a basis for our description of the mode and site of action of the five groups of antidysrhythmic agents.

D. **Electrophysiologic action** (3–5). In the resting state, the heart is "polarized" due to ionic gradients across the cell membrane. The cardiac cell has a higher potassium inte-

TABLE 37-2A. *Classification and electrophysiologic action*

Class and generic trade name	Mechanism of action
Class IA—Indications: SVT, VT, and venticular premature beats	
Moricizine (high mortality, 2.3–0.3%)	1. Fast sodium channel blockade
Quinidine	2. Moderately depresses rate of depolarization of action potential (phase 0) >QRS, >QTc, Torsades de pointes
Sulfate (Cinquin)	3. Prolongs repolarization of action potential (phase 2 and 3)
Gluconate (Quinaglute)	4. Anticholinergic (disopyramide)
Polygalaaerate (Cardioquin)	5. Reduced myocardial contractility
Procainamide (Pronestyl)	6. Slows conduction velocity
Disopyramide (Norpace)	7. Decreases automaticity
	8. Alpha-adrenergic blocking (quinidine)
Class IB—Indications: VT, VF, ventricular premature beats	
Lidocaine (Xylocaine)	1. Minimally depresses rate of depolarization of action potential (phase 0)
Phenytoin (Dilantin)	2. Shorten repolarization of action (phase 2 and 3) potential in normal, but increases in ischemic tissue
Tocainide (Tonocard)	3. No change in conduction through AV node
Mexiletine (Mexitil)	4. Does not increase QRS duration,
	5. Does not shorten or alter QTc
	6. Increases Ven fibrillation threshold
Class IIC—Indications: life-threatening VT or VF, refractory SVT	
Flecainide (Tambocor)	1. Block sodium and potassium channels
Encainide (EnKad)	2. Marked slowing of depolarization of action potential (phase 0)
Lorcainide[a]	3. Little effect on repolarization
Indecainide[a]	4. Prolongs PR, QRS, QT duration; slows or blocks conduction in accessory bypass tracts
Propafenone (Rythmol)	
Class II—Indications: SVT, may prevent AF	
Propranolol (Inderal) (prototype)	1. Inhibit sympathetic (beta) activity (Downs syndrome impaired metabolism of propranolol); depresses AV node
	2. Prolongs PR interval
	3. Quinidine-like effect depresses contractility and conduction
	4. No change in ORS interval; shortens OT
Class III—Indications: amiodarone for refractory VF and VT; sotalol for VT; bretylium for VF, VT	
Amiodarone (Cordarone)	1. Block potassium channels
Sotalol (Betacardone)	2. Prolongs repolarization
Bretylium (Bretylol)	3. Beta-adrenergic blocker, release iodine
	4. Intravenous prolongs conduction and block at AV (beta-blockade effects) node; oral prolongs conduction of SA and AV node
	5. Prolong duration of action potential QTc prolonged, u wave may be present
	6. Prolongs PR, QRS, QT
	7. Release of catecholamines from nerve endings followed by inhibition (bretylium)
	8. Transient acceleration of sinus rate
	9. No effect on PR, QRS, or QTc; decreases refractory period; gives Sinus bradycardia
Class IV—Indications: SVT and AF with rapid ventricular response, effect on ECG	
Nifedipine (Procardia)	1. Inhibit slow inward calcium channel
Verapamil (Calan)	2. Inhibits fast sodium channel
Diltiazem (Cardizem)	3. Prolongs PR; depresses AV node
	4. Reduced cardiac contractility
	5. Slowed AV node conduction
	6. Depressed sinus node activity

(continued)

TABLE 37-2A. *Continued*

Class and generic trade name	Mechanism of action
Class V Digoxin (Lanoxin)	1. Inhibits Na/K-ATPase pump 2. Inhibit SA and AV nodes 3. Increases PR interval and AV blocks 4. Purkinje fibers: shortens action potential 5. Decreases refractory period, increases slope of phase 4 depolarization 6. Increases automaticity and ectopic activity 7. Ventricular and atrial fibers: shortens refractory period and duration of action potential 8. Shortens QT interval Digitalis intoxication does not cause widening of the QRS

[a] Not available in the United States.

SVT, supraventricular tachycardia; VT, ventricular tachycardia; VF, ventricular fibrillation; AV, artial ventricular; SA, sino-atrial.

Modified from refs. 167 and 168.

rior which is negative ($-$) and higher sodium exterior which is positive ($+$). This is maintained by the Na/K ATPase pump. If the cell is adequately stimulated, there is a rapid inward **movement of sodium** through specific channels with loss of interior negativity called **"depolarization"** (Phase 0). This corresponds to the QRS complex on the surface ECG. During **Phase 0,** the transmembrane potential rapidly changes from negative to positive. In **Phase 1, sodium enters at a reduced rate** and marks early rapid repolarization. In **Phase 2,** the **slow calcium channel opens** while the fast sodium channels are still open resulting in a plateauing of the action potential curve. Finally both sodium and calcium currents decline and **"rapid repolarization"** (**Phase 3 and 4**) occurs as a result of **potassium efflux.** In Phase 4, the ATP—dependent sodium-potassium active transport pump restores the large extracellular sodium and intracellular potassium concentrations.

IV. **General facts about antidysrhythmic drug intoxications**
   A. All of the agents used to treat rhythm disorders have the potential for major adverse effects. It has been hypothesized that by slowing conduction antidysrhythmic agents may enhance susceptibility to reentry and precipitate ventricular tachydysrhythmias (4,5).
   B. **General management principles** of antidysrhythmic intoxications are as follows:
      1. Determine **vital functions** and administer **supportive care** as needed. Immediate attention should be given to the airway and assisted ventilation, controlling convulsions and life threatening dysrhythmias. Consideration to electrical assistance of pacemaker or external overdrive and intraaortic baloon.
      2. **Gastrointestinal (GI) decontamination** should generally consist of activated charcoal and cathartics within 4 h postingestion. **Vomiting induced by ipecac syrup** may stimulate vagal reflexes and worsen bradydysrhythmias. We **do not recommend** this for acute overdoses of these agents. Before insertion of a **gastric tube** for lavage, it is important to perform an electrocardiogram to ensure no dysrhythmias are present and to monitor ECG while inserting the tube when these agents are ingested. **Atropine** has been suggested prior to insertion of the

TABLE 37-2B. *Electrophysiologic action of antidysrhythmic agents*

	Conduction velocity	Refractory period	Automaticity	AV nodal conduction
Ia				
Quinidine/procainamide	<<	>>	<<	↔
Disopyramide	<<	>>	<<	>
Moricizine	0/<	0	0/<	0
Ib				
Lidocaine				
Normal tissue	0	c	<	0
Ischemic tissue	<<	>	<<	0
Phenytoin				
Normal tissue	0	<	<	>
Ischemic tissue	0	>	>>	>
Mexiletine/tocainide	0	<	<	0
Ic				
Encainide/flecainide	<<	0	<	0
II				
Propranolol	<	< acute	0	<<
III				
Amiodarone	0/<	>>	>/0	>/0
Bretylium	0	<<	>/0	>/0
Sotalol	<	>>	<	<
IV				
Diltiazem/verapamil	0	0	0	>>

Modified from ref. 169.

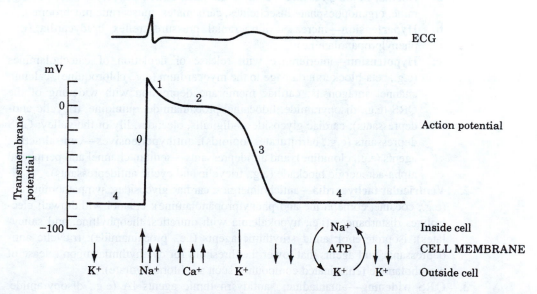

FIG. 37-1. Myocardial cell action potential.

orogastric tube to protect against possible vagal effects. **Activated charcoal** initially with a cathartic and in repeated doses every 3 to 6 h may enhance the elimination of certain antidysrhythmic agents like digoxin or quinidine. There is no data on multiple repeated doses of activated charcoal. **Whole bowel irrigation** with a polyethylene glycol electrolyte lavage solution (PEG/ELS) is recommended for sustained release preparations because they are a significant gut burden of drug. PEG/ELS is administered as 1 to 2 L/h orally in an adult or as 500 mL/h in a child. The endpoint is until all agents have been recoverd, or the occurrence of several bouts of diarrheic stools where the consistency is similar to that of the PEG/ELS.

3. In patients with intoxication by any type IA or type IC, QRS prolongation, bradydysrhythmia and hypotension may respond to **sodium bicarbonate** 1 to 2 mEq/kg i.v. to reverse the cardiac depressant effect caused by inhibition of the fast sodium channel.

4. **Hemodialysis and hemoperfusion** are usually ineffective because of large volumes of distribution (V_d's).

5. **Specific therapies** of overdose and poisonings will be discussed under each class of drugs.

6. **Laboratory:** Monitor ECG, blood pressure, liver and renal functions, blood glucose, electrolytes, calcium, magnesium, phosphorous and serum concentrations of the appropriate antidysrhythmic agent. Central hemodynamic monitoring may be needed. Chest x-ray. CBC for the possibility of agranulocytosis.

C. **Differential diagnosis**

1. **Bradycardia**

   a. **Normal blood pressure**—cholinergic agents (i.e., physostigmine, neostigmine, organophosphate insecticides, carbamates, muscarinic mushrooms).

   b. **Hypertension**—increased intracranial pressure; reflex bradycardia (i.e., phenylpropanolamine).

   c. **Hypotension**—interference with release or depletion of catecholamines (e.g., beta-blockers); damage to the myocardium (e.g., chloroquine); calcium channel antagonsits; cardiac membrane depression with widening of the QRS (e.g., disopyramide, lidocaine, procainamide, quinidine, tricyclic antidepressants); cardiac glycosides—digitalis, oleander, lily of the valley; CNS depressants (e.g., barbiturates, opioids); antihypertensives—central acting agents (e.g., clonidine); and antidepressants—sodium channel and peripheral alpha-adrenergic blockade (e.g., tricyclic and cyclic antidepressants).

2. **Ventricular tachycardia**—anticholinergics; cardiac glycosides; sympathomimetics (e.g., cocaine, epinephrine and phenylpropanolamine); ethanol withdrawal; electrolytes disturbances (i.e., hypokalemia with diuretics, theophylline, and salicylates); isoproterenol; antidysrhythmic agents (i.e., procainamide); tricyclic antidepressants; and agents that lower the threshold for dysrhythmias upon release of catecholamine (chlorinated compounds such as chloral hydrate).

3. **QRS widening**—amantadine; *antidysrhythmic agents IA (e.g., disopyramide, procainamide, *quinidine) and IC; *chloroquine; fluoride; electrolyte abnormalities

(hyperkalemia, hypercalcemia, hypomagnesemia); lithium; phenothiazine (thioridazine, mesoridazine); thallium; *tricyclic antidepressants, and potentially cyclobenzaprine and carbamazepine as well (* = most frequently).

4. **Prolonged QT.** Etiologies of prolonged QT interval syndromes include congenital hereditary Jervell-Lange-Nielsen syndrome, which is a triad of prolonged QT interval, syncope and congenital deafness. The Romano-Ward consists of prolonged QT and syncope without deafness, metabolic/electrolyte, central or autonomic nervous system disorders, coronary artery disease, and mitral valve prolapse. **Medications** and toxins include antidysrhythmic agents (e.g., *procainamide, *quinidine), amantadine, disopyramide, fluoride, electrolyte abnormalities (hyperkalemia, hypocalcemia, hypomagnesemia), lithium, *phenothiazine and quinidine, sotalol, thallium, and *tricyclic antidepressants (* = most frequently).

5. **Shortened QT.** Etiology includes beta-adrenergic blockers and hypercalcemia.

6. **Torsades de pointes** (polymorphic ventricular tachycardia). The commonly reported intoxications that produce this are arsenic; anticholinergics (especially atropine); antidysrhythmic agents [IA quinidine* (1% to 8%), disopyramide, procainamide, aprindine; IB mexiletine, tocainide (lidocaine has no effect on QT and does not cause this rhythm); IC encainide, flecainide; III amiodarone*]; chloral hydrate; corticosteroids; diuretics; phenothiazines (especially thioridazine); probucol (Lurselle, a lipid-lowering agent); organophosphates; maprotiline; pentamidine; thallium (3,4); nonsedating antihistamines (e.g., astemizole and terfenidine); high-protein liquid diet; and sotalol (5% in patients with dose of more than 320 mg) (* = most frequently).

7. **Electrolyte and medication effects:**
   Hypocalcemia: prolonged QT interval
   Hypercalcemia: shortened QT
   Hyperkalemia: narrow, symmetrical peaked T waves, prolongation of the PR interval, flattening of the P wave and widening of the QRS wave (which can progress to ventricular fibrillation).
   Hypokalemia: flattened T waves, depression of the ST segment and the appearance of U waves.
   Hypomagnesemia: prolongation of the QT interval
   Hyponatremia: prolongation of both the PR interval and QRS duration.
   Digitalis effect: downward sloping of the ST segment. There is no correlation between the appearance of the ST segment and the degree of clinical toxicity. Toxicity can result in dysrhythmias and conduction disorders.
   Procainamide and quinidine: prolongation of the QT interval, flattening of the T wave, and widening QRS of the wave.

8. **Asystole:** anticholinergics, antidysrhythmic agents, antihypertensive agents, beta-blockers, hyperkalemia, hypothermia, insulin, nitrates, phenothiazines, physostigmine with tricyclic antidepressants, quinidine, and tricyclic antidepressants alone.

9. **Conduction disorders:** barium, beta-adrenergic antagonists (propranolol), calcium channel antagonists (verapamil), carbon monoxide, chloroquine, clonidine, cardiac glycosides, disopyramide, emetine, lidocaine, opioids, methyldopa, nico-

tine, phenothiazines, potassium excess, procainamide, quinidine, quinine, reserpine, thallium, and tricyclic antidepressants.

10. **Junctional rhythm:** digoxin, calcium channel antagonists, and tricyclic antidepressants.

11. **Premature ventricular contractions:** Physiologic, anticholinergics, beta-adrenergic antagonists, calcium channel antagonists, digitalis, nicotine, nitrates, sympathomimetics (caffeine, theophylline, cocaine).

CLASS IA AGENTS: QUINIDINE, PROCAINAMIDE, DISOPYRAMIDE

V. **Quinidine**

A. **Properties of agent**

1. **Source and forms of toxin.** Quinidine, a dextrorotatory isomer of quinine is available as sulfate salt tablets (200, 300 mg), polygalacturonate (275 mg), and gluconate salt [slow release (**SR**) form, 324 mg] and sulfate (SR, 300 mg) (6). For injection, it is supplied in 10-mL vials containing 80 mg/mL.

2. **Mechanism of action and pathophysiology** of class Ia antidysrhythmic agents (quinidine, procainamide, and disopyramide) (Table 37-2A and Table 37-2B).

   a. The principal electrophysiologic properties of the class 1a agents are that they have **local anesthetic properties** and **block fast sodium inward current,** reduce diastolic depolarization in pacemaker cells, increase the threshold of excitability, decrease the rate of rise of Phase 0 of ventricular muscle or Purkinje fibers, decrease conduction velocity, and prolong the effective refractory period of cardiac muscle (3–6).

   b. These drugs have proved most effective in the prevention of premature atrial, nodal, and ventricular contractions and (especially in the case of quinidine) for the maintenance of sinus rhythm after conversion of atrial flutter or fibrillation.

3. **Pharmacology and pharmacokinetics**

   a. The **therapeutic dose** of quinidine **sulfate** in adults is 200 to 600 mg and in children 6 mg/kg every 4 to 6 h, gluconate salt in adults 324 to 972 mg every 8 to 12 h, polygalacturonase in adults is 275 mg 2 to 3 times daily. The **toxic amount of** quinidine in a child is 60 mg/kg; the toxic dose in adults is 1 g or roughly twice the daily dose. Ingestions of 2.5 g may result in serious toxicity. The fatal dose in adults is 2 to 8 g. However survival after acute doses of 21 g and peak serum concentrations of 21.4 mcg/mL have been reported (10).

   b. **Pharmacokinetics** (Table 37-3). Quinidine **sulfate** is a weak base. The salt forms of quinidine and the other Class 1A agents are rapidly and completely absorbed from the GI tract. The bioavailability of quinidine is 70% to 90% (10). The sulfate salt's **onset of action** is within 1 h, **peak concentration** is at 60 to 90 min and **peak action** is 2 to 4 h with a **duration** of 6 to 8 h. The polygalacturonate salt action peak is 5 to 6 h, and the gluconate is 3 to 4 h. The duration of action of quinidine **SR gluconate** is 12 h. The **half-life** ($t_{1/2}$) for the sulfate salt is 3 to 4 h and gluconate 8 to 12 h (11,12). The $t_{1/2}$ is prolonged in alcoholics. The V_d is 2 to 3 L/kg and protein binding 70% to 80%. The route of elimination is by hepatic hydroxylation into two active metabo-

TABLE 37-3. *Pharmacokinetic data on Class 1a antidysrhythmic agents*

	Quinidine (Duraquin, Quinaglute)	Procainamide (Pronestyl, Procan)	Disopyramide (Norpace)	Moricizine (Ethmozine)
Route	Oral/i.m./i.v.	Oral/i.m./i.v.	Oral	Oral
Absorption	70–90%	75–95%	80–90%	30–40%
Bioavailability	80–90%	85%		
Oral		PA 1–2 h	SR 4.7–5.6 h	1.5 h
Peak level	2–4 h	NAPA 1–8 h	Reg 1–1.5 h	
Protein binding	70–80%	15–25%	50–80%	95%
Volume distribution	2–3 L/kg	2 L/kg	0.8 L/kg	0.8–11.1 L/kg
Duration				
Sulfate	2–3 h	3–6 h	6–12 h	24 h
Gluconate	3–4 h	—	—	—
Sustained release	8–12 h	—	—	—
Polygalacturonate	5–6 h	—	—	—
Elimination $t_{1/2}$	3–16 h	3–6 h	4–8 h	1.5–3.5 h
Elimination				
Hepatic	60–85%	30–40%	15–25%	Feces 56%
Active metabolite	Yes	Yes	Yes	Urine 39%
Renal	15–40%	50–60%	40–60	—
Metabolites	(NAPA $t_{1/2}$ 10 h)			
In urine unchanged	10–20%	40–60%	50%	<1%
Clear L/kg h	0.388	0.552	0.78	N/A
Daily therapeutic dose: gluconate				
Child	p.o. 10–20 mg/kg	p.o. 15–50 mg/kg	p.o. 6–30 mg/kg	NA
Adult	p.o. 1,000–2,000 mg	1,000–4,000 mg	400–800 mg	600–900 mg
Toxic amount				
Child	60 mg/kg	NA	NA	NA
Adult	1 g	2.5 g	2.5 g	NA
Serum concentration therapeutic preparations	1–6 µg/mL	NAPA: 15–25 µg/mL; PA: 4–10 µg/mL	2–4 µg/mL	NA
Quinidine		Caps and tab	Tab 100, 150 mg	Tab 150, 200, 250
Sulfate	200, 300 mg	250, 375, 500 mg	Caps CR 100 mg,	300 mg
Gluconate	SR 300, 324 mg	SR 250, 375		
Polygalacturonate	275 mg	500, 750, 1,000 mg		
References	10–28	38–53	54–65	66–71

lites. About 10% to 20% is excreted unchanged in the urine within 24 h. About 20% is excreted in the urine unchanged but the amount excreted is pH dependent, enhanced in an acid urine. If the **urinary pH** is increased from 6 to 7 to 7 to 8, it may decrease renal clearance by 50% (13). Quinidine passes through the placenta and is found in the breast milk (10,11).

c. **Interactions.** Quinidine's action is **enhanced** by concurrent administration of amiodarone (14), cimetidine (15), and ketoconazole (15). Verapamil may cause a 25% to 35% decrease in the elimination of quinidine and can lead to toxicity (16). It is **decreased** with administration of barbiturates, phenytoin, or rifampin (17,18). Quinidine may significantly increase **digoxin** concentrations (19,20) and potentiate polar and nonpolar muscle relaxants (21), anticholinergic drugs, antihypertensive agents, and warfarin anticoagulants (22).

B. Clinical presentation

1. The **onset of symptoms** begin in 1 to 3 h. GI symptoms are often the initial effects. Significant overdose causes profound hypotension due to vasodilation, myocardial depression and disturbances in cardiac rhythm and conduction as the major life threatening effects (23–28). Death may ensue within a few hours. In large overdoses toxic effects of quinine and quinidine may be indistinguishable. **Quinine** is more likely to produce oculotoxicity (29–32), **and quinidine** is more likely to result in cardiotoxicity (23–28).

2. **Cinchonism** mainly occurs with quinine usually of more than 8 mcg/mL but may occur with quinidine intoxication as well (30). It was originally described as **tinnitus, vertigo, headache, deafness, and visual disturbances** but now is considered a wider diversity of symptoms that includes

   a. **CNS**—headache, vertigo, syncope, confusion (more common than with salicylate poisoning), delirium, ataxia, choreoathetosis, mutism, seizures, and generalized weakness.

   b. **GI**—nausea, vomiting.

   c. **Auditory**—tinnitus, deafness. Deafness maybe an early sign of quinine overdose but hearing deficits resolve within 48 to 72 h.

   d. **Ophthalmologic disturbances**—The ocular manifestations may be delayed for hours to days. The visual and auditory effects are **uncommon with quinidine** and not seen with other type IA antidysrhythmic toxicity. This is much more likely to occur with **quinine** (29–32). Pallor of the optic disc, retinal artery spasm, arteriolar constriction may be seen within 15 to 30 min or may be delayed for hours to days (usually occurs within 10 h postingestion). The initial ophthalmologic examination may be negative and should be followed by frequent subsequent examinations for several days. A cherry red spot, retinal macular edema, fixed dilated pupils have been reported. Fundoscopic exam may show arterial spasm and narrowing of the retinal blood arteries and retinal edema but the cause is a direct effect on ganglion cells by quinine. Central vision usually returns but the visual fields may remain permanently constricted (30). Visual loss lasts from 24 h to weeks and may be permanent. Of 165 cases of quinidine intoxication in one series, 19 developed permanent blindness and five died (31).

2. **Cardiovascular effects** (31)

   a. Myocardial depression, tachycardia, dysrhythmias, disturbances in conduction (AV block and intraventricular block), and hypotension or hypertension. **The ECG changes** may consist of prolongation of PR, although the PR is usually normal (10), widening of the QRS, prolongation of the Q-T intervals, S-T segment depression, depressed AV conduction (most frequent), T wave inversion and Torsades de pointes may occur. **A widening of the QRS by 25%** is noted at therapeutic doses, however widening by 50% is likely to be toxic. Dysrhythmias may occur at high therapeutic concentrations (8,26,33).

   b. **"Quinidine syncope"** was originally believed due to vasodilation secondary the alpha-adrenergic blocking properties of quinidine, however some cases are now considered to be due to dysrhythmias, especially Torsade de pointes, and an idiosyncratic reaction (33).

3. In severe cases of **CNS intoxication** confusion, dementia, psychosis, seizures, and coma may occur. The CNS, GI and auditory effects occur first.

4. **Anticholinergic** effects have been occurred with disopyramide and rarely with quinidine.

5. **Renal failure** has been reported from myoglobinuria/rhabdomyolysis. Black, brown urine has been reported. (25,30)

6. **Dermatologic effects**—A variety of skin rashes and flushing are noted (23).

7. **Hematologic effects**—Hemolysis in G-6-PD deficiency patients may occur. Hypoprothrombinemia and fatal thrombocytopenia has been reported (32). Hemolysis/hemolytic anemias, agranulocytosis, leukopenia, and systemic lupus has been reported.

8. **Metabolic**—Hypoglycemia (due to insulin release) has been reported especially with disopyramide. Hypokalemia, and metabolic acidosis have been noted.

9. Chronic therapy with procainamide can cause a **lupus-like syndrome.**

10. **Adverse reactions of quinidine:** Cardiac—QRS widening, hypotension, QT prolongation, Torsades de pointes cinchonism, GI disorder, hypersensitivity reaction, and fever (25).

C. **Laboratory evaluation**

1. **General tests** (see **IX.A** under general management of Class IA agents)

2. **Toxin specific levels** (Table 37-3). The **therapeutic** plasma concentration for quinidine range from 2 to 6 mcg/mL. **Toxicity** usually occurs if the concentration is greater than 8 mcg/mL. There is high risk of auditory and ocular toxicity when the plasma concentration is more than 10 mcg/mL. A total of 65% of patients will have cardiotoxicity when the concentration is more than 14 mcg/mL, and fatalities have occurred at concentrations of more than 16 mcg/mL.

D. **Management** (see **X** and Fig. 37-2 for algorithm). Due to the similarity of quinidine with the other Class IA agents the managements of each of these agents are discussed together in this section.

E. **Disposition.** Hospitalize all patients with ingestion of a toxic amount or toxic plasma concentration. **Intensive care monitoring and cardiac consult** is required in any symptomatic patient with an overdose since ventricular pacing may be needed.

VI. **Procainamide (PA)**

A. **Properties of agent**

1. **Sources and forms.** Procainamide is available in capsule and tablets containing 250, 375, and 500 mg; and sustained release tablets of 250, 375, 500, 750, and 1,000 mg. Procainamide hydrochloride injection is supplied in 10-mL vials containing 100 mg/mL and 2-mL vials containing 500 mg/mL suitable for i.m. and i.v. injection.

2. **Mechanism of action.** Like quinidine, procainamide causes **prolongation of the repolarization and effective refractory period and reduction in automaticity** (see **V**). In addition, PA decreases the blood pressure by ganglionic blockade resulting in peripheral vasodilation (38). NAPA has primarily class III antidysrhythmic action delaying repolarization.

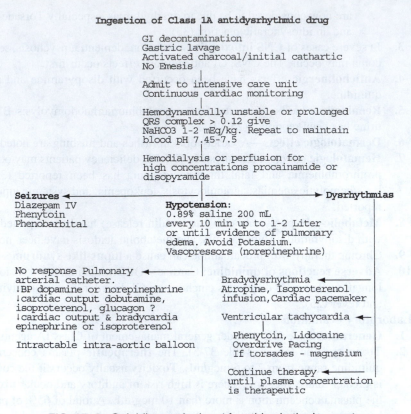

FIG. 37-2. Quinidine and other 1A antidysrhythmic agents.

3. **Pharmacology and pharmacokinetics** (Table 37-3)

   a. Adult oral **therapeutic** loading dose for atrial and ventricular tachycardia is 1000 mg over 2 h in 2 divided doses. Oral maintenance is 50 mg/kg/day or 1 to 4 g/day in 4 to 6 divided doses. Intravenous loading 1 to 1.5 g at 20 to 50 mg/min. Reduce doses in patients with liver or renal impairment, and in the elderly.

   b. Children's oral dose is 15 to 50 mg/kg/day in divided doses every 3 to 6 h; maximum daily dose is 4 g i.v. 10 to 15 mg/kg over 30 min and maintenance 20 to 80 ug/kg/min infusion; i.m. 20 to 30 mg/kg/day in 4 to 8 divided doses, to a maximum of 4 g/day.

   c. **Toxic** oral doses in adults may be as low as twice the daily adult or greater than 1 g. Ingestions of 2.5 g may produce serious toxicity. However survivals of 77 g are reported (39). Toxicity is observed as low as serum concentrations of 10 mcg/mL but this might be due to coexisting active metabolite, *N*-acetyl-procainamide (NAPA) (38,39).

    d.   **Pharmacokinetics** (Table 37-3). Procainamide is a weak base pK_a 9.23. Gut bioavailability is 75% to 95%. **Onset of action:** oral administration is within 1 h (sustained released preparations are delayed); i.m. route is about 1 h; and the i.v. route is almost immediate. The **duration** of action is usually 3 to 6 h. Oral and i.m. **peak** plasma concentrations are reached in 1 to 2 h, but may be delayed after myocardial infarction. Protein binding is 15% to 25%. **Plasma half-life** of PA is 1 to 2 h and is prolonged up to 20 h with renal failure. V_d is 2 L/kg. PA is eliminated by hepatic metabolism (30%) and renal excretion (50% to 70%). In the liver PA is **acetylated** (the rate of acetylation is genetically determined; rapid acetylators are 80% to 90% Eskimos and orientals, slow acetylators are observed in 50% to 60% of caucasians) into *N*-acetylprocainamide (NAPA), which is as active as the parent compound (NAPA is under investigation as an Class III antidysrhythmic agent). Approximately 50% of PA excreted in the urine unchanged. PA excretion is through the proximal renal tubules and partially reabsorbed. Its excretion is directly related to creatinine clearance but minimally influenced by the urinary pH. PA clearance is 8.6 to 9.8 mL/min (38,41). NAPA is 10% protein bound, V_d is 1.6 L/kg, has a therapeutic plasma concentration of 15 to 25 mcg/mL, plasma $t_{1/2}$ is 1 to 8 h and is delayed up to 40 h in renal failure. Elimination is almost entirely by the kidneys (85%) and its rate of clearance (3.1 mL/min) is lower than PA (38,41).

    e.   **Drug interactions** have not been a major problem with procainamide therapy. Some interactions **increase** procainamide toxicity when administered concurrently, these include amiodarone (mechanism unknown) (14), cimetidine (due to increased renal excretion) (45), and ranitidine (46,47). Additive depression of AV conduction may occur when procainamide is given to patients with **digoxin** toxicity (38). A synergistic depressant effect on cardiac contractility may occur when procainamide and lidocaine are given concomitantly, a concern especially in the coronary care unit (38). **Procainamide may aggrevate myesthenia gravis.**

B. Clinical presentation

    1.   Physical examination. The major cardiac effects of procainamide are similar to those of quinidine: hypotension, decreased cardiac output, asystole, AV block, and ventricular tachycardias (e.g., Torsades de pointes) (48,49). Like quinidine, many of the toxic cardiac effects of procainamide are manifested by progressive QT and QRS interval lengthening (49). **Toxicity is suspected if the corrected QT (QTc) is prolonged greater than 25% or the QRS is prolonged by 50% or more (widening of the QRS by 25% is considered therapeutic). Torsades de pointes** has been reported more likely to be caused by NAPA than PA (39,49,50). However, the incidence of sudden death or recurrent syncope due to ventricular tachycardia (especially Torsades de pointes) is greater with quinidine use (40,48,49).

    2.   **Side effects.** Procainamide use has been associated with the development of a **lupus erythematosus-like syndrome** (arthralgias, fever, myocarditis with antinuclear antibodies) in as many as 30% to 40% of patients (51,52). The syndrome may appear as early as 2 weeks after the initiation of therapy, is more likely to occur in slow

acetylators of procainamide, and is not associated with elevations of serum NAPA levels (51,52). Chronic administration of procainamide and especially toxic doses have been commonly associated with anorexia, nausea, vomiting, and diarrhea (51). Rarely, agranulocytosis has been associated with procainamide use (53).

3. **Differential diagnosis** (see **IV**)

C. **Laboratory analysis**
   1. **General tests** (see **IX**)
   2. **Toxin-specific levels** (Table 37-3). **If procainamide** (PA) is involved also obtain a plasma level for NAPA. **Therapeutic** plasma concentrations of **PA** are 4 to 10 mcg/mL. The therapeutic plasma range of **NAPA** is 15 to 25 mcg/mL. Therapeutic and toxic plasma levels of PA and NAPA overlap (40). Plasma concentrations must be interpeted in light of the clinical situation. Toxicity is exacerbated by other antidysrhythmics in the same class.

D. **Management** (see **X** and algorithm in Fig. 37-2)

E. **Disposition.** Hospitalize all patients with ingestion of a toxic amount or toxic plasma concentration. **Intensive care monitoring and cardiac consult** is required in any symptomatic patient with an overdose since ventricular pacing may be needed.

VII. **Disopyramide**
   A. **Properties of agent**
      1. **Sources and forms.** Disopyramide is available in immediate-acting and sustained-release capsules of 100 and 150 mg.
      2. **Mechanism of action.** Disopyramide is similar to quinidine in its antidysrhythmic action; however, it a more potent depressor of myocardial function, has peripheral vasoconstrictor action, and has more anticholinergic activity. It may precipitate or worsen cardiac failure (54–56).
      3. **Pharmacology and pharmacokinetics** (Table 37-3)
         a. The **therapeutic** adult dose is 400 to 800 mg/day or 6 to 30 mg/kg/day in children. The therapeutic blood concentration is 2 to 4 mcg/mL. The **toxic** dose is unknown in children, but ingestions of more than 1.5 g have resulted in severe toxicity in adults in a series of 106 overdoses (65). The mortality rate was 12.2% in these overdoses.
         b. **Pharmacokinetics** (54–58). Rapidly absorbed from the GI tract. The bioavailability is 50% to 80%. The **onset of action** is within a 15 to 30 min. **Peak** concentrations are 1 to 1.5 h. The **duration** of action is 6 to 12 h. The **half-life** is 4 to 8 h. V_d is 0.8 L/kg and protein binding is 50% to 80%. Elimination: 15 to 25% is hepatic metabolism with active metabolites, and 40% to 60% is renally eliminated unchanged in the urine.
         c. **Drug interactions.** Disopyramide should be used with extreme caution with **beta-adrenergic blockers,** as the additive effects of these drugs on contractility and blockade of compensating reflexes could precipitate cardiac failure (59). Use of disopyramide with **warfarin** results in an increased anticoagulant effect due to decreased warfarin metabolism (60). Concomitant use of procainamide with phenytoin and rifampin can result in a decreased disopyramide effect owing to increased disopyramide metabolism (61).

    B. Clinical presentation
        1. **Cardiac toxicity** of disopyramide intoxication is similar to that of quinidine, but greater anticholinergic toxicity may result. Cardiovascular collapse can occur without ECG warning, followed by dysrhythmias, apnea, and death (62,63).
        2. **Respiratory depression or arrest** and **coma** have been reported.
        3. Most **noncardiac side effects** of disopyramide are related to its anticholinergic activity: dry mouth, urinary hesitancy, constipation, blurred vision, and dry eyes, nose, and throat (55). Uterine contractions, glaucoma, cholestatis, hypoglycemia, and metabolic acidosis have also been reported (65).
    C. Laboratory analysis
        1. **General tests** (see **IX**)
        2. **Toxin specific levels** (Table 37–3). The **therapeutic** blood concentration is 2 to 4 mcg/mL. **Toxic** effects have been reported with plasma levels above 3.6 mcg/mL.
    D. Management (see **X** and algorithm in Fig. 37–2)
    E. Disposition. Hospitalize all patients with ingestion of a toxic amount or toxic plasma concentration. **Intensive care monitoring and cardiac consult** is required in any symptomatic patient with an overdose since ventricular pacing may be needed.
VIII. Moricizine hydrochloride (Ethmozine)
    A. Properties of agent
        1. **Sources and forms.** Moricizine is available in 200-, 250-, and 300-mg tablets.
        2. **Mechanism of action.** Moricizine is a derivative of phenothiazine which is approved for the treatment of malignant ventricular arrhythmias (66). It is a potent local anesthetic with **myocardial membrane stabilizing** effects and is indicated for documented cases of life-threatening ventricular dysrhythmia (66). It is the fourth and newest member of class Ia agents. It is unique in the fact that it has characteristics of class Ia, Ib, and Ic. Moricizine reduces the fast inward current of sodium ions like Ia but differs from Ia agents because it shortens Phase I and Phase II repolarization, resulting in decreased action potential duration and effective refractory period in the ventricles.
        3. **Pharmacology and pharmacokinetics** (Table 37–3)
            a. The therapeutic dose is 600 to 900 mg in three divided doses.
            b. **Pharmacokinetics.** Rapidly absorbed from the GI tract. The bioavailability is 30% to 40%. This indicates it undergoes extensive first pass metabolism. The **onset of action** is within 15 to 30 min. The **peak plasma** concentration of moricizine occurs approximately 1.5 h after the administration of a single oral dose (67). The mean peak moricizine plasma level was 0.66 mcg/mL in patients receiving moricizine 10 mg/kg/day in 3 divided doses (68). The **duration of** action is up to 24 h. The **half-life** in patients with ventricular ectopy is 1.5 to 3.5 h. However, longer half-lives have been observed. The mean elimination half-life of moricizine in cardiac patients with dysrhythmias was estimated to be 10 h (range, 6.4 to 13.1 h) (69,70). One cardiac patient with renal insufficiency had an estimated elimination half-life of 47.5 h (70). V_d is 8.3 to 11.1 L/kg and protein binding is 95%. Moricizine has a large hepatic first-pass effect (67). Hepatic biotransformation of moricizine

is complex and involves sulfur oxidation, ring hydroxylation, *N*-dealkylation, acetylation, amide hydrolysis, *N*-oxidation, and glucuronide or sulfate conjugation. Moricizine induces its own metabolism. Some **enterohepatic recycling** occurs; 56% is excreted in feces and 39% in urine.

    c. **Drug interactions.** Caution should be used with other antidysrhythmics(66). Concomitant use with digoxin or beta-adrenergic blockers may prolong the PR interval (69). Cimetidine may increase plasma levels. Theophylline serum levels may decrease (71).

  B. **Clinical presentation.** Moricizine has a low incidence of adverse effects (66). Symptoms of toxicity are vomiting, lethargy, coma, syncope, hypotension, conduction disturbances, exacerbation of congestive heart failure, myocardial infarction, arrhythmias, respiratory failure, and death (71).

  C. **Laboratory analysis**

    1. **General tests** (see **IX**)

    2. **Toxin-specific levels**. The Therapeutic and toxic levels are not defined at this time (Table 37-3).

  D. **Management** (see **X** and algorithm in Fig. 37-2)

  E. **Disposition.** Hospitalize all patients with ingestion of a toxic amount or toxic plasma concentration. **Intensive care monitoring and cardiac consult** is required in any symptomatic patient with an overdose since ventricular pacing may be needed.

IX. **Laboratory analysis of intoxication with Class Ia agents**

  A. **General tests.** Monitor **vital functions, electrolytes**, serum glucose, serum glucose, liver/renal function tests, CBC and platelet count and **ECG** for QT, QRS, or PR prolongation. A 12-lead ECG should be obtained to evaluate the PR, QRS, and QT duration intervals. Obtain a chest radiograph and arterial blood gases if depressed level of consciousness or serious dysrhythmias develop. If signs of **disseminated intravascular coagulation (DIC)** monitor platelets, fibrin degradation products, and fibrinogen.

  B. **Toxin-specific tests.** Blood concentration should be monitored because there is a good correlation with toxicity for these agents (Table 37-3).

X. **Management of Class 1A antidysrthmic agents** (see Fig. 37-2 for algorithm). It is important to **determine if the product is a sustained release formulation.**

  A. **General management**

    1. **Establish immediate vascular access and maintain vital functions.** Obtain a 12-lead ECG as soon as possible. Treat hypotension with Trendelenburg positioning and i.v. fluids and vasopressors, if necessary. **Cautiously monitor the fluids** because of compromised inotropic action of the heart. Continuous cardiac monitoring for dysrhythmias and if unstable, central hemodynamic monitoring may be necessary. Obtain an **immediate cardiology consultation** should these events occur. Electrophysiologic support of the heart should readily available.

    2. **GI decontamination** with immediate **gastric lavage** in asymptomatic patients. **Whole bowel irrigation** may be useful for ingestions involving sustain-release prepartions. Administer **activated charcoal/cathartic** initially and follow with multiple doses of activated charcoal (MDAC), which have been shown to alter the $t_{1/2}$ but its effect on clinical course is not clear (36). Gastric lavage may be indicated for several hours (3–6) postingestion, especially with disopyramide because of its anticholinergic action. **Avoid emesis** because of rapid onset of seizures and coma.

3. **Obtain ophthalmologic and otologic consultation** for symptoms related to quinidine toxicity.

4. **Treat convulsions with diazepam** 5 to 10 mg repeated every 5 to 15 min up to 30 mg at rate 2.5 mg/min in adults; 0.2 to 0.5 mg/kg up every 5 to 15 min to 5 mg in infants and young children (1 month to 5 years) and up to 10 mg in children more than 5 years at a rate 1 mg/min. Phenytoin i.v. 10 to 15 mg/kg at a rate 25 to 50 mg/min. Blood pressure, cardiac and respiratory monitoring is necessary during i.v. anticonvulsant administration.

5. **Avoid the administration of potassium** since moderate hypokalemia (3 to 3.5 mEq/L) has shown to be beneficial and appears to be protective in quinidine intoxication (10).

B. **Cardiovascular effects**

1. **Dysrhythmias and blocks. Avoid Class IA antidysrhythmic agents, beta-adrenergic blockers and bretylium.** Lidocaine may be used.

   a. **Serum alkalinization** with hypertonic sodium bicarbonate has been recommended for patients if hemodynamically unstable or rhythm disturbance with prolonged QRS complex (greater than 0.1 s). The therapeutic effects of sodium bicarbonate are competitive antagonism of sodium channel blockade and promotion of unbinding of drug from the myocardium.

   b. Alkalinization with hypertonic **sodium bicarbonate** 1 to 2 mEq/kg bolus every 5 to 10 min may help overcome the cardiotoxicity of quinidine by making sodium available for the fast sodium channel. The **serum is maintain between a pH of 7.45 and 7.55** (8,10,25,29). Monitor the serum sodium and potassium.

   c. **Markedly impaired conduction or high-degree AV block** unresponsive to sodium bicarbonate therapy, complete AV dissociation, and Torsades de pointes are indications for insertion of a cardiac pacemaker (12).

   d. **Ventricular tachycardia (VT).** Unresponsive ventricular dysrhythmias or VT with hypotension are an indication for cardioversion and its availability should be assured before attempts to terminate any form of VT with any drug. **Lidocaine** 1 mg/kg i.v. bolus over 1 min followed by an infusion of 1 to 4 mg/min or 20 to 50 mcg/kg/min should be used to maintain the blood concentration of 1 to 5 mcg/mL. Lidocaine acts in 60 to 90 sec and lasts 10 to 20 min (contraindications to lidocaine are nodal or third degree blocks). Other antidysrhythmic drugs such as phenytoin may also be tried. **Phenytoin** is administered as a bolus of 5 to 15 mg/kg i.v. at a rate not to exceed 50 mg/min or 1 mg/kg/min. Phenytoin acts within 1 h and has the advantage of increasing the AV conduction. Bretylium prolongs repolarization but it may aggravate the hypotension.

   e. **Torsades de pointes** is a polymorphic ventricular tachycardia with QRS twisting around the isoelectric line and prolonged PR interval of more than 0.5 s (33). Torsades de pointes is treated with **magnesium sulfate** ($MgSO_4$) which facilitates the influx of potassium into the cells through its effect on the ATPase pump, blocks calcium and elevates the threshold stimulus for ventricular fibrillation. MgSO$_4$ is administered as a 2-g dose in adults (10,34, 35,39) or 25 to 50 mg/kg in children by i.v. bolus over 2 to 3 min. If no response in 10 min, the initial dose can be repeated once (10,35). Atrial and ventricular overdrive pacing to shorten the QT interval may be needed. Monitor serum magnesium levels. Isoproterenol has also been effective but may aggravate the hypotension.

   f.   Electrophysiologic support. Transthoracic DC cardioversion requires administration of general anesthetic and ventricular overpacing generally requires percutaneous transvenous placement of an electrode; both are usually effective but time consuming and not without risk.

2.   Hypotension may require Trendelenburg positioning, i.v. fluids, vasopressors (norepinephrine), and central hemodynamic monitoring.

   a.   An **intraaortic balloon pump** has been successful in one case.

   b.   **Glucagon** may be useful for its chronotropic and inotropic actions, but it has not been scientifically evaluated. Glucagon reverses the negative inotropic effects more effectively than the chronotropic effects. The effect occurs in 1 to 3 min and the duration of action is 15 to 30 min. The initial **loading** dose of glucagon in **children** is 50 to 100 ug/kg (0.05 to 0.1 mg/kg) followed by a maintenance infusion of 0.07 mg/kg/h or in **adults** 5 to 10 mg i.v. over 1 min followed by a maintenance infusion of 1 to 5 mg/h and titrated to response. Use D5W to reconstitute the glucagon rather than the manufacturer's diluent which contains phenol. The adverse reactions of glucagon are: nausea, vomiting, hyperglycemia, slight hypokalemia. Isoproterenol has been used in conjunction with glucagon. The only contraindication to glucagon is hypersensitivity reactions.

C.   Enhanced elimination

1.   Acid diuresis has not been shown to be clinically useful for quinidine poisoning and may increase cardiotoxicity. Acid diuresis would also interfere with sodium bicarbonate administration to counteract quinidine membrane depressant effect (30).

2.   Charcoal hemoperfusion has been reported successful in severe cases but needs further clinical evaluation. Quinidine has a large V_d and high tissue distribution so dialysis is not expected to be effective (17). Disopyramide, *N*-acetylprocainamide (NAPA), and procainamide have smaller V_d's and dialysis and hemoperfusion may be effective in severe cases. In one case hemodialysis was reported to remove the active metabolite NAPA by two- to fourfold (39). In another case report, the treatment of *N*-acetylprocainamide intoxication was successfully treated with a combined use of hemodialysis and charcoal hemoperfusion. This resulted in a 50% increase in the clearance over that obtainable by high-efficiency hemodialysis alone (72). Renal failure is an indication for hemodialysis (24).

D.   Disposition. Hospitalize all patients with ingestion of a toxic amount or toxic plasma concentration of a type 1a antidysrhythmic agent. **Intensive care monitoring and cardiac consult** is required in any symptomatic patient with an overdose of an agent in this group since ventricular pacing may be needed.

CLASS IB AGENTS: LIDOCAINE, PHENYTOIN, TOCAINIDE HCL, MEXILETINE HCL

XI. Lidocaine

  A. Properties of agent

  1. Sources and forms of toxin. Lidocaine is available for Injection 0.5% 50 mL; 1%: 2, 5, 10, 20, 30, 50 mL; 1.5%: 20 mL; 2%: 2, 5, 10, 20, 25, 30, 50 mL; 4%: 5 mL; 10%: 3, 5, 10 mL; 20%: 10, 20 mL; premixed with D_5W 2, 4, and 8 mg/mL; topical solution 2, 4%; jelly 2%; ointment 2.5%, 5%; viscous solution 2% (20 mg/mL).

  2. Physical and chemical properties. Lidocaine is an amide type local anesthetic, derivative of cocaine, and a parenteral cardiac antidysrhythmic agent. It is considered the drug of choice for emergency i.v. treatment to prevent ventricular dysrhythmias, including ventricular fibrillation and ventricular tachyarrhythmias. Lidocaine is absorbed as a local agent and topical anesthetic (2% Xylocaine). Illicit **"Florida snow"** is 100% lidocaine.

  3. Mechanism of action of lidocaine is **inhibition of fast sodium channels** and the transmembrane shifts of sodium (intracellularly) and potassium (extracellularly) producing a membrane stabilizing effect and inhibiting depolarization (Phase 0) and nerve conduction. In **therapeutic doses** lidocaine acts on the fast cardiac fibers to inhibit the fast sodium channels, depress automaticity within the Bundle of His, depresses spontaneous diastolic depolarization (Phase 4) and prolong the action potential duration. It minimally effects the refractory period in normal tissue but **increases the refractory period in ischemic tissue.** Lidocaine has **little effect on AV conduction** and **does not increase the duration of the QRS interval** at therapeutic doses. It has minimal effects on SA node automaticity or on iontropy or blood pressure at therapeutic doses. Lidocaine suppresses the automaticity of ischemic tissue while minimally interfering with the electrical activity of normal tissue. Therefore lidocaine decreases the occurrance of block and re-entry phenomena.

  4. Pharmacology and pharmacokinetics

  a. Therapeutic dose for cardiac dysrhythmia is a bolus 1 mg/kg i.v. given over 1 min, which produces a blood concentration of 1 to 5 mcg/mL. Maximum is 3 mg/kg over 30 min. This loading dose is usually followed by an infusion of 10 to 40 mcg/kg/min, or 1 to 4 mg/min, in adults (50). The maximum topical dose is 4.5 mg/kg and 7 mg/kg with epinephrine (51). Topical doses should not be repeated for 2 h. The administration by endotracheal spray of 480 to 720 mg before bronchoscopy resulted in blood concentrations of 1.9 to 7.4 mcg/mL. The **endotracheal route** produces more rapid onset of action and two- to threefold longer duration than i.v.

  b. Pharmacokinetics (Table 37-4). Lidocaine is a weak base with a pK_a 7.8. It is absorbed well from the oral, nasal or esophageal mucosa and undergoes a large hepatic first pass. The **absorption** is enhanced in the presence of inflammated mucosal surfaces. The large hepatic first pass limits intestinal bioavailability to about 35% (73). **Onset of action** i.v. is 45 to 90 s. **Peak blood concentration** occurs 1 h after ingestion. Lidocaine may be significantly absorbed from mucosal surfaces and open wounds. **Oral mucosal** absorption has an immediate onset of action similar to i.v. administration and a duration

TABLE 37-4. *Pharmacokinetic data on class 1b antidysrhythmic agents*

	Phenytoin (Dilantin)	Lidocaine (Xylocaine)	Tocainide (Tonocard)	Mexiletine (Mexitil)
Route	Oral/i.v.	Oral/i.v.	Oral	Oral
Absorption	Slow	Complete	—	—
Bioavailability	80–95%	35–40%	90–100%	80–90%
Oral peak level	8–32 h	1 h	30 min	2 h
Protein binding	95%	60–70%	10–20%	70%
Volume distribution	0.6–1.0 L/kg	1.3 L/kg	2–3 L/kg	5–12 L/kg
Duration	Varies	10–20 min	12–24 h	8–16 h
Elimination $t_{1/2}$	0–30 h	1–1.5 h	9–15 h	6–12 h
Elimination				
Hepatic	Hepatic	Hepatic	Hepatic	Hepatic
Active metabolite renal	Yes	Yes	?	?
Metabolites				
In urine unchanged	5%	10%	40–50%	10–20%
Daily therapeutic dose:				
Child	p.o. 15–20 mg/kg (maintenance 5–8 mg/kg/d)	NA	Not established	15–25 mg/kg/d
	i.v. 15–20 mg/kg (maintenance 5–8 mg/kg/d)	1 mg/kg (max 5 mg/kg)	—	—
Adult	p.o. 15–20 mg/kg (maintenance 5–6 mg/kg/d)	NA	Load 600 mg, then 400 mg at 2 h; avg. maint. dose 1.2–2.4 g/d in 2–3 divided doses of 8–12 h	Load 400–600 mg; Avg. maint. dose 600–1200 mg/d in 3 divided doses
	i.v. 15–20 mg/kg (maintenance 5–6 mg/kg/d)	1 mg/kg q 5 min (max. 5 mg/kg maint. dose 1–4 mg/min)	None	None
Toxic amount				
Child	>20 mg/kg	5 mg/kg	?	?
Adult	>1 g	—	2 g	>1.8 g
Serum concentration				
Therapeutic (mcg/ml)	10–20	1.5–6	3–10	0.5–2
Toxic (mcg/ml)	>25	>6	>10	?
Preparations	Caps 30, 100 Tab 50 mg Sus 30, 125 mg	Viscus 2% Oint 2.5%, 5% Jelly 2% Inj 0.5%, 1%, 2%, 2.4%	Tab 400, 600 mg	Cap 100, 200 250 mg
References	—	72–78	85–91	92–97

of 35 to 60 min. The onset **i.m.** is 10 min with a duration of 3 h (73,74). Viscus lidocaine does not produce toxic blood concentrations when swallowed by adults in doses of 300 mg/kg given every 3 h for 8 doses (73). About 60% to 80% is protein bound to alpha-1 acid glycoprotein. V_d is .3 L/kg, but it is higher in the elderly and premature infants and in pediatric overdose 2.2 L/kg. The alpha **half-life** ($t_{1/2}$) i.v. is 8 to 10 min, i.m. 12 to 28 min and beta elimination $t_{1/2}$ is 80 to 108 min and it may be prolonged in myocardial infarction to 3.2 h, in congestive heart failure and in liver disease to 5.5 to 6.6 h and in newborns 3.5 h. Patients with left to right shunting of blood such as Tetralogy of Fallot may get elevation of lidocaine plasma concentrations due to decreased lidocaine uptake by the lungs. Elimination is 95% by **hepatic metabolism** into **two active metabolites** monoethylglyinexylexylidide (**MEGX**) and glycinexylidide (**GX**) with half-lives of about 10 h. The metabolites may be responsible for neurotoxic effects and they possess antidysrhythmic properties. **MEGX has strong convulsive properties** and is 83% as toxic as the parent drug. Decreased hepatic blood flow such as in congestive heart failure, shock and liver impairment or when propranolol is administered decreases lidocaine clearance. Lidocaine clearance is 10 mL/min/kg and less than 3% is excreted unchanged (73–75).

    c.   **Drug interactions. Propranolol,** when administered with lidocaine, inhibits clearance of the drug (possibly due to decreased hepatic flow and enzyme inhibition), thereby increasing lidocaine levels and toxicity. The metabolism of lidocaine may also be decreased with concomitant use of cimetidine (76). Bupivacaine has been shown to displace protein-bound lidocaine, thereby increasing plasma levels of the drug (77). Finally, concomitant use of tocainide with lidocaine may result in seizures (78).

B.   **Clinical presentation**

    1.   **Mild manifestations** have been reported at blood concentrations of 6 to 9 mcg/mL: vertigo, drowsiness, dysarthria, perioral numbness, muscle twitching, confusion, and tinnitus (79,80).

    2.   **Major manifestations** in severe cases reported include psychosis and status epilepticus resulting in metabolic acidosis. Oral ingestions of more than 5 mg/kg may produce toxicity.

        a.   Severe **CNS** toxicity may occur with coma, and respiratory depression may be seen when blood concentrations exceed 9 mcg/mL (79,80). An oral ingestion of 15 mL of 2% lidocaine produced prolonged seizures and a blood concentration of 10.7 mcg/mL 1 h after ingestion in a 3-year-old (52).

        b.   **Cardiovascular** toxicity resembles antidysrhythmic type 1a quinidine-like toxicity, producing severe bradycardia, sinus arrest, arteriovenous heart block, tachyarrhythmias, and widening of the QRS complex.

    3.   **Methemoglobinemia** has been reported.

C.   **Laboratory analysis**

    1.   **General tests. ECG monitoring** and a 12-lead ECG for abnormalities of intervals and waves are useful. If neuromuscular blockers are used, **EEG monitoring** must be undertaken if seizure disorders are of concern. **Blood gas** monitoring and **methemoglobin** levels are useful, especially if the patient appears cyanotic or the blood is brown.

    2.   **Toxin-specific tests.** The **therapeutic concentration** is 1.5 to 5 mcg/mL although minor CNS symptoms may occur at 4 to 5 mcg/mL and serious intoxication occurs at more than 9 mcg/mL. Monitor lidocaine level every 12 h if congestive heart failure, myocardial infarction or liver dysfunction.

D.   **Management** for lidocaine intoxication should focus on the treatment of seizures, methemoglobinemia, and cardiovascular collapse (80–84).

1. Establish and maintain **vital functions.**
2. Treat **seizures** initially with **diazepam** 0.3 to 0.5 mg/kg i.v. slowly at a rate less than 1 mg/min in a child up to 10 mg, or 5 to 10 mg i.v. slowly at a rate less 2.5 mg/min up to 30 mg in an adult. Lorazepam may also be used. Diazepam may be followed by phenobarbital if necessary. **Phenobarbital** is administered in doses of 15 to 20 mg/kg i.v. slowly over 20 min or less than 25 mg/min in a child, if necessary repeat 5 to 10 mg every 20 min up to 40 mg/kg. In adults 300 to 800 mg i.v. slowly followed by 120 to 240 mg until seizure is controlled or a total of 1 to 2 g is given. **Avoid phenytoin** because of its possible synergic cardiac effects. The seizures may be refractory and require **neuromuscular blocking agents,** intubation, and ventilation. Convulsions may continue even with therapeutic blood concentration of lidocaine due to the action of active metabolites MEGX and GX.
3. The **cardiac dysrhythmias** may require pacing and cardioversion. Lidocaine is rapidly cleared if hepatic blood flow can be restored. Intraoperative cardiopulmonary bypass has successfully been used during intraoperative overdose. Hypertonic sodium bicarbonate if the toxicity is accompanied by QRS widening. If symptomatic bradydysrhythmias occur, use atropine 0.15 mg/kg or a pacemaker. Cardiopulmonary bypass and cardiac pacing has been utilized.
4. **Hypotension** responds to i.v. fluids, and Trendelenburg position and if refractory, vasopressors such as norepinephrine and an intra aortic balloon pump.
5. Treat **acidosis** by controlling seizures and correcting hypotension. If the acidosis persists, consider the use of sodium bicarbonate.
6. Treat **methemoglobinemia** with 100% oxygen initially, then administer methylene blue if symptomatic (dyspnea, altered mental status, or metabolic acidosis when blood level is more than 30%).
   a. The dose of methylene blue (1% solution) for an adult or child is 0.1 to 0.2 mL/kg i.v. (1 to 2 mg/kg) slowly over 5 min. The dose may be repeated in 1 h if necessary up to total of 7 mg/kg.
   b. **Adverse effects** include GI distress, headache, hypertension, dizziness, mental confusion, restlessness, dyspnea, hemolysis, dysuria, burning sensation in the vein, and blue saliva, urine, and skin.
   c. **Contraindications** include renal insufficiency and G6PD deficiency.
7. **Decontamination**
   a. **GI** Decontamination is performed if the drug was ingested, with activated charcoal and a cathartic. Avoid emesis because of rapid onset of symptoms.
   b. **IV administration:** pneumatic tourniquet inflation when the agent has been administered by infiltration or regional injection.
8. **Extracorporeal methods.** Hemodialysis is ineffective but charcoal hemoperfusion may be useful especially after massive overdose or when metabolic elimination is impaired (81).
E. **Disposition.** Hospitalize all patients with ingestion of a toxic amount or toxic plasma concentration. **Intensive care monitoring and cardiac consult** is required in any symptomatic patient with an overdose.

XII. Phenytoin (DPH, Dilantin) (see Chapter 49)

XIII. Tocainide hydrochloride

    A. Properties of agent

        1. **Sources and form of toxin.** Tocainide is available in 400- and 600-mg tablets.

        2. **Mechanism of action and pathophysiology.** Tocainide, an amide local anesthetic, has electrophysiologic actions similar to those of lidocaine and mexiletine. It is given orally to prevent or treat ventricular ectopy and tachycardia.

        3. **Pharmacology and pharmacokinetics.** The usual loading dose is 600 mg followed by 400 mg 2 h later. The maintenance dose ranges from 1.2 to 2.4 g/day in 2 or 3 divided doses every 8 to 12 h.

            a. **Kinetics** (Table 37-4). Tocainide is 90% to 100% bioavailable with negligible first pass metabolism unlike lidocaine. (85–90). **Peak** concentrations occur in 30 min to 2 h. About 10% to 20% is protein bound. Its oral **onset** of action is 1 to 2 h, but may be delayed with food. **Duration** of action is 12 to 24 h. V_d equals 2 to 3 L/kg. About 40% to 50% of drug is excreted unchanged in urine and 50% to 60% is metabolized hepatically to inactive metabolites and eliminated. Renal clearance is dependent on urine pH. The **half life** ranges from 9 to 15 h and may be prolonged if renal insufficiency.

            b. **Drug interactions.** Other antidysrhythmic agents are additive. No other significant drug interactions have been noted for tocainide. A case report of paranoia induced by concomitant use of tocainide and propranolol has been reported (91).

    B. Clinical presentation. Generally the drug is well tolerated.

        1. **Neurologic** toxicities occur in 30% to 50% of patients and include tremor, ataxia, drowsiness, confusion, and paresthesias. Psychosis and seizures have been reported.

        2. **GI toxicity** includes nausea, vomiting, and anorexia.

        3. **Cardiac toxicity.** Underlying ventricular dysrhythmias or conduction disturbances may be exacerbated by tocainide. **QRS and QT remain normal.** AV block, asystole, and hypotension may occur.

        4. Other effects reported after long-term use include agranulocytosis, pulmonary fibrosis, rash, and fever.

    C. Laboratory analysis

        1. **General tests.** Monitor ECG and tocainide level. WBC counts should be performed frequently especially during first several weeks of therapy.

        2. **Toxin-specific tests.** The therapeutic range is 3 to 10 mcg/mL, although it is not well correlated with therapeutic or toxic effects.

    D. Management. See that for lidocaine (see **XI**).

    E. Disposition. Hospitalize all patients with ingestion of a toxic amount or toxic plasma concentration. **Intensive care monitoring and cardiac consult** is required in any symptomatic patient with an overdose.

XIV. Mexiletine hydrochloride

    A. Properties of agent

        1. **Sources and form of toxin.** Mexiletine is available as 100-, 150-, 200-, and 250-mg capsules.

2. **Mechanism of action and pathophysiology.** Mexiletine has electrophysiologic actions similar to those of lidocaine and tocainide. It is a sodium channel antagonist, used for the treatment of ventricular arrhythmias.

3. **Pharmacology and pharmacokinetics**
   a. The usual oral **adult loading dose** is 400 to 600 mg, and the maintenance dose is 200 to 300 mg q8h. Maximum dose is 1200 mg/day. **Pediatric dose** is 15 to 25 mg/kg/day, although the safety and efficacy have not been established. **Therapeutic blood concentration** is 0.5 to 2 mcg/mL, although toxicity has been reported within this range.
   b. **Kinetics** (Table 37-4). Mexiletine is 80% to 90% bioavailable and undergoes less than 10% first-pass hepatic elimination (94). About 70% is protein bound. V_d is large and variable 5 to 12 L/kg. It is predominantly metabolized by the liver to inactive metabolites, 10% to 20% excreted unchanged in urine, depending on urine pH. The **onset** of effect averages 2 h and lasts for 8 to 16 h. The **half-life** ranges from 6 to 12 h.

B. **Clinical presentation** (see **XI**). Manifestations are similar to lidocaine and tocainide and include **convulsions**, cardiovascular toxicity with hypotension and respiratory depression. Ingestions of 1.8 to 2.4 g have resulted in only mild CNS manifestations. In a recent case report of a 41 year-old woman who had ingested 90 of her 200-mg mexiletine tablets, she developed a grand mal seizure in the emergency department without any cardiovascular abnormalities (92). The patient responded to 100 mg of i.v. diazepam, 1 g of phenobarbital, and 5 g of pyridoxine. Status epilepticus occurred 1 h later and she required an additional 40 mg of diazepam and a loading dose of phenobarbital. During the entire time, no electrocardiograph abnormalities were present. Blood levels showed a concentration of 20 mcg/mL. Toxic deaths usually result from hypotension and bradycardia (92). The largest mexiletine overdose reported in patient who survived was an ingestion of 12.4 g (93).

C. **Laboratory analysis**
   1. **General tests.** Monitor ECG and obtain a 12-lead ECG to detect interval and wave abnormalities.
   2. **Toxin-specific tests.** Blood concentrations of 0.5 to 2.0 mcg/mL are therapeutic.

D. **Management**
   1. Same as that for lidocaine (see **XI**) (95–97).
   2. Acidification of urine with ammonium chloride may be theoretically helpful (95), but it has not been evaluated clinically and not recommended.

E. **Disposition.** Hospitalize all patients with ingestion of a toxic amount or toxic plasma concentration. **Intensive care monitoring and cardiac consult** is required in any symptomatic patient with an overdose.

CLASSIC AGENTS: FLECAINIDE ACETATE, ENCAINIDE, PROPAFENONE

Both Lorcainide and Indecainide are also considered in this class but are no longer used in the United States.

XV. **Flecainide acetate (Tambocor)**
   A. **Properties of agent**
      1. **Sources and forms of toxin.** Flecainide is available in 100-mg tablets. An i.v. preparation is available only for investigational use.

2. **Physical and clinical properties.** Flecainide is a benzamide derivative local amide anesthetic. Flecainide was the first of the class 1c drugs to be approved in the United States for treatment of ventricular dysrhythmias (98). Recently, the U.S. Food and Drug Administration (FDA) has advised that both flecainide and encainide be avoided in patients with non–life-threatening ventricular dysrhythmias.

3. **Mechanism of action and pathophysiology.** Like other class 1c agents, flecainide produces minimal effects on repolarization as compared with class 1a drugs, which prolong the total action potential duration, and class 1b drugs, which decrease the relative refractory period. Class 1c compounds exert local anesthetic properties that depress myocardial contractility (99–107).

4. **Pharmacology and pharmacokinetics**

   a. **Initial oral dosage** in adults is 50 to 100 mg twice daily and may be adjusted every 4 to 5 days not to exceed 400 mg/day. The range of therapeutic concentration for flecainide is 0.2 to 1.0 mcg/mL, however trough levels greater than 0.7 mcg/mL have been associated with increased adverse effects. Few data are available on overdoses. An AV block and QRS prolongation was reported in a patient with a flecainide concentration of 3 mcg/mL (100).

   b. **Pharmacokinetics:** Flecainide is approximately 95% bioavailable (98,102). **Peak** plasma levels occur within 2 to 3 h. The apparent V_d is 9 L/kg and protein binding is 37% to 50%. The elimination **half-life** in an adult is 14 h (range 7 to 26 h) and in children (ages 3 to 13) ranges from 7 to 10 (103). Flecainide is metabolized to two mildly active metabolites, meta-O-dealkylated flecainide and itslactam, which are conjugated in plasma. Flecainide clearance is prolonged in patients with CHF and renal failure. The half-life of elimination averages approximately 19 h in CHF and as much as 58 h in end-stage renal failure patients. Acid urine pH increases the excretion of flecainide.

   c. **Drug interactions.** When flecainide and **propranolol** are administered concomitantly, an increase in plasma levels of 20% for flecainide and 30% for propranolol was noted (99). Other antidysrhythmic agents (beta-blockers, amiodarone, disopyramide, and verapamil) may have an additive negative inotropic effect (100). Use of digoxin with flecainide may result in a slight increase in **digoxin** levels (15). Also, an increase in flecainide toxicity may occur with concomitant administration of amiodarone (102). Cimetidine decreases both renal and nonrenal clearance of flecainide.

B. **Clinical manifestations**

   1. **Proarrhythmic activity** leading to ventricular tachycardia is the primary toxicity. ECG changes reported are **increased PR and QT intervals, and widening of the QRS complex.** Decreased ectopic action and hypotension may be noted. Overdose may produce bradycardia, AV block, asystole, and hypotension.

   2. **Visual disturbance** (including blurred vision, photophobia, and spots before the eyes) is a common side effect.

   3. **Respiratory depression** has been noted in fatal animal poisonings but has not been noted in human overdose to date.

C.   **Laboratory:** The therapeutic trough concentration range for flecainide is 0.2 to 1.0 mcg/mL, however trough levels greater than 0.7 mcg/mL have been associated with increased adverse effects (98).

D.   **Management**
1.   Establish and maintain the vital functions.
2.   Cardiac dysrhythmias such as ventricular tachycardia should be treated with common antidysrhythmic agents, cardioversion and ventricular pacing. Hemodynamic support including intraaortic pump may be needed. There are two cases reported on the primary and secondary detoxification in severe flecainide intoxications (104). In case one, the plasma concentration was 6,500 ng/mL (therapeutic=200 to 980 ng/mL). The patient survived with a pacemaker and catecholamine support. In the second case, hemoperfusion terminated the need for emergency resuscitation during the initial phase but was unsuccessful 3 h later. Both cases had a rapid onset of symptoms because of high bioavailability. The authors recommended the prophylactic use of a pacemaker and gastric suction. Hemoperfusion has not been proven useful (104).

E.   **Disposition.** Hospitalize all patients with ingestion of a toxic amount or toxic plasma concentration. **Intensive care monitoring and cardiac consult** is required in any symptomatic patient with an overdose.

XVI.   **Encainide (Enkaid)**
A.   **Properties of agent**
1.   **Sources and forms of toxin.** Encainide is available as 25-, 35-, and 50-mg capsules. In December 1991, encainide was withdrawn from the market and is now available from the manufacturer only for life threatening dysrhythmias.
2.   **Mechanism of action and pathophysiology**
a.   Encainide, an analogue of lysergic acid is a benzananilide derivative. Encainide blocks the sodium channels of the myocardium and Purkinje fibers producing dose related slowing of the Phase 0 depolarization. Sodium channel blockage prolongs the QRS interval and slows intraventricular conduction.
b.   Encainide is similar to flecanide and has the same indication of use. It is not recommended for non–life-threatening dysrhythmias.
3.   **Pharmacology and pharmacokinetics**
a.   In adults, the **therapeutic dose** range is 75 to 150 mg/day. Dosages greater than 200 mg/day require hospitalization of the patient. Minor transient side effects occur in 30% to 60% of patients at therapeutic doses but occur more frequently at doses in excess of 200 mg/day.
b.   **Pharmacokinetics** (Table 37-5). Encainide is well absorbed after oral dosing and has a variable V_d. It is up to 70% to 80% protein bound. It undergoes **extensive hepatic metabolism** within 30 min to 4 h in adults to the **active metabolites** O-dimethyl encainide (ODE) and 3-methoxy-*o*-dimethyl encainide (3-MODE), both of which are more active antidysrhythmic agents than the parent drug, and inactive *N*-dimethylencainide (108). About 7% of the general population has a genetic deficiency in encainide metabolism and their half-life is 8 to 22 h. The half-lives of elimination of encainide, ODE and 3-MODE are 1.9 h, 4 h, and 11.4 h respec-

TABLE 37-5. *Class IC*

	Flecainide (Tambacor)	Encainide (Enkaid)	Propafenone (Rythmol)
Route	Oral	Oral	Oral
Absorption			
bioavailable	90–100%	7–82%	4.8–23.5%
Oral peak level	2–3 h	0.5–2 h	2–3 h
Protein binding	37–50%	70–80%	77–95%
Vol distribution	8–10 L/kg	Small	0.7–3 L/kg
Duration	12–30 h	8 h	—
Elimination $t_{1/2}$	7–26 h	1–3 h (metabolites: ODE 3–4 h; 6–12 h MODE[a])	2–10 h
Elimination	Hepatic	Hepatic	Hepatic
Active metabolite	Yes	Yes	Yes
In urine unchanged	10–50%	10%	<1%
Therapeutic dose			
Child	Not established 100 mg q	Not established 25 mg q 8 h	Not established
Adult	12 h initially, then increase in increments of 50 mg q 12 h q 4–7 d to a maintainence dose of 100–200 mg q 12 h max 400 mg/d	adjusted at 3–5 d intervals to 35 mg q 8 h and then 50 mg q 8 h	600–900 mg/day
Toxic amount			
Child	?	?	133 mg/kg
Adult	?	?	9 g (fatal)
Blood concentration			
Therapeutic	200–1,000 ng/ml	>15–100 ng/ml	120–1000 ng/mL
Toxic	>1,000 ng/ml	?	>3,000 ng/ml
Preparations	Tab 100 mg	Cap 25, 35, 50 mg	Tab 150, 300 mg
References	98–104	108–113	114–119

[a] For details, see text (section V.3. b).

tively. Ninety percent of the population are extensive metabolizers so that ODE and 3-MODE are primarily responsible for the antidysrhythmic effects. ODE is 55% to 65% and MODE is 90% protein bound. In 10% of patients who have a genetic defect and are poor metabolizers and in patients with chronic liver or renal disease, encainide has a longer half-life (5.8 to 13.8 h) and as much as 50% of the drug is eliminated unchanged in the urine (108). Encainide and metabolites are excreted mainly in the urine. About 30% are excreted in the feces.

    c. **Drug interactions.** Concomitant use of encainide and **cimetidine** results in a significant increase (30%) in the levels of encainide and its metabolite ODE and 3-MODE (110). Other antidysrhythmic agents concomitantly may increase cardiac effects.

B. Clinical presentation

    1. With **acute overdose,** cardiac and CNS manifestations, including seizures, bradycardia, hypotension, and ECG changes (prolonged QRS, QTC, and PR intervals, AV dissociation, and asystole), have been reported. These effects have occurred within 2 h after ingestion. ECG changes persisted for more than 2 days (113). An acute overdose of 3 to 4 g in an adult produced manifestations similar to

those seen with class 1a agents. A single 25 mg tablet ingested by a 6 month old infant caused a **wide complex sinus tachycardia** within 30 min. Electroshock cardioversion was performed but the ventricular tachycardia returned. Intraosseous fluids, sodium bicarbonate and phenytoin were administered and defibrillation performed. The encainide plasma levels were over 180 ng/mL of parent drug (normal adult 15 to 100 ng/mL) (108). In the cardiac antidysrhythmic suppression trials (CAST) encainide and flecainide were associated with excess deaths from dysrhythmias (109).

2. Encainide, like flecainide, exerts a **proarrhythmic effect.** In a study of 1245 patients, a proarrhythmic effect was noted in 9.2% (112). In contrast to flecainide, encainide does not exert a negative inotropic effect.

3. The principal **noncardiac side effects** noted in the study of 1245 patients by Soyka were dizziness (26%), blurred vision (19%), metallic taste (4%), and tremor (3%) (112).

C. **Laboratory analysis**

1. **General tests.** Monitor ECG and obtain a 12-lead ECG to detect interval and wave abnormalities.

2. **Toxin-specific tests. Therapeutic** plasma concentrations are 15 to 100 ng/mL (108).

D. **Management**

1. Same as for class 1a agents (see **X**).

2. Active metabolites of encainide are excreted in the urine. Extracorporeal techniques are not useful because of the high protein binding and large V_d.

3. Hypertonic sodium bicarbonate or saline may be useful in managing the cardiac toxicity but there are no scientific studies in humans, although it has been successful in dogs (113). Adverse effects of hypertonic saline include hypernatremia, hypokalemia hyperosmolality, hypocalcemia, and hyperphosphatemia.

E. **Disposition.** Hospitalize all patients with ingestion of a toxic amount or toxic plasma concentration. **Intensive care monitoring and cardiac consult** is required in any symptomatic patient with an overdose.

XVII. **Propafenone (Rythmol)**

A. **Properties of agent**

1. **Sources and forms of toxin.** Available in 150- and 300-mg tablets.

2. **Physical and chemical properties.** Propafenone has been approved by the FDA as a class 1c agent. It has been used for the treatment of supraventricular and ventricular dysrhythmias, including those associated with Wolff-Parkinson-White syndrome (114,118,120,121).

3. **Mechanism of action and pathophysiology.** Propafenone blocks the fast sodium channel in myocardial cells. It has mild beta-blocking activity and weak calcium antagonist properties. It is classified as a 1c antidysrhythmic agent.

4. **Pharmacology and pharmacokinetics**

a. In adults the **therapeutic range** is 600 to 900 mg/day.

b. **Kinetics** (Table 37–5). Over 95% of propafenone is absorbed, but bioavailability is 3.4% with 150 mg and 10.6% with 300 mg (range was 4.8% to 23.5%) because of significant first pass. **Onset** within 3 h. **Peak plasma**

concentrations occur 2 to 3 h after an oral dose. V_d ranges from 0.7 to 3 L/kg with a protein binding to glycoprotein of 77% to 95%. Propafenone undergoes hepatic P450 oxidative metabolism to form 5-hydroxy and *N*-depropyl metabolites (116,117). The extent of hydroxylation is genetically determined poor and extensive metabolizers. About 7% of caucasians are poor metabolizers. The elimination **half-life** is 2 to 10 h (average 4 h) after single dose to 2 to 30 h at steady state. About 10% of patients and those taking quinidine (inhibits one of propafenone pathways) metabolize the drug more slowly and the half lives can be 10 to 32 h. Only about 1% is excreted in the urine unchanged (116).

    c. **Drug interactions.** Concomitant use with **digoxin** has been reported to increase the digoxin concentration 35% to 83% (118). Quinidine and cimetidine interferes with metabolism and increases half-life. Propafenone may increase the plasma concentrations of beta-blockers and warfarin (118–121).

B. **Clinical presentation**

    1. Symptoms usually develop within 3 h postingestion, although the reported onset is 30 to 120 min (116).

    2. **Overdoses** have been rare, as the agent is still relatively new. Primary manifestations include GI distress, mild CNS depression, and ventricular tachyarrhythmias. Hypotension, bradycardia, conduction defects, ventricular dysrhythmias, and seizures have been reported. Myoclonus and acidosis have been noted. A 2-year-old child ingested 133 mg/kg (1800 mg) and developed severe cardiac and neurologic toxicity (115). An adult who ingested a mixed overdose of 9 g of propafenone with amitriptyline and benzodiazepines died (116).

    3. **ECG changes. Prolongation of the PR interval and QRS duration** have occurred with therapeutic doses greater than 450 mg. Prolonged QT interval is seen in overdose reflecting delays in ventricular conduction (116).

C. **Laboratory analysis**

    1. **General tests.** Same as for class 1A agents (see **IX**). Monitor ECG and obtain a 12-lead ECG to detect interval and wave abnormalities.

    2. **Toxin-specific tests.** The **therapuetic blood concentration** is 120 to 1000 ng/mL, most intoxications are associated with blood concentrations greater 3000 ng/mL (116)

D. **Management**

    1. Same as for class 1A agents (see **X**). However, bolus doses of sodium bicarbonate did not narrow the wide QRS (116). Temporary internal pacemaker and epinephrine may be required.

    2. **Cardiac dysrhythmias** such as ventricular tachycardia should be treated with common antidysrhythmic agents, cardioversion, and ventricular pacing (119).

E. **Disposition.** Hospitalize all patients with ingestion of a toxic amount or toxic plasma concentration. **Intensive care monitoring and cardiac consult** is required in any symptomatic patient with an overdose.

CLASS II AGENTS

Beta-adrenergic drugs are widely used in medicine for the treatment of hypertension, dysrhythmias, angina pectoris, open-angle glaucoma, prophylaxis against sudden death after myocardial infarction, and treatment of migraine. A full discussion of their major toxicity and management is discussed in Chapter 36.

CLASS III AGENTS: SOTALOL, AMIODARONE, BRETYLIUM

XVIII.   Sotalol (Betacardone, Sotacor, Betapace)

   A.   Properties of agent

   1.   Source and form of toxin. Sotalol is available in 80, 160, and 240 mg tablets.

   2.   Physical and chemical properties. Sotalol is 70% water soluble. It was originally approved for life-threatening ventricular tachycardias but is efficient for supraventricular tachycardias (122). Unlike other beta-adrenergic blockers, it is the only oral agent in this class used strictly for its antidysrhythmic properties and is not indicated for the treatment of hypertension. Contraindications to use are asthma, bradycardia, blocks, prolonged QT syndromes, congestive heart failure, and with quinidine.

   3.   Mechanism of action and pathophysiology Sotalol is a unique water soluble, nonselective, beta-blocker in that it has properties of both **class II and class III** agents (123). The class II effect is nonselective beta-adrenergic antagonism and the class III effect is prolonging the monophasic action potential duration in all cardiac tissues. This results in less left ventricular depression than propranolol and a lower incidence of toxicity (124). Sotalol has risen as the prototype of class III antidysrhythmics (125,147–149). It delays cardiac repolarization by inhibiting the delayed potassium current, having lesser effects on the inward potassium current and little or no effect on the inward calcium of sodium currents. This causes a prolongation of repolarization and an increase in the effective refractory period not due to the blockade of beta-adrenergic receptors (122,123). Unlike other beta-blocking agents, it prolongs the duration of the action potential in the cardiac tissue, increases refractory period and **lengthens the QT** interval of the ECG at plasma concentrations of 2.6 mcg/mL and can produce ventricular tachycardia and fibrillation (122). As a Class III antidysrhythmic, sotalol has no membrane-stabilizing activity, no intrinsic sympathomimetic activity, and no preferential actions on beta-1 or beta-2 receptors. According to one study, sotalol reduces the heart rate to a greater degree than propranolol and causes significantly less cardiac suppression than propranolol at a given heart rate (126). Beta-adrenergic blockade is evident in doses as low as 25 mg/day and the class III effects are seen in doses above 160 mg.

   4.   Pharmacology and pharmacokinetics

   a.   The oral **therapeutic dose** is 80 to 480 mg. It can prolong the QT interval and may produce Torsades de pointes (122–125). The dose should not be increased earlier than every 2 to 3 days. Maximum daily dose is 480 mg/day. The manufacturer advises that the intiation of therapy with sotalol be in a setting where the patient can be monitored (122).

   b.   **Pharmacokinetics** (Table 37-6). It is orally administered and is 90% to 100% bioavailable. **Onset of action** is 1 to 2 h. **Peak plasma** concentration occurs 2 to 4 h after administration. It is not bound to plasma proteins or metabolized, but more than 90% is excreted unchanged in the urine. V_d is 0.7 to 2.4 L/kg. Plasma **half-life** is 15 h (range 5 to 13). In

TABLE 37-6. *Class III agents*

	Amiodarone (cordarone)	Bretylium (Britylol)	Sotalol (betacardone)
Route	p.o. I.V. (200-mg tabs)	i.v./i.m.	p.o.
Bioavailability	Mean 65%; range 22–100%	12–37%	90–100%
Oral peak level	3–8 h	i.m. 1 h i.v. 2 min	2–4 h
Protein binding	96%	1–6%	0%
Volume distribution	60 L/kg	3.4 L/kg	0.7–2.41/kg
Duration	20 h	—	—

Elimination $t_{1/2}$	Liver
	Acute use (p.o. 3.2–80 h);
	  chronic use (p.o. 14–52 d;
	  average 30 days)
		Renal
		
		7–11 h
			Renal
			
			5–13 h

Active metabolite desethylamiodarone chronic use $t_{1/2}$	60–90 d	?	No
In urine unchanged	<1.%	100%	>90%
Therapeutic dose child maintenance (6 wk to 10 yr)	2.5–34 mg/kg/d	5 mg/kg over 8–10 min	N/A
Loading infants (1–4 months)	50–150mg/d	May be repeated at 16 mg/kg	
Adult			
Loading	600–2,000 mg/d given t.i.d. × 7–14 d	5–10 mg/kg or continuous infusion	80–480 mg/d
Maintain	400–2,000 mg/d, given o.d.	1–2 mg/min	
Toxic dose			
Child	?	?	?
Adult	?	?	>480 mg
Blood concentration			
Therapeutic	1–2.5 mg/L	—	500–4,000 mg/L
Toxic	>2.5 mg/L	—	?
Preparations	Tab 200 mg	2 mg/ml/50 mg/ml	Tab 80, 160, 240 mg
References	150–162	163–166	132–149

[a] The toxic dose for amiodarone (Cordarone) is 5 g/Kg in animals.

end stage renal insufficiency its elimination half-life is 41 h and intervals between doses of 24 to 48 h are recommended.

c. **Drug interactions.** It is not recommended to use sotalol in conjunction with any class Ia or class III agents because of their ability to prolong refractoriness. The combined use of sotalol plus **quinidine** or **procainamide** causes a prolongation of ventricular refractoriness and slows induced ventricular tachycardia in a high number of patients (127). Concomitant use of sotalol with **digoxin** appears to increase proarrhythmic effects. Calcium channel blockers (class IV) should be used with caution in sotalol patients because of the possible additive effects on atrioventricular conduction or ventricular function. Insulin and oral hypoglycemic agents may need to be adjusted after the addition of sotalol because of possible hyperglycemia. Caution is suggested in the discontinuation of clonidine while receiving sotalol or other beta-blockers because of reflexive hypertension. Caution should be used when administering sotalol with any drug that may prolong the QT interval such as tricyclic antidepressants, astemizole, amiodarone, sematilide, phenothiazines, and class I antidysrhythmics.

B. Clinical presentation.

1. The **adverse effects** of sotalol include Torsades de pointes and other ventricular arrhythmias, fatigue, bradycardia, dyspnea, asthenia, and dizziness. Rare cases of new or worsening congestive heart failure have been reported (129). The manufacturer advises that the intiation of therapy with sotalol be in a setting where the patient can be monitored (122).

2. In **overdose** it produces serious cardiac toxicity with a very **prolonged QT** and a risk of **Torsades de pointes** especially if predisposing factors are present such as hypokalemia, bradycardia and concomittant drug use (130). Torsades de pointes occurred in 24 patients or 2% of patients in clinical trials which is similar to quinidine. Reports of multifocal PVCs, bigeminy, ventricular tachycardia appear in the literature (122). The most common manifestations of poisonings are bradycardia, congestive heart failure, hypotension, bronchospasm, and hypoglycemia. In massive overdoses (2 to 16 g), hypotension, bradycardia, ventricular tachycardia, cardiac asystole, prolongation of the QT interval, Torsades de pointes, and premature ventricular complexes occur (130). In a recent overdose of 6.72 g of sotalol reported in a 70-year-old woman, the patient survived despite having two episodes of asystole (128).

C. Laboratory

1. **General:** Continuous cardiac monitoring and a 12-lead ECG for symptomatic patients or a substantial ingestion, blood glucose, electrolytes especially potassium, lactate levels, BUN, creatinine, and transaminases. Arterial blood gases and chest rardiograph if respiratory symptoms develop. In severe cases, central hemodynamic monitoring may be necessary. Cardiac consultation is recommended if symptomatic.

2. **Toxin-specific analysis:** Therapeutic blood concentrations are 500 to 4,000 ng/mL (122).

D. Management

1. **Establish and maintain vital functions.** All patients should have cardiac monitoring, a 12-lead ECG analysis, frequent monitoring of vital signs, and vascular access established with a large-bore i.v. line even if stable.

2. **Examination** should focus on the cardiopulmonary system (blood pressure, bradycardia and conduction disturbances) but the neurologic system and evaluation of renal and hepatic function is also important (131).

3. **Symptomatic patients.** If bradycardia and hypotensive, administer i.v. fluid therapy, beta-adrenergic agonists, vasopressors and consider glucagon. **If unconsciousness** is present, hypoglycemia may be the cause. Perform a blood reagent glucose strip analysis and consider the administration of i.v. glucose. If **endotracheal intubation** is necessary, i.v. atropine 0.01 mg/kg with minimum dose of 0.02 mg in a child or 0.5 mg i.v. in an adult should be on hand or administered to inhibit vagal effects of the procedure.

4. **In patients that are hemodynamically unstable or comatose,** cardiac consultant is advisable since these patients may need cardiac pacing, intraaortic balloon or cardiopulmonary pump support (132,133). Monitoring the heart rate and blood pressure alone is often inadequate for these patients. They often need pulmonary wedge pressure monitoring, observation for renal failure, shock liver, or lactic acidosis (131).

5. **Medical evaluation and GI decontamination** should be considered if a child ingests 1 mg/kg or a healthy adult two times the therapeutic dose or if a patient with cardiac disease ingests any amount more than the prescribed therapeutic dose.

    a. Correct any life threatening manifestation first.

    b. **Avoid induced emesis** because of early onset of altered mental state, apnea, seizures that pose the danger of aspiration, and vagal stimulation that may increase bradycardia. It has also been implicated in the genesis of seizures (131,134).

    c. **Gastric lavage** should be performed first within a few hours after ingestion with precautions to protect the airway and correct dysrhythmias. **Activated charcoal** 1 g/kg and a cathartic initially (sorbitol 1 g/kg in adults and magnesium citrate 4 mL/kg in a child) can be administered after the patient is stabilized. Repeated doses of activated charcoal 0.5 g/kg oral every 4 to 6 h are recommended for symptomatic patients, sustained release preparations and enterohepatic circulation (135–137). **Pretreatment of gastric lavage with atropine** 0.02 mg/kg child and 0.5 mg adult has been suggested to decrease vagal effects in patients with bradycardia or significant intoxications, others feel it should be available (131,138,139). **Whole bowel irrigation** should be considered in sustained release preparations but there are no studies and it may cause desorption of the drug from activated charcoal.

6. **Treat metabolic disturbances** hypoglycemia, hyperkalemia, and seizures appropriately.

7. **Cardiovascular management.** The goal is to restore membrane adenyl cyclase and preserve intracytoplasmic cAMP. Monitor ECG and periodically obtain 12-lead ECG for cardiovascular manifestations.

    a. **Bradycardia and a normal blood pressure.** Oral activated charcoal and close monitoring is all that is necessary. Pharmacologic intervention is indicated only for the symptomatic patient.

    b. **Bradycardia and hemodynamic instability.** Atropine 0.5 to 2 mg in adults, 50 mcg/kg in children i.v. (131), and/or dobutamine, or a cardioselective beta agonist. However, these agents may be ineffective. Use **glucagon** as for refractory hypotension (see below). **A temporary transvenous or an external pacemaker** may be necessary but often evokes a drop in blood pressure and cardiac output. This may be beneficial in treating Torsades de pointes associated with sotalol intoxication (131,138–140). Isoproterenol i.v. initially in a metered infusion of 1 to 5 mg/h in adults and 5 to 20 mg/h may be needed in the first few hours. Isoproterenol has potent vasodilator effects that may limit its efficacy and make a vasoconstrictor necessary (131).

    c. **Hypotension: Volume expanding fluids** 20 mL/kg in children or 500 mL 0.9% saline to produce a systolic blood pressure of more than 100 mm Hg are recommended. In cases of advanced age, cardiomyopathy, hypertension or aortic valve lesions raise the blood pressure upward to restore adequate visceral perfusion. Adequate renal perfusion is indicated by urinary output of at least 0.5 mL/kg/h; myocardial perfusion by the disappearance of signs of coronary insufficiency and pulmonary edema; cerebral perfusion by improvement in mental state; cutaneous perfusion by disappearance of cyanosis and mottling; laboratory by correction of lactic acidosis, hyperkalemia, and hypoglycemia.

    d. Although beta agonists and **vasopressors** may be administered, doses of several times their usual therapeutic doses may be required. To avoid the toxicity of these agents at high doses, consider using glucagon.

    e. **Glucagon** is the choice drug for treatment of beta-adrenoreceptor antagonists intoxication. It improves the inotropic effect more than the chronotropic effect. **Indications:** Symptomatic bradycardia and/or conduction abnormalities, hypotension due to beta-adrenergic blocker toxicity. **Dose:** The i.v. **loading** dose for hypotension is 5 to 10 mg (average is 5 mg) in an adult as a bolus over 1 min or 0.15 mg/kg (150 mcg/kg) in a child. Response is expected within 5 to 10 min. This amount may repeated as a bolus in 10 to 30 min. If no response is observed after the first 10 mg, then alternative therapy must be considered. Therapeutic response with glucagon must be followed by a continuous infusion because of this agent's short half-life and duration of action. A **continuous infusion** is started as 1 to 5 mg/h in an adult or 0.05 to 0.1 mg/kg/h (50 to 100 mcg/kg/h) in a child and titrated to response. Cumulative dose up to 100 mg/24 h have been reported (141–144). **To reconstitute glucagon for infusion use D5W. Do not** use the **Eli Lilly diluent**, which contains 0.2% phenol because of theoretical risk of phenol toxicity if doses of less than 2 mg are used, **or saline solutions** which may cause crystal precipitation (8,143). Since glucagon may cause vomiting, take precautions to avoid aspiration. It may also result rarely in allergic reactions.

    f. **Ventricular tachycardia** or serious premature venticular contractions is managed by lidocaine or phenytoin or overdrive pacing. The administration of magnesium i.v. and isoproterenol may also be effective. Use cardioversion if patient is unstable. Wide complex QRS dysrhythmias may respond to alkalinization with sodium bicarbonate.

    g. Diazepam should be considered if the QRS is greater than 0.12 sec as in the analogy of chloroquine poisoning (140).

    h. **Torsades de pointes** is treated with magnesium sulfate. In adults, this is administered as 2 g by i.v. bolus over 1 to 2 min, if no response in 10 min the dose may be repeated once (143). The dose in children is 25 to 50 mg/kg initially and maintenance is 30 to 60 mg/kg/24 h (0.25 to 0.50 mEq/kg/24 h) up to 1,000 mg/24 h. Magnesium should be administered with cardiac monitoring and calcium gluconate on hand. A pacemaker may be necessary.

i. **Myocardial depression and hypotension:** Correct dysrhythmias, Trendelen-burg positioning, and volume expanding fluids. Hypertonic **sodium bicar-bonate** 1 to 2 mEq/kg in boluses as for tricyclic antidepressant overdose is recommended. A combination of dopamine and dobutamine or isoproterenol has been successful in animal models. This setting requires central hemo-dynamic monitoring with a pulmonary arterial wedge pressure (**PAWP**) catheter. If low cardiac output with low PAWP, give more fluids. If low cardiac output with normal PAWP, use an inotrope (e.g., glucagon). **Vaso-pressors** such as norepinephrine or epinephrine may be needed if the patient fails to respond to correction of the bradycardia, volume resuscitation, and inotropes. **Avoid Class 1a antidysrhythmic agents** (quinidine, pro-cainamide, and disopyramide) and bretylium.

j. **Investigational therapies. Beta-1 adrenergic agonist,** prenalterol, has suc-cessfully reversed both bradycardia and hypotension but is not available in the United States (130). **Phosphodiesterase inhibitors:** Theophylline or amrinone stimulate catecholamine release by inhibiting enzyme inactivation of cyclic AMP by phosphodiesterase and have a synergistic effect with glucagon in canine studies (145). The use of theophylline has been reported in two patients (140). At the present time we are not advocating theophylline because the dose that it inhibits the enzyme inactivation is much higher than the therapeutic dose and can cause toxicity. **Amrinone (Inocor),** a bipyridine derivative, was first introduced into the United States in 1984 as an inotropic agent and vasodilator. It was used in one patient who overdosed on labetalol (146). It should only be considered as a possible last resort in severe cases unresponsive to conventional therapy. Hypotension may limit its usefulness. Its established indications are in adults with chronic congestive heart failure and myocardial dysfunction associated with sepsis. There are two methods to increase the intracellular cyclic AMP, by stimulating the beta-adrenergic receptor or inhibiting phosphodiesterase. The mechanism of action of amri-none is inhibition of phosphodiesterase isoenzyme III specifically in cardiac muscle and vascular smooth musculature. It produces an increase in cyclic AMP subsequently activating protein C which results in phosphorylation of the calcium channels and an increase in calcium influx. This may reverse the negative inotropic effect of a beta-blocker or calcium channel blocker on the heart. In the smooth muscle of the vasculature it decreases the intracellular calcium producing peripheral vasodilation. Amrinone is primarily metabo-lized by a genetic determined rate to N-acetylamrinone and subsequently oxidized to N-glycolylamrinone. Approximately 10% to 40% of it is excreted in the urine unchanged. The **recommended dose** is 0.75 to 2.0 mg/kg (0.15 to 0.4 mL/kg) by i.v. bolus followed by a drip of 5 to 10 mcg/kg/min (see Table 37-7). **Adverse effects** of amrinone are hypotension, dysrhythmias, GI upset, reversible thrombocytopenia, and hepatic enzyme elevation. The prin-cipal side effect is thrombocytopenia probably mediated by N-acetyl-amrinone.

TABLE 37-7. *Amrinone dosage*

	Weight (Kg)									
	30	40	50	60	70	80	90	100	110	120
Loading dose 0.75 mg/kg undiluted of 5 mg/ml concentration										
Dosage, mL (5 mg/mL)	4.5	6.0	7.5	9.0	10.5	12.0	13.5	15.0	16.5	18.0
Infusion rate mL/h of 2.5 mg/mL concentration										
5 µg/kg/min	4	5	6	7	8	10	11	12	13	14
7 µg/kg/min	5	7	9	11	13	14	16	18	20	22
10 µg/kg/min	7	10	12	14	17	19	22	24	26	29

To prepare 2.5 mL concentration for infusion, mix amrinone with equal parts of diluent.—i.e., to mix three 20-mL ampules: 3×20 mL = 60 mL with 60 mL diluent for total volume of 120 mL of 2.5 mg/mL solution.

7. **Bronchospasm:** Administer nebulized bronchodilators (e.g., albuterol). Aminophylline may increase adenyl cyclase and stimulate diaphragmatic action.

8. **Extracorporeal measures. Charcoal hemoperfusion** may be considered for unresponsive patients with sotolal because of its water-solubility, particularly if there is evidence of renal failure (140). There is limited documentation of effectiveness of these methods in removal of beta-blockers because of large V_d and high protein binding (18). Circulatory assistance may be the only solution in intractable circulatory failure. Placement of an intraaortic balloon pump for 48 h was successful in one patient (134,140). **Extracorporeal membrane oxygenation** which has been shown to be useful in severe cases of tricyclic antidepressant overdoses may have a role in this setting.

E. **Disposition.** Hospitalize all patients with ingestion of a toxic amount or toxic plasma concentration. **Intensive care monitoring and cardiac consult** is required in any symptomatic patient with an overdose.

XIX. **Amiodarone (Cordarone)**

A. **Properties of agent**

1. **Sources and forms of toxin.** Amiodarone is available in 100- or 200-mg tablets and for injection as 50 mg/mL in 3-mL ampuls.

2. **Physical and clinical properties.** Amiodarone is a diiodinated benzofuran derivative that is structurally similar to thyroxine. Administered orally or i.v., clinical investigations indicate that it is useful for long-term treatment of unstable supraventricular or ventricular tachycardia or fibrillation that is life-threatening or refractory to other medication. It may be useful for management of atrial fibrillation associated with Wolff-Parkinson-White syndrome (150).

3. **Mechanism of action and pathophysiology**

a. Amiodarone is a group III antidysrhythmic agent, in the same class as bretylium. It functions by prolonging the action potential and Phase 3 of cardiac cell depolarization.

b. It decreases automaticity and conduction velocity. Thus the duration of the action potential is prolonged, as is the refractory period.

  c. It has also been shown to noncompetitively inhibit alpha- and beta-adrener-gic activity (151).

 4. **Pharmacology and pharmacokinetics**

  a. **Therapeutic loading doses** may be as high as 2,000 mg/day in adults and 2.5 to 34.0 mg/kg in children.

  b. **Pharmacokinetics** (Table 37-6). Absorption from the GI tract is variable and incomplete. This is most probably due to a first pass hepatic effect. Bioavailability ranges from between 225 to 86%. **Absorption** from the GI tract continues for up to 15 h and a **peak plasma** level is achieved in 3 to 8 h (154). During long-term administration, the drug is reported to have a **half-life** between 25 to 100 days (155). Amiodarone is distributed throughout the body and accumulates in muscle and fat. This results in a large V_d of 60 L/kg. It is 96% protein bound. The drug is metabolized in the liver and presently only one major metabolite has been identified, desethylamiodarone (DEA). This metabolite has achieved steady state levels similar to that of amiodarone. Its significance is unclear. Less than 1% of amiodarone or its metabolite can be found in the urine. However, both compounds have been found to cross the placenta and to be excreted in breast milk. A **therapeutic level** in the serum is considered to be between 1.0 to 2.5 mcg/mL.

  c. **Drug interactions.** Amiodarone has been shown to potentiate the effects of **warfarin** and to increase the serum levels of **digoxin, quinidine, procainamide,** mexiletine, and propafenone. Beta-blockers and calcium channel blockers may cause marked depression of sinus or atrioventricular nodal function if used concomitantly with amiodarone (156). Torsades de pointes, heart block, and bradyarrhythmias resistant to atropine have occurred when amiodarone has been used with a class I antidysrhythmic.

B. **Clinical presentation**

 1. **Ocular.** Benign yellow brown **corneal microdeposits** have occurred in 76% to 100% of persons undergoing chronic therapy. Visual disturbances such as blurred vision, colored halos, and photophobia are also common (up to 70% of patients) (157). Corneal microdeposits are reversible upon reduction of the dose or drug discontinuation.

 2. **Cardiac.** Overdose of 2.5 to 8.0 g in adults has produced bradycardia and prolonged QT intervals, noted 2 to 4 days after ingestion (152,153). Rapid i.v. infusion has caused hypotension. Dysrhythmias occur in approximately 57% of patients and chronic usage has resulted in Torsades de pointes (157).

 3. **Pulmonary.** The most serious adverse effects are pulmonary **fibrosis** and **pneumonitis.** This condition occurs in 1.4% to 6.0% of patients and can be fatal (158,159). It is manifested by pleuritic chest pain, nonproductive cough, low-grade fever, and dyspnea on exertion. Chest roentgenograms show bilateral pulmonary infiltrates, and laboratory studies reveal leukocytosis. The pulmonary injury has been hypothesized to be due to impairment of normal phospholipid catabolism. It usually occurs in patients receiving more than 400 mg daily. However, it has been reported in patients receiving less but with large loading doses (160).

4. **Thyroid.** Amiodarone is approximately 34% iodine. It is reported to reduce the peripheral transformation of thyroxine (T_4) to triiodothyronine (T_3). It can induce hypo- or hyperthyroidism (1% to 5% of patients) (161).

5. **Hepatic.** Amiodarone can cause a transient elevation of liver function tests (up to 55% of patients) and has caused at least one known case of fatal cirrhosis (162).

6. **Other.** Amiodarone has been shown to cause a peripheral neuropathy, tremor, nausea, vomiting, metallic taste, headaches, sleeplessness in various patients (151). Several cases of blue gray discoloration of the skin have been reported, which are most likely related to lipofuscin deposits rather than melanin and pigment (169).

C. **Laboratory**

1. **General:** Continuous cardiac monitoring and a 12-lead ECG for symptomatic patients or a substantial ingestion, blood glucose, electrolytes especially potassium, lactate levels, BUN, creatinine, and transaminases. Arterial blood gases and chest radiograph if respiratory symptoms are present. In severe cases central hemodynamic monitoring may be necessary. Cardiac consultation is recommended if symptoms are present.

2. **Toxin-specific analysis:** A therapeutic level in the serum is considered to be between 1.0 to 2.5 mcg/mL.

D. **Management**

1. **GI decontamination** with activated charcoal and gastric lavage should be undertaken. Multiple doses of activated charcoal, though not proved, may be useful because of the prolonged half-life of amiodarone.

2. **Treat hypotension and bradydysrhythmias** with conventional measures as for class 1a agents (see **X**).

3. **Hemodialysis or hemoperfusion** does not appear useful based on the kinetics of amiodarone.

E. **Disposition.** Hospitalize all patients with ingestion of a toxic amount or toxic plasma concentration. **Intensive care monitoring and cardiac consult** is required in any symptomatic patient with an overdose.

XX. **Bretylium**

A. **Properties of agent**

1. **Source and forms of toxin.** It is available as a 10-mL ampule

2. **Physical and clinical properties.** Bretylium tosylate is an antidysrhythmic useful for refractory ventricular tachydysrhythmias (163). It is currently administered i.v. or i.m., and studies are ongoing to determine oral efficacy.

3. **Mechanism of action and pathophysiology.** The exact mechanism of action is not known, but the drug causes prolongation of the refractory period by lengthening the action potential duration. No decrease in automaticity is noted in the Purkinje fibers, but a striking prolongation of the repolarization phase is found. Bretylium hyperpolarizes depressed fiber membrane and improves membrane responsiveness, which may explain the catecholamine release induced by the drug. There is also an increase in the threshold for ventricular fibrillation.

4. **Pharmacology and pharmacokinetics**

a. The optimal **therapeutic dose** schedule has not been determined because of a possible delay in the onset of action. The initial dose is 5 mg/kg as an i.v.

bolus. If unresponsive, the dose may be increased to 10 mg/kg at 15 to 30 min intervals up to a total dose of 30 mg/kg. For continuous infusion, dilute an ampule of bretylium (500 mg/10 mL) in 50 mL D5W or normal saline administered at 1 to 2 mg/min.

    b. **Kinetics** (Table 37-6). **Peak** plasma concentration occur approximately 1 h following IM injection (163). Only 12% to 37% is absorbed from the GI tract (164). Minimal binding to serum proteins is found, 15 to 6% (165). The V_d is 3.4 L/kg. Bretylium is not metabolized but is excreted almost unchanged in urine. The **half-life** is reported from 7 to 11 h.

    c. **Drug interactions:** Concomitant use of tricyclic antidepressants and bretylium has been reported to interfere with the therapeutic effects of this agent. Guanethidine has also been reported to interfere with the antidysrythmic effects of bretylium (165).

B. Clinical presentation

    1. **ECG effects** include decreased sinus rate and increased PR and QT intervals. Initially it may cause an increased heart rate (166). Hypotension is common.

    2. Rapid administration may cause **nausea and vomiting** (may be prevented by administering the drug over a longer than 8-min period).

    3. **Headache,** vertigo, dizziness, lightheadedness, syncope, and hyperthermia have been reported.

    4. **Parotitis** has been reported after chronic use.

C. Laboratory analysis of intoxication

    1. **General tests** (see **IX**)

    2. **Toxin-specific levels.** Not specified.

D. Management (see **X** and algorithm in Fig. 37-2)

E. Disposition. Hospitalize all patients who receive above the recommended dose. **Intensive care monitoring and cardiac consult** is required in any symptomatic patient with an overdose.

CLASS IV AGENTS

Calcium channel blocking agents reduce the influx of calcium ion into cardiac and vascular smooth muscle cells by blocking the slow calcium channel. They are used in the therapy of hypertension, dysrhythmias, angina, and peripheral vascular disease. Their toxicity and management are discussed in detail in Chapter 40.

CLASS V AGENTS

Digoxin, a cardiac glycoside, is widely used as a positive inotropic agent for treatment of congestive heart failure and for controlling rapid ventricular response to atrial fibrillation and flutter. Digitalis intoxication may occur after overdose or chronic therapy. This topic is discussed in detail in Chapter 42.

References

1. Hine LK, Gross TP, Kennedy DL. Outpatient antiarrhythmia drug use from 1970 through 1986. *Arch Intern Med* 1989;149:1524.

2. Litovitz TL, Felberg L, Soloway RA, et al. 1994 Annual report of the American Association of Poison Control Centers national data collection system. *Am J Emerg Med* 1995;13:551–597.

3. Vaughan-Williams EM. A classification of antidysrhythmic action reassessed after a decade of new drugs. *J Clin Pharmacol* 1984;24:129.

4. Rosen MR, Horodof AJ. Mechanism of arrhythmias. In: Roberts NK, Gelband H, eds. *Cardiac arrhythmias in neonate, infant, and child.* Norwalk, CT: Appleton-Century-Crofts, 1977:111.

5. Gelband H, Rosen MR. Pharmacologic basis for the treatment of cardiac arrhythmias. *Pediatrics* 1984;55:59.

6. Roden DM, Woosley RL. Class I antidysrhythmic agent quinidine, procainamide and *N*-acetylprocainamide, disopyramide. *Clin Pharmacol Ther* 1989;23:179.

7. Pickoff AS, Singh S, Gelband H. The medical management of cardiac arrhythmias. In: Roberts NK, Gelband H, eds. *Cardiac arrhythmias in the neonate infant and child.* Norwalk, CT: Appleton-Century-Crofts, 1983:1–200.

8. Mofenson HC, Caraccio TR, Schauben J. Poisoning by antidysrhythmic drugs. *Pediatr Clin North Am* 1986;33:725.

9. Karagueuzian HS, Singh BN, Mandel WJ. Antidysrhythmic drugs: mode of action, pharmacokinetic properties and clinical application. In: Mandel WJ, ed. *Cardiac arrhythmias: their mechanisms, diagnosis and management.* Philadelphia: JB Lippincott Co, 1987:697–737.

10. Covinsky JO, et al. Relative bioavailability of quinidine gluconate and quinidine sulfate in healthy volunteers. *J Clin Pharmacol* 1979;19:261.

11. Ueda CT, et al. Disposition kinetics of quinidine. *Clin Pharmacol Ther* 1976;19:30.

12. Kim SY, Benowitz NL. Poisoning due to class IA antidysrhythmic drugs quinidine, procainamide and disopyramide. *Drug Safety* 1990;5:393–420.

13. Qchs HR, Greenblatt DJ, Woo E. Clinical pharmacokinetics of quinidine. *Clin Pharmacokinet* 1980;5:150.

14. Kim Saal A, et al. Effects of amiodarone on serum quinidine and procainamide levels. *Am J Cardiol* 1984;53:1264.

15. Rizack MA, Hillman CD. Handbook of adverse drug interactions 1987. *Med Lett* 1987;1.

16. Trohman RG, et al. Increased quinidine pharmaconcentrations during administration of verapamil; a new quinidine-verapamil interaction. *Am J Cardiol* 1986;57:706.

17. Data JL, et al. Interaction of quinidine with anticonvulsant drugs. *N Engl J Med* 1976;294:699.

18. Bussey HI, et al. The influence of rifampin on quinidine and digoxin. *Arch Intern Med* 1984;144:1021.

19. Doering W. Digoxin-quinidine interaction: pharmacokinetics, underlying mechanism and clinical implications. *N Engl J Med* 1979;301:400.

20. Leahy EB, et al. The effect of quinidine and other oral antidysrhythmic drugs on serum digoxin. *Ann Intern Med* 1980;92:605.

21. Schmidt JL, et al. The effect of quinidine on the action of muscle relaxants. *JAMA* 1963;183:669.

22. Koch-Weser J. Quinidine induced hypoprothrombinemic hemorrhage in patients on chronic warfarin therapy. *Ann Intern Med* 1968;68:511.

23. Lughi RJ, Helwig J Jr, Conn HL Jr. Quinidine toxicity and its treatment. *Am Heart J* 1963;65:340.

24. Gaudreault P. Quinidine. *Clin Toxicol Re. 1982;4:1.*

25. Bateman DN, et al. Quinidine toxicity. *Adverse Drug React* 1986;4:215.

26. Deliocchio T, Pailli F, Testa O, et al. Accidental quinidine poisoning in two children. *Pediatrics* 1976;58:288–290.

27. Swlyn S, Kim SS. Quinidine-induced syncope. *Arch Intern Med* 1983;143:314–316.

28. Gratton-Smith TM, Gillis RJ, Kilham H. Quinidine poisoning in children. *Med J Aust* 1987;147:93–95.

29. Bland ME, Roper SM, Henry JA. Complications of quinine poisoning. *Lancet* 1985,1:384–385.

30. Wolf LR, Otten EJ, Spadafora MP. Cinchonism: two case reports and a review of acute quinine toxicity and treatment. *J Emerg Med* 1992;10:295–301.

31. Smilkstein MJ, Kulig KW, Rumack BH. Acute toxic blindness: unrecognized quinine poisoning. *Ann Emerg Med* 1987;16:98–101.

32. Freiman JP. Fatal quinine-induced thrombocytopenia. *Ann Emerg Med* 1990;112:308.

33. Bauman JL, Bauerfiend RA, Hoff JV, et al. Torsades de pointes due to quinidine: observations in 31 patients. *Am Heart J* 1984;107:425–430.

34. Tzivoni D, et al. Magnesium therapy for Torsades de pointes. *Circulation* 1988;77:392.

35. Piccone, et al. Magnesium infusion in treatment of Torsades de pointes. *Am Heart J* 1986;112:847.

36. Prescott LR, Hamilton AR, Heyworth R. Treatment of quinidine overdose with activated charcoal. *Br J Clin Pharmacol* 1989;27:95–97.

37. Haapanen EJ, Peliinen TJ. Hemoperfusion in quinidine intoxication. *Acta Med Scand* 1981;210:515–516.

38. Koch-Weser J. Pharmacokinetics of procainamide in man. *Ann NY Acad Sci* 1971;178:370.

39. Nguyen KP, Thomsen G, Liem B, et al. *N*-Acetylprocainamide, Torsades de pointes and hemodialysis. *Ann Intern Med* 1986;104:283.

40. Koch-Weser J. Serum proicainamide ievels as the therapeutic quide. *Clin Pharmacokinet* 1977;2:389–402.

41. Karisson E. Clinical pharmacokinetics of procainamide. *Clin Pharmacokinet* 1978;3:97–107.

42. Graffner C, Johnsson G, Sjogren J. Pharmacokinetics of procainamide intravenously and orally as conventional slow-release tablets. *Clin Pharmacol Ther* 1975;17:414.

43. Gibson TP, et al. Acetylation of procainamide in man and its relationship to isonicotinic acid hydrazide acetylation phenotype. *Clin Pharmacol Ther* 1975;17:395.
44. Jaillon P, Winkel RA. Electrophysiological comparative study of procainamide and *N*-acetylprocainamide in anesthetized drugs: concentration-response relationships. *Circulation* 1979;60:1385.
45. Christian CD Jr, et al. Cimetidine inhibits renal procainamide clearance. *Clin Pharmacol Ther* 1984;36:221.
46. Somogyi A, Bocher F. Ranitidine and procainamide absorption. *Br J Pharmacol* 1985;20:182.
47. Martin BK. Effects of ranitidine on procainamide disposition. *Br J Pharmacol* 1985;19:858.
48. Strasberg B, et al. Procainamide-induced polymorphous ventricular tachycardia. *Am J Cardiol* 1981;47:1309.
49. Stratmann HG, Walter KE, Kennedy HL. Torsades de pointes associated with elevated *N*-acetylprocainamide levels. *Am Heart J* 1986;109:375.
50. Connolly SJ. Procainamide toxicity and hemodialysis. *Clin Pharmacol Ther* 1982;7:206–220.
51. Blomgren SE, Coudemi JJ, Vaughan JH. Procainamide-induced lupus erythematosus: clinical and laboratory observations. *Am J Med* 1972;52:338.
52. Uetrect JP, Woosley RL. Acetylator phenotype and lupus erythematosus. *Clin Pharmacokinet* 1981;6:118.
53. Konttinen YP, Tuominen L. Reversible procainamide-induced agranulocytosis twice in one patient. *Lancet* 1971; 2:925.
54. Koch-Weser J. Disopyramide. *N Engl J Med* 1979;300:957.
55. Heel RC, et al. Disopyramide: a review of its pharmacological properties and therapeutic use in treating cardiac arrhythmias. *Drugs* 1978;15:331.
56. Hordof A, Mark J, Steeg C. Treatment of cardiac arrhythmia with disopyramide (Worpace). *Pediatr Res* 1981;15:405.
57. Garrett ER, Hingerling PH. Pharmacokinetics of disopyramide in healthy human subjects [Abstract]. *Clin Pharmacol Ther* 1975;17:234.
58. Willis PW. The clinical scope of disopyramide seven years after introduction—an overview. *Angiology* 1987;38:165.
59. Blonde J. Atenolol inhibits the elimination of disopyramide. *Eur J Clin Pharmacol* 1985;28:41.
60. Haworth E, and Burroughs A. Disopyramide and warfarin interaction. *BMJ* 1977;2:866.
61. Aitio ML, et al. The effect of enzyme induction on the metabolism of disopyramide in man. *Br J Clin Pharmacol* 1981;11:279.
62. O'Keefe B, et al. Cardiac consequences and treatment of disopyramide intoxication; experimental evaluation in dogs. *Cardiovasc Res* 1979;13:630.
63. Haler AM, Holt DW, O'Keefe B. Treatment of disopyramide overdosage. *Med J Aust* 1978;1:234.
64. Anonymous. Treatment of cardiac arrhythmias. *Med Lett* 1986;28:111.
65. Jaeger A, Sauder P, Tempe JD, et al. Intoxications aigues par le disopyramide. Etude multicentrique de 106 observations. *Nouv Presse Med* 1981;10:2883–2887.
66. Vanerio G, Maloney JD. Moricizine: pharmacodynamic, pharmacokinetic, and therapeutic profile of a new antidysrhythmic. *Cleve Clin J Med* 1992;59:79–86.
67. Woosley RL, Morganroth J, Fogoros RN, et al. Pharmacokinetics of moricizine HCl. *Am J Cardiol* 1987;60:35F–39F.
68. Pratt CM, Young JB, Francis MJ, et al. Comparative effect of disopyramide and ethmozine in suppressing complex ventricular arrhythmias by use of a double-blind, placebo-controlled, longitudinal crossover design. *Circulation* 1984;69:288–297.
69. Salerno DM. Review: antidysrhythmic drugs: 1987. Part III: class IC antidysrhythmic drugs—a review of their pharmacokinetics, electrophysiology, efficacy, and toxicity. *Electrophysiology* 1987;1:435–465.
70. Morganroth J, Pearlman AS, Dunkman WB, et al. Ethmozin: a new antiarrthmic agent developed in the U.S.S.R.: efficacy and tolerance. *Am Heart J* 1979;98:621–628.
71. *Drug facts and comparisons.* St. Louis: Facts and Comparisons. 1995:669–677.
72. Kar PM, et al. Combined high-efficiency hemodialysi and charcoal hemoperfusion in severe *N*-acetylprocainamide intoxication. *Am J Kidney Dis* 1992;20:403–406.
73. Benowitz NL, Meister W. Clinical pharmacokinetics of lignocaine. *Clin Pharmacokinet* 1978;3:177–201.
74. Finholt OA, Stirt JA, DiFazio, et al. Lidocaine pharmacokinetics in children during general anesthesia. *Anesth Analg* 1986;55:279–282.
75. Gonzolez del Rey J, Wason S, Druckenbrod RW. Lidocaine overdose: another preventable case? *Pediatr Emerg Med* 1994:10:344–346.
76. Feely J. Increased toxicity and reduced clearance of lidocaine by cimetidine. *Ann Intern Med* 1982;96:592.
77. Goolkasien DL. Displacement of lidocaine from serum alpha-1 acid glycoprotein binding sites by basic drugs. *Eur J Clin Pharmacol* 1983;25:413.
78. France E. A seizure induced by concurrent lidocaine-tocainide therapy—is it just a case of additive toxicity? *Drug Intell Clin Pharm* 1986;20:56.
79. Hess GP, et al. Seizures secondary to oral viscous lidocaine. *Ann Emerg Med* 1988;17:735.
80. Mofenson HC, et al. Lidocaine toxicity from topical mucosal application. *Clin Pediatr* 1983;22:190.

81. Noble J, Kennedy DJ, Latimer RD. Massive lignocaine overdose during cardiopulmonary bypass. Successful treatment with cardiac pacing. *Br J Anesth* 184;56:1439–1441.

82. Edgren B, Titelli J, Gehrz K. Intravenous lidocaine overdose in a child. *Clin Toxicol* 1986;24:51–58.

83. Amitai Y, et al. Death following accidental lidocaine in overdose in a child. *N Engl J Med* 1986;314:182.

84. Garrettson LK, McGee EB. Rapid onset of seizures following aspiration of viscous lidocaine. *J Toxicol Clin Toxicol* 1992;30:413–422.

85. Roden DM, Woosley RL. Drug therapy: tocainide. *N Engl J Med* 1986;315:41–45.

86. Kreeger RW, Hammil SC. New antidysrhythmic drugs: tocaimide, mexilative, flecainide, encainide and amiodarone. *Mayo Clin Proc* 1987;62:1033–1050.

87. Morganroth J, Nestico PF, Horowitz LN. A review of the use and limitiations of tocainide—a class 1 B antidysrhythmic agent. *Am Heart J* 1985;110:856–863.

88. Roden DM, Woosley RL. Drug therapy: tocainide. *N Engl J Med* 1986;315:41.

89. Kreeger RW, Hammil SC. New antidysrhythmic drugs: tocainamide, mexilative, flecainide, encainide and amiodarone. *Mayo Clin Proc* 1987;62:1033.

90. Morganroth J, Nestico PF, Horowitz LN. A review of the use and limitations of tocainide—a class IB antidysrhythmic agent. *Am Heart J* 1985;110:856.

91. Rubino M, Jackson E. Severe paranoia with concomitant tocainide and propranolol therapy. *Clin Pharm* 1982;1:177.

92. Nelson LS, Hoffman RS. Mexiletine overdose producing status epilepticus without cardiovascular abnormalities. *J Toxicol Clin Toxicol* 1994;32:731–736.

93. Frank SE, Snyder JT. Survival following severe overdose with mexiletine, nifedipine, and nitroglycerine. *Am J Emerg Med* 1991;9:43–46.

94. Woolsey RL, Wang T, Stone W, et al. Pharmacology, electrophysiology, and pharmacokinetics of mexiletine. *Am Heart J* 1984;107:1058–1063.

95. Mitchell BG, et al. Mexiletine disposition: individual variation in response to urine acidification and alkalinization. *Br J Clin Pharmacol* 1983;16:281.

96. Nelson LS, Hoffman RS. Mexiletine overdose producing status epilepticus without cardiovascular abnormalities. *J Toxicol Clin Toxicol* 1994;32:731–736.

97. Frank SE, Snyder JT. Survival following severe overdose with mexiletine, nifedipine, and nitroglycerine. *Am J Emerg Med* 1991;9:43–46.

98. Anderson IB, Olson KR. Fatal flecainide poisoning in an infant. *Vet Hum Toxicol* 1994;36:369.

99. Roden DM, Woosley RL. Drug therapy: flecainide. *N Engl J Med* 1986;315:36.

100. Holmes B, Heel RC. Flecainide: a preliminary review of its pharmacodynamic properties and therapeutic efficacy. *Drugs* 1985;29:1.

101. Koppel C, Oberdisse U, Munne G. Clinical course and outcome in class 1c antidysrhythmic overdose. *Clin Toxicol* 1990;28:433–444.

102. Samberg JC, Tepper D. Flecainide: a new antiarrythmic agent. *Am Heart J* 1986;112:808–813.

103. Till J, Holt D, Shinebourne EA, et al. Efficacy and pharmacokinetics of flecainide acetate in the treatment of supreventricular tachycardia in children. *J Am Coll Cardiol* 1987;9:129.

104. Gotz D, et al. Primary and secondary detoxification in severe flecainide intoxication. *Intensive Care Med* 1991;17:181–184.

105. Winkelmann BR, Leinberger H. Life-threatening flecainide toxicity: a pharmacodynamic approach. *Ann Intern Med* 1987:106:807–814.

106. Holmes B, Heel RC. Flecainide: a preliminary review of its pharmacodynamic properties and therapeutic efficacy. *Drugs* 1985;29:1–33.

107. Samberg JC, Tepper D. Flecainide: a new antidysrhythmic agent. *Am Heart J* 1986;112:808.

108. Mortensen ME, Bolon CE, Kelley MT, et al. Encainide overdose in an infant. *Ann Emerg Med* 1992;21:998–1001.

109. Cardiac Arrhythmic Suppressive (CAST) Trial investigators. Preliminary report: effect of encainide and flecainide on mortality in a randomized trial of arrhythmic suppression after myocardial infarction. *N Engl J Med* 1989;321:406–412.

110. Somberg JC, et al. Encainide: a new and potent arrhythmias. *Am J Med* 1986;114:826.

111. Gardner ML, Brett-Smith H, Batford WP. Treatment of encainide proarrhythmia with hypertonic saline. *PACE* 1990;13:1232–1235.

112. Soyka LF. Safety of encainide for the treatment of ventricular arrhythmias. *Am J Cardiol* 1986;58:96C–103C.

113. Pentel PR, et al. Effect of hypertonic sodium bicarbonate in encainide overdose. *Am J Cardiol* 1986;57:878.

114. Hartel G. Efficacy of oral propafenone in chronic ventricular arrhythmias: a placebo controlled cross-over exercise study. *Eur Heart J* 1985;6:123.

115. McHugh TP, Perina DG. Propafenone ingestion. *Ann Emerg Med* 1987;16:437.

116. Furet Y, et al. Intoxication mortelle par association propafenone-amitriptyline: a propos d'un cas [Abstract]. *J Toxicol Clin Exp* 1988;8:63.

117. Kates RE, Yee YG, Winkle RA. Metabolite accumulation during chronic propafenone dosing in arrhythmia. *Clin Pharmacol Ther* 1985;37:610–614.
118. Hodges M, Salerno D, Granrud G. Double-blind placebo-controlled evaluation of propafenone in suppressing ventricular ectopic activity. *Am J Cardiol* 1984;54:45D.
119. Kearns W, English B, Ford M. Propafenone overdose. *Ann Emerg Med* 1994;24:90–103.
120. Siddoway LA, Roden DM, Woosley RL. Clinical pharmacology of propafenone: pharmacokinetics, metabolism and concentration-response relationships. *Am J Cardiol* 1984;54:9D–12D.
121. Hodges M, Salerno D, Granrud G. Double-blind placebo-controlled evaluation of propafenone in suppressing ventricular ectopic activity. *Am J Cardiol* 1984;54:45D–50D.
122. Hohnloser SH, Woosley RJ. Sotalol. *N Engl J Med* 1994;331:31–38.
123. Frishman, Cavusoglu E. Sotalol: a new beta-adrenergic blocker for ventricular arrhythmias. *Prog Cardivasc Dis* 1995;37:423–440.
124. Dunnington CS. Sotalol hydrochloride (Betapace): a new antidysrhythmic drug. *Am J Crit Care* 1993;2:397–406.
125. Singh BN. Electrophysiologic basis for the antidysrhythmic actions of sotalol and comparison with other agents. *Am J Cardiol* 1993;72:8A–18A.
126. Antonaccio MJ, Gomoll A. Pharmacologic basis of the antidysrhythmic and hemodynamic effects of sotalol. *Am J Cardiol* 1993;72:27A–37A.
127. Dorian P, et al. Sotalol and type Ia drugs in combination prevent recurrence of sustained ventricular tachycardia. *J Am Coll Cardiol* 1993;22:106–113.
128. Adlerfliegel M, et al. Sotalol poisoning associated with asystole. *Intensive Care Med* 1993;19:57–58.
129. Kirschenbaum HL, Rosenberg JM. Clinical experience with sotalol in the treatment of cardiac arrhythmias. *Clin Ther* 1994;16:346–364.
130. Heath A. β-Adrenergic blocker toxicity. Clinical features and therapy. *Am J Emerg Med* 1985;2:518.
131. Taboulet P, Cariou A, Berdeaux A, et al. Pathophysiology and management of self poisoning with beta-blockers. *Clin Toxicol* 1993;31:531–551.
132. Kenyon CJ, Aldinger GE, Joshipura P, et al. Successful resuscitation using external cardiac pacing in beta-adrenergic antagonist-induced brady-asystolic arrest. *Ann Emerg Med* 1988;17:711–713.
133. Lewis RV, McDevitt DG. Adverse reactions and interactions with β-adrenergic blocking drugs. *Med Toxicol* 1986;1:343–361.
134. Lane AS, Woodward AC, Goldman MR. Massive propranolol overdose poorly responsive to pharmacologic therapy. *Ann Emerg Med* 1987;16:1381–1383.
135. Du Souich P, Caille G, Larcchelle P. Enhancement of nadolol elimination by activated charcoal and antibiotics. *Clin Pharmacol Ther* 1983;33:585–590.
136. Takahashi H, Ohashi N, Motokawa K, et al. Poisoning by combine ingestion of nefidipine and metoproterolol. *Clin Toxicol* 1993;31:631–637.
137. Karkkaimen S, Neuvonen PJ. Effect of oral activated charcoal and urine pH on satolol pharmacokinetics. *Int Clin Pharmacol Ther* 1984;22:441–446.
138. Weinstein RS. Recognition and management of poisoning with beta-adrenergic blocking agents. *Ann Emerg Med* 1984;13:1123–1131.
139. Soni N, Baines D, Pearson IY. Cardiovascular collapse and propranolol. *Med J Australia* 1983;2:629–630.
140. Kerns W II, Kline J, Ford M. β-Blocker and calcium channel blocker toxicity. *Emerg Clin North Am* 1994;12:365–390.
141. Aqua ED, Wexler LF, Witzburg RS. Massive propranolol overdose: treatment with high dose isoproterenol and glucagon. *Am J Med* 1986;80:755–757.
142. Lagerfelt J, Matell G. Attempted suicide with 5.1 g of propranolol, a case report. *Acta Med Scand* 1979;199:517–518.
143. Mofenson HC, Caraccio TR. Glucagon for propranolol overdose. *JAMA* 1986;255:2025.
144. Henry MA, Kay MM, Vicellio P. Cardiogenic shock associated with calcium channel blockers and beta-blockers. Reversal with intravenous calcium chloride. *Am J Emerg Med* 1985;3:334.
145. Sugg MF, Latham RD, Bruce JE, et al. Potentiation of glucagon by theophylline in intact canine model with complete beta adrenoreceptor blockade by propranolol. *Ann Emerg Med* 1987;16:482.
146. Kollef MH. Labetalol overdose successfully treated with amrine and alpha-adrenergic receptor agonists. *Chest* 1994;105:626–627.
147. Honsloser SH, Woosley RL. Sotalol. *N Engl J Med* 1994;331:31–38.
148. Sung RJ, et al. Intravenous sotalol for the termination of supraventricular tachycardia and atrial fibrillation and flutter: a multicenter, randomized, double-blind, placebo controlled study. *Am Heart J* 1995;129:739–738.
149. Cui G, et al. Effects of amiodarone, sematilide, and sotalol on QT dispersion. *Am J Cardiol* 1994;74:896–900.
150. Mason JW. Amiodarone. *N Engl J Med* 1987;316:455.
151. Lim PK, et al. Neuropathy and fatal hepatitis in a patient receiving amiodarone. *BMJ* 1984;288:1638.
152. Bonati M, et al. Acute overdosage of amiodarone in a suicide attempt. *Clin Toxicol* 1983;20:181.

153. Oreto G, et al. Intoxication aigue par l'amiodarone. *Arch Mal Coeur* 1980;73:857.
154. Pourbaix S, et al. Absolute bioavailability of amiodarone in normal subjects. *Clin Pharmacol Ther* 1985;37:118.
155. Latini R, Tognoni G, Kates RE. Clinical pharmacokinetics of amiodarone. *Clin Pharmacokinet* 1984;9:136.
156. Podrid PJ. Amiodarone: re-evaluation of an old drug. *Ann Intern Med* 1995;122:689–700.
157. Kingele TG, Alves LE, Rose EP. Amiodarone keratopathy. *Ann Ophthalmol* 1984;16:1171.
158. Marchlinski FE, et al. Amiodarone pulmonary toxicity. *Am J Med* 1982;97:837.
159. Dusman RE, Stanton MS, Miles WM, et al. Clinical features of amiodarone induced pulmonary toxicity. *Circulation* 1990;82:51.
160. Rubin A, McAllister A, Sorbera C, et al. Subacute pulmonary toxicity from amiodarone. *NYS J Med* 1991;91: 4403–4405.
161. Mazonson PD, et al. Myxedema coma during long-term amiodarone therapy. *Am J Med* 1984;77:751.
162. Simon JB, et al. Amiodarone hepatotoxicity simulating alcoholic liver disease. *N Engl J Med* 1984;311:167.
169. Trimble JW, Mendelson DS, Fetter BF, et al. Cutaneous pigmentation secondary to amiodarone therapy. *Arch Dermatol* 1983;119:914–918.
163. Romhilt DW, et al. Bretylium tosylate for treatment of premature ventricular contractions. *Clin Pharmacol Ther* 1972; 13:151.
164. Cooper JA, Frieden J. Bretylium tosylate. *Am Heart J* 1971;82:703.
165. Rapeport WG. Clinical pharmacokinetics of bretylium. *Clin Pharmacokinet* 1985;10:248.
166. Bacaner MB. Treatment of ventricular fibrillation and other acute arrhythmias with bretylium tosylate. *Am J Cardiol* 1968;21:530.
167. Roden DM. Risks and benefits of antidysrhythmic therapy. *N Engl J Med* 1994;331:785–791.
168. Katz AM. Cardiac ion channels. *N Engl J Med* 1993;326:1244–1250.
169. Mofenson HC, Caraccio TR. Poisoning by antidysrhythmic drugs. In: Viccellio P, ed. *Handbook of medical toxicology*. Boston: Little, Brown, and Company, 1993.

Emergency Toxicology, Second Edition,
edited by Peter Viccellio.
Lippincott–Raven Publishers, Philadelphia © 1998.

38

Angiotensin Converting Enzyme Inhibitors

Kimberle F. Capes

Lifespan Poison Center, Rhode Island Hospital, Providence, Rhode Island 02903

I. Introduction

    A. Angiotensin-converting enzyme inhibitors (ACEIs) are used in the management of hypertension and congestive heart failure, and have been shown to decrease postmyocardial infarction mortality. Also, ACEIs have been used to prevent worsening of microalbuminuria in diabetic nephropathy. Although several potentially severe side effects have been seen with therapeutic doses, these agents are not widely reported in acute overdose. The most frequently occurring clinical effect in the overdose setting is hypotension.

II. Available sources

    A. ACEI products currently available in the United States are benazepril (Lotensin), captopril (Capoten), enalapril oral and enalaprilat i.v. (Vasotec), fosinopril (Monopril), lisinopril (Prinivil, Zestril), moexipril (Univasc), quinapril (Accupril), and ramipril (Altace).

III. Pharmacology and properties of agent

    A. Mechanisms of action and toxicity

        1. Therapeutic

            a. These agents are valuable in hypertension and heart failure for their actions on the reduction of both preload and afterload. Total peripheral resistance is decreased by the specific inhibition of peptidyldipeptide carboxyhydrolase (kininase II), the enzyme which converts angiotensin I to angiotensin II, a potent vasoconstrictor. The blockade of angiotensin II also inhibits aldosterone release, resulting in fluid volume reduction and a potential increase in serum potassium.

        2. Toxicologic

            a. Some toxic effects of ACEIs are **exacerbations of their therapeutic effects,** such as hypotension. This is also true when decreases in arterial blood pressure and glomerular filtration precipitate acute renal failure in patients with bilateral renal artery stenosis or renal artery stenosis in a solitary kidney (1).

            b. Toxic effects of ACEIs may be attributed to their **effects on the bradykinin-prostaglandin system** in addition to those related to the **renin-angiotensin-aldosterone system.** Chronic dry cough may affect as many as one-third of patients taking ACEIs. The mechanism of this effect probably involves airway accumulation of prostaglandins, bradykinin, or substance P, which normally are degraded by angiotensin converting enzyme. This is not an acute toxic effect, but it may be seen in the ED, and early consideration of this etiology and recognition of its relationship to current drug therapy may prevent unnecessary diagnostic testing (2,3).

    c.   The mechanism of ACEI-induced **angioedema** may involve autoantibodies, bradykinin, or complement-system components. It is currently **believed to be due to inhibition of bradykinin breakdown.**

B. Pharmacokinetics

    1.   **Absorption** is rapid and the onset of therapeutic action is within 1 h for all agents, with peak serum levels at up to 8 h. The absorption of some products is diminished by the presence of food in the stomach or concomitant administration of antacids.

    2.   Benazepril, fosinopril, and quinapril are highly (more than 95%) bound to plasma protein. Captopril, moexipril, and ramipril undergo protein binding to a lesser degree.

    3.   With the exceptions of lisinopril and enalaprilat which are excreted unchanged in the urine, all ACEIs undergo hepatic metabolism to some extent and are excreted in both urine and feces.

    4.   In patients with normal renal function, the half-life of a therapeutic dose of captopril, unchanged enalapril, or quinapril is less than or equal to 2 h; metabolites may extend the actual duration of effects, and half-lives may be increased in overdose. Half-lives for the other agents in this class range from 10 to 15 h. Impaired renal function results in prolonged half-lives for all ACEIs (4).

C. Pertinent drug-drug interactions

    1.   Concurrent administration of ACEIs with **potassium supplements** or potassium-sparing diuretics may result in **hyperkalemia.** ACEIs may **increase plasma digoxin** levels and **serum lithium** levels, resulting in toxic symptoms of these drugs. Additive hypotensive effects can be seen when ACEIs are combined with diuretics and other antihypertensive drugs, and with phenothiazine antipsychotic agents.

    2.   Generally, nonsteroidal antiinflammatory drugs (NSAIDs) decrease the hemodynamic effectiveness of ACEIs by interfering with prostaglandin synthesis. Ketorolac has been reported to cause renal impairment in patients on ACEIs. The combination of ACEIs and cyclosporine also has resulted in decreased renal function.

IV. Clinical presentation

    A.   Patients with underlying congestive heart failure, volume depletion, chronic renal failure, hyperkalemia, or those with mixed ingestions are at greater risk of significant toxicity in ACEI overdose.

    B.   The only acute overdose symptom with ACEIs is **hypotension,** which **should be apparent within 1 h of ingestion.** The peak effect occurs in 1 (captopril) to 6 (lisinopril) h, depending on the pharmacokinetics of the individual product. The duration of effect is likely to be prolonged in overdose. Electrolyte disorders, including hyperkalemia, and renal failure also may be precipitated by ACEI overdose.

    C.   **Angioedema,** a vascular reaction resulting in edema of the face, lips, tongue, and glottis has been reported with ACEIs at a low incidence (0.1 to 0.2 %), but the sequelae may be severe, at times progressing to respiratory distress and death. This reaction can occur at any time in the course of therapy—usually within the first week, but it has been reported years after the initiation of drug therapy. If the etiology is unrecognized, the patient may continue on the drug, with repeat occurrences of life-threatening symptoms. Oropharyngeal swelling may prevent the procurement of an accurate and complete history from the patient.

D. The **differential diagnosis** for acute ACEI overdose includes the ingestion of other drugs which may cause hypotension:

1. Antihypertensive agents—diuretics, beta-adrenergic blockers, calcium channel blockers, vasodilators (e.g., nitrates)
2. Antidysrhythmic agents
3. Psychiatric drugs—cyclic antidepressants, phenothiazines, lithium, monoamine oxidase inhibitors
4. Central nervous system depressants—barbiturates, opioids, chloral hydrate, ethchlorvynol
5. Disulfiram combined with ethanol

E. It should be noted that, while not an acute toxic occurrence, ACEIs have been shown to cause **severe fetal abnormalities** when administered to pregnant women during the second and third trimesters.

V. **Laboratory findings**

A. **Electrolytes and BUN/creatinine** should be measured on presentation and serially as needed if symptoms occur. Renal function may be affected even with therapeutic use. Hyperkalemia may occur due to decreased aldosterone secretion.

B. **Hypoglycemia** requiring hospital admission has been reported in patients with diabetes mellitus (insulin-dependent or on oral antihyperglycemics) concurrently prescribed ACEIs. These drugs may affect insulin sensitivity or glucose metabolism, but no conclusive mechanism has been shown. It is possible that this effect is a result of the increased use of ACEIs in diabetic patients with hypertension, congestive heart failure, or proteinuria, at a time when tight glucose control is also encouraged (5).

C. ACEI **levels** have been measured, but **do not correlate** with the toxic effects of these drugs. A wide range of levels have been reported in symptomatic overdose patients.

VI. **Management**

A. **General**

1. **Accidental ingestion:** Although not studied prospectively, it has been suggested that children under 6 years old with a confirmed history of ingestion of the usual adult therapeutic dose, or less, may be managed at home with telephone follow-up for 4 to 6 h (6).

2. For **intentional ingestion** of large or unknown quantities
   a. **Gastrointestinal decontamination**—gastric lavage for early presentation; oral activated charcoal and cathartic—use saline cathartics with caution in patients with renal dysfunction.
   b. Basic **supportive measures** and stabilization of hemodynamic parameters. Treat hypotension with i.v. normal saline boluses (avoid Lactated Ringer's due to potassium content), and place patient in the Trendelenberg position. If vasopressors are necessary, dopamine 2 to 5 mcg/kg/min is the drug of first

choice, and then norepinephrine 0.1 to 0.2 mcg/kg/min, titrated to effect. ECG monitoring is recommended for patients with chest pain or hypotension.

B. **Specific**

   1. **Angiotensin infusion** (available as angiotensin amide, Hypertensin) has reversed hypotension in overdoses of enalapril and lisinopril where fluids and traditional vasopressor agents failed. In the first case, doses ranging from 3 to 18 mcg/min were used; in the second, 9 mcg/min was effective (7,8). To prepare the infusion, product information from the manufacturer recommends adding 2.5 mg (contents of one vial) to 500 mL physiologic saline or glucose solution. Begin i.v. administration at 0.5 mL/min, and increase gradually to achieve the desired blood pressure effect. Due to the potential for hypertension and cardiac arrhythmias, vital signs and ECG should be monitored continuously during infusion.

   2. **Naloxone** has been shown in animal studies and reported in some human cases to block the antihypertensive effects of captopril. Increased vasopressor response may be mediated by the inhibitory effect of naloxone on endogenous opioids which inhibit angiotensin II (9,10). In one overdose, naloxone was ineffective for this purpose (9). Effective reversal has been reported at doses of 1.6 to 2 mg. If a favorable response is obtained, continuous i.v. infusions in the concentrations used for reversal of narcotic toxicity (0.4 mg/h) may be useful to avoid repeat bolus doses, though these infusions have not been studied in ACEI overdoses (10).

   3. Treatment of **angioedema** includes airway protection and administration of epinephrine, antihistamines (e.g., diphenhydramine, cimetidine), and corticosteroids. However, because the reaction is unlikely to be IgE-mediated, drug therapies may be ineffective, and emergency surgical intervention may be required. Oral antihistamines and corticosteroids should be continued for several days after the acute reaction, and the antihypertensive therapy changed to another class of agents. ACEIs should never be resumed in a patient who has had an episode of related angioedema (2,11,12).

C. **Enhanced elimination**

   1. Hemodialysis would be expected to enhance removal of ACEIs from the body, but its use for this purpose has not been reported.

VII. **Disposition**

   A. Vital signs of overdose patients should be monitored for 6 to 8 h. If related signs or symptoms occur, such as hypotension or changes in laboratory values, the patient is to be admitted. Patients with cardiac manifestations warrant a cardiac monitored bed.

References

1. Kamper AL. Angiotensin converting enzyme inhibitors and renal function. *Drug Safety* 1991;6:361–370.
2. Israili ZH, Hall WD. Cough and angioneurotic edema associated with angiotensin-converting enzyme inhibitor therapy—a review of the literature and pathophysiology. *Ann Intern Med* 1992;117:234–242.
3. Simon SR, Black HR, Moser M, et al. Cough and ACE inhibitors. *Arch Intern Med* 1992;152:1698–1700.
4. Varughese A, Taylor AA, Nelson EB. Consequences of angiotensin-converting enzyme inhibitor overdose. *Am J Hypertens* 1989;2:355–357.
5. Herings RMC, deBoer A, Stricker BHC, et al. Hypoglycaemia associated with use of inhibitors of angiotensin converting enzyme. *Lancet* 1995;345:1195–1198.

6. Spiller HA, Udicious TM, Muir S. Angiotensin converting enzyme inhibitor ingestion in children. *Clin Toxicol* 1989;27:345–353.
7. Jackson T, Corke C, Agar J. Enalapril overdose treated with angiotensin infusion. *Lancet* 1993;341:703.
8. Trilli LE, Johnson KA. Lisinopril overdose and management with intravenous angiotensin II. *Ann Pharmacother* 1994;28:1165–1167.
9. Barr CS, Payne R, Newton RW. Profound prolonged hypotension following captopril overdose. *Postgrad Med J* 1991;67;953–954.
10. Varon J, Duncan SR. Naloxone reversal of hypotension due to captopril overdose. *Ann Emerg Med* 1991;20:1125–1127.
11. Finley CJ, Silverman MA, Nunez AE. Angiotensin-converting enzyme inhibitor-induced angioedema: still unrecognized. *Am J Emerg Med* 1992;10:550–552.
12. Thompson T, Frable MAS. Drug-induced, life-threatening angioedema revisited. *Laryngoscope* 1993;103:10–12.

Emergency Toxicology, Second Edition,
edited by Peter Viccellio.
Lippincott–Raven Publishers, Philadelphia © 1998.

39

Beta-Blockers

*Mark C. Henry, *Peter Viccellio, and †Jason Yuan

*Department of Emergency Medicine, State University of New York at Stony Brook,
Stony Brook, New York 11794-7400; †West Orange, New Jersey 07052*

I. Pharmacology

A. Competitive inhibitors of beta-adrenergic receptors. Beta-blockers competitively inhibit the beta-adrenergic receptors. Through review of the adrenergic nervous system, the effects of beta-blockers and the signs and symptoms of beta-blocker overdose can be anticipated.

1. **Adrenergic receptors.** Catecholamines stimulate alpha- and beta-receptor sites within the adrenergic nervous system. A review of the responses of selected effector organs to autonomic nerve impulses is shown in Table 39-1. The beta-receptors are further broken down to beta-1 (mostly in the myocardium) and beta-2 (in smooth muscle and sites outside the myocardium).

2. **Beta-1 receptors.** Beta-1 receptors stimulate the heart and increase contractility, automaticity, and conduction velocity. Beta-blockers decrease all of the above, and in excess lead to bradycardia, hypotension, and heart block. The hypotension appears more due to depressed inotropy than decreased chronotropy.

3. **Beta-2 receptors.** Stimulation of beta-2 receptors has widespread effects; including relaxation of bronchial and other smooth muscle, increased contractility of skeletal muscle, and glycogenolysis and gluconeogenesis. Blocking beta-2 receptors can lead to bronchoconstriction, increased motility and tone of the GI tract, and blunting of the "fight or flight" response seen with stress and exercise.

4. **Alpha receptors** have some opposing effects to the beta receptors, including vascular smooth muscle contraction, and contraction of genitourinary smooth muscle. Epinephrine and norepinephrine stimulate both alpha and beta receptors. In the setting of beta-blockers, catecholamine release may manifest with a predominant alpha stimulation picture, which is seen in settings such as pheochromocytoma or cocaine overdose, where use of a beta-blocker can result in unopposed alpha stimulation and intense vasoconstriction. Alternatively, the presence of beta-blockers can blunt the classic fight or flight reaction noted by the increased heart rate and blood pressure, redistribution of blood flow from gut and skin to the skeletal muscles, increase in glucose, and dilation of bronchioles and pupils.

B. Available agents. Beta-blockers are classified according to several properties, including selectivity, intrinsic stimulatory activity, lipid solubility, preparation duration, and other pharmacologic properties.

TABLE 39-1. *Responses of selected effector organs to autonomic nerve impulses*

| Effector organs | Adrenergic impulses | | Cholinergic impulses |
	Receptor type	Responses[a]	Responses[a]
Eye			
Radial muscle, iris	α_1	Contraction (mydriasis) ++	—
Sphincter muscle, iris	—	—	Contraction (miosis) +++
Ciliary muscle	β_2	Relaxation for far vision +	Contraction for near vision +++
Heart[b]			
SA node	β_1	Increase in heart rate ++	Decrease in heart rate; vagal arrest +++
Atria	β_1	Increase in contractility and conduction velocity ++	Decrease in contractility, and shortened AP duration ++
AV node	β_1	Increase in automaticity and conduction velocity ++	Decrease in conduction velocity; AV block +++
His-Purkinje system	β_1	Increase in automaticity and conduction velocity +++	Little effect
Ventricles	β_1	Increase in contractility and conduction velocity, automaticity, and rate of idioventricularpacemakers +++	Slight decrease in contractility claimed by some
Arterioles			
Coronary	$\alpha_1, \alpha_2; \beta_2$	Constriction +; dilatation[c] ++	Constriction +
Skin and mucosa	α_1, α_2	Constriction +++	Dilatation[d]
Skeletal muscle	$\alpha; \beta_2$	Constriction ++; dilatation[c,e] ++	Dilatation[f] +
Cerebral	α_1	Constriction (slight)	Dilatation[d]
Pulmonary	$\alpha_1; \beta_2$	Constriction +; dilatation[c]	Dilatation[d]
Abdominal viscera	$\alpha_1; \beta_2$	Constriction +++; dilatation[e] +	—
Salivary glands	$\alpha_1; \alpha_2$	Constriction +++	Dilatation ++
Renal	$\alpha_1, \alpha_2; \beta_1, \beta_2$	Constriction +++; dilatation[c] +	—
Veins (systemic)	$\alpha_1; \beta_2$	Constriction ++; dilatation ++	—
Lung			
Tracheal and bronchial muscle	β_2	Relaxation +	Contraction ++
Bronchial glands	$\alpha_1; \beta_2$	Decreased secretion; increased secretion	Stimulation +++
Kidney			
Renin secretion	$\alpha_1; \beta_1$	Decrease +; increase ++	—
Urinary Bladder			
Detrusor	β_2	Relaxation (usually) +	Contraction +++
Trigone and sphincter	α_1	Contraction ++	Relaxation ++
Skin			
Pilomotor muscles	α_1	Contraction ++	—
Sweat glands	α_1	Localized secretion[g] +	Generalized secretion +++
Adrenal Medulla		—	Secretion of epinephrine and norepinephrine (nicotinic effect)
Skeletal Muscle	β_2	Increased contractility; glycogenolysis; K^+ update	—
Liver	$\alpha; \beta_2$	Glycogenolysis and gluconeogenesis +++	—
Pancreas			
Acini	α	Decreased secretion +	Secretion ++
Islets (β cells)	α_2	Decreased secretion +++	—
	β_2	Increased secretion +	—

1. **Selectivity.** Some agents are nonselective; that is, they have equal affinity for both beta-1 and beta-2 sites. Propranolol is the classic example of the "nonselective" beta-blocker. Other beta-blockers show a greater affinity for the beta-1 sites (e.g., metoprolol, atenolol), and these agents are used when the main goal is to blunt cardiac adrenergic stimulation. Beta-1 blockers are also preferable for patients with asthma or other bronchospastic disorders as well as diabetics. The selectivity is relative, not absolute. Some beta-blockers (i.e., labetalol) also show some alpha-1 blocking activity.

2. **Intrinsic stimulatory activity.** Some beta-blockers (e.g., pindolol) have both beta-blocking and intrinsic sympathomimetic activity. The agonist effect is thought to be useful for certain individuals who are prone to bradycardia.

3. **Lipid solubility.** Some agents (e.g., propranolol, alprenolol, oxprenolol) have a relatively high lipid solubility. Such agents are more likely to have CNS effects and to be less amenable to dialysis in the overdose situation. On the other hand, atenolol, sotalol, and nadolol have relatively low lipid solubility and may be more effectively removed by dialysis.

4. **Preparation duration.** Some beta-blocker preparations have longer half-lives (Table 39-2). Additionally, certain agents are being marketed in long-acting sustained-release forms (e.g., metoprolol-SR, propranolol-SR). Ingestion of such long-acting preparations will require additional treatment measures.

5. **Other pharmacologic properties.** Some agents show membrane-stabilizing or quinidine-like class I antiarrhythmic effects in high doses. They include propranolol, labetalol, and pindolol. Sotalol in high doses exhibits class III antiarrhythmic activity with prolongation of the action potential and refractory period. All beta-adrenergic receptors stimulate adenyl cyclase and lead to an accumulation of intracellular cyclic AMP. Table 39-2 reviews some beta-blockers and their characteristics.

6. Beta-blockers are commonly **prescribed** for hypertension, angina, ischemic heart disease, cardiac dysrhythmias, migraine headaches, and as eyedrops for the control of glaucoma.

7. Beta-blockers can be given i.v., orally, and as ophthalmic preparations. Timolol eyedrops have caused systemic toxicity and side effects including bronchospasm, congestive heart failure, and respiratory arrest.

---

[a]Responses are designated + to +++ to provide an approximate indication of the importance of adrenergic and cholinergic nerve activity in the control of the various organs and functions listed.
[b]Heart also contains α_1 and β_2 receptors, but they are less important for physiologic responses.
[c]Dilatation predominates in situ due to metabolic autoregulatory phenomena.
[d]Cholinergic vasodilatation at these sites is of questionable physiologic significance.
[e]Over the usual concentration ranges of physiologically released, circulating epinephrine, β-receptor response (vasodilatation) predominates in blood vessels of skeletal muscle and liver: α-receptor response (vasoconstriction), in blood vessels of other abdominal viscera. The renal and mesenteric vessels also contain specific dopaminergic receptors, activation of which causes dilatation.
[f]Sympathetic cholinergic system causes vasodilatation in skeletal muscle, but this is not involved in most physiologic responses.
[g]Palms of hands and some other sites ("adrenergic sweating").
Source: Adapted from BB Hoffman, RJ Lefkowitz, and P Taylor. Neurohumoral Transmission: The Autonomic and Somatic Motor Nervous Systems. In AG Gilman, et al, *Goodman and Gilman's The Pharmacologic Basis of Therapeutics* (8th ed). New York: Pergamon Press, 1990. Pp. 89–90.

TABLE 39-2. *Pharmacologic characteristics of selected β-adrenergic antagonists*

Compound	Intrinsic sympathomimetic activity	Membrane-stabilizing activity	Lipid solubility (LOG Kp)[a]	Oral bioavailability (%)	Half-life in plasma (hours)[b]
Nonselective β- (β + β₂) adrenergic antagonists					
Propranolol	0	++	3.65	~25	3–5
Nadolol	0	0	0.7	~35	10–20
Timolol	0	0	2.1	~50	3–5
Pindolol	++	±	1.75	~75	3–4
Labetalol[c]	—	±	—	~20	4–6
Selective β₁-adrenergic antagonists					
Metoprolol	0	±	2.15	~40	3–4
Atenolol	0	0	0.23	~50	5–8
Esmolol	0	0	—	—	0.13
Acebutolol	+	+	1.9	~40	2–4

[a]Kp refers to the octanol: water partition coefficient; propranolol and stenolol are at the lipophilic extremes, respectively.

[b]The duration of effect, in general, is longer than might be expected from the plasma.

[c]Labetalol is also a potent α₁-adrenergic antagonist

Source: From BB Hoffman, and RJ Lefkowitz. Adrenergic Receptor Antagonists. In AG Gilman, et al, *Goodman and Gilman's The Pharmacologic Basis of Therapeutics* (8th ed). New York: Pergamon Press, 1990. p. 234. With permission from McGraw-Hill.

II. Clinical presentation

A. **Cardiac effects.** Bradycardia, AV block, and hypotension are classic findings in overdose situations. The initial ECG may show evidence of conduction disturbances including sinus bradycardia, first-degree block, widening of the QRS complex, peaked T-waves, and ST changes. Bradydysrhythmias are usually low junctional or ventricular. This can rapidly progress to complete heart block and asystole. Tachycardia has been reported with agents having intrinsic sympathomimetic activity but is an unusual finding. Usually it is the combination of bradycardia and decreased contractility that leads to decreased cardiac output and hypotension. Elderly patients or those with limited cardiac reserve will usually manifest hypotension earlier and often without significant bradycardia. Sotalol with its class III antiarrhythmic activity can cause prolongation of the QT interval with ventricular premature beats, ventricular tachycardia, Torsades de pointes, ventricular fibrillation, and asystole.

B. **Neurologic effects.** One can see altered mental status, from delirium to coma. Seizure activity has been reported. These effects are more likely to be seen if the drug has a high lipid solubility. Seizures are often preceded by cardiac conduction disturbances, and in most cases may be secondary to hypoperfusion associated with hypotension and bradycardia.

C. **Pulmonary effects.** Bronchospasm, although it can occur, is not usually seen.

D. **Unstable diabetics** may have hypoglycemic reactions. With an overdose, children have been hypoglycemic. The reflex tachycardia accompanying hypoglycemia is often absent.

E. **Renal and hepatic** dysfunction can occur secondary to decreased perfusion. Urinary output may be decreased.

F. Beta-blockers are rapidly absorbed from the stomach. Toxicity after oral overdose can occur within 20 min of ingestion.

III. **Laboratory evaluation.** Qualitative and quantitative levels of beta-blockers are not readily available to guide initial treatment. Therefore indirect measures of beta-blocker effects are sought through the ECG, cardiac monitoring, blood levels of electrolytes and glucose, and tests for renal and liver function. Radiographic studies for evidence of ingestion of sustained-release preparations may also be helpful. The minimum range of toxicity has not been clearly established. Co-ingestions, especially with calcium channel blockers, have led to toxicity with documented therapeutic levels of both drugs.

IV. **Treatment**

A. **General measures. Supportive care** is the focus of treatment. In severe beta-blocker intoxications, early **mechanical ventilation** at the first signs of airway or breathing compromise may improve prognosis. Consider pretreatment with **atropine** before intubation. Because of the rapidity of gastrointestinal absorption and abrupt appearance of cardiovascular symptoms, **gastric lavage** is preferred over emesis. Emesis should generally be avoided. Some experts advocate the use of **atropine** before gastric lavage to prevent increased vagal tone aggravating depression of the heart. **Charcoal** should be given as well as **cathartics,** with repeat doses of charcoal in the setting of atenolol, sotalol, and nadolol. Multiple-dose activated **charcoal and whole bowel irrigation (WBI)** have both been used in symptomatic ingestion of long-acting sustained-release preparations. The superiority of either, or combination of both, has not been established, although WBI is preferred by many specialists in the treatment of ingestion of long-acting preparations. **Polyethylene glycol-electrolyte lavage solution (PEG-ELS)** should be given for WBI in a dose of 1 to 2 L/h p.o./NGT to an endpoint of (1) progression of KUB findings (if initially present) demonstrating elimination of pills, (2) clinical resolution, or (3) the rectal effluent appears the same as the administered PEG-ELS solution. More recent data suggests that the appearance of clear rectal effluent may not serve as an indicator of bowel decontamination; however, the necessary dose beyond this point has not been established. Indications for use of PEG-ELS for asymptomatic ingestion of sustained-release preparations have not yet been established, but again is recommended by many toxicologists.

B. **Specific and antidotal measures.**

1. To counteract the **cardiac effects** of beta-blockade, remedies include atropine, catecholamines, and glucagon. It is usually the cardiac effects of beta-blocker overdose that cause death. The main focus is on treating the bradycardia and hypotension. **Bronchospasm,** if present, can be treated with a beta-2 aerosol and aminophylline if needed.

   a. **Glucagon,** which increases myocardial cyclic AMP and therefore cardiac inotropy and chronotropy by mechanisms not dependent on beta receptors, **is a first-line drug** for both **bradycardia and hypotension** due to beta-blocker overdose. Its onset of action should be within 10 min with a duration of 15 to 30 min, and dosages are higher than in other clinical settings. It may be given at an initial bolus dose of 3 to 10 mg i.v. Repeat boluses may be administered at a dose of 5 mg every 15 to 30 min or an i.v. infusion started at a rate of

1 to 5 mg/h and titrated up to 10 mg/h for severe ingestions. The glucagon should be reconstituted in normal saline, sterile water, or D5W instead of the standard phenol diluent provided by the manufacturer due to the high doses. Glucagon enhances myocardial contractility, heart rate, and atrioventricular (AV) conduction. Deaths have occurred from failure to stock adequate doses of glucagon for treatment of beta-blocker overdose. In serious ingestions, a total of 30 mg or more of glucagon may be needed.

b. For **symptomatic bradycardia,** the initial treatment is to give **atropine** at an initial dose of 0.5 mg i.v. to adults followed by repeat doses up to a cumulative dose of 3.0 mg. The efficacy of atropine in the treatment of bradycardia appears limited to mild beta-blocker intoxications, with about 25% of patients responding.

c. For bradycardia unresponsive to atropine and glucagon, **isoproterenol** may be given by drip at a rate of 2 to 20 mcg/min to counteract the beta-blocker effect on the heart rate. Although theoretically isoproterenol would appear to be the perfect antidote for beta-blocker toxicity, its clinical effectiveness has been quite limited. Isoproterenol infusion rates as high as 200 mcg/min have been described. However, with isoproterenol, one must be aware of the potential to increase vasodilation and hypotension.

d. **Other catecholamines** with beta-1 selective properties (dobutamine) or combined alpha- and beta-agonist properties (epinephrine, norepinephrine, dopamine) may be necessary. An initial 0.5 to 1 mg of epinephrine i.v. bolus, followed by a continuous infusion of 2 to 10 mcg/min up to as high as 250 mcg/ min has been suggested for treatment of both bradycardia and hypotension. Renal dose dopamine may be used in conjunction to maintain renal perfusion. Pressors should be titrated upwards and may exceed usual dosages.

e. Phosphodiesterase inhibitors such as aminophylline and amrinone can help maintain intracellular cyclic AMP levels. This enhances cardiac contractility and may be useful in normotensive patients with signs of congestive heart failure. However, the number of successfully treated cases is limited, and more study is needed.

f. A **pacemaker** may be necessary if there is high-degree heart block and no response to pharmacological therapy. In sotalol overdose, overdrive pacing, i.v. magnesium sulfate, and lidocaine may be necessary for treatment of ventricular tachydysrhythmias.

g. **Fluid replacement** may be necessary in the face of hypotension. It should be given cautiously and guided by central venous pressure, arterial pressure and Swan-Ganz monitoring.

h. There are case reports of recovery following heroic efforts, including prolonged cardiopulmonary resuscitation, intra-aortic balloon pump, and bypass.

2. Use diazepam for **seizures** and, if necessary, phenytoin or phenobarbital. If **hypoglycemia** is present, use an infusion of glucose and possibly glucagon.

3. For agents with a small volume of distribution, low protein binding, and high level of urinary excretion, **charcoal hemoperfusion and dialysis** may be indicated. This

TABLE 39-3. *Treatment for beta-blocker overdose*

General
 ABCs (consider pretreatment with atropine before intubation)
 Gastric lavage (consider pretreatment with atropine), charcoal, cathartics
 Multiple-dose charcoal and whole bowel irrigation with PEG-ELS for long-acting sustained release preparations
 Consider charcoal hemoperfusion and dialysis
 Glucose if hypoglycemia
Bradycardia
 Atropine 0.5 mg i.v. repeat dose 0.5–1.0 mg i.v.
  End point (3 mg) or resolution of bradycardia
 Glucagon 3–10 mg i.v. repeat 5 mg q 15–30 min or i.v. infusion 1 mg/h and titrate upwards
 Isoproterenol 2 mcg/min i.v. infusion and titrate upwards
  End point: resolution of bradycardia; with hypotension consider need for beta-1 selective agent
  (dobutamine) or combined alpha and beta agent (epinephrine)
 Pacemaker if high-degree heart block or no response (overdrive pacing, i.v. magnesium, and lidocaine for
  sotalol-induced ventricular tachydysrhythmias)
Hypotension
 Fluid replacement, cautiously if needed with monitoring
  End point: CVP 8–12 mm Hg or pulmonary wedge pressure 15–18 mm Hg
 Glucagon (as for bradycardia)
 Dopamine 5 mcg/kg/min i.v. infusion titrate up to 20 mcg/kg/min
  End points: monitor BP PWP, urine output, EKG
 Epinephrine 2 mcg/min i.v. infusion and titrate upwards
  End points: monitor BP, PWP, urine output, EKG
 Dobutamine 2.5 mcg/kg/min i.v. infusion titrate up to 15 mcg/kg/min
  End points: monitor BP, PWP, urine output, EKG
 Intraaortic balloon pump
Seizures
 Diazepam and, if necessary, phenytoin or phenobarbital
Bronchospasm
 Beta-2 adrenergic aerosol
 Aminophylline 5.6 mg/kg i.v. infusion over 15–20 min, then 0.9 mg/kg/h infusion; monitor serum levels

treatment may be necessary after toxicity due to agents such as atenolol, sotalol, nadolol, and acebutolol. Progression of symptoms despite alternative treatment measures in this situation is a strong indication for hemoperfusion and dialysis.

 4. Treatment options are summarized in Table 39-3.

V. Disposition and follow-up. All patients with ingestion of sustained-release preparations must be admitted. Symptomatic patients should be admitted to the intensive care unit. Asymptomatic patients with sustained-release ingestions may be admitted to a monitored setting with expectant management. These patients can be medically cleared if they remain asymptomatic for 24 h.

Selected Readings

Agura ED, Wexler LF, Witzburg RA. Massive propranolol overdose: successful treatment with high-dose isoproterenol and
 glucagon. *Am J Med* 1986;80:755.
Barsan WG, Jastremski MS, Syverud SA. *Emergency drug therapy.* Philadelphia: WB Saunders, 1991.
Cox J, Wang RY. Critical consequences of common drugs: manifestations and management of calcium-channel blocker and
 beta-adrenergic antagonist overdose. *Emerg Med Rep* 1994;15:83.

Ellenhorn MJ, Barceloux DG. *Medical toxicology: diagnosis and treatment of human poisoning.* New York: Elsevier Science, 1988.

Frishman W, et al. Clinical pharmacology of the new beta- adrenergic blocking drugs. Part 8. Self-poisoning with beta-adrenoceptor blocking agents: recognition and management. *Am Heart J* 1979;98:798.

Gilman AG, et al. *Goodman and Gilman's. The pharmacological basis of therapeutics.* 8th ed. New York: Pergamon Press, 1996.

Goldfrank LR, et al. *Goldfrank's toxicologic emergencies.* 5th ed. East Norwalk, CT: Appleton & Lange, 1994.

Heath A. β-Adrenoceptor blocker toxicity: clinical features and therapy. *Am J Emerg Med* 1984;2:518.

Henry M, Kay MM, Viccellio P. Cardiogenic shock associated with calcium-channel and beta blockers: reversal with intravenous calcium chloride. *Am J Emerg Med* 1985;3:334.

Kerns W, Kline J, Ford MD. Beta-blocker and calcium channel blocker toxicity. *Emerg Med Clin North Am* 1994;12:365.

Lane AS, Woodward AC, Goldman MR. Massive propranolol overdose poorly responsive to pharmacologic therapy: use of the intra-aortic balloon pump. *Emerg Med* 1987;16:103.

Rumack BH, ed. *Poisindex information system.* Denver: Micromedex, 1995.

Taboulet P, et al. Pathophysiology and management of self-poisoning with beta-blockers. *J Toxicol Clin Toxicol* 1993;31:531.

Weinstein RS. Recognition and management of poisoning with beta-adrenergic blocking agents. *Ann Emerg Med* 1984;13:79.

Emergency Toxicology, Second Edition,
edited by Peter Viccellio.
Lippincott–Raven Publishers, Philadelphia © 1998.

40

Calcium Channel Blockers

*Peter Viccellio, *Mark C. Henry, and †Jason Yuan

*Department of Emergency Medicine, State University of New York at Stony Brook,
Stony Brook, New York 11794-7400; †West Orange, New Jersey 07052*

I. **Pharmacology and properties of agents.** The selective calcium channel blockers include the following: **phenylalkylamines**—verapamil, gallopamil; **dihydropyridines**—nifedipine, nicardipine, nimodipine, isradipine, amlodipine; **benzothiazepines**—diltiazem; **diphenylpiperazines**—cinnarizine and flunarizine. These agents block membrane influx of calcium through "slow channels" during the excitation-contraction phase in smooth muscle. Cardiac muscle, vascular smooth muscle, and the cardiac conduction system are affected. The various calcium channel blockers vary in their effect on these cells. As such, their clinical utility may vary according to their dominant properties.

A. **Verapamil's** greatest effect is on the conduction system, with depression of the sinus node and of conduction through the atrioventricular (AV) node; its effects on the myocardium and peripheral vasculature are less marked. Pretreatment with calcium blocks verapamil-induced peripheral vasodilation at clinical doses but does not appear to block the effect at the AV node. Binding of verapamil at the AV node is greater than at other sites. Verapamil crosses the placenta and has the potential for slowing the fetal heart rate, the clinical significance of which action is unknown. The negative inotropic effect, particularly of verapamil, may precipitate congestive heart failure or pulmonary edema.

B. **Nifedipine** is a peripheral vasodilator at therapeutic doses, without depressing conduction or inotrope. Overdose with nifedipine is less likely to cause bradydysrhythmias, but this has occurred with serious ingestions. Orthostatic hypotension is frequently seen and is usually primarily due to peripheral vasodilation. Patients typically develop a reflex tachycardia. Sublingual nifedipine causes a drop in the blood pressure within 5 min. A dermatologic flushing is not uncommon.

C. **Diltiazem** is intermediate in its effects between verapamil and nifedipine.

D. **Nimodipine** is similar to nifedipine in action, with a special affinity for the cerebral vasculature. Nimodipine decreases ischemic neurologic complications associated with subarachnoid hemorrhage despite angiographically demonstrated cerebral vasospasm.

E. These agents, other than nimodipine, have been used for the treatment of hypertension and angina. Verapamil is also used for both acute treatment and chronic control of supraventricular dysrhythmias. Other potential uses currently under study include irritable bowel syndrome, migraine, arterial peripheral vascular disease, Raynaud's phenomena, and asthma.

II. **Clinical presentation.** Calcium channel blocker overdose is often precipitous, with **sudden and profound deterioration of vital signs.** Symptoms usually occur 1 to 5 h after oral ingestion, although they may be delayed over 24 h with long-acting sustained-release (SR) oral preparations. Symptoms occur within seconds to minutes after intravenous administration. Patients who respond to initial treatment frequently experience subsequent deterioration. Symptoms will usually resolve by 48 h, but have been reported to persist as long as 7 days. Agents for which SR preparations are available include diltiazem-SR, nicardipine-SR, nifedipine-SR, and verapamil-SR. Additional treatment measures and monitoring are required with these preparations.

   A. **Hallmarks** of calcium channel blocker overdose include the following.
      1. **Bradydysrhythmias.** Sinus bradycardia, narrow-complex junctional bradycardia, sinus arrest, and varying degrees of AV block have been described.
      2. **Myocardial depression** has resulted in hypotension, congestive failure, or frank cardiogenic shock.
      3. **Peripheral vasodilation, hypotension, and syncope.** Symptoms depend on the amount, route, and type of calcium channel blocker ingested. Sensitivity to these agents may be modified by disease (particularly cardiovascular disorders) in the host, as well as the presence of other drugs. In the presence of beta-blockers, patients may experience toxicity at lower doses of calcium channel blockers. Orthostatic hypotension in particular is a manifestation of nifedipine's effect. Hypotension without nifedipine ingestion will require additional monitoring until its resolution.

   B. **Other manifestations** of overdose from these agents include the following.
      1. **Nausea, vomiting,** and ileus
      2. **CNS depression, confusion,** lethargy, and coma
      3. **Seizures**—whether from direct effect of the drug or a consequence of hypoperfusion is unknown. Also, nonhemorrhagic cerebral infarction has been reported. However, seizures are relatively rare, and additional workup may be required.
      4. **Hyperglycemia.** In some reported cases, it has been a major complication of ingestion. The mechanism, as has been shown for verapamil and diltiazem, probably is related to blocking calcium entry into pancreatic islet beta cells, resulting in impairment of insulin release. However, exogenous insulin is rarely required.
      5. **Metabolic acidosis,** likely secondary to hypoperfusion is well-described.

   C. **Differential diagnosis.**
      1. **History and clinical suspicion** are the only immediate modalities available to the physician confronting this diagnosis.
      2. The characteristic presentation of hypotension and sinus or junctional bradycardia, sinus arrest, or varying degrees of AV block are characteristic of calcium channel blocker overdoses but also of several other drug reactions, including **beta-blocker** and **digoxin** overdoses. Beta-blocker overdose in particular causes a syndrome virtually indistinguishable from that due to calcium channel blocker overdose.

III. **Laboratory evaluation**
   A. Routine analysis should include **electrolytes, arterial blood gases, ECG, and cardiac monitoring.** Calcium levels are typically normal. **ECG changes** other than varying

degrees of sinus and AV block and bradydysrhythmias include prominent u-waves, low-voltage T-waves, and nonspecific ST-T wave changes. AV block has been reported up to 24 h after presentation. QT prolongation, though described, is not a usual finding with calcium channel blocker overdoses. Radiographic plain films can help confirm ingestion of some SR preparations.

B. The need for routine **toxicologic screening** should be determined by the treating physician. Most patients require intervention long before the results of such screens can be obtained. Many routine toxicologic screenings do not test for calcium blocking agents, although they may be useful for determining the presence of other agents. Levels of specific agents may be obtained for retrospective confirmation, if desired. Serum levels only approximate clinical manifestations.

IV. Management and treatment

A. **General management.** The treating clinician must keep in mind the potential for precipitous change in clinical status. The patient should be kept in a monitored environment, with equipment and drugs available for airway management and treatment of hypotension and bradydysrhythmias.

B. **Evacuation and elimination**

1. **Ipecac.** Given the possibility of emetic agents having their peak effect in the face of abrupt deterioration, the hazards of the use of emetics outweigh their usefulness, and so they generally should be avoided. In addition, emetics enhance vagal activity and could possibly worsen bradydysrhythmias. It is possible that ipecac may have some clinical utility if given immediately after ingestion.

2. **Gastric lavage** may have some use, particularly if performed within the first 30 min. Vagal stimulation from esophageal intubation may worsen the clinical picture. Meticulous attention to **airway protection** is mandatory. Lavage, if performed, should be done early in clinically symptomatic patients or with ingestion of long-acting preparations, *after* establishing a secure airway. Consider pretreatment with atropine prior to intubation and lavage.

3. **Multiple-dose activated charcoal** is increasingly recommended for all suspected calcium channel blocker overdoses and especially with long-acting SR preparations until clinical symptoms have resolved. A **cathartic** is administered with the first dose and subsequently on an as-needed basis.

4. **Whole-bowel irrigation (WBI).** Given the prolonged absorption and delayed clinical symptoms with ingestions of **long-acting SR preparations,** WBI is recommended with any significant or symptomatic ingestion of these agents. **Polyethylene glycol-electrolyte lavage solution (PEG-ELS)** is administered PO/NGT at 1 to 2 L/h until progression of KUB findings (if initially present) demonstrating clearance of radiopaque material; clinical resolution; or the rectal effluent appears the same as the PEG-ELS solution. Recent evidence suggests that appearance of clear rectal effluent may not be an adequate indicator of bowel decontamination. WBI should also be used if there is any suspicion of **gastric concretions.** Repeat activated charcoal may be administered after WBI. The efficacy of WBI versus charcoal versus both in combination has not been clearly established.

5. **Dialysis.** Reports have described the use of dialysis and charcoal hemoperfusion, but it is not an established or recommended practice. Given the large volume of distribution and significant protein binding of these agents, hemoperfusion would not be expected to play a major role in treatment.

C. **Specific and antidotal measures**

 1. **Hypotension and bradycardia**

 a. **Calcium chloride,** 10% with 10 to 20 mL for adults (10 to 30 mg/kg in children (0.10 to 0.30 mL/kg), administered by slow intravenous push over several minutes, represents the mainstay first-line therapy for calcium channel blocker toxicity. Calcium gluconate has also been used but does not produce as predictable a clinical effect as does calcium chloride. Dosage is empirically based on clinical responses in case reports. Aggressive therapy with calcium chloride may be required to correct conduction defects. Recommendations include intravenous administration of 1 g of calcium chloride over 5 min, repeated every 10 to 20 min up to four times. However, with some massive overdoses, calcium therapy appears less effective. Currently unknown is whether failure to respond to calcium signifies resistance to calcium or merely inadequate dosage. Side effects include peripheral vasodilation with hypotension, primarily with rapid bolus injection; dysrhythmias, particularly in patients taking digoxin; and local tissue necrosis due to intravenous infiltration. Particular care should be exercised if digoxin overdose is suspected, given the propensity for calcium to worsen heart block in this setting. Symptoms of hypercalcemia have not been described following intravenous administration in this setting, and the utility of monitoring calcium levels is unclear, although recommended. Subsequent deterioration, if the patient has shown a response, should be treated with repeat dosages of calcium chloride or continuous calcium infusion; an initial infusion rate of 20 to 50 mg/kg/h for adults has been used with success. If a calcium drip is used, extreme caution must be exercised. Monitoring the QT interval is an inaccurate method for determining calcium serum concentrations.

 b. **Intravenous fluids** (0.9% sodium chloride) may reverse hypotension; but given the potential for calcium channel blocker-induced myocardial depression and congestive heart failure, they should be administered cautiously.

 c. **Atropine** in doses of 0.5 to 1.0 mg (0.01 mg/kg in the pediatric population) should be used initially to treat symptomatic bradydysrhythmias. Bradydysrhythmias and heart block in this setting are not predominantly vagally mediated, however, and success is infrequent with this agent.

 d. **Vasoactive and inotropic agents.** Although the patient may respond dramatically to calcium, many overdoses require treatment with additional agents such as **dopamine, epinephrine, norepinephrine,** and **isoproterenol.** It is possible that in combination these agents are synergistic. Intracellular release of calcium from the sarcoplasmic reticulum of cardiac muscle can be triggered by beta-agonists through mechanisms independent of the transmembrane calcium channels. This pathway is not affected by calcium channel blockade and allows an alternate pathway for enhancing contractility. Similarly, alpha-1 receptors can stimulate contraction of vascular smooth muscle in the face of calcium channel blockade.

e. **Dopamine** has been used in patients who have had inadequate response to calcium chloride at doses as high as 50 mcg/kg/min. It appears to be more effective than **dobutamine,** which lacks significant vasopressor effect. Also, **epinephrine, norepinephrine, phenylephrine,** and **isoproterenol** infusions have been used with success. Epinephrine may be given as an initial 1 mg intravenous bolus, followed by a 2 to 10 mcg/min infusion. Epinephrine infusions as high as 100 mcg/min have been described. Stimulation of peripheral alpha receptors by alpha agents such as phenylephrine and norepinephrine may be critical for reversing the calcium channel blocker-induced peripheral vasodilation. The maximal appropriate dose of these agents in the face of a significant ingestion has not been established. However, the use of these agents in dosages beyond those normally recommended has been commonly reported in the literature without reports of complications from therapy per se.

f. In patients with known **idiopathic hypertrophic subaortic stenosis (IHSS), alpha-agonists** may be of particular use, whereas beta agents may worsen the hemodynamic status. **Alpha-agonists** increase afterload and left ventricular end-diastolic volume, thereby decreasing the obstruction seen in IHSS.

g. **Glucagon** has been used with some success for treatment of heart block and myocardial depression secondary to calcium channel blockade. A standard dosing regimen has not been established, but intravenous boluses of 2 to 10 mg with doses as high as 17 mg have been reported. This can be followed by an infusion starting at 1 to 5 mg/h and titrated upwards to 10 mg/h. If an infusion is used, the glucagon should be reconstituted in normal saline, sterile water, or D5W to avoid phenol toxicity from the standard manufacturer's diluent. The mechanism of action involves pathways independent of calcium channels, most likely secondary to glucagon-induced stimulation of intracellular cyclic AMP production.

h. **Amrinone,** which increases cyclic AMP and calcium influx, thereby improving myocardial contractility, has been described in case reports to have a positive effect. In vascular smooth muscle, amrinone may exacerbate hypotension by decreasing intracellular calcium and causing peripheral vasodilation. Amrinone has been dosed as an initial 0.75 to 2 mg/kg intravenous bolus followed by a 5 to 10 mcg/kg/min infusion. However, the literature on its usage is limited.

i. **4-aminopyridine** directly opposes the effects of verapamil by facilitating calcium influx. Some animal studies have found immediate reversal of calcium channel blockade by the infusion of 4-aminopyridine, and reports of dramatic reversal of toxicity exist in the medical literature. However, other animal studies show no efficacy and no improvement in survival when compared to standard treatment. 4-aminopyridine is currently available in the United States for investigational purposes only.

      j.   **Transvenous or external pacing** should be considered early for patients not responding to initial pharmacologic treatments. Also, **monitoring of pulmonary wedge pressures** and **cardiac output** may be necessary, especially with persistent hypotension. **Intra-aortic balloon counterpulsation** may also be helpful.

      k.   Should a patient with accessory conduction pathways, as with Wolff-Parkinson-White or Lown-Ganong-Levine syndrome, receive verapamil for treatment of a supraventricular tachydysrhythmia, the latter may worsen owing to antegrade conduction down the accessory pathway. Treatment of such dysrhythmias includes **cardioversion, procainamide,** and possibly **lidocaine.** There is little experience with the use of calcium in this particular setting; its utility is unknown.

  2. **Seizures** due to calcium channel blockers are treated in standard fashion with **benzodiazepines** initially. **Phenytoin** or **phenobarbital** may be added if seizures persist. Seizures are probably a consequence of hemodynamic instability rather than a specific CNS effect.

  3. **Hyperglycemia,** may be treated in standard fashion.

V. **Range of toxicity.** The minimum range has not been established and depends on the drug, co-ingestions, and the underlying host.

VI. **Disposition and follow-up.** Symptoms of toxicity can recur hours after the patient appears stable. All SR ingestions must be admitted. Patients with significant or symptomatic ingestions should be admitted to an intensive care setting. Asymptomatic SR ingestions can be admitted to monitored beds. Patients should be observed for 24 h after all their symptoms have completely resolved.

Selected Readings

Adelstein RS, Sellers JR. Effects of calcium on vascular smooth muscle contraction. *Am J Cardiol* 1987;59:4B–10B.

Antman EM, et al. Calcium channel blocking agents in the treatment of cardiovascular disorders. Part I. Basic and clinical electrophysiologic effects. *Ann Intern Med* 1980;93:875.

Cox J, Wang RY. Critical consequences of common drugs: manifestations and management of calcium-channel blocker and beta-adrenergic antagonist overdose. *Emerg Med Rep* 1994;15:83.

Ellenhorn MJ, Barceloux DG. *Medical toxicology: diagnosis and treatment of human poisoning.* New York: Elsevier Science, 1988.

Enyeart JJ, Price WA, Hoffman DA. Profound hyperglycemia and metabolic acidosis after verapamil overdose. *J Am Coll Cardiol* 1983;2:1228.

Gilman AG, et al. *Goodman and Gilman's. The pharmacological basis of therapeutics.* 8th ed. New York: Pergamon Press, 1996.

Godfraind T. Classification of calcium antagonists. *Am J Cardiol* 1987;59:11B.

Goenen M, et al. Treatment of severe verapamil poisoning with combined amrinone-isoproterenol therapy. *Am J Cardiol* 1986;58:1142.

Goldfrank LR, et al., eds. *Goldfrank's toxicologic emergencies.* 5th ed. East Norwalk, CT: Appleton & Lange, 1994.

Henry M, Kay MM, Viccellio P. Cardiogenic shock associated with calcium-channel and beta blockers: reversal with intravenous calcium chloride. *Am J Emerg Med* 1985;3:334.

Herrington DM, Insley BM, Weinmann GG. Nifedipine overdose. *Am J Med* 1986;81:344.

Hofer CA, Smith JK, Tenholder MF. Verapamil intoxication: a literature review of overdoses and discussion of therapeutic options. *Am J Med* 1993;95:431.

Horowitz BZ, Rhee KJ. Massive verapamil ingestion: a report of two cases and a review of the literature. *Am J Emerg Med* 1989;7:624.

Kerns W, Kline J, Ford MD. Beta-blocker and calcium channel blocker toxicity. *Emerg Med Clin North Am* 1994;12:365.

Mitchell LB, Schroeder JS, Mason JW. Comparative clinical electrophysiologic effects of diltiazem, verapamil and nifedipine: a review. *Am J Cardiol* 1982;49:629.

Morris DL, Goldschlager N. Calcium infusion for reversal of adverse effects of intravenous verapamil. *JAMA* 1983;249:3212.

Proano L, Chiang WK, Wang RY. Calcium channel blocker overdose. *Am J Emerg Med* 1995;13:444.

Ramoska EA, Spiller HA, Myers A. Calcium channel blocker toxicity. *Ann Emerg Med* 1990;19:649.

Ramoska EA, et al. A one-year evaluation of calcium channel blocker overdoses: toxicity and treatment. *Ann Emerg Med* 1993;22:196.

Rumack BH, ed. *Poisindex information system.* Denver: Micromedex, 1995.

Salerno DM, et al. Intravenous verapamil for treatment of multifocal atrial tachycardia with and without calcium pretreatment. *Ann Intern Med* 1987;107:623.

Snover SW, Bocchino V. Massive diltiazem overdose. *Ann Emerg Med* 1986;15:1221.

Spiller HA, et al. Delayed onset of cardiac arrhythmias from sustained-release verapamil. *Ann Emerg Med* 1991;20:201.

Stone PH, et al. Calcium channel blocking agents in the treatment of cardiovascular disorders. Part II. Hemodynamic effects and clinical applications. *Ann Intern Med* 1980;93:886.

Whitebloom D, Fitzharris J. Nifedipine overdose. *Clin Cardiol* 1988;11:505.

Wolf LR, Spadafora MP, Otten EJ. Use of amrinone and glucagon in a case of calcium channel blocker overdose. *Ann Emerg Med* 1993;22:1225.

Wolff F, et al. Prenatal diagnosis and therapy of fetal heart rate anomalies: with a contribution on the placental transfer of verapamil. *J Perinat Med* 1980;8:203.

Zaritsky AL, Horowitz M, Chernow C. Glucagon anatagonism of calcium channel blocker-induced myocardial dysfunction. *Crit Care Med* 1988;16:246.

Emergency Toxicology, Second Edition,
edited by Peter Viccellio.
Lippincott–Raven Publishers, Philadelphia © 1998.

41

Clonidine

†Jonathan Rudolf and °Peter Viccellio

†*Department of Emergency Medicine, Shore Memorial Hospital, Somers Point, New Jersey
08244;* °*Department of Emergency Medicine, State University of New York at Stony Brook,
Stony Brook, New York 11794-7400*

I. **Properties of agents and pharmacology**

    A. Clonidine (Catapres) is a widely used **antihypertensive agent.** It is an alpha-adrenergic agonist with both central and peripheral effects. Therefore, its spectrum of toxic manifestations can be divergent.

    B. There are two physiologic subclasses of alpha-adrenergic receptors. The alpha-1 type predominates in the periphery, acting on smooth muscle and other effectors to cause local vasoconstriction. The alpha-2 receptors are mainly found centrally, at presynaptic nerve terminals, but also on platelets, adipose cells, and smooth muscle. Clonidine lowers blood pressure through a dominant alpha-2 effect. By stimulating the receptors on the presynaptic neuron, the drug inhibits that neuron from releasing norepinephrine, thereby decreasing peripheral sympathetically mediated vasoconstriction, as well as inotropy and chronotropy. At normal dosages the effect of direct stimulation of alpha-1 receptors by clonidine is negligible compared to the central alpha-2 inhibition, although transient hypertension following i.v. injection has been reported. Clonidine may also act on medullary opiate receptors to decrease sympathetic outflow and has been used to treat symptomatic narcotic withdrawal.

    C. Clonidine is supplied in tablets of 0.1, 0.2, and 0.3 mg and as transdermal patches that deliver 0.1, 0.2, or 0.3 mg/day. Rapidly and nearly completely absorbed from the gastrointestinal (GI) tract, the drug has a usual onset of action of 0.5 hr, making it useful for the treatment of hypertensive urgency. Peak antihypertensive effect occurs 2 to 4 h after ingestion. Clearance is primarily by the kidney, with 50% excreted unchanged daily in the urine. The half-life in otherwise healthy patients is approximately 10 h. The normal dose is 0.1 mg q12h, titrated upward for therapeutic effect.

II. **Clinical presentation** of clonidine poisoning is marked by fluctuating blood pressure followed by persistent hypotension, with bradyarrhythmias and respiratory and CNS depression. The onset of toxic effects is rapid, beginning in almost all patients 30 min to 4 h after ingestion. No clear linear correlation has been shown between the dose and any toxic effects. Because severe symptoms have developed in children who received as little as 0.1 mg, any ingestion should be regarded as significant. There have been several reports of toxicity from the transdermal preparations, primarily as a result of oral ingestion by children.

    A. **Hypotension** is frequent, and peak effect is usually 2 to 4 h following a rapid onset. Commonly it is accompanied by **bradycardia.** All degrees of **atrioventricular (AV)**

heart block have been reported. Paradoxical hypertension from peripheral alpha stimulation may also occur, most commonly early after ingestion. Although early fluctuation of blood pressure is common, the hypotensive phase, once established, generally persists.

B. **Respiratory depression** is common, particularly in children. Frank apnea or irregular respiratory patterns with periods of apnea have been reported. Usual onset of respiratory symptoms is within 1 h.

C. **CNS manifestations** are seen with nearly all ingestions. Altered mental status ranges from mild drowsiness (the most common effect) to lethargy is coma. This change in mental status occurs rapidly and without warning in many cases. Seizures are a rare symptom. Hypotonia and hyporeflexia, sometimes with any abnormal Babinski test, may occur. Pupils are frequently affected and can be miotic, mydriatic, or unresponsive at any size.

D. **Miscellaneous effects** include irritability, skin pallor, cool extremities, diarrhea, visual hallucinations, and depression. Hypothermia, if present, is usually mild and self-limited.

III. **Diagnosis and workup**

A. **History and clinical suspicion** are the only immediate modalities available to the physician confronting this diagnosis. Respiratory depression with or without characteristic pupillary changes should lead the physician to administer naloxone, which may be effective for either narcotic or clonidine overdose. The presentation of hypertension and seizures suggests the picture of sympathomimetic agents. Persistent hypotension, with or without CNS and respiratory depression, can be caused by any of a large number of other agents.

B. **Laboratory analysis**

1. **Routine** laboratory testing should include electrolytes, arterial blood gases, and an ECG. The need for general or specific toxicologic screening should be determined by the treating physician; most patients with serious overdose require intervention prior to the availability of results of this testing.

2. No **specific** laboratory tests are indicated for clonidine per se. Clonidine levels are not clinically useful. For particular co-ingestions, specific laboratory confirmation may or may not be useful. For altered mental status, glucose level and oxygenation must be checked.

IV. **Management and treatment**

A. **General measures**

1. **Basic and advanced life support** should be immediately available. An intact airway must be ensured, and the patient should be continuously monitored. A large-bore i.v. line should be placed immediately. Naloxone is given to patients with respiratory or CNS depression as part of the standard "coma cocktail." Should the patient not respond to this intervention, mechanical ventilation is necessary. Careful blood-pressure monitoring is essential.

2. **Evacuation and elimination**

a. **Emesis.** Because the rapid onset of CNS depression may quickly lead to an unprotected airway, the use of induced emesis is contraindicated.

b. **Gastric lavage** may be useful in those patients who present shortly after the ingestion. The airway should be protected by having the patient positioned in the left lateral decubitus and Trendelenburg position, with suction readily available. If the patient is not awake and alert, endotracheal intubation is necessary.

    c. **Activated charcoal** given at the usual dosage is standard therapy and effective at preventing absorption. It should be accompanied by a cathartic agent, such as sorbitol or magnesium citrate. Oil-based cathartics are not recommended because of aspiration risk. There are no data comparing single- versus multiple-dose charcoal administration for clonidine poisoning.

    d. **Dialysis.** There is no documented benefit from diuretic use or dialysis because of the relatively fast urinary excretion of the drug. The half-life is not known to change in the setting of overdose.

B. Treatment of specific manifestations

    1. **Hypotension.** Administer isotonic **fluids** rapidly and place the patient in Trendelenburg position. If the blood pressure does not respond to these measures, consider pressors. **Dopamine** is the agent most frequently reported to be effective, beginning with 2 to 5 µg/kg/min, with incremental increases to 10 µg/kg/min if necessary. Consider **tolazoline** or **naloxone** (see **IV.C.1.2**). Other pressors may be effective, but experience is limited.

    2. **Hypertension.** Because it may be transient, it is preferable to use a short-acting agent such as **sodium nitroprusside** starting at 0.5 µg/kg/min titrated up to 10 µg/kg/min as necessary. Blood pressure should, of course, be carefully monitored, preferably by arterial line. Treatment may not be necessary, as the hypertension is commonly of short duration, but it should be commenced if hypertension is severe or symptomatic.

    3. **Bradycardia.** Although **atropine** is the agent most often recommended, it is frequently not effective in reversing bradycardia. Doses of 0.5 mg initially for adults and 0.02 mg/kg (minimum 0.1 mg) for children are routinely used and may be repeated at 5-min intervals up to three times. **Temporary pacing** should be used (external or transvenous) should the patient not respond to atropine. Consider **tolazoline** or **naloxone** (see below). Other arrhythmias have been successfully treated with conventional antiarrhythmic agents.

    4. **Seizures** are usually limited and respond to usual anticonvulsant therapy with **diazepam** or **lorazepam. Phenytoin** and **phenobarbital,** when given in the usual loading doses, are also appropriate if seizures should persist.

    5. **CNS depression. Naloxone** may be useful for reversing CNS depression (see below).

    6. **Respiratory depression** should be managed with supplemental oxygen and assisted ventilation. Patients may respond to **naloxone.**

C. Antidotal therapy

    1. **Tolazoline.** Generally tolazoline is not recommended unless the hypotension or bradycardia is unresponsive to conventional therapy (above). A relatively alpha-2–selective, competitive blocker of alpha-adrenergic receptors, tolazoline has been touted as an antidote for hypotension and bradycardia caused by the structurally

similar clonidine. In practice, it has not been shown to be particularly effective, and side effects of the drug can complicate management of the patient. Its side effects include marked hypertension, tachycardia, and other cardiac arrhythmias. Because of the lack of documented efficacy as well as potentially harmful side effects, this drug should be considered only in extreme circumstances. If given, dosage is 1 mg/kg i.v. up to a maximum of 10 mg and can be repeated at 5- to 10-min intervals to a total dose of 40 mg.

2. **Naloxone.** Administer to severely symptomatic patients with hypotension or respiratory or CNS depression. Naloxone has not been definitively shown to be effective in controlled studies, although the reported response rate in retrospective studies is around 50%. Clonidine overdose has several manifestations that are clinically similar to those of opiates. Clonidine has been used as treatment for opiate withdrawal and vice versa. Naloxone is regarded as free of adverse effects, though some patients treated in this setting have been reported to develop hypertension. With adequate hemodynamic monitoring it is unlikely that a patient will suffer a significant adverse effect from naloxone administration. Dosage is 0.4 to 2.0 mg i.v. (0.01 mg/kg for pediatric patients) and may be repeated every 2 to 3 min with careful monitoring. Those who respond may require multiple doses because of its short half-life; and a continuous infusion titrated to therapeutic effect may be used. Higher doses (up to 10 mg as a bolus) may have greater effect but have not been formally studied.

V. Disposition. Symptoms are nearly always present within 4 h of ingestion. All asymptomatic patients must be monitored in the hospital for at least 4 h, and those with symptoms should be admitted and observed until all symptoms are resolved. Most symptomatic patients require intensive care unit observation for 24 to 48 h after ingestion. In virtually all cases, symptoms cease by 24 h (mean duration 9 to 10 h).

Selected Readings

Anderson RJ, et al. Clonidine overdose: report of six cases and review of the literature. *Ann Emerg Med* 1981;10:107–112.
Artman M, Boerth RC. Clonidine poisoning: a complex problem. *Am J Dis Child* 1983;137:171–174.
Fiser DH, Moss MM, Walker W. Critical care for clonidine poisoning in toddlers. *Crit Care Med* 1990;18:1124–1128.
Heidemann SM, Sarnaik AP. Clonidine poisoning in children. *Crit Care Med* 1990;18:618–620.
Schieber RA, Kaufman ND. Use of tolazoline in massive clonidine poisoning [Letter]. *Am J Dis Child* 1981;135:77–78.
Wiley JF, et al. Clonidine poisoning in young children. *J Pediatrics* 1990;116:654–658.

Emergency Toxicology, Second Edition,
edited by Peter Viccellio.
Lippincott–Raven Publishers, Philadelphia © 1998.

42

Digoxin

*William David Binder and *†William J. Lewander

**Department of Emergency Medicine, †Department of Pediatrics, Rhode Island Hospital,
Providence, Rhode Island 02903*

I. **Introduction.** The cardiac glycosides, of which digitalis is the most commonly known, have an extensive history in pharmacotherapy. Squill, mentioned in the Ebers papyrus, and derived from the sea onion (*Urginea maritima*) was commonly used by the Egyptians and Greeks in their therapeutics. William Withering published his classic *Account of the Foxglove and Some of its Medical Uses* in 1785, remarking upon his experience with digitalis in a series of 163 patients over 9 years. Indians in South America have utilized cardiac glycosides in their dart poisons. Digitalis toxicity was well known in previous centuries, and it has been suggested that toxic visual symptoms may have played a role in Van Gogh's use of swirling greens and yellows (1,2,3,4). Current indications for cardiac glycosides such as digoxin include use in CHF, where they increase cardiac index and improve left sided diastolic and systolic dysfunction, and in atrial fibrillation, where they assist in rate control and improved inotropy.

II. **Available preparations**

   A. Digitalis and related compounds are terms that generally encompass cardiac glycoside inotropic and chronotropic drugs. These compounds are very often derived from **plants** such as foxglove, or Digitalis purpurea Linne (digitoxin, digitalis, gitalin), Digitalis lanata Erhart (digoxin, lanatoside C, deslanoside), Strophanthus gratus (ouabain), and Acokanthera schimperi (ouabain). Other sources of plant glycosides, or cardenolides, include lily of the valley, oleander, and hellebore (one study from Australia identified cross reacting cardiac glycosides in 27 species from 20 genera of plants) (3,5,6,7).

   B. The Chinese have used Yixin Wan, a cardiotonic agent extracted from toad venom and skin, for centuries. Yixin Wan contains **bufadienolides,** which are naturally occurring cardioactive steroids with digoxin-like effects. Recently, several deaths in New York City have been reported in association with the ingestion of a purported topical aphrodisiac. The product, marketed under the name of "Stone," "Lovestone," "Rock Hard," and other names is, in fact, identical to Chan Su, a traditional Chinese medication used which also contains several bufadienolides. These herbal medications are sold in grocery stores and by street vendors and have been distributed both legally and by drug traffickers throughout the United States (8).

   C. Endogenous sources of cardiac glycosides exist, as well, and these may act in a paracrine or autocrine fashion.

D.   Digoxin is the most commonly used cardiac glycoside in the United States and is available as an oral tablet, as the Lanoxicap, a gel tab form with increased bioavailability, an elixir containing 0.05 mg/mL, and as an intravenous preparation. Digitoxin, or crystodigin, is available in tablet form as 0.1 or 0.2 mg concentrations.

III.   **Pharmacology and properties**

A.   **Mechanism of Action.** The glycoside structure consists of an aglycone (or genin) group, which consists of a steroid nucleus and a lactone ring at the C17 positions, coupled with from one to four sugar molecules. The pharmacologic action resides with the aglycone moiety, but the attached sugars (usually at a C3 hydroxyl group) modify solubility and potency. The aglycone is chemically related to bile acids, sterols, and steroid hormones.

1.   **Intracellular calcium:** Calcium enters the normal myocyte by slow calcium channels, which are indirectly activated by the voltage sensitive fast sodium channel. Sodium inflow through the channel mediates the upstroke of the cardiac action potential and leads to depolarization of the sarcolemmal membrane, which results in the release of Ca^{2+} from the sarcoplasmic reticulum into the cytosol. The calcium influx activates contractile proteins, thus allowing actin and myosin to interact in the thin and thick filaments. Intracellular calcium homeostasis is maintained by a Na^+/Ca^{2+} exchanger which mediates transarcolemmal movement in a $3:1$ ratio. This exchanger allows both inward and outward movement of calcium and sodium, and will tend toward equilibrium. The activity of the Na^+/Ca^{2+} exchanger is influenced by the Na^+/K^+ ATPase pump. This crucial pump regulates intracellular sodium by extruding Na^+ while pumping K^+ into the cell in a $3:2$ ratio (3). Cardiac glycosides inhibit the Na^+/K^+ ATPase pump, leading to a transient increase in intracellular sodium and extracellular potassium. The Na^+/Ca^{2+} exchanger responds to the increase in sodium by both mediating an exchange for calcium as well as reducing calcium extrusion, causing a relative increase in intracellular calcium. This results in increased contractility. While therapeutic levels of digitalis cause only small increases in intracellular calcium, it appears that diastolic and systolic levels rise appreciably under toxic conditions. This contributes to oscillatory disturbances of membrane potential which results in the membrane after depolarizations that are believed to trigger dysrhythmias (1,3,9). Cardiac glycosides also have other mechanisms of action. The digoxin induced increase in intracellular Ca^{2+} concentration is accompanied by a fall in the intracellular pH, which leads to activation of a Na/H exchange pump. This results in extrusion of H^+, an increase in intracellular sodium, and greater inotropy (9).

2.   **Electrophysiologic effects:** Digoxin's therapeutic importance is also related to its electrophysiologic effects. Cardiac glycosides slow conduction and increase the refractory period in specialized cardiac conducting tissue by stimulating vagal tone. Digitalis has parasympathetic properties which include hypersensitization of carotid sinus baroreceptors and stimulation of central vagal nuclei. Clinically, this manifests itself as a reduced ventricular rate and increased refractoriness in the AV node and junctional tissue. Digoxin also appears to have variable effects on sympathetic tone, depending on the specific cardiac tissue involved (10).

3. **Vasomotor effects:** Digoxin and the other cardiac glycosides cause direct vaso-constriction in the arterial and venous system through inhibition of the Na^+/K^+ ATPase pump in vascular smooth muscle as well as by stimulating afferent, central and efferent neural mechanisms. The clinical significance of this property is controversial. In patients with vascular insufficiency, digoxin can lead to mesenteric ischemia and infarction. Furthermore, vasoconstrictor effects of digitalis-like compounds may theoretically cause a decline in cardiac output due to an acute increase in left ventricular afterload, resulting in angina and pulmonary edema (10). However, other studies demonstrate that patients with moderate to severe left ventricular dysfunction show an improvement in hemodynamics without an increase in myocardial oxygen consumption. It is likely that the clinically significant vasoconstrictive effects of digoxin are variable, with normal subjects demonstrating an increase in vascular resistance secondary to digoxin, while patients with impaired left ventricular function given digoxin show a decrease in vascular resistance (11).

B. **Pharmacokinetics**

1. **Absorption/bioavailability.** Up to 60% to 80% of tablet preparations are absorbed from the GI tract. Encapsulated gelcaps have improved bioavailability to 90 to 100%. Intravenous **digoxin** has a rapid onset of action; most of its inotropic effect is reached within 1 h. After oral administration the serum concentration of digoxin reaches a peak in 2 to 3 h. The maximum effect is apparent after 4 to 6 h, and the elimination half life is about 1 to 2 days (12). Factors that influence digoxin absorption include drugs that affect gastrointestinal (GI) motility (e.g., anticholinergics, opioids, and motility stimulants such as metoclopramide). Digoxin malabsorption can occur with small bowel disorders including edematous bowel of patients with chronic CHF, pancreatitis, or any other cause of malabsorption. Furthermore, 10% of the population in the United States carries the intestinal bacterium *Eubacterium lentum* which hydrolyzes digoxin to the inactive metabolite dihydrodigoxin. This is more common in urban dwellers. Antibiotic therapy which affects this bacterium can increase the concentration of serum digoxin (1,2,12,13). Digoxin and **digitoxin** are the two most commonly used oral cardiac glycosides. While these agents differ by only 1 hydroxyl group on their steroid nucleus, they have strikingly different pharmacokinetic properties based on the difference in polarity. Digoxin is a polar compound. It is less lipid soluble, less well absorbed and is incompletely bound to serum albumin. Digoxin's renal tubular reabsorption is minimal. This results in predominantly urinary elimination of the drug and a shorter half life, which is affected by renal function (12,13). Digitoxin's bioavailability is approximately 100%. Its onset of action is slower in comparison to digoxin; intravenous administration yields an apparent maximum effect after 6 h while the oral preparation's maximum effect occurs over about 24 h. The elimination half life of digitoxin is 7 days. Digitoxin is 95% bound by albumin and thus it has negligible renal excretion and is primarily metabolized in the enterohepatic circulation. Factors which affect digoxin absorption also influence digitoxin bioavailability (12,13).

2. **Distribution.** The distribution of digoxin is described by a two compartment pharmacokinetic model. There is an initial rapid decrease in concentration due to dilution in blood (this takes minutes), followed by distribution where the drug equilibrates between peripheral (skeletal muscle and myocardium) and central (plasma and liver and kidneys) compartments. Distribution is affected by physiologic and pathophysiologic factors. Binding of digoxin to the Na^+/K^+ ATPase receptor is directly related to serum potassium concentrations; hypokalemia stimulates binding, and hyperkalemia inhibits binding. Binding is reversible and consequently potassium administration may cause reversal of digoxin toxicity in hypokalemic patients. Other electrolyte abnormalities will affect digitalis' effect; hypomagnesemia, hypercalcemia, and acid/base imbalance will all increase an individual's sensitivity to the cardiac glycosides (13). Skeletal muscle is the largest storage depot of digoxin. Up to 50% of total body digoxin distributes into the peripheral compartment. This has great clinical significance in the digoxin toxic patient. Serum levels may fall after stopping digoxin intake, yet tissue levels may lag behind and remain elevated, and thereby cause continued toxicity. Conversely, the skeletal muscle component is particularly important in the **elderly** patient as their skeletal muscle decreases with age, predisposing them to toxicity. Similarly, physical activity can lower serum digoxin levels by as much as 33% by increasing binding sites in muscle. While skeletal muscle serves as a reservoir for digoxin, the drug's concentration per cell in myocardium is much greater than in skeletal muscle. The extensive binding of digoxin leads to a large and highly variable apparent volume of distribution (Vd) of digoxin, ranging from 3 to 10 L/kg of body weight (1). Distribution is also affected by factors which can alter the availability of binding sites. Increasing age and hypothyroidism lead to fewer binding sites, while pregnancy and hyperthyroidism increase the number of digoxin binding sites. Adipose does not bind digoxin, and thus lean body mass should be used when calculating dosages. Digoxin distributes across placenta and into breast milk (2,13,14).

3. **Elimination and metabolism.** Digoxin is predominantly **renally** excreted, although newer evidence suggests that hepatic metabolism can be extensive (see below). The elimination **half life** of digoxin varies between 26 to 45 h in healthy adult controls, and from 11 to 50 h in children. Any intervention or pathologic state that impairs the kidney's function will result in decreased excretion and increased digoxin levels. Intrinsic disease, aging, excessive diuretics, severe CHF, and drugs such as indomethacin, cyclosporine, spironolactone, quinidine and other antiarrhythmic agents will increase digoxin serum concentration by their direct effect on the kidney and/or by decreasing elimination. Vasodilators, conversely, will enhance renal excretion (1,2,13,14). Digitoxin, on the other hand, is primarily metabolized by hepatic microsomal enzymes. Its half life is 7 days, and this is not appreciably changed by hepatic disease. Drugs that induce microsomal enzymes can accelerate metabolism, as well as drugs which displace digitoxin from its serum albumin binding sites. These include phenylbutazone, warfarin, tolbutamide, sulfadimethoxine, clofibrate and others. Enterohepatic metabolism can be

extensively interrupted by nonabsorbable resins, such as cholestyramine, and by activated charcoal (2).

C. **Drug-digoxin interactions.** Numerous drugs interact with digoxin in a variety of mechanisms. Table 42-1 lists drug interactions (2,12,14,15,16).

IV. **Clinical manifestations of toxicity.** Prior to the 1980s cardiac glycoside toxicity was extremely common. Digoxin toxicity was frequently reported to be anywhere from 15% to 30% in numerous studies. Reasons for this included incomplete understanding of drug absorption, non-standardized drug formulations, and prior to 1969, no accurate means of testing serum digoxin levels. In 1969 a sensitive radioimmune assay was developed for measuring serum digoxin concentrations. Since the late 1970s the reported incidence of digoxin toxicity has fallen to approximately 2% to 4%. The reasons are multi-factorial and include the development of new classes of drugs for the treatment of SVT and CHF, a broad recognition of drug interactions, widespread availability of digoxin level testing, and importantly, a higher incidence of under dosing (17,18). Patient characteristics have changed as well. In 1971 of those receiving long term digoxin therapy, greater than 70% had coronary artery disease and 60% had a previous MI. In a 1990 study by Mahdyoon, these numbers were 35% and 20%, respectively (17).

A. **Patients at risk for digoxin toxicity:** (10,13,14,19,20)

1. Renal insufficiency
2. Ischemic heart disease (digitalis enhanced Purkinje fiber automaticity may be exacerbated by ischemia) as well as those with other forms of cardiac disease (e.g. amyloid cardiomyopathy).
3. Patients with electrolyte abnormalities.
4. Hypothyroidism and hyperthyroidism (increased sensitivity of tissue to digoxin).
5. Advanced pulmonary disease and hypoxia (hypoxia and right sided heart disease increase myocardial sensitivity to digoxin because of its proarrhythmic state).

TABLE 42-1. *Drug-digoxin interactions*

Mechanism	Drug	Serum digoxin level
Decreased GI absorption	Neomycin, cholestyramine, colestipol, activated charcoal, metoclopromide antacids, eathartics	Lower
Increased hepatic clearance due to enzyme induction	Rifampin	Lower
Increased GI absorption	Omeprazole, propantheline, erythromycin, tetracycline	Higher
Decreased renal excretion due to decreased GFR	Hydralazine, guanethiadine, alpha methlydopa, thiazide diuretics, furosemide, ethacrynic acid	Higher
Decreased distribution and clearance	Quinidine, quinine, spironolactone, amiodarone, verapamil	Higher
Unknown mechanism	Alprazolam, diazepam	Higher
Cardiac sympathetic tone		
Increased receptor sensitivity	Beta-adrenergic agonist, theophylline, succinylcholine	Increase
Decreased receptor sensitivity	Beta-adrenergic blockers, bretyllium	Decrease

   6. Patients taking other drugs leading to pharmacokinetic and pharmacodynamic interactions.

   7. Extremes of age.

B. Cardiac and vasomotor manifestations of toxicity.

   1. Dysrhythmias: Death from digoxin toxicity is attributed to cardiac rhythm disorders. In the absence of renal failure, most fatalities due to acute digoxin poisoning occur in the first 24 h upon ingestion. There are no dysrhythmias diagnostic of digoxin toxicity. However, the simultaneous phenomena of increased automaticity and depressed AV conduction are characteristic of digoxin intoxication. Some dysrhythmias are suggestive of digoxin toxicity and include (4,17,22,23):

     a. Atrial tachycardia with variable conduction at the AV node (PAT with block).

     b. Accelerated junctional rhythm especially in the setting of atrial fibrillation (abrupt regularization of atrial fibrillation).

     c. Fascicular tachycardia

     d. Ventricular bigeminy with alternating right and left axis deviation

     e. Bidirectional ventricular tachycardia

     f. Multiform PVCs during atrial fibrillation

   2. Atrial effects: At toxic levels digoxin has varying effects at the different specialized cardiac tissue. Digoxin can cause sinus arrest or sinus exit block due to a direct drug effect on the sinus node. While therapeutic levels of digoxin does not seem to profoundly affect atrial myocardium, toxic levels do result in automatic impulse initiation in the atria. This can lead to increased automaticity, which may result in atrial arrhythmias. AV junctional block and increased ventricular automaticity is perhaps the most common manifestation of digoxin toxicity. First degree AV block may merely indicate that digoxin is effective; higher degrees of block, however, are evidence of toxicity. Second degree type I block is associated with toxicity; rarely does one see a Mobitz Type II pattern associated with digoxin toxicity. Third degree heart block is nearly always transient and does not require permanent pacing (2,10,17,23).

   3. Ventricular tissue and the Purkinje system: At the Purkinje fibers and in ventricular muscle, digoxin toxicity commonly causes premature ventricular beats of varying morphology by altering action potentials. Spontaneous depolarizations due to previous action potentials, or delayed after depolarizations, may lead to PVCs and possible ventricular arrhythmias, including ventricular tachycardia and fibrillation. Hypokalemia and hypercalcemia can enhance the arrhythmogenic nature of digoxin, by altering the electrochemical milieu of the cell (10,17).

C. Extracardiac manifestations (Table 42-2) (9,12,14,17,21,24). Signs and symptoms of extracardiac manifestations of digitalis toxicity are well delineated. The following signs and symptoms are probably the most common:

   1. GI: In acute and chronic toxicity anorexia nausea, vomiting, abdominal pain, and diarrhea may occur. Mesenteric ischemia is a rare but potentially disastrous acute complication of rapid intravenous infusion.

   2. Central nervous system: Drowsiness, lethargy, fatigue, neuralgia, headache, dizziness, and confusion may occur.

TABLE 42-2. *Acute versus chronic digoxin toxicity*

Manifestations	Acute	Chronic
Age	Young	Elderly
Intent	Purposeful	Accidental
Gastrointestinal	Nausea, vomiting, anorexia, diarrhea, abdominal pain; mesentric ischemia may occur from rapid i.v. infusion.	Less pronounced
Central nervous system	Less pronounced	Headache, fatigue, weakness, dizziness, confusion, and coma; visual changes may occur.
Renal/electrolytes	Hyperkalemia normal renal function	Normal to low serum potassium, hypomagnesemia, renal insufficiency
Cardiac	Bradydysrhythmia, SVT with conduction abnormality, and, less commonly, ventricular dysrhythmias	Ventricular dysrhythmias

3. Ophthalmologic: Visual aberrations are often some of the earliest indications of chronic digitalis intoxication. Yellow green distortions are most common but red, brown, blue and white also occur. Drug intoxication may also cause snowy vision, photophobia, photopsia, and decreased visual acuity.

4. Many extracardiac toxic manifestations of cardiac glycosides are neurally mediated. While GI symptoms may be due, in part, to local irritation, they are primarily mediated by chemoreceptors in the area postrema of the medulla.

V. **Laboratory evaluation**

   A. **Digoxin levels**

      1. One of the major advancements in diagnosing digoxin toxicity was the development of a radioimmunoassay (RIA) in 1969. The therapeutic and toxic ranges for digoxin were initially defined by extensive trials on patients with CHF at only a few medical centers. Therapeutic levels vary with the lower limit ranging from 0.6nmol/L to 1.3 nmol/L, while the upper limit is generally agreed upon to be 2.6nmol/L (25). Serum concentrations associated with toxicity overlap between therapeutic and toxic ranges because of the myriad of factors potentiating digoxin toxicity.

      2. Because of digoxin's delayed onset of action, at least 6 h must elapse between dosage and drawing a digoxin level specimen (some authors prefer 12 h, with the patient at rest 1 h prior to collection) in order to prevent spuriously elevated levels. Strict adherence to levels without regard to clinical manifestations can result in inappropriate and costly interventions.

      3. Other confounding variables include digoxin metabolites, drugs, and **endogenous digoxin like factors.** While most patient metabolize less than 20% of digoxin, 10% of the population will metabolize up to 55% of digoxin to initially active metabolites. Not all routinely used RIAs measure each of these metabolites (19). Additionally, the antibodies used in digoxin immunoassays can cross react with numerous compounds including steroids and other drugs (spironolactone, for example). Finally, serum from neonates, pregnant women, patients with renal and hepatic failure, and patients with essential hypertension may cross react with the

digoxin antibody due to endogenous digitalis like factors produced by these individuals. These substances may account for 50% of serum digoxin measured by RIAs in particular patients (4,13,19).

   B. Electrolyte evaluation

    1. Hyperkalemia: In the acute setting hyperkalemia is common due to the inactivation of the Na^+/K^+ ATPase pump.

    2. Hypokalemia: Chronic digoxin users are very often hypokalemic because of concurrent diuretic use.

    3. Hypomagnesemia: Chronic digoxin users are often hypomagnesemic secondary to diuretic usage. Intracellular magnesium depletion may occur in chronic diuretic use despite normal serum magnesium levels (26). Importantly, magnesium is a cofactor of the Na^+/K^+ ATPase pump and alterations of its concentration will affect the pump's actions.

VI. Management (Fig. 42-1).

    A. Effective management and treatment of digitalis toxicity relies on early recognition that a dysrhythmia and/or non cardiac manifestation may be related to digitalis intoxication.

    1. General principles of management include assessment of the severity of the problem and the etiology of toxicity—diminished renal clearance, dose mediated, concurrent medications, and whether there has been accidental vs. intentional overdosage. Factors which influence treatment include age, medical history, chronicity of digoxin intoxication, existing heart disease and/or renal insufficiency, and importantly, ECG changes.

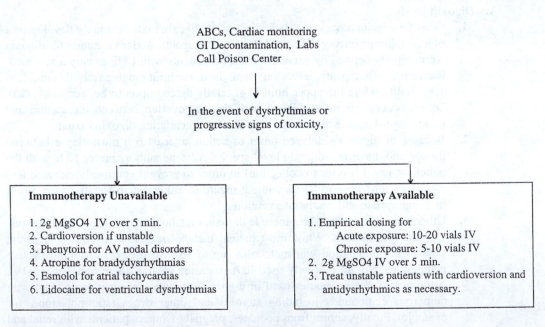

FIG. 42-1. Management of digoxin overdose.

2. First, apply the ABCs. Generally, cardiac glycosides do not cause respiratory compromise; they clearly can cause dysrhythmias and in the digoxin toxic patient with a history of CHF and/or cardiac disease respiratory failure can certainly complicate the clinical picture.

3. Early stabilization and supportive measures remain the cornerstone of initial treatment. Continuous hemodynamic assessment including 12-lead ECG and cardiac monitoring will often direct management. Intravenous access needs to be established immediately.

4. Atrial blocks and dysrhythmias rarely require emergent intervention. Unstable ventricular rhythms require immediate and aggressive interventions. These will be discussed below.

5. Electrolyte levels including potassium, calcium, and magnesium, as well as serum creatinine and digoxin levels should be sent to the laboratory promptly. It is important to recognize that serum digoxin levels shortly after an acute overdosage may not be accurate and relying upon them may result in costly and unnecessary interventions.

B. **GI decontamination/enhanced elimination. First line treatment in an acute ingestion is gastric lavage and activated charcoal with repeat dosings.** These have been shown to reduce gastric absorption and the latter can interrupt enterohepatic circulation. Repeated administration of activated charcoal to healthy volunteers increased digoxin clearance by almost 50% (28). Gastric lavage may increase vagal tone and lead to worsening of AV block or bradycardia (and can cause asystole), and consequently pretreatment with atropine has been recommended (4). Binding resins such as cholestyramine and colestipol hydrochloride can also interrupt enterohepatic circulation of digitoxin and digoxin metabolites, and can be used as adjuncts to activated charcoal, although these are less frequently used in practice (20,29). Cholestyramine is probably more appropriately utilized in **chronic toxicity with renal insufficiency.**

C. **Electrolyte imbalance**
   1. **In the acute setting,** hyperkalemia is commonly observed due to the inactivation of the Na^+/K^+ ATPase pump. Standard treatment for hyperkalemia (when indicated by ECG and potassium level) including bicarbonate, glucose and insulin are all useful in this setting. Ion exchange resins such as sodium polystyrene sulfonate (Kayexalate) can be utilized as well. However, if digoxin antibody therapy is anticipated then these other forms of treatment for hyperkalemia is not necessary. This is because the antibody will reactivate the Na^+/K^+ ATPase pump and potassium will redistribute normally. The use of **calcium** can be disastrous, because digoxin toxicity causes an enormous influx of calcium into the cell. Adding additional calcium can lead to delayed after-depolarizations and be pro-arrhythmogenic. In patients with uncontrolled hyperkalemia, it may be necessary to institute hemodialysis.

   2. **In chronic digoxin ingestion,** toxicity is more insidious. Chronic users are generally hypokalemic and hypomagnesemic due to concurrent diuretic use. The importance of serum potassium concentration cannot be overstated—a drop in serum potassium from 3.5mEq/L to 3.0 mEq/L will be accompanied by an increase in car-

diac sensitivity to digoxin by approximately 50% (19). Hypokalemia should be corrected and caution should be duly noted in the renally insufficient patient.

Magnesium is an essential electrolyte as well. Initially, 2 g of intravenous MgSO$_4$ should be given to the symptomatic digoxin toxic patient over 5 min. Magnesium is safe and should be used in patients who are hypokalemic, have ECG changes, and demonstrate any other digoxin related toxicities. In the patient with renal failure MgSO$_4$ should be used cautiously (26).

D. Antidysrhythmics

1. If the patient with an acute or chronic ingestion develops a digitalis-induced dysrhythmia the management of the arrhythmia is directed toward the cause of the rhythm disturbance. Aside from correcting obvious electrolyte abnormalities, an antidysrhythmic may be indicated, especially in the absence of, or delay in administering, immunotherapy.

2. **Phenytoin** and **lidocaine** are the antiarrhythmic drugs of choice. The former improves AV nodal conduction and can suppress PVCs and sustained VT. Lidocaine can also be used for ventricular dysrhythmias, although it does not enhance AV node conductivity (14).

3. **Atropine** is recommended for improving AV nodal conduction and is used in bradyarrhythmias.

4. **Quinidine, procainamide**, and **bretylium** are **contraindicated.** Both quinidine and procainamide worsen AV, SA, and His-Purkinje conductivity. Additionally, quinidine reduces digoxin tissue binding and renal clearance, thereby worsening digoxin levels. Bretylium can precipitate a worsening ventricular dysrhythmia (4,14,17).

5. Beta adrenergic blockers can decrease automaticity and slow conduction velocity induced by a catecholamine surge from digitalis intoxication, and can shorten the refractory period of atrial and ventricular muscle. Because of the potential toxicity to the SA and AV nodes, esmolol, a short acting beta blocker, is recommended in rapid atrial conduction (14,17).

6. Intravenous **magnesium sulfate,** 2 g over 5 min (repeat doses over 30 min may be used with the caveat being that magnesium toxicity is the obvious endpoint) has been shown to terminate digoxin-toxic cardiac arrhythmias in patients with and without overt cardiac disease. Aside from successful replacement of intracellular magnesium, it may also act as an indirect antagonist of digoxin at supraphysiologic levels (26).

7. **Temporary pacing** is a viable alternative for patients with nodal blocks, and this should be made readily available in high grade blocks before any other medical interventions are attempted (one study, however, suggests that pacing may increase adverse outcomes in some patients and suggests immunotherapy should be attempted prior to initiating pacemaker activity) (30,31).

E. Electrical cardioversion

1. Cardioversion for severe dysrhythmias due to digitalis overdose is hazardous and can precipitate ventricular fibrillation and asystole. However, if the patient is hemodynamically unstable and has a wide complex tachycardia, and if a fascicular tachycardia has been ruled out, cardioversion will need to be used early.

2. If the history is consistent with digitalis intoxication, it is best to use a minimal effective dose. Some clinicians have suggested using 10 to 25 joules initially

in VT/VF presenting to the ED, but most clinicians suggest starting at from 50 to 100 joules for a wide complex ventricular tachycardia, rather than the recommended 200 joules found in the ACLS protocol (4).

F. Immunotherapy. Immunotherapy is probably the most valuable recent addition to the treatment of digoxin and digitoxin intoxication. In both stable and unstable patients it is a first line therapy, and some authors feel that it is inappropriate to pronounce a patient in a code situation until digoxin-specific Fab fragments have been administered.

1. Introduced in 1976 but not commercially available until a decade later, **digoxin-specific Fab fragments** are the product of papain digestion of sheep IgG produced in response to an antigenic carrier protein couple to digoxin. The Fab fragments are small and eliminated through glomerular filtration rather than through reticuloendothelial degradation. The Fab fragments (commercially known as Digibind) are rapid and effective—onset of action ranges from 20 to 90 min—and they irreversibly remove digoxin from the myocardium and other specific binding sites. A complete response generally occurs within 4 h (32). Fab fragments utility in digitoxin toxicity has been documented. While the binding affinity of digoxin-specific Fab fragments to naturally occurring plant cardiac glycosides has not been thoroughly examined, Digibind's efficacy in oleander toxicity as well as in numerous other plants containing glycoside compounds has been demonstrated (33,34,35).

2. Over the past decade a review of the numerous cases of digoxin intoxication treated with **digoxin-specific Fab fragments** has revealed impressive results. Antman et al.'s landmark study published in 1990 examined 150 patients with potentially life threatening toxicity who were treated with digoxin-specific antibody fragments. Of the 150 patients, 80% demonstrated a complete response to the antibody, 10% were partial responders, and 10% showed no response. Partial and nonresponders were primarily due to heart disease as the true etiology of arrhythmia, improper dosing of Fab therapy, and moribund status at the time of dosing. Remarkably, of the 56 patients who suffered cardiac arrest in this study, 30 (54%) survived hospitalization after treatment with digoxin-specific Fab fragments (32).

3. Independent **indications** for using Digibind include the following (4,14,21,36,37):
   a. Ingestion of massive quantities of digitalis
      (i) Children more than 4 mg or 0.1 mg/kg
      (ii) Adults more than 10 mg, although some authors cite 3 to 15 mg as reasons for Digibind use, depending on age and extent of underlying cardiac disease. Note that these are rough guidelines. The history offered is notoriously inaccurate and one must handle each case individually. (Always consult your local poison control center.) The varying dose suggests that no definitive study has been undertaken, and that the clinical situation should take precedence.
   b. Hyperkalemia (more than 5 mEq/L)
   c. Digoxin-induced ventricular dysrhythmias or high grade AV block.
   d. Rapidly progressive signs and symptoms of digoxin toxicity.
   e. Cardiac arrest or cardiogenic shock in a patient with suspected digoxin intoxication.

   f.   Post distribution serum digoxin levels more than 5 ng/mL (Note that while some authors suggest more than 10 ng/mL in adults, elevated mortality has been seen in patients with levels more than 5 ng/mL).

4.   Dosing of Digibind:

   a.   This is based on the **total body load (TBL)** of digoxin and can be calculated by the following equations:

   i.   TBL = digoxin serum level (ng/mL) × 5.6 L/kg × body weight in kg.

   ii.   Number of vials of Fab = TBL/0.6mg. (A 40-mg vial of Digibind will bind 0.6mg of digoxin.) These equations should be used when the level is drawn greater than 6 h after an ingestion. For levels of less than 6 h after ingestion, one can multiply the dose ingested by 0.8 to approximate the TBL (14,21,36).

   b.   If an **unknown** dose has been ingested **acutely** and the patient is to be treated empirically, some authors suggest 10 to 20 vials of Digibind should be used. In a **chronic** ingestion 5 to 10 vials of Digibind will be appropriate in well over 90% to 95% of cases, although in practice a reduced dose may be adequate (4).

   c.   For patients who have ingested bufadienolides (as seen in traditional Chinese herbal medicines and in street drugs) and other plant cardiac glycosides empiric administration of 10 vials of Digibind should be given to symptomatic patients (8).

   d.   Digoxin-specific Fab fragments can be administered as a bolus over 5 min if cardiac arrest is imminent. Otherwise, this agent is to be given IV over 20 to 30 min through a 0.22 micron Millipore filter (32).

5.   Post immunotherapy treatment

   a.   **Digoxin levels:** After treatment with Fab fragments, the serum digoxin level will rise considerably, reflecting digoxin-Fab complexes from the extravascular compartment (i.e. skeletal muscle). Consequently, serum digoxin level cannot be used as a guide to treatment after administration of the Fab fragments. Free digoxin levels can be used, but most hospitals do not have this assay available (38,39).

   b.   **Adverse affects**

   (i)   The elimination half life of the digoxin Fab complex is between 20 to 30 h, although clearance is directly related to the glomerular filtration rate and is consequently prolonged in renal insufficiency. It is possible to have **recrudescence** of digoxin toxicity since the Fab complexes are eliminated more rapidly than digoxin's release from tissue binding sites (40).

   (ii)   Significantly, in a chronic user who requires Fab treatment for digoxin toxicity, administration can precipitate worsening **heart failure** by removing digoxin's beneficial inotropic activity, hypokalemia, and **atrial arrhythmia with rapid ventricular response. Hypokalemia** occurred in patients who were treated with standard therapy as well as Fab fragments. Clinically adverse phenomena have occurred in less than 10% of patients treated with immunotherapy (21,32,40,41,42,43).

   (iii)   Other untoward effects of digibind include anaphylaxis and serum sickness, as it is a foreign protein. These reactions are quite uncommon, and in one study of 717 patients only 0.8% had evidence of an allergic reaction, none of which were serious. Allergy to Fab fragments are associated with patients who have multiple allergies (17,32).

G. Hemodialysis. Hemodialysis and peritoneal dialysis do not effectively treat digoxin overdose due to the drug's large volume of distribution and its molecular weight, nor do they effectively remove Fab-digoxin complexes because of their large complex size. Digitoxin is not dialyzed well because of its extensive serum protein binding. In some studies continuous arteriovenous hemofiltration has been reported to decrease digoxin levels, but because of the availability and ease of using Digibind, it is probably unnecessary (41).

H. Specific patient populations

   1. Renal failure

      a. As noted above digoxin and digoxin-Fab complex excretion is directly related to the glomerular filtration rate (GFR). As GFR decreases, the elimination half life of both digoxin and Fab fragments are prolonged. In renal failure, recrudescence of digoxin toxicity can extend up to 14 days after Fab fragments are administered. **Retreatment** may be necessary.

      b. Electrolyte levels are always of great concern in renal patients exhibiting dysrhythmias. Potassium, calcium and magnesium levels should be checked. As an indicator of significant toxicity, the serum potassium if of less value in this setting than in a patient with normal renal function. Standard therapeutics for hyperkalemia should be instituted in the end staged renal patient. Digoxin-specific Fab fragments will decrease serum potassium in digoxin intoxication. Hemodialysis may need to be considered. Magnesium should be administered judiciously, if at all, in the patient with renal failure.

   2. Pediatric patients

      a. Digoxin is commonly used in the treatment of SVTs and CHF in infants and children and has been utilized successfully in both direct and indirect treatment of sustained fetal tachycardia. Because of both dose variations of digoxin in different age groups as well as accidental overdosage (especially in children under 6 years of age), the pediatric population is at risk for toxicity. The pediatric history is notoriously inaccurate and treatment with digoxin-specific Fab complexes should be based on the criteria noted above (see **VI.F.3**).

      b. Treatment of digoxin toxicity in infants and children is similar to that of adults. Children with healthy hearts appear to be more resistant than adults to digoxin toxicity, and children who do become ill either have taken massive overdoses or have preexisting cardiac disorders.

      c. Therapy is not unlike that in adults—GI decontamination (lavage, charcoal) and supportive care are the initial stages of management. Frequent vital signs, serial ECGs, and measurement of electrolytes and renal function should be undertaken. Antidysrhythmics and pacemaker therapy have been used in the pediatric population. Fab fragments can be administered safely, although hypokalemia following administration may occur. An ingestion of greater than 0.3 mg/kg or a total of 4 mg probably portends a life threatening illness. In adolescents and children with preexisting heart disease a lower threshold for digoxin-specific Fab treatment can be used (37,45,46).

3. **Digoxin in pregnancy.** Digoxin is widely used in the acute management and prophylaxis of fetal paroxysmal SVT as well as in rate control of atrial fibrillation. It is a **Category C** drug. Increased digoxin dosage may be necessary during pregnancy because of enhanced renal clearance and expanded blood volume. No series has been published regarding toxicity in the pregnant female. Digoxin-specific Fab fragments can be used in pregnancy, with the caveat that careful monitoring of the fetus must be maintained (47,48).

VII. **Disposition**

A. **Admission** criteria for patients with digoxin toxicity should include anyone with the following:

1. Rising digoxin levels
2. ECG conduction abnormalities associated with digoxin
3. Dysrhythmias
4. Any symptomatic patient with or without a toxic serum digoxin level
5. Any patient who has received digoxin-specific Fab fragments. This includes patients with mild, chronic toxicity who respond to treatment in the Emergency Department.
6. There is no absolute digoxin level requiring admission; however, elevated serum digoxin levels without associated symptoms may require hospitalization and central telemetry because a proven steady state level may require 12 h of observation. Poison control should be contacted.

B. Hospitalized patients will require frequent vital signs, close monitoring of serum electrolytes and renal function, serial ECGs and a monitored bed. **ICU** admission is appropriate in acute ingestions, an unclear diagnosis, or if Fab fragment use is anticipated. As noted above, digoxin levels may be misleading if Fab fragments have been administered and in many hospitals Fab use will require an ICU admission. These criteria are for both the adult and pediatric population. Step down units with central telemetry may be utilized for patients suffering chronic toxicity and who are merely bradycardic but otherwise hemodynamically stable.

C. In chronic digoxin users, patients can be safely redigitalized after it can be demonstrated by serum measurements that digoxin-specific Fab fragments have been eliminated and that there is no ECG or clinical evidence of a recrudescence of toxicity. This will require several days to 2 weeks in a patient with impaired renal function and up to 1 week in a patient with normal renal function.

D. Patients can be **medically cleared** from the Emergency Department if they demonstrate both a lack of clinical manifestations *and* a falling digoxin level within a therapeutic range. Generally, one must wait 6 to 12 h until one can demonstrate an accurate steady state level. Patients can be discharged from inpatient status if they similarly demonstrate a falling and therapeutic level, as well as no systemic toxicity.

References

1. Soldin SJ. Digoxin—issues and controversies. *Clin Chem* 1986;32:5–12.
2. Smith TW, Antman EM, Friedman PL, Blatt CM, Marsh JD. Digitalis glycosides: mechanisms and manifestations of toxicity. Part 1. *Prog Cardiovasc Dis* 1984;26:413–458.

3. Rose A, Valdes R Jr. Understanding the sodium pump and its relevance to disease. *Clin Chem* 1994;40:1674–1685.
4. Bayer MJ. Recognition and management of digitalis intoxication: implications for emergency medicine. *Am J Emerg Med* 1991;9:29–34.
5. Kwan T, Paiusco AD, Kohl L. Digitalis toxicity caused by toad venom. *Chest* 1992;102:949–950.
6. Kelly R, Smith TW. Is ouabain the endogenous digitalis? *Circulation* 1992;86:694–697.
7. Radford DJ, et al. Immunological detection of cardiac glycosides in plants. *Aust Vet J* 1994;71:236–238.
8. Deaths associated with a purported aphrodisiac—New York City, February 1993 to May 1995. *JAMA* 1995;274:1828–1829.
9. Smith TW. Digitalis: mechanisms of action and clinical use. *N Engl J Med* 1988;318:358–365.
10. Smith TW, Antman EM, Friedman PT, Blatt CM, Marsh JD. Digitalis glycosides: mechanisms and manifestations of toxicity—part 2. *Prog Cardiovasc Dis* 1984;26(5):495–540.
11. Vitarelli A, et al. A reexamination of the hemodynamic effects of digitalis relative to ventricular dysfunction. *Cardiology* 1995;86:94–101.
12. Gilman AG, Rall TW, Nies AS, Palmer T, ed. *The pharmacological basis of therapeutics*. New York: Pergamon Press, 1990.
13. Lewis RP. Clinical use of serum digoxin concentrations. *Am J Cardiol* 1992;69:97G–107G.
14. Krisanda TJ. Digitalis toxicity. *Postgrad Med* 1992;91:273–282.
15. Piergies AA, Worwag EM, Atkinson AJ. A concurrent audit of high digoxin plasma levels. *Clin Pharmacol Ther* 1994;55:353–358.
16. Magnani B, Malini P. Cardiac glycosides: drug interactions of clinical significance. *Drug Safety* 1995;12:97–109.
17. Kelly RA, Smith TW. Recognition and management of digitalis toxicity. *Am J Cardiol* 1992;69:108G–119G.
18. Kernan WN, et al. Incidence of hospitalization for digitalis toxicity among elderly Americans. *Am J Med* 1994;96:426–431.
19. Aronson JK, Hardman M. Digoxin. *BMJ* 1992;305:1149–1152.
20. Lip GYH, Metcalfe MJ, Dunn FG. Diagnosis and treatment of digoxin toxicity. *Postgrad Med J* 1993;69:337–339.
21. Taboulet P, Baud FJ, Bismuth C. Clinical features and management of digitalis poisoning—rationale for immunotherapy. *J Toxicol Clin Toxicol* 1993;31:247–260.
22. Moorman JR, Pritchett EL. The arrhythmias of digitalis intoxication. *Arch Intern Med* 1985;145:1289–1292.
23. Marchlinski FE, Hook BG, Callans DJ. Which cardiac disturbances should be treated with digoxin immune Fab (ovine) antibody? *Am J Emerg Med* 1991;9:24–28.
24. Smith H, Janz TG, Erker M. Digoxin toxicity presenting as altered mental status in a patient with severe chronic obstructive lung disease. *Heart Lung* 1992;21:78–80.
25. Howanitz PJ, Steindel SJ. Digoxin therapeutic drug monitoring practices. *Arch Pathol Lab Med* 1993;117:684–690.
26. Kinley S, Buckley, N. Magnesium sulfate in the treatment of ventricular arrhythmias due to digoxin toxicity. *Clin Toxicol* 1995;33:55–59.
27. Arsenian MA. Magnesium and cardiovascular disease. *Prog Cardiovasc Dis* 1993;35:271–310.
28. Ibanez C, et al. Activated charcoal increases digoxin elimination in patients. *Int J Cardiol* 1995;48:27–30.
29. Pieroni RE, Fisher JG. Use of cholestyramine resin in digitoxin toxicity. *JAMA* 1981;245:1939–1940.
30. Taboulet P, Baud FJ, Bismuth C, Vicaut E. Acute digitalis intoxication—is pacing still appropriate? *J Toxicol Clin Toxicol* 1993;31:261–273.
31. Woolf A. Editorial comment: revising the management of digitalis poisoning. *J Toxicol Clin Toxicol* 1993;31:275–276.
32. Antman EM, et al. Treatment of 150 cases of life-threatening digitalis intoxication with digoxin-specific Fab antibody fragments. *Circulation* 1990;81:1744–1752.
33. Rich SA, Libera JM, Locke RJ. Treatment of foxglove extract poisoning with digoxin-specific Fab fragments. *Ann Emerg Med* 1993;22:1904–1907.
34. Clark RF, Selden BS, Curry SC. Digoxin-specific Fab fragments in the treatment of oleander toxicity in a canine model. *Ann Emerg Med* 1991;20:1073–1077.
35. Cheung K, et al. Plant cardiac glycosides and digoxin Fab antibody. *J Paediatr Child Health* 1991;27:312–313.
36. Bosse GM, Pope TM. Recurrent digoxin overdose and treatment with digoxin-specific Fab antibody fragments. *J Emerg Med* 1994;12:179–185.
37. Woolf AD, Wenger TL, Smith TW, Lovejoy FH. Results of multicenter studies of digoxin-specific antibody fragments in managing digitalis intoxication in the pediatric population. *Am J Emerg Med* 1991;9:16–20.
38. Ujhelyi MR, et al. Influence of digoxin immune Fab therapy and renal dysfunction on the disposition of total and free digoxin. *Ann Intern Med* 1993;119:273–277.
39. Smith TW. Review of clinical experience with digoxin immune Fab (ovine). *Am J Emerg Med* 1991;9:1–6.
40. Wenger TL. Experience with digoxin immune Fab (ovine) in patients with renal impairment. *Am J Emerg Med* 1991;9:21–23.
41. Robert S, Ujhelyi MR, Zarowitz BJ. Reinstitution of digoxin after digoxin Fab antibody therapy in a hemodialyzed patient. *Crit Care Med* 1993;21:1585–1587.
42. Clark RF, Barton ED. Pitfalls in the administration of digoxin-specific Fab fragments. *J Emerg Med* 1994;12:233–234.

43. Hickey AR, et al. Digoxin immune Fab in the management of digitalis intoxication: safety and efficacy results in an observational surveillance study. *J Am Coll Cardiol* 1991;17:590–598.

44. Nuwayhid N, Johnson GF. Digoxin elimination in a functionally anephric patient after digoxin-specific Fab fragment therapy. *Ther Drug Monit* 1989;11:680–685.

45. Lewander WJ, et al. Acute pediatric digoxin ingestion. *Am J Dis Child* 1986;140:770–773.

46. Woolf AD, Wenger T, Smith TW, Lovejoy FH. The use of digoxin-specific Fab fragments for severe digitalis intoxication in children. *N Engl J Med* 1992;26:1739–1744.

47. Cox JL, Gardner MJ. Treatment of cardiac arrhythmias during pregnancy. *Prog Cardiovasc Dis* 1993;36:137–178.

48. van Engelen AD, et al. Management outcome and follow-up of fetal tachycardia. *J Am Coll Cardiol* 1994;24: 1371–1375.

Emergency Toxicology, Second Edition,
edited by Peter Viccellio.
Lippincott–Raven Publishers, Philadelphia © 1998.

43

Disulfiram

†Maria Micalone and *Rosemarie Carnevale

*†Department of Emergency Medicine, *Pharmacy, Rhode Island Hospital, Providence,
Rhode Island 02903*

I. Introduction

A. Disulfiram is a thiuram disulfide compound that has long been used in the rubber industry and in the treatment of ethanol addiction. First used in the 1950s as an aversive in the treatment of alcoholism, there are currently over 200,000 people prescribed this medication annually.

B. Pure disulfiram overdose is rare and usually inoffensive; however, it can occasionally prove problematic. The most common and serious encounters with disulfiram toxicity result from its interaction with ethanol (1).

II. Available preparations

A. Pharmacological: Disulfiram (Antabuse) is available as a scored tablet in two strengths, 250 and 500 mg. It is used as an alcohol deterrent and has also been advocated in the treatment of nickel dermatitis.

B. Industrial: Thiurams are used by the rubber industry in vulcanization as an accelerator and by the agricultural industry in various fungicides, insecticides, and seed disinfectants. These agents are effective as pesticides because their metabolite, isothiocyanate, inhibits enzyme systems by inactivating sulfhydryl groups.

III. Pharmacology and properties

A. Mechanism of action

1. In ethanolism: Disulfiram alters the intermediary metabolism of ethanol by inhibiting aldehyde dehydrogenase. Ethanol is metabolized to acetaldehyde predominantly in the liver by three enzymatic pathways: alcohol dehydrogenase, microsomal ethanol oxidizing system and catalase. Acetaldehyde is then metabolized by aldehyde dehydrogenase to acetate which in turn can be converted to acetyl coenzyme A to enter the Kreb cycle. This conversion to acetate requires NAD as a cofactor. Disulfiram irreversibly competes with NAD for binding sites on aldehyde dehydrogenase and slows the rate of metabolism of acetaldehyde. The inhibition of aldehyde dehydrogenase is irreversible and recovery of activity requires the synthesis of new enzyme. Acetaldehyde levels may rise five to 10 times higher than normal and result in the adverse effects seen in the "disulfiram-ethanol" reaction (DER) (2,3).

2. Various antihistamine and decongestant preparations, aftershaves, and mouthwashes contain enough ethanol to trigger a reaction. Skin cleansers, shampoos,

lotions or perfumes, which often contain ethanol, may also precipitate a mild systemic reaction or dermal reaction with topical application. Blood ethanol levels as low as 5 mg/dL may induce a reaction (4).

3. In toxicity: Diethyldithiocarbamate (DDC), the major metabolite of disulfiram, chelates copper and other metals which can inhibit several biologic metalloenzymes. An example is dopamine beta-hydroxylase, which, if inhibited, will lead to a reduction in norepinephrine synthesis and an increase in levels of dopamine in the brain. In acute ingestions, this can lead to altered patterns of behavior (e.g., depression, schizophrenia), and hypotension. DDC also inhibits cytochrome P450, which can alter the metabolism of drugs dependent on this system (i.e., phenytoin, barbiturates) (5,6).

4. Carbon disulfide is another metabolite of disulfiram, and is believed to be responsible for the neurologic manifestations seen with chronic disulfiram use and overdose. This metabolite is known to cause pyridoxine depletion which ultimately causes a reduction in GABA activity. This may result in seizures and peripheral neuropathies. Catatonia and parkinsonism suggesting basal ganglia dysfunction has also been described (7).

B. Absorption and distribution

1. The initial dosing regimen is 500 mg daily for 2 weeks followed by a maintenance dose of 125 to 250 mg/day. Therapy should not be initiated until the patient has abstained from alcohol for at least 12 h.

2. Disulfiram is approximately 80% absorbed from the gastrointestinal (GI) tract. Due to its high lipid solubility, it is uniformly distributed into body fats. Disulfiram and its metabolites are highly protein bound.

3. The peak serum level is achieved 6 to 8 h after a dose is taken. The time to peak effect (maximal reaction with ethanol) is approximately 8 to 12 h, when fat and serum equilibrium are reached. The clinical efficacy of disulfiram persists for 7 to 14 days after the last dose.

C. Metabolism and elimination. The majority of disulfiram is converted rapidly to DDC and diethylamine by glutathione reductase located in erythrocytes and the liver. About 50% to 70% of the drug is excreted as metabolites via the kidneys, and up to 20% is eliminated unchanged in the feces. A small percentage of carbon disulfide is eliminated via the lungs (8).

IV. Clinical manifestations. Reports of toxicity from disulfiram have been few despite the large number of patients that are prescribed this medication on an annual basis. The clinical manifestations will vary according to the nature of the ingestion.

A. Acute disulfiram overdose. Disulfiram overdose is rarely deleterious. However, toxic reactions have been described with disulfiram in the absence of other agents. CNS depression and minor GI effects are the most prominent symptoms. Cardiovascular and dermatologic effects as outlined below occur less frequently.

1. **CNS:** The primary manifestations are somnolence and headaches. Neuropathy, paresthesias, peripheral neuritis, and polyneuritis are reported less frequently. Ataxia, dysarthria, dizziness, confusion, and amblyopia may also be seen. In rare cases, coma and death have occurred.

2. **Psychiatric:** Psychiatric manifestations include depression, personality disorders, decreased libido, disorientation, hallucinations, psychosis, and amnesia. These are much more common in patients who have or have had psychiatric disturbances in the past.

3. **GI:** Diarrhea, epigastric pain, and vomiting are the most common presenting symptoms. There may be a sulfur odor or garlic taste in the breath due to the carbon disulfide metabolite.

4. **Cardiovascular:** Hypotension may result from either GI fluid loss or norepinephrine depletion (9).

B. **Disulfiram and children.** Children manifest a symptom complex that is distinct from adults in acute disulfiram overdose. The clinical picture includes increased lethargy, blurred vision, somnolence, difficulty walking, hypotonia, and absent or diminished deep tendon reflexes. These may resemble the encephalopathy seen in Reye's syndrome. Children are very susceptible to the CNS effects and can progress to coma with smaller mg/kg doses than adults. Severe effects may occur with as little as 3 g (8 pills or less). Vomiting, with resultant dehydration and ketosis can occur rapidly. Any symptomatic child, should be admitted for observation because of the potential for delayed reactions (a lag time of 12 h from time of ingestion to onset of symptoms is common) and the tendency for a worse prognosis than adults (10).

C. **Chronic toxicity.** Four organ systems have shown evidence of chronic toxicity, which are partially to fully reversible upon discontinuation of the drug. In the cases studied, treatment with disulfiram ranged from days to years.

1. **Liver:** Minor elevations in transaminases are common, but overt liver failure is rare and idiosyncratic. Maximal effects are seen within the first 6 months of treatment and reversible upon discontinuation. Death from fulminant liver failure has been reported (11).

2. **Neurologic:** This is the most commonly affected system. The incidence slowly increases with treatment periods greater than six months. Toxicities manifest as optic neuritis, headaches, dizziness, ataxia, paresthesias, confusion, polyneuropathy, Parkinsonism, catatonia, and encephalopathy. Partial to full recovery is expected upon discontinuation (7,12).

3. **Dermatologic:** Reactions are seen early with a peak incidence at seven days. Reported effects include exfoliative dermatitis, dermatitis, rash, urticaria, and pruritis.

4. **Psychiatric:** Reported diagnoses are psychoses, memory impairment, sleep disorders, paranoid ideas, emotional lability, and delusions (9,13).

D. **Reproductive.** Disulfiram is pregnancy category X due to reports of congenital anomalies and spontaneous abortion. It is contraindicated in women who are or wish to become pregnant.

E. **Disulfiram–ethanol reaction (DER)**

1. There is no correlation between the amount of ethanol ingested and the severity of the disulfiram-ethanol reaction. The reaction typically begins 5 to 15 min after ingestion of ethanol, but can be delayed for as long as 1 to 2 h. Maximum severity is seen in 20 to 30 min, and recovery is usually within 2 to 4 h. Delayed reac-

tions starting 12 h after ingestion have been reported. A DER may occur up to two weeks after the last dose of disulfiram is taken.

2. Initial symptoms include facial flushing, dizziness and a throbbing headache. With ethanol doses of greater than 0.2 g/kg (48 mL of 80 proof distilled spirits in the average 70 kg man) and a therapeutic disulfiram dose, significant manifestations including protracted vomiting and hypotension may occur and last for up to 90 min. Shock, coma, and death have been reported.

3. EKG findings include sinus tachycardia with occasional PVC's and PACs, and T wave flattening with ST depression.

4. Most DERs are self-limiting, unless secondary complications arise such as dehydration, myocardial infarction, intracranial hemorrhage, or cardiopulmonary collapse. Complications may ultimately lead to coma, seizure, and death if not anticipated and addressed rapidly (14).

F. **Drug-drug interactions.** Concurrent use of disulfiram and metronidazole should be avoided due to reports of visual and auditory hallucinations. The metabolism of paraldehyde and phenytoin is decreased and the biotransformation of warfarin, isoniazid, rifampin, diazepam, and chlordiazepoxide is inhibited. These aforementioned drugs should be used with caution, and the patient should be closely monitored with appropriate laboratory tests (15). For mechanisms of the above interactions (16), see Table 43-1.

G. **Differential Diagnosis**

1. The manifestations of disulfiram overdose are often nonspecific and therefore the differential is broad. One of the most common manifestations is flushing, which may also be seen with allergic reactions, monosodium glutamate ingestion, food poisoning (e.g., scombroid), and certain medications (e.g., niacin, nitrates) (Table 43-2).

2. It is important to make the distinction between a disulfiram overdose, DER, chronic toxic effects of disulfiram. and other substances that may produce disulfiram-like reactions. A large number of drugs cause reactions similar to DER when ingested with ethanol. Most commonly seen disulfiram-like reactions occur with

TABLE 43-1. *Disulfiram-drug interactions*

Drug	Mechanism
Antipyrine	Inhibits hepatic mixed-function oxidase, catalyzed hydroxylation
Benzodiazepines	Decreases clearance, leading to drug accumulation
Coumarin derivatives	Prolongs prothrombin time by decreasing biotransformation of coumarin
Ethylene dibromide	High levels of carcinogenicity and unexplained mortality of rats
Isoniazid	Unknown, leading to neurotoxicity
Metronidazole	Visual and auditory hallucinations
Opioids (morphine, meperidine)	Increase toxicity of central-acting agents
Paraldehyde	Metabolism of this acetaldehyde polymer is blocked at acetaldehyde phase
Phenytoin	Inhibits metabolism, leading to phenytoin toxicity
Primidone	Enhances primidone conversion to phenobarbital
Rifampin	Prolongs half-life of disulfiram

From ref. 16, with permission.

TABLE 43-2. *Drugs that mimic portions of the disulfiram reaction*

Status	Example	Effects
Normotensive	Niacin overdose (without alcohol)	Similar flush without effect on the cardiovascular system
Hypertensive	MAO inhibitors with tyramine (Chianti wine or aged cheese); INH combined with Swiss cheese	Increased stores of norepinephrine
Hypotensive	Chloryl hydrate with ethanol	Vasodilation and tachycardia

Adapted from ref. 16.

metronidazole (up to 24%), cephalosporins, and oral hypoglycemic agents, for which the mechanism is unknown. Sulfonamides and griseofulvin have also been implicated. For a more complete listing (17), see Table 43-3.

3. Other less common precipitants of disulfiram-like reactions include certain mushroom strains (e.g., *Coprinus atramentarius*), pesticides, and industrial chemicals (e.g., trichloroethylene).

4. A review of the drug-drug interaction profile in patients who are on numerous medications and suspected of having a reaction is crucial (18).

V. **Laboratory evaluation.** The diagnosis of disulfiram toxicity or DER is based on clinical and historical data. There is little help to be found through the use of laboratory tests. Disulfiram, its metabolites and acetaldehyde are not readily measured. In studies of disulfiram and DERs, no correlation was found between levels, reaction severity or patient prognosis.

TABLE 43-3. *Agents producing disulfiram-like reactions with ethanol*

Antimicrobial agents
    Cephalosporins (cefoperazone, cefotetan)
    Chloramphenicol
    Diethylthiocarbamate (Imuthiol)
    Furazolidone
    Griseofulvin
    Metronidazole (Flagyl)
    Quinacrine, nitrofurantoin
Industrial agents
    Carbon disulfide
    Hydrogen sulfide
    Tetraethyl lead
    Tetramethylthiuram disulfide
    Trichloroethylene
Oral hypoglycemic agents
    Acetohexamide (Dymelor)
    Chlorpropamide (Diabinese)
    Glipizide (Glucotrol)
    Tolazamide (Tolinase)
    Tolbutamide (Orinase)
Miscellaneous
    Mushrooms (e.g., *Coprinus atramentarius, Clitocybe clavipes*)

From ref. 16, with permission.

However, ethanol levels should be obtained to confirm a DER. Liver function tests should be monitored for chronic exposures. An EKG is necessary in evaluating overdoses and DERs. Electrolytes should be monitored in patients with significant GI fluid loss.

VI. **Management**

A. As with any potentially unstable patient the airway, breathing, and circulation (ABCs) deserve primary assessment and stabilization. Supportive care is the mainstay of treatment in disulfiram overdose and ethanol induced reactions as no antidotes are available. Hypotension is treated with intravenous fluid boluses and norepinephrine in refractory situations (19). Hypotensive patients are unlikely to respond adequately to dopamine because disulfiram inhibits dopamine beta-hydroxylase and prevents its conversion to norepinephrine.

B. Vitamin C and antihistamine therapy have been investigated and are not recommended in therapy.

C. In an acute overdose of disulfiram alone, routine decontamination is recommended. Ipecac is not recommended because it contains a small amount of ethanol which can precipitate a DER. Lavage is recommended if the ingestion is within 2 h. Disulfiram is adsorbed to activated charcoal and its administration is routinely recommended. Activated charcoal and gastric lavage is not recommended in the setting of a DER metoclopramide (adult: 10 mg i.v. every 30 min, max. 1 mg/kg/24 h; pediatric: 0.1 mg/kg i.v. every 30 min, max. 1 to 3 mg/kg/24 h) may be effective in controlling protracted vomiting with a DER.

D. Seizures are to be treated with benzodiazepines, and if uncontrolled, with phenytoin or phenobarbital. Pyridoxine, 1 g i.v., has been used when signs of neurotoxicity (e.g., paresthesias, polyneuropathies, and ataxia) are present. Its efficacy is yet unproven.

E. Methylpyrazol (4-MP) is an inhibitor of alcohol dehydrogenase and may potentially have a role in controlling the symptoms of a DER. Acetaldehyde levels are significantly lower in 4-MP treated patients since the conversion of ethanol to acetaldehyde is inhibited. This agent is currently under investigation for methanol and ethylene glycol poisonings.

F. Enhanced elimination through hemodialysis, hemoperfusion, and forced diuresis is not indicated in the management of these patients.

VII. **Disposition**

A. In disulfiram overdoses without alcohol, all adult patients should be observed for at least 12 h because of the potential for delayed toxicity. They can then be discharged if they remain asymptomatic. All children should be admitted for overnight observation regardless of symptoms because of the higher incidence of both delayed and serious effects (10,20).

B. In DERs, patients should be observed until all clinical effects have cleared, which usually occurs in about 4 h. Any cardiovascular events would mandate admission to a monitored bed.

C. Upon discharge, disulfiram-overdosed and DER patients should be instructed to avoid ethanol use for 14 days. If DER patients wish to restart disulfiram treatment, therapy should not commence for at least 12 h. Psychiatric consultation should be considered when indicated.

References

1. Fuller RK, et al. Disulfiram treatment of alcoholism—a Veterans Administrative Cooperative Study. *JAMA* 1986;256:1449.
2. Rall TW. Hypnotics and sedatives: ethanol. In: Gilman AG, Goodman LS, eds. *The pharmacological basis of therapeutics.* 8th ed. New York: McGraw-Hill, 1990:378–379.
3. Lieber CS. Metabolism and metabolic effects of alcohol. In: Geokas MC, ed. Ethyl alcohol and disease. *Med Clin North Am* 1984;68:3.
4. Becker C. The alcoholic patient as a toxicologic emergency. In: Haddad LM, Winchester JF, eds. *Clinical management of poisoning and drug overdose.* Philadelphia: WB Saunders, 1983.
5. Eneanya DI, et al. The actions and metabolic fate of disulfiram. *Ann Rev Pharmacol Toxicol* 1981;21:575–579.
6. Sellers EM, Naranjo CA, Peachey JE. Drugs to decrease alcohol consumption. *JAMA* 1981;21:1255–1261.
7. Laplane D, et al. Lesions of the basal ganglia due to disulfiram neurotoxicity. *J Neurol Neurosurg Psychiatr* 1992;55:925–929.
8. Johansson B. A review of the pharmacokinetics and pharmacodynamics of disulfiram and its metabolites. *Acta Psychiatr Scand* 1992;86:15–26.
9. Enghusen PH, et al. Disulfiram therapy—adverse drug reactions and interactions. *Acta Psychiatr Scand* 1992;86:59–66.
10. Benitz WE, Tatro DS. Disulfiram intoxication in a child. *Pediatrics* 1984;105:487.
11. Forns X, et al. Disulfiram-induced hepatitis. Report of four cases and review of the literature. *J Hepatol* 1994;21:853–857.
12. Borrett D, et al. Reversible, late-onset disulfiram-induced neuropathy and encephalopathy. *Ann Neurol* 1985;17:396–399.
13. Daniel DG, Swallows A, Wolff F. Capgras delusion and seizures in association with therapeutic dosages of disulfiram. *South Med J* 1987;12:1577–1579.
14. Linden CH, Kulig K, Rumack BH. Disulfiram. *Top Emerg Med* 1984;6:30.
15. Hansten PD. *Drug interactions.* 3rd ed. Philidelphia: Lea & Febiger, 1976:156–161.
16. Goldfrank LR, et al. Disulfiram and disulfiram like reactions. In: Goldfranks LR, et al., eds. *Goldfrank's toxicologic emergencies.* 5th ed. Norwalk, CT: Appleton & Lange, 1994:903.
17. Rosa DA. Interactions between drugs and nutrients. *Med Clin North Am* 1979;63:985–1007.
18. Goldfrank LR, et al. Disulfiram. In: Goldfrank LR, et al., eds. *Goldfrank's toxicologic emergencies.* 3rd ed. East Norwalk, CT: Appleton-Century-Crofts, 1986:475–480.
19. Motte S, et al. Refractory hyperdynamic shock associated with alcohol and disulfiram. *Am J Emerg Med* 1986;4:323.
20. Ellenhorn MJ, Barceloux DG. Disulfiram. In: Ellenhorn MJ, Barceloux DG, eds. *Medical toxicology—diagnosis and treatment of human poisoning.* New York: Elsevier Science, 1988.

Emergency Toxicology, Second Edition,
edited by Peter Viccellio.
Lippincott–Raven Publishers, Philadelphia © 1998.

44

Antihistamines

†Adam J. Singer, °Warren L. Fisher, *Diane Sauter, and †Peter Viccellio

*†Department of Emergency Medicine, State University of New York at Stony Brook, University Hospital, Stony Brook, New York 11794-7400; °Seattle, Washington 98103; *Metropolitan Hospital, New York, New York 10029*

I. **Introduction.** Antihistamines are among the most commonly used medications in the world. To date, three histamine receptors have been described: H1 receptors play an important role in inflammation and allergic reactions, H2 receptors are important in gastric acid secretion, and H3 receptors are involved in the feedback control of histamine synthesis and release (1,2). Histamine receptors have been cloned and shown to belong to the superfamily of G protein-coupled receptors. Generally, poisoning from the antihistamines presents as two common forms: peripheral or central anticholinergic toxicity, or cardiovascular toxicity. The specific agent and the route of delivery will determine which of these findings will be paramount. With first generation H1 antagonists, central and peripheral anticholinergic toxicity predominates; rarely, a wide-complex tachycardia occurs. Major toxicity from second generation H1 antagonists results from QTc prolongation and Torsades de pointes. Toxicity with H2 antagonists is rare. However, bradycardia and hypotension have been reported with i.v. administration of high doses. Currently, H3 antagonists are available only for research purposes. Although most exposures to antihistamines are benign, serious toxicity and death have occurred (3,4). During the years 1985 to 1994, there were 104 deaths among 244,727 cases of antihistamine ingestion reported to the American Association of Poison Control Centers, of which 19 were isolated ingestions (5).

II. **Available preparations**

A. Antihistamines are divided into two main categories, H1-receptor-blocking agents and H2-receptor-blocking agents. H1 antagonists are used for treating allergic states, as sedatives, as antinauseants, and for preventing motion sickness (1,2). H2 antagonists are used to reduce stomach acidity, and recently have been increasingly utilized in the treatment of allergic reactions (6).

B. Antihistamines are found in many over-the-counter (OTC) preparations in combination with analgesics, sympathomimetics, caffeine, anticholinergics, and ethanol. Various combinations of these drugs are packaged as cough syrups, common cold remedies, and sleep medications. Parenteral forms are available for diphenhydramine, hydroxyzine, brompheniramine, and chlorpheniramine as well as all of the H2 antagonists.

C. Classification of the antihistamines appears in Table 44-1.

III. **Pharmacology and properties**

A. **Mechanism of action**

1. **H1 antagonists** are competitive antagonists of histamine at the H1 receptor site. Their major therapeutic effects are alleviation of histamine induced allergic reactions

TABLE 44-1. *Classification and characteristics of antihistamines*

Drug	Preparations	Duration	Major characteristics
First generation agents			
Ethanolamines			Anticholinergic effects, sedation,
Carbinoxamine	Oral	3–4 h	weak GI effect
Clemastine	Oral		
Dimenhydranate	Oral, injection	4–6 h	
Diphenhydramine	Oral, injection, topical	4–6 h	
Ethylenediamines			Strong GI effects, weak CNS effects
Pyrilamine	Oral	4–6 h	
Tripelennamine	Oral	4–6 h	
Alkylamines			CNS stimulation
Bropheniramine	Oral, injection	4–6 h	
Chlorpheniramine	Oral, injection	4–6 h	
Piperazines			Antiemetic effects, CNS depression
Cyclizine	Oral, injection	4–6 h	
Meclizine	Oral	12–24 h	
Hydroxyzine	Oral, injection	6–24 h	
Phenothiazines			Significant anticholinergic effects
Promethazine	Oral, injection, rectal	4–6 h	
Second generation agents			
Piperadines			Nonsedating, cardiotoxic
Astemazole	Oral	>24 h	
Terfenadine	Oral	12–24 h	
Loratidine	Oral	24 h	
Levocabastine	Topical	16–24 h	
Piperazines			Prolonged duration of action,
Cetrizine	Oral	12–24 h	antiemetic effects
Alkylamines			
Acrivastine	Oral	6–8 h	—

and sedation. The toxic effects of the H1 antagonists include the anticholinergic syndrome and cardiac membrane stabilization. First generation H1 antagonists may also affect cholinergic, serotonergic, and alpha-adrenergic receptors.

    a. **Allergic reactions** H1 receptor antagonists block histamine's ability to cause bronchoconstriction, vasodilation, edema, and pruritis (1).

    b. **CNS** effects include both stimulation and depression. Therapeutic doses typically result in sedation, whereas toxic levels may result in central excitation and psychomotor agitation. The mechanism by which antihistamines produce these effects is not well understood. H1 antagonists have been shown to be effective in countering motion sickness, possibly due their muscarinic blocking activity. The low central nervous system effects of the second generation H1 antagonists is probably due to inability of these agents to penetrate the blood brain barrier (7).

    c. **Anticholinergic effects.** Many H1 antagonists inhibit muscarinic acetylcholine (ACh) receptors. Second generation agents, such as terfenadine and astemizole, have no effect on muscarinic ACh receptors (7).

2. **H2 antagonists** are competitive antagonists of histamine at the H2 receptor site. Their major therapeutic effects include inhibition of gastric acid secretion and alleviation of histamine induced allergic reactions. The toxic effects of the H2 receptor antagonists are essentially limited to their cardiotoxic effects. These include inhibition of atrial H2 receptors, inhibition of H2 mediated coronary vasodilation, and unopposed H1 cardiac activity (1). These agents may also cause confusion, particularly in the elderly.

   a. **Gastric secretion.** H2-receptor antagonists are reversible, competitive antagonists of the actions of histamine on H2 receptors of gastric parietal cells (6). They cause suppression of daytime and nocturnal basal gastric acid secretion. They also inhibit gastric acid secretion stimulated by food, histamine, pentagastrin, caffeine, and insulin (8). The H2-receptor antagonists have no consistent effect on the rate of gastric emptying, pressure of the lower esophageal sphincter, or pancreatic secretion (9).

   b. **Allergic reactions.** These drugs have also been shown to be effective for the treatment of allergic reactions (10).

B. **Pharmacokinetics** (Table 44-1)

   1. **H1 antagonists** are well absorbed by mouth. Peak concentrations are achieved within 2 to 3 h. Effects usually last 4 to 6 h but may be much longer for meclizine, hydroxyzine, and the second generation H1 antagonists due to active metabolites. H1 antagonists are widely distributed throughout the body. Antihistamines are converted to active or inactive metabolites in the liver and excreted mainly in the urine. In children drug elimination is more rapid; in liver disease it is prolonged. The second generation H1 antagonists are agents with greatly reduced CNS penetration and a prolonged duration of action.

   2. **H2 antagonists** have little to no effect on H1 receptors. They are well absorbed by mouth, with peak concentrations reached within 1 to 2 h. The half-life for cimetidine, famotidine, and ranitidine is 2 to 3 h. Renal excretion is the major route of elimination of H2-receptor antagonists. Cimetidine and, to a lesser extent, ranitidine undergo hepatic metabolism as well. Severe liver dysfunction may result in a prolonged elimination half-life.

C. **Drug interactions**

   1. Use of macrolide antibiotics and antifungal imidazoles increase the levels of terfenadine and astemazole and may increase the risk of Torsades de pointes (11,12). Concurrent use of alcohol or benzodiazepines enhances the sedative effect of H1 antagonists (13).

   2. Cimetidine and other H2 antagonists inhibit the cytochrome P450 system, thereby prolonging the half-life of drugs dependent on cytochrome P450 breakdown, including warfarin, phenytoin, theophylline, phenobarbital, benzodiazepines, digitoxin, propranolol, ketoconazole, and tricyclic antidepressants (14,15).

IV. **Clinical presentation**

A. **H1 antagonists**

   1. **General.** H1 antagonists are rarely ingested for suicidal purposes and have a high therapeutic/toxic dose ratio. However, a large number of OTC preparations sold as

sedative-hypnotics contain antihistamines with significant anticholinergic activity. These are readily available in large amounts and are a common source of accidental intoxications in children. Since many of the antihistamines are part of a mixed preparation (i.e., contain aspirin, acetaminophen, or alcohol), it is sometimes more important for the physician to exclude these toxicities than to evaluate antihistamine toxicity.

   a. The most frequent toxic effect, sedation (16,17), is common to all first generation H1 antagonists (7). Concurrent ingestion of alcohol or other CNS depressants produces an additive sedating effect (13). Onset of symptoms is usually between 30 min and 2 h after ingestion. Interestingly, there have been reports of anticholinergic withdrawal presenting as cholinergic toxicity in patients who have stopped taking antihistamines (18).

   b. High doses of the second generation H1 antagonists have rarely been associated with quinidine-like effects, including QT interval prolongation, and Torsades de pointes (19–20). Concomitant use of macrolide antibiotics (erythromycin and troleandomycin) and imidazole antifungals, which inhibit the hepatic cytochrome P450 enzyme system, has resulted in toxic levels of terfenadine and astemazole with resulting Torsades de pointes (11,12). Massive ingestions of diphenhydramine have rarely been reported to cause wide-complex tachycardias and circulatory collapse (21).

   c. Inappropriate use of topical Caladryl® lotion (diphenhydramine 1%, alcohol 2%, and menthol 2%) for a rash has rarely caused an acute organic psychosis in children (22,23).

2. **Symptoms** range from mild CNS excitation and psychomotor agitation (more common in children) to CNS depression, hyperpyrexia, convulsions, and death. Convulsions are ominous, as the convulsant dose is near the lethal dose. Adults usually present with lethargy followed by CNS excitation. Patients may also complain of symptoms referable to anticholinergic effects, including blurred vision, diplopia, dry mouth, chest tightness, nausea, constipation, and urinary retention. Patients who develop Torsades de pointes may present with syncope.

3. **Physical examination**

   a. **Anticholinergic effects.** Findings are similar to those seen with an anticholinergic overdose. Vital signs may show hyperpyrexia due to psychomotor agitation, tachycardia, and hypertension. Urinary retention, delirium, fixed and dilated pupils, blurred vision, diplopia, and dry mouth and nose are other manifestations.

   b. **CNS effects** may include either sedation, coma, psychomotor agitation, or seizures. Signs of CNS excitation (including seizures) are more common in young children. Dystonic reactions, dyskinesia, and choreoathetosis have also been reported (24–26). Cyproheptadine, which has antiserotonergic effects as well as predominantly central anticholinergic effects, possess significant potential for CNS toxicity.

   c. **GI effects.** Although nausea, vomiting, and diarrhea all may be seen with antihistamine overdose, the most significant toxic effect is adynamic ileus.

      d. Cardiovascular effects. Massive diphenhydramine overdose has been reported to cause myocardial depression and QRS widening presenting with syncope (21). QT prolongation resulting in Torsades de pointes with loss of consciousness has been described with ingestion of terfenadine and astemazole particularly in patients taking erythromycin, ketoconazole, or another cytochrome P450 enzyme inhibitor (11,12,19,20).

B. H2 antagonists

    1. H2 antagonists have not been implicated in suicide fatalities and most ingestions are benign (27,28). Ingestion of up to 20 g of cimetidine has produced only mild to moderate toxic manifestations (29). One death due to ingestion of 24 g of cimetidine in a 39-year-old woman has been reported (30).

    2. Significant cardiotoxicity, including bradycardia, hypotension, and even sinus arrest have been reported with several H2 receptor antagonists, especially with i.v. administration of high doses (31,32).

    3. CNS symptoms are rare but appear to be more common among the elderly and those with hepatic and renal disease. Symptoms include a spectrum from drowsiness and lethargy to agitation, hallucinations, and seizures.

    4. Rarely, cimetidine use has been associated with reversible bone marrow suppression, hepatitis, and anaphylaxis. Experience with the other H2 antagonists is more limited, however, adverse effects are similar to those described with cimetidine.

C. Differential diagnosis. When a patient is encountered with the clinical presentation described, the list of possible offending agents is long and includes all agents that may cause sedation or anticholinergic effects (cyclic antidepressants, antiparkinsonian drugs, antipsychotics, antispasmodics, belladona alkaloids, mydriatics, skeletal muscle relaxants). One must also always consider the possibility of ingestion of multiple drugs, mushrooms, or other toxic plants (e.g., *Datura stramonium*). In young children with presumed febrile seizures without a clear source of infection, one should consider the ingestion of an antihistamine. Careful patient or family history may reveal such an ingestion as the cause of these clinical findings.

V. Laboratory evaluation

A. Electrocardiographic monitoring, especially in patients ingesting a second generation H1 antagonist is essential. Supraventricular as well as ventricular dysrhythmias may be observed. Particular attention should be paid to the QT and QRS intervals.

B. Arterial blood gas results depend on the extent of the intoxication and may show profound metabolic acidosis secondary to hypotension or psychomotor agitation.

C. CBC values are nonspecific, although there are rare reports of antihistaminic ingestion associated with hemolytic anemia and agranulocytosis (33).

D. Rhabdomyolysis has been seen following diphenhydramine and doxylamine ingestions. The effect is attributed to excessive use of muscles from agitation, and/or direct toxicity to the striated muscle by these agents (34,35). Therefore, the presence of myoglobin in the urine should be evaluated with a urine reagent strip.

E. Specific chromatographic assays have been developed to measure blood and urine concentrations of antihistamines but are usually not readily available. Therefore, although confirmatory, blood levels are not helpful for guiding therapy.

F. Assays for commonly co-ingested agents, such as aspirin and acetaminophen, should be considered since most antihistamine products are mixed preparations.

VI. **Treatment.** In general, treatment is supportive. After initial assessment and stabilization, treatment is targeted at reducing the amount of absorbable toxin.

A. In symptomatic patients and those with a history of recent ingestion, **gastric lavage** procedures may be helpful. Due to the anticholinergic effects of antihistamines which decrease gastrointestinal motility, gastric lavage may be useful even beyond the first hour after ingestion. Patients who are not alert enough to protect their airway should have a cuffed endotracheal tube placed prior to gastric lavage.

B. **Activated charcoal and a cathartic** in standard doses should be given to all symptomatic patients and those ingesting a significant amount of any antihistamine.

C. **Psychomotor agitation and seizures** should be treated with a benzodiazepine such as diazepam or lorazepam. If seizures and agitation recur or cannot be controlled with a benzodiazepine, phenytoin or phenobarbital are indicated. Physostigmine should be considered for extreme cases unresponsive to standard therapy.

D. **Dysrhythmias. Sinus tachycardia,** the most common dysrhythmia, requires treatment only in the hemodynamically unstable patient. Initial management is with fluids since many patients are dehydrated. Psychomotor agitation, which contributes to the degree of tachycardia, should be addressed with benzodiazepines prior to initiating treatment with specific antidysrhythmics. Other supraventricular tachyarrhythmias should be managed with standard therapy. Supraventricular tachyarrhythmias resistant to standard medical therapy may respond to physostigmine as described in section G below. Magnesium sulfate 2 g i.v. in adults or 25 to 50 mg/kg in children should be given over 2 to 3 min for **Torsades de pointes.** If no response is observed within 10 min, this dose may be repeated and followed by a continuous infusion of 5 to 10 mg/min in adults and 30 to 60 mg/kg/24 h in children. Isoproterenol, cardioversion, and overdrive pacing may all be required to treat this potentially lethal dysrhythmia. Symptomatic **bradycardia** should be managed with atropine in standard doses or a pacemaker.

E. **Conduction abnormalities.** Patients with QRS interval prolongation (more than 100 ms) should be treated with i.v. boluses of sodium bicarbonate 1 mEq/kg to maintain a serum pH of greater than 7.45 to 7.55 (21).

F. **Hypotension** should be managed with i.v. fluid boluses or vasopressors in refractory states.

G. **Severe anticholinergic toxicity** has rarely been treated with physostigmine, a reversible acetylcholinesterase inhibitor. Indications for physostigmine administration include seizures, hallucinations, psychomotor agitation, and supraventricular tachyarrhythmias unresponsive to other measures. However, physostigmine has significant inherent toxicity and may cause seizures, bronchoconstriction, and asystole. Therefore, physostigmine is to be avoided in patients with either ingestions of agents that can cause cardiac conduction defects (e.g., TCAs), or evidence of QRS/QT prolongation on the ECG. Also, patients with asthma, cardiovascular disease, mechanical bowel obstruction, or active gangrene are not to receive this antidote. Physostigmine should never be used just to keep a comatose patient awake. In adults, physostigmine 2 mg is given i.v. slowly over 5 min. In children 0.02 to 0.05 mg/kg (up to 0.5 mg in children younger than 5) may be given i.v. cautiously. The patient must be on a cardiac monitor and atropine available to reverse symptomatic bradycardia. A second dose of physostigmine may be attempted in patients who fail to respond to the first dose. The administration of physostigmine should be immediately discontinued if the physician observes bradycardia or the patient complains of abdominal pain.

H. Enhanced elimination. For severe, toxic overdoses of H1 antagonists not responding to conventional treatments, various extracorporeal clearance methods, such as hemodialysis, hemoperfusion, peritoneal dialysis, and exchange transfusion, have been attempted. However, true efficacy is questionable given the large volume of distribution of most antihistamines. Hemodialysis and hemoperfusion have been shown to remove significant amounts of cimetidine and ranitidine in experimental overdose settings.

VII. Disposition

A. Admission criteria. All patients with cardiac dysrhythmias (including persistent sinus tachycardia which does not resolve with standard treatment and observation), seizures, or persistently depressed mental status beyond a 6-h observation period should be admitted until symptoms resolve. Adults who ingest more than twice the recommended daily dose of a second generation nonsedating H1 antagonists and children who ingest any amount of the nonsedating antihistamines should be admitted for cardiac monitoring for 24 h regardless of symptoms.

B. Discharge criteria. Patients who are asymptomatic after an observation period, and who have not ingested a significant amount of the nonsedating H1 antagonists may be discharged to home. For the second generation agents, a second ECG at 6 h is required before medical clearance. Admitted patients that have been observed for 24 h and have no evidence of either CNS or cardiovascular toxicity may be medically cleared of this exposure. The regional poison control center or medical toxicologist may be consulted for further questions.

References

1. Babe KS, Serafin WE. Histamine, bradykinin, and their antagonists. In: Hardman JG, Limbird LE, eds. *Goodman and Gilman's. The pharmacological basis of therapeutics.* 9th ed. New York: Pergamon Press, 1996:581.
2. Simons EF, Simons KJ. The pharmacology of the H1 receptor antagonists. *N Engl J Med* 1994;320:1663–1669.
3. Krenzelock EP, Anderson GM, Mirick M. Massive diphenhydramine overdose resulting in death. *Ann Emerg Med* 1982;11:212–213.
4. Winn R, McDonnell KP. Fatality secondary to massive overdose of diphenhydramine. *Ann Emerg Med* 1993; 22:1481–1484.
5. Litovitz TL, Felberg L, Soloway RA, Ford M, Geller R. The 1994 annual report of the American Association of Poison Control Centers Toxic Exposure Surveillance System. *Am J Emerg Med* 1995;13:551–597.
6. Brunton LL. Agents for control of gastric acidity and treatment of peptic ulcers. In: Hardman JG, Limbird LE, eds. *Goodman and Gilman's The pharmacological basis of therapeutics.* 9th ed. New York: Pergamon Press, 1996:901.
7. Kaliner MA. Nonsedating antihistamines: pharmacology, clinical efficacy and adverse effects. *Am Fam Physician* 1992;45:1337–1342.
8. Ostro MJ. Pharmacodynamics and pharmacokinetics of parenteral histamine receptor antagonists. *Am J Med* 1987; 83:15–22.
9. Dobrilla G. H2-antagonists and motility of the upper gastrointestinal tract in man. *Hepatogastroenterology* 1988; 35:30–33.
10. Bleehen SS, Thomas SE, Graves MW, et al. Cimetidine and chlorpheniramine in the treatment of chronic idiopathic urticaria: a multi-centre randomized double blind study. *Br J Dermatol* 1987;117:81–88.

11. Honig PK, Wortham DC, Zamani K, Conner DP, Mullin JC, Cantilena LR Jr. Terfenadine-ketoconazole interaction. *JAMA* 1993;12:1513–1518.
12. Honig PK, Woosley RL, Zamani K, Conner DP, Cantilena LR. Jr. Changes in the pharmacokinetics and electrocardiographic pharmacodynamics of terfenadine with concomitanat administration of erythromycin. *Clin Pharmacol Ther* 1992;52:231–238.
13. Moser L, Huther KJ, Koch-Weser J, Lundt PV. Effects of terfenadine and diphenhydramine alone or in combination with diazepam or alcohol on psychomotor performance and subjective feelings. *Eur J Clin Pharmacol* 1978;14:417–423.
14. Powell JR, Donn K. Histamine H2-antagonist drug interactions in perspective: mechanistic concepts and clinical implications. *Am J Med* 1984;77:56–84.
15. Sedman AJ. Cimetidine-drug interactions. *Am J Med* 1984;76:109–114.
16. Koppel C, Ibe C, Tenczer J. Clinical symptomatology of diphenhydramine overdose: an evaluation of 136 cases in 1982 to 1985. *J Toxicol Clin Toxicol* 1987;25:53–70.
17. Carruthers SG, Shoeman DW, Hignite CE, Azarnoff DL. Correlation between plasma diphenhydramine level and sedative and antihistamine effects. *Clin Pharmacol Ther* 1978;23:375–382.
18. Gualtieri JF, Sioris LJ. Withdrawal syndrome in a child with chronic Bromfed-PD use [Abstract]. *Vet Human Toxicol* 1994;36:348.
19. Craft TM. Torsades de pointes after astemazole overdose. *BMJ* 1986;292:660.
20. Monahan BP, Ferguson CL, Killeavy ES, Lloyd BK, Troy J, Cantilena LR Jr. Torsades de pointes occurring in association with terfenadine use. *JAMA* 1990;264:2788–2790.
21. Clark RF, Vance MV. Massive diphenhydramine poisoning resulting in a wide-complex tachycardia: successful treatment with sodium bicarbonate. *Ann Emerg Med* 1992;21:318–321.
22. Filloux F. Toxic encephalopathy caused by topically applied diphenhydramine. *J Pediatr* 1986;108:1018–1020.
23. Patranella P. Diphenhydramine toxicity due to topical application of Caladryl. *Clin Pediatr* 1986;25:163.
24. Favis GR. Facial dyskinesis related to antihistamine? *N Engl J Med* 1976;294:730.
25. Lavenstein BL, Cantor FK. Acute dystonia: an unusual reaction to diphenhydramine. *JAMA* 1976;236:291.
26. Samie MR, Ashton AK. Choreoathetosis induced by cyproheptadine. *Mov Disord* 1989;4:81–84.
27. Sawyer D, Conner CS, Scalley R. Cimetidine: adverse reactions and acute toxicity. *Am J Hosp Pharmacol* 1981;38:188–197.
28. Krenzelok EP, Litovitz TL, Lippold KP, McNally CF. Cimetidine toxicity: an assessment of 881 cases. *Ann Emerg Med* 1987;17:1216–1221.
29. Illingforth RN, Jarvie DR. Absence of toxicity in cimetidine overdosage. *BMJ* 1979;1:453–454.
30. McMillan MA, Ambis D, Siegel JH. Cimetidine and mental confusion. *N Engl J Med* 1978;298:284.
31. Litovitz TL, Schmitz BF, Baily KN. 1989 annual report of the American Association of Poison Control Centers National Data Collection System. *Am J Emerg Med* 1990;8:394–442.
32. Balestrazzi P, Gregori R, Bevenasconi S, Giovannelli G. Bradycardia and neurologic disorders associated with ranitidine in a child. *Am J Dis Child* 1985;139:442.
33. Hulisz DT, Welko JR, Heiselman DE. Sinus arrest associated with continuous-infusion cimetidine. *Pharmacotherapy* 1993;13:64–67.
34. Hardin AS, Padilla F. Agranulocytosis during therapy with a bromopheniramine-medication. *J Ark Med Soc* 1978; 75:206–208.
35. Koppel C, Ibe K, Oberdisse W. Rhabdomyolysis in doxylamine overdose. *Lancet* 1987;1:442.
36. Hampel G, Horstkotte K, Rumpf KW. Myoglobinuric renal failure due to drug-induced rhabdomyolisis. *Hum Toxicol* 1983;2:197–201.

Emergency Toxicology, Second Edition,
edited by Peter Viccellio.
Lippincott–Raven Publishers, Philadelphia © 1998.

45

Hypoglycemic Agents

Gregory L. Almond

Metropolitan Hospital Center, New York, New York 10029

I. **Introduction.** Oral hypoglycemic medications and insulin are occasionally used in suicide attempts. Although side effects of these medications present commonly, this chapter will specifically address the toxicity of these agents resulting from intentional or nonintentional overdose.

II. **Available preparations.** The sulfonylureas and biguanides comprise the class of medications known as oral hypoglycemic agents. Insulin is the only parenteral agent available for the treatment of hyperglycemia. The sulfonylureas are classified as first- or second-generation agents depending upon potency. The first-generation sulfonylureas include tolbutamide, acetohexamide, tolazamide, and chlorpropamide. The second-generation sulfonylureas include glyburide and glipizide. The potency of these second-generation agents results in an increased risk of severe hypoglycemia. The biguanides include phenformin, metformin, and buformin. Phenformin was once available in the United States, but was removed by the U. S. Food and Drug Administration in 1977 because of its assocation with severe lactic acidosis. Metformin is now available in the United States. Biguanides remain available in other countries. Insulin is available in various preparations and is classified according to onset, peak, and duration of action.

III. **Pharmacology and properties**

A. **Mechanism of action.** The presence of some endogenous insulin is necessary for the hypoglycemic action of the sulfonylureas. All of the toxic effects of the sulfonylureas result from an excess of insulin. Serum insulin levels will be elevated. Sulfonylureas increase the permeability of the cell-membrane to the potassion ion and enhance calcium flux. This results in the depolarization of the β-cell membrane and the release of insulin from the pancreas (1). Sulfonylureas are known to potentiate adenylate cyclase and to inhibit phosphodiesterase in the pancreatic islet cell (2). Hepatic gluconeogenesis is inhibited (3). Insulin sensitivity is enhanced in the peripheral tissues. Suppression of the release of glucagon and somatostatin from the A- and D-cells may indirectly increase insulin secretion (4). Glucose is deposited as glycogen in the liver. Biguanides also require endogenous insulin for their effects, but do not result in an increased insulin level. They induce an increase in peripheral glucose utilization (5) and less glucose absorption from the intestinal tract (6,7). Hepatic gluconeogenesis is decreased (8). A severe lactic acidosis resulting in a mortality of 50% to 70% may occur with the routine use of the biguanides. The mechanisms for the production of lactic acid from biguanides is poorly understood. Lactic acidosis occurs more frequently with phenformin. Most cases of metformin-associated lactic acidosis occur in patients with renal impairment as metformin does not undergo extensive metabolism (9). Insulin produces hypoglycemia by facilitating the transport of glucose into cells. Insulin binds to receptors, which propagate signals that interact with enzymes and glucose transport proteins. It stimulates peripheral glycolysis, inhibits gluconeogenesis, stimulates lipogenesis, inhibits lipolysis and free fatty acid release from adipose cells, stimulates protein synthesis and the metabolism of ketone bodies. Insulin results in hypokalemia as potassium is transported inside the cell with glucose. Counterregulatory hormones including glucagon and epinephrine have opposite effects. Glucagon is released during periods of hypoglycemia or stress and results in the stimulation of cyclic AMP and promotion of glycogenolysis, gluconeogenesis, and ketogenesis.

B. **Absorption and distribution.** The sulfonylureas are rapidly absorbed from the GI tract. They are highly protein bound. All sulfonylureas except chlorpropamide undergo extensive hepatic metabolism. The duration of action varies between 6 and 24 h, except for that of chlorpropamide, which is from 36 to 60 h (Table 45-1). Hypoglycemia is more likely to be fatal when caused by agents with a prolonged half-life (chlorpropamide), with active metabolites (including but not limited to hydroxyhexamide from acetahexamide) (10), or with unusual properties (glibenclamide accumulates progressively in islet tissues) (11). The biguanides are only partially absorbed from the gastrointestinal tract and are less than 20% protein bound in the blood stream. Phenformin is the only biguanide which is metabolized by the liver. The metabolite is inactive. Phenformin is excreted 33% to 66% unchanged, versus buformin and metformin which are excreted 100% unchanged (3). Insulin is rapidly absorbed after parenteral administration. It is distributed throughout extracellular fluid. Approximately 50% of the dose is metabolized by the liver. Less than 2% is excreted unchanged.

C. **Metabolism and elimination.** Even though some sulfonylureas are excreted in bile, chlorpropamide does not undergo extensive enterohepatic recirculation (12). Chlorpropamide is a weak acid, with a pK_a of 4.8. Renal clearance is pH dependent. This explains the variability in the elimination kinetics of chlorpropamide among individuals

TABLE 45-1. *Oral hypoglycemic agents available in the United States*

	Trade name	Duration of Action (h)
First-generation sulphonylureas		
Acetahexamide	Dymelor	12–18
Chlorpropamide	Diabinase	24–72
Tolazamide	Tolinase	16–24
Tolbutamide	Orinase	6–12
Second-generation sulphonylureas		
Glipizide	Micronase, DiaBeta	16–24
Glyburide	Glucotrol	18–24
Biguanides		
metformin	Glucophage	12[a]

[a]From Bristol Meyers and Squibb, Pharmaceutical Division, P.O. Box 4500, Princeton, NJ 08543-4500.

(13,12). Drug interactions are common with the oral agents, but less likely with the second-generation sulfonylureas. These agents have different protein binding sites and displacement by coumarins, heparins, or phenylbutazone is less likely. The disulfiram-ethanol-like reaction does not occur with the second-generation sulfonylureas. Sulfonylureas range in half-life from 3 to 48 h and have a duration of action ranging from 6 to 72 h. Biguanides have shorter half-lives, from 1 to 15 h. Rapid acting insulin preparations have a 5- to 16-h duration of action, intermediate preparations last 18 to 24 h, and long-acting preparations last 24 to 36 h (14).

IV. **Clinical presentation.** Prolonged hypoglycemia may occur with relatively small doses of sulfonylureas in patients with defective metabolic or excretory mechanisms or in those with decreased glycogen stores or in conditions of prolonged and excessive insulin secretion (14). Following an overdose with a hypoglycemic agent, many patients will present with an altered mental status. The appearance of hypoglycemia may be delayed. The physician may be unable to obtain an accurate history. If the mental status is normal and the patient is cooperative, the specifics of the ingestion must be obtained. Any past medical history of liver or kidney disease and substance abuse including alcohol must be obtained. The nutritional status is important for the evaluation of glycogen stores. A list of current medications will allow assessment of possible drug interactions. The combined ingestion of chlorpropamide and alcohol may result in a reaction that is clinically similar to the disulfiram-alcohol-like reaction. Cutaneous flushing with a feeling of warmth spreading from the face to the trunk may occur. The initial signs and symptoms of hypoglycemia result from autonomic hyperactivity and include tremulousness, sweating, and palpitations. Cerebral dysfunction follows with alterations in behavior. The presence of nausea, vomiting, food intolerance, abdominal pain, diaphoresis, and dyspnea is common. The airway may be obstructed as a result of coma, seizure activity or the presence of vomitus. Respiratory function will vary. Tachypnea may be observed early in the course with agonal respirations preterminally. The presence of Kussmaul's respirations may be evidence of an underlying metabolic acidosis. The circulatory status depends on the length and severity of the hypoglycemic insult. The patient's mental status may range from normal (even with abnormally low serum glucose levels) to coma. A hyperactive, agitated, confused, and uncooperative state is common. Crying and poor feeding may be the only symptoms in pediatric exposures. Pupillary changes are variable and focal neurologic findings may be present. However, oculovestibular and oculocephalic reflexes will not be affected. Other manifestations include lethargy, slurred speech, athetoid movements, dysarthria, ataxia, the absence of deep tendon reflexes, and clonus. Seizures are common. Diabetes insipidus may complicate sulfonylurea ingestions (15). Hepatomegaly from glycogen deposition has been reported several days after an acute ingestion of chlorpropamide (16). Drugs which result in displacement from plasma protein binding sites, inhibit hepatic microsomal enzymes, decrease urinary excretion of sulfonylureas, or block the physiologic response to hypoglycemia cause an increased hypoglycemic effect of the sulfonylureas. Those that induce hepatic enzyme systems or inhibit insulin release and action decrease the hypoglycemic effects of sulfonylureas (14).

V. **Differential diagnosis.** Emotionally disturbed persons (EDPs) present to the Emergency Department because of their irrational, agitated, or violent behavior that may be a result of acute hypoglycemia. The psychiatric evaluation should follow an adequate period of observation. Other causes of altered mental status including hypovolemia, head trauma, sedative hypnotic ingestion, infection, uremia, adrenal suppression and cerebrovascular accident must be considered. There are no absolute criteria to distinguish one form of metabolic coma from another (17). Salicylates, alcohol, endocrine abnormalities, tumors, hepatic disease, and other etiologies of hypoglycemia must be considered. Alcoholic hypoglycemia is very common and may occur without the ingestion of hypoglycemic agents. The oxidative metabolism of ethanol results in a decreased NAD/NADH ratio. This altered redox state of the liver results in impaired gluconeogenesis (17). These patients are at a greater risk of hypoglycemia than the normal population when taking hypoglycemic agents.

VI. Laboratory analysis. Frequent measurement of the serum glucose level is mandatory in all patients who overdose with hypoglycemic agents, even those who are initially asymptomatic patients. The presence of glycosuria does not adequately exclude hypoglycemia (17). Electrolytes should be carefully monitored, with hypokalemia being the most common abnormality. The electrocardiogram (EKG) may be consistent with hypokalemia. An overdose of a sulfonylurea may present with hypokalemic metabolic acidosis. Serum ketone levels are usually low as a result of high insulin levels secondary to inhibited fatty acid metabolism. A complete blood count with a leukocytosis as high as 20,000 may be present as a result of stress and catecholamine release. An electroencephalogram (EEG) may be necessary to exclude posthypoglycemic encephalopathy for patients who have a persistently abnormal mental status following treatment with i.v. glucose. CSF glucose may be low for several hours after the serum glucose has returned to normal. Serum levels of various hypoglycemic agents are available but are useful only for confirmation of the ingestion. The clinical status may not correlate with serum levels. Patients who are injecting themselves with insulin may develop antibodies to insulin within 2 months. While not a part of the acute evaluation, testing for antibodies to insulin will be useful to evaluate for factitious hypoglycemia. Exogenous insulin-induced hypoglycemia is diagnosed if C-peptide levels are less than 0.5 ng/mL. Patients with hypoglycemia secondary to insulinoma will have the presence of C-peptide levels, as will patients with hypoglycemia secondary to sulfonylurea-stimulated insulin production.

VII. Management. Unless adequately treated, a significant overdose of any hypoglycemic agent may result in coma and death. In those that survive, permanent neurological deficits may occur consistent with delayed treatment. All patients with abnormalities of the vital signs require immediate stabilization. Assessment of the ABCs must include assessment for hypoglycemia. Any patient with altered mental status should be treated immediately with 50 cc of 50% glucose i.v. bolus after blood has been drawn for a dextrostick and serum glucose level. Thiamine (100 mg i.v. push) should be given concurrently. Pregnancy is not a contraindication to the administration of thiamine. Respiratory insufficiency or coma with pinpoint pupils may be treated with naloxone (0.5 to 2.0 mg i.v. push). Hypotension can be treated by placing the patient in Trendelenburg's position with the administration of isotonic intravenous fluids, followed by dopamine or norepinephrine if needed. Hypothermia is common with hypoglycemia. If the hypothermia is mild, active rewarming is not necessary (17). Seizures require the intravenous administration of diazepam. If seizures are caused by hypoglycemia, glucose is the drug of choice. Evaluation for structural and systemic metabolic disorders responsible for altered mental status and seizures is necessary.

Glucagon 1 to 2 mg i.m. should be considered for patients with difficult i.v. access or with severe pronounced hypoglycemia not responding to intravenous dextrose. Glucagon promotes glycogen breakdown and the release of glucose from the liver. Patients with inadequate glycogen stores (malnutrition, alcoholism, defective carbohydrate metabolism) may not benefit from glucagon (17). The use of glucagon in patients with sulfonylurea overdoses is controversial because glucagon's effects are short-lived and it may later increase insulin secretion (18). If a large ingestion has occurred, consider gastric lavage with a 40-French orogastric tube in the adult after the airway is secured. Activated charcoal at 1 g/kg with a cathartic should be administered orally or by nasogastric tube. Since most sulfonylurea drugs are poorly soluble at the normal gastric pH, charcoal should be administered even if the time since ingestion has been several hours. The more potent second-generation sulfonylureas may require a larger initial dose of charcoal to prevent saturation of the adsorption sites on the charcoal (19). Enterohepatic circulation of chlorpropamide has been demonstrated (20), therefore repeated doses of activated charcoal might benefit the symptomatic patient. D10W should be infused peripherally to keep the serum glucose levels normal. If higher concentrations of dextrose solution are needed, a central line access must be used to prevent the thrombophlebitis associated with these hyperosmolar fluids. Severely hypoglycemic patients may require D20 supplemented with boluses of D50 (17). Once the patient is able to tolerate food, he should be placed on a high carbohydrate diet. The i.v. fluids should be tapered to D5W as serum levels allow (17). Diazoxide (Hyperstat) is an antihypertensive agent that was noted to cause hyperglycemia and has been used for patients with sulfonylurea overdoses. It is indicated for patients with oral hypoglycemic agent overdose with hypoglycemia refractory to dextrose therapy. Diazoxide inhibits the release of insulin from the pancreas and raises the concentration of glucose in the plasma (21). Diazoxide can be given 300 mg p.o. q4h in the noncritical adult patient. Pediatric patients should receive 1 to 3 mg/kg/dose i.v. to a maximum dose of 150 mg. In the critical patient, the same dose can be given i.v. over 30 min q4h (18). The slow i.v. infusion of diazoxide should not result in hypotension (22). Adrenal suppression may cause hypoglycemia and is treated with 100 mg of hydrocortisone sodium succinate i.v. bolus. Alkalinization of the urine enhances the elimination of chlorpropamide by ion trapping. Such therapy is indicated in symptomatic exposures. With an adequate urine flow and a urine pH of 8, the half-life of chlorpropamide can be shortened to 5 to 10 h. Sulfonylureas cross the placenta and result in hypoglycemia in the newborn after delivery. Frequent glucose monitoring is indicated.

VIII. **Disposition.** The following patients presenting with hypoglycemia must be admitted (17): oral hypoglycemic agent, ethanol, or long-acting insulin; medical history for hepatic or renal failure; malnutrition; and of unknown etiology. Any patient who presents for a second time for hypoglycemia from any agent should be admitted for further metabolic evaluation. All suicide attempts, victims of attempted homicide, and child abuse cases should be admitted. Individuals with potentially self-induced factitious hypoglycemia must be admitted, as well. Any massive insulin overdose must be admitted even when serum glucose levels are normal. Uncomplicated nonintentional short-acting and intermediate-acting insulin overdoses do not require admission after an adequate period of observation and treatment. Patients with oral hypoglycemic ingestions may be medically cleared only after prolonged observation (at least 24 h) if they then have no signs of hypoglycemia.

References

1. Campbell RK, Hansten PD. Metabolism of chlopropamide, correspondence. *Diabetes Care* 1981;4:332.
2. Pendergast BD. Glyburide and glipizide. Second-generation oral sulfonylurea hypoglycemic agents. *Clin Pharm* 1984;31:473–485.
3. Asmal AC, Marble A. Oral hypoglycaemic agents. An update. *Drugs* 1984;28:62–78.
4. Melander A, Wahlin-Boll E. Clinical pharmacology of glipizide. *Am J Med* 1983;75:41–45.
5. Butterfield WJH, Whichelow JJ. The hypoglycemic action of phenformin. Effect of phenformin on glucose metabolism in peripheral tissues. *Diabetes* 1962;11:281–286.
6. Czyzyk A, Tawecki J, Sadowski J, et al. Effect of biguanides on intestinal absorption of glucose. *Diabetes* 1968; 17:492–498.
7. Schafer G. Some new aspects on the interaction of hypoglycemia producing biguanides with biological membranes. *Biochem Pharmacol* 1976;25:2015–2034.
8. Haeckel R, Haeckel H. Inhibition of gluconeogenesis from lactate by phenylethylbiguanide in the perfused guinea pig liver. *Diabetologia* 1972;8:117–124.
9. Campbell IW. Metformin and the sulphonylureas: comparative risks. *Hormone Metab Res* 1985;15:105–111.
10. Ferner RE, Chaplin S. The relationship between the pharmacokinetics and pharmacodynamic effect of oral hypoglycaemic drugs. *Clin Pharm* 1987;12:379–401.
11. Hellman B, Sehlin J, Taljedal IB. Glibenclamide is exceptional among hypoglycaemic agents in accumulating progressively in B-cell rich pancreatic islets. *Acta Endocrinol* 1984;105:385–390.
12. Neuvonen PJ, Kärkkäinen S. Effects of charcoal, sodium bicarbonate and ammonium chloride on chlorpropamide kinetics. *Clin Pharmacol Ther* 1983;33:386–393.
13. Neuvonen PJ, Kannisto H, Hirvisalo EL. Effect of activated charcoal on absorption of tolbutamide and valproate in man. *Eur J Clin Pharmacol* 1983;24:243–246.
14. Ellenhorn MJ, Barceloux DG. Hypoglycemics and insulin. In: Ellenhorn MJ, Barceloux DG, eds. *Medical toxicology*. New York: Elsevier Science, 1988. pp 440–461.
15. De Troyer A, Ectors M, Hubert JP. Chlorpropamide poisoning and diabetes insipidus. *Lancet* 1975;2:514.
16. Greenberg B, Weihl C, Hug G. Chlorpropamide poisoning. *Pediatrics* 1968;41:145–147.
17. Goldfrank LR. Hypoglycemic agents. In: Goldfrank LR, Flomenbaum NE, Lewin NA, Weisnan RS, Howland MA, Hoffman RS, eds. *Goldfrank's toxicologic emergencies*. 5th ed. Norwalk, CT: Appleton & Lange, 1994, pp 577–588.
18. Johnson SF, Schade DS, Peake GT. Chlorpropamide-induced hypoglycemia. Successful treatment with diazoxide. *Am J Med* 1977;63:799–804.
19. Kannisto H, Neuvonen PJ. Adsorption of sulfonylureas onto activated charcoal in vitro. *J Pharm Sci* 1984;73:253–255.
20. Huupponen R, Lammintausta R. Chlorpropamide and glibenclamide serum concentrations in hospitalized patients. *Ann Clin Res* 1982;14:119–122.
21. Larner J. Insulin and oral hypoglycemic drugs; glucagon. In: Gilman AG, Goodman LS, Gilman A, eds. *The pharmacological basis of therapeutics*. 6th ed. New York: Macmillan, 1980.
22. Sellers EM, Koch-Weser J. Protein binding and vascular activity of diazoxide. *N Engl J Med* 1969;281:1141.

Emergency Toxicology, Second Edition,
edited by Peter Viccellio.
Lippincott–Raven Publishers, Philadelphia © 1998.

46

Skeletal Muscle Relaxers

†William L. Haith and †*Jeffrey M. Cox

*†Department of Emergency Medicine, *Department of Surgery, Rhode Island Hospital,
Providence, Rhode Island 02903*

I. Introduction

A. **Skeletal muscle relaxants (SMRs)** are a heterogeneous group of agents used for the relief of skeletal muscle spasms or spasticity. They work by a variety of mechanisms, including central neurologic depression, and direct skeletal muscle relaxation. In 1994, 10,000 SMR exposures were reported to the American Association of Poison Control Centers (5).

B. Centrally acting SMRs frequently become drugs of abuse, especially in combination with other drugs such as alcohol or opioids. There are many reports of their use in attempted suicide attempts, some successfully.

II. Available preparations

A. The SMRs are classified by their site of action in the neuromuscular system: CNS, spinal cord, and skeletal muscle. These are all synthetic chemicals that are prescription medications. All come in oral form, while dantrolene, baclofen, methocarbamol, and orphenadrine are also available parentally.

B. There are many dosages and forms available (Table 46-1).

C. Several SMRs are frequently compounded with aspirin, acetaminophen, caffeine, or codeine. This significantly increases their toxic potential.

III. Pharmacology and properties

A. Mechanism of action and toxicity

1. Therapeutic

a. The mode of action of the centrally acting SMRs is not well understood. These agents do not directly relax skeletal muscles and are not neuromuscular blocking agents. It is not clear that any of these agents offer a therapeutic advantage over benzodiazepines for the treatment of acute muscle spasms.

b. **Carisoprodol (Soma), chlorphenesin carbamate (Maolate), chlorzoxazone (Parafon Forte), cyclobenzaprine (Flexeril), metaxalone (Skelaxin), methocarbamol (Robaxin),** and **orphenadrine (Norflex)** are centrally acting SMRs commonly used for the treatment of acute muscle spasms. Their major effect is CNS depression, which accounts for their therapeutic efficacy and toxicology effects. Carisoprodol is structurally related to and metabolized to meprobamate—a prescribed sedative/hypnotic agent. Additional CNS depression is related to this byproduct. Cyclobenzaprine is a tricyclic

TABLE 46-1. *Pharmacology and toxicology of skeletal muscle relaxants*

	Baclofen (Lioresal)	Carisoprodol (Reta, Soma, Soridol)	Chlorphenesin (Maolate)	Chlorzoxasone (Paraflex, Strifon Forte, Paraton Forte)	Cyclobenzaprine (Flexeril)	Dantrolene (Dantrium)	Metaxalone (Skelaxin)	Methocarbamol (Robaxin)	Orphenadrine (Norflex, Dispal)
Doses available (p.o.)	10, 20 mg	350 mg	400 mg	250, 500 mg	10 mg	25, 50, 100 mg	400 mg "Compound": 200 mg with 325 mg aspirin Soma compound with codeine: 200 mg with aspirin 325 mg and codeine 16 mg	500, 750 mg Robaxisal: 400 mg with 325 mg aspirin	100 mg Norgesic, Orphenegesic: 25 mg with aspirin 385 mg and caffeine 30 mg double all amounts if "Forte" form
Metabolism	Liver, enterohepatic recirculation	Liver	Liver	Liver	Liver	Liver	Liver	Liver	Liver
Elimination	Urine	Urine	Urine	Urine	Urine	Urine	Urine	Urine	Urine
Half-life (h)	3–4	8	2–5	1	1–3	9	2–3	1–2	14
Therapeutic effects	Sedation, GABA-nergic activity	Sedation	Sedation, analgesia	Sedation	Sedation, anticholinergic	Decreased muscle tone, spasm	Sedation	Sedation	Stimulation, anticholinergic, antihistaminic, analgesia
Toxicologic effects	Sedation, cardiovascular and respiratory depression, hepatotoxicity, hypothermia, hyporeflexia, seizures, coma, death	Sedation, respiratory depression, coma, death	Sedation, agitation	Sedation, respiratory depression, hypotension, hepatotoxicity	Sedation, hallucinations, agitation, arrhythmias, seizures, coma, death	Weakness, respiratory depression, sedation	Sedation, lowers seizure threshold	Sedation, hyperthermia, hypotension, seizures, coma	Stimulation, anticholinergic, apnea, hypotension, shock, arrhythmias, hepatotoxicity, seizures, coma, death
ED management	Supportive, AC, atropine if bradycardic, consider forced diuresis; anticipate delayed second peak; admit to ICU for symptoms	Supportive, AC, consider hemodialysis	Supportive, AC	Supportive, AC, check LFTs	Supportive AC, monitor EKG, i.v. bicarbonate for QRS > 0.1 s; admit to ICU for symptoms	Supportive, AC, check LFTs, saline diuresis	Supportive, AC	Supportive, AC	Supportive, AC, check LFTs, physostigmine for life threats[a]; admit to ICU for symptoms

[a] Life threats may include unstable arrythmias, bradycardia, hypotension, seizures, and coma.
AC, activated charcoal.

amine, similar in structure to amitriptyline, and was originally marketed as an antidepressant. It acts in the CNS at the brain stem level to produce SMR activity. Other pharmacological properties include peripheral and central anticholinergic effects, norepinephrine release or potentiation, reserpine antagonism, and sedation. Orphenadrine possesses both anticholinergic and antihistaminic actions.

    c. **Benzodiazepines** are also commonly used for their central effects. They are discussed in Chapter 60.

    d. **Baclofen** (Lioresal) is another centrally acting SMR that is a structural analog of gamma-aminobutyric acid (GABA). It is used for the treatment of muscle spasticity associated with multiple sclerosis, spinal cord diseases, and spinal cord injuries. It is not recommended for the acute management of muscle spasm. Acting on spinal cord GABA receptors, baclofen depresses nerve transmissions, reduces postsynaptic potentials, and possibly reduces release of neurotransmitter. This drug also has CNS depressant properties.

    e. **Dantrolene** (Dantrium) is a direct acting SMR and is useful for the treatment of muscle spasticity due to various uppermotor neuron and spinal cord disorders. Dantrolene produces muscle relaxation by direct actions on skeletal muscles by interfering with the release of calcium from the sarcoplasmic reticulum; decreasing the action of the excitation-contraction complex. CNS depression may also be observed with this agent.

  2. **Toxicologic.** The primary toxicologic action of the centrally acting SMRs is their depression of the CNS. Orphenadrine and cyclobenzaprine also exhibit significant anticholinergic effects. Overdoses of orphenadrine may present with manifestations of cardiotoxicity, e.g., conduction defects, dysrhythmias, and hypotension. Despite its structural similarity to amitriptyline, cyclobenzaprine has rarely, if at all, exhibited serious cardiotoxic effects. Fatal and nonfatal hepatocellular damage have resulted from the use of orphenadrine, baclofen, dantrolene, and chlorzoxaxone. These occurrences are attributed to either idiosyncratic or hypersensitivity reactions, usually with chronic use. Reactions range from transient transaminitis to fulminant failure.

C. **Pharmacokinetics**

  1. Gastrointestinal **absorption** is rapid and complete for all centrally acting SMRs, except for cyclobenzaprine. The anticholinergic effects of this agent delays gastric emptying and gut absorption. Orphenadrine's effect on gastrointestinal motility is less pronounced. Dantrolene is incompletely and slowly absorbed from the gastrointestinal tract. **Distribution** of the SMRs is essentially to all tissues. Their volume of distribution is large (V_d greater than 1 L/kg), but has not been measured. Baclofen concentrates in fat, possibly accounting for its prolonged toxicity. Live **metabolism** is universal, mostly by the microsomal enzymes. Chlorphenesin is conjugated to a glucuronide before elimination.

  2. The **half-lives** are all in the range of 1 to 4 h, except for orphenadrine (14 h), and cyclobenzaprine (1 to 3 days). Orphenadrine undergoes enterohepatic circulation, and a large portion is excreted in the feces. Repeat doses of activated charcoal could then reduce toxic levels through interruption of enterohepatic circulation.

These drugs are excreted in the urine as parent within 4 to 6 h and have a half-life of 9 h. They are slowly metabolized by the liver and excreted in the urine.

3.   Specific **SMR interactions** with other drugs are not known, except that we know that all sedative effects are exacerbated by alcohol, opioids, and sedative-hypnotic drugs. Propoxyphene may add to orphenadrine's CNS effects, causing confusion, tremors, and anxiety. This may be due to an additive hypoglycemic activity of the two drugs. MAO inhibitors should not be used in conjunction with cyclobenzaprine since it is a tricyclic amine and will be less effectively metabolized, increasing active drug levels. Orphenadrine may decrease the effectiveness of phenothiazines and haloperidol.

IV.   **Clinical presentations**

   A.   **At risk population.** SMR toxicity occurs most frequently as a result of intentional overdoses. Drug abusers may unintentionally become toxic when using these agents in combination with other CNS depressants, especially alcohol and opioids. Carisoprodol is popular amongst drug abusers for the effects of its metabolite, meprobamate. The elderly seem to have a poor tolerance for baclofen. One case series reported orphenadrine overdoses in young males given the drug to relieve side effects of their antipsychotic medications (8).

   B.   The major **toxicologic effect** of the centrally acting SMRs is CNS depression. Toxicities to SMRs usually manifest as only minor or moderate symptoms. General findings include dizziness, confusion, headache, nausea, and vomiting. Decreased muscle strength, weakness, and tone, along with decreased reflexes have been reported. In severe cases, respiratory depression, coma, seizure, cardiac dysrhythmias and death may occur. Severe toxicities are usually seen with large overdoses of baclofen, carisoprodol, cyclobenzaprine, methocarbamol, and orphenadrine. Cyclobenzaprine and orphenadrine poisonings may present with agitation and hallucinations secondary to their anticholinergic properties.

      1.   **Cyclobenzaprine** toxicity will present with an anticholinergic syndrome. Because of the similarity in structure to the tricyclic antidepressants, cyclobenzaprine may also ECG QT and QRS prolongation (see Chapter 55). Case reports with conduction defects were only in combination with other cardiotoxic drugs.

      2.   **Baclofen** has demonstrated delayed toxicity and deaths. The general syndrome includes depression of the CNS, cardiovascular, and respiratory systems. Hypothermia, mild hepatotoxicity, seizures, coma, and death may also result. A second peak in serum concentration occurs at about 8 h postingestion and is attributed to either enterohepatic circulation or delayed absorption. This would cause delayed or prolonged clinical effects. Since this agent has unique effects at the level of the spinal cord, there are characteristic clinical findings of muscular hypotonia and absent limb reflexes. Respiratory depression is a common cause of death.

      3.   **Orphenadrine** is the most toxic of the SMRs. Deaths have been reported with as few as 10 or 20 pills (1 to 2g). Rapid intoxication is manifested by an anticholinergic syndrome. Direct cardiotoxicity includes decreased contractility, hypotension, and tachyarrhythmias e.g., SVTs. This drug is potentially hepatotoxic, causing an elevation of liver transaminases in both chronic and acute exposures.

4. **Carisoprodol** overdoses are uncommon but may produce prolonged CNS depression resulting from its active metabolite, meprobamate.

5. **Methocarbamol** overdoses have resulted in respiratory depression, coma, and death.

C. **Differential diagnosis.** All agents affecting the CNS are to be considered when evaluating a patient with a SMR overdose. The sedative/hypnotics (e.g., meprobamate, alcohols, methaqualone, barbiturates, benzodiazepines, chloral hydrate, ethchlorvynol) and opioids can cause lethargy and respiratory compromise. Tricyclic antidepressants, antihistamines, phenothiazines, and antispasmodics are some classes of drugs that contain anticholinergic properties.

V. **Laboratory evaluation**

A. Routine studies are to be obtained to establish a baseline and to investigate for coingestants. These include CBC, electrolytes, BUN, Cr, serum glucose, urine analysis, and EKG. Salicylate and acetaminophen levels are important because of the frequency of SMRs compounded with these two drugs. Liver function studies should be obtained for suspected baclofen, orphenadrine, dantrolene and chlorzoxazone ingestions. Check the ECG for evidence of cardiac dysrhythmias or conduction disorders (e.g., QT or QRS prolongation) in cyclobenzaprine and orphenadrine overdosing.

B. Specific **drug levels** are not helpful in the immediate evaluation and management of these patients. The toxic doses for these drugs are ill-defined and based largely on case reports. Treatment should rely on the clinical presentation and course.

VI. **Management**

A. **General.** The approach to a SMR overdose is largely supportive. The ABCs are assessed and stabilized. All symptomatic patients should be followed with continual oxygen saturation monitoring. Recent ingestions require gastric lavage and at least one dose of oral activated charcoal for all exposures. Repeat charcoal for symptomatic baclofen, cyclobenzaprine, and orphenadrine.

B. **Cardiac.** Cyclobenzaprine toxicity is to be managed similarly to that of tricyclic antidepressants (see Chapters 55 and 56). EKG evidence of QRS prolongation greater than 0.1 s warrants alkalinization of the serum to a pH of 7.45 to 7.55. This can be accomplished with sodium bicarbonate as a loading dose of 1 to 2 mEq/kg and maintenance dose of 0.2 to 0.4 mEq/kg/h. Symptomatic bradycardia resulting from baclofen toxicity should be initially managed with atropine.

C. Hemodialysis has been used successfully with carisoprodol overdose. Hemoperfusion has been used to enhance elimination of meprobamate. Its use would only be recommended with otherwise unmanageable life-threatening toxicity. Forced diuresis with mannitol or a loop diuretic may increase excretion of baclofen. Ensure a good urine output to prevent crystalluria with dantrolene overdoses (2 mL/kg/h).

D. **Antidotes.** Although there are reports of successful use of physostigmine to reverse both baclofen and orphenadrine toxicity, the potential consequences of this therapy outweighs its benefits. Similar to its use in tricyclic antidepressant overdoses, physostigmine could reverse the anticholinergic effects, but at the expense of increasing cardiotoxicity. Thus, physostigmine is not recommended in the management of SMR toxicity.

VII. **Disposition.** Most single drug SMR overdoses can be managed in the ED. Monitor for cardiorespiratory depression and admit those patients with continued sedation, significant toxic coingestions, or psychiatric issues. Admission to intensive care monitoring is recommended for symptomatic overdosing that involves orphenadrine, cyclobenzaprine, and baclofen. These agents are the most toxic of this class. They exhibit toxicities other than sedation, have delayed effects and can rapidly deteriorate. Other patients with overdoses can be observed in the ED for at least 4 to 6 h and discharged if not clinically intoxicated and not suicidal.

References

1. Crabbe N. Skeletal muscle relaxers. *Clin Tox Rev* 1987;10:1.
2. Elenbaas JK. Skeletal muscle relaxers. *Am J Hosp Pharm* 1980;37:1313.
3. Elder NC. Abuse of skeletal muscle relaxers. *Am Fam Physician* 44(4):1223–6, 1991 Oct.
4. Linden CH. Cyclobenzaprine overdose. *J Toxicol* 1983;20:81.
5. McEvoy G, ed. *American hospital formulary service 95*. Bethesda, MD: American Society of Health System Pharm, 1995.
6. O'Riordan W. Overdose of cyclobenzaprine, the tricyclic muscle relaxant. *Ann Emerg Med* 1985;15:592.
7. Snyder BD. Orphenadrine overdose treated with physostigmine (Letter). *N Engl J Med* 295(25):1435, 1976 (Dec 16).
8. Sorensen HC. Death caused by orphenadrine poisoning. *Zeitschrift fur Rechtsmedizin* (Journal of Legal Medicine) 1986;97(2):133–139.
9. Spiller H. Five-year multicenter retrospective review of cyclobenzaprine toxicity. *J Emerg Med* 1995;13:781.

Emergency Toxicology, Second Edition,
edited by Peter Viccellio.
Lippincott–Raven Publishers, Philadelphia © 1998.

47

Colchicine

†Richard E. Westfal and °James P. Morgan

†*Department of Emergency Medicine, New York Medical College, Saint Vincents Hospital,
New York, New York 10011; °Department of Internal Medicine, Loyola University—Chicago,
Maywood, Illinois 60153*

I. **Introduction.** In 1994 alone, there were 125 reported cases of colchicine toxicity according to the "Annual Report of the American Association of Poison Control Centers." This represents about a 15% higher incidence compared to 1993 data (1,2). Emergency physicians ought to be familiar with the clinical presentation and management of this drug's toxicity.

II. **Uses.** Colchicine is derived from the *Colchicum autumnale* (autumn crocus) plant. Its primary use has been for the acute attack of gouty arthritis (3), though it has also been used in treatment of alcoholic liver disease (4), primary biliary cirrhosis (5), Behcet's syndrome (6), pseudogout (chondrocalcinosis) (7), and familial Mediterranean fever (familial paroxysmal polyserositis) (8).

III. **Pharmacology**
   A. Colchicine binds reversibly to microtubules and therefore causes mitotic arrest in metaphase. Bizarre nuclear configuration (sometimes called "colchicine figures") ensues, and the cells frequently die (9).
   B. Colchicine is rapidly absorbed after oral administration, with peak plasma levels reached within 30 min to 2 h; its serum half-life is just 20 min. Because enterohepatic circulation is prominent, a significant amount of the drug is absorbed by the intestinal tract. The most common initial signs of toxicity are nausea, vomiting, diarrhea, and abdominal pain (10).
   C. Colchicine has a wide volume of distribution (three to four times the total amount of body water) and is not removed from the body by hemodialysis.
   D. The drug is metabolized hepatically, and is excreted in the bile and urine. It is also secreted in breast milk (11).
   E. Intravenous colchicine may exhibit toxicity at significantly lower doses, especially in patients with hepatic or renal insufficiency (12).

IV. **Clinical presentation**
   A. Colchicine toxicity is uncommon, but when it occurs it usually results from intentional overdose and rarely from long-term administration. Toxicity is also seen in the setting of hepatic or renal dysfunction.
   B. Signs and symptoms of colchicine intoxication have been delegated to three stages (13), as outlined in Table 47-1.

V. **Diagnosis and appropriate work-up**. The diagnosis of colchicine toxicity is confirmed by the history, presence of empty vials, or acute therapeutic administration.

TABLE 47-1. *Signs and symptoms of colchicine intoxication*

Stage I: GI stage (0–12 h)	Stage II: multisystem damage/failure stage (24–72 h)	Stage III: recovery (7–10 d)
Abdominal pain	Cardiovascular	Alopecia
Nausea	Cardiogenic shock	Rebound leukocytosis
Vomiting	Hypovolemic shock	
Diarrhea	Cardiac dysrhythmias	
Volume depletion	Decreased myocardial contractility	
Leukocytosis	Pulmonary	
	Respiratory muscle weakness	
	ARDS	
	Metabolic	
	Electrolyte disorders	
	Acidosis	
	Hepatic insufficiency	
	Renal	
	Acute renal failure secondary to hypovolemia	
	Rhabdomyolysis	
	Neuromuscular	
	Diffuse weakness	
	Coma	
	Papilledema	
	Seizures	
	Hematologic	
	leukopenia (potentially life-threatening)	
	Anemia, thrombocytopenia	
	Disseminated intravascular coagulation	

VI. **Management**

  A. General measures include the following:

    1. Complete physical examination.

    2. Gastric lavage to remove all tablets.

    3. Activated charcoal followed by cathartic.

  B. Specific measures

    1. Fluid administration/monitoring: Patients who have manifested acute GI losses secondary to vomiting and diarrhea require aggressive fluid administration. However, because of the additional complications of depressed cardiac contractility and acute renal failure, it is essential that fluid administration and possible vasopressor agents be administered with hemodynamic monitoring.

    2. Antidote: Several investigators have demonstrated the efficacy of anticolchicine Fab fragments in animal models (14,15). A recent case report has shown dramatic reversal of life threatening colchicine overdose using goat antiserum. The patient would have otherwise likely died. As of 1996, a commercially prepared antidote is not yet available, though one appears to be on the horizon (16).

    3. Respiratory insufficiency due to myopathy and neuropathy causing respiratory depression, ARDS, hypotension and shock: The patient must be followed carefully with repeated examinations and serial arterial blood gases (ABGs) to identify onset of respiratory insufficiency. Such patients require endotracheal intubation and ventilatory support.

4. Metabolic monitoring must be repeated several times daily, including sodium, potassium, bicarbonate, glucose, BUN, creatinine, calcium, phosphorus, magnesium, and creatinine phosphokinase; additionally, urine myoglobin levels and serum lactate levels may be helpful.

5. Neuromuscular assessment. Serial neurologic assessments with the institution of seizure precautions and endotracheal intubation are performed if coma or respiratory compromise intervenes.

6. Hematologic/coagulopathy surveillance. With the onset of myelosuppression due to mitotic arrest of active precursor cells and the development of a consumptive coagulopathy, it is essential that a CBC, APTT, PT, fibrinogen level, and fibrin degradation products be determined twice daily. The patient may require transfusions of packed red blood cells and platelets, as well as the administration of vitamin K and fresh frozen plasma.

VII. **Disposition.** Patients need to be assessed based upon the time and the amount of colchicine taken, the route of administration, and their clinical status. Those reliable patients with only mild intoxication may be discharged provided good follow-up is available. However, in cases of clinical evidence for more severe intoxication or when follow-up is in question, hospital admission is necessary and aggressive supportive care mandated.

References

1. Litovitz TL, et al. 1994 annual report of the American Association of Poison Control Centers Toxic Exposure Surveillance System. *Toxicology* 1994:586.
2. Litovitz TL, et al. 1993 annual report of the American Association of Poison Control Centers Toxic Exposure Surveillance System. *Toxicology* 1993:579.
3. Roberts W, et al. Colchicine in acute gout. Reassessment of risks and benefits. *JAMA* 1987;257:1920.
4. Kershenobich D, et al. Colchicine in the treatment of cirrhosis of the liver. *N Engl J Med* 1988;318:1709.
5. Bodenheimer H Jr, et al. Evaluation of colchicine therapy in primary biliary cirrhosis. *Gastroenterology* 1988;95:124.
6. Moutsopoulos H. Behcet's syndrome. In: Isselbacher et al., eds. *Harrison's principles of internal medicine.* 13th ed. New York: McGraw-Hill, 1994:1669.
7. Alvarellos A, et al. Colchicine prophylaxis in pseudogout. *J Rheumatol* 1986;13:804.
8. Zemer D, et al. Colchicine in the prevention and treatment of the amyloidosis of familial Mediterranean fever. *N Engl J Med* 1986;314:1001.
9. Borisy GG, et al. The mechanism of action of colchicine. *J Cell Biol* 1967;34:525.
10. Hardman JG, Gilman A, Limbard LE, eds. *The pharmacological basis of therapeutics.* 9th ed. New York: McGraw-Hill, 1996:647–649.
11. Guillonnean M, et al. Colchicine is excreted high concentrations in human breast milk. *Eur J Obstet Gynecol Reprod Biol* 1995;61:177.
12. Wallace SL, Singer JZ. Systemic toxicity associated with intravenous administration of colchicine. Guidelines for use. *J Rheumatol* 1988;15:495.
13. Stapezynski JS, et al. Colchicine overdose: report of two cases and review of the literature. *Ann Emerg Med* 1981; 10:364.
14. Urtizberea M, et al. Reversal of murine colchicine toxicity by colchicine-specific Fab fragments. *Toxicol Lett* 1991;58:193.
15. Sabouraud A, et al. Dose-dependent reversal of acute murine colchicine poisoning by goat colchicine-specific Fab fragments. *Toxicology* 1991;68:121.
16. Baud FJ, et al. Treatment of severe colchicine overdose with colchicine-specific Fab fragments. *N Engl J Med* 1995; 332:642.

Emergency Toxicology, Second Edition,
edited by Peter Viccellio.
Lippincott–Raven Publishers, Philadelphia © 1998.

48

Isoniazid

†Richard E. Westfal, °John S. Yuthas, and *Peter Viccellio

†*Department of Emergency Medicine, New York Medical College, Saint Vincents Hospital,
New York, New York 10011; °Noble, Oklahoma 73701; *Department of Emergency Medicine,
State University of New York at Stony Brook, Stony Brook, New York 11794-7400*

I. **Introduction.** Isoniazid (INH) is in widespread use worldwide for treatment and prophylaxis of mycobacterial infections. In 1994, 458 cases of INH poisoning were reported in the United States. Of 1,150 patients treated in health care facilities from 1992 to 1994, 21.9% had complications regarded as minor, 16.6% as moderate, and 15.0% as severe after INH exposure (1–3). There were five deaths. INH is also one of the most common causes of seizures in overdose (4). The populations at risk for exposure are numerous because use of the drug is so widespread. Native Americans, Asian Americans, especially Cambodians (5), and more recently, acquired immunodeficiency syndrome (AIDS) patients are particularly at risk, due to the higher incidence of treatment with INH in these groups. Sievers et al. (6) claimed that 150 cases of INH exposure occurred over the course of a decade of their experience in the Indian Health Service System.

II. **Available preparations**

  A. Numerous formulations for INH exist. Most commonly, INH is available in a 300-mg white scored tablet. It is also available in 100- and 50-mg round scored tablets, as a syrup of 50 mg/mL, and in combination packets with rifampin (150 mg INH + 300 mg rifampin). A parenteral form (100 mg/mL) is available, as is an oral dosage "kit" containing 300 mg INH and two 150-mg rifampin tablets.

  B. Dosage.

    1. There are several recommended dosage regimens for INH. Currently, recommended adult prophylactic dosage after skin test conversion is 300 mg/day p.o. with concurrent pyridoxine therapy. An alternative schedule of 900 mg twice a week is also used. In children, the dosage for prophylaxis is 10 mg/kg/day up to 300 mg or 15 mg/kg/dose twice weekly up to a 900-mg dose (7).

    2. With active tuberculosis, the dosage is less standardized. Generally, INH 5 to 20 mg/kg/day is given with another antimycobacterial agent (8).

III. **Pharmacology and properties**

  A. **Physical properties**

    1. INH is a water-soluble agent that is rapidly absorbed from the GI tract, predominantly the small bowel. With a nontoxic dosage, absorption is complete within 1 to 2 h.

    2. After a 15 mg/kg dose of INH, peak levels (10 to 15 mcg/mL) occur at 1 to 2 h. The rate of absorption is increased in an empty stomach and may be somewhat

decreased if it is administered concomitantly with aluminum hydroxide antacids (9,10).

3. INH appears to be distributed to the total body water and is found in highest concentration in the skin and lungs. It also rapidly enters the cerebrospinal fluid (CSF), peripheral nerves, pleural fluids, and saliva. INH rapidly crosses the placenta and has been found in breast milk in nonhuman primates (9).

B. **Metabolism and elimination.** INH is metabolized to at least eight major intermediate compounds. The dominant first step is its acetylation to the inactive intermediate acetyl isoniazid by acetyl coenzyme A-dependent hepatic *N*-acetyltransferase. Following acetylation, most of a single dose is eliminated in the urine along with a small percentage of unchanged INH. There is a distinct bimodal distribution in rate of elimination in humans due to two separate phenotypes. Rapid acetylators (elimination half-life 35 to 110 min) eliminate INH at five to six times the rate of slow acetylators (half life of 140 to 300 min) (9).

   1. Weber and Hein (9) have exhaustively reviewed the phenotypic characters of various races and found that Northern Europeans, U.S. Caucasians, Egyptians, and Israelis were predominantly slow acetylators. U.S. Hispanic, African-Americans, and most African Blacks were about 50% slow acetylators, whereas Asians, Japanese, Native Americans, and some Alaskan Eskimos were predominantly rapid acetylators.

   2. Single doses of INH undergo a significant first-pass effect, which is marked in rapid acetylators (9). Approximately 25% to 30% of an INH dose is eliminated unchanged by slow acetylators, compared to 10% to 15% by fast acetylators.

   3. Several factors interfere with rapid inactivation and elimination of INH. Moderate renal disease is relatively unimportant in inactivation. Severe renal disease may be associated with increased acute toxicity (11,12). There are reports of INH toxicity at therapeutic dosages of INH in patients using chronic ambulatory peritoneal dialysis (12); however, the mechanism of toxicity seems to be pyridoxine deficiency associated with renal disease. Hepatic insufficiency may prolong the half-life of INH. The amount of prolongation correlates roughly with the serum bilirubin concentration. Drug interactions that may prolong half-life occur between **para-aminosalicylic** acid, procainamide, chlorpromazine, and **phenyramidol** (9). There are case reports suggesting that ethanol is frequently co-ingested during suicide attempts and may decrease INH half-life but increase its acute toxicity (13). The mechanism and clinical relevance of this phenomenon are not known.

C. **Mechanism of toxicity**

   1. **Acute toxicity.** Symptoms of toxicity will sometimes occur after an acute ingestions as small as 10 mg/kg. At 30 mg/kg, seizures may occur, and death may occur at ingestions of 50 mg/kg. The most dramatic and severe toxic effect of INH occurs in the CNS. INH is believed to impair the production of gamma-aminobutyric acid (GABA), an inhibitory neurotransmitter. The toxicity of INH is believed to result from pyridoxine (vitamin B_6) depletion. The active form of pyridoxine (pyridoxal-5′-phosphate) is required for the production of GABA by L-glutamic acid decarboxylase (14). The result of rapid vitamin B_6 depletion is GABA depletion,

followed by neural excitation and **seizures.** Such seizures are refractory to hydantoins or barbiturates but are believed to respond to **benzodiazepines.** Benzodiazepines are believed to increase **GABA-mediated inhibition** by acting on the GABA receptor indirectly (14).

2. **Chronic toxicity.** INH has been associated with chronic toxicity to the liver and peripheral nerves. Chronic elevation of SGOT (ALT) is seen in 10% to 20% of patients taking INH. The mechanism of hepatotoxicity is not known; however, a derivative of INH, acetylhydrazine, may be responsible (15). The elderly, alcoholics, and patients with underlying hepatic disease are more predisposed to hepatotoxicity (14). Rarely, acute pancreatitis has been reported as a manifestation of chronic toxicity (16,17). Peripheral neuritis has also been demonstrated to result from chronic use of INH. It appears to be dose-related and is mediated by pyridoxine deficiency. Thus, alcoholics, the malnourished elderly and young, patients with chronic renal failure, slow acetylators, and individuals receiving INH at more than 6 mg/kg/day are at greatest risk (14,18,19).

IV. **Clinical presentation**

    A. **History.** History of exposure is the key to diagnosis of acute toxicity. Typically, patients present with a history of INH ingestion due to either suicidal intention or accidental exposure. However, INH toxicity should be suspected in any patient on INH who presents with a seizure. In some studies, a disconcertingly large percentage of toxic patients took someone else's INH (5,20). As such, the diagnosis of INH toxicity should be considered in anyone presenting with seizures of unknown cause.

    B. **Symptoms**

        1. **Acute.** After the ingestion of a toxic dose of INH, patients are usually asymptomatic for 30 to 180 min. Toxicity may begin with generalized seizure, profound acidosis, and coma; or these symptoms may be heralded by nausea, vomiting, slurred speech, abdominal pain, sensation of warmth, lethargy, or disorientation. Progression of symptoms can be quite rapid (20–33). Seizures will generally occur within 6 h of ingestion of INH. Most patients seize repeatedly or continuously, and many progress to a state of coma even with treatment. During the interictal period, patients often demonstrated hyperreflexia, suppressed gag, plantar extension, and hypotension. Postictal hypotension may be profound and associated with evidence of shock (28).

        2. **Chronic toxicity**

            a. Mild neuropathy with daily regimens of 10 mg/kg/day is relatively common. It most frequently presents as an ascending peripheral neuropathy (34). The syndrome involves both the sensory and motor neural elements with sensory predominating. Symptoms include paresthesias, burning, numbness, weakness, and hyporeflexia, generally beginning in the feet (34).

            b. A clinical syndrome of asymptomatic elevation of SGOT and SGPT occurs in about 10% of patients taking INH. It usually occurs during the first few weeks of therapy, although it may begin at any time during treatment. In most of these patients enzyme levels will return to normal in 3 to 4 weeks whether the drug is continued or not. About 1% of patients taking INH will develop a syndrome of chemical hepatitis which is similar to viral hepatitis (35). Gastro-intestinal symptoms predominate (anorexia, nausea, vomiting). On physical exam approximately one third of patients have hepatomegaly, and some liver edge tenderness. Fever of more than 37.8°C (100°F) is unusual. On laboratory analysis, elevations of SGOT and SGPT are noted. About 25% of patients will have marked hyperbilirubinemia (more than 20 mg/dcl) which is associated with poor prognosis. One in 10 patients with INH-induced hepatitis (0.1% of all the patients taking INH) will progress to fulminate hepatic necrosis and death (15,36).

    c. Arthritis, with swollen tender, stiff joints has been described and generally occurs during the first 2 months of therapy (19).

V.   Laboratory studies

  A. Laboratory studies obtained during seizures demonstrate the consequences of sustained or repeated INH-induced seizures: anion gap metabolic acidosis, elevated serum lactate, mildly elevated or normal white blood cell count, normal to markedly elevated serum potassium. With prolonged apnea or respiratory embarrassment, respiratory acidosis may be superimposed on the metabolic acidosis, as noted by Chin et al. (37). Severe acidemia (pH less than 7.2) is not expected in asymptomatic patients who have not yet seized, even in large INH exposures.

  B. Hyperglycemia (glucose 200 to 400 mg/dL), often with associated glycosuria, is a common laboratory finding (5) and, when associated with profound acidosis, may lead to erroneous diagnosis of DKA in comatose or seizing patients for whom no history is available.

  C. Clinical INH toxicity correlates with a serum INH concentration greater than 10 mcg/mL, a level greater than 3.2 mcg/mL at 2 h after ingestions, or greater than 0.2 mcg/mL at 6 h postingestion (38).

VI.   Treatment

  A.   Prevention of absorption

    1. Ipecac is contraindicated in INH exposures. INH may rapidly induce coma or seizure and complicate the use of emetics.

    2. Gastric lavage may be useful if begun early. In general, rapid absorption of INH occurs, and attempts to lavage more than 1 to 2 h after ingestion of the drug may fail to recover significant amounts. Care should be taken to protect the airway against the event of seizure or coma. Placing awake patients in leftlateral decubitus position in Trendelenburg is preferred for gastric lavage.

    3. Activated charcoal appears to effectively absorb INH in studies when the two are given concomitantly (25); however, rapid absorption of INH in the GI tract may limit the effectiveness of charcoal. When used, an activated charcoal dose of 1 g/kg with sorbital 1 to 2 g/kg (up to 150 g) or magnesium citrate 4 mL/kg (up to 300 mL) is recommended (39).

  B. The cornerstones of management of acute severe toxicity are control of seizures and basic resuscitation. The physician should be prepared for sudden changes in the patient's clinical status. The use of pyridoxine and diazepam are indicated in any nonallergic patient who has taken a known toxic dose of INH or who has manifestation of severe

INH toxicity (seizures, history of seizures, protracted postictal state, coma) after a known exposure. Concerns about the toxicity of acute high-dose pyridoxine are probably not warranted. In one study reporting the treatment of two cases of false morel toxicity, pyridoxine doses of 2 g/kg (total doses of 132 and 183 g of pyridoxine) had been given during a three day period before toxicity, in the form of irreversible sensory loss and ataxia, was manifested (40). There is some concern that prophylactically treating otherwise nontoxic doses of INH with pyridoxine could precipitate INH toxicity and seizures (41). Prophylactic treatment of nontoxic acute INH exposures with pyridoxine is not recommended.

1. The seizures induced by INH are the result of acute pyridoxine deficiency and subsequent GABA deficiency, and they are poorly responsive to phenytoin, phenobarbital, pentobarbital, or diazepam alone. In animal studies of INH toxicity diazepam and pyridoxine, used together, exhibit clear synergism, and may prevent both seizures and mortality when given early and in adequate amounts (42). Diazepam alone is poorly effective in controlling seizures. In studies of dogs, doses of diazepam 1 mg/kg were ineffective in preventing seizures or mortality (43). Prevention of seizures by curarization does not prevent death in animal studies (37).

2. **Pyridoxine availability.** Ninety five percent of hospitals surveyed in one study (55/58) stocked less than 5 g of i.v. pyridoxine (44). When the i.v. form of pyridoxine is not available oral tablets can be ground and given as an NG slurry (19). The efficacy of this method of treatment is not known with certainty. Pyridoxine for i.v. use is cheap ($3 to $4 per 3-g vial) and has a long shelf life (up to 24 months). It should be made readily available in large amounts.

C. **Pyridoxine dosing**

1. **Dosing when amount of INH is known.** In patients with mild symptoms or no symptoms of toxicity who have taken a toxic dose of INH in a known amount, initially 1 g of pyridoxine per 1 g of INH ingested should be given over 30 to 60 min (40 to 70 mg/kg in children). In seizing patients this initial dose may be given much more rapidly (over 3 to 5 min i.v. push). It may be repeated in the first hour (with doses of diazepam) if needed to control seizures. The maximum dose of pyridoxine is not known, but it has been given successfully in doses as high as 357 mg/kg (21) and 52 g total dosage (13).

2. **Empirical dosage in INH exposures of unknown amount.** If the quantity of INH taken is not known, the generally recommended initial pyridoxine dosage is 5 g i.v. over 30 to 60 min. For seizing or severely symptomatic patients, 5 g pyridoxine may be given by i.v. push over 3 to 5 min. This dose may be repeated in the first hour if seizures recur. In children, a dose of 40 mg/kg is recommended for initial treatment of suspected toxicity or active seizure, again, the dose may be repeated if needed to control seizures (45). The recommendations for giving pyridoxine are based on success with INH toxicity resuscitation by Europeans (46). This pyridoxine regimen was shown to provide effective seizure control in dogs by Chin et al. (42).

D. **Diazepam dosing.** Diazepam 0.25 to 0.40 mg/kg/dose (child) or 5 to 10 mg (adult) slow push is recommended (28,39) in conjunction with high-dose pyridoxine. This dose may be repeated if needed, and additional pyridoxine may be given if INH toxicity is clearly responsible. Seizures not readily controlled by diazepam may be treated with **phenobarbital** 15 to 20 mg/kg i.v. in 60 mL of normal saline over 15 min.

E. If seizures continue unremittingly or are only transiently broken by pyridoxine, diazepam, and phenobarbital, consideration should be given to hemodialysis, general anesthesia, or both. Peritoneal dialysis has been used effectively (47) but is not preferred over hemodialysis. When general anesthesia is induced with thiopental for seizure control, an electroencephalography (EEG) monitor should be used to verify cessation of seizure activity. As in other patients with altered mental status care should be taken to exclude other causes of seizures, particularly falls, intracranial infections, alcohol withdrawal, and presence of other toxins. **A poor response to adequate treatment for INH toxicity should increase the clinician's index of suspicion for other causes of AMS.**

F. **Use of bicarbonate.** Severe acidosis often accompanies INH toxicity. A pH of 6.49 was documented in one patient who subsequently recovered fully (31). Studies in dogs indicated that acidosis in INH toxicity is the direct result of prolonged seizures, and the best preventive medicine for acidosis in controlling seizure activity (37). Seizure-induced lactic acidosis usually clears rapidly on its own after cessation of seizures. With acidosis where the pH is less than 7.2, treatment with sodium bicarbonate (1 to 3 mEq/kg initially) may improve the efficacy of diazepam and pyridoxine (37). It is not uncommon for multiple doses of sodium bicarbonate to be required during prolonged seizures (39). This may be worth consideration if stores of pyridoxine prove inadequate to control seizures and dialysis is not available. The safety of bicarbonate administration has not been established.

G. Hypotension as a result of INH toxicity has been observed with some frequency. Generally, it is responsive to fluid challenge with normal saline 10 to 20 mL/kg. **Vasopressor agents** such as dopamine (beginning at 2 to 5 µg/kg/min) and norepinephrine (initially 0.1 to 0.2 µg/kg/min) have been used successfully and are recommended for treating hypotension refractory to fluid bolus (39).

H. **Chronic toxicity**

   1. **Neuropathy.** The treatment for chronic peripheral neuropathy due to INH is coadministered oral pyridoxine (10 to 50 mg/day). Renal dialysis patients may require larger doses of 100 mg/day (18). Patients who fail to respond to oral pyridoxine usually respond to discontinuation of INH.

   2. **Hepatitis.** Transient mild asymptomatic elevations of SGOT and SGPT do not generally require treatment. These patients should be observed closely for clinical signs and symptoms of hepatitis. The initial treatment for patients with clinical evidence of hepatitis due to INH is immediate discontinuation of the INH therapy (48). Supportive care should be instituted as needed.

VII. **Disposition**

   A. **Acute toxicity**

      1. In patients with deliberate or accidental polyingestions including INH no clear recommendations can be made. Delayed toxicity in polyingestion of INH with other substances has not been well studied. It is likely that coingestion of INH with ethanol will delay the onset of seizures (43); however, there is no agreement concerning its effect on INH toxicity.

2. Know Quantities of INH. When INH has been ingested alone, in a quantity known with certainty, as a single dose, disposition should be based on the amount ingested. A person ingesting only a therapeutic biweekly dose of INH (900 mg or 10 mg/kg in children) can be discharged to home or psychiatric service after a brief period of observation. Therapeutic doses of INH are rapidly absorbed, and peak levels occur within 3 h in most healthy subjects (9), therefore late complications would not be expected in this group. Asymptomatic patients with a history of known toxic ingestion should be treated as if they have severe toxicity.

3. Severe toxicity, even with a rapid response to treatment, requires admission. Delays in toxicity and absorption of INH during treatment are poorly understood. Recurrence of seizures after treatment, even with resolution of symptoms in the interictal period, is well documented.

4. Asymptomatic patients with ingestion of an unknown amount of INH. The literature suggests that symptoms of INH toxicity are usually manifested within 3 h. Indeed, the most common presenting symptoms in severe toxicity are seizure, lethargy, or coma. However, the period of observation required to rule out toxicity is not clear. When the quantity of INH ingested is unknown, prolonged observation (6 h) or admission would seem to be the most prudent course.

B. **Chronic toxicity**
1. **Neuropathy.** Mild chronic neuropathy can be treated without hospitalization. Severe cases associated with ataxia and weakness may require admission.
2. **Hepatitis.** There is no clear recommendation for disposition in the literature. Patients with clinical evidence of hepatitis due to INH have an expected mortality of 10%, most within the first two weeks of diagnosis. In a large study of INH-related hepatitis, about half of the patients with clinically suspected hepatitis were admitted (15,36). Patients who are diagnosed late in the course of INH therapy and those with markedly elevated bilirubins (more than 20 mg/dcl) have a poor prognosis and should probably be routinely admitted. Any patient with evidence of fulminant hepatic necrosis or failure who can be transported should be admitted to a center capable of liver transplant.

References

1. Litovitz TL, et al. 1992 annual report of the American Association of Poison Control Centers Toxic Exposure Surveillance System. *Am J Emerg Med* 1993;11:494–455.
2. Litovitz TL, et al. 1993 annual report of the American Association of Poison Control Centers Toxic Exposure Surveillance System. *Am J Emerg Med* 1994;12:546.
3. Litovitz TL, et al. 1994 annual report of the American Association of Poison Control Centers Toxic Exposure Surveillance System. *Am J Emerg Med* 1995;13:551.
4. Olson K, Benowitz N, Pentel P. Survey of causes and consequences of seizures during drug intoxication. *Vet Hum Toxicol* 1982;24:281.
5. Blanchard PD, et al. Isoniazid overdose in the Cambodian population of Olmsted County, Minnesota. *JAMA* 1986; 256:3131.
6. Sievers ML, et al. Treatment of isoniazid overdose. *JAMA* 1982;247:583.
7. The use of preventative therapy for tuberculous infection in the United States. *MMWR* 1990;39:9.
8. American Hospital Formulary Service. Isoniazid. In: McEvoy GK, ed. *Drug information.* Bethesda, MD: American Society of Hospital Pharmacists. 362–365, 1992.

9. Weber WW, Hein DW. Clinical pharmacokinetics of isoniazid. *Clin Pharmacokinet* 1979;4:401.

10. Hearse DJ, Weber WW. Multiple *N*-acetyltransferases and drug metabolism: tissue distribution, characterization and significance of mammalian *N*-acetyltransferase. *Biochem J* 1973;132:519.

11. Cheung WC, et al. Isoniazid-induced encephalopathy in dialysis patients. *Tubercle Lung Dis* 1993;74:136.

12. Asnis DS, Bhat JG, Melchert AF. Reversible seizures and mental status changes in a dialysis patient on isoniazid preventative therapy. *Ann Pharmacother* 1993;27:444.

13. Sievers ML, Herrier RN. Treatment of acute isoniazid toxicity. *Am J Hosp Pharm* 1975;32:202.

14. Synder IS, Finch RG. Drugs used in the treatment of tuberculosis and leprosy. In: Craig CR, Stitzel RE, eds. *Modern pharmacology*. 2nd ed. 707–719.

15. Mitchell JR, et al. Isoniazid liver injury: clinical spectrum, pathology, and probable pathogenesis. *Ann Intern Med* 1976;84:181.

16. Chan KL, et al. Recurrent acute pancreatitis induced by isoniazid. *Tubercle Lung Dis* 1994;75:383.

17. Rabassa AA, et al. Isoniazid-induced acute pancreatitis. *Ann Intern Med* 1994;121:433.

18. Siskind MS, Thienemann D, Kirlin L. Isoniazid-induced neurotoxicity in chronic dialysis patients: report of three cases and a review of the literature. *Nephron* 1993;64:303.

19. Osborne H. Antitubercular agents. In: Goldfrank LR, et al., eds. *Toxicologic emergencies*. 5th ed. Norwalk, CT: Appleton & Lange, 1994:627–635.

20. Cameron WM. Isoniazid overdosage. *Can Med Assoc J* 1978;118:1413.

21. Wasen S, LaCouture PG, Lovejoy FH. Single high-dose pyridoxine treatment for isoniazid overdose. *JAMA* 1981;246:1102.

22. Brown A, et al. Acute isoniazid intoxication: reversal of CNS symptoms with large doses of pyridoxine. *Pediatr Pharmacol* 1984;4:199.

23. Ducobu J, et al. Acute isoniazid, ethambutol, rifampicin overdosage. *Lancet* 1982;1:632.

24. Orlowski JP, Paganini EP, Pippenger CE. Treatment of a potentially lethal dose isoniazid ingestion. *Ann Emerg Med* 1988;17:73.

25. Siefkin AD, Albertson TE, Corbett MG. Isoniazid overdose: pharmacokinetics and effects of oral charcoal in treatment. *Hum Toxicol* 1987;6:497.

26. Goldin JG, Linton DM, Potgieter PD. Isoniazid poisoning. *S Afr Med J* 1987;72:223.

27. Nolan CM, Elarth AM, Barr HW. Intentional isoniazid overdosage in young Southeast Asian refugee women. *Chest* 1988;93:803.

28. Bredeman JA, Krechel SW, Eggers GWN. Treatment of refractory seizures in massive isoniazid overdose. *Anesth Analg* 1990;71:554.

29. Hankins DG, et al. Profound acidosis caused by isoniazid ingestion. *Am J Emerg Med* 1987;5:165.

30. Miller J, Robinson A, Percy AK. Acute isoniazid poisoning in childhood. *Am J Dis Child* 1980;134:290.

31. Terman DS, Teitelbaum DT. Isoniazid self-poisoning. *Neurology* 1970;20:299.

32. Watkins RC, et al. Isoniazid toxicity presenting as seizures and metabolic acidosis. *J Natl Med Assoc* 1990;82:57.

33. Yarbrough BE, Wood JP. Isoniazid overdosage treated with high-dose pyridoxine. *Ann Emerg Med* 1983;12:303.

34. Goldman AL, Braman SS. Isoniazid: a review with emphasis on adverse effects. *Chest* 1972;62:71.

35. Kopanoff DE, Snider DE, Caras GJ. Isoniazid-related hepatitis: a U.S. Public Health Service cooperative surveillance study. *Am Rev Respir Dis* 1978;117:991.

36. Black M, et al. Isoniazid-associated hepatitis in 114 patients. *Gastroenterology* 1975;69:289.

37. Chin L, et al. Convulsions as the etiology of lactic acidosis in acute isoniazid toxicity in dogs. *Toxicol Appl Pharmacol* 1979;49:377.

38. Shah BR, et al. Acute isoniazid neurotoxicity in an urban hospital. *Pediatrics* 1995;95:700.

39. Rumack B. *Poisindex information system*. Denver: Micromedex, 1989.

40. Albin RL, et al. Acute sensory neuropathy-neuropathy from pyridoxine overdose. *Neurology* 1987;37:1729.

41. De'Clari F. The paradoxical anticonvulsive and awakening effect of high-dose pyridoxine treatment for isoniazid intoxication. *Arch Intern Med* 1992;152:2346.

42. Chin L, et al. Evaluation of diazepam and pyridoxine as antidotes to isoniazid intoxication in rats and dogs. *Toxicol Appl Pharmacol* 1978;45:713.

43. Chin L, et al. Potentiation of pyridoxine by depressants and anticonvulsants in the treatment of acute isoniazid intoxication in dogs. *Toxicol Appl Pharmacol* 1981;58:504.

44. Scharman EJ, Rosencrance JG. Isoniazid toxicity. A survey of pyridoxine availability. *Am J Emerg Med* 1994;12:386.

45. Howland MA, Kulberg AG. Antidotes in depth. In: Goldfrank LR, et al., eds. *Toxicologic emergencies*. 4th ed. Norwalk, CT: Appleton-Century-Crofts, 1990:325–326.

46. Brown CV. Acute isoniazid poisoning. *Am Rev Respir Dis* 1972;105:206.

47. Cocco AE, Pazourek LJ. Acute isoniazid intoxication—management by peritoneal dialysis. *N Engl J Med* 1963;269:852.

48. Davidson PT, Le HQ. Drug treatment of tuberculosis—1992. *Drugs* 1992;43:651.

Emergency Toxicology, Second Edition,
edited by Peter Viccellio.
Lippincott–Raven Publishers, Philadelphia © 1998.

49

Anticonvulsants

Bruce Sanderov

Department of Emergency Medicine, Winthrop University Hospital, Mineola, New York 11501

The anticonvulsant drugs constitute a diverse group of frequently prescribed medications whose adverse effects are both multisystem and nonspecific. In the setting of toxicity, the clinician is often called on to determine if the patient's presenting signs and symptoms are nonlethal, drug-related side effects that will abate spontaneously with supportive management or portend a protracted clinical course with possible life-threatening complications. Table 49-1 summarizes some key properties of the major anticonvulsants. With the exception of certain caveats, the treatment of antiepileptic toxicity or overdose is symptomatic and employs the same basic modalities used for many overdoses. These principles have been outlined in Part II in this book. In most cases, clinical judgment can guide the physician as to which patients should be hospitalized for careful monitoring and which may simply require a period of observation followed by discharge.

PHENYTOIN

I. **Introduction.** Phenytoin (diphenylhydantoin, DPH) has been available commercially since 1938. It has been shown to effectively control a variety of seizure disorders, including status epilepticus. It is used also to treat disturbances of cardiac rhythm, especially those associated with digitalis toxicity. Although the reported incidence of side effects ranges from 15% to 45%, when given orally phenytoin is usually a safe drug, as most adverse reactions are not life-threatening. This situation is in contrast to the severe hemodynamic instability that can result from improper intravenous use.

II. **Available preparations.** Preparations vary with regard to bioavailability, rate of absorption, and duration of action. Phenytoin is available as 50-mg tablets, 30- and 100-mg capsules, and as a solution in a solvent for parenteral use (50 mg/mL). **Extended release preparations** (Kapseals) are also available in 100- and 30-mg capsules and in a 125-mg suspension form. A pediatric **chewable tablet** (Infatabs) containing 50 mg of phenytoin is also on the market. It should be noted that the free acid form of phenytoin is used in the suspension and Infatabs. Since the free acid form results in an 8% increase in drug content over the sodium salt, serum levels should be carefully monitored when these preparations are used.

III. **Pharmacology and properties**

   A. **Phenytoin absorption** and its time to peak serum concentration after an oral dose are highly dependent on product formulation, the amount of drug ingested, as well as other concomitantly ingested drugs. Once absorbed, it is 90% to 95% protein-bound. Concurrently administered drugs that are highly protein-bound may enhance the metabolism of phenytoin by displacing it from serum proteins. This displacement may cause

TABLE 49-1. *Pharmacologic properties of anticonvulsants*

	Phenytoin	Carbamazepine	Valproic acid	Ethosuximide	Phenobarbital	Primidone
Therapeutic range	10–20 µg/mL	6–12 µg/mL	30–100 µg/mL	40–100 µg/mL	10–35 µg/mL	Variable*
Time to peak level after dose	3–12 h	Up to 72 h	1–4 h	3–7 h	Variable	3 h
Plasma half-life	6–60 h	15–54 h	7–20 h	30–50 h	80–120 h	Primidone 8–12 hr PEMA metabolites 16–36
Acute toxic dose	20 mg/kg	10 mg/kg	200 mg/kg	NA	6–10 g	NA
Major manifestations of toxicity	Lethargy, vertigo, seizures, coma, anticholinergic symptoms	Lethargy, vertigo, seizures, coma, myocardial depression, hypotension, heart block, anticholinergic symptoms	Confusion, agitation, lethargy, nystagmus, hepatotoxicity	Nausea, vomiting, anorexia, lethargy, headache	Lethargy, coma, slurred speech, hypotension	Similar to phenobarb

Ranges and values above will vary with anticonvulsant drug formulation, other ingested medication, and whether intoxication is acute/chronic.
*Reference to phenobarbital metabolite may be useful.
NA, no reference available.

a decrease in total (measured) serum phenytoin with an increase in the percentage of free (unmeasured) phenytoin, resulting in toxicity. A mechanism such as this may be responsible for the elevated levels seen in patients taking a newly formulated slow release valproate (Depakene R) (23). Table 49-2 lists drugs that may influence phenytoin metabolism.

B. Phenytoin is **metabolized** in the liver by parahydroxylation. At low serum concentrations of phenytoin of less than 18 mcg/mL, the rate of metabolism demonstrates first-order kinetics, with a *given percent* metabolized per unit time. At higher levels, the enzyme necessary for metabolism is saturated and elimination becomes zero-order. Drug is now metabolized at a constant amount per unit of time. Along with altered kinetics, drug half-life is prolonged with increasing serum levels. Thus, if the dose of administration is not adjusted with elevated serum concentrations, toxicity can easily occur.

C. The half-life of phenytoin within the normal therapeutic range is about 1.5 days, whereas in patients with toxic levels the half-life can be as long as 3 to 5 days.

IV. Clinical presentation

A. Oral toxicity. The most common **signs** following an acute ingestion are nystagmus, dysphasia, and cerebellar ataxia; the most common **symptoms** are dizziness, tremor, and visual disturbances, including double vision. Nystagmus, which may be horizontal and vertical, occurs when serum levels exceed 20 to 30 mcg/mL. Above 30 mcg/mL, about 75% of patients exhibit nystagmus (1). Nausea and vomiting may be seen, possibly secondary to GI irritation due to phenytoin preparations. Other CNS symptoms develop at higher levels, including drowsiness, delirium, and bizarre behavior. Although paradoxical seizures have been described with phenytoin toxicity, it should be noted

TABLE 49-2. *Drug interactions with phenytoin*

Inhibit phenytoin metabolism
  Antituberculous drugs—isoniazid, paraamino salicylic acid, cycloserine
  Antibiotics: chloramphenicol, sulfonamides (sulfamethizole, sulfaphenazole, trimethoprim)
  Antipsychotics: phenothiazines, trazodone
  Anticoagulants: bishydroxycoumarin (Dicumarol)
  Sedative/hypnotics: phenobarbital, ethanol, diazepam, chlordiazepoxide
  Others: disulfiram, ? valproic acid, phenylbutazone, cimetidine, tolbutamide, estrogens
Drugs displacing phenytoin from plasma protein-binding (drugs that increase the free phenytoin fraction)
  Phenylbutazone, salicylates, sulfonamides, paraamino salicylic acid, and chlorothiazide
Enhance phenytoin metabolism
  Carbamazepine, ? theophylline, folic acid, molindone, small amounts of ethanol, and phenobarbital
    (at therapeutic doses)
Phenytoin inhibits the metabolism of
  Warfarin, phenobarbital
Phenytoin enhances metabolism of
  Bishydroxycoumarin, corticosteroids, doxycycline, metyrapone, ? oral contraceptives, methadone,
    theophylline

From ref. 41, with permission.

that these patients had poorly controlled seizures (3). Death, although rare, has been reported, especially in children (2). The recognition of phenytoin toxicity in patients on long-term therapy may be difficult. Its onset can be insidious. Reports of the development of choreoathetosis and other movement disorders in the absence of nystagmus have appeared. Chronically high levels may produce encephalopathy or a schizophrenic-like psychosis (1). The well-known and well-reported gingival hyperplasia, also a result of chronic therapy, is directly related to dose and the tissue titer of the drug. Reports also indicate that among epileptic patients, relatively mild intoxication can lead to cerebellar degeneration, with magnetic resonance images showing moderate to severe cerebellar atrophy. There is no correlation between the degree of atrophy and severity of symptoms and serum phenytoin levels (24,25).

B. Intravenous toxicity. Oral phenytoin can be administered in large initial doses without significant side effects (4). In contrast, when given intravenously, phenytoin must be administered cautiously, no faster than 50 mg/min, and patients should undergo continuous blood pressure and ECG monitoring. Adverse effects from improper intravenous use of phenytoin have been well documented and include hypotension, decreased myocardial contractility, prolonged atrioventricular (AV) conduction, and prolongation of the PR interval and QRS complex. Phenytoin should be given more slowly (20 mg/min) to patients with bradycardia or high degrees of AV nodal block (5). Propylene glycol, the agent used to solubilize phenytoin, is the cause of many of these side effects. The mechanism for the abnormalities induced by this compound are thought to be both direct myocardial and vagally mediated effects.

C. Fetal hydantoin syndrome. The fetal hydantoin syndrome pertains to a variety of birth defects associated exposure to phenytoin during pregnancy. It occurs in 10% to 30% of infants born to females taking 100 to 800 mg/day during at least the first trimester of gestation. An excellent review of the subject can be found in the paper by Adams (27). The syndrome is defined by various combinations of abnormalities including cranial-facial defects, growth deficiency, impaired cognitive function, microcephaly, deformed nasal bridge, cleft lip/palate, and limb defects. Research is ongoing as to the exact cause of this syndrome and the genotypic, phenotypic, or enzymatic markers that may place a female at risk.

   D. **Differential diagnosis.** Important **entities to exclude** for any patient thought to have phenytoin toxicity are cerebellar hemorrhage, hypoglycemia, alcohol withdrawal or intoxication, and sedative-hypnotic overdose. The list of agents that may cause neurologic findings similar to those due to phenytoin is extensive (6). In most cases the patient provides a history of having taken phenytoin. Difficulties arise with obtunded or confused patients, in whom unless one specifically considers phenytoin toxicity the diagnosis may be missed. Patients without obvious reasons for toxicity will require further investigations for underlying acute metabolic disorders (e.g., liver disease) and the possibility of drug-drug interactions.

 V. **Laboratory evaluation. Normal therapeutic range** for phenytoin is 10 to 20 µg/mL. Levels above this range are considered toxic. The diagnosis of phenytoin toxicity must rest on correlation of the clinical and laboratory findings, especially in patients on chronic therapy. Since the concentration of free (active/unbound) drug in a patient will vary with the degree of protein binding, total serum concentrations which may result in toxicity may also vary. Patients, for example, with renal and liver disease, may experience toxicity in spite of a total plasma concentration of phenytoin within the normal range. In these cases, the concentration of free phenytoin should be measured.

VI. **Management**

   A. **Initial management** for acute phenytoin intoxication is similar to that followed for other toxic substances.

   B. For patients who arrive soon after ingestion and are not vomiting on presentation, **gut evacuation** should be accomplished with proper protection of the patient's airway. Oral activated charcoal is indicated in the acutely and chronically toxic patient because it can not only limit drug absorption but, also enhance drug elimination (7,8,26). If antiemetics are needed, **metoclopramide** is recommended because of its low incidence of dystonic reactions.

   C. **Intravenous hydration** should be started and routine blood work performed with special attention to serum glucose and ethanol levels. An **ECG** is important for the evaluation of potential conduction disturbances. **Dextrose** and **thiamine** should be considered in patients with an altered sensorium. **Naloxone** may be given if the patient demonstrates signs and symptoms of opiate toxicity and is hypoventilating.

   D. **Complete physical examination** is performed with emphasis on the neurologic component. The presence of focal findings mandates an emergency head **computed tomography (CT) scan** to exclude structural abnormalities.

   E. **Treatment of arrhythmias** is difficult. Most side effects can be prevented if the solution is administered properly. There is some evidence that atropine may be useful for abolishing the bradycardia and AV conduction blocks (5). Intravenous fluid bolus and direct acting vasopressors (i.e., norepinephrine) are indicated in the hypotensive patient.

   F. **Other modalities of treatment,** including dialysis and forced diuresis have not been found to be effective for the treatment of overdoses because of the extensive protein binding of phenytoin.

VII. Disposition. Not all patients require admission. If all other serious illnesses have been ruled out, disposition depends on the patient's clinical status. Patients on chronic therapy with mildly elevated levels and minimal symptoms may be discharged assuming the patient is reliable, protected from falls due to ataxia, and close follow-up is available. Patients with acute ingestions, especially with persistent vomiting, ataxia, or confusion require admission or observation until their symptoms abate and their level has declined into the theraputic range. Similarly, those on other medications which are also highly protein bound warrant closer observation. Cardiac monitoring is unnecessary in most cases.

CARBAMAZEPINE (CBZ)

I. Introduction. First used in the treatment of trigeminal neuralgia, carbamazepine in now used in the treatment of all seizures except absences. Other uses include it use for manic depression where lithium is not effective.

II. Preparations. Carbamazepine (Tegretol) is available in 200-mg tablets, 100-mg chewable tablets, and in suspension form at 100 mg per 5 mL.

III. Pharmacology and properties. CBZ, a **benzodiazepine derivative,** is pharmacologically and structurally similar to both meprobamate (9) and the tricyclic antidepressants. This similarity accounts for many of its adverse effects. CBZ is poorly soluble and is absorbed slowly and erratically from the GI tract, with peak levels reached in 64 h. The drug may form a compact mass in the stomach, delaying absorption and signs of toxicity up to 72 h. **Delayed absorption** is further promoted by its ability to decrease GI mobility, as seen with the tricyclic drugs. CBZ **metabolism** follows first-order kinetics. The main metabolite is carbamazepine-10-epoxide (CBZ-E), which has anticonvulsant properties and is present at about 15% of the level of the parent compound at steady state. The epoxide makes a significant contribution to the toxicity of the CBZ. Much of CBZ undergoes enterohepatic recycling and is excreted in the bile (10). The **half-life** of CBZ and the epoxide is 18 to 54 h after a single dose and 16 to 20 h in patients who receive chronic therapy. This decrease in the half life occurs because CBZ induces its own metabolism. When administered with other medications, several types of **drug-drug interaction** may occur. CBZ may induce the metabolism of other antiepileptic drugs—phenytoin, primidone, valproic acid (VA), and ethosuximide. Commonly encountered interaction associated with CBZ therapy occurs in patients who become acutely ill and receive macrolide antibiotics, i.e., erythromycin or clarithromycin (28). These drugs are competitive inhibitors of the hepatic microsomal drug enzyme system. After 3 to 5 days of antibiotics these patients develop classic signs of CBZ intoxication and elevated levels. This toxicity is rapidly reversible if either drug is discontinued. A similar effect can be found with cimetidine and propoxyphene (11).

IV. Clinical presentation. Estimates of the incidence of **adverse reactions** associated with CBZ treatment range from 33% to 50% (12). Most of these effects are mild and reversible if the dosage is reduced. They include nausea, drowsiness, vertigo, blurred vision, and slurred speech. More severe reactions from an acute overdose of CBZ may result in profound respiratory depression, seizures, cerebellar dysfunction, and coma (29). Since CBZ is also structurally related to the TCA imiprimine, **anticholinergic** and **cardiovascular** manifestations of toxicity may occur. Seizures, disorientation, ataxia, abnormal deep tendon reflexes, mydriasis, myoclonus, nystagmus, and sinus tachycardia have all been reported (13). Cardiac complications have been reported and include profound myocardial depression with bradycardia, hypotension, and conduction disorders (e.g., AV block, QT and QRS prolongation) (14). **Idiosyncratic** reactions have been noted, including agranulocytosis, aplastic anemia and leukopenia. Stevens-Johnson syndrome, hepatic failure, and water retention. The latter may be secondary to the syndrome of inappropriate antidiuretic hormone secretion (15) or alteration of the sensitivity of osmol receptors (30). **Intrauterine effects,** including neural tube defects and spina bifida have been reported although additional studies are needed (31,32). **Deaths** after CBZ overdose are rare but may result from severe cardiovascular effects, status epilepticus, hepatitis, or aplastic anemia. Among patients on chronic therapy, the occurrence of seizures and total CBZ dose greater than 24 g may be an indicator of a fatal outcome (29).

V. **Differential diagnosis.** No single group of signs or symptoms is characteristic of CBZ overdose. This ingestion should be included in the differential diagnosis of unexplained seizures. If the patient presents comatose, sedative-hypnotic toxicity must also be considered. Likewise, dilated pupils, tachycardia, and disorientation raise the possibility of tricyclic antidepressants or other anticholinergic drug ingestion.

VI. **Laboratory evaluation.** Due to patient variability and erratic drug absorption, **serial monitoring** of CBZ levels are necessary in the setting of an acute ingestion. Maximal plasma concentrations may occur as late as 72 h after ingestion. The assay is not part of routine toxicologic screening for most laboratories, and measurements must be requested on a serum sample. Although CBZ levels do not clearly correlate with clinical outcome or symptoms, some studies advise that patients (especially pediatric) with levels greater than 28 µg/mL are at a higher risk for severe adverse reactions and should be admitted to intensive care (33,36). Others have suggested that a level of approximately 24 µg/mL requires close observation, while those with levels greater than 36 µg/mL require intensive support (34).

VII. **Management.** Care of acute CBZ toxicity is **mainly supportive.** It should be emphasized that after an acute overdose the absorption of CBZ may be impaired due to delayed gut motility or mass formation in the stomach. Late development of toxicity should be anticipated. **Emesis** is not recommended for CBZ exposures because unexpected clinical deterioration may occur. **Gastric lavage** may prove unsuccessful in removing all of the drug. One study recommended that if mass formation is considered likely, gastroscopic decontamination should be performed (9). Repeat doses of **activated charcoal** is indicated to limit delayed gut absorption and to interupt enterohepatic drug recylcing. While this may increase clearance of the drug, its effect on clinical outcome is questionable (35). **Charcoal hemoperfusion** has been found to be effective, and is recommended for patients with life-threatening manifestations of toxicity, such as ventricular arrhythmias refractory to standard therapy or status epilepticus. Hemodialysis and peritoneal dialysis are not effective in this overdose management. Some reports show that CBZ overdose has been successfully treated with **flumazenil,** although it is not approved for this clinical use (39).

VIII. **Disposition.** Because of CBZ's erratic absorption and potential for delayed toxicity, all patients with significant acute CBZ intoxications should be admitted until serum concentrations are clearly declining and in the therapeutic range. Patients with an altered sensorium warrant a cardiac monitored bed. Patients on chronic therapy who exhibit mild signs of toxicity may be managed by discontinuation of CBZ and close outpatient follow-up.

VALPROIC ACID

I. **Introduction.** VA was introduced for clinical use in 1978. It is unique among the anti-epileptic drugs in that it is a simple branched-chain carboxylic acid. Studies have found it useful for controlling both generalized and partial seizures. The most common side effect is hepatic necrosis, which occurs unpredictably.

II. **Available preparations.** VA (Depakene) is available in 250-mg capsules and in a syrup containing the sodium salt containing 250 mg of VA per 5 mL. A long-acting preparation is not currently available in the United States.

III. **Pharmacology and properties.** VA tablets are rapidly **absorbed** from the GI tract, with peak levels occurring 1 to 4 h after a single dose. VA acts by raising brain's level of the inhibitory neurotransmitter gamma-aminobutyric acid (GABA) (16). The drug has a **half-life** of 7 to 15 h. Active **metabolites** of VA are produced by oxidation and hydroxylation. They all have some tendency to increase seizure threshold but less than VA itself. The majority of VA is excreted in the urine in the conjugated form. Urinary excretion also occurs in the form of ketone bodies, which may produce a false-positive test in the urine of diabetics (10). **Most interactions** between VA and other drugs occur because VA is sensitive to enzyme induction and has a high affinity for proteins. Concomitant administration with other enzyme-inducing antiepileptic drugs—CBZ, phenytoin, and phenobarbital (PB)—tends to lower serum VA levels.

IV. **Clinical effects**

A. **Acute toxicity.** Acute VA poisoning occurs infrequently and most patients experience a benign course. The most common symptom is drowsiness, with unconsciousness occurring only with large ingestions (more than 200 mg/kg) (17). Ataxia, nystagmus, altered behavior, confusion, seizures, hypernatremia, metabolic acidosis, hypocalcemia, and hyperthermia have also been observed (18). Other findings may include pinpoint pupils, hypotension, nausea, vomiting, and diarrhea. Acute pancreatitis has occurred in patients receiving therapeutic doses. Gross movement disorders are rare. Less common side effects in patients on chronic therapy include hematologic abnormalities, asymptomatic hyperammonemia, weight gain, and hair changes (19,20).

B. **Hepatotoxicity.** VA causes two types of hepatotoxicity. The more common type is a mild form which is asymptomatic, dose-related, reversible and limited to a transaminitis. The less common idiosyncratic reaction, leads to **hepatic failure.** This is more serious because of its unpredictability and potential for fatal consequences. Patients primarily at risk for hepatic failure are children less than 2 years old who have associated medical problems and receiving multiple anticonvulsants. Hepatic failure has never been reported in patients over age 10 years and on monotherapy. Onset of severe hepatic illness is not immediate and occurs within the first 3 months of therapy. Clinical signs of hypersensitivity—fever, rash, eosinophilia—are not present. The most common symptoms are nausea, vomiting, anorexia, lethargy, and jaundice. It is believed that liver failure may be due to aberrant cytochrome P450-dependent metabolism of VA, which produces a toxic metabolite similar in structure to agents that can produce a Reye's-like syndrome in animal models (20,21). Recommendations for reducing the risk of serious hepatic toxicity with VA were outlined by Dreifuss et al. (21). Despite increased clinical use of the drug, reported cases of fatal hepatic failure have declined owing to greater awareness, recognition of risk factors, and closer patient monitoring.

C. Intrauterine effects. Intrauterine effects, including a "fetal valproate syndrome", has been described in infants born to mothers who are prescribed this drug. These malformations, related to dosage during the first trimester, are mostly congenital heart disease (37).

D. Differential diagnosis. The GI and nonspecific adverse effects of VA may initially resemble an early acetaminophen overdose. In patients less than 2 years old with GI complaints, coma, or both, Reye's syndrome should be considered. Finally, opiate overdose, sedative/hypnotic toxicity, and alcohol ingestion may also present with coma.

V. Laboratory analysis. Results of **serum VA** determinations reflect total levels (bound and unbound) and do not correlate well with CNS effects. Free VA levels are not readily available and have not been shown to be useful for management of the overdosed patient. **Liver function** tests, serum **amylase** levels, and **complete blood counts** should be monitored. **Abnormal bleeding and coagulation times** may be present. Serum **ammonia** may be elevated in patients with hepatitis and an altered mental status. It should be noted that abnormalities in liver enzymes in cases of fatal hepatotoxicity are reported to vary significantly and may not correspond to apparent clinical toxicity or predict outcome.

VI. Management. Supportive treatment is the mainstay of VA overdose. Activated charcoal can limit gut absorption when administered early and enhance drug elimination when given in a repeated fashion. Although highly protein bound, at high concentrations free VA may be subject to removal by hemodialysis and hemoperfusion (38). The use of these modalities is dependent on the patient's clinical status. If there are any questions, it is recommended to consult with the regional poison center.

VII. Disposition. Disposition of a patient with a VA overdose should rest on clinical evaluation. Patients who present with an altered mental status or coma should be admitted. Likewise, a child on VA who has symptoms of "gastroenteritis" warrants close observation. Patients with acute ingestions **without symptoms** should be observed for at least 7 h from the time of ingestion, which coincides with the time of the peak plasma concentration. Patients remaining asymptomatic should recieve another dose of activated charcoal before medical clearance.

ETHOSUXIMIDE

I. Introduction. Ethosuximide (ETX) is one of a class of drugs called succinimides that are useful for treatment of absence (petit mal) seizures. It is relatively free of side effects, and there are few reports of acute intoxication. Other succinimides, such as methsuximide and phensuximide are not available in the United States.

II. Available preparations. Ethosuximide (Zarontin) is availble as 250-mg capsules and as a syrup as 250 mg per 5 mL.

III. Pharmacology and properties. ETX **peak plasma levels** are reached within 3 to 7 h after a single oral dose and blood levels may remain elevated for up to 24 h. There is minimal protein binding. After absorption, the drug is **metabolized** in the liver by the hepatic microsomal enzyme system. ETX has no active metabolites and an elimination **half-life** of 40 h. Methsuximide has a plasma **half-life** of about 2 h. Its active metabolized product, *N*-demethylmethsuximide, has a half-life of 40 h. The long half-life of this metabolite should be measured in management of methsuximide toxic patients.

IV. Clinical toxicity. Clinical toxicity does not correlate well with plasma levels. Levels over 100 mcg/mL have been reported without adverse reactions (10). GI and psychiatric complaints are the most frequently reported side effects, although prolonged lethargy or coma can occur with an acute overdose. Other adverse reactions include insomnia, rash, severe headaches, and a systemic lupus erythematosus (SLE)-type syndrome. In chronic toxicity, hematologic abnormalities, including leukopenia, eosinophilia, thrombocytopenia, pancytopenia, and aplastic anemia have been observed. Paradoxical seizures may also occur (15).

V. Treatment. Treatment of ETX overdose is supportive. Because of its long half-life, close observation may be warranted. Patients who present in coma require hospitalization in an intensive care unit. There is some indication that charcoal hemoperfusion may be of use in the treatment of methsuximide overdose, as it increases the clearance of its active metabolite, *N*-demethylmethsuximide (40).

PHENOBARBITAL AND PRIMIDONE

I. Introduction. PB is the oldest antiepileptic agent. Primidone is a desoxy derivative of PB. PB is also an active metabolite of primidone. Adverse effects and treatment of overdoses are similar for the two compounds.

II. Preparations. PB is available in a variety of tablet and dosage forms and as an elixir. Preparations are also available for parenteral use. Primidone (Mysilone) is available as 50- and 250-mg tablets and a suspension of 50 mg per 5 mL.

III. Pharmocology and properties. PB structure lends itself to be classified as a **long-acting barbiturate.** PB has a short side chain substituted onto the barbituric acid ring. It is less potent, less lipid-soluble, and more protein bound than the short-acting barbiturates. In general, the more lipid soluble a barbiturate, the (a) shorter the duration of action and time to onset of action, (b) greater and faster its rate of hepatic elimination, and (c) greater its hypnotic activity. Thus, short acting barbiturates, i.e., thiopental and amobarbital have a more rapid onset of action and a shorter duration of action than PB. Because PB is a **weak acid,** concentrations of the drug are affected by local pH. PB has a low pKa which allows it to be mostly in the ionized state at physiologic blood pH. When the pH is lowered, more nonionized PB is available. Since cell membranes are selectively permeable to nonionized structures, the pH of the environment can determine drug distribution and elimination. The **half-life** of PB ranges from 80 to 140 h (6). **Primidone** is totally **metabolized** in the liver to the active metabolites PB and phenylethylmalonamide (PEMA). The **half-life** of Primidone is 8 to 12 h after a single dose, shorter after chronic administration. The half-life of **PEMA metabolite** is 29 to 36 h (10).

IV. Clinical effects. The potentially lethal, acute adverse effects of both PB and primidone are **respiratory depression** and **coma.** Depending on the level of coma, the patient may have decreased deep tendon reflexes and fixed dilated pupils. Cutaneous plaques, blisters, or bullae may be seen with PB overdose but are not specific for it. Shock can occur secondary to medullary and myocardial depression and venodilation. Other adverse effects include nausea, vomiting, nystagmus, ataxia, Steven-Johnson syndrome, and hematologic abnormalities (6,15). **Long-term intoxication** of barbiturates can result in physiological tolerance and physical dependence. In such patients, **withdrawal** symptoms can develop within 24 h of discontinuance of the drug. Symptoms of withdrawal include nausea and vomiting, insomnia, agitation, abdominal cramps, tremor, and sweating. More severe symptoms include hallucination (usually auditory) and grand mal seizures.

V.   **Differential diagnosis.** A number of drugs can cause CNS depression, including alcohols, opiates, phenothiazines, sedative-hypnotics, tricyclics, and anticonvulsants. Trauma, and endocrinologic and metabolic abnormalities should also be excluded.

VI.   **Laboratory analysis. Plasma PB levels** are helpful for making a diagnosis but of little value when predicting the severity of the overdose. As with ethanol, chronic users of PB may have elevated serum levels with little CNS depression. When evaluating a patient after a primidone overdose, one should measure serum levels of the metabolites PB and PEMA. Massive crystalluria due to the precipitation of primidone indicates severe poisoning, which may occur at levels over 80 µg/mL (10).

VII. **Management**
      A.   **General measures:** As with other ingestions, basic principles of management of the overdosed patient should be followed. Because of the potential for CNS depression, the patient's mental status should be carefully assessed prior to GI decontamination. **Intubation and ventilatory support** may be necessary in the patient with profound CNS depression. **Emesis or lavage** is important, as barbiturates decrease GI motility and can form concretions in the stomach. Repeated doses of activated **charcoal** are critical, as it has been shown to hasten toxin removal by increasing nonrenal elimination and decreasing serum half-life (22).
      B.   **Toxin-specific measures.** Because PB is a weak acid, increased urinary elimination can be achieved through alkaline diuresis. Intravenous sodium barbonate is administered to maintain a urine pH between 7.5 and 8.0. Symptomatic patients with an elevated PB level warrant alkaline diuresis. When alkaline diuresis is not possible (e.g., renal failure, noncardiogenic pulmonary edema, congestive heart failure), hemodialysis or hemoperfusion should be used to remove PB in the severely toxic patient. Refractory hypotension is another indication for extracorporeal elimination.

VIII. **Disposition.** Because of the long half-life of PB and its potential for profound CNS depression, close observation of all patients is advised. Peak serum levels are achieved in 6 to 8 h after an oral theraputic dose. The patient who presents in coma may require hospitalization for several days in an intensive care facility.

References

1. Kooiker JC, Sumi SM. Movement disorders: a manifestation of diphenylhydantoin intoxication. *Neurology* 1974;24:68.
2. Laubscher FA. Fatal DPH poisoning. *JAMA* 1966;198:1120.
3. Masdeu J, Stillman N. Incidence of seizures with Dilantin toxicity. *Neurology* 1988;35:1769.
4. Osborn HH, Zisfein J, Sporano R. Single dose oral phenytoin loading. *Ann Emerg Med* 1987;16:407.
5. Voigt G. Death following intravenous sodium dilantin. *Johns Hopkins Med J* 1968;123:153.
6. Goldfrank LR, Breswitz EA. Phenytoin. In: Goldfrank LR, ed. *Toxicologic emergencies.* Norwalk, CT: Appelton-Century-Crofts, 1986.
7. Weichbrodt GD, Elliot DP. Treatment of phenytoin toxicity with repeated doses of activated charcoal. *Ann Emerg Med* 1987;16:1387.
8. Stack L, et al. Enhancement of phenytoin elimination by multiple dose-activated charcoal. *Ann Emerg Med* 1987;16:407.
9. Coutselinis A. An unusual case of carbamazepine poisoning with a near fatal relapse after two days. *Clin Toxicol* 1980;16:385.
10. Ellenhorn MJ, Barceloux DG. *Medical toxicology—diagnosis and treatment of human poisoning.* New York: Elsevier Science, 1988.

11. Pippenger CE. Clinically significant carbamazepine drug interactions: an overview. *Epilepsia* 1987;28:S71.
12. Pellock JM. Carbamazepine side effects in children and adults. *Epilepsia* 1987;28:S64.
13. Sullivan JB, Rumack BH, Peterson RG. Acute carbamazepine toxicity resulting from overdose. *Neurology* 1981;31:621.
14. Leslie PJ, Heyworth R, Prescott LF. Cardiac complications of carbamazepine: treatment by hemoperfusion. *BMJ* 1983; 286:1018.
15. Pellock JM. Efficacy and adverse effects of antiepileptic drugs. *Pediatr Clin North Am* 1989;36:435.
16. Nau H, Loscher W. Valproic acid and metabolites: pharmacological and toxicological studies. *Epilepsia* 1984;29:514.
17. Garnier R, Boudignat O, Fournier PE. Valproate poisoning. *Lancet* 1987;2:97.
18. Alberto G, et al. Central nervous system manifestations of a valproic acid overdose responsive to Narcan. *Ann Emerg Med* 1989;18:889.
19. Schmidt D. Adverse effects of valproate. *Epilepsia* 1984;25:S44.
20. Dreifuss F, Langer DH. Side effects of valproate. *Am J Med* 1988;84:34.
21. Dreifuss FE, et al. Valproic acid hepatic fatalities: retrospective review. *Neurology* 1987;37:379.
22. Berg M, et al. Acceleration of body clearance of phenobarbital by oral activated charcoal. *N Engl J Med* 1982;307:642.
23. Suzuki Y, et al. Interaction between vapproate formualtion and phenytoin concentration. *Eur J Clin Pharm* 1995;48: 61–63.
24. Luef G, et al. Phenytoin overdosage and cerebellar atrophy in epileptic patients. *Eur Neurol* 1994;34:79–81.
25. Ney GC, et al. Cerebellar atrophy in patients with long term phenytoin exposure and epilepsy. *Arch Neurol* 1994;51:767–771.
26. Howard CE, et al. Use of multiple dose-activated charcoal in phenytoin toxicity. *Ann Pharmacother* 1994;28:201–203.
27. Adams J, et al. Developmental neurotoxicity of anticonvulsants: human and animal evidence on phenytoin. *Neurotoxicol Teratol* 1990;12:203–214.
28. O'Connor NK, et al. Clarithromycin-carbamazepine interaction in a clinical setting. *J Am Board Fam Pract* 1994;7: 489–492.
29. Schmidt S, et al. Signs and symptoms of carbamazepine overdose. *J Neurol* 1995;242:169–173.
30. Gandelman MS. Review of carbamazepine hyponatremia. *Prog Neuropsychopharmacol Biol Psychiatry* 1994;18: 211–233.
31. Gladstone DJ, et al. Course of pregnancy and fetal outcome following maternal exposure to carbamazepine and phenytoin: a prospective study. *Reprod Toxicol* 1992;6:257–261.
32. Kallen AJ. Maternal carbamazepine and infant spina bifida. *Reprod Toxicol* 1994;8:203–205.
33. Macnab AJ, et al. Carbamazepine poisoning in children. *Pediatr Emerg Care* 1993;9:195–198.
34. Tibballs J. Acute toxic reaction to carbamazepine: clinical effects and serum concentrations. *J Pediatr* 1992;121: 295–299.
35. Wason S, et al. Carbamazepine overdose—effects of multiple dose-activated charcoal. *J Toxicol Clin Toxicol* 1992;30: 39–48.
36. Stemski ES, et al., Pediatric carbamazepine intoxication. *Ann Emerg Med* 1995;25:624–630.
37. Thisted E, et al. Malformations, withdrawl manifestations, and hypoglycemia after exposure to valproate in utero. *Arch Dis Child* 1993;69:288–291.
38. Yank JE, et al. Simultaneous "in series" hemodialysis and hemoperfusion in management of valproic acid overdose. *Am J Kidney Dis* 1993;22:341–344.
39. Martens F, et al. Clinical experience with the benzodiazepine antagonist flumazenil in suspected benzodiazepine or ethanol poisoning. *Clin Toxicol* 1990;28:341–343.
40. Baehler RW, et al, Charcoal hemoperfusion in the therapy of methsuximide and phenytoin overdose. *Arch Intern Med* 1980;140:1466–1468.
41. Goldfrank LR, et al. *Goldfrank's toxicologic emergencies.* 4th ed. Norwalk, CT: Appleton & Lange, 1990.

Emergency Toxicology, Second Edition,
edited by Peter Viccellio.
Lippincott–Raven Publishers, Philadelphia © 1998.

50

Methylxanthines: Theophylline and Caffeine

†Lisa Torraca and °Richard Y. Wang

†*Department of Emergency Medicine, Central Maine Medical Center, Lewiston, Maine 04240;*
°*Department of Emergency Medicine, Rhode Island Hospital, Providence, Rhode Island 02903*

I. Introduction

A. The methylxanthines are naturally occurring alkaloids found in plants with a wide geographic distribution. As far back as Paleolithic humans, these plants have been brewed into beverages that were believed to stimulate the mind, elevate mood, decrease fatigue, and increase capacity for work (1). Theophylline (1,3-dimethylxanthine) and caffeine (1,3,7-trimethylxanthine) are two of the most common methylxanthines found in both pharmaceuticals and in ordinary beverages. They are closely structurally related and exert similar physiologic effects on the CNS, gastrointestinal (GI), smooth muscle, metabolic, and cardiovascular systems.

B. The number of exposures to theophylline reported to the American Association of Poison Control Centers in 1994 was 4,033 (2). Over 2,000 of these cases arrived to health care facilities for aid, and 32% of them became ill. Death was the outcome in 35 cases. Theophylline toxicity affects multiple organ systems and can progress rapidly. Since no antidote is available, physicians must be able to recognize the disease early and institute appropriate therapy so that their patients may have an improved outcome.

II. Available preparations

A. Theophylline comes in many chemical forms, including its free anhydrous state, and salt compounds (oxtriphylline) and complexes (aminophylline). Combining theophylline with other agents increases its solubility; however, when dissolved in aqueous solution, these complexes dissociate to yield anhydrous theophylline. Theophylline can be dispensed as tablets, capsules, liquids, or suppositories. It can be the only agent or combined with other ingredients. More important in the overdosed setting is the availability of **sustained-release** (SR) formulations. These preparations, and whether they are granular or tabular form, will have direct implications in terms of effectiveness of gastric lavage and delayed symptoms. There are multiple SR formulations, and only the common ones available in tablet form are listed in Table 50-1.

B. Caffeine is found in a variety of beverages such as coffee, tea, and soft drinks. The average cup of brewed coffee has between 85 and 99 mg; tea has between 30 and 75 mg; and soft drinks have between 40 and 60 mg per glass. There are also several prescription and over-the-counter (OTC) preparations which contain caffeine, including Cafergot, Darvon, Fiorinal, Anacin, and Excedrin.

TABLE 50-1. *Common sustained release theophylline tablets that may not be recovered by gastric lavage*

Constant T	Theochron
Duraphyl	TheoDur[a]
LaBID	Theolair
Quibron T/SR[a]	Theo-Time
Respbid[a]	Uniphyl
Sustaire	

[a] Available in both capsules and tablets.

C. These agents are currently used in the management of apnea of prematurity, bronchial asthma, and migraine headaches.

III. **Pharmacology and properties**

A. **Mechanisms of action.** The physiologic effects of the methylxanthines are relaxation of smooth muscles, stimulation of the central nervous and cardiovascular system, promotion of gastric acid secretion, and renal diuresis. These actions are achieved through the following mechanisms:

1. They act as **adenosine antagonists** by blocking adenosine receptors, which mediate a variety of responses. Adenosine causes bronchiolar smooth muscle constriction, peripheral vasodilatation, elevation of seizure threshold, and diminished cardiac pacemaker discharge.

2. They promote the **release of endogenous catecholamines** and lead to elevated plasma levels of epinephrine and norepinephrine (3). Excess stimulation of adreno-receptors causes positive inotropic and chronotropic cardiac activity, peripheral vasodilatation and metabolic changes. These include hypokalemia, hyperglycemia, and lactic acidosis.

3. They directly stimulate the respiratory and vasomotor center of the brain to increase the rate and depth of breathing.

4. They **inhibit phosphodiesterases**, which increases cAMP to inhibit the release of IgE-mediated bronchoconstricting agents. This action, however, is only significant at serum levels 1,000 times the therapeutic range (1).

B. **Pharmacokinetics**

1. Methylxanthines are rapidly and efficiently absorbed from the GI tract with peak levels of immediate release theophylline preparations occurring within 2 h, and SR forms within 6 h from time of ingestion. These time intervals will be prolonged to 6 and 12 h, respectively, in the overdosed setting because of altered absorptive characteristics. Under therapeutic conditions, caffeine is more rapidly absorbed than theophylline with maximal serum concentrations occurring within 1 h.

2. Theophylline and caffeine have similar volumes of **distribution,** averaging between 0.4 to 0.6 L/kg. Methylxanthines cross the placenta and pass into breast milk. At therapeutic levels, theophylline is approximately 60% protein bound. This percentage decreases with higher plasma concentrations.

3. The methylxanthines are primarily **metabolized** by the cytochrome P450 oxidase system in the liver. This enzyme system can be saturated at elevated drug levels,

such that small doses can result in marked elevation of serum concentrations. The metabolism of theophylline in **preterm neonates** differs markedly from that of adults. Nearly 50% of theophylline is excreted unchanged in the urine in these patients, while 25% to 30% is metabolized to caffeine. In patients up to 4 weeks of age, both theophylline and caffeine levels should be drawn when theophylline toxicity is suspected to monitor the degree of toxicity and guide management.

4. The average **half-life** of theophylline and caffeine in healthy, nonsmoking adults is 5 to 8 h. The clearance of methylxanthines in preterm neonates is significantly prolonged, with half-lives of theophylline and caffeine to 20 h and 50 h, respectively.

5. The cytochrome P450 enzyme system determines hepatic clearance for the methylxanthines and is affected by factors that can either enhance or retard drug metabolism (Table 50-2). This can result in higher or lower serum drug concentrations.

IV. **Clinical manifestations**

A. Theophylline and caffeine toxicity present similarly and can affect multiple organ systems. At therapeutic levels, these agents can cause gastritis, tremulousness, and insomnia. Toxicity should be suspected in those who develop nausea, vomiting, tachydysrhythmias, agitation, or seizures. Patients at risk for either toxicity or a poor outcome are those with extremes of age, compromised health due to preexisting disease, and the use of medications affecting drug clearance.

B. There are two syndromes of toxicity with methylxanthines: the acute and the **chronic exposures.** Acute events are defined by a single ingestion of a toxic quantity of theophylline in a person not regularly taking the preparation. Chronic exposures are defined by a toxic serum theophylline concentration resulting after more than 24 h of theophylline use, without the ingestion of a single toxic quantity (4). Table 50-3 summarizes the clin-

TABLE 50-2. *Factors affecting theophylline clearance*

Decrease clearance	Increase clearance
Drugs	
Cimetidine	Carbamazepine
Enoxacin	Isoniazid
Erythromycin	Isoproterenol
Propranolol	Pentobarbital
Quinolones	Phenobarbital
Troleandomycin	Phenytoin
	Secobarbital
	Sulfinpyrazone
Diseases	
CHF	Cystic fibrosis
COPD	Hyperthyroidism
Cor pulmonale	
Hepatic Insufficiency	
Influenza	
Pneumonia	
Other conditions	
High-carbohydrate diet	Cigarette/marijuana smoking
	High-protein diet

TABLE 50-3. *Clinical differences between acute and chronic ingestions.*

Acute	Chronic
The young	The elderly
Serum levels correlate better with severity of illness	More severe symptoms at lower serum levels
Supraventricular dysrhythmias	Ventricular dysrhythmias
Hypokalemia, hyperglycemia, metabolic acidosis	

ical manifestations of these two syndromes. Patients who present with chronic toxicity are at higher risk for more severe manifestations and complications at serum concentrations lower than those with acute toxicity. This phenomenon may be related to the underlying state of health of the patient. Patients arriving to the emergency department (ED) soon after an acute exposure may progress to more severe manifestations of toxicity because of continual drug absorption. However, in patients with a chronic exposure, it is unlikely for them to deteriorate significantly upon admission.

C. **GI.** Nausea and vomiting occur in 60% to 100% of patients with serum levels greater than 20 mcg/mL (5). Diarrhea is a less common finding in methylxanthine overdoses. Upper GI bleeding has been reported in severe acute theophylline toxicity, and is attributed to catecholamine induced gastric acid secretion (6). It is important to note that the absence of GI symptoms does not exclude serious toxicity, and they may not present before more severe CNS or cardiac manifestations.

D. **Central nervous system.** The CNS effects of theophylline and caffeine toxicity include headache, tremulousness, agitation, confusion, lethargy, psychosis, and intractable seizures. Seizures are most concerning because they are associated with increased mortality (7). In acute overdoses they usually occur with serum levels greater than 80 mcg/mL, and in the chronic setting, with levels above 40 mcg/mL (8). The initial sign of toxicity may be a seizure, which is typically nonfocal and can progress to either stupor, coma, or status epilepticus. Prolonged seizures can contribute to rhabdomyolysis.

E. **Cardiovascular**
   1. The most common cardiac manifestation of methylxanthine toxicity is sinus tachycardia. This is invariably present in all significant toxicities. Supraventricular dysrhythmias are more common than ventricular types, and they occur more often in the younger population. Ventricular tachycardias are associated with severe toxicity and usually occur in the elderly and in those with underlying cardiac disease. Patients with chronic lung disease are predisposed to multifocal atrial tachycardias (MAT). Other factors contributing to dysrhythmias are hypoxia, metabolic acidemia, and electrolyte disorders.
   2. Hypotension is a more common manifestation in acute exposures. This may occur from either excessive catecholamine stimulation of beta-2 adrenergic receptors or volume depletion.

F. **Metabolic.** Metabolic derangements in methylxanthine toxicity include a lactic acidosis (secondary to seizure activity, agitation, or hypotension), hypokalemia, hyperglycemia, hypercalcemia, hypomagnesemia, and hypophosphatemia. Catecholamine stimulation, renal wasting, and vomiting are responsible for these effects. These effects increase the risk of dysrhythmias and seizures.

G. **Differential diagnosis.** Agents that can present in a similar fashion to either theophylline or caffeine toxicity are those causing an anion gap metabolic acidosis (especially iron, salicylates); other beta-2 adrenergic agonists (e.g., tertbutaline, albuterol) and other methylxanthines [e.g., theobromine, pentoxifylline (Trental)]. Pentoxifylline is used in the treatment of intermittent claudication. Although the occurrence of significant toxicity from methylxanthines other than theophylline is rarely reported, the management would be the same.

V. **Laboratory evaluations**

A. The laboratory manifestations of toxicity are respiratory alkalosis, metabolic acidosis, leukocytosis, hypokalemia, hyperglycemia, hypercalcemia, hypomagnesemia, and hypophosphatemia. These findings are more common in acute than chronic exposures. The EKG will most often show a sinus tachycardia. In more serious cases, supraventricular and ventricular dysrhythmias may be seen.

B. Serum theophylline levels correlate better with toxic symptoms in exposures that are acute rather than chronic. Minimal toxicity is expected at levels between 20 to 40 mcg/mL, moderate toxicity at 40 to 100 mcg/mL, and severe toxicity at serum levels over 100 mcg/mL. In chronic exposures, clinical manifestations are expected to occur at concentrations lower than these.

C. The time to peak drug level can be delayed because of SR formulations and altered pharmacokinetics in the toxic setting. Frequent monitoring of levels (e.g., every 1 to 2 h) may be necessary to guide management.

IV. **Management.** Patients presenting after a methylxanthine overdose can be severely ill and warrant immediate attention. All patients require i.v. access, cardiac monitoring, and baseline laboratory studies. These include a theophylline level, electrolytes, glucose, BUN, creatinine, complete blood count, arterial blood gas, and electrocardiogram. Upon stabilization of the ABCs, the method of GI decontamination is to be considered. For an outline of the management of the theophylline intoxication, see Fig. 50-1.

A. **Decontamination**

1. **Ipecac.** Induced emesis with ipecac is reserved only for ingestions of SR tablets (Table 50-1) in the following setting: arrival to a health care facility within 1 h of ingestion, the patient is not currently on a theophylline preparation, and no prior emesis has occurred. These conditions maximize the chance of pill recovery and minimize any untoward events to the patient. Otherwise, gastric ravage should be performed.

2. **Gastric lavage.** Gastric lavage with a 40-French orogastric tube is indicated in all exposures presenting within 1 h of ingestion, or with life-threatening manifestations of toxicity. Prior emesis and ingestion of SR tablets may limit the efficacy of lavage. The role of gastric lavage is more important with theophylline than other types of exposures because of the amount of drug involved. Large exposures to theophylline may consist of drug quantities that would exceed the amount of activated charcoal that can be practically administered to a patient in a given period of time. If the patient ingested 30 g of theophylline, then 300 g of activated charcoal would be necessary to bind this amount of drug. Since the patient will not be able to tolerate this amount of charcoal at one time, other means (e.g., gastric lavage) to decrease the drug burden will be necessary.

All Patients
1. Initial stabilization—ABC's
2. Cardiac monitor
3. Treat life-threatening arrhythmias
4. Establish IV line
5. IV $D_{50}W$, naloxone, and thiamine for altered mental status
6. Stat theophylline level and routine laboratory tests including Ca, PO_4, CPK
7. Rapid physical exam
8. OAC 30–40g q2–4h with cathartic initially (then PRN)
9. Repeat theophylline levels every 2 hours

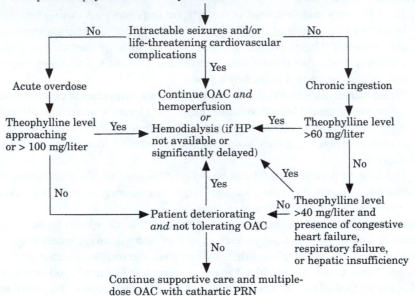

FIG. 50-1. Algorithm for the management of theophylline overdose.

3. **Activated charcoal.** Charcoal is extremely effective in limiting gut absorption of theophylline (9) and an initial dose of charcoal (1 g/kg p.o.) is indicated in all exposures. If diarrhea is not present, one dose of a cathartic can be administered as well. Repeat dose activated charcoal has been shown to enhance the elimination of theophylline with immediate and SR (10) preparations, and in parenteral overdoses (11). Even in toxic patients with delayed presentations, repetitive dose charcoal is indicated (12). The dosing of charcoal for repeat administration varies from 0.5 to 1 g/kg, every 2 to 4 h. In severe exposures, the amount of charcoal given will be greater and more frequent. Subsequent doses of cathartics are not indicated.

4. It is imperative that the patient maintains the oral doses of charcoal because this is the only medical therapy, aside from enhanced elimination, that has been shown to effectively limit the absorption and enhance the elimination of theophylline. Nasogastric tube administration of charcoal and aggressive use of i.v. antiemetics may be necessary. Ranitidine or famotidine may also be considered in the patient with GI distress.

5. **Whole bowel irrigation (WBI).** Clinical data is limited regarding the efficacy of polyethylene glycol electrolyte lavage (e.g., GoLytely, CoLytely) versus repeat dose activated charcoal therapy. Despite this, WBI therapy is indicated when there is a rising level despite attempts at enhanced elimination (e.g., repeat dose charcoal, hemodialysis, hemoperfusion), or when a significant ingestion of an SR preparation is suspected. The dose for the adult patient is 1 to 2 L/h, orally, until the stool is clear and theophylline levels are decreasing. Activated charcoal can be mixed with the WBI preparation.

B. **Antiemetics.** Protracted vomiting should be aggressively treated with metoclopramide. The dose is 0.1 mg/kg i.v., every 15 to 30 min (maximum 1 to 3 mg/kg/24 h). Ondansetron in a dosage of 0.15 mg/kg i.v. every 4 to 8 h may also be used in patients with refractory vomiting.

C. **Cardiovascular**

1. Common manifestations of toxicity are hypotension and tachydysrhythmias. Initial management should include the administration of an i.v. fluid bolus and the correction of hypoxemia, metabolic acidemia, and electrolyte imbalances. Adenosine is not recommended in controlling methylxanthine induced tachydysrhythmias because these agents impede the therapeutic effects of adenosine.

2. **Supraventricular tachycardia (SVT).** Therapy will depend on the patient's age, and hemodynamic and cardiac response. In the young patient with an adequate blood pressure and no evidence of cardiac ischemia on an ECG, supportive therapy would be recommended. The success of pharmacotherapeutic attempts in controlling drug induced tachycardia is uncertain and may contribute to adverse effects. Thus, in the stable patient, conservative therapy is warranted. In the elderly patient who may not be able to tolerate the rapid rate, or has evidence of cardiac ischemia on an ECG, and a stable blood pressure, then rate control with a calcium channel blocker (e.g., verapamil) or a short acting beta-1 adrenergic blocker (e.g., esmolol) can be used. Caution must be exercised in using any beta adrenergic blocker in patients with a history of reactive airway disease.

3. Patients with SVT and hypotension should initially receive an i.v. fluid bolus (10 to 20 mL/kg NS) for presumed dehydration resulting from toxicity. Electrical cardioversion in the unstable patient may be effective; however, its effects would be temporary as the drug toxicity will persist. An alpha adrenergic agonist (e.g., phenylephrine 100 to 200 mcg i.v., every 10 to 15 min until effect; then a maintenance infusion of 40 to 180 mcg/min) is recommended because it will not only raise the blood pressure, but also decrease the heart rate by causing a reflex bradycardia. Calcium channel blockers and esmolol are considerations; however, the contributory effects of these agents to hypotension and bronchospasm need to be weighed.

4. **Ventricular tachycardia.** In the hemodynamically stable patient, administer lidocaine. The efficacy of procainamide and bretylium in this setting is less well supported. Bretylium may enhance toxicity by increasing catecholamine levels. If the patient is hemodynamically unstable, electrocardioversion, lidocaine, and procainamide are indicated. In refractory situations where excessive catecholamine

stimulation may be contributing to the ventricular tachydysrhythmia, the cautious use of esmolol may be considered.

D. Seizures represent significant toxicity and should be aggressively managed. Initial treatment with benzodiazepines and then barbiturates is indicated. General anesthesia is required in refractory states. Phenytoin is not effective in controlling methylxanthine induced seizures, and has been demonstrated in animal studies to enhance mortality in this setting (13).

E. Metabolic

  1. Hypokalemia can result from GI loss and catecholamine-induced intracellular shifting. It should be repleted; the urgency depends on the level and condition of the patient.

  2. Metabolic acidosis. This is usually the result of an inciting event (e.g., hypotension, agitation, seizure) and will resolve if the primary condition is corrected.

F. Enhanced elimination

  1. The expeditious removal of the methylxanthine is indicated in certain situations to limit morbidity and mortality resulting from the exposure. Hemoperfusion is the preferred method because it clears theophylline more effectively than hemodialysis. However, when hemoperfusion is not available, hemodialysis would be indicated. Peritoneal dialysis is a poor alternative and is not recommended.

  2. Criteria for enhanced elimination are based on absolute levels and clinical manifestations. They include theophylline levels of greater than 100 mcg/mL in acute exposures and 50 mcg/mL in chronics (regardless of symptoms); severe clinical manifestations including seizures, uncontrollable dysrhythmias or refractory hypotension; or a rising level despite attempts at aggressive gut decontamination with charcoal. The endpoint for hemoperfusion/dialysis is when the serum concentration falls below 20 mcg/mL.

  3. Early consultation with a nephrologist is recommended when enhanced elimination is being considered. When the situation is unclear, the regional poison center or medical toxicologist can be consulted for assistance.

VII. Disposition

  A. All theophylline exposures must be observed until the trend of the serum concentration and its peak has been determined. If this can not be accomplished within 6 h, the patient should be admitted for further monitoring. All patients with rising serum theophylline levels over 20 mcg/mL or who have signs and symptoms of toxicity are to be admitted for continuous cardiac monitoring and serial levels drawn every 2 to 4 h to confirm elimination. Repeat doses of activated charcoal (0.5 to 1 g/kg) should be given every 2 to 4 h until the serum level is less than 20 mcg/mL and declining. Patients requiring hemoperfusion or hemodialysis should be stabilized and transferred to a facility with this capability and admitted to the intensive care unit.

  B. Patients who have declining theophylline levels below 20 mcg/mL can be considered for outpatient management. One dose of activated charcoal should be administered prior to discharge if an SR preparation is involved. If there is no significant electrolyte or EKG abnormalities, and other organic causes have been evaluated for, then the patient may be medically cleared of their exposure. Psychiatric consultation would be necessary as indicated.

References

1. Rall TW. Drugs used in the treatment of asthma. In: Goodman LS, Gilman A, eds. *Goodman and Gilman's The pharmacological basis of therapeutics*. 8th ed. New York: Pergamon Press, 1990:619–630.
2. Litovitz T, et al. 1994 annual report of the AAPCC Toxic Exposure Surveillance System. *Am J Emerg Med* 1995;13:551–597.
3. Vestal RE, Eriksson CE Jr, Musser B, Ozaki LK, Hafter JB. Effect of intravenous aminophylline on plasma levels of catecholamines and related cardiovascular and metabolic responses in man. *Circulation* 1983;67:162–171.
4. Shannon M, Lovejoy FH. Hypokalemia after theophylline intoxication. The effects of acute vs. chronic poisoning. *Arch Intern Med* 1989;149:2725–2729.
5. Paloucek FP, et al. Evaluation of theophylline overdoses and toxicities. *Ann Emerg Med* 1988;17:135–138.
6. Foster LJ, Trudear WL, Goldman AL. Bronchodilator effects on gastric acid secretion. *JAMA* 1979;241:2613–2615.
7. Zwillich CW, Sutton FD, Neff TA, Cohn WM, Matthay RA, Weinberger MM. Theophylline-induced seizures in adults. *Ann Intern Med* 1975;82:784–787.
8. Olson KR, Benowitz NL, Woo OF, Pond SM. Theophylline overdose: acute, single ingestion versus chronic repeated overmedication. *Am J Emerg Med* 1985;3:386–394.
9. Neuvonen PJ, Vartiainem M, Tokila O. Comparison of activated charcoal and ipecac syrup in prevention of drug absorption. *Eur J Clin Pharm* 1983;24:557–562.
10. Minton NA, Henry JA. Prevention of drug absorption in simulated theophylline overdose. *Clin Toxicol* 1995;33:43–49.
11. Berlinger WG, Spector R, Goldberg MJ, Johnson GF, Quee CK, Berg MJ. Enhancement of theophylline clearance by oral activated charcoal. *Clin Pharm Ther* 1983;33:351–354.
12. Lim DT, Singh P, Nourtsis S, Dela Cruz R. Absorption inhibition and enhancement of elimination of sustained-release theophylline tablets by oral activated charcoal. *Ann Emerg Med* 1986;15:1303–1307.
13. Blake KV, Massey KL, Hendeles L, Nickerson D, Neims A. Relative efficacy of phenytoin and phenobarbital for the prevention of theophylline-induced seizures in mice. *Ann Emerg Med* 1988;17:1024–1028.

Emergency Toxicology, Second Edition,
edited by Peter Viccellio.
Lippincott–Raven Publishers, Philadelphia © 1998.

51

Quinine

†Diane Sauter and °Richard Y. Wang

†Metropolitan Hospital, New York, New York 10029; °Department of Emergency Medicine,
Rhode Island Hospital, Providence, Rhode Island 02903

I. Introduction

A. Quinine is a major alkaloid of the bark of the cinchona tree, which is indigenous to various parts of South America. Cinchona, used since the seventeenth century as an antipyretic, contains more than 20 alkaloids, among which quinine and quinidine are perhaps the most familiar. These two agents are optic isomers and have similar properties.

B. Quinine is currently used as an antimalarial and in 1994 there were 221 exposures of this class reported to the American Association of Poison Control Centers (1). Fifty-eight percent of these patients were treated in a health care facility and there were two deaths attributed to quinine.

II. Available preparations

A. The oral preparation, quinine sulfate, is available in 120-, 200-, or 325-mg capsules or 260- and 325-mg tablets (2). Quinine dihydrochloride was available for parenteral use; however, it has been replaced by quinidine gluconate (80 mg/mL).

B. Quinine can also be found in tonic water. One liter contains about 100 to 200 mg of quinine.

III. Pharmacology and properties

A. The currently accepted use of quinine is in the treatment of chloroquine-resistant strains of *Plasmodium falciparum* (3). Quinine was used for the relief of nocturnal leg cramps, but is now replaced by other antimalarial agents. It has been demonstrated to be effective in myotonia congenita patients and has been used as a sclerosing agent for treatment of varicose veins. Quinine has achieved historical notoriety as an abortifacient. It is also found as an adulterant in heroin (4).

B. Mechanism of action

1. Quinine has local anesthetic action through the inhibition of sodium channels. However, pain, edema, and a reactive fibrosis occur at concentrations slightly higher than those necessary to achieve anesthesia (5).

2. It is a severe local irritant and when ingested causes nausea, vomiting, and abdominal pain. Subcutaneous or intramuscular injection, as occurs with heroin abuse, causes pain and can lead to the formation of skin abscesses. Its irritant property leads to vascular thrombosis when injected by vein and is the basis for the use of quinine as a sclerosing agent.

       3. Quinine exerts a curare-like effect on skeletal muscle. It decreases motor end-plate excitability.

  C. Pharmacology

       1. Quinine is readily absorbed when given orally. Absorption occurs in the proximal small intestine. Peak plasma concentrations occur within 1 to 3 h of ingestion. After discontinuation of therapy, plasma levels fall rapidly and are negligible after 24 h. Approximately 70% of plasma quinine is protein-bound.

       2. Quinine has a wide volume of distribution and is metabolized largely by the liver. Less than 5% of the unaltered form is excreted in the urine. Acid diuresis may enhance quinine renal elimination by ion trapping; however, the potential for increasing cardiac toxicity by promoting tissue binding lessens the appeal of this therapy.

       3. Dosage adjustment is required in the presence of renal failure, as its metabolites are excreted in the urine.

       4. The elimination half-life of quinine is prolonged in states of toxicity and can be as long as 26 h. The therapeutic elimination half-life is 11 h.

       5. Quinine does cross the placenta (6).

IV. **Clinical manifestations**

  A. Quinine has been called a "general protoplasmic poison" because it affects nearly every biologic system.

  B. Therapeutic doses of quinine—those used to treat malaria—may produce a set of symptoms to which the term cinchonism is applied. In its mildest form tinnitus, headache, altered auditory acuity, blurred vision, abdominal pain, nausea, and diarrhea occur. These symptoms may appear after a single dose or with accumulated low-dose therapy. There is marked individual variability of tolerance to quinine, but when small doses cause toxic manifestations the individual is probably hypersensitive and the drug should not be used.

  C. The daily ingestion of 1 L of tonic water (100 to 200 mg quinine) for 2 weeks has also resulted in mild toxicity with symptoms including blurred vision and difficulty with positional sense (7,8)

  D. Quinine toxicity occurs most commonly as a complication of attempts at abortion, suicide attempts, and accidental ingestions. Heroin abusers may present with signs and symptoms of quinine toxicity. After a single large ingestion or repeated high doses, more severe symptoms can occur, affecting particularly the GI tract, CNS, and cardiovascular systems (9). Ocular damage is characteristic.

  E. No clear lethal dose of quinine has been identified. Adverse effects occur with ingestions of 2.5 g or more. Death has occurred with ingestions of 8 g in adults, but the lethal dose may lie between 2 and 8 g; 900 mg has been fatal in children.

  F. Signs and symptoms

       1. GI symptoms occur with both mild and severe forms of toxicity and appear within 6 h of ingestion. The local irritant effects of quinine result in nausea, vomiting, pain, and diarrhea. A central action on the medulla contributes to the vomiting that occurs.

       2. Although the actions of quinine and quinidine on cardiac muscle are qualitatively similar, the effects of quinine are less intense (10). In general, quinine has few cardiac effects at therapeutic dosages. Serious cardiotoxicity following overdose has rarely been reported (11). The cardiac effects of quinine in overdose are probably secondary to the dysrhythmic properties it shares with quinidine. Conduction delays include prolongation of the PR and QT intervals, and QRS duration. Other abnormalities noted on the EKG are minor ST depression, T wave flattening or inversion, and the presence of U waves. Tachycardia following an overdose may result from vagal blockade. Significant hypotension has occurred with the use of quinine, particularly by the i.v. route. It is secondary to vasodilation and possibly to decreased myocardial contractility. Intravenous preparations should be appropriately diluted and administered slowly. Those deaths that occurred have resulted from intractable dysrhythmias (e.g., Torsades de pointes) or cardiovascular collapse. Plasma levels above 16 mg/L are associated with cardiac dysrhythmias.

3. With severe toxicity, CNS symptoms may include headache, apprehension, confusion, and delirium. Respiratory depression and coma may ensue. Tinnitus, decreased auditory acuity, and vertigo result from temporary impairment of the eighth nerve. Large overdoses have resulted in temporary deafness, but no case of permanent impairment has been reported. Seizures may occur and are observed more frequent in children (12).

4. Other than cardiotoxicity, the most severe toxic effects are ocular.

   a. Ocular toxicity is characterized by symptoms that include clouding of vision, abnormal color vision, photophobia, constriction of peripheral fields, diminution of central acuity, and in some cases complete blindness (13).

   b. Loss of vision usually occurs after 2 to 4 h but may be delayed for 1 to 2 days. The mechanism of this injury has been an area of controversy. Upon physical examination the pupils are found to be dilated and unreactive. The funduscopic appearance is normal at the onset of visual deterioration and may remain so, but in some individuals the examination has revealed marked retinal arteriolar constriction, pale disks, and edema following the onset of blindness (14). The latter findings are the basis for the controversy that exists. For many years the ocular damage has been attributed to this arteriolar spasm and associated ischemia. More recent research has implicated direct neural injury to the retina. Electroretinographic changes suggest that quinine initially affects the photoreceptor and ganglion cell layers (15). Electroculographic changes also suggest a toxic effect on the photoreceptor cells or retinal pigment epithelium. Arteriolar constriction is thought to be a secondary occurrence, but its exact role in the pathogenesis of retinal impairment remains uncertain. Complete blindness is usually not permanent. Visual defects resolve or improve over several hours (i.e., 12 to 18 h) to days or, in some cases, weeks (16). Individuals who experience the greatest degree of impairment are usually left with abnormal color vision, night-blindness, or constricted peripheral fields.

   c. Plasma quinine concentrations above 15 mg/L within 10 h of ingestion or 10 mg/L after 10 h of ingestion are associated with an increased risk of permanent ocular damage.

5. Hematologic toxicity includes acute hemolysis, hypoprothrombinemia, thrombocytopenic purpura, and agranulocytosis. A quinine-induced immunologic thrombocytopenia results from quinine-dependent antiplatelet antibodies (17).

6. Dermatologic symptoms include pruritus, with or without rash, erythema multi-forme, and angioedema. Photosensitivity has been reported in individuals on low doses of quinine (18,19).

7. Renal damage has been reported with the development of uremia and anuria.

8. A high incidence of hypoglycemia has been observed in patients receiving i.v. quinine for severe cases of malaria. The mechanism is thought to be the stimulation of pancreatic beta cells, resulting in insulin release (20). Patients receiving i.v. quinine are seriously ill, usually comatose, and should therefore undergo attentive monitoring for this complication. Administration of the drug in glucose solutions may be necessary. Those at increased risk include malnourished individuals, pregnant women, children, and those who are already hypoglycemic. Quinine does cross the placenta and can stimulate the fetal pancreas in the same manner.

9. Quinine has been used to induce abortion. Toxicity to the patient often occurs before abortion, and its use as an abortifacient should not be condoned. Quinine crosses the placenta, and there are some anecdotal case reports of congenital abnormalities, including optic atrophy in children exposed to quinine in utero. In a review, home use of quinine as an abortifacient was associated with 59% congenital anomalies and 15% maternal deaths (21).

10. Quinine has been shown to increase serum digoxin levels to cause toxicity by decreasing renal drug clearance (22). The production of vitamin K dependent clotting factors is diminished by quinine, which can potentiate the effects of oral anticoagulants (23).

G. Differential diagnosis. Other drug-induced disorders that need to be considered in the setting of quinine toxicity are those affecting hearing, vision, and cardiac conduction.

1. Salicylates, NSAIDs, aminoglycosides, antineoplastics, heavy metals (mercury and arsenic), and loop diuretics can present with altered hearing acuity.

2. Diminished vision can result from methanol, ergotamines, and cocaine toxicity.

3. Common agents that can cause cardiac membrane stabilizing effects are tricyclic antidepressants, Type IA and IC antidysrhythmics, carbamazepine, and cyclobenzaprine.

V. Laboratory evaluation. Quinine may be detected in urine. This test has been used for drug abuse screening, as quinine is a common adulterant of illicit drugs. Some institutions can measure plasma quinine levels by modifying the test for quinidine. Plasma levels may be useful early to predict the potential for ocular toxicity. Levels more than 10 mg/L have been associated with an increased risk of permanent ocular damage. Death is associated with levels of more than 16 mg/L (10,11). There is no correlation between plasma levels and the duration of the QT interval on the ECG.

VI. Management

A. The initial approach towards a quinine overdose consists of early gastric emptying, oral administration of activated charcoal, and supportive measures for the various complications. The use of activated charcoal for quinine poisoning has not been studied.

B. Cardiac dysrhythmias associated with a prolongation of the QRS duration may respond to serum alkalinization with sodium bicarbonate to a pH 7.45 to 7.55. This can be accomplished by administering sodium bicarbonate i.v. in the following manner: loading dose 1 mEq $NaHCO_3$/kg and maintenance infusion 0.2 to 0.4 mEq $NaHCO_3$/kg/h. In the setting of quinine toxicity, the serum should be alkalinized when the QRS is greater than 0.1 s and continued until this effect is no longer apparent. Resistant cardiac dys-rhythmias or those unassociated with conduction delays are best managed with lidocaine and correction of electrolyte abnormalities. Magnesium may be used in the presence of Torsades de pointes. Type IA antidysrhythmics (e.g., quinidine and procainamide) are contraindicated in the management of quinine-induced cardiotoxicity.

C. Treatment of ocular toxicity with stellate ganglion blockade, retrobulbar injection, and the use of oral and i.v. vasodilators has been advocated (24). None of these techniques have been demonstrated to be effective. The risks associated with stellate ganglion blockade or other vasodilator therapies outweigh the benefits, and their use is no longer advocated (25). There is presently no known treatment for the ocular neural damage.

D. Techniques for enhancement of drug excretion, including forced acid diuresis, hemo-dialysis, peritoneal dialysis, exchange transfusion, and charcoal hemoperfusion, have generally been found to be ineffective. The limitations are the drug's large volume of distribution and high protein binding. There have been a few case reports of clinical improvement in patients treated with hemoperfusion. Charcoal hemoperfusion does effectively lower serum levels at least temporarily and may be beneficial in severely ill patients. However, redistribution from tissue to the vascular compartment occurs and the patient will likely experience the return of symptoms after cessation of treatment. Ulti-mately, hemoperfusion may be of most benefit in patients who present early after an overdose and before tissue distribution has occurred. None of these techniques has been adequately studied, and to date none has been shown to be of any benefit in the preven-tion of the ocular manifestations of toxicity. Acidification of the urine, although demon-strated to increase urinary excretion of quinine, is not recommended because cardio-toxicity may be enhanced.

VII. **Disposition**

A. All patients with suspected quinine toxicity should be evaluated in a health care facility. During the assessment period, it is necessary to obtain an initial EKG and to maintain the patient on a continuous cardiac monitor.

B. If the patient remains asymptomatic (i.e., no GI manifestations, and normal repeat ECG) after 6 h of observation, the patient may be medically cleared of their exposure.

C. Symptomatic patients are to be admitted to a cardiac monitored bed for further observa-tion and management. Patients with either cardiovascular or CNS findings warrant an intensive care unit bed. Periodic funduscopic examinations should be performed by an ophthalmology consultant.

D. The regional poison control center can be consulted for further assistance.

References

1. Litovitz TL, et al. 1994 annual report of the American Association of Poison Control Centers Toxic Exposure Surveil-lance System. *Am J Emerg Med* 1995;13:551.
2. *AMA drug evaluations*. 5th ed. Chicago: AMA, 1983.
3. Henry J. Quinine for night cramps. *BMJ* 1985;291:3.

4. Goldfrank LR, Osborn M. Quinine. In: Goldfrank LR, et al., eds. *Goldfrank's toxicologic emergencies*. East Norwalk, CT: Appleton & Lange, 1990:337–340.
5. Webster LT. Drugs used in the chemotherapy of protozoal infections. In: Goodman LS, Gilman A, eds. *Goodman and Gilman's. The pharmacological basis of therapeutics*. 8th ed. New York: Pergamon Press, 1990:991–994.
6. Looareesuwan S, et al. Quinine and severe falciparum malaria in late pregnancy. *Lancet* 1985;2:4.
7. Berglund F. Toxicity of quinine. *Toxicology* 1989;58:237.
8. Satjchuk JT, et al. Electronystagmographic findings in long-term low-dose quinine ingestion. *Arch Otolaryngol* 1984; 110:788.
9. Boland ME, Brennand Roper SM, Henry JA. Complications of quinine poisoning. *Lancet* 1985;1:384.
10. Dyson EM, et al. Death and blindness due to overdose of quinine. *BMJ* 1985;291:31.
11. Bateman DN, et al. Pharmacokinetics and clinical toxicity of quinine overdosage: lack of efficacy of techniques intended to enhance elimination. *Q J Med* 1985;54:125.
12. Grattan-Smith TM, Gillis J, Kilham H. Quinine poisoning in children. *Med J Aust* 1987;147:93.
13. Smilkstein MJ, Kulig KW, Rumack BM. Acute toxic blindness: unrecognized quinine poisoning. *Ann Emerg Med* 1987;16:98.
14. Bacon P, Spalton DJ, Smith SE. Blindness from quinine toxicity. *Br J Ophthalmol* 1988;72:219.
15. Moloney JB, Hillery M, Fenton M. Two year electrophysiology follow-up in quinine amblyopia. *Acta Ophthalmol (Copenh)* 1987;65:731.
16. Canning CR, Magne S. Ocular quinine toxicity. *Br J Ophthalmol* 1988;72:23.
17. Christie DJ, Diad-Aruzo M, Cook J. Antibody mediated platelet destruction by quinine, quinidine and their metabolites. *J Lab Clin Med* 1988;117:631.
18. Ljunggren B, Sjovall P. Systemic quinine photosensitivity. *Arch Dermatol* 1986;122:909.
19. Ferguson J, Addo HA, Johnson BE. Quinine-induced photosensitivity: clinical and experimental studies. *Br J Dermatol* 1987;117:631.
20. Rizack MA, Hillman CD, eds. *The* Medical Letter *handbook of adverse drug interactions*. New Rochelle, NY: Medical Letter, 1985:68.
21. Dannenberg AL, Dorfman SF, Johnson J. Use of quinine for self-induced abortion. *South Med J* 1983;76:846.
22. Aronson JK, Carver JG. Interaction of digoxin with quinine. *Lancet* 1981;1:1418.
23. Okitolonda W, et al. High incidence of hypoglycemia in African patients treated with intravenous quinine for severe malaria. *BMJ* 1987;295:716.
24. Dyson EM, Proudfoot AT, Bateman DN. Quinine amblyopia: is current management appropriate? *Clin Toxicol* 1986; 23:571.
25. Bateman DN, et al. Stellate ganglion block and quinine overdose. *Anesthesia* 1984;39:71.

Emergency Toxicology, Second Edition,
edited by Peter Viccellio.
Lippincott–Raven Publishers, Philadelphia © 1998.

52

Ergot Alkaloids

†Michael T. Handrigan and °Richard Y. Wang

*†San Antonio, Texas 78247-5902; °Department of Emergency Medicine, Rhode Island Hospital,
Providence, Rhode Island 02903*

I. **Introduction.** The ergot alkaloids are byproducts of metabolism of the fungus Claviceps (1). Epidemic intoxication has occurred from the ingestion of rye grain contaminated by this fungus. The first reference to the clinical syndrome of ergot toxicity, or "ergotism," was in the 9th century A.D. (2) and became known as "St. Anthony's Fire." Victims that consumed the affected grain complained of paresthesias of the hands and feet, and developed gangrene of the extremities. Several compounds have been identified from the grain, including histamine, histidine, tyramine, tyrosine, tryptophan, choline, acetylcholine, and ergosol (3). The most recent grain-related epidemic occurred in Ethiopia in 1978. Strict agricultural controls have virtually eliminated such risks in the United States. Today, in the United States, ergot toxicity most commonly occurs as a result of the therapeutic use of these agents in the treatment of vascular headaches. Chronic use and overuse of these agents is most often the case; however, toxicity can occur following a single therapeutic dose.

II. **Available preparations**

    A. The ergot alkaloids are classified into two categories, according to their side chain substituents. They are the amine alkaloids and the ergopeptides. The majority of the available preparations are used in the **treatment** of acute migraine headache. These contain a standard amount of either ergotamine or dihydroergotamine. Many **preparations** also contain caffeine, belladonna alkaloid, and phenobarbital. Caffeine enhances both the rapidity and completeness of ergotamine absorption. The belladonna alkaloid is used to decrease the emetic effects of the ergots. Other uses for these agents are postpartum bleeding, inhibition of lactation, Parkinsonism, dementia, and narcolepsy.

    B. Table 52-1 summarizes the available ergot alkaloids with respect to their dosing, indication, and primary toxicity.

III. **Pharmacology and properties**

    A. **Mechanisms of action**

        1. The ergot alkaloids exert their primary effects by **stimulating adrenergic receptors,** both peripherally and centrally. Each of the ergot alkaloids has a variable degree of agonist-antagonist activity at serotonergic, dopaminergic, and alpha- and beta-adrenergic receptor sites (4). These agents also directly stimulate smooth muscle fibers. The result is a combination of peripheral and central vasoconstriction, myometrial contraction, and stimulation of emesis. Hypotension may also

TABLE 52-1. *Available ergot preparations*

	Maximum dose	Principal action	Primary toxicity
Amine alkaloids			
Metherginine (methylergonon-vine, 0.2-mg tab)	0.2 mg i.v., i.m., q 24 h 0.2 mg p.o. q 4 h	Smooth muscle stimulation	Hypertension followed by hypotension
Sandsert (methysergide, 2-mg tab)	4–8 mg p.o. daily	Serotonin blockade	Tissue fibrosis, vasospasm, ischemia
Ergopeptides			
Bellergal (each tab contains 0.3–0.4 mg ergota-mine, 40 mg phenobarbitol, 0.2 mg bella-donna alkaloid)	1 p.o. b.i.d.	Vasoconstriction, proemetic, myometrial contraction	Combined toxicity of all three constituents, though there has been no reported overdose
Cafergot (each tab contains 1 mg ergotamine tar-trate, 100 mg caffeine; each suppository (spp.) contains 2 mg ergotamine tartrate, 100 mg caffeine)	6 tabs or 2 spp. per headache; or 10 tabs or 5 spp. per week	Vasoconstriction, proemetic, myometrial contraction	Vasospasm, cardia ischemia, hypertension, CNS depres-sion, seizure, and general-ized tissue fibrosis
Ergostat, Wigraine, Ergomar (2 mg ergotamine tartrate)	1 tab s.l. q 30 min × 3 (max daily dose 6 mg; max weekly dose 10 mg)	Vasoconstriction, proemetic, myometrial contraction	Vasospasm, cardia ischemia, hypertension, CNS depres-sion, seizure, and general-ized tissue fibrosis
DHE 45 (1 mg dihydroergotamine)	1 mg i.m./i.v. q 1 h (max 2 mg i.v., 3 mg i.m.; max weekly dose 6 mg	Alpha-adrenergic blockade, vasoconstriction	Vasospasm, cardia ischemia, hypertension, CNS depres-sion, seizure, and general-ized tissue fibrosis
Hydergine (0.5–1 mg ergoloid mesylate)	1 mg t.i.d. p.o./s.l.	Unknown mechanism	Lingual irritation, nausea, vomiting; no vasocon-striction
Parlodel (2.5–5 mg bromocriptine)	100 mg/d (Parkinsonism); 2.5–15 mg/day (inhibition of lactation)	Alpha-adrenergic blockade, proemetic	Mainly CNS depression and adrenergic instability; no vasoconstriction

occur because of central sympatholytic activity in combination with peripheral adrenergic blockade.

2. The **amine alkaloids** (e.g., methysergide) have potent myometrial contractile properties and minimal alpha-adrenergic and serotonergic receptor activities.

3. The **ergopeptides** have more potent alpha-adrenergic activity. Ergotamine is the most potent agent in this class with respect to vasopressor and emetic activities. Dihydroergotamine has strong alpha-adrenergic blocking and weak serotonergic and emetic effects.

4. Bromocriptine is mainly an alpha-adrenergic blocker and an emetic, and has no serotonergic and myometrial activity.

B. **Pharmacokinetics.** The pharmacokinetics of the ergot alkaloids have been studied in healthy volunteers given therapeutic doses. No information exists regarding the pharmacokinetic behavior of these agents in the toxic setting.

    1. **Absorption.** The ergots are poorly absorbed and have variable bioavailability by either the gastrointestinal or i.m. route of administration. Caffeine is commonly added in the formulations of the ergot alkaloids because it enhances water solubility of the ergot alkaloids and hence increases both the amount absorbed and the rate of absorption of these agents (5). The oral route yields lower peak plasma concentrations than the rectal route because of hepatic metabolism from the first pass effect. The time to peak plasma concentrations is usually achieved within 1 h by oral dosing and 2 to 3 h by rectal dosing. The half-life of ergotamine is approximately 2 h, whereas that of dihydroergotamine is as long as 13 h (6). These agents are rapidly distributed to the tissues and are concentrated in the liver, lungs, kidney, and heart. Slow release from tissue stores may result in a delayed elimination. Although the specific metabolic pathways have not been described, it is likely that active metabolites are present since prolonged clinical effects may persist in spite of nondetectable ergotamine levels (7). **Intravenous** administration results in a rapid peak plasma concentration and a plasma half life of less than 1 h. The i.m. route is less favored because of erratic absorption. Nevertheless, peak plasma levels may be achieved in 15 min. The volume of distribution is 2 L/kg.

    2. **Metabolism.** The ergot alkaloids are metabolized by the liver, and only 10% of the parent compound is excreted renally unchanged. Biliary elimination accounts for 80% to 90% of drug elimination.

IV. **Clinical manifestations.** "Ergotism" is an old term used to describe the constellation of findings due to ergot toxicity. This is comprised of nausea, vomiting, and ischemia. However, as more types of alkaloids became available for therapeutic use, the manifestations of ergot toxicity became less well-defined. Individual agents have selective pharmacologic activity which contribute to a varied clinical presentation in the toxic setting. Patients who are **predisposed** to toxicity include those with a history of coronary artery disease, peripheral vascular disease, thyrotoxicosis, hypertension, asthma, active hepatic or renal disease, sepsis, and pregnancy. **Chronic** therapeutic use or overuse result mainly in peripheral and organ ischemia. **Acute** intoxication has a more dramatic presentation with multiple system involvement. In general, the patient will manifest nausea, vomiting, hypertension and/or hypotension, tissue and organ ischemia/infarction, and spontaneous abortion.

A. **CNS.** Central nervous system depression including lethargy and coma may occur. Seizure, cerebral infarction, and psychosis have been reported following acute overdose (8). Nonspecific symptoms include anxiety, euphoria, insomnia, depression, dizziness, and dysarthria. Headache may occur in the setting of chronic overuse, acute overdose, or from withdrawal of an ergotamine after chronic therapy. Withdrawal symptoms may necessitate a slow wean from therapeutic use of these agents. Cortical atrophy and focal neurologic deficits have been reported following long-term therapy (9).

B. **Cardiovascular.** Hypertension and reflex bradycardia may occur from peripheral vasoconstriction. In the presence of a beta-adrenergic blocker (e.g., propranolol), this effect may be exaggerated because of unopposed alpha-adrenergic stimulation. Hypotension can result from the combined effects of central sympatholytic activity and peripheral alpha blockade. Tachycardia and bradycardia have been reported. Prolonged vasospasm may lead to limb ischemia, which would be evidenced by pain, pallor, coolness, paresthesias, and the lack of pulses. Complete arterial occlusion may occur leading to a gangrenous extremity or organ. While the lower extremities are most often affected, any vascular bed may be susceptible. Other manifestations of acute toxicity include coronary artery spasm, myocardial infarction, ventricular ectopy, dysrhythmia, mesenteric ischemia, Raynaud's phenomenon, pseudoaneurysm, and deep venous thrombosis. Long-term use is associated with intermittent claudication and peripheral neuropathies (10).

C. **Respiratory.** Severe bronchospasm may develop in patients with a known history of asthma secondary to direct stimulation of bronchial smooth muscle (11).

D. **Gastrointestinal.** Nausea, vomiting, and abdominal pain are associated with overdoses and the therapeutic use of these agents. Enteric vascular insufficiency progressing to bowel infarction can occur. The pancreas and liver are other organs susceptible to ischemia. Chronic therapy resulting in portal vein fibrosis can lead to portal hypertension. Rectal stenosis can occur with long-term suppository use.

E. **Renal.** Renal failure may result from chronic vascular insufficiency.

F. **Pregnancy.** Spontaneous abortion, intrauterine fetal demise, postpartum CVA, puerperal psychosis and birth deformities are associated with these agents. The ergots are classified by the FDA as Category X.

G. **Specific agents**
    1. **Ergotamine tartrate/dihydroergotamine.** The amino acid alkaloids have the most potent vasoconstrictive properties of all the ergots. They are, not only, extremely effective in treating vascular headaches, but also, the most likely to cause significant toxicity. Chronic therapeutic use or misuse can lead to vascular changes, including thickening of the elastic interna, subintimal and medial fibrosis, and thrombosis. Limb ischemia, especially of the lower extremities, may occur and present days after exposure. Other vascular beds commonly involved are the heart, kidneys, mesentery, eyes, tongue, and brain (12).
    2. **Methysergide** is primarily a serotonin antagonist. Although it shares some of the effects of ergotamine, it has less vasoconstrictive and direct smooth muscle activity. Chronic use may result in vascular changes similar to ergotamines. There is a higher incidence of tissue fibrosis associated with the long-term use with methysergide than with other agents in this class. Fibrosis of heart valves, great vessels, retroperitoneum, lung, and pleura have been reported in the literature (13).
    3. **Bromocriptine** toxicity is limited to CNS depression, nausea, and vomiting (14). There are no vasoconstrictive effects associated with its use. The potential for hemodynamic or autonomic instability from bromocriptine ingestion is small.

H. **Differential diagnosis.** All causes of hypertension, increased adrenergic states, primary causes of tissue ischemia (e.g., myocardial infarction, stroke), and hypercoagulable states should be considered.

V. **Laboratory**
    A. Serum concentrations of the ergot alkaloids are not helpful in determining the therapeutic course of the patient. Necessary interventions are based on the clinical assessment and the presence of objective evidence of toxicity.

B. Serum chemistries, including cardiac enzymes and lactic acid levels, may demonstrate evidence of end organ ischemia. An electrocardiogram is necessary to evaluate for any cardiac involvement. Abdominal radiographs may show thickened bowel walls, thumb printing, and adynamic ileus as evidence of bowel ischemia. If there is evidence of limb ischemia, angiography is recommended to confirm its presence, and to determine its location, nature (thrombotic, embolic, vasospastic), and extent of involvement. Color flow Doppler has been helpful in following the efficacy of treatment and in delineating coexistent deep venous thrombosis. A baseline prothrombin and partial thromboplastin time is necessary if heparin therapy is anticipated. A computer tomography scan can assist in the evaluation of cerebral and renal infarctions.

VI. Management (Fig. 52-1)

   A. General. Patients presenting with an altered sensorium need to be initially managed by stabilizing their airway, breathing, and circulatory status. All patients presenting with an altered mental status should receive standard doses of thiamine, naloxone, and 50% dextrose, for presumed hypoglycemia, hypoxemia, opioid toxicity, and thiamine deficiency. Acute overdose with ergots warrants gastric lavage and the administration of activated charcoal. Emesis with ipecac is not recommended because of the potential for altered mental status and uncontrolled blood pressure. Patients with chronic toxicity should have these agents discontinued.

   B. Specific. The mainstay of therapy in ergot intoxication involves cardiovascular stabilization and supportive care. The general principles of treatment are outlined in Fig. 52-1. Those patients in whom you suspect an acute ingestion, and patients with a chronic exposure who present with evidence of vascular insufficiency, require continuous cardiac monitoring and an i.v. access.

      1. For patients presenting with evidence of **organ or limb ischemia,** a peripheral vasodilator is recommended to reverse any vasospasm. Intravenous and intra-arterial nitroglycerin have been used with good results (15–17). A nitroglycerin infusion, beginning at 2 to 5 mcg/kg/min, can be titrated to effect. **Heparin** and low molecular weight dextran are useful in preventing thrombosis caused by vascular stasis. Anticoagulation with heparin (5,000 U i.v. bolus followed by a constant infusion of 800 to 1,000 U/h) may be of benefit when arterial insufficiency is present (18). The incidence of arterial thrombus formation is low in ergot intoxication, however, when documented by arteriography, **thrombolytic agents** such as streptokinase or urokinase should be considered. When medical management fails to reestablish vascular flow, surgical revascularization with angioplasty or arthrectomy may be indicated. Hyperbaric oxygen therapy has also been used successfully in treating ergot induced ischemia refractory to medical therapy. A peripheral vasodilator is recommended for the management of uncontrolled **hypertension. Nitroglycerin** (0.4 mg SL, or an i.v. infusion to begin at 5 mcg/min and titrated to effect) and nitroprusside (begin at 1 to 5 mcg/kg/min i.v.) may be used for emergent situations. Caution is to be exercised in using oral or sublingual nifedipine because of the difficulty in titration. For less urgent situations, oral therapy with prazosin (1 mg q8h) (19), captopril (50 mg p.o. t.i.d.) (20), and nifedipine (10 mg p.o. t.i.d.) have shown some clinical benefit. The use of beta adrenergic blocking agents is not

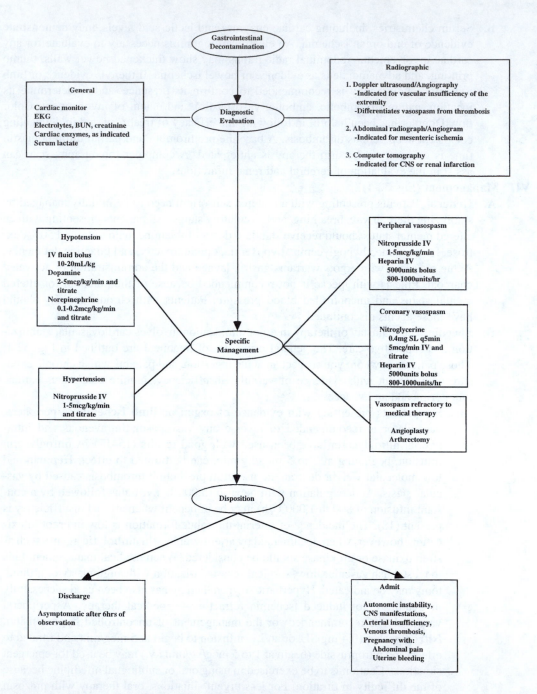

FIG. 52-1. Management of ergotamine toxicity.

recommended because of the potential for unopposed alpha-adrenergic effects. Hypotension can initially be managed with 10 to 20 mL/kg normal saline bolus and Trendelenburg positioning. Refractory hypotension can be treated with vasopressors, such as **dopamine** (starting at 2 mcg/kg/min i.v.) or norepinephrine (starting at 0.1 to 0.2 mcg/kg/min i.v.).

2. Persistent **abdominal pain** may represent visceral arterial occlusion. Angiography is currently the gold standard in evaluating mesenteric ischemia and should be considered in all such patients. In the presence of elevated creatinine, hematuria, or decreasing urine output, an abdominal CT is indicated to rule out renal artery occlusion or renal infarct.

3. Benzodiazepines are recommended for the management of **psychomotor agitation** and **seizures.** For refractory or recurrent seizures, phenytoin and/or phenobarbital are indicated. A head CT is indicated to define a cerebrovascular accident or subarachnoid hemorrhage. If there is no evidence of intracranial blood, heparin anticoagulation is recommended if there is clinical evidence for cerebrovascular occlusive disease. An i.v. peripheral vasodilator can be used for blood pressure control and to promote distal blood flow.

C. **Enhancing elimination.** Repeat dose activated charcoal may enhance biliary elimination of these agents because 90% of the drug is cleared by this route. These agents have large volumes of distribution and are not amenable to either hemodialysis or peritoneal dialysis.

VII. **Disposition**

A. **Admission.** All patients exhibiting evidence of adrenergic instability, (e.g., hypertension, hypotension, and cardiac dysrhythmias), limb ischemia, or altered mental status mandate admission to a centrally monitored bed for further management. Pregnant patients with abdominal pain are to be admitted for fetal monitoring with an obstetrical consultation.

B. **Discharge.** Patients who are asymptomatic on arrival and for 6 h of observation can be medically cleared of this ingestion. Consultation with psychiatry should be obtained as needed. Patients admitted to the hospital may be discharged when all evidence of toxicity has resolved. In all other situations, the regional poison center or medical toxicologist are to be consulted for further recommendations.

References

1. Merrhof GC, Porter JM. Ergot toxicity. *Ann Surg* 1974;180:773–779.
2. Barger G. *Ergot and ergotism.* London: Gurney and Jackson, 1931.
3. Henry LG, et al. Ergotism. *Arch Surg* 1975;110:929–932.
4. Ellenhorn JM, Barceloux BD, eds. *Medical toxicology: treatment of human poisoning.* New York: Elsevier Science, 1988.
5. Aellig WH, Nuesch E. Comparative pharmacokinetic investigations with tritium labeled ergot alkaloids after oral and intravenous administration in man. *Int J Clin Pharmacol* 1977;15:106–112.
6. Tfelt-Hansen P, Paalzow L. Intramuscular ergotamine: plasma levels and dynamic activity. *Clin Pharmacol Ther* 1985;37:29–35.
7. Orton DA, Richardson RJ. Ergotamine absorption and toxicity. *Postgrad Med J* 1982;58:6–11.
8. Senter HJ, Lieberman AN, Pinto R. Cerebral manifestations of ergotism. *Stroke* 1976;7:88–92.

9. Finchman RW, Perdue Z, Dunn VD. Bilateral focal cortical atrophy and chronic ergotamine abuse. *Neurology* 1985;35: 720–722.

10. Harrison TE. Ergotaminism. *JACEP* 1978;7:162–169.

11. Talwar KK, Kothari SS, Bhatia ML. Bronchospasm following ergotamine testing for coronary spasm. *Am Heart J* 1985;109:1415.

12. Galer BS, et al. Myocardial ischemia related to ergot alkaloids: a case report and literature review. *Headache* 1991;31: 446–450.

13. Orlando RC, Richardson RJ. Methysergide therapy and constrictive pericarditis. *Ann Intern Med* 1978;88:213–214.

14. Vermund SH, et al. Accidental bromocriptine ingestion in childhood. *J Pediatr* 1984;105:838–839.

15. Husum B, et al. Nitroglycerine infusion for ergotism. *Lancet* 1979;2:794.

16. Dierckx RA, et al. Intra-arterial sodium nitroprusside infusion in the treatment of severe ergotism. *Clin Neuropharmacol* 1986;9:542–548.

17. Eurin B, Samii K, Rorby JJ. Ergot and sodium nitroprusside. *N Engl J Med* 1978;298:632–633.

18. Harrison TE. Ergotism after a single dose of ergotamine tertrate. *J Emerg Med* 1984;2:23–25.

19. Cobaugh DS. Prazosin treatment of ergotamine-induced peripheral ischemia. *JAMA* 1980;244:1360.

20. Zimran A, Ofed B, Hershko C. Treatment with captopril for peripheral ischemia induced by ergotamine. *BMJ* 1984; 288:364.

21. Kemerer VF, Dagher FJ, Osher PS. Successful treatment of ergotamine with nifedipine. *AJR* 1984;143:333–334.

Emergency Toxicology, Second Edition,
edited by Peter Viccellio.
Lippincott–Raven Publishers, Philadelphia © 1998.

53

Thyroid Hormones

Adam J. Singer

Department of Emergency Medicine, University Hospital and Medical Center,
State University of New York at Stony Brook, Stony Brook, New York 11794-7400

I. **Introduction.** Thyroid hormones are used as replacement therapy in hypothyroidism and as suppressant therapy in goiters and certain thyroid neoplasms. These agents have an effect on a wide range of actions, including growth and development, oxygen consumption, basal metabolism, and heat generation. Hypothyroidism is a relatively common endocrine disorder that affects between 1% and 7% of the adult population (1). Despite wide availability, severe toxicity from thyroid hormone ingestion is relatively rare. Even massive ingestions may have a benign course (2–6). During the years 1985 to 1994, there were three deaths among 34,582 cases of thyroid hormone ingestion reported to the American Association of Poison Control Centers. All of these deaths were attributed to a coingestant. An acute overdose of thyroid hormone, alone, has never been reported to cause death; however, serious toxicity—especially in patients with underlying cardiovascular disease—may result. Excessive intake in chronic users of thyroid hormone has resulted in sudden death (7).

II. **Available preparations**
  A. Natural sources such as thyroid extract or desiccated thyroid hormone are available, but are no longer widely prescribed. Their average daily dose is 1 grain or 65 mg.
  B. Synthetic preparations are most commonly prescribed.
   1. Levothyroxine or tetraiodothyronine (T4) is available as Synthroid, Cytolen, or Levoid. The average daily dose is 0.1 mg or 100 mcg. Levothyroxine is also available in an injectible form as Levoid and Synthroid.
   2. Liothyronine sodium or triiodothyronine (T3) is available as Cytomel. The average dose is 25 mcg.
  C. Potency equivalents. The dose equivalents for the various commercial hormone preparations are approximately 1 g (60 mg) of the crude thyroid extract for 0.1 mg of L-thyroxine and 30 mcg of L-triiodothyronine (8). Liotrix contains a 4:1 mixture of T4 and T3 and is dispensed in grain equivalents of the crude extract.

III. **Pharmacology and properties of agents**
  A. **Physiology.** L-Tetraiodothyronine (T4) and L-triiodothyronine (T3) are synthesized within thyroglobulin, which is a large protein molecule stored within the lumen of the thyroid gland follicles. The thyroid hormones are iodine containing derivatives of the amino acid thyronine. Iodine is absorbed in the gut in the reduced form of iodide. It is then taken up by the thyroid gland where it is oxidized and attached to tyrosine residues of thyroglobulin (organification) to form monoiodotyrosine (MIT) or diiodotyrosine

(DIT). The coupling of MIT and DIT forms T3, and the coupling of two molecules of DIT forms T4. The synthesis and release of thyroid hormones are controlled by pituitary thyrotropin (TSH) which in turn is controlled by a delicate balance between the stimulatory effect of hypothalamic TSH-releasing hormone (TRH) and the inhibitory feedback effect of free thyroid hormone. Most of the actions of thyroid hormone at the cellular level are mediated by T3. T4 is active through its conversion to T3 in the peripheral tissues which takes 3 to 4 days to occur.

B. **Mechanism of action**

1. Thyroid hormones regulate several activities in the body, including growth, calorigenesis, lipolysis, and carbohydrate metabolism. These actions are primarily attributed to increase protein synthesis, which results from thyroid hormone stimulation of gene transcription.

2. These agents can also enhance metabolism by increasing the number and activity of mitochondrias, and promoting the active transport of ions across the cell membrane. Uncoupling of oxidative phosphorylation can occur at high concentrations of thyroxine and cause an excess amount of heat generation (9).

3. The positive chronotropic and ionotropic effects of thyroid hormones on the heart are mediated by an increase in number of cardiac beta-adrenergic receptors and the regulation of myosin chain synthesis. The production of more heavy chain alpha myosin and less heavy beta myosin results in increased myocardial contractility through the enhancement of Ca^{2+}-ATPase activity.

C. **Pharmacokinetics**

1. Absorption from the stomach occurs within 1 to 2 h. The oral bioavailability of T3 is approximately 95% (10), whereas the bioavailability of T4 is 30% to 90% (11). Peak levels for T3 are attained after 24 h; those of T4 are achieved in less than 12 h. More than 99% of thyroid hormones are protein bound.

2. Metabolism of both hormones is mainly by peripheral deiodonation. About 20% of the hormone is excreted in the feces unchanged or as a conjugated liver metabolite. The elimination half-life of T3 is 2 days or less and of T4 is 5 to 7 days (12). In children, the half-life of T4 is slightly less (13).

3. Time of onset and duration. T3 usually produces clinical effects within several hours. T4, which requires peripheral conversion to T3, yields delayed clinical effects that can appear up to 7 days (usually 3 to 4 days) after ingestion. Preparations containing T3 and T4 can have both early and delayed effects.

IV. **Clinical presentation.** Thyroid hormone ingestions are usually seen in patients and close contacts of patients on chronic thyroid hormone replacement therapy. Ingestions may also be seen in health care workers.

A. **Manifestations** are principally due to sympathomimetic effects, increased metabolism, and increased motor activity. The earliest signs of toxicity are tachycardia, hyperactivity, and fever (5,14–16). Children appear to be more resistant to the toxic effects of thyroid hormones than adults (2,3,5,6,15,16).

1. Sympathomimetic effects. Tachycardia, hypertension, mydriasis, diaphoresis, dysrhythmias (particularly atrial fibrillation), chest pain (secondary to myocardial ischemia or infarction), and rarely circulatory collapse.

2. Neurologic effects. Agitation, tremor, dizziness, headaches, seizures, and coma.
3. GI effects. Vomiting and diarrhea.
4. Other effects include fever and thyrotoxicosis. Fever is the result of psychomotor agitation and uncoupling of oxidative phosphorylation. Thyrotoxicosis is a syndrome consisting of tachycardia, anxiety, insomnia, diarrhea, weight loss, heat intolerance, flushed skin, and muscle wasting. Angina, cardiac dysrhythmias, and cardiac failure may be seen in the elderly. Seizures, psychosis, and coma have also been described. This disorder caused by thyroid hyperfunction and rarely occurs after an acute ingestion of thyroid hormones.

B. **Differential diagnosis** includes ingestion of other sympathomimetic agents such as cocaine, amphetamines, and phenylpropanolamine as well as states of withdrawal from sedative hypnotic agents.

V. **Laboratory evaluations.** Elevated levels of T3 and T4 may confirm ingestion, however they are poorly correlated with the degree of clinical toxicity. The delayed availability of these test results limit their clinical utility. Elevated values of T4 (more than 25 mcg/dL) 6 h after ingestion require clinical assessment for at least 10 days due to delayed effects.

VI. **Management**

A. **General.** Although most authorities agree that ingestions of less than 0.5 to 2.0 mg of T4 do not require any GI decontamination in the asymptomatic child or adult (5,16–18), it has recently been suggested that ingestions of up to 5 mg do not require decontamination (15). In a recent review of the literature, no major toxicity following ingestions of 5 mg or less of thyroid hormone was reported (15). Accidental ingestions of less than 2 to 5 mg of thyroxine require only home observation and close follow-up for 10 days. All intentional and accidental ingestions of greater than 2 to 5 mg of thyroxine or 0.75 mg of triiodothyronine require GI decontamination and evaluation in a health care facility. Children who ingest any amount of T3 should also receive GI decontamination and evaluation. Activated charcoal and cathartics should be given in conventional doses. Since thyroid hormones may undergo enterohepatic recirculation, repeat doses of activated charcoal may be helpful in large ingestions and in symptomatic patients.

B. **Specific measures**

1. Monitor blood pressure and cardiac function.
2. Beta adrenergic blockers should be given to control significant hypertension and tachycardia. Propranolol 1 mg i.v. over 1 min, for every 2 to 5 min up to a maximum of 5 mg may be given in adults. Children should receive 0.01 to 0.02 mg/kg i.v. (maximum of 1 mg/dose) over 1 min, for every 2 to 5 min. Simple tachycardia may be managed orally by propranolol 0.25 mg/kg every 6 h. Esmolol or metoprolol may be used alternatively in standard doses.
3. Life threatening dysrhythmias should be managed with antidysrhythmic agents or cardioversion as indicated.
4. Fever may be controlled with cooling blankets.
5. Agitation should be managed with benzodiazepines, which may assist in the control of blood pressure, heart rate, and temperature.
6. Seizures should be controlled with standard anticonvulsant medications.

7. The limited clinical experience with inhibitors of thyroid hormone metabolism, e.g., sodium ipodate (19), propylthiouracil (20,21); exchange transfusion (22); plasmapheresis (23); and charcoal hemoperfusion (24) in this setting prevents any specific recommendations. Hemodialysis and diuresis are not effective due to the extensive protein binding of thyroid hormones.

VII. Disposition

A. Admission criteria. All symptomatic patients are to be admitted. Patients with intentional ingestions for whom psychiatric evaluation cannot immediately be arranged should also be admitted.

B. Discharge criteria. Asymptomatic patients with accidental ingestions may be discharged after GI decontamination and a brief period of observation. Patients who ingest T3 should be observed for 6 to 12 h prior to discharge. Patients who ingest T4 should have close telephone follow-up for at least 10 days to ensure that they remain asymptomatic.

References

1. Sawin CT. Hypothyroidism. *Med Clin North Am* 1985;69:989–1004.
2. Tenebein M, Dean HJ. Benign course after massive levothroxine ingestion. *Pediatr Emerg Care* 1986;2:15–17.
3. Tenebein M, Dean HJ. Benign course after massive levothroxine ingestion. *JAMA* 1985;254:2190.
4. Nystrom E, Lindstedt G, Lundberg PA. Minor signs and symptoms of toxicity in a young woman in spite of massive thyroxine ingestion. *Acta Med Scand* 1980;207:135–136.
5. Golightly LK, Smolinski SC, Kuly KW, et al. Clinical Effects of accidental levothroxine ingestion in children. *Am J Dis Child* 1987;141:1025–1027.
6. Mandel SH, Magnusson AR, Burton BT, Swanson R, LaFranchi SH. Massive levothroxine ingestions: conservative management. *Clin Pediatr* 1989;28:374–376.
7. Bhasin S, Wallace W, Lawrence JB, Lesch M. Sudden death associated with thyroid hormone abuse. *Am J Med* 1981; 71:887–890.
8. Refetoff S. Thyroid hormone therapy. *Med Clin North Am* 1975;59:1147–1163.
9. Guyton AC. *Medical physiology.* 8th ed. Philadelphia: WB Saunders, 1991:834–835.
10. Hays MT. Absorption of triodothyronine in man. *J Clin Endocrinol* 1970;30:675–677.
11. Hays MT. Absorption of thyroxine in man. *J Clin Endocrinol* 1968;28:749–756.
12. Hyanes RC Jr Thyroid and antithyroid drugs. In: Gilman AG, et al., eds. *Goodman and Gilman's The pharmacological basis of therapeutics.* 8th ed. New York: Pergamon Press, 1990:1361–1383.
13. Hadad HM. Rates of I-131–labeled thyroxine metabolism in euthyroid children. *J Clin Invest* 1960;39:590.
14. Lewander WJ, Lacouture PG, Silva JE, Lovejoy FH. Acute thyroxine ingestion in pediatric patients. *Pediatrics* 1989;84: 262–265.
15. Tunget CL, Clark RF, Turden SG, Manoguerra AS. Raising the decontamination level for thyroid hormone ingestions. *Am J Emerg Med* 1995;13:9–13.
16. Gorman RL, Chamberlain JM, Rose SR, et al. High anxiety–low toxicity: a massive T4 ingestion. *Pediatrics* 1988;82: 666–669.
17. Rumack BH, ed. *Poisondex information system.* Denver: Micromedex, 1995.
18. Lotovitz TL, White J. Levothroxine ingestions in children: an analysis of 78 cases. *Am J Emerg Med* 1985;3:247–300.
19. Berkner PD, Starkman H, Person N. Acute L-thyroxine overdose; therapy with sodium ipodate: evaluation of clinical and physiological parameters. *J Emerg Med* 1991;9:129–131.
20. Lehrner LM, Weir MR. Acute ingestion of thyroid hormones. *Pediatrics* 1984;73:313–317.
21. Lewander WJ, Silva JE, Lancoutre PG, et al. Acute pediatric thyroxine ingestions, abstracted. *Vet Hum Toxicol* 1985; 28:295.
22. Gerard P, Malvaux P, DeVisscher M. Accidental poisoning with thyroid extract by exchange transfusion. *Arch Dis Child* 1972;47:980–982.
23. May ME, Mintz PO, Lowery P, et al. Plasmapheresis in thyroxine overdose—a case report. *J Toxicol Clin Toxicol* 1983; 20:517–520.
24. Candrina R, Di Stefano O, Spandrio S, et al. Treatment of thyrotoxic storm by charcoal plasmaperfusion [Letter]. *J Endocrinol Invest* 1989;12:133–134.

PART V

Psychiatric Drugs

Emergency Toxicology, Second Edition,
edited by Peter Viccellio.
Lippincott–Raven Publishers, Philadelphia © 1998.

54

Antipsychotic Agents

†David S. Rosen and °Paul M. Wax

*†Department of Emergency Medicine, Medical College of Pennsylvania, Philadelphia,
Pennsylvania 19129; °Department of Emergency Medicine, University of Rochester
Medical Center, Rochester, New York 14642*

I. Introduction

   A. **History.** First discovered and utilized in France in the early 1950s, antipsychotic medications, also known as neuroleptics, have revolutionized the management of schizophrenia. Since their introduction, the number of psychiatric hospital admissions has
   decreased dramatically. Because of their sedative properties, these drugs were initially
   used to prolong and augment clinical anesthetics. Increased sedation without significant
   alteration of consciousness made them ideal adjuncts to potentiate anesthetic agents.
   Subsequent research uncovered their ability to decrease arousal and treat psychoses.
   Irreversible extrapyramidal symptoms (EPS) and the potentially lethal consequences of
   neuroleptic malignant syndrome (NMS) has decreased the enthusiasm by which clinicians initially embraced the neuroleptics. Newer antipsychotic medications such as
   clozapine (Clozaril) and risperidone (Risperdal) hold promise for the treatment of refractory schizophrenia with fewer permanent side effects, but are not without risk. Aging
   demographic shifts and HIV disease are expected to increase the number of emergency
   department (ED) visits for antipsychotic related disorders over time.

   B. **Present indications.** The antipsychotic agents are used for a large number of psychiatric
   disorders as well as an increasing number of nonpsychiatric disorders. Psychiatric indications for these agents include schizophrenia, schizophreniform disorder, organic psychoses, schizoaffective disorder, mood disorders with psychotic features, and behavior
   problems. Nonpsychiatric disorders include Gilles de la Tourette syndrome, nausea,
   Huntington's disease, intractable hiccups, alcoholic hallucinosis, migraine headache,
   dysreflexia, chemotherapy-induced emesis, and porphyria.

   C. **Toxicity overview.** Overdose with antipsychotic medications is common and often
   benign. Commonly prescribed drugs with potential for abuse include "hidden" dopamine
   antagonists such as prochlorperazine (Compazine), promethazine (Phenergan), cisapride
   (Propulsid), and metoclopramide (Reglan). Due to the high therapeutic index of the
   antipsychotics, fatalities from overdose are rare: In 1994, there were 12,000 neuroleptic
   overdoses reported to the American Association of Poison Control Centers and only
   24 deaths. Acute overdose most often results in CNS and cardiovascular toxicity. At therapeutic doses, hypotension is the most common side effect of the neuroleptics. Movement disorders (i.e., EPS), however, may account for the most common neuroleptic-

related visit to the ED. Neuroleptic malignant syndrome most often occurs during therapeutic dosing, and while rare, it is a life-threatening emergency.

II. Pharmacology and properties of agents

A. Nomenclature/structure. Phenothiazines are the oldest class, most widely studied, and most widely prescribed of the antipsychotic drugs. They have a basic three-ring structure consisting of two benzene rings with a nitrogen/sulfur linkage. Drugs in this class include chlorpromazine (Thorazine), mesoridazine (Serentil), perphenazine (Trilafon), trifluoperazine (Stelazine), fluphenazine (Prolixin), and thioridazine (Mellaril). The commonly used antiemetic, prochlorperazine (Compazine), is also a phenothiazine compound. Other classes are noted in Table 54-1. While the chemical structures of these various antipsychotic groups may differ, they tend to have similar pharmacologic properties and therapeutic effects. Newer antipsychotics, such as clozapine (a tricyclic

TABLE 54-1. *Important antipsychotics*

Class	Comments
Phenothiazines	
Aliphatic	
Chlorpromazine (Thorazine)	The prototype low-potency drug, anticholinergic effects, ileus, coma, decreased seizure threshold, impaired gag reflex, EKG changes, EPS. Miosis is common.
Piperidines	
Thioridazine (Mellaril)	Impaired consciousness, arrhythmias (torsades, V tach, AV block, long QT); potent anticholinergic effects, hypotension. Mydriasis is common.
Mesoridazine (Serentil)	A metabolite of thioridazine. EKG changes, arrhythmias (wide QRS), respiratory depression.
Piperazines	
Trifluoperazine (Stelazine)	High-potency, EPS, confusion, seizures, EKG changes.
Fluphenazine (Prolixin)	Available in long-acting decanoate and enanthate forms.
Perphenazine (Trilafon)	—
Prochlorperazine (Compazine)	—
Dibenzoxazepines	
Loxapine (Loxitane)	Tricyclic structure related to amoxapine, may cause prolonged seizures.
Dihydroindolones	
Molindone (Moban)	—
Thioxanthenes	
Thiothixene (Navane)	Akathisia
Butyrophenones	
Haloperidol (Haldol)	High-potency, high incidence of EPS, long-acting decanoate form available.
Diphenylbutylpiperidines	
Pimozide (Orap)	Tourette syndrome
Dibenzodiazepine	
Clozapine (Clozaril)	Sedation, dizziness, seizures with doses > 600 mg/d, fever, agranulocytosis, sialorrhea
Benzisoxazole	
Risperidone (Risperdal)	Decreased concentration, sedation, hypotension, asthenia, weight gain, galactorrhea, amenorrhea
Benzamide	
Remoxipride	Fatigue, insomnia, tremor, decreased concentration, akathisia

dibenzodiazepine), risperidone (a benzisoxazole derivative), and remoxipride (a substituted benzamide), are often referred to as atypical neuroleptics because of their distinctive mechanisms of action.

B. **Pharmacokinetics**

1. **Absorption.** Oral absorption is erratic and may be impaired by concomitant ingestion of antacids. Intramuscular dosing may increase the bioavailability by four to 10 times due to the lack of first-pass metabolism. Anticholinergic effects may slow gastric emptying.

2. **Distribution.** These compounds are highly lipophilic, have a large volume of distribution ($\sim$ 20 L/kg), and are greater than 90% bound to albumin. These factors limit the utility of hemodialysis and hemoperfusion in drug removal. Antipsychotics may easily enter the fetal circulation.

3. **Metabolism.** There is a big first-pass effect associated with oral dosing. Plasma levels peak within 2 to 4 h. Biotransformation occurs in the liver and the phenothiazines such as chlorpromazine (Thorazine) and thioridazine (Mellaril) have many active metabolites. In contrast, butyrophenones such as haloperidol (Haldol) have few active metabolites. Half-lives of antipsychotic drugs are variable and may range from 20 to 40 h. Elimination of parenteral decanoate formulations such as fluphenazine may take 7 to 10 days. Many preparations have long lasting biologic effects up to 24 h and are therefore dosed on a once a day basis.

4. **Elimination.** Antipsychotics are excreted by the kidneys and through enterohepatic circulation. Hydrophilic metabolites are eliminated in the urine.

C. **Mechanism of action.**

1. **Receptor blockade.** The antipsychotics exert an inhibitory effect at several important receptors.

   a. **Dopamine blockade.** Their most important inhibitory effect is at dopaminergic receptors in the limbic system and basal ganglia. Dopamine blockade in the basal ganglia plays an important role in regulating postural tone and involuntary movement. The potency of the antipsychotics appears to be directly related to their affinity for D_2 and to a lesser extent, D_1 receptors. In general, drugs with low potency (i.e., weak affinity for dopamine receptors) have strong sedative and anticholinergic effects; those with higher potency (i.e., haloperidol) are more likely to produce movement disorders. Neuroendocrine pathways involving dopaminergic neurons are located in the hypothalamus, terminate in the pituitary, and are believed to be responsible for increases in serum prolactin levels seen with use of antipsychotic agents.

   b. **Other receptors.** In addition, these drugs have inhibitory effects at alpha, cholinergic (muscarinic), histamine, and serotonergic receptors.

2. **Newer drugs** such as clozapine, risperidone, and remoxipride have different mechanisms of action (described below).

   a. **Clozapine** (Clozaril), which is chemically similar to the benzodiazepines, has a strong affinity for the D_4 receptor with lesser effects at D_1 and D_5 receptors. Its preferential activity at limbic rather than striatal dopamine receptors may explain its relative lack of EPS. It is also a potent alpha, histamine, and muscarinic antagonist.

b. **Risperidone** acts at central serotonergic 5-HT$_2$ receptors with some effect at alpha-1, alpha-2, and D$_2$ receptors.

c. **Remoxipride** is a weak dopamine receptor antagonist with affinity for extrastriatal D$_2$ receptors. Its affects are minimal at cholinergic, adrenergic, histamine, and serotonin receptors.

III. **Clinical presentation**
  A. **Acute overdose**
    1. **Lethality.** Deaths as a result of toxic ingestion of antipsychotics are relatively uncommon. When they do occur, they are most often associated with thioridazine, mesoridazine or multiple drug ingestions. Most serious toxic effects are due to cardiac arrhythmias and severe hypotension. Lethal exposures are not well established and vary widely. Deaths have been reported with chlorpromazine (Thorazine) doses of 9 grams in an adult and 350 mg in a child. A thioridazine (Mellaril) ingestion of 3 grams, mesoridazine (Serentil) ingestion of 2.5 gms, and clozapine (Clozaril) ingestion of 2.5 grams have also resulted in fatalities.
    2. **CNS effects.**
      a. **Altered mental status.** Impaired consciousness is common and dose-related. Some patients may be agitated and confused. Coma, while reported with chlorpromazine (Thorazine) and thioridazine (Mellaril), is uncommon, even at high doses.
      b. **Lowered seizure threshold.** Seizures may occur with low potency drugs such as chlorpromazine (Thorazine), and thioridazine (Mellaril), as they tend to lower the seizure threshold. Loxapine (Loxitane) has been associated with recurrent seizures. Haloperidol (Haldol) may also lower the seizure threshold. The annual incidence of seizures in patients taking clozapine (Clozaril) is 5%.
      c. **Extrapyramidal reactions.** Dystonic reactions may occur in up to 15% of patients taking antipsychotics at therapeutic doses with onset one to five days after ingestion. The exact incidence of dystonic reactions after antipsychotic overdose is unknown although they do occur. Diffuse CNS motor signs such as hyperreflexia or dorsiflexion of toes may also be present. Suppression of the gag reflex is a common side effect of phenothiazines and has important implications for airway management.
    3. **Cardiovascular effects**
      a. **Conduction disturbances/arrhythmias.** Sinus tachycardia is common. Cardiotoxic effects are most pronounced among patients on thioridazine (Mellaril) and its active metabolite, mesoridazine (Serentil). Sudden death due to cardiac arrest has been reported. Conduction abnormalities (prolonged QTc and PR intervals, a wide QRS), supraventricular and ventricular tachyarrhythmias, torsades de pointes, and EKG changes (blunt T waves, right axis deviation, and prominent U waves) have been reported. In acute ingestions, EKG findings may be normal for up to 10 h after an ingestion. Up to 1/2 of patients with an acute thioridazine (Mellaril) overdose may develop an arrhythmia

and/or EKG abnormalities. Arrhythmias may persist for several days following ingestion. Syncope may occur secondary to cardiac arrhythmias.

    b. **Blood pressure**

        (1) **Hypotension.** Hypotension is a common and potentially serious side effect, occurring in up to 10% to 15% of toxic overdoses. Blood pressure may fall due to the peripheral alpha-blocking and central effects of these drugs in the hypothalamus or midbrain. Abnormal ventricular function may appear late and appears to be dose related. Among the most concerning of the antipsychotics with regard to hypotension is chlorpromazine (Thorazine) which has a direct negative inotropic action and is a potent vasodilator.

        (2) **Hypertension.** Transient elevated blood pressures have also been reported.

4. **Impaired thermoregulation.**

    a. **Hypothermia** is common, especially in the elderly, due to central effects at the anterior hypothalamus and peripheral vasodilatation.

    b. **Hyperthermia** may also occur and is due to the anticholinergic effects leading to impaired heat dissipation and increased motor activity. Neuroleptic malignant syndrome can result in severe hyperpyrexia. Interactions with other drugs may also produce heat stress and are potentially dangerous (Table 54-2).

5. **Respiratory effects.** Respiratory depression is uncommon. Up to 10% of acute phenothiazine overdoses may experience respiratory complications. Pulmonary edema may also occur. Upper airway obstruction may occur secondary to swelling of the glottis.

TABLE 54-2. *Antipsychotic drug interactions*

Alcohol	Increased sedation. ? Increased EPS.
Anticholinergics	Low-potency antipsychotics (chlorpromazine, thioridazine, clozapine) may have additive effects.
Anticonvulsant	Induced microsomal P450 system with a decrease in serum plasma level of antipsychotics (except Valproate), increased plasma levels of anticonvulsant. ? Increased delirium. ? Increased sedation.
Antidiarrheals	? Impaired absorption.
Antidepressants	Increased serum plasma levels of antipsychotics. ? Increased EPS with fluoxetine. ? Increased delirium with clozapine.
Antihypertensives	Increased hypotension. ? Hypoglycemia.
Antivirals	Decreased effect of antipsychotics with rifampin.
Benzodiazepines	Sedation, ataxia, syncope, sialorrhea, cardiac arrest (especially with clozapine).
H2 blockers	Increased clozapine levels with cimetidine.
Lithium	Mental status changes, neurotoxicity, increased risk of EPS, NMS, hyperthermia, pyramidal, and cerebellar signs have been reported, especially with haloperidol, thioridazine, fluphenazine, thiothixene.
Opioids	Increased respiratory depression with meperidine.
Tobacco	Increased clearance of antipsychotics, especially with clozapine. Experimentally increases dopamine levels. May theoretically increase risk of Parkinsonism with abrupt smoking cessation.

6. **Anticholinergic effects.** Decreased bowel sounds, ileus, dry mucous membranes, decreased sweating, urinary retention (rare, except in prostatism) and mydriasis are seen most commonly with clozapine (Clozaril) and with low potency drugs such as thioridazine (Mellaril) and mesoridazine (Serentil). Miosis is common with chlorpromazine (Thorazine) due to its alpha blocking effects.

7. **Miscellaneous effects.** Other clinical effects that have been reported with antipsychotic overdose include cholestatic and/or hepatocellular jaundice, acute renal failure following NMS and rhabdomyolysis, hypo or hyperglycemia and priapism.

B. **Therapeutic dosing.** The following effects have been noted after therapeutic dosing of neuroleptics: sedation, dizziness, headache, irritability, constipation, dry mouth, decreased sweating, urticaria, decreased gag reflex, swallowing difficulties, hyperpyrexia, hypothermia (especially in the elderly), altered seizure threshold, hypotension, tachycardia, nonspecific Q and T wave abnormalities, syncope, priapism, jaundice, agranulocytosis, leukocytosis, leukopenia, eosinophilia, anemia, thrombocytopenic purpura, and increased prolactin levels. Hypertension, nausea and vomiting, mood changes, insomnia, and abdominal pain have been reported with abrupt discontinuation of antipsychotic medications.

C. **Atypical antipsychotics.** Less data is available on the clinical effects seen in overdose of these drugs since they have only recently become available.

1. **Clozapine** overdose has been associated with tachycardia, sialorrhea, hypotonicity, somnolence, confusion, ataxia, agitation, myoclonic jerking, and seizures. At therapeutic dosing the most prominent adverse effect is agranulocytosis. Sedation, sialorrhea, tachycardia, eosinophilia, and seizures may also occur at therapeutic dosing.

2. **Risperidone** overdose has also been associated with tachycardia, drowsiness, slurred speech, altered mental status, and agitation. EPS, hypertension, and QRS and QTc prolongation has also been reported.

3. **Remoxipride** overdose is infrequently reported but has been associated with orthostasis, drowsiness, sedation, and seizures.

IV. **Laboratory findings**

A. **Plasma drug levels** of neuroleptics are not useful in determining toxic ingestions. Since there may be a ten-fold variation in serum plasma levels seen among individuals on identical drug regimens, relevant therapeutic levels have been difficult to establish. Urine drug screens may detect some of the neuroleptics but such qualitative assessment rarely influences management.

B. A serum **CPK** should be drawn in cases where NMS is clinically suspected.

C. Continuous **cardiac monitoring** with serial EKG's is essential, especially in cases of thioridazine and mesoridazine overdose. QRS and QTc intervals should be closely monitored.

D. **Abdominal radiographs** may be useful to detect the presence of unabsorbed drug since antipsychotic preparations are often radiopaque although a negative x-ray does not preclude an antipsychotic ingestion.

V. **Management**

A. **Overview:** As always, a careful history of toxic ingestion should be obtained. Simultaneous ingestion of more than one antipsychotic medication, or ingestion in the setting of drug and alcohol abuse may precipitate a more malignant clinical course. Because of the delayed onset and long half-lives of these medications, initial CNS and cardiotoxic effects may appear 10 to 15 h postingestion. Treatment is primarily supportive.

B. Initial evaluation and gastrointestinal decontamination

1. **ABCs.** As always, airway, breathing, and circulation must be initially assessed. Identification of concomitant drug/alcohol ingestions is essential as these patients have the potential to experience a more dangerous clinical course.

2. **Syrup of ipecac** is contraindicated. Do not attempt to induce emesis as increased sedation, decrease or loss of gag reflex and dystonic reactions may predispose to aspiration and compromise the airway.

3. **Gastric lavage** performed with a large bore orogastric tube (adult, 36- to 40-French; child, 24- to 32-French) may be warranted with a large overdose of a particularly toxic antipsychotic such as thioridazine or mesoridazine if the patient presents within 1 to 2 h after ingestion.

4. **Activated charcoal** should routinely be administered after neuroleptic overdose. Repeated doses administered every 4 to 6 h may offer some benefit in enhancing drug elimination although definitive proof is lacking.

5. **Hemodialysis** is not recommended since antipsychotics are highly lipophilic with a large volume of distribution.

C. Management of complications

1. **Hypotension**

   a. **Trendelenburg position and intravenous fluids** (10 to 20 mg/kg LR or normal saline) are sufficient to manage hypotension in most patients.

   b. **Dopamine** (2 to 5 µg/kg/min and increasing to 5 to 10 µg/kg/min p.r.n.) is the first line treatment of choice in refractory hypotension from antipsychotic medication.

   c. **Alpha agonists** such as norepinephrine, phenylephrine, or metaraminol should be used if dopamine is ineffective.

2. **Arrhythmias**

   a. **Sodium bicarbonate.** Due to similarities between thioridazine/mesoridazine and the tricyclic antidepressants on cardiac conduction, sodium bicarbonate may be useful in the treatment of arrhythmias from these phenothiazines.

   b. **Lidocaine** may also be considered for the treatment of ventricular tachyarrhythmias although its efficacy in this situation has not been studied.

   c. **Direct current cardioversion** should be attempted if the arrhythmia is refractory to drug therapy.

   d. **Pacing** may be appropriate in the presence of AV block.

   e. **Avoid type 1A** antiarrhythmics such as quinidine, procainamide, and disopyramide due to their similar mode of action on sodium channels.

   f. **Correction** of underlying electrolyte abnormalities is essential.

   g. **Treatment for torsade** includes cardioversion in unstable patients, atrial overdrive or ventricular pacing, and treatment with magnesium sulfate or isoproterenol.

   3. **CNS toxicity**

       a. **Seizures** should be treated with diazepam or lorazepam. If refractory or recurrent, phenobarbital should be administered.

       b. **Coma** requires no specific intervention other than supportive measures as needed.

       c. **Physostigmine** should be avoided since the risks of seizures and arrhythmias from its use outweighs the potential benefits.

VI. Disposition

   A. Hospitalize. Patients with CNS or cardiovascular toxicity following antipsychotic overdose should be admitted for 24 h observation.

   B. Discharge from ED. Patients who remain asymptomatic for 6 h and have not been exposed to a sustained-release (SR) or depot preparation may be medically cleared for psychiatric evaluation.

VII. Movement disorders

   A. Overview: Movement disorders are common, troubling, and potentially lethal side effects of antipsychotic therapy (Table 54-3). Several syndromes have been described. They are thought to arise from the disruption of a delicate balance between dopaminergic and cholinergic receptors in the nigrostriatal pathways in the basal ganglia. Collectively, these movement disorders are referred to as EPS, because their origin stems from CNS processes within the basal ganglia, "extra," or outside of the pyramidal tracts that

TABLE 54-3. *Treatment of extrapyramidal symptoms*

Dystonic reactions
  Immediate
    Adults and older children
      Cogentin 1–2 mg i.v.
      Diphenhydramine i.v. 1 mg/kg, max 50 mg/dose × 2 doses
      Diazepam 0.1 mg/kg i.v.
    Children
      Diphenhydramine 1 mg/kg/dose i.v. over 2 min, max 5 mg/kg/d
  Long term
    Adults
      Cogentin 1–2 mg b.i.d. × 2 days
      Artane 2 mg t.i.d. × 2 days
      Diphenhydramine 50 mg q.i.d. × 2 days
    Children
      Diphenhydramine maintenance dose for 2 days
Akathisia
  Immediate
    Decrease dose of antipsychotic or change to a different drug
    Propranolol 20–80 mg/d
Parkinsonism
  Anticholinergics
  Decrease antipsychotic dosage
  Add antiparkinsonism agent
Tardive dyskinesia
  Increase dose of neuroleptic
  Change neuroleptic to one with minimal anticholinergic effects
  Anticholinesterase, choline, lecithin, reserpine

are involved in voluntary movements. The prevalence of movement disorders in HIV-infected patients on neuroleptics is as high as 50%.

B. **Acute dystonic reactions** are the earliest occurring of the movement disorders. These spasms may involve the muscles of the neck (torticollis), face, tongue, jaw, eyes (upward gaze paralysis), lips, abdomen (tortipelvis), and spine (opisthotonos). Patients typically present between 48 and 72 h after initiation of therapy and can occur after a single dose. They occur most commonly in children and affect men greater than women. Drugs often implicated include the mid to high potency agents such as haloperidol (Haldol), fluphenazine (Prolixin), trifluoperazine (Stelazine), and prochlorperazine (Compazine). When they affect the musculature surrounding the larynx and pharynx, they may be deadly. These symptoms often subside within several hours of discontinuing the offending drug. In mild cases, reassurance is often sufficient therapy. More severe cases are usually treated with anticholinergic medications. Symptoms often resolve within several hours after treatment. It is postulated that dystonic reactions are due to dopaminergic blockade with subsequent higher acetylcholine receptor density in the basal ganglia. Thus, anticholinergics are usually effective treatment (Table 54-3). Antihistamines and benzodiazepines are also effective.

C. **Akathisia,** or extreme motor restlessness, usually presents in older patients within the first two months after initiation of antipsychotic therapy. Patients often cannot sit still and may complain of muscle discomfort and/or insomnia. These symptoms often disappear spontaneously. Clinicians must be vigilant to recognize restlessness as a neuroleptic side effect rather than a treatment failure for psychotic agitation as increasing the medication may worsen symptoms. Treatment options include decreasing the dosage of antipsychotic, changing to a different drug or adding additional medications such as propranolol or diazepam.

D. **Parkinsonism** (akinesia) is a common side effect of antipsychotics, affects up to one half of elderly women, and generally occurs within one week to two months after antipsychotic therapy. Cardinal features include resting tremor (usually of the upper extremities), muscular rigidity, bradykinesia (slowness and poverty of movement), decrease in postural stability and a shortened and uncontrollable acceleration of gait (festinating). Additional features include masked facies, shuffling gait, pill-rolling, muscle weakness and monotony of speech. These symptoms are usually controlled by decreasing drug dosage, changing to another antipsychotic, or adding an anti-Parkinsonian agent for two to three months with reevaluation at that time.

E. **Tardive dyskinesia** (TD), a late (after months or years of treatment) and potentially irreversible side effect of antipsychotic medications, may occur in up to 10% to 30% of patients on long-term neuroleptic therapy. Tardive dyskinesia is characterized by involuntary, repetitive movements of the face, tongue, and lips. Choreiform movements of the extremities may also be seen. Movements disappear during sleep. The elderly, especially women, are commonly affected. Depot preparations are often implicated and the syndrome may be seen after attempts to decrease dosages after long-term therapy. It is theorized that a chronic blockade of dopamine receptors leads to increased dopamine secretion and hypersensitivity of dopamine receptors in the nigrostriatal pathway. Among patients receiving levodopa, reduction of the dosage tends to decrease or eliminate TD.

Decreasing antipsychotic dosages may improve or worsen the movement disorder and should be tried as an initial treatment. Occasionally, an increase in drug dose is needed to block the unregulated receptors. TD is worsened by anticholinergics, and generally unaffected by cholinergic agents. By depleting dopaminergic stores presynaptically, reserpine and tetrabenazine have been used successfully to decrease TD. Although, benzodiazepines, calcium channel blockers, B-blockers, clonidine, bromocriptine, and valproic acid have also been used with varying success, definitive benefit of any of these agents has not been demonstrated.

F. **Differential diagnosis** of the movement disorders includes tetanus, strychnine, focal seizures, progressive supranuclear palsy, olivopontocerebellar atrophy, Shy-Drager syndrome, corticobasal ganglionic degeneration, Alzheimer's Disease, Wilson's disease, Huntington's Disease, infarction or vasculitis of basal ganglia, carbon monoxide, manganese, methanol, MPTP, mercury, methanol, cyanide, alpha-methyldopa, metoclopramide, CNS infections, CNS neoplasms, and hysteria.

VIII. **Neuroleptic malignant syndrome**

A. **Overview.** Neuroleptic malignant syndrome (NMS) is a poorly understood complication of antipsychotic therapy. Clinical and laboratory observations suggest an acute decrease in dopamine activity, often associated with systemic risk factors such as dehydration, exhaustion, or agitation may precipitate NMS. While relatively uncommon (incidence estimates vary from 0.1% to 2% of patients on antipsychotic medications) its lethality makes early recognition and treatment imperative. Onset is unpredictable and may occur at any time during antipsychotic drug therapy, with the withdrawal of antipsychotic or antiparkinsonian medications, or by the additional administration of sedative drugs. Greater than 90% of cases occur during the first 2 weeks of drug therapy. Symptoms have a relatively slow onset from one to three days and may last up to three weeks. Predisposing factors include a recent change in drug regime and dehydration. While NMS is seen in all age groups, it is most common in young men, mean age of 40. In cases of acute antipsychotic overdose, NMS is rare.

B. **Etiologic agents.** Fluphenazine decanoate is most often implicated although NMS has been reported with use of trifluoperazine, thioridazine, haloperidol, and chlorpromazine. Clinicians should be on the outlook for patients who have been taking common medications such as metoclopramide (Reglan), cisapride (Propulsid), prochlorperazine (Compazine), hydroxyzine (Vistaril), and promethazine (Phenergan)—all dopamine antagonists.

1. **Clinical features.** The syndrome is characterized by four cardinal features: mental status changes, muscle rigidity, hyperthermia, and autonomic instability. Up to 1/2 of patients will fail to exhibit all of these "classic" signs at initial presentation.

2. **Mental status changes** may include fluctuating levels of alertness, agitation, and coma.

3. **Muscle rigidity** involves mostly the face and trunk in adults and tends to be more generalized in children. Increased chest wall compliance with subsequent hypoventilation, tracheal spasm, dysphagia, and increased heat production may also occur.

4. **Hyperthermia.** Elevated temperatures to 41 degrees C or more may occur.

5. **Autonomic disturbances** include tachycardia, labile hypertension, pallor, profuse diaphoresis, drooling, and incontinence.

C. **Differential diagnosis.** NMS is a diagnosis of exclusion and other common causes of mental status changes, fever, rigidity and autonomic instability should be ruled out. Differential diagnosis includes meningitis, encephalitis, sepsis, tetanus, mass lesions, trauma, seizures, hyperthyroidism, hypocalcemia, heatstroke, anticholinergic or strychnine toxicity, drug or alcohol withdrawal, interaction with MAOI's, lethal catatonia, malignant hyperthermia, or severe dystonia.

D. **Complications** include shock, cardiovascular collapse, renal failure due to rhabdomyolysis, disseminated intravascular coagulation, pulmonary embolus, aspiration pneumonia. Death is usually attributed to respiratory failure.

E. **Laboratory findings.** The majority of patients with NMS have elevated serum creatinine phosphokinase (CPK) levels. Leukocytosis is common. Serum iron is low. Hypocalcemia has been reported in 1/2 of patients with NMS.

F. **Management.** Treatment should be aimed at correcting the underlying mechanism of disease (attributed to dopamine blockade in the basal ganglia), symptomatic control, and supportive therapy.

   1. Antipsychotic medications should be stopped.

   2. Rapid cooling with ice packs or mist and a fan, and cool humidified oxygen, should be instituted in patients with significant hyperthermia.

   3. Airway compromise, aspiration, or hypoventilation may require intubation. Fluids and electrolytes should be monitored and abnormalities corrected.

   4. Patient monitoring in an ICU is recommended.

   5. Forced diuresis and dialysis are generally ineffective in eliminating antipsychotics and are not recommended.

   6. **Drug therapy.**

      a. **Bromocriptine,** a central acting dopamine agonist, should be considered in any patient who presents with significant manifestations of NMS, particularly if they have evidence of autonomic instability. A dose of 5 mg p.o. or via nasogastric tube every 8 h is recommended.

      b. **Dantrolene,** an agent that has a direct effect on the contractile response of skeletal muscle, may be useful in patients with severe muscular rigidity, although its role here remains controversial. Although dantrolene is the agent of choice for malignant hyperthermia (a genetically inherited disorder of skeletal muscle precipitated by inhalational anesthetics or depolarizing muscle relaxants), NMS is an entirely different disease entity and is characterized by a CNS process. Hepatic toxicity has been reported with dantrolene. If dantrolene is used, the recommended dose is 2.5 mg/kg i.v. q6h; 1 mg/kg p.o. q12h; maximum 50 mg/dose or 100 to 200 mg p.o./day.

      c. **Benzodiazepines** are a good first line agent for any condition that presents with muscle rigidity, especially in the setting of hyperthermia.

      d. **L-dopa and carbidopa** may be of some benefit in patients presenting with NMS following withdrawal of Parkinsonian drugs, since these drugs may increase availability of central dopamine stores.

      e. **Amantadine,** a glutamate receptor antagonist, has been used with varying efficacy to treat NMS.

G. Outcome. Mortality may be as high as 20% if the condition goes unrecognized or is undertreated. Although carefully controlled clinical trials are lacking, treatment with bromocriptine, dantrolene, or amantadine may decrease the mortality rate from NMS to approximately 5%. Because of the high rate of recurrence of NMS (30%), antipsychotic therapy with the same class of drug is not recommended.

Selected Readings

Baldessarini RJ. Drugs and the treatment of psychiatric disorders: psychosis and anxiety. In: Hardman JG, et al., eds. *Goodman and Gilman's. The pharmacological basis of therapeutics.* 9th ed. New York.: McGraw-Hill, 1996;399–430.

Buckley NA, Whyte IM, Dawson AH. Cardiotoxicity more common in thioridazine overdose than with other neuroleptics. *J Toxicol Clin Toxicol* 1995;33:199–204.

Caroff SN, Mann SC. Neuroleptic malignant syndrome. *Med Clin North Am* 1993;77:185–202.

Goff DC, Baldessarini RJ. Drug interactions with antipsychotic agents. *J Clin Psychopharm* 1993;13:57–67.

Kane, JM. Newer antipsychotic drugs: a review of their pharmacology and therapeutic potential. *Drugs* 1993;46:585–593.

Le Blaye I, Donatini B, Hall M, Krupp P. Acute overdosage with thioridazine: a review of the available clinical exposure. *Vet Hum Toxicol* 1993;35:147–150.

Lewin, NA, Wang RY. Neuroleptic agents. In: Goldfrank LR, et al., eds. *Goldfrank's toxicologic emergencies.* 5th ed. Norwalk, CT: Appleton & Lange, 1994;739–749.

Emergency Toxicology, Second Edition,
edited by Peter Viccellio.
Lippincott–Raven Publishers, Philadelphia © 1998.

55

Tricyclic Antidepressants

†King F. Hom and °Paul M. Wax

†Pediatric Practice, Intermountain Health Care, Ogden, Utah 84403; °Department of Emergency Medicine, University of Rochester Medical Center, Rochester, New York 14642

This chapter focuses on the diagnosis and management of the first generation tricyclics as well as amoxapine and maprotiline. Consideration of the newer agents will be taken up in the next chapter.

I. **Introduction**

  A. **History.** The prototypic tricyclic antidepressant (TCA), imipramine hydrochloride, was originally introduced in 1948 as a sedative-hypnotic agent. An analog of the phenothiazines, it was subsequently investigated for its antihistaminic and antipsychotic properties. The first report on the effectiveness of imipramine as a treatment for endogenous depression appeared in 1958 and by 1959, the first cases of TCA overdose and toxicity were reported in the literature (1,2).

  B. **Present indications.** Although often replaced by the serotonin reuptake inhibitors as first line therapy, the TCAs are still among the most frequently prescribed pharmacologic agents for the treatment of both endogenous and reactive depression. Additionally, imipramine is approved for the treatment of enuresis in children over 6 years of age while other TCAs are used for migraine prophylaxis in adults, chronic pain syndromes, and acute cocaine withdrawal.

  C. **Toxicity overview.** Despite the changing prescribing patterns of TCAs, overdoses of these drugs are common and deadly. Sudden cardiovascular deterioration is the hallmark of toxicity. Seizures and the ensuing acidemia may markedly worsen the clinical situation. Altered mental status in the setting of normal cardiac conduction is less problematic. While no true antidote exists for TCA toxicity, the infusion of sodium bicarbonate may be life saving.

II. **Pharmacology and properties of agents**

  A. **Nomenclature/structure** (Table 55-1)

   1. **First generation TCAs.** There are seven compounds classified as first generation TCAs, each containing the characteristic three-ringed nucleus: two benzene rings joined by a central ring. These seven compounds are further differentiated into tertiary and secondary tricyclic amines depending on whether there are three or two carbon groups attached to the nitrogen atom of the aminopropyl side chain.

     a. **The tertiary amines** are imipramine, amitriptyline, doxepin, and trimipramine.

     b. **The secondary amines** consist of protriptyline, desipramine, and nortriptyline, the latter two being demethylated metabolites of imipramine and amitriptyline, respectively.

TABLE 55-1. *Classification of antidepressants*

First generation TCAs	Second generation TCAs	Newer agents
Imipramine (Tofranil)	Amoxapine (Asendin)	Bupropion (Wellbutrin)
Amitriptyline (Elavil)	Maprotiline (Ludiomil)	Trazodone (Desyrel)
Desipramine (Norpramin)		nefazodone (Serzone)
Doxepin (Sinequan)		Fluoxetine (Prozac)
Nortriptyline (Aventyl)		Paroxetine (Paxil)
Protriptyline (Vivactil)		Sertraline (Zoloft)
Trimipramine (Surmontil)		

TCA = tricyclic antidepressant.

2. **Second generation TCAs.** A second generation of cyclic antidepressants, **maprotiline** and **amoxapine,** were introduced in the 1980s. Maprotiline is a tetracyclic compound, while amoxapine, a demethylated metabolite of loxapine, is a tricyclic dibenzoxazepine compound. Compared with traditional TCA overdoses, maprotiline exhibits similar cardiotoxicity with a slight increase in the incidence of seizures while amoxapine is also associated with a greater incidence of seizures but has fewer cardiotoxic effects.

3. **Newer antidepressants,** specifically the serotonin reuptake inhibitors (e.g., fluoxetine, paroxetine, and sertraline), and bupropion have recently been introduced into clinical use. These agents bear very little resemblance to the traditional TCAs in terms of molecular structure and pharmacodynamics.

    a. **Serotonin reuptake inhibitors** have enjoyed substantial growth in popularity due to fewer side effects at therapeutic doses and less toxicity in overdose.

    b. **Bupropion** use has been limited by concerns about seizures at therapeutic doses.

    c. **Trazodone** and more recently, **nefazodone,** both of which have similar inhibitory effects on the serotonin receptors, are also increasingly used in the treatment of depression.

B. **Pharmacokinetics**

1. **Orally administered TCAs** are rapidly absorbed with peak serum concentrations occurring anywhere from 2 to 8 h after a therapeutic dose. Once absorbed, these lipophilic drugs are widely distributed throughout the body with high concentrations in the brain, liver, kidney, lung and myocardium. The tissue:plasma concentration ratios easily exceed 10:1 with a ratio as high as 40:1 reported in brain tissue. Protein binding is usually 90% or greater. These properties give TCAs a large apparent volume of distribution, usually in the range of 10 to 50 L/kg.

2. **Metabolism.** TCAs are extensively metabolized in the liver. Tertiary amines are demethylated to form pharmacologically active metabolites such as some of the secondary amines. These compounds are further demethylated and hydroxylated to form inactive metabolites which are eliminated after a final step of glucuronide conjugation. A very small fraction appears unchanged in the urine. Therapeutic half-lives for the different TCAs are variable, ranging from about 18 h for imipramine to 80 h for protriptyline.

C. **Mechanism of action and toxicity**
   1. **Neurotransmitter reuptake** inhibition. The TCAs efficacy in treating depression is believed to be largely due to their ability to inhibit neurotransmitter reuptake at various strategic sites in the central nervous system. This blockade results in increased neuronal synaptic concentrations of neurotransmitters including norepinephrine, dopamine, and serotonin. During TCA overdose, this peripheral increase in norepinephrine may contribute to the sinus tachycardia and an initial transient hypertensive effect. Increased cardiac concentrations of catecholamines may also contribute to the development of ventricular arrhythmias.
   2. **Receptor blockade.** TCAs are competitive antagonists of muscarinic cholinergic receptors, α-adrenergic receptors, serotonin receptors, histaminic H_1 and H_2 receptors and GABA receptors. In particular, cholinergic and α-adrenergic blockade are responsible for many annoying side effects at therapeutic doses and more problematic symptoms during overdose.
      a. **Anticholinergic blockade.** The most common clinical manifestations of peripheral anticholinergic blockade are sinus tachycardia, hyperthermia, mydriasis, ileus and urinary retention. The most serious complications of central nervous system anticholinergic blockade are agitation, delirium, hyperthermia, coma, and seizures.
      b. **α-Adrenergic blockade.** Inhibition of α-adrenergic receptors may result in significant peripheral vasodilatation contributing to the often severe hypotension and the tachycardia seen in TCA overdose.
   3. **Myocardial membrane depressant effects.** The most important mechanism of TCA toxicity is a depressant effect on the myocardial membrane resulting in delayed depolarization and impairment of cardiac conduction. These effects, often described as **"quinidine-like"** effects, can cause lethal cardiac arrhythmias and are responsible for most of the fatalities associated with TCA overdoses. Myocardial membrane depressant effects result from specific TCA inhibition of predominantly fast inward sodium channels, with some calcium channel inhibition noted as well. Impaired sodium entry corresponding to phase 0 of the action potential leads to various degrees of conduction delays predisposing the heart to various arrhythmias, especially reentry type ventricular tachycardias. As intracellular calcium release is also dependent on phase 0 sodium entry, one of the other major effects on the myocardium is decreased contractility, further contributing to the hypotension seen in TCA overdose. This effect on the sodium channels can be modified by manipulation of extracellular pH and sodium concentration, explaining the efficacy of sodium bicarbonate. Other myocardial effects include delays in phase 3 repolarization and phase 4 spontaneous depolarization. The clinical implications of these changes include a prolonged QT interval with possible development of Torsades de pointes and decreased automaticity with suppression of ventricular escape rhythms and possible bradycardia and asystole.

III. **Clinical presentation**
   A. **Epidemiology.** Early reviews from the 1960s showed a mortality rate between 15% to 20% for hospitalized TCA overdose cases. Case series since 1979 have placed the over-

all mortality rate for TCA overdose closer to less than 2% (3). Data from the 1994 AAPCC annual report (4) showed that there were nearly 20,000 cases of cyclic antidepressant exposures, accounting for 2.3% of all drug exposures. The mortality rate for overdoses was 0.7% with cyclic antidepressant fatalities accounting for 16.3% of all reported drug overdose fatalities. Along with analgesics, TCAs accounted for the greatest number of drug overdose fatalities.

  B. **Manifestations of toxicity.** The most common sequelae of a toxic TCA ingestion involve the cardiovascular system, the central nervous system and the parasympathetic nervous system. Cardiotoxic manifestations, specifically ventricular arrhythmias and depressed myocardial contractility, are the most common immediate causes of mortality.

   1. **Cardiovascular**
      a. **Sinus tachycardia.** The most common finding is due largely to anticholinergic effects. Other contributing factors include peripheral vasodilatation secondary to α-adrenergic inhibition and increased concentrations of catecholamines secondary to reuptake inhibition. The presence of sinus tachycardia indicates toxicity but is not helpful in prognosticating the eventual level of cardiotoxicity.
      b. **Conduction delays.** Due to "quinidine-like" effects on myocardial membranes. Prolonged PR, QRS and QTc intervals may occur. Prolonged QRS (more than or equal to 0.10 s) may help in identifying patients at risk for serious complications, especially arrhythmias and seizures. Prolonged QTc is less prognostic.
      c. **Ventricular arrhythmias.** Reentry type secondary to conduction delays. Ventricular tachycardia is the most common. Ventricular fibrillation is usually terminal. PVCs are rare. It is often difficult to differentiate ventricular tachycardia from sinus tachycardia or SVT with aberrancy when the QRS is widened and P waves are not obvious.
      d. **Depressed inotropy.** Secondary to calcium channel blockade. Contributes to hypotension.
      e. **Hypotension.** Due to α-adrenergic block and decreased inotropy. Often orthostatic but may be severe.
      f. **Hypertension.** Usually transient and occurs early in the course of overdose. Due to increased levels of circulating catecholamines resulting from synaptic reuptake inhibition. Usually not clinically significant.
      g. **Atrioventricular block.** Prolonged PR interval common while second and third degree blocks are rare.
      h. **Torsades de pointes.** Uncommon.
      i. **Bradycardia.** Usually only seen as terminal event.
   2. **Central nervous system**
      a. **Depression of mental status and coma.** Usually self-limiting but may last as long as 3 days in nonfatal ingestions. Glasgow Coma Score of less than 8 during initial period of observation may have predictive value for serious complications (5).
      b. **Delirium; altered sensorium.** Due to central cholinergic blockade.

    c. **Seizure.** Usually generalized, brief and self-limited. May develop early in course and cannot be predicted by general mental status. Associated with QRS of more than or equal to 0.10 s. Can exacerbate acidosis, hypoxia and hyperthermia contributing to further cardiotoxicity. Particularly problematic with amoxapine and maprotiline.

    d. **Myoclonus.** Sometimes difficult differentiating from seizures. May occur in awake patients.

    e. **Nonspecific cerebellar and extrapyramidal signs.** Nystagmus, choreo-athetosis, dysarthria and ataxia may be observed.

3. **Parasympathetic**

    a. **Dry skin and mucosa, ileus, urinary retention, and mydriasis.** Common peripheral anticholinergic signs not contributing significantly to morbidity by themselves. Varies depending on particular TCA. Not helpful in prediction of serious complications from overdose.

    b. **Hyperthermia.** Due to decreased sweating and impaired ability to dissipate heat. Seizures, myoclonus and general agitation may also contribute. May also occur in patients on therapeutic doses of tricyclics in setting of heat stress.

C. **Incidence** of the more significant clinical signs in 2,536 TCA overdose cases as reported in a 1987 review by Frommer et al. (6) can be seen in Table 55-2.

D. **Differential diagnosis** should include those agents that can exert similar anticholinergic effects, similar cardiac conduction disturbances or seizure (Table 55-3).

IV. **Laboratory findings**

A. **Plasma drug levels** show poor correlation with severity of toxicity and are not very useful in the acute management of overdoses. Additionally, it is not a test that is routinely available in most laboratories.

B. **Qualitative urine toxicology screens** can be used as well to detect TCAs in instances where diagnosis is uncertain. The test may also be helpful in cases where coingestions are suspected. However, a prolonged turn-around time commonly limits the toxicology screen's utility in the initial management of TCA overdoses.

C. **Electrocardiogram** (Fig. 55-1)

1. **The classic EKG finding** in TCA toxicity is a prolonged QRS interval (more than 0.10 s). A hallmark study by Boehnert and Lovejoy in 1985 (7) showed that seizures and arrhythmias were unlikely when the QRS interval was less than 0.10 s. With a QRS interval between 0.10 and 0.16 s, the risk for arrhythmias continues to be negligible while the risk for seizures increases into the moderate range. The highest risk for seizures and life-threatening arrhythmias was associated with a QRS interval greater than 0.16 s. The duration of the QRS interval is presently the most commonly used clinical indicator for initiating alkalinization to reduce the risk of arrhythmias.

2. **A second EKG finding** commonly associated with TCA toxicity is a rightward shift of the terminal 40 ms frontal plane QRS axis to values between 130 to 270 degrees (8). This finding is fairly specific for TCA toxicity but its absence does not preclude toxicity. Additionally, it has not been shown to have much prognostic value. A right-

TABLE 55-2. *Frequency of clinical findings seen with TCA overdose*

Clinical finding	Percentage
Sinus tachycardia (HR > 100 beats/min)	51
Coma	35
QRS ≥ 0.10 sec	21
Hypotension (SBP < 90 mm Hg)	14
Seizure	8.4
Arrhythmias (ventricular and supraventricular)	6.2

TCA = tricyclic antidepressant.

ward axis shift is evidenced by a negative final deflection of the QRS complex in lead I and aVL and a positive terminal deflection in lead aVR. Other possible EKG findings associated with TCA overdose include prolonged PR and Qtc intervals, AV blocks, nonspecific ST-T wave changes and various levels of ectopy.

   D. **Serum electrolytes** and blood gases to follow serum pH should be obtained in cases of moderate to severe toxicity.

V.   **Management** (Fig. 55-2)

   A. **General Considerations**

      1. **Initial presentations** of severe intoxications may be quite variable, ranging from no symptoms to death. Nearly all serious complications will develop within the first 6 h and can appear quite suddenly in an otherwise well-appearing patient. Catastrophic deterioration, manifested by rapid onset of wide complex dysrhythmia, hypotension or seizures, most commonly occurs within 1 to 2 h after a toxic TCA ingestion. Cases of delayed complications after 24 h or relapse after initial recovery are rare and have all been associated with inadequate initial gut decontamina-

TABLE 55-3. *Differential diagnosis of major clinical findings seen with TCA overdose*

Anticholinergic effects	Conduction abnormalities	Seizures
Antiparkinson agents (benztropine mesylate)	Hyperkalemia	Theophylline
Antihistamines	Beta-blockers	Cocaine
Phenothiazines	Class IA agents (e.g., procainamide)	Isoniazid
Belladonna alkaloids (jimson weed)	Class IC agents (e.g., flecainide)	Antihistamine
Mydriatics	Quinine	Phenothiazine
	Chloroquine	Carbamazepine
	Terfenadine	Pyrethrins
	Astemizole	Organophosphates
	Phenothiazine	Camphor
	Thioridazine	Caffeine
	Amantadine	Salicylates
	Cocaine	Methanol
	Cyclobenzaprine	Methylphenidate
	Carbamazepine	Lithium
	Bretylium	Heavy metals
	Amiodarone	Cyanide
	Arsenic	

TCA = tricyclic antidepressant.

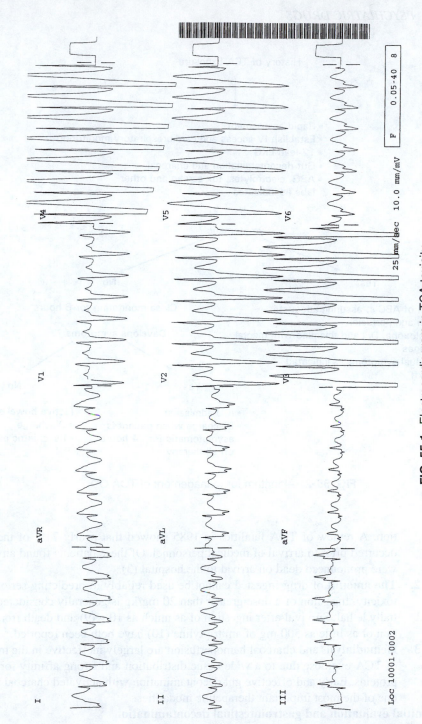

FIG. 55-1. Electrocardiogram in TCA toxicity.

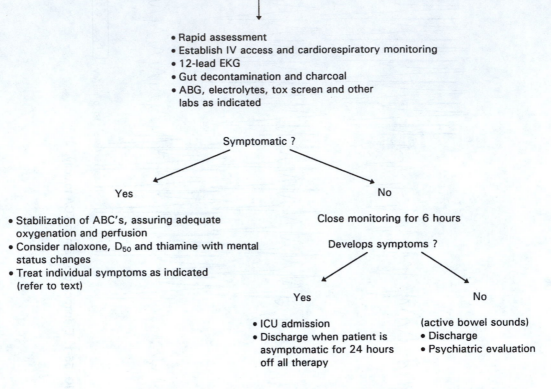

FIG. 55-2. Algorithm for management of TCA OD.

tion. A review of TCA fatalities in 1985 showed that nearly 71% of the deaths occurred prior to arrival of medical personnel. Of these patients found alive, 44% were pronounced dead on arrival to the hospital (3).

2. **The amount** of drug ingested cannot be used reliably in predicting serious TCA toxicity. Ingestion of a dose greater than 20 mg/kg is generally considered potentially lethal. Survival after ingestion of as much as 10 g (9) and death from ingestion of as little as 500 mg of amitriptyline (10) have both been reported.

3. **Hemodialysis** and charcoal hemoperfusion are largely ineffective in the treatment of TCA overdose due to a wide tissue distribution and strong affinity for plasma proteins. Early and effective gut decontamination with activated charcoal remains one of the most important therapeutic modalities.

B. **Initial evaluation and gastrointestinal decontamination**
   1. **Rapid assessment** and stabilization of ABC's as needed.
   2. **Establish i.v. access** and cardiorespiratory monitoring

3. **Obtained 12-lead EKG** and determination of maximal QRS duration. Arterial blood gas, electrolytes, toxicology screens, serum levels, CXR, and other labs as indicated.
4. **Gut decontamination.**
   a. **Syrup of ipecac**–induced emesis should be avoided because of the dangers of abrupt seizure activity or deterioration in mental status with concomitant risk of aspiration.
   b. **Gastric lavage** using a large bore orogastric tube should be performed as soon as possible.
   c. **Activated charcoal** (50 to 100 g in adults) and a cathartic should be promptly administered following lavage.
   d. **Repeated doses of activated charcoal** (25 g q4h) may be helpful in severe cases but its efficacy is probably limited.
5. **Naloxone, D_{50} and thiamine** may all be considered in cases of mental status changes.

C. **Treatment of conduction disturbances/arrhythmias**
1. **Sodium bicarbonate** is the single most effective agent for treatment of conduction disturbances and arrhythmias associated with significant TCA toxicity.
   a. **Mechanism.** Both alkalinization and increased plasma sodium concentration appear to play important roles. An effect on increased protein binding of TCAs appears to be negligible.
   b. **Indication.** The use of $NaHCO_3$ is indicated for all cases in which the QRS interval exceeds 0.1 s with or without arrhythmias.
   c. **Dose.** One to 2 mEq/kg boluses of $NaHCO_3$ can be used to alkalinize the blood followed by a continuous $NaHCO_3$ infusion (100 to 150 mEq $NaHCO_3$/1 L D_5W at one to two times maintenance) after the initial boluses to maintain alkalinization.
   d. **Endpoint.** The serum pH should be maintained between 7.45 and 7.55. Therapy can be stopped when patient is stable with narrowing of QRS interval.
   e. **Risks.** The potential risks from $NaHCO_3$ therapy include impaired oxygen delivery due to a leftward shift of the oxygen-hemoglobin dissociation curve, extreme alkalosis, paradoxical CNS acidosis, hyperosmolarity, fluid overload, hypokalemia, and hypocalcemia.
2. **Lidocaine** may be considered for control of refractory ventricular arrhythmias although evidence for its efficacy is lacking. Toxic doses of lidocaine must be avoided as high doses may cause conduction disturbances and precipitate seizures.
3. **Bretylium** should be avoided.
4. Attempts at **cardioversion** are often futile due to continuing drug effect.

D. **Treatment of hypotension**
1. **Fluids.** Mild to moderate hypotension will often respond to crystalloid or colloid fluid boluses (20 mL/kg).
2. **Sodium bicarbonate** may also be useful in the treatment of hypotension. It appears to increase blood pressure by increasing myocardial contractility.
3. **Vasopressors.** For persistent hypotension, vasopressors should be added. Since much of the hypotension is the result of α-adrenergic block, greater success may

be achieved using agents with more selective α-adrenergic activity such as norepinephrine and phenylephrine. Additional agents that may be considered include dobutamine and dopamine. The efficacy of dopamine may be limited by the catecholamine depletion associated with TCA toxicity.

    4. **Mechanical support.** Further therapy for severe hypotension may include mechanical support such as intra-aortic balloon pump and cardiopulmonary by-pass.

E. **Treatment of seizures.** Seizure activity can lead to increasing acidosis and hypoxia, worsening TCA-induced cardiotoxicity. Recurrent or protracted seizure activity must be treated aggressively.

    1. Intravenous **diazepam or lorazepam** is the logical first choice.

    2. Additional seizure control can be achieved using **phenobarbital.**

    3. The use of **phenytoin is usually avoided** due to an association with increased incidence of arrhythmias and hypotension.

    4. Refractory seizures may require administration of **general anesthesia or paralytic agent** therapy.

F. **Other treatment considerations**

    1. **Coma/alteration in mental status.** If the respiratory status is stable, only close monitoring and supportive therapy are required. The coma may last for several days. Mental status changes also do not require any specific therapy other than close observation. A thorough evaluation for other potentially treatable etiologies should be performed. Empiric use of naloxone, D_{50} and thiamine can be considered. Flumazenil should never be used in patients with suspected TCA overdose.

    2. **Sinus tachycardia.** By itself, sinus tachycardia does not require any specific therapy other than observation.

G. **Contraindicated therapeutic agents**

    1. **Ipecac.** The abrupt onset of seizures and/or mental status deterioration precludes the use of ipecac for gut decontamination. Additionally, effective therapy with activated charcoal can be significantly delayed.

    2. **Physostigmine.** Both the central and the peripheral anticholinergic effects of TCA toxicity may be temporarily reversed with an acetylcholinesterase inhibitor such as physostigmine. However, these anticholinergic effects are usually not serious and do not always require specific therapy. On the other hand, the often life-threatening cardiac complications such as conduction disturbances and arrhythmias, are not anticholinergic in origin and do not improve with physostigmine. The use of physostigmine has also been associated with an increased incidence of seizures (11), bradycardia and asystole (12). Animal studies also suggest that overall mortality rate may be higher in cases of TCA toxicity when physostigmine is used (13). Complications of excessive cholinergic stimulation such as hypersalivation and bronchospasm may also become problematic. Because of its uncertain therapeutic benefit and the potential complications, the use of physostigmine for treatment of TCA toxicity is not recommended.

    3. **Type 1A and 1C antiarrhythmic agents.** The membrane stabilization effects of antiarrhythmic agents such as quinidine, procainamide, and flecainide are similar to

those produced by TCA toxicity. Consequently, their use for TCA-induced arrhythmias is contraindicated as cardiotoxicity may be significantly exacerbated.

4. **Phenytoin.** It has been speculated that phenytoin may be effective in treating TCA toxicity by improving cardiac conduction and prophylaxing for or treating seizures. However, recent animal studies have not substantiated any significant clinical efficacy (14) and have actually demonstrated an increased incidence of ventricular tachycardia with phenytoin prophylaxis (15). With additional concerns over phenytoin-induced hypotension, the use of phenytoin for TCA toxicity is not recommended.

5. **Beta-blockers.** The use of β-adrenergic blocking agents such as propranolol has been associated with significant hypotension and cardiac arrest in patients with TCA toxicity (16). These outcomes are most likely related to the negative inotropic and chronotropic effects of the β-blocking agents and their use is also not recommended.

6. **Flumazenil,** a competitive antagonist for the benzodiazepine receptors, has been associated with an increased incidence of seizures when used in coingestions of benzodiazepines and TCAs (17). Its use is contraindicated in any instance where TCA ingestion is suspected.

VI. **Disposition**

A. **Asymptomatic patients** should be monitored closely for 6 h in the Emergency Department. If no symptoms develop within this observation period, bowel sounds are active and appropriate gut decontamination has been performed, the patient may then be discharged for psychiatric evaluation. Patients with isolated sinus tachycardia that improves with volume or time may also be discharged for psychiatric evaluation after the 6-h observation period.

B. **Symptomatic patients,** including patients with persistent sinus tachycardia (HR of more than 100 to 120), should be monitored in the Intensive Care Unit once vital signs are stabilized in the Emergency Department. Specific therapeutic modalities should be initiated and maintained during hospitalization. Monitoring is necessary until patient is asymptomatic for 24 h after being off all therapy. Late onset of life-threatening arrhythmias has been reported but is very rare and always associated with inadequate gut decontamination.

References

1. Kuhn R. The treatment of depressive states with G223JJ (imipramine hydrochloride). *Am J Psychiatry* 1959;115; 459–464.
2. Mann Am, Catterson AG, McPherson AS. Toxicity of imipramine: Report of serious side effects and massive overdosage. *CMA J* 1959;81:23–28.
3. Callaham M, Kassel D. Epidemiology of fatal tricyclic antidepressant ingestion: implications for management. *Ann Emerg Med* 1985;14:1–9.
4. Litovitz TL, Felberg L, et al. 1994 annual report of the American Association of Poison Control Centers toxic exposure surveillance system. *Am J Emerg Med* 1995;13:551–597.
5. Emerman CL, Connors AF, Burma GM. Level of consciousness as a predictor of complications following tricyclic overdose. *Ann Emerg Med* 1987;16:326–330.
6. Frommer DA, Kulig KW, et al. Tricyclic antidepressant overdose. *JAMA* 1987;257:521–526.
7. Boehnert M, Lovejoy FH. Value of the QRS duration versus the serum drug level in predicting seizures and ventricular arrhythmias after an acute overdose of tricyclic antidepressants. *N Engl J Med* 1985;313:474–479.

8. Niemann JT, Bessen HA, Rothstein RJ, et al. Electrocardiographic criteria for tricyclic antidepressant cardiotoxicity. *Am J Cardiol* 1986;57:1154–1159.
9. Manoguerra A, Weaver L. Poisoning with tricyclic antidepressant drugs. *Clin Toxicol* 1997;10:149–158.
10. Burks J, et al. Tricyclic antidepressant poisoning. *JAMA* 1974;230:1405–1407.
11. Newton R. Physostigmine salicylate in the treatment of tricyclic antidepressant overdosage. *JAMA* 1975;231:941–943.
12. Pentel P, Peterson CD. Asystole complicating physostigmine treatment of tricyclic antidepressant overdose. *Ann Emerg Med* 1980;9:588–590.
13. Vance MA, Ross SM, Millington WR, Blumberg JB. Potentiation of tricyclic antidepressant toxicity by physostigmine in mice. *Clin Toxicol* 1977;11:413–421.
14. Mayron R, Ruiz E. Phenytoin: does it reverse tricyclic antidepressant–induced cardiac conduction abnormalities? *Ann Emerg Med* 1986;15:876–880.
15. Callaham M, Schumaker H, Pentel P. Phenytoin prophylaxis of cardiotoxicity in experimental amitriptyline poisoning. *J Pharmacol Exp Ther* 1988;245:216–220.
16. Freeman JW, Loughhead MG. Beta-blockade in the treatment of tricyclic overdose. *Med J Aust* 1973;1:1233–1235.
17. Spivey WH. Flumazenial and seizures; analysis of 43 cases. *Clin Ther* 1992;14:292–305.

Emergency Toxicology, Second Edition,
edited by Peter Viccellio.
Lippincott–Raven Publishers, Philadelphia © 1998.

56

New Antidepressants

†John D. Markman and °Paul M. Wax

*†Department of Neurology, Harvard University Medical School, Cambridge, Massachusetts
02238; °Department of Emergency Medicine, University of Rochester Medical Center,
Rochester, New York 14642*

I. Introduction

    A. History. The introduction of fluoxetine into widespread use for the treatment of depression in 1988 launched a new era in antidepressant therapy. These and other newer antidepressants have been variously categorized as "atypical," "heterocyclic," "second generation," or "third generation." They are easily distinguished from their predecessors, the tricyclic antidepressants (TCAs) and monoamine oxidase inhibitors (MAOIs), by the selectivity of their pharmacologic actions and a more heterogeneous chemical structure. This chapter will primarily focus on the specific serotonin reuptake inhibitors (SSRIs) fluoxetine (Prozac), sertraline (Zoloft), paroxetine (Paxil), and fluvoxamine (Luvox). Trazodone (Desyrel) and nefazodone (Serzone), bupropion (Wellbutrin), and venlafaxine (Effexor) will be discussed separately due to their distinctive chemical structure and action.

    B. Present indications. These newer antidepressants have become the most commonly prescribed antidepressant replacing the older TCAs as first-line therapy in the treatment of depression. Other indications for these new medications include obsessive-compulsive disorders and eating disorders.

    C. Toxicologic overview. Experience to date suggests that overdose of these newer antidepressants are considerably more benign than an overdose of TCAs or MAOIs. Their high specificity for the serotonergic family of receptors confers a wide therapeutic index with fewer adverse effects. The SSRIs, as well as trazodone and nefazadone, appear to cause little serious toxicity in overdose. Significant morbidity and/or mortality with these drugs seems limited to polydrug overdoses involving the combination of these drugs with more toxic agents. Bupropion and venlafaxine overdose may result in seizures but do not appear to cause the life-threatening cardiac conduction disturbances and dysrhythmias associated with the TCAs. The most alarming toxic aspect of these drugs appears to be their role in precipitating the life-threatening serotonin syndrome.

II. Specific serotonin reuptake receptors

    A. Pharmacology and properties of agents

        1. Nomenclature/structure. The SSRIs share a common mode of biologic action, but they have distinct molecular structures and pharmacokinetic profiles. Fluoxetine is a phenylpropylamine derivative in contrast to sertraline, a naphthalenamine derivative and paroxetine, a phenylpiperidine derivative. They have demonstrated nearly equivalent efficacy as antidepressant therapies.

2. **Pharmacokinetics**

   a. **Absorption.** They are all well absorbed through the GI tract and have maximum biologic activity between 4 and 8 h after administration.

   b. **Metabolism.** These agents are hepatically metabolized by the P450 enzyme system. Fluoxetine has the longest half-life (approximately 50 h) and its active metabolite norfluoxetine may persist for 2 to 3 days. The other three agents have significantly shorter half-lives: on average 20 h.

   c. **Elimination.** SSRIs are predominantly hepatically metabolized to inactive metabolites excreted in the urine.

B. **Mechanism of action and toxicity**

   1. **Mechanisms**

      a. **Serotonin reuptake inhibition.** By definition, the SSRIs are all very specific for the serotonergic pathways. These agents are thought to work by inhibiting neuronal reuptake of serotonin thereby increasing synaptic levels of this neurotransmitter. Although toxicity from acute overdose is rather low, excessive serotonin states, as manifested by the serotonin syndrome, can result in significant morbidity.

      b. **No receptor blockade.** Unlike the TCAs, SSRIs do not cause significant blockade of cholinergic or adrenergic receptors.

      c. **No "quinidine-like" effects.** SSRIs also do not produce myocardial membrane depressant effects on sodium channels that may result in conduction disturbances and arrhythmias.

   2. **Adverse effects at therapeutic doses**

      a. **CNS**

         (1) **Headache, nervousness, insomnia, and drowsiness** are the most commonly reported adverse effects of fluoxetine.

         (2) **Seizures.** The incidence of seizures with fluoxetine is comparable with other antidepressant therapies at 0.2% of all patients treated with the drug.

         (3) **Serotonin syndrome.** The constellation of mental status, neuromuscular, and autonomic effects that comprise the serotonin syndrome represents the most concerning adverse effects of this group of agents. (see below)

      b. **Gastrointestinal.** Aside from the CNS, the other major systemic effects of the SSRIs are seen in the GI tract with commonly reported associated symptoms of nausea, anorexia, dry mouth, and diarrhea.

      c. **Reproductive.** Five percent of patients complain of impaired sexual functioning (anorgasmia, impotence, delayed ejaculation) associated with fluoxetine use.

   3. **Drug interactions** account for many instances of adverse effects due to SSRIs as well as induction of the serotonin syndrome. The most commonly implicated agents are the MAOIs, which when combined with the SSRIs synergistically increase brainstem and spinal cord levels of serotonin. Due to its long half-life, fluoxetine should not be taken for 5 weeks before initiating MAO therapy. For the

other agents in this group, a 2-week washout interval is sufficient. Fluoxetine relies heavily on the P450 system and may prolong the hepatic metabolism of other CNS agents including carbamazepine, valproic acid, clozapine, haloperidol, perphenazine, diazepam, lithium, and TCAs.

C. Clinical presentation

1. **Overview.** Most of the data concerning acute toxicity of the SSRIs involves fluoxetine. Significant morbidity and mortality from fluoxetine overdose generally occurs in the setting of a multiple drug overdose. When there have been no coingestants, the symptoms have been mild and transient. In several different emergency department studies more than half of patients who ingested supratherapeutic doses did not complain of any symptoms.

2. **Cardiovascular effects.** The most common cardiovascular effect is tachycardia. ST depression, junctional arrhythmias, and prolonged QTc syndrome has also been reported but appears to be uncommon.

3. **CNS effects** are typically limited to drowsiness, dizziness, ataxia, anxiety, and tremor. Although uncommon, seizures may also occur up to 5 to 10 h after ingestion.

4. **Gastrointestinal.** Nausea, vomiting, and diarrhea are less frequently seen and usually present as part of a "flu-like" syndrome.

D. Laboratory findings

1. **Plasma levels.** Obtaining plasma levels of fluoxetine and its active metabolite, norfluoxetine, do not influence the management of fluoxetine overdose, and therefore, are not recommended.

2. **Urine toxicology screens** may detect fluoxetine and possibly some other newer antidepressants, but such testing should not change management of these patients.

3. **EKG.** In case of possible coingestion with TCAs, an EKG should be obtained to rule *out* the typical conduction disturbances seen with these more toxic drugs.

E. Management

1. **Initiate** basic life support measures as needed.

2. **Establish i.v. access.**

3. **GI decontamination.** Activated charcoal should probably be administered if the ingestion occurred within 4 h of presentation. Certainly this is most important if any concomitant ingestion is suspected. Gastric lavage is not necessary.

4. **Period of observation.** Although an optimal time period of observation has not been determined for asymptomatic patients who present after SSRI overdose, given the relative rapid absorption of these drugs, a 4-h period of observation to monitor for tachycardia and any change in level of consciousness should suffice.

5. **Complications.** In the unlikely case of seizure onset, diazepam or lorazepam should be administered.

III. Bupropion (Wellbutrin)

A. Pharmacology and properties of agents

1. **Nomenclature/structure.** Bupropion is a unicyclic antidepressant that was introduced into the North American market in 1989. It is structurally unrelated to other antidepressants and is usually classified as an atypical antidepressant. Its aminoketone structure resembles amphetamine.

2. **Pharmacokinetics**
   a. **Absorption.** Bupropion is easily absorbed from the GI tract. The peak plasma concentration is achieved within 2 h after ingestion and the average half-life is 12 h.
   b. **Metabolism.** Hydroxybuproprion is the only active metabolite, with a half-life of about 24 h.
   c. **Elimination.** 90% of the drug is excreted in the urine, mostly as metabolites.

B. **Mechanism of action and toxicity**
   1. **Biogenic amine reuptake inhibition.** The mechanism of action appears to be reuptake inhibition of biogenic amines. Although studies of its effects on the various neurotransmitter systems remain inconclusive bupropion appears to have weak inhibitory effects on serotonin and norepinephrine reuptake activity. While it does block the reuptake of dopamine, there is no reported effect on dopaminergic transmission. There are also no anticholinergic, antiadrenergic or quinidine-like effects.
   2. **Adverse effects at therapeutic doses.** Therapeutic doses have been associated with vomiting, agitation, visual and auditory hallucinations, and catatonia. An increased incidence of seizures at high therapeutic doses is a major concern.
   3. **Drug interactions.** Combination of bupropion therapy with fluoxetine, lithium, phenelzine, or levodopa are likely to lower the seizure threshold. Concurrent or recent (within 14 days) use of MAOIs and bupropion places the patient at risk for a hypertensive crisis.

C. **Clinical presentation**
   1. **Overview.** While overdoses of bupropion cause somewhat more toxicity than pure SSRI antidepressant overdoses, life-threatening toxicity is usually not seen. Outcomes of overdoses are generally benign with full neurologic recovery.
   2. **CNS.** Seizures occur in approximately one-third of reported cases of acute overdose. Seizure activity usually manifests within 1 to 4 h following ingestion. Tremor is the other widely reported CNS symptom.
   3. **Cardiac.** Sinus tachycardia is common.
   4. **Other.** There are no clinically significant anticholinergic or other cardiotoxic effects.

D. **Laboratory findings**
   1. **Plasma levels of bupropion and urine toxicology screens** are not generally useful in the management of bupropion overdose
   2. **EKG.** Should be obtained to check for TCA findings in case of polydrug overdose.

E. **Management**
   1. **GI decontamination**
      a. **Gastric lavage** may be warranted if patients present within 1 h after a large overdose in an attempt to limit drug absorption and decrease seizure incidence.
      b. **Activated charcoal** should be given regardless of whether lavage has been performed.
   2. **Seizure control.** Administer diazepam or lorazepam i.v. bolus to control seizure activity.

IV. Venlafaxine (Effexor)

  A. Pharmacology and properties of agents

    1. Nomenclature/structure venlafaxine is among the newest nonspecific amine uptake inhibitors indicated for the treatment of depression. Venlafaxine has the unique bicyclic structure of a cyclohexanol hydrochloride.

    2. Pharmacokinetics

      a. Absorption. Venlafaxine is well absorbed through the GI tract (92%). Peak serum levels are achieved within 2 h; the agent has a half-life of approximately 5 h.

      b. Metabolism. Venlafaxine is metabolized in the liver by the P450 enzyme system to its active metabolite *O*-desmethylvenlafaxine. The half-life of this metabolite is 11 h.

      c. Elimination. Venlafaxine and metabolites are predominantly eliminated in the urine.

  B. Mechanism of action and toxicity

    1. Biogenic amine reuptake inhibition. The inhibitory effects of venlafaxine on neuronal amine reuptake mechanisms influence both serotonergic and noradrenergic pathways. It is a weak inhibitor of dopamine reuptake. It does not affect muscarinic or alpha-adrenergic receptors or possess MAO inhibitory activity.

    2. Adverse effects at therapeutic doses. Therapeutic doses have been associated with anxiety, nausea, headache, hypertension, insomnia, somnolence, dizziness, and sweating.

    3. Drug interactions. Recent discontinuation or concurrent use with an MAOI place the patient at risk for hypertensive crisis, hyperthermia, rigidity, myoclonus, and autonomic instability. As with other agents affecting serotonergic pathways, a 2-week washout period should be undertaken before initiating MAOI therapy. Concurrent use with cimetidine results in a significantly (43%) reduction in clearance of venlafaxine.

  C. Clinical presentation

    1. Overview. Initial reports of venlafaxine toxicity show it to be a relatively benign agent when taken in excess.

    2. CNS findings predominate in the case reports of overdose with venlafaxine. The most commonly noted effect is somnolence. There also have been a few reports of seizure activity.

    3. Cardiac. Sinus tachycardia and palpitations are the most commonly observed cardiac manifestations.

  D. Management

    1. GI decontamination

      a. Gastric lavage may be warranted if patients present within 1 h after a massive overdose in an attempt to limit drug absorption and decrease seizure incidence.

    2. Activated charcoal should be given regardless of whether lavage has been performed.

    3. Seizure control. Administer diazepam or lorazepam i.v. bolus to control seizure activity.

V.   Trazodone (Desyrel) and nefazodone (Serzone)

   A.   Pharmacology and properties of agents

      1.   Nomenclature/structure. Trazodone is a triazolpyridine derivative whose triazole moiety is thought to be critical to its efficacy as an antidepressant. Its structure does resemble certain side chain components of TCAs. It has been shown to be a moderately effective anxiolytic. Nefazodone is a phenylpiperazine analogue of trazodone.

      2.   Pharmacokinetics

        a.   Absorption. Trazodone is well absorbed through the GI tract. On an empty stomach, peak blood levels are achieved after 1 h; when taken with food, peak levels are reached in 2 h. Elimination follows a biphasic pattern; the early phase lasts hours while the second, slower phase averages 5 to 9 h.

        b.   Metabolism. The active metabolite, *m*-chlorophenylpiperazine (m-CPP) has an extended half-life of 4 to 14 h with highest levels reached in the brain. Nefazodone shares the m-CPP metabolites and has a second derivative (hydroxynefazodone).

        c.   Elimination. 75% of the active metabolite is excreted in the urine.

   B.   Mechanism of action and toxicity

      1.   Direct 5-HT receptor agonist activity and reuptake inhibition. Trazodone exhibits direct serotonin receptor antagonist activity in addition to relatively weak, though very specific, serotonin reuptake inhibition. Trazodone's potent antagonism of postsynaptic alpha-1 adrenergic receptors probably explains its tendency to cause orthostatic hypotension. There are no anticholinergic effects. Nefazodone has short-term norepinephrine reuptake blockade with little known clinical effect. Significantly, nefazodone lack antagonist activity at alpha-adrenergic receptors and giving it a more favorable side effect profile than trazodone.

      2.   Adverse effects at therapeutic doses. Therapeutic doses have been associated with orthostatic hypotension and consequent dizziness as well as sedation, seen most commonly in the elderly. Priapism is a notable side effect most likely to occur during the first month of treatment at doses lower than 150 mg/day. There is frequently associated nausea and vomiting. Ten percent of patients experience peripheral edema at therapeutic doses.

      3.   Drug interactions. Combination therapy with other agonists of the serotonergic pathways may predispose to the Serotonin Syndrome. Trazodone has been shown to increase plasma TCA levels. Augmentation of hypotension may result when trazodone is used in combination with antihypertensives or phenothiazines. Interaction with MAOIs is less likely than with other SSRIs, and they are commonly administered together to offset the insomnia associated with MAOI use.

   C.   Clinical presentation

        a.   Overview: Overdoses of trazodone are mostly benign. Reported fatalities have occurred in the context of patient's taking other drugs. Nefazodone is not yet widely used in North America so a significant data base about its presentation has yet to be compiled. There are no clinically significant respiratory or cardiotoxic effects.

      b.   **CNS.** Drowsiness, lethargy, and ataxia are the most commonly described symptoms. There are rare reports of coma and seizures. The drug's effects are heightened by concomitant alcohol use.

      c.   **Cardiovascular.** Hypotension and bradycardia has been reported.

      d.   **GU.** Priapism is not associated with toxic levels of trazodone, but it does represent a medical emergency as 40% to 50% of patients with this symptom will become impotent as a result if treatment is delayed 4 to 6 h.

D.   **Laboratory findings**

    1.   **Plasma levels of trazodone and nefazodone** are not useful in the management of overdose.

    2.   **EKG.** Should be obtained to check for TCA findings in the context of polydrug overdose

E.   **Management**

    1.   **GI decontamination.** Activated charcoal should be given but gastric lavage is not warranted.

    2.   **Hypotension.** Administer i.v. fluids and place in Trendelenburg position. Atropine may be indicated if significant heart block or bradycardia is present.

    3.   **Priapism.** Urological consultation and irrigation of the corpus cavernosa with an alpha agonist such as metaraminol (Aramine) or epinephrine (Adrenalin) may be required.

VI.   **Serotonin syndrome**

A.   **Overview.** With the introduction into widespread use of the SSRIs for the treatment of major depression, the incidence of cases of serotonergic hyperstimulation known as the "serotonin syndrome" has risen. This drug-induced syndrome is characterized by simultaneous alteration of mental status and behavior, neuromuscular function, and autonomic tone and occurs at therapeutic drug dosing not overdose.

    1.   **Mechanism.** These symptoms are associated with an increased concentration of serotonin and heightened stimulation of 5-HT_{1A} receptors on brain stem and spinal cord neurons.

    2.   **Precipitants and time course.** The syndrome typically develops within hours to days following the introduction of a second generation antidepressant (fluoxetine, clomipramine, sertraline, trazodone) or after recent discontinuation of a serotonin-enhancing agent (lithium or MAOI).

    3.   **Severity.** While the majority of these cases have been benign and self-limiting, a small number have been fatal.

B.   **Clinical presentation.** There is a wide spectrum of symptoms, some of which mimic neuroleptic malignant syndrome. Symptoms from each of the following three groups must be present.

    1.   **Mental status changes** range from the more common agitation and confusion to drowsiness and coma.

    2.   **Neuromuscular abnormalities** include myoclonus, rigidity, hyperreflexia (legs greater than arms), and tremor.

    3.   Features of **autonomic instability** are low-grade fever, nausea, vomiting, diarrhea, tachycardia, and diaphoresis.

4. **Other.** In rare instances, the syndrome has been associated with seizures, high fever, nystagmus, oculogyric crises, dysarthria, paraesthesias, Babinski signs, renal failure and DIC.

C. **Diagnostic evaluation.** The diagnosis of serotonin syndrome is made on clinical grounds. The diagnosis rests solely on the constellation of symptoms, agents, and timing of the medication history. The exclusion of other etiologies including substance abuse or withdrawal and infectious etiologies should be undertaken. Electrolytes, CSF studies, and brain imaging all tend to be normal. The serotonin syndrome most closely resembles neuroleptic malignant syndrome in that both may have characteristic alteration in mental state, autonomic instability, rigidity, and hyperpyrexia. Some authorities have suggested that serotonin syndrome is actually a variant of neuroleptic malignant syndrome

D. **Management**
   1. **Aggressive supportive therapy** should be provided as needed.
      a. **Cooling** with ice water bath and/or cool mist and fans may be necessary to quickly decrease the body temperature when it exceeds 105°F. If a toxic ingestion took place within 4 h of presentation, gastric decontamination with 50 g of activated charcoal is indicated.
      b. **Close observation** should be performed until spontaneous resolution of symptoms occurs. This usually occurs within 24 h since the syndrome is typically short-lived.
   2. **Withdrawal of the causative agent** should be performed.
   3. **Antidotes.** Serotonin receptor antagonists (methysergide, cyproheptadine) and muscle antagonists have not been shown to alter the course of the condition. In the rare cases with a protracted course, methysergide, and propranolol have been administered as accessory treatments, but their effect has not been definitively assessed.

Selected Readings

Banerjee AK. Recovery from prolonged cerebral depression after fluvoxamine overdose. *Br Med J* 1988;296:1774.

Borys DJ, Setzer SC, Ling LJ, et. al. Acute fluoxetine overdose: a report of 234 cases. *Am J Emerg Med* 1992;10:115–120.

Braithers G, Curry SC. Seizure in isolated fluoxetine overdose. *Ann Emerg Med* 1995;26:234–237.

Fantaskey A, Burkhart KK. A case report of venlafaxine toxicity. *Clin Toxicol* 1995;33:359–361.

Gamble DE, Peterson IG. Trazodone overdose: four years of experience from voluntary reports. *J Clin Psychiatry* 1986;47:544–546.

Garnier R, Azoyan P, Chataigner D, et al. Acute fluvoxamine poisoning. *J Int Med Res* 1993;21:197–208.

Henry JA, Ali CJ, Caldwell R, et al. Acute trazodone poisoning: clinical signs and plasma concentrations. *Psychotherapy* 1984;17:77–81.

Hofmon M, Liu JK. Conduction abnormalities and ventricular tachyarrhythmia associated with fluoxetine overdose. *Vet Hum Toxicol* 1994;36:371.

Kaminski CA, Robbins MS, Weibley RE. Sertraline intoxication in a child. *Ann Emerg Med* 1994;23:1371–1374.

Myers LB, Dean BS, Krenzelok EP. Paroxetine (PAXIL): overdose assessment of a new selective serotonin reuptake inhibitor. *Vet Hum Toxicol* 1994;36:370.

Rickels K, Schweizer E. Clinical overview of serotonin reuptake inhibitors. *J Clin Psychiatr* 1990;51:9–17.

Rudorfer MV, Manji HK, Potter WZ. Comparative tolerability profiles of newer versus older antidepressants. *Drug Safety* 1994;10:1846.

Spiller HA, Ramoska EA, Krenzelok EP, et al. Bupropion overdose: a 3-year multicenter perspective analysis. *Am J Emerg Med* 1994;12:43–45.

Sporer KA. The serotonin syndrom: implicated drugs, pathophysiology and management. *Drug Safety* 1995;13:94–104.

Sternbach H. The serotonin syndrome. *Am J Psychiatr* 1991;148:705–713.

Stower AB. Bupropion overdose and seizure. *Am J Emerg Med* 1994;12:183–184.

Emergency Toxicology, Second Edition,
edited by Peter Viccellio.
Lippincott–Raven Publishers, Philadelphia © 1998.

57

Monoamine Oxidase Inhibitors

Daniel J. Cobaugh

Department of Emergency Medicine, University of Rochester Medical Center, Rochester, New York 14608

I. **Introduction**

    A. **History.** Monoamine oxidase inhibitors (MAOIs) were the first antidepressant drugs introduced during the 1950s. Although their use declined with the introduction of the tricyclic antidepressants (TCAs) in the 1960s, a resurgence in their use has been noted over the past 10 years. Since 1990, the American Association of Poison Control Centers has reported 3,761 cases of possible MAOI poisoning and 31 deaths due to these agents (1).

    B. **Present indications.** MAOIs are predominantly utilized in the treatment of atypical and refractory depression. They have also been used in the treatment of certain anxiety disorders such as panic attacks, narcolepsy, and bulimia. Selegiline has been used as an adjunct in the treatment of Parkinson's disease.

    C. **Toxicity overview.** MAOI toxicity may result from acute overdose, or drug-drug or food-drug interactions. Life threatening events, especially hypertension, agitation and hyperpyrexia, and cardiovascular collapse may occur. Onset of symptoms usually occurs within the first few hours after exposure to the interacting substance, but may be considerably delayed in the acute overdose setting.

II. **Properties of agent**

    A. **Structure.** Structurally, the MAOIs are either hydrazines (phenelzine), hydrazides (isocarboxazid), or amines (tranylcypromine, pargyline).

    B. **Preparations.** Commercially available MAOIs and initial daily dosage

        1. Phenelzine (Nardil)—15 mg t.i.d.

        2. Tranylcypromine (Parnate)—10 mg t.i.d.

        3. Selegiline (Eldepryl)—5 mg b.i.d. (used only in Parkinson's disease)

III. **Mechanism**

    A. **Inhibits monoamine oxidase enzyme.** The primary pharmacologic and toxicologic mechanism for the MAOIs is their ability to inhibit catabolism of monoamine neurotransmitters such as dopamine, norepinephrine, epinephrine, and serotonin. This interference with monoamine oxidase enzymes results in the accumulation of excessive amounts of neurotransmitters, particularly norepinephrine and serotonin. Two types of monoamine oxidase (MAO) enzymes, MAO-A and MAO-B, have been identified. MAO-A is responsible for catabolism of norepinephrine and serotonin (5-hydroxytryptophan) and MAO-B deaminates phenylethylamine. Dopamine and tyramine are catabolized by both types of the enzyme (2,3) (see Fig. 57-1).

B. **Other suggested pharmacologic mechanisms** include increased release of norepinephrine from nerve terminals and metabolism to amphetamine and amphetamine derivatives (4).

IV. **Pharmacokinetics**

A. **Absorption.** MAOIs are rapidly and completely absorbed from the gastrointestinal (GI) tract. Extensive first-pass metabolism has been reported with some MAOIs.

Catecholamine Pathways

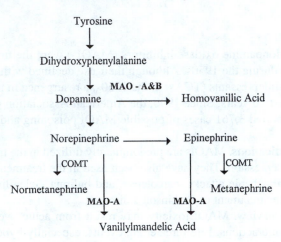

Serotonin Pathway

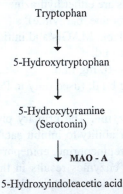

FIG. 57-1. Metabolism of catecholamines and serotonin.

B. **Distribution.** Reported volumes of distribution range from 1 to 3 L/kg. Protein binding ranges from 50% to 94%.

C. **Metabolism.** The MAOIs are metabolized primarily in the liver. Metabolites include amphetamine and methamphetamine.

D. **Elimination.** Renal elimination of inactive metabolites occurs. Elimination half-lives range from 0.15 to 2.5 h. Clinical effects persist for a considerably longer time period due to the continued inhibition of MAO.

V. **Clinical presentation (5–8).** Signs of toxicity may be due to accidental poisoning, overdose, drug-drug interactions and drug-food interactions. The incidence of common clinical findings is listed in Table 57-1 (9). The hallmark of MAOI toxicity is hyperadrenergic and hyperserotonergic stimulation due to the excess of available neurotransmitters at the synapse.

A. **Acute overdose**

1. **Onset of effect.** Following acute overdose, the signs of MAOI toxicity may be delayed for 6 to 12 h after ingestion. Toxicity which has been delayed to 29 h after ingestion has been reported. This delayed onset of clinical effects necessitates observation and monitoring for 24 h after MAOI overdose even if the patient initially presents asymptomatic.

2. **Neurologic** effects may include irritability, drowsiness, confusion, and hallucinations. Early neuromuscular effects, in part due to a hyperserotonergic state, include hyperreflexia, fasciculations, rigors, involuntary limb movement, myoclonus, and trismus. Late signs of toxicity may include coma, opisthotonus, decerebrate and decorticate posturing, and seizures. Headache, often severe, may occur secondary to hypertension.

TABLE 57-1. *Common clinical findings following in MAOI toxicity*

Clinical finding	Percentage incidence
Excitement/agitation	67
Sinus tachycardia	67
Mydriasis	58
Muscle rigidity	58
Coma	50
Hyperthermia	50
Sweating	42
Hyperreflexia	33
Nystagmus	33
Writhing/grimacing	25
Tachypnea	17
Seizures	17
Hypotension	17
Hypertension	17
Cardiac arrest	17
Hallucinations	8
EKG changes (peaked T waves)	8
Papilledema	8

Data from ref. 9.

3. **Ocular** findings may include dilated pupils which are not reactive to light as well as oscillating or rolling eye movements.

4. **Cardiovascular** changes associated with increased catecholamine effect include tachycardia and hypertension. These can be followed by hypotension, ventricular dysrhythmias, bradycardia, conduction disturbances, and asystole. Dysrhythmias are usually preterminal events associated with vascular collapse.

5. **Temperature.** Significant hyperpyrexia may also present following overdose. This is due to severe agitation and muscle rigidity. This hyperpyrexia may advance to malignant proportions rapidly. Even in the absence of hyperpyrexia, diaphoresis may be quite prominent.

6. **Renal** failure secondary to rhabdomyolysis and myoglobin release may occur following excessive neuromuscular activity and elevations in temperature.

7. **Pulmonary** effects include pulmonary edema and difficulty in maintaining ventilation due to muscle rigidity. Hypercarbia and acidosis may ensue.

8. **Hematologic** changes including leukocytosis and leukopenia have been reported following MAOI overdose. Hemolysis and disseminated intravascular coagulation (DIC) may also occur in severe cases.

9. **Hepatic** toxicity may also occur as a complication of the hyperpyrexia.

B. **Food and drug interactions**

1. **Overview.** Numerous food and drug interactions have been reported with the MAOIs (10–15) (Tables 57-2 and 57-3). Although some of the clinical characteristics of these food and drug interactions are similar to those seen with overdose, significant differences do exist. The specific clinical presentation is determined, in part, by which neurotransmitter is most affected by the interaction.

2. **Drug interaction mechanisms**
   a. Increased availability of norepinephrine, e.g., amphetamine
   b. Increased availability of serotonin, e.g., meperidine
   c. MAOI inhibition of hepatic oxidative metabolism, e.g., morphine

3. **Food interaction mechanism**
   a. Foods containing significant amounts of tyramine cause increased availability of norepinephrine.

4. **Onset of effect.** Unlike MAOI toxicity, the clinical effects of an interaction of an MAOI with a drug or food usually occur soon after ingestion of the interacting food or medication. Food and drug interactions can occur for several weeks after discontinuation of an MAOI due to prolonged inhibition of MAO.

5. **Hypertension,** secondary to increased alpha-1 stimulation, is the primary clinical effect manifested following coadministration of MAOIs and medications that increase norepinephrine availability. Similarly, foods which contain tyramine also produce significant hypertension when coingested with MAOIs.
   a. **Severe headache,** accompanied by diaphoresis and flushing, is often associated with increases in blood pressure. While the actual blood pressure measurement may not be very high, a significant change in blood pressure from a previously normal baseline may be the harbinger of sudden clinical deterioration.

TABLE 57-2. *MAOI–drug interactions*

Mechanism and agents	Severity classification
Increased norepinephrine release	
Amphetamines/anorexiants	Major
Amphetamine, benzamphetamine, dextroamphetamine, diethylpropion, fenfluramine, mazindol, methamphetamine, phendimetrazine, phenmetrazine, phentermine	
Sympathomimetics	Major
Phenylephrine, cocaine, dopamine, ephedrine, mephentermine, metaraminol, phenylpropanolamine, pseudoephedrine	
Tricyclic antidepressants	Major
Amitriptyline, amoxapine, clomipramine, desipramine, doxepin, imipramine, nortriptyline, protriptyline, trimipramine	
Increased dopamine	
Levadopa	Major
Methyldopa	Moderate
Increased serotonin	
Dextromethorphan	Major
Meperidine	Major
Selective serotonin reuptake inhibitors	Major
Fluoxetine, paroxetine, sertraline	
L-Tryptophan	Major
MAOI inhibition of hepatic metabolism	
Morphine	Moderate
Sulfonamides	Moderate
Other	
Guanethidine (interference with amine uptake)	Moderate
Insulin (simulation of insulin secretion and gluconeogenesis)	Moderate
Unknown	
Barbiturates	Moderate
Beta-blockers	Minor
Cyproheptadine	Moderate
Sulfonylureas	Moderate

TABLE 57-3. *Common MAOI–food interactions*

Cheese/dairy products	Stilton	Bananas
American processed	Yogurt	Fava beans
Blue	Meat/fish	Figs
Boursault	Beef liver	Raisins
Brick, natural	Chicken liver	Sauerkraut
Brie	Tenderized meats	Soy sauce
Camembert	Fermented sausages	Miso soup
Cheddar	Game meat	Bean curd
Emmenthaler	Meat extracts	Alcoholic beverages
Gruyere	Dried fish (salted herring)	Imported beer and ale
Mozzarella	Pickled herring	(including nonalcoholic)
Parmesan	Shrimp paste	Red wine (especially Chianti)
Romano	Fruits/vegetables	Sherry
Roquefort	Avocados	Chocolate
Sour cream	Yeast extracts	

      b. **Hypertensive crisis,** secondary to these drug and food interactions, can precipitate intracranial hemorrhage. Some authors suggest that at least 6 mg of tyramine is necessary for moderate increases in blood pressure to occur. Ingestion of 20 mg or more of tyramine can result in profound hypertension.

    6. **Agitation/muscle rigidity/hyperpyrexia.** Increases in serotonin, following coadministration of agents such as meperidine and fluoxetine, can result in agitation, hyperreflexia, hyperpyrexia, coma, and death.

VI. **Laboratory analysis**

  A. **Not helpful**

    1. **MAOI serum concentrations,** which are not readily obtainable, have little if any value in the diagnosis and management of the patient with MAOI toxicity. Elevation of catecholamines and concurrent decreases in catecholamine metabolites may occur in MAOI overdose. Increases in neuromuscular activity may lead directly to increases in catecholamine levels.

    2. **Urine drug tests.** Since most urine drug screens are not capable of detecting the presence of MAOIs, a negative urine drug screen may be misleading as it does not preclude the presence of MAOIs.

  B. **Other laboratory tests** which may be helpful include BUN, serum creatinine, CK, urine myoglobin, WBC, ABGs, and LFTs.

VII. **Differential diagnosis**

  A. Other drug overdoses, including stimulants—i.e., amphetamines, cocaine, phencyclidine, caffeine, and over the counter diet medications—should be considered.

  B. Serotonin syndrome

  C. Neuroleptic malignant syndrome

  D. Malignant hyperthermia

  E. Thyroid storm

  F. Drug withdrawal

  G. Tetanus

  H. Pheochromocytoma

  I. Dystonic reaction

  J. Encephalitis

VIII. **Treatment**

  A. **No specific antidotes for the MAOIs exist.** Therefore treatment should include prevention of absorption and supportive care.

  B. **Prevention of absorption**

    1. **Syrup of ipecac** induced emesis should not be induced due to the potential for changes in neurologic status.

    2. **Gastric lavage** should be reserved for ingestion of significant amounts of an MAOI that occurs within 1 h of presentation to the emergency department (ED).

    3. **Activated charcoal** effectively adsorbs MAOIs in the stomach and intestines. A single dose of activated charcoal, with or without a cathartic, should be administered in those patients that present to the ED beyond 1 h and as an adjunct to gastric lavage. There is no evidence that multiple doses of activated charcoal enhance MAOI clearance or improve outcome.

4. **Whole bowel irrigation** with a polyethylene glycol electrolyte lavage solution has limited value in the setting of MAOI ingestion.

C. **Enhancing elimination.** Efforts to enhance the elimination of MAOIs, including urinary pH manipulation and hemodialysis, are not effective.

D. **Management of specific toxicities**

1. **ABCs.** Airway compromise may require intubation and mechanical ventilation. Ventilation may become difficult due to excessive neuromuscular activity. Acidosis should be treated with adequate ventilation and sodium bicarbonate.

2. **Agitation/seizures**

    a. **Benzodiazepines.** CNS excitation can be managed with benzodiazepines (i.e., midazolam) and barbiturates (i.e., amobarbital) which have rapid onset and short duration of effect. Longer acting agents (lorazepam, diazepam) may also be required. Paralysis may be necessary if excessive neuromuscular activity occurs. Although phenothiazines such as chlorpromazine have been recommended to decrease neuromuscular activity, they should be avoided due to their ability to cause decreases in LOC, hypotension, and lowering of the seizure threshold. Seizures can be treated with benzodiazepines (i.e., lorazepam), or barbiturates (i.e., phenobarbital).

3. **Hyperthermia** should be treated aggressively. Lack of cooling can rapidly result in severe morbidity and death.

    a. **Cooling blankets, cool compresses, and mist and fan techniques** can be used to treat mild to moderate hyperthermia.

    b. **Ice baths.** Severe hyperthermia, i.e., temperatures of greater than 40°C, should be treated with ice baths.

    c. **Benzodiazepines** should be optimized to control any neuromuscular activity that is producing heat.

    d. **Paralytic agents** may be required if excessive neuromuscular activity can not be otherwise controlled.

    e. **Dantrolene.** Although its use is controversial, the direct acting skeletal muscle relaxant dantrolene, has been used to control hyperthermia in MAOI toxicity. Dantrolene in doses of 2.5 mg/kg/day administered every 6 h has been used (20). It should not be considered a first-line agent.

4. **Hypertension** should be treated with vasodilators.

    a. **Nifedipine.** Case reports exist in which sublingual nifedipine has been effective in the management of mild hypertension associated with the MAOIs (21). Intravenous vasodilators should be used for more significant hypertension.

    b. **Phentolamine.** The alpha-1 blocker phentolamine has been used in doses of 2 to 5 mg i.v. push, repeated as necessary.

    c. **Sodium nitroprusside** has also been used at initial doses of 0.5 mcg/kg/min with dose titrated to clinical response.

5. **Hypotension,** which may present later in the clinical course, should be treated with vasopressors.

    a. **Norepinephrine.** Direct acting agents such as norepinephrine are preferred over indirect acting agents such as dopamine. Indirect acting agents depend on release of norepinephrine which will most likely be depleted in this stage of toxicity. Norepinephrine should be used cautiously and at low doses given the possibility for an exaggerated pressor response. Initial dose of 1 mcg/min titrated to clinical effect are recommended.

6. **Dysrhythmias,** other than sinus tachycardia, may be preterminal events. Management is dependent on the type of dysrhythmia that is present. Lidocaine, procainamide and phenytoin appear to be safe agents for the management of ventricular dysrhythmias. Bretylium should be avoided due to its ability to interfere with norepinephrine reuptake and subsequent norepinephrine depletion. Atropine, epinephrine and a pacemaker can be utilized for bradydysrhythmias and conduction disturbances. Epinephrine should be used carefully due to potential for an exaggerated response.

7. **Rhabdomyolysis** should be treated with termination of neuromuscular hyperactivity, management of hyperthermia, hydration and urinary alkalinization. Sodium bicarbonate, 132 mEq (3 amps) in 1 liter of D5W administered at a rate of 2 to 2.5 times maintenance can be utilized to alkalinize the urine. Urinary and arterial pH should be monitored.

IX. **Disposition.** All MAOI overdoses should be admitted to a monitored bed for 24 h. Patients presenting after the ingestion of a potentially interacting drug or food product should be observed in the ED for 4 to 6 h.

References

1. Litovitz TL, Felberg L, White S, et al. 1995 annual report of the American Association of Poison Control Centers Toxic Exposure Surveillance System. *Am J Emerg Med* 1996;13:487–537.
2. Leiberman JA, Kane JM, Reife R. Neuromuscular effects of monoamine oxidase inhibitors. *J Clin Psychopharmacol* 1985;4:221–228.
3. Lipkin D, Kushnick T. Pargyline hydrochloride poisoning in a child. *JAMA* 1967;201:57–58.
4. McEvoy GK. *AHFS 96 drug information.* Bethesda, MD: American Society of Health-System Pharmacists, 1996.
5. Linden CH, Rumack BH, Strehike C. Monoamine oxidase inhibitor overdose. *Ann Emerg Med* 1984;13:1137–1144.
6. Myrenfors PG, Eriksson T, Sandstedt CS, Sjoberg G. Moclobemide overdose. *J Intern Med* 1993;223:113–115.
7. Breheny FX, Dobb GJ, Clarke GM. Phenelzine poisoning. *Anesthesia* 1986;41:53–56.
8. Matter BJ, Donat PE, Brill ML, Ginn Jr HE. Tranylcypromine sulfate poisoning. *Arch Intern Med* 1965;116:18–20.
9. Meredith TJ, Vale JA. Poisoning due to psychotropic agents. *Adverse Drug React Acute Poisoning Rev* 1985;4:83–122.
10. Olin BR. *Drug facts and comparisons.* St. Louis: Facts and Comparisons, 1996.
11. Tatro DS. *Drug interaction facts.* St. Louis: Facts and Comparisons, 1996.
12. Tollefson GD. Monoamine oxidase inhibitors: a review. *J Clin Psychiatry* 1983;44:280–288.
13. Blackwell B. Adverse effects of antidepressant drugs. *Drugs* 1981;21:201–219.
14. Wells DG, Bjorksten AR. Monoamine oxidase inhibitors revisited. *Can J Anaesth* 1989;36:64–74.
15. Ragheb M. Drug interactions in psychiatric practice. *Int Pharmacopsychiatry* 1981;16:92–118.
16. Verrilli MR, Salanga VD, Kozachuk WE, Bennetts M. Phenelzine toxicity responsive to dantrolene. *Neurology* 1987; 37:865–867.
17. Clary C, Schweizer E. Treatment of MAOI hypertensive crisis with sublingual nifedipine. *J Clin Psychiatry* 1986;48: 249–250.

Emergency Toxicology, Second Edition,
edited by Peter Viccellio.
Lippincott–Raven Publishers, Philadelphia © 1998.

58

Lithium

†P. N. Galaska and °Paul M. Wax

*†Department of Emergency Medicine, °Virginia Commonwealth University, Medical College
of Virginia, Richmond, Virginia 23233; Department of Emergency Medicine, University of
Rochester Medical Center, Rochester, New York 14642*

I. Introduction

A. **History.** Lithium was first used in medicine in the 1800s; lithium urate was employed in the treatment of gout, and lithium bromide was used as an anticonvulsant and a sedative. In the 1940s and 1950s, patients on a sodium-restricted diet used lithium chloride as a salt substitute. Subsequent deaths in cardiac patients on this regimen curtailed the practice. Lithium has been utilized in psychiatry since the late 1940s for the treatment of mania, but concerns about its safety delayed FDA approval for this indication until 1970.

B. **Present indications.** Lithium is utilized mainly in the treatment of psychiatric illnesses, most commonly affective disorders. These include acute mania, major depression, bipolar disorder, schizo-affective, and schizophrenic disorders. Other uses of lithium include the treatment of alcohol dependence, neutropenia, and anemia.

C. **Toxicity overview.** Lithium toxicity most prominently affects the CNS, kidneys, and gastrointestinal (GI) tract. Chronic lithium intoxication is more common than acute intoxication. Increase in the maintenance dosage, altered pharmacokinetics or renal impairment may all contribute to the development of chronic lithium toxicity. Chronic toxicity also tends to be more serious because it may be initially unrecognized, and, if left untreated, lead to long term neurological sequelae. Acute overdose presentations tend to be more benign. Treatment of lithium intoxication, especially chronic, is often problematic. The goal of treatment should be reversal of the toxic effects and prevention of chronic neurological sequelae.

II. Pharmacology and properties of agent

A. **Nomenclature/structure.** Lithium is a monovalent cation, lightest of the alkali metals, has an atomic number of 3, and a molecular weight of 6.94 Daltons. It shares similar ionic properties with those of sodium and potassium. It may substitute for sodium, potassium, as well as magnesium and calcium at various cellular sites, and influence the synthesis and function of intracellular messengers.

1. **Preparations.** In the United States, lithium is available for pharmacological use as lithium carbonate or lithium citrate.

   a. **Lithium carbonate** (Li_2CO_3) contains 8 mEq of lithium per 300 mg of carbonate salt.

       (1) Available forms
         (a) Regular release
           (i) Eskalith 300-mg capsules
           (ii) Lithonate 300-mg capsules, Lithotabs 300-mg tablets
           (iii) Lithium carbonate 100-, 150-, and 600-mg capsules, and 300-mg tablets
         (b) Sustained release
           (i) Eskalith CR 450-mg tablets
           (ii) Lithobid SR 300-mg tablets

     b. **Lithium citrate** ($C_6H_5Li_3O_7$-$4H_2O$) contains 8 mEq of lithium per 5 ml of citrate liquid.

  2. **Usual dosage:** 900 to 1,800 mg/day.

  3. **Therapeutic lithium serum concentration:** 0.6 to 1.2 mEq/L. Since lithium has a low therapeutic index, lithium serum concentration monitoring is necessary to determine the appropriate dosage schedule.

B. Pharmacokinetics

  1. **Absorption.** Lithium is administered orally. Complete absorption requires 6 to 8 h, and peak plasma levels occur 2 to 4 h after ingestion. Sustained release preparations have a slower rate of absorption.

  2. **Distribution.** The volume of distribution of lithium is 0.6 to 1.0 L/kg. The distribution is uneven with the cerebrospinal fluid compartment containing only 40% to 60% of the plasma concentration. Lithium does not bind to proteins. Its ability to transverse cell membranes is characteristically slower than that of other cations. Since lithium entry into the brain is particularly slow, the CNS effect may lag behind peak blood levels after acute ingestion. At the recommended doses it usually takes 7 to 10 days before an equilibrium is established between the plasma and CSF and the therapeutic effect can be achieved. In patients with chronic lithium toxicity, improvement in CNS symptoms may lag considerably behind falling lithium levels due to the slow movement of lithium across cellular membranes and out of the CSF compartment.

  3. **Metabolism and elimination.** Lithium does not undergo metabolism. Approximately 95% of lithium is eliminated through the renal system, 4% to 5% in perspiration, and approximately 1% in feces. The half-life is 18 to 26 h. Two-thirds of a single dose are excreted initially during 6 to 12 h, and the remaining one-third undergoes slow elimination over the following 10 to 14 days. Following glomerular filtration about 80% of the filtered lithium is reabsorbed in the proximal tubule along with sodium. Sodium depletion will result in a compensatory attempt of the proximal tubule to increase the reabsorption of sodium. Increased sodium reabsorption will result in increased lithium reabsorption and retention. This process may ultimately lead to development of lithium intoxication. Elderly patients have a decreased GFR and therefore decreased lithium excretion and are more vulnerable to intoxication.

C. Mechanism of action and toxicity. The exact mechanism of lithium action is still unknown. Lithium, a monovalent cation, acts competitively against other monovalent and divalent cations (sodium, potassium, calcium, magnesium) at the level of cell membranes and neuronal synapses. It has the ability to pass through sodium channels and can block potassium channels at higher concentrations. Lithium is also capable of inhibiting adenyl cyclase and as a result decrease the intracellular level of cAMP. It can also inhibit the calcium dependent release of dopamine and norepinephrine in neuronal tissue, and thus, possibly decrease the responsiveness of neurons to stimuli.

III. **Clinical presentation**
   A. **Overview.** The adverse effects and toxicity of lithium most commonly involve the CNS, renal, and GI systems. The most serious and debilitating effects involve the CNS. **The hallmark of lithium intoxication is neuromuscular irritability.** A marked tremor, hyperreflexia and ankle clonus are characteristic of significant lithium toxicity. The absence of these findings decreases the likelihood of severe lithium intoxication. Toxicity occurs at lower serum levels in chronic ingestions and higher serum levels in acute ingestions. Older patients are at higher risk of developing chronic lithium intoxication secondary to their decreased renal function. Side effects from lithium seen at therapeutic blood concentrations and signs and symptoms of lithium intoxication associated with high lithium concentrations form a continuum (Table 58-1).

   B. **Factors predisposing to toxicity**
      1. Poor oral intake, gastroenteritis, heat stress, sodium depletion, and congestive heart failure may all cause dehydration and lead to lithium retention. **Lithium-induced nephrogenic diabetes insipidus** may also contribute to this process.
      2. **Drug interactions.** There are a number of drug interactions between lithium and other drugs. Of particular concern is the effect of diuretics causing dehydration and subsequent lithium retention. Interaction between neuroleptics and lithium, and serotonin reuptake inhibitors and lithium may be quite problematic and have been associated with the development of neuroleptic malignant syndrome and serotonin syndrome (Table 58-2).

   C. **Correlation of severity of toxic effects with serum level in chronic therapy**
      1. Mild to moderate 1.5 to 2.5 mEq/L
      2. Serious 2.5 to 3.0 mEq/L
      3. Critical 3 to 4 mEq/L

      After an acute ingestion of lithium serum levels may be significantly higher without evidence of serious side effects.

   D. **Manifestations of toxicity**
      1. **CNS.** Mild CNS symptoms may be present in approximately 40% to 50% of patients that are started on lithium therapy. These may include symptoms of fatigue, lethargy, headache, confusion, muscle weakness, and tremor. Most symptoms will usually subside with continued treatment.
         a. **Mental status changes** in the setting of lithium intoxication are often subtle. Initially the patient may appear only slightly confused or lethargic. Changes that may appear minor to the physician who does not know the patient's baseline mental state may be more noticeable to family and friends who have continued contact with the patient.
         b. **Neuromuscular irritability.** Evidence of coarse tremor, significant hyperreflexia, and ankle clonus is indicative of moderate to severe lithium intoxication.

TABLE 58-1. *Side effects and symptoms of lithium toxicity*

Organ system	Side effects	Mild toxicity	Moderate toxicity	Severe toxiciy
Neurologic	Fatigue, lethargy, impaired memory, impaired concentration, tremor, polyneuropathy	Tremor (fine), weakness, hyperreflexia, fatigue	Tremor (coarse), ataxia, dysarthria, tinnitus, hypertonia, myoclonus, extrapyramidal symptom	Fasciculations, spasticity, rigidity, choreoathetosis, stupor, coma, seizures, paralysis, pseudotumor cerebri, EEG slowing
GI	Nausea, vomiting, diarrhea, abdominal pain, dry mouth	Nausea, vomiting, diarrhea, abdominal pain	Nausea, vomiting, diarrhea, abdominal pain	Nausea, vomiting, diarrhea
Renal	Polydipsia, polyuria, DI, albuminuria, glycosuria, glomerular sclerosis, tubular atrophy, interstitial fibrosis	—	—	—
Cardiovascular	T wave changes, sinus node dysfunction, AVN dissociation	T wave changes, sinus node dysfunction, AVN dissociation	Hypotension, CV collapse	—
Endocrine	Hypothyroid, goiter, myxedema coma, thyrotoxicosis, hyperglycemia, hypercalcemia, hypermagnesemia	—	—	—
Dermatologic	Edema, dermatitis, stomatitis, psoriasis	—	—	—
Ophthalmologic	Tearing, burning, nystagmus, papilledema	—	—	—
Hematological	Neutrophilia, eosinophilia	—	—	—

   c. **Chronic sequelae** may include cerebellar ataxia, dysarthria and peripheral neuropathy.

2. **GI.** About 10% to 30% of patients will experience some gastrointestinal disturbances with the onset of therapy that usually subside with the continuation of treatment. These most commonly include **nausea, vomiting, diarrhea,** abdominal discomfort, and dry mouth. These same symptoms will be present during intoxication.

3. **Renal.** Symptoms of polyuria and polydipsia will occur in 30% to 50% of patients on chronic maintenance therapy and may persist in 10% to 20% of patients. If renal concentrating ability is significantly impaired, diabetes insipidus may occur. In certain cases, renal effects may progress to albuminuria, glycosuria, glomerular sclerosis, tubular atrophy, and interstitial fibrosis. Renal effects from lithium are more commonly a result of chronic use rather than intoxication.

TABLE 58-2. *Important drug–lithium interactions*

Reduce renal clearance	Increase renal clearance	Increase lithium toxicity at therapeutic levels
Diuretics	Acetazolamide	Amitriptyline
Thiazide	Cisplatin	Pancuronium
Potassium sparing	Sodium bicarbonate	Carbamazepine
	Theophylline	Neuroleptics
NSAIDs	Verapamil	Succinylcholine
Ibuprofen		
Naproxen		
Ketoprofen		
Others		
Tetracycline		
Methyldopa		
Phenytoin		

4. **Endocrine.** Lithium therapy may induce hypothyroidism, goiter, and even progress to myxedema coma. Lithium may also effect the parathyroid gland leading to hypercalcemia. Transient hyperglycemia may also occur.

5. **Cardiovascular.** In 20% to 30% of patients on lithium therapy, T wave changes may occur on the ECG. Conduction disturbances and arrhythmias are less common. Lithium may also lead to sinus node dysfunction resulting in sinus bradycardia or sinoatrial block, and also affect the AV node leading to AV node dissociation and junctional rhythms. Peripheral edema may also develop. In rare cases hypotension and cardiovascular collapse may occur.

6. **Hematological.** Lithium may lead to elevated neutrophil and eosinophil counts.

7. **Dermatological.** Patients may experience psoriasis, dermatitis, and edema.

8. **Ophthalmological.** Patients may develop excessive tearing, burning, nystagmus, exophthalmos, and even papilledema.

IV. **Laboratory analysis**

A. **What to order.** In all cases of suspected lithium intoxication, a **quantitative blood lithium level should be obtained.** Lithium is not detected on most urinary toxicology screening tests. A normal urinary toxicology screen may mislead the clinician away from a diagnosis of lithium intoxication.

B. **Blood quantitative levels** are measured by atomic absorption.

C. **Interpreting blood levels**

1. **Acute intoxication.** Due to slow blood-tissue distribution of lithium and slow blood-CNS distribution of lithium the clinical presentation of acute lithium intoxication may not correlate well with the blood level. In particular, a high level drawn within 2 to 4 h after an acute overdose may not be associated with significant clinical toxicity due to incomplete distribution of lithium to the cells. In acute ingestions significant symptoms may not develop until the level is above 4.0 mEq/L.

2. **Chronic intoxication.** Given lithium's low therapeutic index, a patient with chronic intoxication may have significant symptoms with only a mild elevation in the serum lithium level. This is particularly true of elderly patients. It is therefore

important to monitor very closely both the serum level as well as the clinical condition of the patient. Since the cells are already saturated with lithium, toxicity will occur with a slight rise in the serum level and onset will be more rapid. In the setting of a chronic ingestion, toxicity may occur in patients with a level as low as 1.2 mEq/L. A falling level in chronic lithium toxic patients may be associated with continued clinical deterioration due to progressive cellular toxicity and a lag in the redistribution of lithium from the CNS to the blood and renal system.

D. **Renal function tests** are also useful to obtain. A BUN to creatinine ratio of more than 20:1 would indicate the presence of azotemia, likely from dehydration. Such a situation often responds to aggressive intravenous rehydration. An elevated creatinine with a BUN to creatinine ration of 10:1 would be more consistent with an intrinsic renal process, less likely to improve with fluids and more likely to require hemodialysis.

E. An **ECG** should also be obtained.

V. **Treatment.** The goal in treating lithium toxicity should be to decrease the serum lithium concentration, reestablish fluid and electrolyte balance and prevent the occurrence of chronic neurological sequelae. **There is no known antidote for lithium.** Any patient with an acute ingestion of lithium should be initially evaluated and treated as any other ingestion.

A. **Airway.** The patient's airway must be assessed and protected as necessary.

B. **GI decontamination.** In the case of an acute ingestion of lithium, GI decontamination should be performed as soon as possible.

   1. With early presentation (less than 2 h) of acute lithium ingestion the patient should undergo GI decontamination with **syrup of ipecac** or **gastric lavage.** Ipecac should be avoided in cases of CNS depression or impending CNS depression from coingestants.

   2. **Activated charcoal** does not adsorb lithium. Activated charcoal should still be administered if there is any concern of possible toxic coingestants.

   3. **Whole bowel irrigation** with a balanced electrolyte solution, such as polyethylene glycol (PEG) solution, may also be performed. It may be particularly useful in overdose cases of **sustained release preparations.** The recommended rate of administration is 2 L/h in an adult and 500 mL/h in children. It is performed until the rectal effluent is clear.

C. **Fluids.** Patients with lithium intoxication will often be volume depleted and may have electrolyte imbalances. Hydration should be initiated with normal saline solution to restore intravascular volume and improve impaired GFR. Rehydration by itself may result in marked clinical improvement.

   1. **How much.** The infusion of several liters of isotonic fluid may be required in patients with significant intravascular fluid depletion. Once the patient is adequately rehydrated, fluid administration should be continued until toxicity is resolved.

   2. **Type of fluid.** Changing from normal saline to one half normal saline may be preferred once initial rehydration is completed because of concerns of hypernatremia from the use of normal saline in patients with possible concentrating defects.

   3. In a patient with **compromised renal function** hemodialysis should be considered as an early option for treatment.

D. Diuretics

1. **Thiazide (e.g., hydrochlorothiazide) and loop diuretics (e.g., furosemide)** are not recommended in the treatment of lithium toxicity. Their use may result in dehydration and sodium depletion likely to further lithium retention.

2. Although **osmotic diuretics (e.g., mannitol), carbonic anhydrase inhibitors (e.g., acetazolamide), and phosphodiesterase inhibitors (e.g., theophylline)** will initially lead to increased lithium secretion, they also may lead to dehydration and worsening intoxication and have not been shown to be useful in the treatment of lithium intoxication.

3. A beneficial effect for urinary alkalinization with **sodium bicarbonate** has not been shown.

E. Hemodialysis. Often it is difficult to determine which patients may benefit from aggressive treatment of lithium toxicity with the use of hemodialysis. Both the laboratory data and clinical condition of the patient have to be considered. In the severely lithium toxic patient who presents with significant dehydration, fluid resuscitation should take precedence over the immediate initiation of hemodialysis. Patients who clinically improve after rehydration may not require hemodialysis.

1. **Indications**

   a. **Compromised renal function.** Any patient with compromised renal function, should be considered for hemodialysis since the only significant route of elimination is renal. This also includes elderly patients whose GFR is decreased.

   b. **Significant symptoms.** Patients with significant symptoms, especially neurological symptoms warrant consideration for hemodialysis. The onset of hyperreflexia and clonus is an indication that lithium is exerting toxic effects which could potentially be irreversible.

   c. **Lithium level.** The lithium level may be helpful in determining the need for hemodialysis, but must be considered along with the clinical status of the patient.

      (1) **In acute ingestions,** consideration of hemodialysis is warranted in significantly symptomatic patients with levels of more than 4.0 mEq/L at 6 h. Since many acutely intoxicated patients with high levels will recover uneventfully without hemodialysis, patients exhibiting fewer signs of toxicity can usually be managed more conservatively.

      (2) **In chronic ingestions** successful management requires consideration of hemodialysis in any patient with a level above the therapeutic range who manifests significant toxicity. Patients presenting initially with mild symptoms may quickly progress to seizures, coma and even cardiovascular failure. Permanent neurological sequelae are more likely to occur the longer the tissues are exposed to a high lithium burden.

2. **Endpoint.** The goal of hemodialysis is to shorten the duration of tissue exposure to elevated lithium concentrations and to bring the serum lithium level as low as possible, preferably to less than 1.0 mEq/L. Usually there is a significant rebound effect after hemodialysis once equilibrium is reestablished between the intra and

extracellular compartment. Prolonged dialysis of 8 to 12 h duration may be useful but most nephrologists initially prefer 3 to 6 h dialysis runs. A lithium level needs to be rechecked 6 to 8 h after hemodialysis to assess the extend of the rebound effect. Usually, multiple runs of hemodialysis have to be performed to maintain the lithium level in a nontoxic range. Once again, due to extensive distribution of lithium to the brain, despite clearance of the blood by hemodialysis, clinical recovery may lag behind decreasing serum lithium levels.

F. Other Treatments. Peritoneal dialysis has been employed in the treatment of lithium toxicity but has been found to be inefficient and with significant complications. There is a report of successful treatment of lithium intoxication with continuous arteriovenous hemofiltration, but experience with this modality is limited.

VI. Disposition. After an acute overdose of a regular release lithium preparation, patients who remain asymptomatic and have a nontoxic lithium level 4 to 6 h postingestion can be medically cleared. Patients ingesting sustained release preparations should be observed for a longer period of time. The presence of significant symptoms or an elevated lithium level require admission and appropriate therapeutic interventions. Patients presenting with chronic lithium intoxication should be admitted to the medical service for appropriate intravenous hydration and monitoring. Subsequent psychiatric admission may be necessary.

Selected Readings

Amdisen A. Clinical features and management of lithium poisoning. *Med Toxicol* 1988;3:18–32.

Bejar JM. Cerebellar degeneration due to acute lithium toxicity. *Clin Neuropharmacol* 1985;8:4:279–381.

Brust JC, Hammer JS, Challenor Y, et al. Acute generalized polyneuropathy accompanying lithium poisoning. *Ann Neurol* 1979;6:360–362.

Gadallah M, Feinstein EI, Massry SG. Lithium intoxication: clinical course and therapeutic considerations. *Mineral Electrolyte Metab* 1988;14:146–149.

Groleau G. Lithium toxicity. *Emerg Med Clinics North Am* 1994;12:511–531.

Hansen HE, Amidsen A. Lithium intoxication (report of 23 cases and review of 100 cases from the literature). *Q J Med* 1978; 47:123–144.

Hauger RL, O Connor KA, Yudofsky S, et. al. Lithium toxicity: when is hemodialysis necessary? *Acta Psychiatr Scand* 1990; 81:515–517.

Jaeger A, Kopferschmitt SJ, Jaegle ML. Toxicokinetics of lithium intoxication treated by hemodialysis. *Clin Toxicol* 1985; 23:501–517.

Okusa M, Crystal LJ. Clinical manifestations and management of acute lithium intoxication. *Am J Med* 1994;97:383–389.

Schou M. Long-lasting neurological sequelae after lithium intoxication. *Acta Psychiatr Scand* 1984;70:594–602.

Smith SW, Ling LJ, Halstenson CE. Whole-bowel irrigation as a treatment for acute lithium overdose. *Ann Emerg Ed* 1991; 20:536–539.

von Hartitzsch B, Hoenich NA, Leigh RJ, et al. Permanent neurological sequelae despite haemodialysis for lithium intoxication. *BMJ* 1972;4:757–759.

PART VI

Drugs of Abuse

Emergency Toxicology, Second Edition,
edited by Peter Viccellio.
Lippincott–Raven Publishers, Philadelphia © 1998.

59

Opioids

Oliver L. Hung

New York City Poison Control Center; Department of Emergency Medicine, Bellevue Hospital Center, New York University Medical Center, New York, New York 10016

I. **Introduction.** Opioids are among the most common causes of drug-related emergency department (ED) visits in the United States. In 1994, there were 6,173 reported visits to health care facilities for opioid exposure that resulted in 52 fatalities (1). According to the "Drug Abuse Warning Network" (DAWN), ED visits for heroin usage have increased from 1978 to 1992, by 50% (2). Thus, it appears that opioid abuse will continue to be widespread, necessitating continued ED vigilance for toxicity and adherence to appropriate management and care.

   A. **Terminology and classification** (Table 59-1). Opioids are a broad class of alkaloid compounds that have opium or morphine-like activity. They are subdivided into natural, semisynthetic, synthetic, and mixed agonist/antagonist subclasses. Unlike the term "opioid," "narcotic" describes any substance that has abuse potential or sedative properties and is too nonspecific to be useful in the pharmacologic or toxicologic lexicon (3). The term "opiate" refers to naturally occurring opium agonists such as morphine and codeine and the semisynthetic opioids. Like the term "narcotic," its usage is also considered obsolete. Opium, a naturally occurring substance with over 20 constituents, is derived from the sap of the poppy plant, *Papaver somniferum*. The word opium is derived from the Greek name for juice (3). Morphine and codeine are the only two naturally occurring opium alkaloid derivatives. Semisynthetic opioids are derived from the structural alteration of the morphine alkaloid. Examples of semisynthetic opioids include heroin, hydromorphone, oxymorphone, and oxycodone. Synthetic opioids are produced completely by laboratory synthesis. Examples of synthetic opioids include meperidine, methadone, diphenoxylate, fentanyl, and propoxyphene. Opioids with mixed agonist and antagonist properties include buprenorphine, nalorphine, and pentazocine.

   B. **Pharmacology.** The opioids exert their pharmacologic effects by interacting with specific opioid receptors in the CNS (4). The three main opioid receptor types are classified as mu, kappa, and delta. All three mediate analgesia effects. A fourth receptor sigma is no longer considered to be an opioid receptor because it cannot be antagonized by naloxone. The mu receptor has two subtypes, mu_1 and mu_2. The mu_1 receptor is considered the most important receptor for supraspinal analgesic effects, while the mu_2 receptor is postulated to mediate respiratory depression, gastrointestinal (GI) actions, and cardiovascular effects (5). The kappa receptors, which include three subtypes, and the delta receptors, which include two subtypes, appear to primarily mediate spinal analgesic effects. The mu_1, $kappa_3$, and $delta_2$ receptors are located in the brain. The mu_2, $kappa_1$, and $delta_1$ receptors

TABLE 59-1. *Chemical classification of opioids*

Opioid	Common trade name
Natural opium derivative	
Codeine	—
Morphine	—
Opium (dry or tincture)	—
Paragoric (camphorated tincture or opium)	Pantopon
Semisynthetic agents	
Buprenophine	Buprenex
Butorphanol	Stadol
Dextromethorphan	Delsym
Drocode (dihydrocodeine)	Synalgos-DC
Heroin (diacetylmorphine)	—
Hydrocodone	Hycodan
Hydromorphone	Dilaudid
Levorphanol	Levo-Dromoran
Nalbuphine	Nubain
Oxycodone	Percodan, Percocet
Oxymorphone	Numorphan
Synthetic agents	
Meperidine and related	
Alfentanil	Alfenta
Alphaprodine	Nisentil
Diphenoxylate	Lomotil
Fentanyl	Submilaze
Loperamide	Imodium
Meperidine (pethidine)	Sufenta
Methadone and related	
Dextromoramide	Palfium
Dipipanone	Diconal
Methadone	Dolophine
Propoxyphene	Darvon
Other	
Pentazocine	Talwin

Adapted from previous edition.

are located in the spinal cord (6). Opioids are commonly used clinically as analgesics and anesthetic agents, but are also available illicitly as drugs of abuse. Absorption of opioids may occur via parenteral, oral, or inhalational routes. Intravenous preparations have an onset of action within 0.5 h. Most oral preparations have an onset of action within 1 h; however, several oral preparations may have delayed effects. Methadone's peak effects occur 4 h after ingestion. Because of the anticholinergic effect of atropine, the opioid effects of lomotil (diphenoxylate/atropine) can be delayed up to 12 h after ingestion (7).

C. **History.** In many cases of opioid overdose, it may be impossible to obtain a clear history from the patient because of CNS depression, coma, or lack of cooperation. A directed history is essential because it may provide sufficient clues to better guide patient care. The history may alert the physician to the seriousness of the exposure. An inconsistent history may alert the physician to the possibility of other toxicologic syndromes or perhaps other pathological processes (e.g., trauma, infectious diseases). With the conscious patient, it is important to determine the type and amount of opioid used, time of

TABLE 59-2. *Classification, potency, and characteristics of opioid agonists*

	Receptor	Analgesic dose equal to 10 mg MSO$_4$ (s.c.)	Analgesic duration (h, s.c.)	Volume of distribution (L/kg)	Half-life (h)
Natural (opium)					
Morphine	μ_1, μ_2, κ, σ	10	4–5	3.3 ± 0.9	1.4–2.4
Codeine	μ_1, μ_2, κ, σ	120	4–5 (p.o.)	2.6 ± 0.3	2.2–3.6
Semisynthetic					
Heroin	—	5	4–5	—	0.5
Hydromorphone	μ_1, μ_2, κ, σ	1.3	4–5	—	2–3
Oxymorphone	—	1.0	4–6	—	2–3
Oxycodone	—	10–15	4–5	—	—
Synthetic					
Meperidine	—	75–100	2–4	4.4 ± 0.9	2.4–4.0
Methadone	—	10	4–5	3.8 ± 0.6	24–48
Levorphanol tartrate	μ_1, μ_2, κ, σ	2	4–5	—	12–16
Paregoric	—	25 ml	4–5	—	—
Diphenoxylate	—	40–60	?	—	—
Fentanyl	—	0.125	1	4.0 ± 0.4	3.3–4.1
Propoxyphene	—	240	4–6	—	6–12

Adapted from ref. 21.

use, and route of absorption. Knowledge of the common street names of opioids may be helpful in obtaining this history. It is also important to ascertain whether other medications or drugs of abuse were used by the patient and whether the overdose was actually a suicide attempt. Allied health professionals (such as paramedics) and witnesses may also provide helpful information. They should be asked if the patient was found in an area endemic for drug abuse and if drug paraphernalia was found at the scene. If pharmacologic therapy was administered on route to the hospital, determining its effect on

TABLE 59-3. *Classification, potency, and characteristics of opioid antagonists and agonist-antagonists*

	Predominant receptor		Single dose (mg)	Duration of action (h)	Respiratory depression	Volume of distribution (L/kg)	Half-life (h)
	Agonist	Antagonist					
Mixed							
Buprenorphine	μ_1, μ_2 (partial)	κ	0.4	4–5	Yes	—	5
Nalorphine	κ_1	μ_1, μ_2	5–10	1–4	Yes	—	—
Levallorphan	κ_1	μ_1, μ_2	5–10	1–4	Yes	—	—
Cyclazocine	κ_2	μ_1, μ_2	—	24	Yes	—	—
Pentazocine	κ_1	μ_1, μ_2	50–60	2–3	Yes	7.1 ± 1.4	4.6 ± 1.0
Propiram	κ_1	μ_1, μ_2	25–50	4–6	Yes	—	—
Butorphanol	κ	μ_1, μ_2	2.0	4–6	?	—	2–3
Nalbuphine	κ	μ_1, μ_2	10	4–6	?	3.8 ± 1.1	2.3 ± 1.2
Pure antagonist							
Nalmefene	—	μ_1, μ_2, κ, σ	0.1–2	1–2.5	No	—	10.3–12.9
Naloxone	—	μ_1, μ_2, κ, σ	0.4–10	0.3–1	No	0.8	1
Naltrexone	—	κ, σ	50	24	No	19 ± 5	2.7 ± 1.0

Adapted from ref. 21.

TABLE 59-4. *Slang names of commonly abused opioids*

Drug combination	Street name
Alpha- or 3-methyl fentanyl	China white
Codeine	3s and 4s
Codeine and glutethimide	Loads, Pacs
Heroin	H, horse, junk, smack
Heroin with amphetamine or cocaine	Speedball
Methadone	Dolly
Morphine	M, Emma
MPPP/MPTP[a]	Synthetic meperidine
Oxycodone	Perks
Oxymorphone	Blues
Paregoric and tripelennamine	Blue velvet
Pentazocine and tripelennamine	Ts and blues

[a]Meperidine analogues (1-methy-4-phenyl-propioxonypiperidine and 1-methyl-4-phenyl-1,2,3,6-tetrahydropyridine).
Adapted from previous edition.

the patient is important. Finally, witnesses and family may corroborate suspected drug abuse or a suicide attempt.

D. **Physical examination.** The classic features of opioid poisoning include CNS depression, respiratory depression, and miosis. Other common features include hypothermia, diminished bowel sounds, hypotension, bradycardia, and hyporeflexia. The initial examination should begin with airway evaluation and the adequacy of ventilation. Apnea, shallow respirations, and cyanosis suggest inadequate air exchange, requiring supplemental oxygen or even artificial ventilation. The pulmonary examination may reveal rales or wheezing, which are suggestive of bronchospasm or acute pulmonary edema. The examination should also determine the adequacy of cardiovascular function, since opioid-mediated hypothermia and hypotension may also require acute intervention. Miosis or pinpoint pupils are commonly associated with opioid poisoning but may not be present in certain situations: overdoses of meperidine, morphine, propoxyphene or pentazocine; hypoxia; after the use of naloxone; and the presence of coingestants whose pupillary effects override opioid effects (e.g., sympathomimetics, anticholinergics) (8). Opioid effects on the sensorium may range from euphoria to dysphoria, sedation to coma depending on the amount, type of opioid, and time of exposure (9). Typical symptoms of opioid withdrawal include nausea, vomiting, and abdominal cramping. Distinctive physical signs include mydriasis and piloerection. Opioid withdrawal is self-limiting and life-threatening only in neonatal withdrawal (10).

II. **Management**

A. **Initial management.** Initial management should begin with airway management. Profound CNS depression, apnea, and an impaired gag reflex suggest the potential need for endotracheal intubation for airway control and to protect against aspiration. Patients with mild respiratory depression may only require supplemental oxygen. Intravenous access should be obtained and secured. Patients with altered conciousness should receive intravenous thiamine (100 mg) and glucose (25 g, 50% solution for adults; 1 g/kg, 10% to 25% solution pediatrics) empirically (11).

B. Naloxone. Naloxone, a short-acting "pure" opioid antagonist, can be considered for opioid reversal in those patients with respiratory depression or altered conciousness. It competes with opioids for their receptor sites and rapidly reverses the respiratory depression, analgesia, sedation, miosis, and GI stasis produced by exogenous opioids (12). The onset of action and duration of action of intravenous naloxone are 1 min and 20 min, respectively. "Successful" opioid reversal is both of diagnostic and therapeutic value. Complete resolution of respiratory and CNS depression is diagnostic of opioid intoxication and obviates the need to search for other etiologies or the potential need to intubate the patient. Unfortunately, many opioid-overdose patients presenting to the ED are opioid-dependent. Overadministration of naloxone in these patients may precipitate unwanted opioid withdrawal symptoms including nausea, vomiting, agitation, and violence, in the opioid-dependent patient. Overadministration of naloxone is particularly dangerous in the setting of polydrug intoxication. Administration of naloxone in the opioid-dependent patient with combined opioid and sedative-hypnotic intoxication may produce opioid withdrawal symptoms without improvement in conciousness. Consequently, the patient may vomit and aspirate because of the lack of airway protection. Administration of naloxone in the patient with combined opioid and sympathomimetic (e.g., cocaine, amphetamine) intoxication may theoretically provoke life-threatening manifestations of sympathomimetic toxicity by removing the protective opioid-mediated CNS depressant effects. For the these reasons, naloxone should be administered with caution. For patients with CNS depression or mild respiratory depression, the initial dosage for naloxone should be low, 0.1 mg i.v. Patients with severe respiratory depression should receive a higher initial dose of naloxone, 2 mg i.v. If there is no response after 2 to 3 min, the naloxone dose can be progressively doubled until there is a response or a total dose of 10 mg has been administered. Most patients will respond to 2 mg of naloxone; however, high-potency opioids such as fentanyl and mixed opioid agonist/antagonist may require higher dosages. If there is no response to 10 mg of naloxone, the diagnosis of isolated opioid toxicity is unlikely (13). When intravenous access cannot be obtained, naloxone can also be administered by subcutaneous, intramuscular, intralingual, and endotracheal routes. Intralingual and endotracheal routes are preferable because of comparable rapid onset of effect to that of intravenous administration (14,15). Subcutaneous and intramuscular routes suffer from delayed onset of effect (up to 15 min) and erratic absorption in those patients with poor peripheral perfusion (16). However, intralingual administration of naloxone may be technically difficult and dangerous in the uncooperative or stuporous opioid-overdose patient. Patients who are already intubated do not require naloxone for therapeutic intervention, and it may be advisable to wait until intravenous access has been established before administering naloxone. Continuous naloxone infusion may be required to maintain continued opioid reversal. The hourly infusion rate should equal two-thirds the initial naloxone bolus dose that produced patient arousal (13). A repeat naloxone bolus equal to 50% the initial bolus dose may be necessary 20 to 30 min after beginning the infusion. A new long-acting parenteral opioid antagonist, nalmefene, also exists for the treatment of opioid overdose but at this time its usage remains poorly studied and cannot be recommended (17).

C. GI decontamination. GI decontamination may be an extremely valuable adjunct to the management the opioid-overdose patient. In those patients with a massive opioid ingestion within 1-h duration, gastric lavage with a large-bore orogastric tube should be considered. Endotracheal intubation may be necessary to protect against aspiration before attempting gastric lavage. In one study, orogastric lavage followed by activated charcoal reduced salicylate levels by 48% compared with a 37% and 17% reduction in salicylate levels by gastric lavage and activated charcoal alone (18). All patients overdosed by opioid ingestion should receive activated charcoal (1 g/kg) with a sorbital (0.5 to 1 g/kg) or magnesium sulfate (250 mg/kg up to 30 g) cathartic unless contraindicated. Activated charcoal may also decrease the opioid half-life by adsorbing drugs that undergo enterohepatic recirculation (19,20). Syrup of ipecac should be avoided in patients with decreased level of consciousness or the potential for rapid clinical deterioration. Multiple-dose activated charcoal and whole bowel irrigation should be considered for use in body packers or body stuffers with retained drug packets in the GI tract.

D. Acetaminophen/salicylate levels. Propoxyphene, oxycodone, and codeine preparations are commonly combined with acetaminophen and salicylates. Serum salicylate and acetaminophen levels should be checked in all patients with suspected suicide attempts from combination opioid preparations.

E. Radiological studies. A chest radiograph may be helpful since severe opioid overdose is associated with noncardiogenic pulmonary edema. An abdominal radiograph may be useful in identifying potential body packers or body stuffers.

F. Urine toxicology. Urine toxicological screens are not indicated in the acute management of the opioid poisoned patient.

   1. Search for other possible etiologies. If the patient does not respond to initial management, naloxone, and supportive care including correction of hypoxemia, hypotension, and hypothermia, the physician should quickly begin to search for and treat other diagnoses. These include other toxicologic syndromes (e.g., sedative-hypnotics, organophosphates, phenothiazines, organophosphates or carbamates, and clonidine), head trauma, cerebrovascular accident, seizure with postictal phase, and infectious diseases (21).

G. Complications. Opioid overdose may produce a myriad of pulmonary, neurologic, cardiovascular, and infectious complications. Pulmonary complications include aspiration and noncardiogenic pulmonary edema. The risk of aspiration may be minimized by appropriate airway management. Treatment for aspiration pneumonia remains conservative. Antibiotics should be withheld until definite evidence of infection exists. Noncardiogenic pulmonary edema has been described as a frequent complication of either heroin or methadone overdose and occurs during the first 24 h of presentation (22–24). It has also been reported with the use of morphine and prophoxyphene (25,26). The incidence of NCPE ranges from 2.4% to 48% of all opioid overdoses and the risk is probably greatest for those patients who present with cyanosis or near respiratory arrest (23,27,28). The finding of diffuse pulmonary infiltrates and normal cardiac indices based on pulmonary artery catheter measurements confirm the diagnosis of noncardiogenic pulmonary edema, but it is usually established on clinical grounds. Neurologic complications include seizures and CNS abnormalities secondary to opioid-induced hypoxia or hypoglycemia. Generalized seizures have also been associated with intravenous fentanyl and sufentanil (29,30), prolonged use of meperidine (31), propoxyphene and pentazocine overdose (32,33), and neonates in opioid withdrawal (34). Seizures should be managed with an appropriate benzodiazepine. Hypoxia and hypoglycemia should be corrected. Meperidine merits special consideration. Its active metabolite normeperidine has twice the convulsant activity of meperidine. In one study, neurologic manifestations in patients including nervousness, tremors, myoclonus, and seizures directly correlated with normeperidine levels (31). In the presence of renal failure, sickle cell disease, and neoplasm, normeperidine has a markedly prolonged half-life. The clinical use of meperidine, particularly in repetitive dosing, should be avoided in these circumstances. Opioid overdoses are commonly associated with hypotension and bradycardia. Propoxyphene has additional cardiovascular side effects because of its cardiotoxic metabolite, norpropoxyphene. It has been associated with cardiac dysrhythmias with quinidine-like ECG changes: including heart block, intraventricular conduction delay, ST-T wave abnormalities, and ventricular arrhythmias (35). Naloxone does not reverse the cardiotoxic effect of norpropoxyphene (36,37). In one case report, sodium bicarbonate was successfully used to reverse propoxyphene-induced cardiac dysrhythmia and may be a treatment option for propoxyphene-induced wide QRS dysrhythmias (38).

H. **Admission criteria.** All opioid-overdose patient requiring sustained naloxone infusion or multiple naloxone boluses should be admitted to the hospital. Patients resuscitated from respiratory arrest or who present in near respiratory arrest should also be admitted to the hospital and observed. Patients with overdoses from presumed suicide attempts and young children who are victims of abuse require hospitalization for appropriate psychiatric and social service care. Observation should continue for at least 24 h from the time of overdose for those patients at risk for developing noncardiogenic pulmonary edema. A longer period of observation, 36 to 48 h, may be required for overdoses with long-acting agents such as methadone and should be based on clinical grounds (39). Occasionally, an opioid-overdose patient who has been resuscitated with naloxone may request to leave the hospital against medical advice (AMA). This situation is problematic because the patient may appear alert, awake, and oriented. Because of the definite risk of resedation and respiratory arrest after the effects of naloxone have worn off, it is important to enlist the aid of friends, family, clergy, social services, and psychiatry to persuade the patient to remain in the hospital. If the patient remains unpersuaded, it may be necessary to act in the best interest of the patient and restrain him/her for continued observation until the risk of resedation has passed. In general, the legal system has upheld the right of the physician to restrain a patient who is dangerously disturbed for a short period of time pending evaluation and emergency intervention (40).

References

1. Litovitz TL, Felberg L, Soloway RA, et al. 1994 annual report of the American Association of Poison Control Centers toxic exposure surveillance system. *Am J Emerg Med* 1995;13:551–585.
2. Drug Abuse Warning Network Office of Applied Studies. Substance Abuse and Mental Health Services Administration. Department of Health and Human Services.

3. Jaffe JH, Martin WR. Opioid analgesics and antagonists. In: Gilman AG, Rall TW, Nies AS, et al., eds. *The pharmacological basis of therapeutics.* 8th ed. New York: Pergamon Press, 1990:485–521.
4. Pasternak GW. Pharmacological mechanisms of opioid analgesics. *Clin Neuropharmacol* 1993;16:1–18.
5. Pasternak GW. Multiple morphine and enkephalin receptors and the relief of pain. *JAMA* 1988;259:1362–1367.
6. Chang KJ, Cooper BR, Hazum E, Cuatrecasas P. Multiple opiate receptors: different regional distribution in the brain and differential binding of opiates and opioid peptides. *Mol Pharmacol* 1979;16:91–104.
7. Rumack BH, Temple AR. Lomotil poisoning. *Pediatrics* 1974;53:495–500.
8. Shelly MP, Park GR. Morphine toxicity with dilated pupils [Letter]. *BMJ* 1984;289:1071–1072.
9. Bickell WH, O Benar JD. Life-threatening opioid toxicity. *Prob Crit Care* 1987;1:106.
10. Chiang WK, Goldfrank LR. Substance withdrawal. *Emerg Med Clin North Am* 1990;8:613–632.
11. Hoffman RS, Goldfrank LR. The poisoned patient with altered consciousness. *JAMA* 1995;274:562–569.
12. Martin WR. Naloxone. *Ann Intern Med* 1976;85:765–768.
13. Goldfrank LR, Weisman RS, Errich JK, Lo MW. A dosing nomogram for continuous infusion intravenous naloxone. *Ann Emerg Med* 1986;15:566–570.
14. Maio RF, Griener JC, Clark MR, et al. Intralingual naloxone reveral of morphine-induced respiratory depression in dogs. *Ann Emerg Med* 1984;13:1087–1091.
15. Tandberg D, Abercrombie D. Treatment of heroin overdose with endotracheal naloxone. *Ann Emerg Med* 1982;11:443–445.
16. Handal KA, Schauben JL, Salamone FR. Naloxone. *Ann Emerg Med* 1983;12:438–445.
17. Kaplan JL, Marx JA. Effectiveness and safety of intravenous nalmefene for emergency department patients with suspected narcotic overdose: a pilot study. *Ann Emerg Med* 1992;22:1326–1330.
18. Burton BT, Bayer MJ, Barron L, et al. Comparison of activated charcoal and gastric lavage in the prevention of aspirin absorption. *J Emerg Med* 1984;1:411–416.
19. Karkkainen S, Neuvonen PJ. Effect of oral charcoal and urine pH on dextropropoxyphene pharmacokinetics. *Int J Clin Pharmacol Ther Toxicol* 1985;23:219–225.
20. Baselt RC. *Disposition of toxic drugs and chemicals in man.* 2nd ed. Canton, CT: Biomedical Publications, 1982:536–539.
21. Goldfrank LR, Weisman RS. Opioids. In: Goldfrank LR, Flomenbaum NE, Lewin NA, et al., eds. *Goldfrank's toxicologic emergencies.* 5th ed. Norwalk, CT: Appleton-Century-Crofts, 1994:773.
22. Steinberg AD, Karliner JS. The clinical spectrum of heroin pulmonary edema. *Arch Intern Med* 1968;122:122–127.
23. Duberstein JL, Kaufman DM. A clinical study of an epidemic of heroin intoxication and heroin-induced pulmonary edema. *Am J Med* 1971;51:704–714.
24. Frand UI, Shim CS, Williams MH. Methadone-induced pulmonary edema. *Ann Intern Med* 1972;76:975–979.
25. Bogartz LJ, Miller WC. Pulmonary edema associated with propoxyphene intoxication. *JAMA* 1971;215:259–262.
26. Lusk JA, Maloley PA. Morphine-induced pulmonary edema [Letter]. *Am J Med* 1988;84:367–368.
27. Smith DA, Leake L, Loflin JR, Yealy DM. Is admission after intravenous heroin overdose necessary? *Ann Emerg Med* 1992;21:1326–1330.
28. Brzozowski M, Shih RD, Bania TC, Hoffman RS. Discharging heroin overdose patient after observation [Letter]. *Ann Emerg Med* 1993;22:1638–1639.
29. Rao TLK, Mummaneni N, El-Etr AA. Convulsions: an unusual response to intravenous fentanyl administration. *Anesth Analg* 1982;61:1020–1021.
30. Molbegott LP, Flashburg MH, Karasic HL, et al. Probable seizures after sufentanil. *Anesth Analg* 1987;66:91–93.
31. Kaiko RF, Foley KM, Grabinski PY, et al. Central nervous system excitatory effects of meperidine in cancer patients. *Ann Neurol* 1983;13:180–185.
32. Young DJ. Propoxyphene suicides. Report of nine cases. *Arch Intern Med* 1972;129:62–66.
33. Challoner KR, McCarron MM, Newton EJ. Pentazocine (Talwin) intoxication: report of 57 cases. *J Emerg Med* 1990;8:67–74.
34. Koren G, Butt W, Pape K, et al. Morphine-induced seizures in newborn infants. *Vet Hum Toxicol* 1985;27:519–520.
35. Gary N, Maher JF, DeMyttenaere MH, et al. Acute propoxyphene hydrochloride intoxication. *Arch Intern Med* 1968;121:453–457.
36. Holland DR, Steinberg MI. Electrophysiologic properties of propoxyphene and norpropoxyphene in canine conductive tissue in vitro and in vivo. *Toxicol Appl Pharmacol* 1979;47:123–133.
37. Nickander R, Smits Se, Steinberg MI. Propoxyphene and norpropoxyphene: pharmacologic and toxic effects in animals. *J Pharmacol Exp Ther* 1977;200:245–253.
38. Stork CM, Redd JT, Fine K, et al. Propoxyphene-induced wide qrs complex dysrhythmia responsive to sodium bicarbonate—a case report. *Clin Toxicol* 1995;33:179–183.
39. Waldron VD, Klimt CR, Seibel JE. Methadone overdose treated with naloxone infusion. *JAMA* 1973;225:53.
40. Gonzalez v. State 110 A.D., 2d. 810, 488 N.Y. 2d. 231, 67 N.Y. 2d. 647 (1985).

Emergency Toxicology, Second Edition,
edited by Peter Viccellio.
Lippincott–Raven Publishers, Philadelphia © 1998.

60

Sedative-Hypnotics

†G. Richard Bruno and °Susi U. Vassallo

†Kings County Hospital, Brooklyn, New York 11203; °Department of Emergency Medicine, New York University Medical School, Bellevue Hospital Center, New York, New York 10016

I. **Introduction.** The sedative-hypnotics are a heterogeneous group of compounds prescribed in the treatment of insomnia, anxiety, agitation, muscle rigidity syndromes, seizures, and ethanol/hypnotic withdrawal states. Sedative-hypnotics are also used illicitly and, despite improved regulation and awareness, remain substances with high incidences of abuse and dependence (1). This chapter reviews the pharmacology and toxicology of major sedative-hypnotic agents.

II. **Barbiturates.** The barbiturates have been used extensively as sedative-hypnotics since the introduction of barbital in 1903 (2). Barbiturates are substituted pyrimidine derivatives with a common barbituric acid nucleus. Despite problems with abuse, withdrawal, and overdose; barbiturates continue to have important therapeutic indications. Short-acting barbiturates (thiopental, methohexital, pentobarbital, etc.) are used for sedation and induction of general anesthesia. Longer acting agents with less hypnotic effect (phenobarbital and mephobarbital) are used as anticonvulsants agents (Tables 60-1 and 60-2). Phenobarbital is also found in combination with the anticholinergic (atropine, scopolamine, and hyoscyamine) in the GI antispasmodic (Donnatal). The short-acting barbiturate butalbital, in combination with acetaminophen and caffeine (Fioricet), is prescribed for treatment of some headache syndromes. The use of barbiturates as anxiolytics or hypnotics have largely been replaced by agents with higher therapeutic to toxic ratios.

  A. **Mechanism of action.** Barbiturates have dose related CNS depressant effects. The site of these actions is believed to be primarily in the reticular activating system through "facilitation" of the GABA inhibitory neurotransmitter system (3). In vitro experiments demonstrate that the alpha and beta subunit of the $GABA_A$ receptor are required for barbiturates to exert their effects. Barbiturates binding to the $GABA_A$ receptor results in the GABA dependent chloride channel remaining open longer and increased inhibitory synaptic transmission (4,16). Other properties of barbiturates that may contribute to global CNS depression include inhibition of the glutamate excitatory neurotransmitter system, decreased release of calcium ions into the synaptic junction, and inhibition of calcium dependent action potentials (5).

  B. **Pharmacokinetics.** Therapeutic uses of the different barbiturates are related to their time to onset of action, speed to redistribution, mode of metabolic inactivation, and route of elimination. The barbiturates are generally divided by their clinical pharmacology

TABLE 60-1. *Barbiturates*

	Ultra short	Short	Intermediate	Long
Lipid solubility	++++	+++	++	+
pK_a	7.6–7.9	7.9	7.7	7.2
Onset of CNS effect p.o.	[a]	10–15 min	45–60 min	≥60 min
Onset of CNS effects i.v.	30–60 sec	0.5–2 min	[a]	15–20 min
Redistribution	++++	+++	++	+
Duration of action	0.3 h	3 h	3–6 h	6–12 h
Agents	Thiopental, methohexital, thiamyal	Pentobarbital, secobarbital	Amobarbital, aprobarbital, butabarbital, butalbital	Mephrobarbital, phenobarbital

[a] Data not available.
Data from refs. 61 and 62.

into ultra short, short, intermediate, and long-acting agents. Barbiturates are available in all forms for administration: i.m., i.v., p.o., and rectal.

1. **Onset of action.** The onset of action of the barbiturates is related to their ability to penetrate the CNS. Lipid solubility and pK_a are the two factors that dictate how quickly individual barbiturates are able to induce CNS effects. Highly lipid soluble agents penetrate the CNS most rapidly. Agents with high pK_a's are poorly ionized at physiologic pH's and are able to cross membranes more quickly.

2. **Redistribution.** The highly lipid soluble agents are redistributed widely and rapidly throughout the body's tissues. Agents with high pK_a's are also redistributed more rapidly in body tissue (secondary to increased ablity to cross membranes) than those with lower pK_a's.

3. **Elimination.** Barbiturates are either completely inactivated by metabolism in the liver microsomal enzyme system or partially liver metabolized and subsequently excreted in the urine (phenobarbital, aprobarbital). The requirement of renal elimination contributes to a longer duration of action of the long-acting barbiturates.

III. **Benzodiazepines.** Benzodiazepines are the most commonly prescribed psychotropic drug. They were first used clinically in the United States in 1965 when chloradiazepoxide was introduced (6,7). Benzodiazepines are used in the treatment of anxiety disorders, seizures, insomnia, muscle rigidity syndromes, and alcohol/hypnotic withdrawal states (8–10). They are generally felt to have high therapeutic to toxic indices, which have allowed them to replace the barbiturates and other more toxic agents as first-line anxiolytics and hypnotics. Chronic use of benzodiazepines may lead to tolerance, dependence, and withdrawal symptoms (11,12).

A. **Receptor physiology.** Benzodiazepines are believed to exert their effects through high affinity binding at the now characterized-benzodiazepine receptors (BZ) (13,14). These receptors are found in the CNS and peripheral tissues. Central benzodiazepine receptors are grouped into BZ_1 and BZ_2 receptors and are located at the alpha subunit of the $GABA_A$ receptor complex (15). BZ_1 receptors are more abundant in the CNS than BZ_2

TABLE 60-2. *Benzodiazepines*

Generic name	Trade name	Dose (mg)	Available forms	$t_{1/2}$ (h)	Major active metabolites $t_{1/2}$ (h)	Primary clinical uses
Long-acting						
Chlordiazepoxide	Librium	10	p.o., i.v., i.m.[a]	5–30	Desmethylchlordiazepoxide, Desmoxepam, Desmethyldiazepam (36–200)	Anxiolytic, withdrawal
Diazepam	Valium	5	p.o., i.v., p.r., i.m.[a]	20–100	Desmethyldiazepam (36–200)	Anxiolytic, anticonvulsant, withdrawal, sedation
Flurazepam	Dalmane	15	p.o.	[b]	Desalkylflurazepam (47–100), N-1-hydroxyethylflurazepam (2–4), desmethyldiazepam (36–200), oxazepam (3–21)	Hypnotic
Clorazepate	Tranxene ClorazeCaps	7.5	p.o.	[b]	Desmethyldiazepam (36–200), oxazepam (3–21)	Anxiolytic, withdrawal, hypnotic
Clonazepam	Klonopin	1	p.o.	18–50	None	Anticonvulsant
Prazepam	Centrex	10	p.o.	[b]	Desmethyldiazepam (36–200)	Anxiolytic
Halazepam	Paxipam	20	p.o.	14	Desmethyldiazepam (36–200)	Anxiolytic
Intermediate						
Oxazepam	Serax	15	p.o.	3–21	None	Anxiolytic, withdrawal
Lorazepam	Ativan	1	p.o., i.v., i.m.	10–20	None	Sedation, anticonvulsant
Temezepam	Restoril	15	p.o.	10–20	None	Hypnotic
Alprazolam	Xanax	0.5	p.o.	12–15	None	Anxiolytic
Short-acting						
Midazolam	Versed	1–2.5	I.V., I.M., intranasal	1–12.3	1-Hydroxymethylmidazolam	Sedation
Triazolam	Halcion	0.25	p.o.	1.6–5.4	None	Hypnotic

[a] Intramuscular possible but not recommended.
[b] First-pass metabolism to active form.
Data from refs. 6, 7, 10, 19, 20, and 22.

receptors and are located primarily in the motor/sensory cortex and subcortex. BZ_2 receptors are primarily located in the limbic system, striatum, and spinal cord (16). The net effect of the benzodiazepines on the $GABA_A$ receptor complex is to increase the frequency of opening at the $GABA_A$ chloride channel (17). Peripheral benzodiazepine receptors are located in the mitochondria membranes of many tissues (heart, kidney, platelets, adrenal glands, mast cells, and brain). The functional significance of these receptors have not yet been defined (18).

B. **Pharmacokinetics.** Differences in absorption, redistribution, metabolism, and elimination dictate the therapeutic role of individual benzodiazepines.

1. **Absorption/redistribution.** Benzodiazepines are available for all routes of administration. The oral absorption is rapid in flurazepam, diazepam, clorazepate; intermediate in triazolam and lorazepam; and slow in temazopam and oxazepam (19). Intramuscular absorption is best with midazolam, intermediate with lorazepam, and erratic or unpredictable with diazepam or chloradiazepoxide. Clinically, benzodiazepines have also been utilized rectally and intranasally. All benzodiazepines are highly protein bound and have good CNS penetration. The more lipid soluble agents (diazepam and midazolam) penetrate the CNS more quickly, have a faster onset of sedating effect, and have more rapid redistribution than less lipophilic compounds (lorazepam and chloradiazepoxide) (20,21).

2. **Metabolism/elimination.** All benzodiazepines are highly metabolized in the liver either by the microsomal oxidation system or glucuronic acid conjugation. Many agents (chlordiazepoxide, clorazepate, diazepam, and flurazepam) are metabolized to active intermediates by the microsomal enzyme pathway. Other agents are metabolized to inactive intermediates by glucuronidation (oxazepam, lorazepam, and temazepam). Inactive metabolites are excreted by the kidney (7,22).

3. **Active metabolites.** Active intermediates generated in the microsomal oxidizing system must be considered when developing therapeutic strategies with benzodiazepines. When other drugs compete for the enzymes, in patients with hepatic disease, and in elderly patients, the microsomal oxidizing system may be less effective in benzodiazepine metabolism and prolonged sedation may result. Agents with active metabolites may be advantageous in the treatment of patients with ethanol/hypnotic withdrawal because they provide a prolonged active agent. This may decrease the need for repeat dosing after initial withdrawal symptoms are controlled.

IV. **Other sedative hypnotics**

A. **Bromides** are a historically important class of sedative hypnotic agents that were removed from the U.S. market secondary to their toxicity. Bromides have CNS depressant and anticonvulsants effects. They were used extensively in the early part of the century as anxiolytics and hypnotics. The regular use of bromide containing compounds leads to a chronic condition of bromide intoxication termed bromism. Chronic users present with symptoms of acute psychosis and fluctuating mental status. On physical examination, patients have marked variability in their neurologic function and may exhibit a characteristic actiniform rash. The insidious onset of symptoms and inconsistency of physical examination makes bromism a difficult diagnosis, and historically many patients were misidentified as suffering from psychiatric disorders (23).

1. **Pharmacology.** Since the bromide ion is similar to the chloride ion, one proposed mechanism of action for bromide as a sedative-hypnotic is substitution for chloride in body tissues (24). Bromide leads to a false elevation of the chloride ion concentration by common laboratory methods. This is the key to diagnosis of bromism (25). Bromide is presumably excreted in all body fluids that contain chloride. The kidneys are responsible for the majority of both chloride and bromide elimination. Preferential reabsorption of bromide over chloride by the kidney contributes to bromide intoxication. Situations that increase chloride reabsorption (i.e., dehydration) increase bromide reabsorption and worsen toxicity.

B. **Chloral hydrate** is a trichloroethane diol that was first introduced in 1869. It is still widely used as a hypnotic in hospitalized adults and for procedural sedation in children (26). Chloral hydrate is said to have a characteristic odor that has been compared to the pear fruit. It is also radiopaque and may be visualized on x-ray examinations in large overdoses. Chloral hydrate is the only chloral containing hypnotic still available in the United States. The continued use of chloral hydrate has come under question secondary to its low therapeutic to toxic ratio and possible carcinogenic potential (27,28).

1. **Pharmacology.** The mechanism of action of chloral hydrate is not fully understood. The active metabolite trichloroethanol is believed to be responsible for the CNS depressant effects of the parent compound. Chloral hydrate is rapidly absorbed after oral or rectal administration, and it is converted to trichloroethanol by alcohol dehydrogenase (ADH) in the liver. Trichloroethanol is further metabolized to inactive glucuronidates and trichloroacetic acid. Both metabolites are mostly excreted in the urine with minimal fecal elimination. Chloral hydrate is believed to sensitize the myocardium to catecholamines and decrease contractility (29). Coingestion of chloral hydrate with ethanol, historically called the "Mickey Finn," is of special interest because the two compounds compete for the alcohol dehydrogenase enzyme. As ethanol is converted to acetaldehyde, the cofactor NADH is produced for use in the chloral hydrate conversion to its active metabolite trichloroethanol (30). The result is potentiation of CNS depression.

C. **Ethchlorvynol** (Placidyl) is a chlorinated tertiary acetylenic alcohol first used in 1955 (31). It was primarily used as a hypnotic agent in the treatment of insomnia, but has been largely replaced by the short-acting benzodiazepines. Ethchlorvynol has a specific plastic or vinyl odor that facilitates its identification.

1. **Pharmacology.** Ethchlorvynol has CNS depressant, anticonvulsant, and muscle relaxant properties (32). The mechanism of action of ethchlorvynol is not well understood (33). Ethchlorvynol is intended for oral use although illicit i.v. use has been reported (34). This agent is rapidly absorbed in the GI tract and is highly lipid soluble. Duration of action is 4 to 5 h at therapeutic dose but may be much longer in overdose (35). It is renally excreted.

D. **Glutethimide** (Doriden) is a piperidinedione derivative introduced in 1954. It was a popular hypnotic that declined in use after a high incidence of dependence and withdrawal symptoms were noted. Coingestion of glutethimide and codeine bearing such names as "Hits," "Loads," or "Fours and Doors" lead to many fatalities in the 1980s (36,37).

1. **Pharmacology.** Glutethimide has CNS depressant effects and anticholinergic effects. It is only moderately well absorbed in the GI tract after oral administration.

In the liver, glutethimide is metabolized by hydroxylation to several metabolites. There is some disagreement in the literature about the importance of the main metabolite [4-hydroxy-2-ethyl-2-phenylglutarimide (4-HG)] in glutethimide toxicity. 4-HG has been hypothesized to be twice as potent as the parent compound, but clinically 4-HG levels have failed to correlate with severity of intoxication or depth of coma (38,39). Prolonged coma, punctuated with periods of apparent recovery and then resedation, characterize massive ingestions. The products of glutethimide metabolism are eventually renal excreted with minimal unchanged glutethimide found in the urine.

E. **Meprobamate** (Miltown, Equagesic, Deprol) is a carbamate derivative introduced in 1955 primarily as an anxiolytic. The use of meprobamate as an anxiolytic decreased secondary to reported toxicity and the availability of safer agents (40). The active metabolite of the common muscle relaxant carisoprodol (Soma) is meprobamate, another source of potential meprobamate toxicity (41).

    1. **Pharmacology.** The mechanism by which meprobamate causes CNS sedation and muscle relaxation is poorly understood. It is rapidly absorbed in the GI tract and has a uniform distribution in body tissues (42). Meprobamate is metabolized in the liver by hydroxylation and glucuronidation. The plasma half-life is 10 to 12 h. Meprobamate has no active metabolites, and undergoes renal excretion. There have been case reports of massive concreation formation after meprobamate overdoses that have lead to death after apparent "lucid intervals" (43).

F. **Methaqualone** (Quaalude, Sopor) is a quinazalinone hypnotic introduced in 1965. From the late 1960s until removal from the U.S. market in 1984, methaqualone experienced a huge following for its euphoric and dissociative properties. Methaqualone is still made outside the United States. There are reports of adulterated street copies available from illicit methaqualone manufacturing and distribution (44–46).

    1. **Pharmacology.** The mechanism of action by which methaqualone causes CNS effects is not well understood. Its primary effects are hypnotic, but it also has pro and anticonvulsant effects (44,47). Methaqualone is rapidly absorbed in the GI tract and is highly protein bound. The liver is the primary site of metabolism with induction of the microsomal enzymes system, and the route of excretion is primarily renal (48).

G. **Over-the-counter (antihistamines).** All over the counter sleep medication available in the United States today are antihistamines H1-receptor antagonist (i.e., diphenhydramine,doxalamine, etc.) (for a full discussion of antihistamine toxicity, see Chapter 44).

V. **New sedative hypnotics.** The two new sedative hypnotics, buspirone and zolpidem, are products of advances in molecular pharmacology and understanding of receptor mechanisms. They may soon replace benzodiazepines as first-line anxiolytics. These new sedative hypnotic agents have more specific mechanisms of actions, and are less sedating.

A. **Buspirone** is a azaspirodecanedione introduced in 1986. It lacks major sedative affects, and is believed to have little abuse or physical dependence potential (49).

    1. **Pharmacology.** The mechanism of action of buspirone is only partially understood. Buspirone does not have $GABA_A$ receptor or benzodiazepine receptor affinity (50). Buspirone has serotonin receptor (5-HT_{1A}) affinity and dopaminer-

gic receptor (D_2) affinity. The interaction with the dopanergic system is believed to be D_2 presynaptic blockade. The serotonin effects of buspirone are probably responsible for its anxiolytic properties. It is thought to be a partial agonist or mixed agonist antagonist at the 5-HT_{1A} receptor (51). Buspirone has been shown to potentiate the serotonergic effects of the serotonin re-uptake inhibitor fluoxetine. There have been recent case reports of acute anxiety and hypertension when used with serotonin re-uptake inhibiting agents. This supports the role of buspirone as an agonist at the 5-HT receptor and raises the question of possible serotonin syndrome in mixed buspirone overdoses (52–54). Buspirone is only available in oral form. In the liver, buspirone undergoes oxidation to its active metabolite 1,2-pyrimidinyl-piperazine. Buspirone is highly protein bound, has volume of distribution of 5.3 l/kg, and a half-life of about 2 to 4 h. It mostly excreted in urine with minor fecal elimination (55).

B. **Zolpidem** (Ambien) is an imidazopyridine derivative hypnotic recently introduced to the U.S. market. It is believed to have less abuse or dependence potential than the benzodiazepines.

1. **Pharmacology.** Zolpidem is a fast acting hypnotic that exerts its action through the BZ_1 receptor of the $GABA_A$ receptor complex. After oral administration, zolipidem is well absorbed in the GI tract. It is highly protein bond and has a volume of distribution of 0.54 L/kg. Zolpidem is metabolized by the liver to active metabolites. Experience in zolpidem overdose and chronic use is limited. In a review of 344 cases, no life-threatening CNS or respiratory depression could be linked to zolpidem ingestion alone (56). The effects of chronic zolpidem administration are believed to be minimal; however, there has been at least one case report of tolerance and mild withdrawal phenomenon in chronic high doses of zolpidem (57,58).

VI. **Clinical presentation**

A. **Toxicology of acute sedative-hypnotic use.** Despite the numerous agents available, intoxication with sedative-hypnotic agents have clinically similar findings. CNS depression, hypotension, and respiratory depression are the hallmarks of toxicity.

1. **CNS.** The sedative-hypnotics have dose related global CNS depressant effects. Symptoms range from ataxia, dysarthria, and mild somnolence to frank coma, loss of corneal reflexes, and centrally mediated respiratory arrest. Other CNS effects include diminished deep tendon reflexes and temperature instability (59,60). The benzodiazepines are less sedating than the barbiturates and older agents, with coma and respiratory arrest rare in benzodiazepine intoxications except with i.v. use or coingestion (61). The duration of the CNS depression varies with dose and specific agents. Prolonged coma, lasting several days, has been noted in meprobamate (Equanil, Miltown), Glutethimide (Doriden), ethchlorvynol (Placidyl), and barbiturate overdoses. In addition to general CNS depression, several sedative hypnotic agent have toxicities that warrant special mention. Glutethimide can cause psychosis, hyperthermia, and mydriasis owing to its anticholinergic properties (39,62). Methaqualone intoxication can lead to paresthesias, hypertonia, and seizures (44). Bromides may present with rapidly

changing neurologic findings, including dramatic fluctuations in consciousness, motor examination, and reflexes (24).

2. **Respiratory.** In sufficient doses, any of the sedative-hypnotics, with the possible exception of buspirone and zolpidem, can lead to respiratory depression. Thus in the early evaluation of the patient with an acute sedative-hypnotic overdose, it is of highest importance to access the risk of aspiration. In a review of barbiturate related morbidity and mortality, pneumonias were the leading cause of death and disability (63). Noncardiogenic pulmonary edema has been noted in sedative-hypnotic overdoses involving ethchlorvynl and meprobamate (35,40).

3. **Cardiovascular.** The cardiovascular manifestations of acute sedative-hypnotic overdose range from normal heart rate and blood pressure, in most oral benzodiazepine ingestions, to mild tachycardia and hypotension characteristic in barbiturate and older sedative-hypnotic overdoses. The hypotension may be profound in severe overdoses and is believed to be related to venous pooling and/or hypovolemia. Sedative-hypnotics are not primary dysrhythmic agents, with the exception of chloral hydrate, but dysrhythmias and cardiac arrest may be terminal events secondary to shock or respiratory depression.

4. **Gastrointestinal.** In general there are not profound GI effects related to sedative-hypnotic overdoses. Nausea and vomiting have been noted after bromide, methaqualone, and chloral hydrate ingestion. In addition chloral hydrate has been reported to cause GI bleeding, perforation, and esophageal strictures. Glutethimide may decrease bowel motility secondary to its anticholinergic effects. Concreation and bezoar formation may be a concern in massive oral overdoses of sedative-hypnotics. Bezoar formation has been reported in bromide and meprobamate intoxications (60,64).

5. **Renal/hepatic.** Sedative-hypnotic agents are not specific hepatic or renal toxins at therapeutic doses; however, there may be secondary organ failure after profound sedative-hypnotic induced hypotensive episodes. Chloral hydrate has been specifically implicated in renal and hepatic failure in massive doses.

6. **Dermatologic.** One of the most interesting clinical findings in sedative-hypnotic toxicity is the skin manifestations. Barbiturate use has the potential for vesicular and bullous formation on the skin which is termed "Barb burns." The mechanism for these drug eruptions is poorly understood (65). Other agents implicated in bullous skin lesions include glutethimidine, meprobamate, and methaqualone (66). Chronic bromide use also has a characteristic cutaneous manifestation, described as a "acne" like dermatitis known as Bromoderma.

B. **Toxicology of chronic sedative/hypnotic use.** Long term use of most sedative-hypnotic agents can lead to tolerance, psychological craving, and physical dependence. Withdrawal symptoms will occur if the agents are stopped acutely in a physically dependent patient,. The mechanism of withdrawal has not been completely elucidated, but is hypothesized to involve rebound hypersensitivity of the $GABA_A$ receptor system and increased catecholamine synthesis and turnover. Clinically, the patient entering withdrawal will experience agitation, autonomic instability (tachycardia, hypertension, hyperthermia, diaphoresis), and even seizures (67). In severe cases, these symptoms may progress to disorientation, delirium, and hallucinations. The onset of withdrawal symptoms correlates with the half-life of the agents. Withdrawal symptoms may be delayed for up to 3 to 6 days or even longer in agents with long half-lifes, such as the benzodiazepines diazepam or chloradiazepoxide (for a full discussion of withdrawal syndromes, see Chapter 70).

C. **Coingestion of sedative hypnotics.** When sedative-hypnotic agents are used together or with alcohol a profound potentiation of their CNS sedation and an exacerbation of respiratory depression, hypothermia, and hypotension may result.

D. **Differential diagnosis.** Sedative-hypnotic intoxication may appear similar to any clinical entity that presents as decreased mental status. A diligent clinical evaluation, including available history, thorough physical examination, laboratory data, and other diagnostic modalities, will help to determine the cause of the altered state of consciousness. The broad differential includes opioid intoxication, ethanol intoxication, CNS events (bleeds, trauma, malignancies, infections), metabolic abnormalities (hyper/hypoglycemia, hyper/hyponatremia hypercalcemia, uremia), hepatic encephalopathy, or other toxins (heavy metals, carbon monoxide, etc.).

VII. **Laboratory evaluation.** The laboratory evaluation of the sedative-hypnotic patient will depend on the clinical presentation of the patient. There are few specific studies that apply in patients with sedative hypnotic-overdoses. Basic toxicological principles should guide laboratory and diagnostic evaluation of sedative-hypnotic overdoses. Diagnostic measures may include fingerstick glucose determination, electrolytes, ECG, ethanol, and acetaminophen level. In the more acutely ill patient, arterial blood gases may be appropriate to monitor the acid/base and ventilatory status. Sedative-hypnotic levels are not part of the initial management of the patient because of irregular correlation of serum levels and clinical status, and the lack of rapid availability (68). The one exception to this rule is phenobarbital intoxication. Phenobarbital levels can influence clinical decisions making (The use of urinary alkalinization, repeat dosing of activated charcoal, or hemoperfusion). Electrolyte measurement may also help exclude other causes of altered mental status, and in the unusual instance of bromide intoxication will suggest the diagnosis with falsely elevated chlorides concentrations and low or negative anion gap.

VIII. **Management of sedative-hypnotic ingestions.** The management of sedative-hypnotic toxicity is rooted in proper supportive care (69). Differences in the safety margins of sedative-hypnotics are important in developing therapeutic strategies in overdoses. The benzodiazepines and newer agents (zolipidem and buspirone) are generally felt to have high therapeutic to toxic indexes with little more than monitoring and proper fluid management necessary in oral, single agent ingestions. In contrast, barbiturate and other sedative-hypnotic ingestions or coingestions may require aggressive management of respiratory depression, hypotension, and coma.

A. **General emergency management principles**

1. **Airway.** Supportive care should begin with airway management. The patient should be evaluated for signs of respiratory depression and endotracheal intubation accomplished if necessary. Long periods of intubation in the ICU have been required after massive ingestion of barbiturates or older agents.

2. **Hypotension.** Barbiturate and other nonbenzodiazepine sedative hypnotic ingestions may present with profound hypotension. Fluid management is an important

aspect of the management of these patients. The hypotension associated with sedative-hypnotic overdoses should be first treated with normal saline boluses. In refractory hypotension, a pressor agent and central venous or pulmonary artery pressure monitoring may be necessary. Dopamine, norepinephrine, or phenylephrine should be tried initially in hypotension unresponsive to fluids. Extracorporeal support of blood pressure by aortic balloon pump is a therapeutic options in extreme cases of sedative-hypnotic induced hypotension.

3. **Gastric decontamination.** The issue of gastric decontamination should be addressed in all sedative-hypnotic overdoses, and basic decontamination principles apply. Despite decreased gastric motility, and case reports of ileus and small bowel obstruction reported after massive barbiturate overdose, repeated doses of activated charcoal is believed to be beneficial in all sedative hypnotic overdoses and generally recommended (70–73). The patient should be checked frequently for bowel sounds. Initially, the patients should receive 1 g/kg of activated charcoal and cathartic (i.e., sorbital) orally or NG tube followed by repeat dosing of 0.5 to 1 g/kg of charcoal every 4 to 6 h. After initial dosing, repeat cathartic is not required.

4. **CNS depression.** The depressed level of consciousness resulting from sedative-hypnotic toxicity may resemble other CNS events (infectious, trauma, metabolic, vascular, or other toxins). In the deeply obtunded patient, basic laboratories, CT, ABG, and LP are all necessary to exclude other or comorbid disease states while basic supportive care is initiated.

B. **Specific management**
   1. **Benzodiazepines**
      a. Patients who present after oral ingestion of benzodiazepines may be moderately obtunded, but severe respiratory depression and marked hypotension are extremely rare. These patients require little more than monitoring and observation. If a patient presents with the history of benzodiazepine ingestion and has hypotension, respiratory depression, and deep coma; coingestion or other etiologies must be explored to explain the vital signs. The principles outlined in **VIII.A.** should be followed.
      b. **Flumazenil (Romazicon).** Flumazenil is a competitive benzodiazepine receptor antagonist that has been discussed as a possible useful antidote for benzodiazepine toxicity. However, flumazenil has a very limited role in acute benzodiazepine intoxication. The therapeutic utility of flumazenil is limited by unreliable reversal of benzodiazepine respiratory depression, induction of withdrawal syndromes in chronic benzodiazepine users, possible seizures in patients with tricyclic coingestions, and the decreased efficacy of further benzodiazepine administration should they be required in cases of induced seizures or withdrawal (74–76). If a patient has respiratory depression secondary to benzodiazepine use, flumazenil should not be substituted for aggressive airway management and proper supportive care. Furthermore, the duration of flumazenil antagonist effects may be as short as 20 to 30 min—much shorter than most oral benzodiazepines. Patients who receive flumazenil still require further observation for signs of resedation. The primary indi-

cation for flumazenil is in the procedure suite or operating room to reverse i.v. benzodiazepine sedation in patients with no history of chronic benzodiazepine use.

2. **Barbiturates**

   a. In contrast, a patient with a significant barbiturate ingestion is often life-threatening; and the respiratory compromise, hypotension, and CNS depression should be managed aggressively in the manner outlined in **VIII.A.**

   b. **Alkalinization.** In cases of intoxication with the long-acting barbiturate phenobarbital it is possible to enhance elimination by alkalinization the urine based on the relatively low pK_a of the agent ($pK_a \leq 7.2$). At higher urine pHs, more of the phenobarbital will exist in the ionized form and renal tubular reabsorption and tissue penetration will be decreased (77). Patients should be given 1 mEq/kg of sodium bicarbonate bolus i.v., and further boluses if needed. This should be followed with a sodium bicarbonate infusion of approximately 88 mEq of sodium bicarbonate/liter of D_5W to maintain a urine pH of 7.5 to 8.0. If the urine can not be alkalinized with the sodium bicarbonate infusion, a serum potassium concentration should be checked and any hypokalemia corrected. Low serum potassium concentrations will prevent urine alkalinization because the potassium/hydrogen ion exchange in the distal renal tubules will reabsorb potassium at the expense of hydrogen ions, in an attempt to normalize serum potassium levels.

   c. **Hemodialysis and hemoperfusion** have been successfully utilized in barbiturate and certain other sedative-hypnotic overdoses with refractory hypotension and dense coma. Hemodialysis and hemoperfusion have been demonstrated to increase the elimination of barbiturates and other sedative hypnotics (not benzodiazepines), but these techniques have not been demonstrated to definitively decrease morbidity and mortality. Hemodialysis and hemoperfusion should be reserved for extreme cases where prolonged coma are anticipated.

3. **Other sedative-hypnotics**

   a. Most of the older nonbarbiturate, nonbenzodiazepine agents can cause life-threatening CNS depression, hypotension, and respiratory depression; and the management principles outlined in **VIII.A** should be followed. As with barbiturate overdoses, dialysis and hemoperfusion may be options in severe cases of chloral hydrate, meprobamate, glutethimide, bromides, ethchlorvynol, and methaqualone overdoses (78–82).

   b. **Chloral hydrate.** In addition to the CNS depression, hypotension, and respiratory depression associated with most sedative-hypnotic, chloral hydrate intoxication may lead to atrial and ventricular arrhythmias resulting from myocardial irritation and increased sensitization to catecholamines. These dysrhythmias can be fatal and should be carefully treated with beta-adrenergic blocking agents.

   c. **Bromides.** While diuresis has little role in the general management of most agents, it is first-line therapy in bromide toxicity. Bromides are preferentially reabsorbed by the kidney or chloride. Diuresis with normal saline and possibly loop diuretics leads to less bromide reabsorption secondary to the overabundance of chloride ions and the overall decreased reabsorption of halide ions due to adequate volume status.

C. **Treating withdrawal.** Withdrawal has been associated with chronic use of most of the sedative-hypnotics. Initial symptoms of diaphoresis, tachycardia, hypertension, and low grade fever can progress to delirium and hallucinations. These patient must receive supportive care and treatment with a cross tolerant drug. A good first agent in the treatment of withdrawal is diazepam because of rapid onset of action and active metabolites. Butryrophenones (haloperidol) and phenothiazines are not cross tolerant drugs with the GABA system and do not have a role in the treatment of acute sedative-hypnotic withdrawal. It is recommended that the patient be given 10 mg of diazepam i.v. initially; followed by repeat 10-mg doses every 2 to 10 min until the patients symptoms improve and sedation is achieved. Experience has demonstrated the patient in withdrawal may require up to 1 to 2 g of diazepam to relieve withdrawal symptoms. The patient who exhibits refractory signs of acute withdrawal after large doses of diazepam may require the addition of a barbiturate and perhaps endotracheal intubation (for a full discussion of withdrawal states, see Chapter 70).

References

1. Nicholi AM. The nontherapeurtic use of psychoactive drugs: a modern epidemic. *N Engl J Med* 1983;308:925–933.
2. Smith MC, Riskin BJ. The clinical use of barbiturates in neurologic disorders. *Drugs* 1991;42:365–378.
3. Staley K. Enhancement of the excitatory actions of GABA by barbiturates and benzodiazepines. *Neurosci Lett* 1992;146:105–107.
4. Sivilotti L, Nistri A. Gaba receptor mechanisms in the central nervous system. *Prog Neurobiol* 1991;36:35–92.
5. Macdonald R, McLean M. Cellular bases of barbiturate and phenytoin anticonvulsant drug action. *Epilepsia* 1982;231:S7–S18.
6. Shader RI, Greenblatt DJ. The use of benzodiazepines in clinical practice. *Br J Clin Pharm* 1981;11:5S–9S.
7. Greenblatt DJ, Shader RI. Benzodiazopines. *N Engl J Med* 1974;291:1011–1015,1239–1243.
8. Gillen JC, Byerley WF. The diagnosis and management of insomnia. *N Engl J Med* 1990;322:239–248.
9. Bird RD, Makela EH. Alcohol withdrawal: what is the benzodiazepine of choice? *Ann Pharm* 1994;28:67–71.
10. Greenblatt DJ, Shader RI, Abernethy DR. Current status of benzodiazipines. *N Engl J Med* 1983;309:354–358,410–414.
11. Busto UB, et al. Withdrawal reaction after long-term therapeutic use of benzodiazepines. *N Engl J Med* 1986;315:854–859.
12. Miller LG, Greenblatt DJ, Barnhill JG, Shader RI. Chronic benzodiazipine administration. *J Pharm Exp Ther* 1988;246:170–181.
13. Meldrum BS, Chapman AG. Benzodiazepine receptors and their relationship to the treatment of epilepsy. *Epilepsia* 1986;27:S3–S13.
14. Snyder SH. Drug and neurotransmitter receptors: new perspectives with clinical relevance. *JAMA* 261:3126–3129.
15. Sanger DJ, et al. Recent developments in the behavioral pharmacology of benzodiazopine receptors: evidence for functional significance of receptor subtypes. *Neurol Behav Rev* 1994;18:355–372.
16. Benavides, et al. Comparative autoradigraphic distribution of central benzodiazipine modulatory site subtypes with high, intermediate and low affinity for zolpidem and alpidem. *Brain Res* 1993;604:240–250.
17. Twyman RE, Rogers CJ, Macdonald RL. Differential regulation of gamma-aminobutyric acid receptor channels by diazepam and phenobarbital. *Neurol Ann Neurol* 1989;25:213–220.
18. Mestrer M, Carriot T, et al. Electrophysiologic and pharmacolgic characterization of peripheral benzodiazipine receptors in a guinea pig heart preparation. *Life Sci* 1984;35:953–962.
19. Greenblatt DJ, Divoll M, et al. Benzodiazepine hypnotics kinetic and therapeutic options. *Sleep* 1982;5:S18–S27.
20. Anonymous. Midazolam. *Med Lett* 1986;28:73–74.
21. Van Der Kleijn E, Vree TB, et al. Factors influencing the activity and fate of benzodiazepines in the body. *Br J Clin Pharm* 1981;11:85S–98S.

22. Greenblatt DJ, Shad4er RI, Divoll M, Harmatz JS. Benzodiazipines: a summary of pharmacokinetic properties. *Br J Clin Pharm* 1981;11:11S–16S.
23. Blaylock JD. Brominism: a persistent peril. *J Ark Med Soc* 1973;70:130–135.
24. Perkins HA. Bromide intoxication. *Arch Intern Med* 195;85:783–794.
25. Blume RS, MacLowery JD, Wolff SM. Limitations of chloride determination in the diagnosis of bromism. *N Engl J Med* 1968;279:593–595.
26. Miller RR, Greenblatt DJ. Clinical effects of chloral hydrate in hospitalized medical patients. *J Clin Pharm* 1979: 669–674.
27. Salmon AG, Kizer KW, et al. Potential carcinogenicity of chloral hydrate—a review. *Clin Toxicol* 1995;33:115–121.
28. Steinberg AD. Should chloral hydrate be banned? *Pediatrics* 1993;92:442–446.
29. Bowyer K, Glasser SP. Chloral hydrate overdose and cardiac arrhythmias. *Chest* 1980;77:232–235.
30. Graham SR, Fulde GW, Lee R, Day RO. Overdose with chloral hydrate: a pharmacology and therapeutic review. *Med J Aust* 1988;149:686–688.
31. Kelner MJ, Bailey DN. ethchlorvynol ingestion: interpretation of blood concentrations and clinical findings. *Clin Toxicol* 1983–4;21:399–408.
32. Winek CL, Bricker JD, Esposito FM. A death due to ethchlorvynol abuse. A case report. *Forensic Sci Int* 1981;17: 219–224.
33. Skoutakis VA, Acchiardo SR. Ethchlorvynol intoxication. *Clin Toxicol Consult* 1982;4:70–79.
34. Schottstaedt MW, Nicotra MB, Rivera M. Placidyl abuse: a dimorphic picture. *Crit Care Med* 1981;9:677–679.
35. Anonymous. Ethclorvynol. *Clin Toxicol Rev* 1980;2.
36. Bailey DN, Shaw RF. Blood concentrations and clinical findings in nonfatal and fatal intoxications involving glutethimide and codeine. *J Toxicol Clin Toxicol* 1985–6;23:557–570.
37. Feuer E, French J. Descriptive epidemiology of mortality in New Jersey due to combinations of codeine and glutethimidine. *Am J Epidemiol* 1984;119:202–207.
38. Hansen AR, Kennedy KA, et al. Glutethimide poisoning: a metabolite contributes to morbidity and motality. *N Engl J Med* 1975;292:250–252.
39. Curry SC, Hubbard JM, et al. Lack of correlation between plasma 4-hydroxyglutethimide and severity of coma in acute glutethimide poisoning. *Med Toxicol* 1987;2:309–316.
40. Allen MD, Greenblatt DJ, Noel BJ. Meprobamate overdosage: a continuing problem. *Clin Toxicol* 1977;22:501–515.
41. Littrell RA, Hayes LR, Stillner V. Carisprodol (soma): a new and cautious perspective on an old agent. *South Med J* 1993;86:753–756.
42. Lin JL, Lim PS, Lai BC, Lin WL. Continuous arteriovenous hemoperfusion in meprobamate poisoning. *Clin Toxicol* 1993;31:645–652.
43. Jenis EH, Payne RJ, Goldbaum LR. Acute meprobamate poisoning: a fatal case following a lucid interval. *JAMA* 1969; 207:361–362.
44. Inaba DS, Gay GR, et al. Methaqualone abuse—luding out. *JAMA* 1973;224:1505–1509.
45. Pascarelli EF. Methaqualone abuse—the quiet epidemic. *JAMA* 1973;224:1512–1514.
46. Gonzalez ER. Methaqualone abuse implicated in injuries, deaths, nationwide. *JAMA* 1981;246:813–819.
47. Brown SS, Goenechea S. Methaqualone: metabolic, kinetic, and clinical pharmacologic observation. *Clin Pharm Ther* 1973;14:314–324.
48. Morris RN, Gunderson GA, et al. Plasma levels and absorption of methaqualone after oral administration to man. *Clin Pharm Ther* 1972;13:719–723.
49. Cole JO, Orzack MH, et al. Assessment of the abuse liability of buspirone in recreational sedative users. *Clin Psych* 1982;43:69–74.
50. Elison AS, Temple DL. Buspirone: review of its pharmacology and current perspectives on its mechanisms of action. *Am J Med* 1986;80:1–9.
51. Tunnicliff G. Molecular basis of buspirone's anxiolytic action. *Pharm Toxicol* 1991;69:149–156.
52. Chignon JM, Lepine JP. Panic and hypertension associated with single dose of buspirone [Letter]. *Lancet* 1989;2:46–47.
53. Norman TR, Judd FK. Panic attacks, buspirone, and serotonin function [Letter]. *Lancet* 1989;2:615.
54. Pols HL, Griez E, Zandbergen J. Does buspirone have anxiogenic properties [Letter]. *Lancet* 1989;2:682–683.
55. Anonymous. Buspirone: a non-benzodiazepine for anxiety. *Med Lett* 1986;28:117–118.
56. Garnier R, Guerault E, et al. Acute zolpidem poisoning: analysis of 344 cases. *Clin Toxicol* 1994;32:391–404.
57. Cavallaro R, Regazzetti MG, Covelli G, Seraldi E. Tolerance and withdrawal with zolpidem [Letter]. *Lancet* 1993;342: 374–375.
58. Gericke C, Ludolph AC. Chronic abuse of zolpidem. *JAMA* 1994;272:1721–1722.
59. Shubin H, Weil MH. Shock associated with barbiturate intoxication. *JAMA* 1971;215:263–268.
60. Setter JG, Maher JF, Schreiner GE. Barbiturate intoxication. *Arch Intern Med* 1966;117:224–236.
61. Katz RL. Sedatives and tranquilizers. *N Engl J Med* 1972;286:757–760.

62. Haddah LM, Winchester JF. *Clinical management of poisoning and drug overdoses*. Philadelphia, 1983.
63. Goodman JM, Bishel MD, Wagers PW, Barbour BH. Barbiturate intoxication: morbitity and mortality. *West J Med* 1976;124:179–186.
64. Iberti TJ, Patterson BK, Fisher CJ. Prolonged bromide intoxication resulting from a gastric bezoar. *Arch Intern Med* 1984;144:402–403.
65. Groschel D, Gerstein AR, Rosenbaum JM. Skin lesions as a diagnostic aid in barbiturate poisoning. *N Engl J Med* 1970; 283:409–410.
66. Slazinski L, Knox DW. Fixed drug eruption due to methaqualone. *Arch Dermatol* 1984;120:1073–1075.
67. Faught E. Methaqualone withdrawal syndrome with photoparoxysmal responses and high amplitude visual evoked potentials. *Neurology* 1986;36:1127–1129.
68. McCarron MM, Schulze BW, et al. Short-acting barbiturate overdoses: correlation of intoxication score with barbiturate concentration. *JAMA* 1982;248:55–61.
69. Skoutakis VA, Acchiardo SR. Toxicologic emergencies:management of nonbarbiturate intoxications. *Clin Toxicol Consult* 1981;3:1–22.
70. Goldberg MJ, Berlinger WG. Treatment of phenobarbital overdoses with activated charcoal. *JAMA* 1982;247: 2400–2401.
71. Pond SM, Olson KR, et al. Randomized study of the treatment of phenobarbital overdoses with repeated doses of activated charcoal. *JAMA* 1984;251:3104–3108.
72. Berg MJ, Berlinger WG, et al. Acceleration of the body clearance of phenobarbital by oral activated charcoal. *N Engl J Med* 1982;307:642–644.
73. Atkinson SW, Young Y, Trotter GA. Treatment with activated charcoal complicated by gastrointestinal obstruction requiring surgery. *BMJ (British Medical Journal)* 1992;305:563.
74. Hoffman RS, Goldfrank LR. The poisoned patient with altered consciousness, controversies in the use of a coma cocktail. *JAMA* 1995;562–569, Vol. 274.
75. Spivey WH. Flumazenil and seizures: analysis of 43 cases. *Clin Ther* 1992;14:292–305.
76. Polland BJ, Masters AP, Bunting P. The use of flumazenil (Anexate, Ro 15-1788) in the management of drug overdoses. *Anesthesiology* 1989;44:137–138.
77. Henderson LW, Merril JP. Treatment of barbiturate intoxication. *Ann Intern Med* 1966;44:876–891.
78. Vaziri ND, Kumar KP, et al. Hemodialysis in treatment of acute chloral hydrate poisoning. *S Med J* 1977;70:377–378.
79. Buur T, Larsson R, Norlander B. Pharmacokinetics of chloral hydrate poisoning treated with hemodialysis and hemoperfusion. *Acta Med Scand* 1988;223:269–274.
80. Lynn RI, Honig CL, et al. Resin hemoperfusion for treatment of ethchlorvynol overdose. *Ann Intern Med* 1979;91: 549–553.
81. Benowitz N, Abolin C, et al. Resin hemoperfusion in ethchlorvynol overdose. *Clin Pharmacol Ther* 198;27:236–242.
82. Baggish D, Gray S, et al. Treatment of methaqualone overdose with resin hemoperfusion. *Yale J Biol Med* 1981;54: 147–150.

Emergency Toxicology, Second Edition,
edited by Peter Viccellio.
Lippincott–Raven Publishers, Philadelphia © 1998.

61

Hallucinogens

Lewis S. Nelson

*Department of Emergency Services, New York University, Bellevue Hospital, New York,
New York 10016*

I. **Introduction.** The term "hallucinogen," although in many cases a misnomer, has received widespread use to describe an agent that alters one's interpretation of the environment. A true hallucination is a false sensory experience that arises de novo, without prompting from the external environment. However, most drugs used with the intent of inducing hallucinations are, in fact, illusionogenic. An illusion is a misinterpretation of normal sensory input, that is, prompted by the external environment. Since most hallucinogens result in multiple perceptual alterations, other more comprehensive descriptive terms have been suggested, including phantasticants, psychedelics, mind expanding drugs, entactogens, and psychotomimetics.

II. **Clinical effects.** Although the pharmacology of each agent may differ, the hallucinogenic effects produced by all of the drugs are remarkably similar; this has been termed the psychedelic syndrome. Sensory perception and thought processes are grossly distorted, and mood is altered. Reality (space, time, bodily dimension) is distorted and a feeling of depersonalization makes the patient feel separated from the situation. Consciousness is maintained and the sensorium is clear; the patient can be brought back to reality, at least temporarily, and should be capable of interaction with the caregiver until redistracted by thought content. Although hallucinations may be tactile, auditory, gustatory or olfactory, the majority of drug-induced hallucinations are visual in nature. Occasionally, blending of sensory modalities (synesthesia) may be observed. Profound philosophical thoughts, deep introspection, self-examination, or religious overtones may be prominent components of the psychedelic experience. Often the hallucinations take the form of gross somatic distortions, and at times these may be deeply disturbing. The setting accompanying the drug use has a dramatic effect on the content of the psychedelic experience. Used in the wrong context, or unknowingly administered, the resulting hallucinations may be psychologically damaging. Common clinical effects include mydriasis, tachycardia, hypertension, and tremor. These effects are shared by both anticholinergic and sympathomimetic agents. The majority of the commonly used recreational psychedelic agents induce mild sympathomimetic findings in their users. Although anticholinergic agents are now infrequently used as recreational psychedelics, such patients often present with a pronounced anticholinergic toxidrome.

III. **Hallucinogenic substances: historical perspectives and modern epidemiology.** The history of hallucinogenic substances parallels the history of native cultures. Although modern civilization has aggressively sought stimulant-type mind altering substances (largely caffeine, nicotine and cocaine), it was not until the later half of the twentieth century that psychedelic substances captured public attention. Most hallucinogenic substances utilized before the 1950s were obtained in their native form (i.e. from plants) and many still are (Table 61-1). Modern psychedelic drugs were widely used in the counterculture of the 1960s, but fell out of favor until their recent resurrection in 1989. From 1988 to 1992, the percentage of high school seniors that had used LSD in the past year rose from 4.8% to 5.6% (1). This coincided with a decrease in cocaine use of 7.9% to 3.1% over the same time period. By 1993, approximately 8.7% of all Americans had used a hallucinogen in their lifetime, with 7.0% using LSD (2). Among the longest used psychedelic substances are mushrooms. Soma, a psychoactive plant alluded to in the Rig-Veda of ancient India (about 1500 B.C.), was probably derived from *Amanita muscaria* (3). This mushroom, also known as fly agaric, is now known to contain ibotenic acid, a glutamate agonist, and muscimol, a GABA agonist. It has been speculated that the same mushroom was responsible for the altered sensory perceptions experienced by Alice in *Through the Looking Glass* (4). This mushroom has no modern psychedelic use in North America. Teonanacatl, a mushroom used for thousands of years in shamanic rituals in Mexican Indian culture, is a pscilocin containing *Psilocybe mexicana* (5). This mushroom genus provides the magic mushrooms which are recreationally consumed in modern North American society (*P. cubensis, P. semilancinanta*). Use of plants containing anticholinergic substances have historical associations dating back to Bacchanalian festivals in ancient Greece. Anticholinergic plants, (*Atropa belladona, Hyoscyamus niger,* and *Mandragora officinarum*) which contain tropane alkaloids such as scopolamine, have also been linked with witchcraft during the middle ages (6). The broomstick may have been used as an applicator; the alkaloids are well absorbed through the mucous membranes of the genitalia

TABLE 61-1. *Some "Old World" hallucinogens (all are plants unless otherwise noted)*

Hallucinogen	Source	Primary constituent	Region of origin
Ayahuasca, yajé, caapi	*Banisteriopsis caapi*	Harmine, harmaline	South America
Syrian Rue	*Peganum harmala*	Harmine, harmaline	Middle East
Bicho de tacuara (bamboo worm)	*Myelobia smerintha* (moth larvae)	—	South America
Cohoba	*Piptadenia (Anadenanthera) peregrina*	DMT, bufotenine	South America
Yopo	*Piptadenia (Anadenanthera) peregrina*	DMT, bufotenine	West Indies
Colorado River Toad	*Bufo alvarius* (toad)	Bufotenine	South America
Hawaiian Baby Wood Rose	*Argyreia nervosa, Ipomoea tuberosa*	Lysergic acid amide	Mexico
Tlitliltzen	*Ipomoea violacea*	Lysergic acid amide	Mexico and South America
Ololiuqui	*Rivea corynbosa*	Lysergic acid amide	Mexico and South America
Hierba de la Virgen (Herb of the Virgin)	*Salvia divinorum*	Salvinorin A	Oaxaca (Mexico)
Iboga	*Tabernanthe iboga*	Ibogaine	Africa
Mescal bean	*Sophora secundiflora*	Cytisine	Mexico
Teonanacatl ("Gods Flesh")	*Psilocybe mexicana*	Psilocin, psilocybin	Central America

DMT, dimethyltryptamine.
Data from refs. 5, 6, and 34.

resulting in hallucinations of flight. Jimson weed (*Datura stramonium*) was responsible for the colonists' victory over the British army in Virginia, when it was inadvertently used by the British soldiers to prepare their meal (6). The resulting hallucinations lasted for over a week. The current recreational use of anticholinergic substances is limited to teenagers who forage for Jimson weed seeking an inexpensive high (7). In addition, unsuspecting i.v. drug users have been sold scopolamine-tainted heroin under the pretense of longer lasting effects (8). Mescaline, found in the peyote cactus (*Lophophora williamsii*), is a naturally occurring amphetamine-like substance. The ritualistic use of the peyote cactus seems rooted in Aztec culture in pre-Columbian Mexico. Peyote was introduced into the southwestern United States in the late nineteenth century. The Native American Church has, in recent times, been granted the right to utilize peyote in their religious services in the United States. Aldous Huxley described his experiences with mescaline in his book *The Doors of Perception* (9). Other naturally occurring structural relatives of amphetamine include myristin and elemicin from nutmeg (*Myristicin fragrans*) and metcathinone (Khat) from *Catha edulis*. Only recently have the synthetic amphetamine derivatives come into vogue. The relative ease by which small functional groups can be added to the basic phenylethylamine structure has accounted for the proliferation of designer drugs. These newly synthesized agents were created to provide enhanced psychoactive effects and, until recently, were able to subvert the law. This changed with the introduction of the Controlled Substance Analog Enforcement Act of 1986 (10), which outlawed designer drugs (Table 61-2). Most of these drugs are made by amateur chemists in clandestine drug laboratories, often in home basements, using chemicals available on the open market. In fact, recipes for constructing designer drugs are available by mail-order and on the internet. MDMA, also known as ecstasy, XTC, or Adam, is a particularly prevalent variety of designer amphetamine in the United States. Although used in the early 1980s as a psychotherapeutic adjunct (11), this drug has achieved its greatest notoriety through illicit use at dance clubs. Individuals attending these parties, called raves, participate in night-long dance sessions, with inadequate fluid intake, often resulting in dehydration and

TABLE 61-2. *Classification of psychedelic substances*

Anticholinergic psychedelics
   Scopolamine (Jimson weed, *Datura stramonium*)
Catecholaminergic psychedelics
   Mescaline (peyote, *Lophophora williamsii*)
   Amphetamine derivatives (MDMA, DOM/STP, MDA, DMA, etc.)
   Myristin, elemicin (nutmeg, *Myristica fragrans*)
Serotonergic psychedelics
   Lysergic acid (Hawaiian baby woodrose, morning glory)
   Lysergic acid diethylamide (*Claviceps purpura*)
   Dimethyltryptamine derivatives
     Bufotenin
     Psilocybin, psilocin (Psilocybe, Panaeolus, Conocybe mushrooms)
Anesthetic psychedelics
   Phencyclidine
   Ketamine
Essential oil pyschedelics
   Tetrahydrocannabinol (Cannabis, marijuana, hashish)

occasionally death (12). The beginning of the modern era of hallucinogenic substance use occurred in 1943 when Albert Hofmann, a Swiss chemist, accidentally ingested a compound which he had synthesized five years earlier during his search for a safe analeptic agent (13). Human investigation of this compound, lysergic acid diethylamide (known as LSD-25), as a model for mental illness began shortly afterward. The drug quickly received attention on college campuses and, with the help of proponents like Dr. Timothy Leary and The Grateful Dead, became a symbol for an entire generation. It is most commonly available now as perforated sheets of paper impregnated with the drug, which are easily torn into unit doses, known as blotter acid. Hofmann synthesized LSD from the alkaloid lysergic acid which had been extracted from the rye fungus *Claviceps purpurea* (ergot). Lysergic acid is a naturally occurring hallucinogen, although only one-tenth as potent as LSD. Ergot tainted bread has been suspect in the epidemics of witchcraft in colonial Salem, Massachusetts (14). Other naturally occurring analogues of LSD have been isolated from many plants used historically as hallucinogens (Table 61-1), as well as from secretions of the Colorado River toad (*Bufo alvarius*). Several of the plants originally used by aboriginal cultures are still utilized today for recreational purposes. During the 1960s several studies utilized hallucinogenic substances (LSD, DMT) as aids to psychotherapy for depressed and sociopathic patients (15). These studies suffered basic design flaws that have limited the applicability of their results. As alluded to earlier, MDMA has been used to enhance the therapeutic relationship (16). Although early studies failed to show a benefit of hallucinogenic agents in combating chronic substance abuse, renewed investigations using ibogaine have yielded potentially promising results (15).

IV. **Classification of hallucinogens.** Classification of hallucinogenic agents is most clinically useful when based on structural homology to the endogenous neurotransmitters that appear to be involved in the production of hallucinations (Table 61-3). Categorization in this manner allows prediction of expected clinical characteristics and potential complications without actually knowing the specific agent used by the patient. Three classes are apparent: acetylcholine-like (anticholinergic), catecholamine-like (catecholaminergic) and serotonin-like (serotonergic). Other classification schemes exist (15) based on pharmacokinetic and pharmacodynamic properties. Anticholinergic agents produce hallucinations by competitive antagonism of acetylcholine at the muscarinic cholinergic receptors. It is unclear precisely why this produces hallucinations. The initial effect of anticholinergic agents is more appropriately termed a toxic delirium, since confusion and lethargy are prominent. This is associated with the many other signs and symptoms which comprise the anticholinergic toxidrome (see appropriate sections). Scopolamine, a prominent alkaloid found in *Datura stramonium* (Jimson weed), has more potent central nervous system effects than atropine, an effect related to its

TABLE 61-3. *Pharmacologic and clinical parameters of some hallucinogenic agents*

Agent	Typical dose	Time to onset (min)	Clinical duration (h)	Toxidrome expected
DMT	1 mg/kg	3–5	1	Mild sympathetic
Psilocybin	20 mg	30–60	6	Mild sympathetic
MDMA	50–100 mg	30	6	Profound sympathetic
Mescaline	5 mg/kg	30–60	10	Moderate sympathetic
LSD	50–100 μg	30	10–12	Mild sympathetic
Scopolamine	2–5 mg	60	24–72	Anticholinergic

higher blood-brain barrier permeability. As the peripheral anticholinergic effects wane, a more pure hallucinatory condition often remains; this has been termed the central anticholinergic syndrome. At this stage the diagnosis of anticholinergic intoxication may be impossible without a reliable history of exposure. It is interesting that atropine and scopolamine are structural analogues of cocaine, yet their receptor specificity, and clinical effects, are markedly different. The serotonergic system is essential in the production of psychedelic effects. Hallucinogenic agents of the indolealkylamine group share structural similarity with serotonin. These substances, including LSD and tryptamine derivatives (psilocin, bufotenine), induce hallucinations through partial agonist effects at the 5-HT$_2$ receptor subtype (17). Their relative affinity for the 5-HT$_2$ receptor is correlated with their hallucinogenic potency (18). Agents capable of blocking the 5-HT$_2$ receptor, such as risperidone and ritanserin, have been able to prevent the expected behavioral changes in animals (19). The neuroanatomical basis for hallucinations and the precise inter-relationship of other serotonin receptor subtypes and the catecholaminergic system remains elusive. Catecholaminergic agents produce a clinical syndrome resembling cocaine or amphetamine due to elevation of the synaptic concentrations of norepinephrine and dopamine. Expected findings include tachycardia, diaphoresis, and mydriasis. However, these agents differ from cocaine and amphetamine by producing hallucinations and other perceptual changes at conventional doses. This group contains many structurally related compounds, each differing from amphetamine (and the endogenous neurotransmitters) by one or several methyl, hydroxy, or methoxy moieties. This structural alteration increases their affinity for 5-HT$_2$ receptors, where these agents function as partial agonists (18,20). As with the indolamines, the potency of these agents is correlated with their binding affinity to these receptors (21). This appears to account for the psychedelic properties of this group. In addition, the enhanced lipophilicity of these agents may enhance the psychedelic effects by permitting penetration into brain regions previously untapped by amphetamine and cocaine.

V. **Differential diagnosis.** In the absence of a clear history of drug use, altered mental status and hallucinations should be initially assumed to be due to another etiology. Hypoglycemia and hypoxia are common, and can be empirically treated or easily excluded with simple laboratory tests. Meningitis, encephalitis or temporal lobe seizures are CNS etiologies of hallucinations. Metabolic etiologies include thyrotoxicosis and Cushings syndrome, as well as hyponatremia and other electrolyte abnormalities. Other drug intoxications may result in hallucinations or similar behavior. Phencyclidine, a dissociative anesthetic, is often sold in forms mimicking blotter acid (LSD) or magic mushrooms (psilocybin). Both acute intoxication with ethanol and ethanol withdrawal (hallucinosis or delirium tremens) are associated with hallucinations. Therapeutic misadventures or intentional misuse of either over-the-counter (OTC) cold or sleeping preparations, may produce typical anticholinergic symptoms. Psychiatric illness often presents with auditory or visual hallucinations. In the absence of a compatible history, patients should have other etiologies evaluated before psychiatric consultation.

VI. **Complications.** The most prevalent complication of hallucinogen use is dysphoria ("bad trip"), occasionally presenting as a panic reaction. This is most commonly attributed to a poor choice of set and setting for drug use. While experienced users may develop bad trips, individuals surreptitiously administered hallucinogenic agents may be at highest risk. Given their high prevalence of use, the hallucinogens as a group are directly responsible for few deaths (22). Although massive LSD overdose has been associated with coma (23), this is a distinctly uncommon event. Overindulgence with amphetamine-like psychedelics may produce toxicity similar to amphetamines or cocaine, including myocardial infarction, cerebrovascular accidents, or rhabdomyolysis. Although prolonged administration of MDMA to rats has resulted in destruction of serotonin neurons (24,25) it is unclear if human neurons are susceptible. Indirect "toxic" effects are responsible for the majority of complications associated with hallucinogenic drugs. As discussed earlier, hyperthermia and dehydration are clearly associated with the use of hallucinogenic amphetamines at rave parties (12). These indirect complications are largely preventable by ambient cooling and sufficient fluid intake. Accidents and suicide appear to be more common during a bad trip (26), and other risky activities (e.g., sun gazing or attempting to fly) are more likely during drug use. Twenty percent of drug-using adolescents reported that they or a friend were involved in an LSD related trauma (26). Patients using certain hallucinogens, particularly the amphetamine derivatives, in combination with other serotonergic agents are at risk for developing the "serotonin syndrome" (27,28). Patients with this syndrome, in which excess intrasynaptic serotonin produces hyperstimulation of the post-synaptic neuron, present with muscle rigidity, hyperthermia, and altered mental status. Unless rapidly cooled and the rigidity alleviated, rhabdomyolysis and death may occur (28). Potential drug interactions resulting in this syndrome include monoamine oxidase inhibitors (several of which are amphetamine derivatives), selective serotonin reuptake inhibitors, tricyclic antidepressants, and L-tryptophan. Acute psychotic reactions may occur when the perceptual experience overwhelms the individuals ability to cope. Exacerbation of an underlying psychosis may also result. Several chronic complications are well described. Hallucinogen persisting perceptual disorder (HPPD), previously known as "flashbacks", is characterized by intermittent, spontaneous, self-limited recurrences of the drug effect (29). The mechanism is unclear, but they may recur for months after the last drug use. In general, flashbacks interfere very little with normal functioning of an individual (30).

VII. **Treatment.** Patients experiencing a dysphoric reaction should receive an explanation of the nature of the hallucinations and assurance of their limited duration (31). However, prolonged "psychotherapy" in the Emergency Department is not practical. In patients not rapidly responding to "talking down," chemical amelioration of threatening hallucinations is indicated. The treatment of choice is a benzodiazepine such as diazepam, 10 to 20 mg po, or 5 to 10 mg i.v., with repetitive dosing as needed. The goal is pacification of the hallucinations, not necessarily complete sedation. It is important to entertain phencyclidine intoxication early in the course of hospital evaluation as the treatment differs markedly. PCP intoxicated patients cannot be expected to respond to rationalization of the psychedelic experience. Without aggressive sedation and restraint, phencyclidine intoxicated patients may injure themselves or their caretakers. Experimentally, risperidone may be effective in blocking the hallucinogenic effects of LSD (19). It is unknown if risperidone is effective in stopping hallucination if given after psychedelic use. Additionally, it is not known if the same effects will be produced in humans. However, no controlled human study has ever been performed. In the past, various neuroleptic agents have been recommended to break the hallucinations. Although most patients are sedated, success in stopping the hallucinations has never been documented. In addition, there may be an increased incidence of HPPD in patients receiving neuroleptic agents (32). In cases of documented anticholinergic drug ingestion resulting in significantly altered mental status or hallucinations, cautious use of the cholinesterase inhibitor physostigmine may be indicated. The return of a delirious patient to their normal baseline mental status may confirm the diagnosis and obviate a prolonged search for other etiologies. In addition, although the patients usually relapse, allowing family members to see the patient while well may allay their concerns. Finally, the psychological effects of prolonged anticholinergic delirium are unknown. Contraindications to use of physostigmine include tricyclic antidepressant overdose, which may produce an anticholinergic toxidrome, and reversible airway disease. If given slowly, over 5 min, an initial dose of 1 mg should produce cholinergic symptoms in patients not intoxicated by an anticholinergic substance. No response to an initial dose is an indication to administer slowly escalating doses until the patient clears or develops cholinergic symptoms. Administration of activated charcoal is generally unnecessary in recreational users. In those with large overdoses or unclear etiologies administration by mouth or via nasogastric tube is recommended unless contraindicated for other reasons. Orogastric lavage or syrup of ipecac administration is not likely to be beneficial. Disposition of most casual psychedelic drug users to the care of a responsible adult is typical. Hospitalization is indicated for patients with unclear diagnoses, persistent hallucinations, or inadequate caretakers. In addtion, patients with signs of hyperthermia or rhabdomyolysis may require hospital admission. Chronic abusers, especially of the amphetamine derivatives, may need acute hospitalization for depression or concomitant medical problems. Those with acute psychotic reactions will need acute psychiatric intervention.

VIII. Laboratory evaluation. All of the hallucinogenic agents described can be identified in the urine if specifically requested, but routine assessment is expensive and not clinically useful. If desired for documentation in children or forensic cases, discussion with the hospital laboratory or the police is suggested. Although no rapid screen is available for LSD, it can be accurately detected and quantitated by GC/MS (33). However, most in-house toxicology laboratories are not equipped to detect these drugs. A rapid amphetamine screen is widely available for use by emergency departments or in-house laboratories. The cross-sensitivity of these screens for amphetamine derivatives is variable and unreliable. Sophisticated forensic and reference laboratories can adequately detect the substances.

References

 1. National Institute of Drug Abuse. *National survey on drug use: monitoring the future study, 1975–1992: National High School Senior Survey.* NIH publication no. 93-3597. Rockville, MD: NIH, 1993.
 2. NHSDA. *Preliminary estimates from the 1994 National Household Survey on Drug Abuse.* Advance report no. 10. Bethesda, MD: U.S. Department of Health and Human Services, Public Health Service, 1995.
 3. Wasson RG. *Soma: The divine mushroom of immortality.* New York: Harcourt Brace Jovanovich, 1971.
 4. Carroll L. *Through the looking glass.* Kingsport, TN: Grosset and Dunlap, 1946.
 5. Schultes RE, Hofmann A. *Plants of the gods.* Rochester, VT: Healing Arts Press, 1992.
 6. Lewis WH, Elvin-Lewis MPF. *Medical botany.* New York: John Wiley & Sons, 1977.
 7. Perrotta DM, Nickey LN, Raid M, et. al. Jimson weed poisoning—Texas, New York, and California, 1994. *MMWR* 1995;44:41–44.
 8. Hamilton R, Perrone J, Meggs WJ, et al. Epidemic anticholinergic poisoning from scopolamine tainted heroin [Abstract]. *J Toxicol Clin Toxicol* 1995;33:502.
 9. Huxley A. *The doors of perception.* New York: Harper & Row, 1954.
10. Anon. Public Law no. 99–570, 21 USC 813.
11. Grinspoon L, Bakalar JB. Can drugs be used to enhance the psychotherapeutic process? *Am J Psychother* 1986;40: 393–403.
12. Henry JA. Ecstasy and the dance of death. *BMJ* 1992;305:5–6.

13. Hofmann A. *LSD: my problem child.* New York: McGraw-Hill, 1980.
14. Caporael LR. Ergotism: the Satan loosed in Salem? *Science* 1976;192:21–26.
15. Strassman RJ. Hallucinogenic drugs in psychiatric research and treatment. *J Nerv Ment Dis* 1995;183:127–138.
16. Riedlinger TJ, Riedlinger JE. Psychedelic and entactogenic drugs in the treatment of depression. *J Psychoactive Drugs* 1994;26:41–55.
17. Glennon RA. Do classical hallucinogens act as 5-HT$_2$ agonists or antagonists? *Neuropsychopharmacology* 1990;3: 509–517.
18. Titeler M, Lyon RA, Glennon RA. Radioligand binding evidence implicates the brain 5-HT$_2$ receptor as a site of action for LSD and phenylisopropylamine hallucinogens. *Psychopharmacology* 1988;94:213–216.
19. Meert TF, de Haes P, Janssen PAJ. Risperidone (R 64 766), a potent and complete LSD antagonist in drug discrimination by rats. *Psychopharmacology* 1989;97:206–212.
20. Glennon RA, Teitler M, Sanders-Bush E. Hallucinogens and serotonergic mechanisms. *NIDA Res Monogr* 1992;119: 131–135.
21. Sadzot B, Baraban JM, Glennon RA, et al. Hallucinogenic drug interactions at human brain 5-HT$_2$ receptors: implications for treating LSD-induced hallucinations. *Psychopharmacology* 1989;98:495–499.
22. Gable RS. Toward a comparative overview of dependence potential and acute toxicity of psychoactive substances used nonmedically. *Am J Drug Alcohol Abuse* 1993;19:263–281.
23. Klock JC, Boerner U, Becker CE. Coma, hyperthermia, and bleeding associated with massive LSD overdose: a report of eight cases. *West J Med* 1974;120:183–188.
24. Ricuarte G, Bryan G, Strauss L, Seiden L, Schuster C. Hallucinogenic amphetamine selectively destroys brain serotonin nerve terminals. *Science* 1985;225:986–988.
25. Battaglia G, Yeh SY, O'Hearn E, et al. 3,4-Methylenedioxymethamphetamine and 3,4-methylenedioxyamphetamine destroy serotonin terminals in rat brain: quantification of neurodegeneration by measurement of [^{3}H]-paroxetine-labelled serotonin uptake sites. *J Pharmacol Exp Ther* 1987;242:911–916.
26. Schwartz RH, Coomerci GD, Meeks JE. LSD: patterns of use by chemically dependent adolescents. *J Pediatr* 1987; 111:936–938.
27. Sporer KA. The serotonin syndrome: implicated drugs, pathophysiology and management. *Drug Safety* 1995;13:94–104.
28. Smilkstein MJ, Smolinske SC, Rumack BH. A case of MAO inhibitor/MDMA interaction: agony after ecstasy. *Clin Toxicol* 1987;25:149–159.
29. American Psychiatric Association. *Diagnostic and statistical manual of mental disorders.* 4th ed. Washington, DC: APA, 1994.
30. Wesson DR, Smith DE. An analysis of psychedelic drug flashbacks. *Am J Drug Alcohol Abuse* 1976;3:425–438.
31. Taylor RL, Maurer JI, Tinklenberg JR. Management of bad trips in an evolving drug scene. *JAMA* 1970;213:422–425.
32. Abraham HD, Aldridge AM. Adverse consequences of lysergic acid diethylamide. *Addiction* 1993;88:1327–1334.
33. Nelson CC, Foltz RL. Chromatographic and mass spectrometric methods for determination of lysergic acid diethylamide (LSD) and metabolites in body fluids. *J Chromatogr* 1992;580:97–109.
34. Weil A, Rosen W. *From chocolate to morphine: everything you need to know about mind-altering drugs.* Boston: Houghton Mifflin Co, 1993.

Emergency Toxicology, Second Edition,
edited by Peter Viccellio.
Lippincott–Raven Publishers, Philadelphia © 1998.

62

Phencyclidine

†Rama B. Rao and °Robert S. Hoffman

*†New York City Poison Control Center, Department of Emergency Medicine, New York
University Medical Center, Bellevue Hospital, New York, New York 10016;
°Department of Surgery and Emergency Medicine, New York University School of Medicine,
New York, New York 10016*

I. **Introduction.** Phencyclidine, or PCP as it is commonly known, is an illicit drug of abuse that was originally used as a dissociative anesthetic agent because it induced anesthesia without producing respiratory or cardiac depression (1–5). It was abandoned for human medical uses in the early 1960s as its use was fraught with emergence reactions and agitation (1–9). Its precursors were easy to obtain, however, and soon PCP was being illegally synthesized in clandestine laboratories (7,10–13). PCP is distributed on the streets in a variety of forms for abuse. It is sold as pills, sprinkled into dried leaves and smoked, liquified and ingested or used as a dip for tobacco cigarettes or marijuana, snorted, used intravenously, or, rarely, used as an i.m. injection (11–19). PCP is also known as angel dust, hog, crystal joints, greens, animal tranquilizer, kay jay, peace pill, rocket fuel, shermans, supercools, and several other street names (12,20–23). Because the production and sale of the drug is relatively simple and profitable, it has been used to adulterate other illicit substances sold as THC, cocaine, mescaline, psilocybin, and LSD, which are replaced in part, or entirely by PCP itself (14,18,24). Since these manufacturing processes are not regulated or standardized, purities and contaminants may vary, and dosages are rarely known by the drug's user. This in turn has led to a paucity of well-controlled studies regarding its clinical effects and management of its toxicity.

II. **Sources.** As mentioned above, illicit manufacture of phencyclidine and its subsequent distribution as a drug of abuse, or to adulterate other drugs of abuse are currently the only sources of this drug.

III. **Pharmacology.** The mechanism of action of PCP is poorly understood. It is a dissociative anesthetic like its derivative ketamine, and demonstrates pharmacological activity (see clinical affects below) at doses of 0.25 mg/kg in the i.v. route (1,3–6). Subjective changes in sensorium reportedly occur with as little as 0.07 mg/kg (3,5). Doses of 0.5 mg/kg cause agitation, and doses near or above 1.0 mg/kg cause frank seizures (1). Phencyclidine is a weak base with a $pK_a = 8.5$, and a volume of distribution of about 6.2 L/kg (25–27). It is soluble in water or ethanol as a hydrochloride salt and has a melting point 234° to 235° (5). Purities of PCP in seized samples range from 10% to nearly 100% pure depending on the form of the substance (14).

A. **Absorption.** Absorption can occur via inhalation, oral, i.v., intranasal, or i.m. routes, and onset of action varies with route (1,2,25,26). The onset of effect of inhaled PCP is from 2 to 5 min, and peak plasma concentrations occur within 5 to 30 min (11,26). There is evidence of a second peak effect with this route, probably due to tissue redistribution

(26,27). However, there is no established correlation of plasma concentration and clinical effect (11,26,27). Effects last between 2 to 6 h with an irregular sensation occurring up to 24 h (1–3,5,11,18). With oral dosing, the onset of action occurs within 15 to 30 min and plasma levels peak at 2.5 h. A similar duration of action has been reported (11,25). The onset of action with intravenous or intranasal use approximates that seen with inhalation. Bioavailability varies with route of ingestion. When given in a trial of subclinical doses oral PCP was estimated to have a mean bioavailability of 72%, which may be significantly lower than when smoked (25). Development of tolerance has not been studied, but it is suggested by animal studies and subjective reports from chronic PCP abusers (18,28).

B. Distribution. Phencyclidine has a volume of distribution of 6.2L/kg. It has been found in the CNS, adipose tissue, perspiration, saliva, placenta, and in animal studies, breast milk (25,26,30–36). PCP is highly protein bound (29).

C. Metabolism. A "first-pass" effect in oral dosing has been suggested, but not well studied (37). Metabolism occurs primarily via hydroxylation in the liver with subsequent urinary excretion. A small percentage is excreted unchanged in the urine, and is pH dependent (25–27). Because PCP is a weak base, it is subject to the effects of "ion-trapping" in an acid milieu. Thus, regardless of the route of administration, PCP may be present in gastric secretions and available for recirculation (25,26,38). Metabolites are poorly studied and are of little clinical effect (21,25,26,37,39). A contaminant generated by manufacture may include PCC, whose labile cyano group can decompose to hydrogen cyanide. Some of the infrequent gastrointestinal (GI) effects have been attributed to this compound (13,40,41).

D. Elimination. Elimination follows first order kinetics even at extremely high doses (42). A half life of between 7 and 46 h has been reported. Metabolism is the primary method of clearance. Renal clearance of unchanged PCP represents approximately 9% of total clearance, and minimal amounts are excreted via the GI tract (25,26). A low urine pH increases the amount of PCP excreted in the urine (34,43). This however, does not necessarily correlate with clinical improvement, or changes in plasma concentration. PCP can usually remain in the urine for 2 to 3 weeks, but up to 4 weeks has been reported (44,45).

E. Drug interactions. When it was used clinically for anesthesia, PCP was given safely with atropine, scopolamine, meperidine, morphine, succinyldicholine, D-tubocurarine, barbiturates, and nitrous oxide (1,2,6). The effects of these drugs on PCP activity or metabolism were not specifically studied, but they did not seem to alter the course of PCP effects. Haloperidol has been studied in a double-blind, placebo-control study with known doses of PCP and had a 93% success rate in relieving the psychotic manifestations (6). In one report, however, haloperidol therapy was discontinued because of seizures. Thus, it is unclear whether the haloperidol played a role in PCP toxicity (46). Clinically, benzodiazepines, antihypertensive medications, as well as medications to control hyperthermia have been used to treat the complications of PCP but not studied for specific interactions (11,19,42,47–52). Of particular concern in management decisions would be the other drugs that the patient may have used such as ethanol, barbiturates, marijuana, cocaine, heroin, hallucinogens, or over-the-counter (OTC) agents.

IV. **Clinical effects of toxicity**

A. **Who uses this drug?** PCP use can be divided into two categories: intentional and knowing exposure, and unintentional exposure. The latter category includes illicit drug users that are not aware that the substance they purchased has been "laced" or adulterated by PCP, body packers who intend to transport the drug by ingesting a package of PCP which subsequently leaks or ruptures, children who ingest any of the forms of the drug, neonates that have been exposed in utero, and, potentially children who have inhaled the smoke-filled air of a room in which PCP was being smoked (18,24,26,31–33,35,42, 47,48,52–59).

B. **Effects.** Anesthesia studies suggest that the effects of PCP are dose related and span a wide range of systemic and neurologic presentations. When used for elective operative procedures, effects were titrated to euphoria, conscious sedation with blank stare, analgesia, amnesia, and a sense of environmental and bodily dissociation (1,2,6). However, some patients rather unpredictably underwent memorable and unpleasant hallucinations, violent agitation, nausea and vomiting, prolonged unconsciousness, seizures, and a prolonged sense of bodily distortion lasting for up to 24 h after PCP administration (1–3,5,6). When used illicitly, any of the same symptoms occur in an often prolonged and exaggerated manner. In addition, psychosis, which is often paranoid in nature, poor ability to concentrate and integrate environmental stimuli, inability to sense danger, bizarre behavior including public nudity, and catatonia may occur (2–5,19,42,46,48,51,52,55,56,60). These derangements in mental status combined with the anesthetic effects of PCP place the patient at high risk for physical injury and significant trauma to which the patient may be completely oblivious (61). The behavioral toxicity of PCP has accounted for significant morbidity and fatalities caused by inadvertent, or purposeful self-inflicted injury (30). Medical effects include hyperthermia, hypertension, seizures, tachycardia, muscle rigidity, focal neurologic changes, dystonias, and sometimes incontinence. The attendant complications reported in the literature include intracranial bleeds, rhabdomyolysis, renal failure, hepatotoxicity, life-threatening hyperthermia, status epilepticus, coma and death (8,11,19,42,47–50,52,57,62–69). Typically, however, patients will present to medical care because of some change in mental status. They can present from agitated but alert with no change in vital signs, to coma with hypertension, tachycardia, and hyperthermia and variable presentations in between these two extremes. Patients have also been described, though rarely, as presenting with a relatively benign course only to undergo a precipitous demise while being observed (47). A more detailed description of the physical findings is discussed below.

C. **Identifying the PCP toxic patient.** Patients may be able to give a history of PCP use. The route of exposure should be determined, and, if possible, the amount used. Although histories are not always reliable, they may yield some valuable information in the cases of large ingestions.

1. **History.** Patients may give a history of vertigo, euphoria, body distortion, numbness, hallucinations, vomiting, and parasthesias. The physician should attempt to get a history of motive (recreational versus suicidal ingestion), underlying psychiatric disorders, and pregnancy status. PCP use should be suspected in patients using any illicit drug who have symptoms and findings consistent with PCP and

inconsistent with the drug they claim to have used. These patients may complain of an unusual or bad "trip" from their usual high.

2. **Examination.** Physical examination also is important in the diagnosis of PCP toxicity.

3. **Vital signs.** Patients can present with hyperthermia, hypertension, tachypnea, and tachycardia. These abnormalities can appear individually or in any combination, and can present in a delayed fashion. Concerns about the airway should be addressed, then hyperthermia prior to proceeding with the remainder of the examination. Depressed respirations are not expected, and hypotension almost never occurs. These findings should alert the physician to institute immediate management and consider other etiologies. Frequent monitoring of all of the vital signs at regular intervals is important. Patients may have vertical, rotatory or horizontal nystagmus. In a case series of 1,000 patients, nystagmus was found in 57% (19). Pupils can be dilated or constricted variably, but are usually equal and reactive. Excessive salivation has occasionally but inconsistently reported in the literature, as has been diaphoresis (11,19). Evidence of head trauma should be sought by careful inspection of the head for bruising, swelling or bony depressions, checking for hemotympanum, or unequal pupils. The lungs are usually clear although bronchospasm has been reported rarely. The heart can be tachycardic, but is often normal with respect to rate. PCP has not been shown to induce bradycardia or dysrhythmias in humans in the absence of extreme hyperthermia or acidosis. The abdomen is rarely tender, however patients may complain of nausea and some vomiting. PCP has no reproducible effects on bowel sounds. Urinary retention has been infrequently reported, and should be checked for by percussion and straight catheterization when feasible. Horizontal and/or vertical nystagmus is the most suggestive finding of PCP toxicity. Patients may also have dystonia, athetoid movements, and increased deep tendon reflexes. Rigidity without cogwheeling, muscle twitching, and seizures may also occur. A diffuse decrease in ability to feel pain will be notable on sensory examination (2,11,19,31,42,47–49,51,52,56,57,63,64,66,68,69). Typically there are no associated skin changes other than signs of trauma, bruises, of wounds of which the patient may be unaware.

D. **Differential diagnosis.** The differential diagnosis of phencyclidine toxicity includes all causes of agitated delerium especially cocaine toxicity, and withdrawal from sedative-hypnotic agents.

V. **Laboratory tests.** Laboratory confirmation of PCP use is neither sensitive, specific or clinically useful and should be discouraged. Quantitative toxicology screening for other drugs such as ethanol, salicylates, and acetaminophen should be obtained as indicated. Blood should be sent for BHCG, renal function, electrolytes, CPK, and liver function.

VI. **General management.** Assess the airway and breathing. If airway protection is indicated in the comatose patient, consider intubation. If respirations are depressed, consider naloxone administration and entertain a new or concomitant diagnosis. Establish intravenous access. Draw blood for SMA-6, serum glucose, ethanol, fingerstick blood glucose. Administer D50W and thiamine as indicated or if fingerstick blood glucose is unavailable. Place the patient on a cardiac monitor and proceed with the physical examination described above. Check vital signs, including temperature, frequently. If the patient is agitated, physical restraints may be necessary to prevent the patient from further injury. These patients may have increased muscle tone and rigidity and may be at risk for rhabdomyolysis and hyperthermia which can be aggravated by restraints (8,50,63,66,69–71). Adjunctive pharmacological therapy is always indicated. Benzodiazepines are recommended as they will provide sedation, produce muscle relaxation, treat the differential of sedative-hypnotic withdrawal and cocaine intoxication if the diagnosis is unclear, and potentially, though never studied, prevent PCP induced seizures. Haloperidol, while used anecdotally, will not treat other conditions, and may carry the theoretical risk of lowering the seizure threshold and impairing heat dissipation.

A. **Decontamination.** Although no studies have proven the efficacy of activated charcoal (AC) in humans, canine studies demonstrated that AC decreases the LD_{50}, the number of seizures, and fatalities from PCP (38). A patent airway with gag reflex and bowel sounds must be present prior to administering the activated charcoal at a dose of 1 g/kg with a cathartic. Patients who cannot drink AC should have nasogastric tubes placed. This may also be of value in multiple ingestions where other harmful drugs may have been taken, or the diagnosis is unclear. Syrup of ipecac is contraindicated. Hemodialysis or hemoperfusion have never proven effective and would not be expected to be useful given PCP's large volume of distribution (25,26,47).

B. **Special management.** Hyperthermia should be promptly and aggressively cooled with submersion in an ice bath or misting and fans and continual rectal monitoring. The mechanism underlying PCP induced hyperthermia is largely agitation and muscle rigidity. Neuromuscular blocking agents have also been used to treat the rigidity and attendant hyperthermia (66). In the setting of severe hyperthermia and muscle rigidity it would be wise to avoid haloperidol or phenothiazines as neuroleptic malignant syndrome may also be in the differential. Consider evaluation for infectious etiologies of fever, including spinal tap for CSF, urine, and chest radiograph. Hypertension will most likely be mild and transient in nature in less severe exposures, however there have been cases of delayed elevations in blood pressure which were severe and associated with fatal intracerebral hemorrhage, although it is unclear which occurred first (47,65). Other authors have reported cases of intracranial bleeding associated with PCP and hypertension, so institution of antihypertensive therapy with frequent blood pressure monitoring and neurologic examinations may be warranted (22,57). No specific agents have been studied for treatment. Sedation of the patient may be efficacious in most cases. Nitroprusside can be used in extreme cases of hypertension from PCP toxicity. Rhabdomyolysis commonly occurs in the setting PCP use, and is most likely secondary to increased isometric muscle contraction. In the extremely agitated or rigid patient, urine should be examined for evidence of rhabdomyolysis. In the patient requiring physical or pharmacologic restraints, or in patients who are comatose, a foley catheter should be placed to monitor urine output. Acute renal failure has been reported and may require hemodialysis. Creatinine phosphokinase (CPK) should be sent, and i.v. fluids should be used to maintain an adequate urine output. If the diagnosis of rhabdomyolysis is made, urine alkalinization with sodium bicarbonate should be instituted if not otherwise contraindicated (8,50,63,66, 69–71). Dystonias usually resolve with benzodiazepines or anticholinergic agents such as diphenhydramine. The latter should not be used in patients with agitation or hyperthermia. Seizures are usually self limited but indicate a significant exposure. Fatal status epilepticus has been reported in a patient with high levels of PCP (68). Benzodiazepines or, if needed, barbiturates should be used for treatment. Airway maintenance and reducing to risk of aspiration are important considerations. A CT scan of the head is indicated to exclude CNS lesions.

C. **Prolonged coma.** Patients with PCP toxicity may have prolonged periods of psychosis for days after use. Coma, however, is rarely prolonged beyond 72 h in the absence of other complications unless a massive ingestion has occurred. In the setting of prolonged coma a ruptured packet of PCP in a body packer, or major suicidal gesture should be considered. Aggressive bowel decontamination with multiple dose AC and with whole bowel irrigation should be administered. Abdominal radiographs should be considered to help diagnose body packing.

D. **Time course and discharge.** Patients with hyperthermia or evidence of end-organ damage may require admission for monitoring or ongoing therapy. Patients should have stable vital signs, no neurologic findings, and some memory of in-hospital events to be certain that they are not still amnestic on discharge. Appropriate mental health evaluation should be arranged, as well as follow-up.

E. **Changes from prior recommendations.** Urine acidification is no longer recommended to enhance elimination of PCP as its clinical benefit has never been proven. Case reports suggest it may be harmful in cases of rhabdomyolysis, and in one pediatric case was associated with profound systemic metabolic acidosis (32). Likewise, alkalinization of urine in the setting of rhabdomyolysis should not be withheld. Continuous gastric suctioning should be avoided as it removes little PCP and may be associated with fluid and electrolyte abnormalities.

F. **Special considerations.** Neonates born to mothers who used PCP during pregnancy have been found to have irritability alternating with lethargy, poor feeding, tremors, and in one case dysmorphism that could not be explained by other metabolic or genetic causes (23,54,56,58,59). Home safety in exposed neonates, or in children with diagnosed PCP intoxication should be carefully evaluated as well as the potential for child neglect. Adolescents voluntarily using PCP should have full mental health evaluations for depression and chronic substance abuse (18,28). Pregnant women should be counselled as to the hazards of PCP use. Pregnant women identified as PCP users should have careful follow-up as nutritional status and regular prenatal care have been compromised in this group of patients (23,72). Fatalities have occured in association with PCP use. Deaths are usually related to associated injuries such as drowning, suicide, or homicide (30). Death has also resulted from hyperthermia, status epilepticus, intracranial bleeding, liver necrosis, hypertensive crisis, pulmonary embolus, and sepsis (47,50,62,65,68). Though these cases are rare, it is important to realize the potential gravity of phencyclidine toxicity and be vigilant in management of these patients.

References

1. Griefenstein FE, DeVault M. A study of 1-aryl cyclo hexyl amine for anesthesia. *Anesth Analg* 1958;37:283–294.
2. Johnstone M, et al. Sernyl (C1-395) in clinical anesthaesia. *Br J Anaesth* 1959;31:433–439.
3. Davies BM, Beech HR. The effect of 1-arylcyclohexylamine (Sernyl) on twelve normal volunteers. *J Mental Sci* 1960;106:912–924.
4. Bakker CB, Amini FB. Observations on the psychomimetic effect of Sernyl. *Comp Psychiatry* 1961;2:269–280.

5. Ban TA, et al. Observations on the action of Sernyl—a new psychotropic drug. *Can Psychiatr Assoc J* 1961;6:150–157.

6. Helrich M, Atwood JM. Modification of Sernyl anesthesia with haloperidol. *Anesth Analg Curr Res* 1964;43:471–474.

7. Shulgin AT, Mac Lean DE. Illicit synthesis of phencyclidine (PCP) and several of its analogs. *Clin Toxicol* 1976;9:553.

8. Hoogwerf B, et al. Phencyclidine-induced rhabdomyolysis and acute renal failure. *Clin Toxicol* 1979;14:47–53.

9. Wright HH, et al. Phencyclidine-induced psychosis: eight-year follow-up of ten cases. *South Med J* 1988;81:565–67.

10. Maddox VH, et al. The synthesis of phencyclidine and other 1-arylcyclohexamines. *J Med Chem* 1965;8:230.

11. Burns RS, et al. Phencyclidine-states of acute intoxication and fatalities. *West J Med* 1975;123:345–349.

12. Lerner SE, Burns RS. Phencyclidine use among youth: history, epidemiology, and acute and chronic intoxication. *NIDA Res Monogr Ser* 1978;20–21:66.

13. Petersen RC, Stillman RC. Phencyclidine: an overview. *NIDA Res Monogr Ser* 1978;20–21:1.

14. Lundberg GD, et al. Phencyclidine: patterns of street drug analysis. *Clin Toxicol* 1976;9:503.

15. Burns RS, Lerner SE. Perspectives: acute phencyclidine intoxication. *Clin Toxicol* 1976;9:477.

16. Burns RS, Lerner SE. Causes of phencyclidine-related deaths. *Clin Toxicol* 1978;12:463–481.

17. Siegel RK. Phencyclidine and ketamine intoxication: a study of four populations of recreational users. *NIDA Res Monogr Ser* 1978;20–21:119.

18. Schwartz RH, et al. Clinical and laboratory observations—use of phencyclidine among adolescents attending a suburban drug treatment facility. *J Pediatr* 1987;110:322–324.

19. McCarron MM, et al. Acute phencyclidine intoxication: incidence of clinical findings in 1,000 cases. *Ann Emerg Med* 1981;10:237–242.

20. Gibson MS. Phencyclidine intoxication. *Ears Nose Throat J* 1983;62:75–80.

21. Domino EF. Neurobiology of phencyclidine—an update. *NIDA Res Monogr Ser* 1978;20–21:18.

22. Sloan MA, et al. Occurrence of stroke associated with use/abuse of drugs. *Neurology* 1991;41:1358.

23. Tabor BL, et al. Perinatal outcome associated with PCP versus cocaine use. *Am J Drug Alcohol Abuse* 16:337–348.

24. Schnoll SH, Vogel WH. Analysis of street drugs. *N Engl J Med* 1971;284:791.

25. Cook CE, et al. Phencyclidine disposition after intravenous and oral doses. *Clin Pharm Ther* 1982;31:625.

26. Cook CE, et al. Phencyclidine and phenycyclohexene disposition after smoking phencyclidine. *Clin Pharm Ther* 1982;31:635–641.

27. Busto U, et al. Clinical pharmacokinetics of non-opiate abused drugs. *Clin Pharmacokinet* 1989;16:1.

28. Fauman MA, Fauman BJ. The psychiatric aspects of chronic phencyclidine use: a study of chronic PCP users. *NIDA Res Monogr Ser* 1978;20–21:183.

29. Giles HG, et al. Plasma protein binding of phencyclidine. *Clin Pharm Ther* 1982;31:77–82.

30. Burns RS, Lerner SE. Causes of phencyclidine-related deaths. *Clin Toxicol* 1978;12:463–481.

31. Golden NL, et al. Angel dust: possible effects on the fetus. *Pediatrics* 1980;65:18.

32. Strauss AA, et al. Neonatal manifestations of maternal phencyclidine (PCP) abuse. *Pediatrics* 1981;68:550–552.

33. Nicholas JM, et al. Phencyclidine: its transfer across the placenta as well as into breast milk. *Am J Obstet Gynecol* 1982;143:143–146.

34. Perez-Reyes M, et al. Urine pH and phencyclidine excretion. *Clin Pharm Ther* 1982;32:635–641.

35. Kautman KR, et al. Phencyclidine in umbilical cord blood: preliminary data. *Am J Psychiatry* 1983;140:450–452.

36. Rayburn WF, et al. Phencyclidine: biotransformation by the human placenta. *Am J Obstet Gynecol* 1984;148:111–112.

37. Woodworth JR, et al. Phencyclidine (PCP) disposition kinetics in dogs as a function of dose and route of administration. *J Pharmacol Exp Ther* 1985;234:654–661.

38. Picchioni AL, Consroe PF. Activated charcoal—a phencyclidine antidote, or hog in dogs. *N Engl J Med* 1979;300:202.

39. Wong LK, Biemann K. Metabolites of phencyclidine. *Clin Toxicol* 1976;9:583.

40. Soine WH, Vincek, W. C. Phencyclidine contaminant generates cyanide. *N Engl J Med* 1979;301:438.

41. Cohen S. Angel dust. *JAMA* 1977;238:515–516.

42. Jackson JE. Phencyclidine pharmacokinetics after a massive overdose. *Ann Intern Med* 1989;111:613–615.

43. Domino EF, Wilson AE. Effects of urine acidification on plasma and urine phencyclidine levels in overdosage. *Clin Pharm Ther* 1977;22:421–424.

44. Khajawall AM, Simpson GM. Peculiarities of phencyclidine urinary excretion and monitoring. *J Toxicol Clin Toxicol* 1982–83;19:835–842.

45. Simpson GM, et al. Urinary phencyclidine in chronic abusers. *J Toxicol Clin Toxicol* 1982–83;19:1051–1059.

46. Rainey Jr JM, Crowder MK. Prolonged psychosis attributed to phencyclidine: report of three cases. *Am J Psychiatry* 1975;132:1076–1078.

47. Eastman JW, Cohen SN. Hypertensive crisis and death associated with phencyclidine poisoning. *JAMA* 1975;231:1270–1271.

48. Liden CB, et al. Phencyclidine—nine cases of poisoning. *JAMA* 1975;234:513–516.

49. McMahon B, et al. Hypertension during recovery from phencyclidine intoxication. *Clin Toxicol* 1978;12:37–40.

50. Patel R, Connor G. A review of thirty cases of rhabdomyolysis-associated acute renal failure among phencyclidine users. *Clin Toxicol* 1985–86;23:547–556.

51. Tong TG, et al. Phencyclidine poisoning. *JAMA* 1975;234:512–513.
52. Young JD, Crapo LM. Protracted phencyclidine coma from an intestinal deposit. *Arch Intern Med* 1992;152:859–860.
53. Golden NL, et al. Phencyclidine use during pregnancy. *Am J Obstet Gynecol* 1984;148:254–269.
54. Golden NL, et al. A practical method for identifying angel dust use during pregnancy. *Am J Obstet Gynecol* 1982; 142:359–360.
55. Karp HN, et al. Phencyclidine poisoning in young children. *J Pediatr* 1980;97:1006–1009.
56. Welch MJ, Correa GA. PCP intoxication in young children and infants. *Clin Pediatr* 1980;19:510–514.
57. Crosley CJ, Binet EF. Cerebrovascular complications in phencyclidine intoxication. *J Pediatr* 1979;94:316–318.
58. Wachsman L, et al. What happens to babies exposed to phencyclidine (PCP) in utero? *Am J Drug Alcohol Abuse* 1989; 15:31–39.
59. Rahbar F, et al. Impact of intrauterine exposure to phencyclidine (PCP) and cocaine in neonates. *J Natl Med Assoc* 1993;85:49–52.
60. Burns RS, et al. Phencyclidine—states of acute intoxication and fatalities. *J West Med* 1975;123:345–349.
61. Grove Jr DE. Painless self-injury after ingestion of "angel dust." *JAMA* 1979;242:655.
62. Armen R, et al. Phencyclidine-induced malignant hyperthermia causing submassive liver necrosis. *Am J Med* 1977; 77:167–172.
63. Barton CH, et al. Rhabdomyolysis and acute renal failure associated with phencyclidine intoxication. *Arch Intern Med* 1980;140:568–569.
64. Barton CH, et al. Phencyclidine intoxication: clinical experience in 27 cases confirmed by urine assay. *Ann Emerg Med* 1981;10:243–246.
65. Bessen HA. Intracranial hemorrhage associated with phencyclidine abuse. *JAMA* 1982;248:585–586.
66. Cogen FC, et al. Phencyclidine-associated acute rhabdomyolysis. *Ann Intern Med* 1978;88:210–212.
67. Jan K, et al. Hot hog: hyperthermia from phencyclidine. *N Engl J Med* 1978;299:722.
68. Kessler GF, et al. Phencyclidine and fatal status epilepticus. *N Engl J Med* 1974;291:979.
69. Lahmeyer HW, Stock PG. Phencyclidine intoxication, physical restraint, and acute renal failure: case report. *J Clin Psychiatry* 1983;44:184.
70. Goode DJ, Meltzer HY. The role of isometric muscle tension in the production of muscle toxicity by phencyclidine and restraint stress. *Psychopharmacologia* 1975;42:105.
71. Goode DJ, et al. Effect of limb restraints on serum creatinine phosphokinase activity in normal volunteers. *Biol Psychiatry* 1977;12:743–755.

Emergency Toxicology, Second Edition,
edited by Peter Viccellio.
Lippincott–Raven Publishers, Philadelphia © 1998.

63

Marijuana

†Sean M. Rees and °Robert S. Hoffman

†*Department of Emergency Medicine, Bellevue Hospital, New York, New York 10016;*
°*Department of Surgery and Emergency Medicine, New York University School of Medicine,*
New York, New York 10016

I. **Introduction.** Marijuana is a psychoactive drug that has been used since ancient times for both its medicinal and recreational effects (1,2). Marijuana is made from the flowering portions of the hemp plant (Cannabis species). Other names for marijuana include Mary Jane, MJ, weed, and pot. Once dried and ground, the plant is smoked either in cigarettes (joints), in pipes, or in water-cooled apparatuses (bongs). Cannabis can also be harvested by scraping the flowering parts to produce another psychoactive compound known as hashish. Hashish can either be in resin or oil form. The potencies of marijuana vary depending on the area in which it is grown, the presence of seeds, and the time of use since harvest. Although marijuana and hashish are predominantly smoked, ingestion is also common. People who use marijuana present to health care in either the acute or chronic phase of abuse. Although lethality is rare, significant morbidity can be associated with both acute and chronic marijuana use.

II. **Sources of agent.** *Cannabis sativa,* an herbaceous annual, consists of two varieties: *indica* and *americana. C. sativa* contains over 400 compounds, approximately 60 of which are cannabinoids. The predominant psychoactive cannabinoid is 1-δ^9-tetrahydrocannabinol (THC). Marijuana contains between 1% and 5% THC (3,4,5). Due to reduced oral bioavailability, three to four times the inhaled dose of marijuana must be ingested in order to achieve the same clinical effect. In addition, the effects of an oral dose are more unpredictable. Hashish is significantly more potent than marijuana. The resin form contains between 5% and 15% THC, and the oil form contains between 30% and 60% THC (4,5). Due to this wide range of potencies, both habitual abusers and marijuana-naive individuals can have unpredictable reactions to THC. Cannabis can be used individually, together (coating joint paper with hashish oil), or with other agents such as PCP to potentiate its effects.

III. **Pharmacology and properties**

  A. **Mechanism of action.** Marijuana and hashish have been used for centuries for their medicinal properties (6). Their pharmacologic effects include the treatment of pain, decreased spasticity and ataxia in multiple sclerosis, decreased intraocular pressure in glaucoma, relief of nausea associated with chemotherapy, and for appetite stimulation in both AIDS and cancer patients with wasting syndrome (7,8,9,10,11). Currently, there is no FDA-approved role for marijuana or hashish; however, a pharmaceutical grade form of THC exists (dronabinol, Marinol, Roxane Laboratories Inc.) and is approved specifically for the treatment of chemotherapy-associated nausea and vomiting, and anorexia associated with AIDS and cancer (8,12–15). Although considerable research exists, the exact mechanism of THC's pharmacology remains only partially understood. Receptors for THC have been found in greatest concentration in the basal ganglia, hippocampus, cerebral cortex, and cerebellum. The specific location of these receptors and THC's ability to increase cerebral blood flow (16) may be responsible for the characteristic CNS effects of THC-containing compounds. Significantly lower concentrations of the receptors exist in the brain stem, and this may explain the low mortality rate (16). The receptor is a G protein coupled receptor; therefore, it inhibits adenylate cyclase activity (16). THC stimulates sympathetic receptors and inhibits parasympathetic receptors in cardiac tissue. This increase in catecholamines may explain the increase in heart rate and augmented left ventricular performance seen in patients who use marijuana (19,20). This increase in catechols may also improve night vision by binding to ciliary adrenoceptors (21). Marijuana smoke also has many adverse effects on pulmonary tissue. Marijuana, like tobacco, is a potential carcinogen (22). Due to the way in which marijuana is smoked, with deep extended inspirations, its pulmonary burden of toxins may be greater than that of tobacco (23,24).

B. Pharmacokinetics. After pyrolysis, the bioavailability of THC is approximately 20%, while after ingestion it falls to approximately 6% (25). The initial effects of inhaled THC are seen in 2 to 3 min and peak at 10 to 20 min. The effect typically lasts from 90 to 120 min. Ingestion of THC produces effects in 30 to 60 min, peaks in 2 to 3 h and lasts for 2 to 5 h (26,27,28). Once in the blood, THC binds to lipoproteins and albumin. These complexes then pass through the liver, where, through hydroxylation and carboxylation they are converted into inactive compounds. The major inactive compound is 11-nor-THC-9 carboxylic acid. THC is extraordinarily lipophyllic and initial plasma levels fall rapidly from distribution into lipid-rich tissues, giving it an apparent volume of distribution of 9 L/kg (630 L for a 70-kg adult). Elimination is via both urine and feces (20% to 35% in urine, 65% to 80% in feces) (4,5,29). Less than 1% of THC is excreted unchanged. The elimination half-life of THC averages between 28 to 56 h, and results predominately from a large terminal elimination half-life ($\beta t_{1/2}$) as the compound is leached from the lipid stores. If used in conjunction with ethanol or other sedatives the effects of THC may be potentiated.

IV. Clinical presentation. For most recreational users of marijuana or hashish, the experience is described as pleasurable or euphoric. Aside from an increased appetite (30), few adverse effects are perceived. However, both the infrequent and frequent abusers of these drugs may present seeking medical attention.

    A. Acute toxicity

        1. Symptoms. Patients with acute toxicity are likely to be seen in the emergency department setting. They can present with symptoms of an acute toxic psychosis with delusions, hallucinations or confusion; feelings of extreme anxiety or panic reactions, feelings of impending doom, extreme depression, paranoia, chest palpitations, chest tightness, dry mouth, irritated eyes, or unsteady gait (31,32,33). Although these symptoms are more frequently seen in the marijuana naive patient, they can occur in anyone as the THC concentration is unpredictable. Psychotic symptoms are usually transient, but can persist even after single usage (34). These symptoms manifest in relation to the concentration of the dose form. Rarely, cases of myocardial infarction (35), urinary retention (36), pneumothorax, pneumomediastinum, and pneumopericardium have been reported. These later effects result from Valsalva maneuvers during deep inspiration which generate pressures great enough to cause the pathology (37). It must be emphasized, that in healthy individuals without preexisting comorbidity, these presentations are uncommon. Although the above morbid events are rarely seen, Cannabis routinely produces other effects. Cannabis has been shown to have detrimental effects on motor function (38), the ability to perform complex tasks (39), and on the ability to track objects (40). Together, these all have a significant effect on the ability to drive and results in motor vehicle accidents. These effects can persist for several hours, but usually resolve by the following day (39,41).

2. **Signs.** Patients may present with tachycardia, disorientation or ataxic gait. Although blood pressure changes are unpredictable, orthostatic hypotension may be seen following large doses. In addition to conjunctival hyperemia, other ocular findings consistent with THC use include diplopia, photophobia, blepharospasm, and impaired accommodation (42). Nystagmus is not routinely seen with THC use, and may suggest concomitant PCP intoxication. The electrocardiogram typically shows sinus tachycardia, but ST segment and T wave changes consistent with ischemia have been rarely reported (35). Marijuana has also been shown to increase metabolic rate and increase minute ventilation (43). Radiographic findings are usually unremarkable although pneumothorax, pneumomediastinum and pneumopericardium should be suspected in patients with chest pain or pulmonary symptoms. Drug smugglers have also been found to have foreign bodies on chest and abdominal radiographs after swallowing drug filled packages. Packages have also been identified in the esophagus on lateral neck radiographs (44). In Great Britain, marijuana has been found lodged in the external auditory canal as individuals attempt to conceal the drug prior to being searched (45).

B. **Chronic toxicity**

1. **Symptoms.** These patients may not have any specific complaints, but may be brought to the attention of a primary care physician for falling academic performance, decreased motivation, impaired memory or impaired motor skills. Chronic abusers may complain of chronic red sore eyes, or chronic cough. Patients may also present seeking rehabilitation.

2. **Signs.** Physical exam may be normal or have subtle signs of use such as conjunctival hyperemia, decreased pulmonary function tests, or chronic bronchitis (46). Heart rate is typically normal (47). THC has complex endocrine interactions in the chronic user. Studies have shown decreases in luteinizing hormone, testosterone and follicle stimulating hormone with prolonged use of marijuana. Although reports suggest a change in ovulatory patterns and spermatogenesis, the effect on reproduction is not clear as hormone levels generally remain within normal limits (48). Patients should routinely be examined and questioned about the use of other recreational drugs as this will affect the evaluation. Pregnant patients should be encouraged to abstain from marijuana use during their pregnancy and seek prenatal care. Extensive research exists on the potential effects of Cannabis on the fetus and neonate in both animal and human studies (49–57). Adverse effects have been shown at the cellular level (52) and with respect to morphologic features at birth such as birth weight and birth length (53–55). Maternal marijuana use also correlates with an increased risk of developing acute nonlymphoblastic leukemia (56). Additional studies however, have conflicting results (49,57,58). Studying the

effects of marijuana on neonatal outcome is challenging because controlling for confounding variables such as additional drug use, genetic and environmental factors is difficult. Conflicting results aside, the potential for adverse outcome is substantial enough to outweigh other speculation.

V.   Laboratory findings (59–63). Metabolites of THC can be found in plasma, feces and urine. Urine is the most frequently tested source, as urine assays can detect many cannabinols. The major urinary metabolite is 11-nor-THC-9 carboxylic acid, which reaches a detectable level 60 min after smoking THC containing compounds. In infrequent users, levels will fall below detectable ranges in 2 to 5 days, but metabolites can be detected for up to 6 to 8 weeks in chronic users. Several methods exist to detect 11-nor-THC-9 carboxylic acid, each with a different sensitivity. The homogeneous enzyme immunoassay (EMIT st and EMIT dau) and the radioimmunoassay (RIA) are typically used for screening. Both will detect 11-nor-THC-9 carboxylic acid but will also detect other cannabinoids. They are inexpensive and have few false positives results. The EMIT system can detect levels as low as 50 ng/mL 95% of the time, and 20 ng/mL 50% of the time. False negatives can be seen if contaminants are added to the specimen, such as lemon juice, vinegar, salt, or detergents. Dilution can also produce falsely negative results. The RIA system has similar sensitivity to the EMIT system and is subject to the same false negative potential with added contaminants. Gas chromatography/mass spectrometry (GC/MS) is the most specific test. GC/MS can detect 11-nor-THC-9 carboxylic acid at 5 ng/mL without cross-reaction, but is expensive and cumbersome. All of the mentioned tests can be used to detect the presence of THC metabolites and confirm recent use of THC containing compounds, but in no way can they be used to imply that the patient was intoxicated at the time of specimen collection. Passive inhalation of marijuana smoke can produce positive urine tests results (64). However, these circumstances must be extreme (i.e., being in an unventilated room with several people smoking for over 1 h). Thus, the validity of such claims should be questioned.

VI.   **Management.** The initial management of patients with marijuana toxicity should be similar to that for any other drug overdose. Upon first presentation, the exact toxin is often unknown and coingestants, or coinhalants, cannot be excluded. After the airway, breathing and circulation have been assessed, the stabilized patient should be placed on a monitor and given supplemental oxygen. A 12-lead electrocardiogram and a rapid blood glucose measurement should also be performed. There is no toxidrome specific for THC toxicity, but an expedient physical examination should be performed in conjunction with the above measures to evaluate for evidence of coingestants or coinhalants that might alter the resuscitation plan. If no life-threatening events are identified and no evidence of additional drugs is present, then only supportive care is typically indicated. Patients who present with acute paranoia or toxic psychosis often benefit from gentle sedation with a benzodiazepine.

VII.   **Disposition.** The majority of patients with single drug presentation can be discharged from the emergency department once in a stable condition. Patients should have adequate support at home to help them through what can be a stressful experience. Patients should have follow-up arranged with a primary care physician to monitor long-term effects and to screen for continued drug use. Referral to a drug rehabilitation program should also be made. Selective referral to psychiatric services may be made on a case specific basis. Patients who show evidence of cardiac ischemia, morbidity from additional overdoses, need of acute psychiatric intervention or insufficient supportive resources should be considered for admission. In addition to drug counseling, the pregnant patient must have obstetric follow-up.

References

1. Parsche F, Balabanova S, Pirsig W. Drugs in ancient populations. *Lancet* 1993;341:503.
2. Mechoulam R, Devane WA, Breuler A, Zahalka J. A random walk through a Cannabis field. *Pharm Biochem Behav* 1991;40:461–464.
3. Ritzlin RS, Gupta RC, Lundberg GD. Delta-9-tetrahydrocannabinol levels in street samples of marijuana and hashish: correlation to user reactions. *Clin Toxicol* 1979;15:45–53.
4. Nahas GG. Cannabis: toxicological properties and epidemiological aspects. *Med J Aust* 1986;145:82–87.
5. Wason S. Cannabis. *Clin Toxicol Rev* 1979;2:1–2.
6. Zias J, Stark H, Sellgman J, et al. Early medical use of Cannabis. *Nature* 1993;363:215.
7. Noyes R, Brunk SF, Baram DA, Canter A. Analgesic effect of delta-9-tetrahydrocannabinol. *J Clin Pharm* 1975;15: 139–143.
8. Synthetic marijuana for nausea and vomiting due to cancer chemotherapy. *Med Lett* 1985;27:97.
9. Meinck HM, Schonle PW, Conrad B. Effect of cannabinoids on spasticity and ataxia in multiple sclerosis. *J Neurol* 1989;236:120–122.
10. Iversen LL. Medical uses of marijuana? *Nature* 1993;365:12–13.
11. Cohen S. Marijuana: does it have a possible therapeutic use? *JAMA* 1978;240:1761–1763.
12. Cat LK, Coleman RL. Treatment for HIV wasting syndrome. *Ann Pharm* 1994;28:595–597.
13. Beal JE, Olson R, Laubenstein L, et al. Dronabinol as a treatment for anorexia associated with weight loss in patients with AIDS. *J Pain Symptom Manage* 1995;10:89–97.
14. Nelson K, Walsh D, Deeter P, Sheehan F, et al. A phase II study of delta-9-tetrahydrocannabinol for appetite stimulation in cancer-associated anorexia. *J Palliat Care* 1994;10:14–18.
15. *Physicians' desk reference.* 49th ed. Montvale, NJ: Medical Economics, 1995.
16. Mathew RJ, Wilson WH. Acute changes in cerebral blood flow after smoking marijuana. *Life Sci* 1993;52:757–767.
17. Musty RE, Reggio P, Consroe P. A reviw of recent advances in cannabinoid research and the 1994 international symposium on Cannabis and the cannabinoids. *Life Sci* 1995;56:1933–1940.
18. Rinaldi L. Marijuana: a research overview. *Alaska Med* 1994;36:107–113.
19. Benowitz NL, Rosenberg J, Rogers W, Bachman J, Jones R. Cardiovascular effects of intravenous delta-9-tetrahydrocannabinol: autonomic nervous mechanisms. *Clin Pharmacol Ther* 1979;25:440–446.
20. Gash A, Karliner J, Janowsky D, Lake C. Effects of smoking marijuana on left ventricular performace and plasma norepinephrine. *Ann Intern Med* 1978;89:448–452.
21. West ME. Cannabis and night vision. *Nature* 1991;351:703.
22. Taylor FM. Marijuana as a potential respiratory tract carcinogen: a retrospective analysis of a community hospital population. *South Med J* 1988;81:1213–1216.
23. Tilles DS, Goldenheim P, Johnson D, Mendelson J, Mello N, Hales C. Marijuana smoking as cause of reduction in single-breath carbon monoxide diffusing capacity. *Am J Med* 1986;80:601–606.
24. Wu TC, Tashkin D, Djahed B, Rose J. Pulmonary hazard of smoking marijuana as compared with tobacco. *N Engl J Med* 1988;318:347–351.
25. Wall Me, Perez-Reyes M. The metabolism of delta 9-tetrahydrocannabinol and related cannabinoids in man. *J Clin Pharm* 1981;21:178s–189s.
26. Isabell H, Gordoetzsky CW, Jasinski D, Claussen U, Spulak F von, Korte F. Effects of delta-9-trans-tetrahydrocannabinol in man. *Psychopharmacology* 1967;11:184–188.
27. Lemberger L, Silberstein SD, Axelrod J, Kopin IJ. Marihuana: studies on the disposition and metabolism of delta-9-tetrahydrocannabinol in man. *Science* 1970;170:1320–1322.
28. Lemberger L, Tamarkin NR, Axelrod J, Kopin IJ. Delta-9-tetrahydrocannabinold: metabolism and disposition in long-term marijuana smokers. *Science* 1971;173:72–74.
29. Jaffe JH. Drug addiction and drug abuse. In: Gilman A, Rall TW, Nies AS, Taylor P, eds. *Goodman and Gilman's: The pharmacological basis of therapeutics.* 8th ed. New York: Pergamon Press, 1990;522–573.
30. Foltin RW, Brady JV, Fischman MW. Behavioral analyis of marijuana effects on food intake in humans. *Pharm Biochem Behav* 1986;25:577–582.
31. Talbolt JA, Teague JW. Marijuana psychosis. *JAMA* 1969;210:299–302.
32. Weil AT. Adverse reactions to marihuana. *N Engl J Med* 1970;282:997–1000.
33. Nahas G, Latour C. The human toxicity of marijuana. *Med J Aust* 1992;156:495–497.
34. Gersten SP. Long-term adverse effects of brief marijuana usage. *J Clin Psych* 1980;41:60–61.

35. Charles R, Holt S, Kirkham N. Myocardial infarction and marijuana. *Clin Toxicol* 1979;14:433–438.
36. Burton TA. Urinary retention following Cannabis ingestion. *JAMA* 1979;242:351.
37. Birrer RB, Calderon J. Pneumothorax, pneumomediastinum, and pneumopericardium following Valsalva's maneuver during marijuana smoking. *NY State J Med* 1984;Dec:619–620.
38. Reeve VC, Grant JD, Robertson W, Gillespie HK, Hollister LE. Plasma concentration of delta-9-tetrahydrocannabinol and impaired motor function. *Drug Alcohol Depend* 1983;11:167–175.
39. Heishman SJ, Huestis MA, Henningfield JE, Cone EJ. Acute and residual effects of marijuana: profiles of plasma THC levels, physiological, subjective and performance measures. *Pharm Biochem Behav* 1990;37:561–565.
40. Barnett G, Licko V, Thompson T. Behavioral pharmacokinetics of marijuana. *Psychopharmacology* 1985;85:51–56.
41. Chait LD, Perry JL. Acute and residual effects of alcohol and marijuana, alone and in combination, on mood and performance. *Psychopharmacology* 1994;115:340–349.
42. Green K, McDonald TF. Ocular toxicology of marijuana: an update. *J Toxicol Cut Ocular Toxicol* 1987;6:309–334.
43. Zwillich CW, Doekel R, Hammill S, Weil JV. The effect of smoked marijuana on metabolism and respiratory control. *Am Rev Respir Dis* 1978;118:885–890.
44. Somjee S. A narcotic foreign body in the throat. *J Laryngol Otol* 1991;105:774–775.
45. Mason J, O'Flynn P, Gibbin K. Cannabis in the external ear. *J Laryngol Otol* 1993;107:444.
46. Tashkin DP, Coulson AH, Clark VA, et al. Respiratory symptoms and lung function in habitual heavy smokers of marijuana alone, smokers of marijuana and tobacco, smokers of tobacco alone, and nonsmokers. *Am Rev Respir Dis* 1987;135:209–216.
47. Perez-Reyes M, White WR, McDonald SA, Hicks RE, Jeffcoat AR, Cook CE. The pharmacologic effects of daily marijuana smoking in humans. *Pharm Biochem Behav* 1991;40:691–694.
48. Hollister LE. Health aspects of Cannabis. *Pharmacol Rev* 1986;38:1–20.
49. Richardson GA, Day NL, McGauhey PJ. The impact of prenatal marijuana and cocaine use on the infant and child. *Clin Obstet Gynecol* 1993;36:302–318.
50. Fried PA. Prenatal exposure to tobacco and marijuana: effects during pregnancy, infancy, and early childhood. *Clin Obstet Gynecol* 1993;36:319–333.
51. Nahas G, Frick HC. Developmental effects of Cannabis. *Neurotoxicol* 1986;7:381–396.
52. Blevins RD, Regan JD. Delta-9-tetrahydrocannabinol: effect on macromolecular systhesis in human and other mammalian cells. *Arch Toxicol* 1976;35:127–135.
53. Quzi QH, Mariano E, Milman DH, Beller E, Crombleholme W. Abnormalities in offspring associated with prenatal marihuana exposure. *Dev Pharm Ther* 1985;8:141–148.
54. Hatch EE, Bracken MB. Effect of marijuana use in pregnancy on fetal growth. *Am J Epidemiol* 1986;124:986–993.
55. Zuckerman B, Frank DA, Hingson R, et al. Effects of maternal marijuana and cocaine use on fetal growth. *N Engl J Med* 1989;320:762–768.
56. Robison LL, Buckley JD, Daigle AE, et al. Maternal drug use and risk of childhood nonlymphoblastic leukemia among offspring. *Cancer* 1989;63:1904–1911.
57. Dreher MC, Nugent K, Hudgins R. Prenatal marijuana exposure and neonatal outcomes in Jamacia. *Pediatrics* 1994;93:254–260.
58. Hingson R, Alpert JJ, Day N, et al. Effects of maternal drinking and marijuana use on fetal growth and development. *Pediatrics* 1982;70:539–546.
59. Schwartz RH, Hawks RL. Laboratory detection of marijuana use. *JAMA* 1985;254:788–792.
60. Ellis GM, Mann MA, Judson BA, Schramm NT, Tashchian A. Excretion patterns of cannabinoid metabolites after last use in a group of chronic users. *Clin Pharm Ther* 1985;38:572–578.
61. Frederick DL, Green J, Fowler MW. Comparison of six cannabinoid metabolite assays. *J Anal Toxicol* 1985;9:116–120.
62. Moyer TP, Palmen MA, Johnson P, et al. Laboratory Medicine: marijuana testing—how good is it? *Mayo Clin Proc* 1987;62:413–417.
63. Bakerman S. *ABC's of interpretive laboratory data*. 3rd ed. Myrtle Beach, SC: Interpretive Laboratory Data, 1994.
64. Law B, Mason PA, Moffat AC, King LJ, Marks V. Passive inhalation of Cannabis smoke. *J Pharm Pharmacol* 1984;36:578–581.

Selected Readings

Goldfrank LR, et al. *Goldfrank's toxicologic emergencies*. 5th ed. Norwalk, CT: Appleton & Lange, 1994.
Hollister LE. Health aspects of Cannabis. *Pharmacol Rev* 1986;38:1–20.
Schwartz RH. Marijuana: an overview. *Pediatr Clin North Am* 1987;34:305–317.

Emergency Toxicology, Second Edition,
edited by Peter Viccellio.
Lippincott–Raven Publishers, Philadelphia © 1998.

64

Amphetamines

Jeanmarie Perrone

*Department of Emergency Medicine, University of Pennsylvania, Philadelphia,
Pennsylvania 19104*

I. **Introduction.** Amphetamines encompass a large class of phenylethylamine derivatives with a long history as substances of abuse. The first synthetic stimulant was produced in 1887 and later marketed as a nasal decongestant (Benzedrine inhaler) in 1932; abuse of the inhaler soon followed (1). Amphetamines were widely prescribed during the 1930s and 1940s for over 40 indications, including head injuries, barbiturate overdose, morphine addiction, heart block, and low blood pressure. Over 200 million amphetamine doses were supplied to U.S. troops during World War II to heighten vigilance and reduce fatigue. Patterns of abuse emerged in the 1950s and 1960s for weight loss and heightened awareness in truck drivers, students, and professionals. "Designer amphetamines" refers to the new hallucinogenic derivatives synthesized in "underground" laboratories, which have fostered a resurgence of amphetamine abuse in the past 30 years.

II. **Sources**

  A. **Licit.** Amphetamines (and derivatives) are available and can be prescribed for the following indications: short-term weight loss, narcolepsy and attention deficit disorder or other behavioral syndromes in children. Methylphenidate (Ritalin, CibaGeneva Pharmaceuticals, Summit, NJ) production tripled from 1990 to 1993 to meet the increased prescribing of this agent (2). Other sources include the abuse of nonprescription agents such as phenylpropanolamine, found in cold medications and diet aids, as well as ephedrine, also available as the herbal product *Ma Huang*.

  B. **Illicit.** Clandestine laboratory synthesis of methamphetamines and other amphetamine derivatives is increasing. DEA seizures of clandestine laboratories increased from 184 in 1981 to 647 in 1987 (3). A new source of an amphetamine derivative in the United States has resulted from the illegal importation of Khat, an East African plant commonly abused in Somalia and Ethiopia, containing cathine (norpseudoephedrine), a compound with 10% activity of D-amphetamine (4). Use of this agent was popularized during the United Nations mission in Somalia.

  C. **Specific agents**

   1. **Amphetamine derivatives:** methamphetamine (ice), phentermine, phenmetrazine, fenfluramine, methylphenidate, phenylpropanolamine, ephedrine.

   2. **"Hallucinogenic amphetamines":** mescaline, methylenedioxyamphetamine (MDA), methylenedioxymethamphetamine (MDMA), methylenedioxyethamphetamine (MDEA), 4-methyl-2-5-dimethoxyamphetamine DOM/STP.

III. **Pharmacology**
  A. **Mechanism.** Amphetamines are sympathomimetic agents which enhance the release and block the reuptake of catecholamines and may also directly stimulate catecholamine receptors (5). At higher doses and with varying structures, they can also induce release of serotonin and affect central serotonin receptors. The serotonergic effects account for the hallucinogenic properties of some amphetamine derivatives (MDMA, MDEA, mescaline) (6). Release of dopamine centrally may modulate typical behaviors (7) and adverse reactions such as choreoathetosis (8).
  B. **Toxicity.** Excess catecholaminergic activity results in cardiovascular and CNS toxicity similar to cocaine. Lethality results from dysrhythmias, seizures, hyperthermia, hypertension (intracranial hemorrhage or infarct), and encephalopathy.
  C. **Pharmacokinetics.** Amphetamines are most commonly abused by ingestion, i.v., or by inhalation (*pyrolysis*, i.e., smoked) or insufflation of a pure preparation of methamphetamine known as "ice." As with cocaine, absorption and peak effects occur rapidly via inhalation, insufflation, and i.v. The clinical effect may last significantly longer, however, and has been reported to be as long as 12 to 24 h following methamphetamine or MDMA use (9). Amphetamines have large volumes of distribution, between 3 to 5 L/kg and up to 11 to 33 L/kg, precluding any role for hemodialysis in removal. Elimination is via hepatic biotransformation or renal filtration depending on the specific agent and the urine pH. Although acidification of the urine was once recommended to increase excretion it should *not* be done due to the increased risk of renal tubular precipitation of myoglobin in the presence of rhabdomyolysis (10). Amphetamine use in a patient taking monoamine oxidase inhibitors can precipitate a profound hypertensive crisis (11).

IV. **Clinical presentation.** Patients with a history of dieting, body image problems, herbal or plant use especially ephedrine *(Ma Huang)* and norpseudoephedrine (cathine or Khat), students, polysubstance abusers, and attendants of "rave" dance parties or concerts may be at risk for amphetamine abuse and complications. Physical examination can be remarkable for life threatening vital sign abnormalities especially hypertension or hyperthermia. The patients generally appear restless, anxious or agitated, but may be combative or obtunded due to an untoward intracranial event. Other findings reflect sympathomimetic excess including tachycardia, mydriasis, diaphoresis, hyperactive bowel sounds, and seizures. Specific physical manifestations may include "track marks" from i.v. use or a rash secondary to vasculitis. Nasal hyperemia and coryza may reflect intranasal abuse. Evidence of bruxism or other repetitive dyskinesias may be a clue to chronic amphetamine abuse.
  A. **Specific agents/syndromes.** Phenylpropanolamine which is principally a peripheral alpha agonist results in the sine qua non *hypertension and reflex bradycardia* (12). Patients who are lethargic or obtunded should get a head CT to exclude intracranial hemorrhage or infarct (13,14). The hallucinogenic amphetamines MDMA, MDEA, mescaline etc. present with varied hallucinations, synesthesias and euphoria or with the complications of hyperthermia, seizures and rhabdomyolysis resulting from rave dance parties. Fatalities have been reported (15). Amphetamine psychosis is a true, paranoid-hallucinatory psychosis resulting most often from the chronic abuse of amphetamines (16,17). Several cases of intracranial hemorrhage resulting from phenylpropanolamine-induced CNS vasculitis have also been reported (18,19). Amphetamine withdrawal may result in abstinence symptoms of anxiety, abdominal cramps, headache, lethargy, and depression.

Inadvertent intraarterial injection or peripheral vasculitis may present with signs of arterial insufficiency (pain, palor, pulselessness, paresthesias) or a petechial rash.

B. **Toxicologic differential diagnosis.** Amphetamine intoxication may be indistinguishable from other sympathomimetic toxidromes including cocaine. The duration of toxicity is significantly longer, however, than with cocaine. Sedative/hypnotic (especially ethanol) withdrawal may manifest similar autonomic hyperactivity and also may be difficult to distinguish from amphetamine intoxication. The diagnosis of neuroleptic malignant syndrome is based on the presence of four criteria following exposure to neuroleptics: altered mental status, neuromuscular rigidity, autonomic hyperactivity, and increased temperature. Essentially all of these findings have been reported following use of hallucinogenic amphetamines in the setting of the "rave" parties (15). The history may be helpful for distinguishing between the two, although the treatment is essentially the same for both disorders. Monoamine oxidase inhibitor/food-drug interactions and excess ergot alkaloid use may present with phenomenon consistent with amphetamine intoxication.

V. **Diagnostic testing.** An electrocardiogram should be done as a screen for hyperkalemia and dysrhythmias. A urine sample should be dipped for blood, and if positive, should be examined for the presence of red blood cells. The absence of red blood cells strongly suggests early rhabdomyolysis and should prompt aggressive i.v. hydration. An electrolyte panel and CPK should be ordered to screen for rhabdomyolysis and early renal insufficiency. A positive urine drug screen may confirm the clinical diagnosis in a patient with the above findings and may help define the duration of toxicity when either methamphetamine or cocaine are suspected. However, since many amphetamine derivatives are not detected, a negative urine drug screen could be misleading.

VI. **Management.** Patients with a history of amphetamine use or positive drug screens not manifesting signs and symptoms of toxicity do not require any specific treatment other than referral for drug counseling. Following stabilization and satisfactory assessment of ABCs in a patient with potential amphetamine toxicity, physical and pharmacologic restraints should be utilized as needed to prevent injury to the patient and others. Patients manifesting agitation or autonomic hyperactivity should be sedated with a rapidly titratable i.v. benzodiazepine such as diazepam, lorazepam, or midazolam. Normalization of vital signs may follow appropriate sedation with benzodiazepines or may require more specific therapy. Hypertension not responding to adequate sedation should be treated with a specific antihypertensive agent (considering the patient's age and probable baseline blood pressure). Phentolamine, a specific alpha antagonist has been used successfully, especially for phenylpropanolamine toxicity: the initial dose can be 5 mg i.v. (12). Nitroprusside can also be used and may be more easily titrated. Beta-blockers should be avoided due to their propensity to exaggerate unopposed alpha agonism and worsen hypertension (20). Patients with altered mental status, lethargy or obtundation should get a CT scan of the brain because both intracranial hemorrhage and infarct have been associated with amphetamine use (13,14,21). Hyperthermia should be immediately treated with rapid cooling in an ice water bath. Benzodiazepines should be used for muscle relaxation. Anticholinergic agents should be specifically avoided due to their ability to interfere with temperature regulation. Dysrhythmia management should follow ACLS guidelines, however, again, beta-blockers should be avoided. Although some literature supports the use of phenothiazines or butyrophenones in the management of amphetamine psychosis, emergency management is best achieved with benzodiazepines until the differential diagnosis (ethanol withdrawal, cocaine intoxication) has been clarified. The management of patients with oral amphetamine overdoses should include gut decontamination primarily with oral or nasogastric tube administration of activated charcoal.

VII. Disposition. Patients requiring ongoing sedation for continued agitation or abnormal vital signs should be admitted to a unit where vital signs will be frequently or continuously monitored. Any patient who presents with hyperthermia or who has evidence of rhabdomyolysis should be hospitalized. Patients in whom toxicity is resolving (vital signs normalized) but who are pharmacologically sedated may be admitted to a less monitored setting. Patients with intentional ingestions who have received a dose of activated charcoal and who have normal vital signs and no symptoms during a 4-h observation period in the emergency department can be discharged (or medically cleared for psychiatric assessment). Other patients who can be considered for discharge are those with marginal vital sign abnormalities initially who have responded to minimal pharmacologic sedation and who are now awake and alert following observation in the emergency department.

References

1. Monroe RR, Drell HJ. Oral use of stimulants obtained from inhalers. *JAMA* 1947;135:909–914.
2. Swanson JM, Lerner M, Williams L. More frequent diagnosis of attention deficit-hyperactivity disorder (ADHD) [Letter]. *N Engl J Med* 1995;333:944.
3. Soine WH. Contamination of clandestinely prepared drugs with synthetic by-products. *NIDA Res Monogr* 1989;95: 44–50.
4. Luqman W, Danowski TS. The use of Khat (*Catha edulis*) in Yemen: social and medical observations. *Ann Intern Med* 1976;85:246–249.
5. Hoffman BB, Lefkowitz RJ. Catecholamines, sympathomimetic drugs and adrenergic receptor antagonists. In: Hardman JG, Limbird LE, Molinoff PB, Ruddon RW, Gilman AG, eds. *Goodman and Gilman's The pharmacological basis of therapeutics.* 9th ed. New York: McGraw-Hill, 1996:219–222.
6. Rudnick G, Wall SC. The molecular mechanism of "ecstasy" [3,4-methylenedioxymethamphetamine (MDMA)]: serotonin transporters are targets for MDMA-induced serotonin release. *Biochemistry* 1992;89:1817–1821.
7. Gold LH, Geyer MA, Koob GF. Neurochemical mechanisms involved in behavioral effects of amphetamines and related designer drugs. *NIDA Res Monogr* 1989;94:101–121.
8. Sperling LS, Horowitz JL. Methamphetamine-induced choreoathetosis and rhabdomyolysis. *Ann Intern Med* 1994;121: 986–987.
9. Cho AK. Ice: a new dosage form of an old drug. *Science* 1990;249:631–634.
10. Curry SC, Chang D, Connor D. Drug- and toxin-induced rhabdomyolysis. *Ann Emerg Med* 1989;18:1068–1084.
11. Smilkstein MJ, Smolinske SC, Rumack BH. A case of MAO inhibitor/MDMA interaction. Agony after ecstasy. *J Toxicol Clin Toxicol* 1987;25:149–159.
12. Pentel P. Toxicity of over-the-counter stimulants. *JAMA* 1984;252:1898–1903.
13. Kase CS, Foster TE, Reed JE, Spatz EL, Girgis GN. Intracerebral hemorrhage and phenylpropanolamine use. *Neurology* 1987;37:399–404.
14. Kikta DG, Devereaux MW, Chandar K. Intracranial hemorrhages due to phenylpropanolamine. *Stroke* 1985;16:510–512.
15. Henry JA, Jeffreys KJ, Dawling S. Toxicity and deaths from 3,4-methylenedioxymethamphetamine ("ecstasy"). *Lancet* 1992;340:384–387.
16. Angrist B, Sathananthan G, Wilk S, Gershon S. Amphetamine psychosis: behavioral and biochemical aspects. *J Psychiatr Res* 1974;11:13–23.
17. Janowsky DS, Risch C. Amphetamine psychosis and psychotic symptoms. *Psychopharmacology* 1979;65:73–77.
18. Fallis RJ, Fisher M. Cerebral vasculitis and hemorrhage associated with phenylpropanolamine. *Neurology* 1985;35: 405–407.
19. Glick R, Hoying J, Cerullo L, Perlman S. Phenylpropanolamine: an over-the-counter drug causing central nervous system vasculitis and intracerebral hemorrhage. *Neurosurgery* 1987;20:969–974.
20. Doshi BS, Kulkarni RD, Dattani KK, et al. Effects of labetalol and propanolol on responses to adrenaline infusion in healthy volunteers. *Int J Clin Pharm Res* 1984;4:29–33.
21. Harrington H, Heller A, Dawson D, Caplan L, Rumbaugh C. Intracerebral hemorrhage and oral amphetamine. *Arch Neurol* 1983;40:503–507.

Emergency Toxicology, Second Edition,
edited by Peter Viccellio.
Lippincott–Raven Publishers, Philadelphia © 1998.

65

Cocaine

Judd E. Hollander

Villanova, Pennsylvania 19085

I. **Introduction**

    A. **Prevalence.** Over 23 million Americans have used cocaine at least once, and 1% of the population uses cocaine each month. Cocaine is the most common illicit drug seen in emergency departments (EDs) for the past decade, and cocaine-related medical complaints continue to increase.

II. **Sources of cocaine**

    A. **Nature.** Cocaine is present in the leaves of **Erythroxylon coca,** a plant indigenous to South America.

    B. **Medicinal use.** First used as a local anesthetic in 1884, cocaine is still popular for otolaryngology procedures since it is well absorbed through the nasal mucosa and causes local anesthesia and vasoconstriction.

    C. **Historical sources.** During the early 20th century, cocaine was transiently used as an ingredient in Coca-Cola.

III. **Pharmacology and properties of cocaine.** Cocaine has sympathomimetic properties, is a strong CNS stimulant, and is a local anesthetic. Most of cocaine's clinical actions are related to the above properties.

    A. **Mechanism of action and toxicity**

        1. **Sympathomimetic properties.** Sympathetic stimulation is caused through inhibition of reuptake of both epinephrine and norepinephrine at presynaptic adrenergic neurons. In the CNS, cocaine also enhances the release of norepinephrine and excitatory amino acids, and blocks the neuronal reuptake of dopamine and serotonin. As a result of increased adrenergic tone, cocaine causes CNS stimulation, tachycardia, hypertension, temperature elevation, arterial vasoconstriction, thrombus formation, and platelet aggregation.

        2. **Local anesthetic effects.** Cocaine is a local anesthetic of the ester group. It blocks the fast inward sodium channel. All local anesthetics may cause depressed left ventricular function; they are proconvulsants and may also be proarrhythmic.

        3. **The Goldfrank-Hoffman model of cocaine toxicity** is shown in Fig. 65-1. This model of cocaine toxicity clarifies the interaction between the peripheral nervous system and CNS effects of cocaine. The blockade of the peripheral effects of cocaine may be associated with enhanced CNS toxicity. On the other hand, treat-

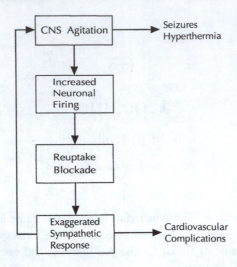

FIG. 65-1. The Goldfrank-Hoffman model of cocaine toxicity.

ment of the CNS toxicity reduces both the central and peripheral manifestations of cocaine toxicity.

B. Pharmacokinetics

   1. **Absorption.** Application of cocaine to the nasal mucosa, ingestion with absorption through the gastrointestinal (GI) mucosa, smoking of crack with pulmonary alveolar absorption, and direct intravenous injection all can result in toxicity. Oral administration has a lag phase of about 30 min but reaches peak concentrations in approximately 60 min. Effects from buccal (chewing) and nasal insufflation begin almost immediately, but are variable due to local vasoconstriction. Peak concentrations are reached within 30 to 60 min. Intravenous and inhalational routes of cocaine use produce near immediate distribution of cocaine to the CNS and system circulation. "Crack" is the direct precipitate of "free base" cocaine that results from alkalinization of aqueous cocaine hydrochloride.

   2. **Distribution.** The biologic half-life of cocaine is 0.5 to 1.5 h; the volume of distribution is 2 L/kg; and the systemic clearance is 2 L/min. Benzoylecgonine and ecgonine methyl ester (EME), the major metabolites of cocaine, have half-lives of 5 to 8 h and 3.5 to 6 h, respectively.

   3. **Metabolism.** Cocaine is hydrolyzed rapidly by liver and plasma esterases to EME, which accounts for 30% to 50% of the parent product. Nonenzymatic hydrolysis results in the formation of the other major metabolite, benzoylecgonine (approximately 40% of the parent product). Other minor metabolites, such as norcocaine and cocethylene, account for the remainder of cocaine's degradation products. The activity of plasma cholinesterase determines the relative concentrations of the various metabolites, and quite possibly affects the degree of toxicity that develops.

4. **Elimination.** Relatively little cocaine is excreted unchanged in the urine (1% to 5%). Benzoylecgonine and EME are also excreted in the urine. Due to a long elimination half-life, assays for cocaine and cocaine metabolites generally will detect benzoylecgonine for up to 48 to 72 h following use.

5. **Drug-drug interactions**
   a. **Ethanol.** When ethanol and cocaine are used concurrently, a unique metabolite, cocethylene, is produced. Cocethylene produces similar psychomotor stimulation to cocaine but produces more depression of left ventricular function than cocaine alone. Lethality may be increased when cocaine and ethanol are used in combination.
   b. **Tobacco.** Tobacco causes an alpha adrenergic mediated coronary vasoconstriction similar to cocaine. When they are used in combination the magnitude of coronary vasoconstriction is greater than when either is used alone.
   c. **Beta-adrenergic antagonists.** These agents are contraindicated in patients with potential cocaine-induced myocardial ischemia. They have been shown to enhance coronary vasoconstriction, worsen left ventricular function, and increase lethality in cocaine toxicity. Labetalol, a combined alpha-beta antagonist does not appear to offer any advantages over pure beta antagonists.

IV. **Clinical presentation.** The complications of cocaine occur in all organ systems. The most common cocaine-associated medical complaints relate to the cardiovascular system, with chest pain being the single most common complaint.

   A. **Effects on vital signs.** Since cocaine is a sympathomimetic stimulant, cocaine-intoxicated patients will frequently have hypertension and/or tachycardia. Hyperthermia and tachypnea are less common. Hyperthermia is one of the major causes of death in cocaine-intoxicated patients.

   B. **Cardiovascular effects.** Acutely, cocaine causes arterial vasoconstriction. Chronic cocaine use can result in accelerated atherosclerosis, left ventricular hypertrophy, and enhanced thrombus formation. These effects can cause myocardial ischemia or infarction. Supraventricular and ventricular arrhythmias may occur either as a direct result of cocaine or as a complication of myocardial ischemia. The negative inotropic effects of cocaine can result in the acute depression of left ventricular function and congestive heart failure. Chronic cocaine use can result in dilated cardiomyopathy. Aortic dissection and rupture occur after use of cocaine.

   C. **Neurologic effects.** Most cocaine-intoxicated patients are anxious or agitated. Bland cerebral infarcts, hemorrhagic infarcts, and subarachnoid hemorrhages occur. Seizures can occur as a direct result of these processes or in their absence. An entity called the "cocaine washed-out syndrome" has been described, where patients remain extremely lethargic and are difficult to arouse for up to 24 h after cocaine use.

   D. **Other ischemic effects.** Mesenteric, renal, pulmonary, and ophthalmic artery ischemia have been noted. The clinician should assume that ischemia of all vascular beds can occur secondary to cocaine.

   E. **Rhabdomyolysis.** Skeletal muscle injury occurs secondary to cocaine. Although patients may have overt clinical signs such as muscle tenderness, they usually present without signs and symptoms of muscle injury.

F. Body packers. Patients with continued toxicity despite treatment, and patients who arrive from the airports or cities that are large exporters of cocaine should be considered possible body packers. Most of these patients will be asymptomatic. Symptomatic patients should be considered a major medical emergency.

V. Laboratory findings

A. Blood tests. Patients with only mild toxicity may not require laboratory evaluation. Electrolytes may reflect the adrenergic effects of cocaine with hyperglycemia and hypokalemia. A mild leukocytosis may also occur. The creatinine may be useful in cases of renal failure or infarction. The creatine kinase is elevated in cases of rhabdomyolysis, and in almost half of patients with chest pain. Creatine kinase MB usually indicates a myocardial infarction, but "false positive" elevations may occur. Troponin I may be useful to confirm a myocardial infarction.

B. Radiography. Chest radiographs may detect pneumothorax, pneumomediastinum, pneumopericardium, pulmonary infarctions, and pneumonia. Abdominal radiography may detect cocaine condoms in body packers. Computerized tomography (CT) should be used to detect cerebrovascular events.

C. Electrocardiography. Myocardial infarction occurs in patients with normal and abnormal electrocardiograms. Normal 12 lead electrocardiography should not be considered sufficient to exclude myocardial infarction. Unfortunately, ST elevations that meet thrombolysis criteria occur in 11% to 43% of patients with cocaine-associated chest pain in the absence of infarction.

D. Toxicology tests. Urine immunoassays for cocaine metabolites generally detect the major metabolite of cocaine, benzoylecgonine at or above concentrations of 300 ng/mL. Usually, the presence of cocaine or its metabolites can be detected for 48 to 72 h after use. Rarely, using more sensitive methods (GC/MS), cocaine metabolites have been detected for up 3 weeks after the last use.

E. Other testing. Additional laboratory or diagnostic testing should be considered depending on the clinical condition. For example, lumbar puncture should be performed in patients with suspected subarachnoid hemorrhage and normal head CT's; ventilation-perfusion scans should be used in patients suspected of pulmonary infarction.

VI. Management

A. General supportive care should be provided with attention to the airway, breathing, and circulatory support.

B. Sinus tachycardia should be treated with observation and anxiolytics. Diazepam 5 to 10 mg. or lorazepam 2 to 4 mg intravenously can be titrated to the desired effect.

C. Supraventricular tachycardia, in hemodynamically stable patients, can be treated with benzodiazepines and calcium channel antagonists (intravenous diltiazem 20 mg or verapamil 5 mg). In cases of atrioventricular reentry, i.v. adenosine 6 to 12 mg can be used. For hemodynamically unstable patients, cardioversion should be used.

D. Ventricular arrhythmias should be treated with i.v. lidocaine 100-mg bolus followed by continuous infusion of 2 mg/min or sodium bicarbonate if hemodynamically stable. Unstable patients should be defibrillated.

E. Hypertension should be treated with observation or benzodiazepines if mild to moderate. For malignant refractory hypertension, i.v. nitroglycerin, nitroprusside, or phentolamine can be used. Beta-adrenergic blockade has not been demonstrated to be useful and may exacerbate myocardial ischemia through unopposed alpha adrenergic stimulation.

F. **Ischemic chest pain** should be treated with benzodiazepines, aspirin 325 mg, and sublingual nitroglycerin 1/150 every 5 min for three tablets. Refractory chest pain can be treated with either morphine sulfate or intravenous nitroglycerin titrated to a 10% reduction in mean arterial pressure. Patients who do not respond to the above regimen can be treated with phentolamine 1 mg i.v. every 5 to 10 min until effect, or verapamil 5 to 10 mg i.v. Patients with unstable angina should receive heparin according to standard doses. Either cardiac catheterization with mechanical reperfusion or thrombolytic therapy should be considered for patients with acute myocardial infarction refractory to medical management. Beta-adrenergic antagonists and mixed alpha-beta antagonists are contraindicated in patients with potential cocaine-induced myocardial ischemia as they increase coronary artery vasoconstriction and decrease myocardial blood flow.

G. **Pulmonary edema** should be treated with diuretics, morphine, and nitroglycerin according to standard protocols.

H. **Hyperthermic patients** should be cooled with restricted activity; tepid, cool or iced water baths; intubation with cool air ventilation; and gastric lavage with iced water depending on the severity of the hyperthermia and clinical status of the patient.

I. **Anxious and agitated patients** should not be physically restrained in the absence of chemical sedation. Inappropriate physical restraints may increase skeletal muscle activity thus exacerbating hyperthermia and rhabdomyolysis. The agents of choice for chemical sedation in the cocaine-intoxicated patient are benzodiazepines, which can be titrated to effect.

J. **Seizures** are usually brief and transient. Patients should be treated with benzodiazepines as necessary for continued or recurrent cocaine-associated seizures. Intracranial hemorrhage should be excluded.

K. Patients with **cerebrovascular ischemia or subarachnoid hemorrhages** should be managed with supportive care.

L. The **cocaine washed-out syndrome** is self-limited, and patients should be allowed to sleep until freely arousable. Occult myocardial infarction has been reported in patients too lethargic to complain of chest pain.

M. **Rhabdomyolysis.** Breakdown of skeletal muscle can occur from cocaine use. Patients with significant elevation of creatine kinase or myoglobinuria should be managed with vigorous hydration to maintain a urine output of at least 3 mL/kg/h; sodium bicarbonate to alkalinize the urine; and hemodialysis if renal failure occurs.

N. **Body packers** should receive activated charcoal to limit cocaine absorption and whole bowel irrigation to increase GI transit. All such patients should be monitored until the cocaine bags have been eliminated, even if they are asymptomatic. In rare cases, surgical removal may be necessary for bowel obstruction or cocaine toxicity.

VII. **Disposition.** Patients with ventricular arrhythmias, congestive heart failure, potentially ischemic chest pain, cerebrovascular ischemia, rhabdomyolysis, and all body packers need hospital admission. Most other complications of cocaine can be managed in the ED and do not require hospital admission. Referral to social services and/or drug rehabilitation programs should be performed, when appropriate.

References

1. Brogan WC, Lange RA, Kim AS, Moliterno DJ, Hillis LD. Alleviation of cocaine-induced coronary vasoconstriction by nitroglycerin. *J Am Coll Cardiol* 1991;18:581–586.
2. Callaway CW, Clark RF. Hyperthermia in psychostimulant overdose. *Ann Emerg Med* 1994;24:68–76.
3. Catravas JD, Waters IW. Acute cocaine intoxication in the conscious dog: studies on the mechanism of lethality. *J Pharmacol Exp Ther.* 1981;217:350–356.
4. Daras M, Tuchman AJ, Marks S. Central nervous system infarction related to cocaine abuse. *Stroke* 1991;22:1320–1325.
5. Goldfrank LR, Hoffman RS. The cardiovascular effects of cocaine. *Ann Emerg Med* 1991;20:165–175.
6. Holland RW, Marx JA, Earnest MP, Renninger S. Grand mal seizures temporally related to cocaine use: clinical and diagnostic feature. *Ann Emerg Med* 1992;21:772–776.
7. Hollander JE, Carter WC, Hoffman RS. Use of phentolamine for cocaine-induced myocardial ischemia. *N Engl J Med* 1992;327:361.
8. Hollander JE, Hoffman RS, Gennis P, et al. Prospective multicenter evaluation of cocaine-associated chest pain. *Acad Emerg Med* 1994;1:330–339.
9. Hollander JE, Hoffman RS, Gennis P, et al. Nitroglycerin in the treatment of cocaine-associated chest pain: clinical safety and efficacy. *J Toxicol Clin Toxicol* 1994;32:243–256.
10. Hollander JE, Hoffman RS, Burstein J, Shih RD, Thode HC, and the Cocaine-Associated Myocardial Infarction Study (CAMI) Group. Cocaine-associated myocardial infarction. Mortality and complications. *Arch Intern Med* 1995;155:1081–1086.
11. Hollander JE, Burstein JL, Shih RD, Hoffman RS, Wilson L, and the Cocaine-Associated Myocardial Infarction Study (CAMI) Group. Cocaine-associated myocardial infarction: clinical safety of thrombolytic therapy. *Chest* 1995;107:1237–1241.
12. Hollander JE. Management of cocaine-associated myocardial ischemia. *N Engl J Med* 1995;333:1267–1272.
13. Landry MJ. An overview of coaethylene, an alcohol-derived, psychoactive cocaine metabolite. *J Psychoactive Drugs* 1992;24:273–276.
14. Lange RA, Cigarroa RG, Yancy CW, et al. Cocaine-induced coronary artery vasoconstriction. *N Engl J Med* 1989;321:1557–1562.
15. Lange RA, Cigarroa RG, Flores ED, et al. Potentiation of cocaine-induced coronary vasoconstriction by beta-adrenergic blockade. *Ann Intern Med* 1990;112:897–903.
16. Negus BH, Willard JE, Hillis LD, et al. Alleviation of cocaine-induced coronary vasoconstriction with intravenous verapamil. *Am J Cardiol* 1994;73:51–513.
17. Shih RD, Hollander JE, Hoffman RS, et al. Lidocaine in cocaine-associated myocardial infarction: clinical safety. *Ann Emerg Med* 1995;26:702–706.
18. Welch RD, Todd K, Krause GS. Incidence of cocaine-associated rhabdomyolysis. *Ann Emerg Med* 1991;20:154–157.

Emergency Toxicology, Second Edition,
edited by Peter Viccellio.
Lippincott–Raven Publishers, Philadelphia © 1998.

66

Alcohol Intoxication

Jeffrey S. Fine

Department of Pediatrics, Pediatric Emergency Medicine, New York University School of Medicine, Bellevue Hospital, New York, New York 10016

I. **Introduction.** Ethanol is the alcohol constituent of "alcoholic" beverages and is a solvent commonly used in medicinal preparations. Ethanol is the most commonly abused intoxicating substance, and 10% of adult Americans suffer from alcohol abuse or dependence. Serious neurologic, gastrointestinal (GI), nutritional, and psychiatric disease accompany chronic alcoholism, and 3% of annual deaths may be attributable to alcohol. The use or abuse of ethanol is highly associated with both major trauma such as motor vehicle collisions, fires, burns, and falls and is also significantly associated with domestic violence, child abuse, and suicide. Acute ethanol intoxication mimics sedative-hypnotic intoxication with altered mental status progressing to a depressed level of consciousness. Chronic intoxication (alcoholism) is marked by numerous chronic health effects and may be complicated by acute intoxication or withdrawal. This chapter deals primarily with the evaluation and management of acute ethanol intoxication and the acute complications of chronic alcoholism.

II. **Definitions and abbreviations**

    A. **Blood alcohol concentration.** Blood alcohol concentration (BAC) is the term most often used in the literature and is used in this chapter to refer to serum ethanol concentration. A *whole blood* ethanol concentration is approximately 15% lower than a spun and separated *serum* ethanol concentration. All the following serum ethanol concentrations are equivalent:

$$100 \text{ mg/dL} = 100 \text{ (mg)} \% = 0.1 \text{ g/dL} = 0.1 \text{ (g)} \% = 1 \text{ g/L}$$
$$100 \text{ mg/dL} = 22 \text{ mM/L}$$

    B. **Reinforcement.** The effects of ethanol that lead to repeat use.

    C. **Alcohol abuse.** Heavy drinking in a nondependent person that leads to social or health consequences.

    D. **Tolerance.** Diminished ethanol effect with repeated use or the requirement for higher serum ethanol concentrations to achieve an effect.

    E. **Physical dependence.** Physiologic requirement for ethanol to prevent symptoms of withdrawal.

    F. **Psychologic dependence.** Craving for ethanol for its pleasurable effects or to avoid discomfort.

    G. **Kindling.** Physiologic sensitization such that successive episodes of withdrawal are worse than previous episodes.

III. **Sources.** Ethanol is found in a wide variety of commercial products (Table 66-1). It is the alcohol of "alcoholic" beverages (beers, wines, and spirits). It is a common vehicle for both prescription and over-the-counter medications. Ethanol also serves as the diluent for many household products such as mouthwashes, colognes, perfumes, and extracts. "Proof" is a term used to describe the ethanol content of alcoholic beverages:

"Proof" = 2 × [alcohol concentration by volume, the percentage alcohol]

IV. **Properties.** Ethanol (ethyl alcohol, CH_3-CH_2-OH) is a 2-carbon, aliphatic alcohol, which is a clear and colorless liquid at room temperature. It has a molecular weight of 46 Daltons, a specific gravity of 790 mg/mL, and yields 7.1 kcal/g when oxidized.

V. **Pharmacology**

    A. **Mechanism of action.** Ethanol has toxic effects on almost every organ system. Although some of these toxic manifestations can be related to effects of the metabolite acetaldehyde or to changes in the redox potential of cells, the mechanism by which ethanol causes "intoxication" is not specifically known. Early work suggested that ethanol interacted with and became integrated into the lipid bilayer of cell membranes, increased membrane "fluidity," and thereby interfered with normal cellular function. These effects may occur at very high ethanol concentrations where ethanol acts as an anesthetic. At lower "intoxicating" concentrations, at least with respect to neurologic effects, ethanol does not have gross membrane destabilizing effects. Although almost every neurotransmitter system is affected by ethanol, there do not appear to be specific receptors for ethanol as there are for opiates or benzodiazepines. Rather, ethanol may interact with specific portions of cell membranes of particular neurons or groups of neurons located in specific regions of the brain. Several neurochemical systems are the focus of current research. GABA is an inhibitory neurotransmitter. Ethanol seems to potentiate the activity of GABA by interacting with the $GABA_a$-receptor chloride channel. Glutamate is an excitatory neurotransmitter. Alcohol appears to inhibit glutamate function at the *N*-methyl-*D*-aspartate (NMDA) receptor which opens calcium channels. Glycine, another inhibitory neurotransmitter that controls calcium channels and which has interactions with both $GABA_a$ and NMDA receptors, is also influenced by ethanol. Through an interaction with the G_s protein, ethanol influences the activity of adenylate cyclase which regulates synthesis of cyclic adenosine monophosphate (c-AMP), a "second messenger" which regulates many intracellular functions. These neurochemical transmitters are involved with acute intoxication as well as chronic effects including reinforcement, tolerance

TABLE 66-1. *Ethanol concentration of some commercial products*

Product	Ethanol concentration(%)	"Proof"[a]
Beer	2–6	4–12
Wine	10–20	20–40
Distilled spirits	40–50	80–100
Cough medicines	3–25	6–50
Mouthwash	16–27	32–54
Colognes	40–60	80–120
Vanilla extract	30–35	60–70

[a]"Proof" generally applies to alcoholic beverages, but it is used here for comparison between products.

and dependence. For instance, at the NMDA receptor, the acute effect of alcohol is inhibitory, while following chronic exposure, up-regulation of the receptor leads to decreased ethanol effect. NMDA and GABA$_a$ receptors are thought to have an etiologic role in the development of withdrawal seizures, related to changes in receptor function after chronic ethanol exposure.

B. **Routes of administration.** The primary route of ethanol administration is oral ("drinking"). Ethanol can also be administered i.v. when used as an antidote for methanol or ethylene glycol intoxication (see Chapter 15).

C. **Absorption.** Eighty percent of ingested ethanol is absorbed from the small intestine; a small amount is absorbed from the mouth, esophagus, and stomach. In fasting healthy adults, peak absorption occurs from 30 to 90 min following intake. The peak level following a dose of ethanol will depend on individual characteristics such as age, gender, weight, and previous experience with alcohol, as well as characteristics of the product ingested; wine is absorbed faster than distilled spirits. If gastric emptying is delayed, absorption will also be delayed. For example, increased gastric contents (food), ileus (from trauma) or decreased GI motility (from toxin or previous surgery) will delay absorption. The peak serum ethanol concentration (mg/dL) can be calculated:

$$= \frac{\left[\text{Dose of Ethanol (mg)}\right]}{\left[\text{Vd (L/kg)} \times 10(\text{dl/L}) \times \text{Body Weight (kg)}\right]}$$

$$= \frac{\left[\text{Volume of Ethanol(mL)} \times \text{Concentration(\%)} \times \text{Specific Gravity(790 mg Ethanol/mL)}\right]}{\left[0.6 \text{ L/kg} \times 10 \text{ dl/L} \times \text{Body Weight (kg)} \times 100 \text{ (\% conversion factor)}\right]}$$

$$= \frac{\left[\text{Volume of Ethanol(mL)} \times \text{Concentration(\%)} \times 1.3\right]}{\left[\text{Body Weight (kg)}\right]}$$

$$= \frac{\left[\text{Volume of Ethanol(mL)} \times \text{Concentration(\%)}\right]}{\left[\text{Body Weight (kg)}\right]}$$

Therefore, 1 mL/kg of 100% ethanol (1 g/kg) will raise the serum ethanol level to approximately 100 mg/dL. Approximately 10 g of ethanol contained in one standard drink (12 oz of beer, 4 oz of wine, or 1 oz of distilled spirits) will raise the BAC 25 to 30 mg/dL. Four to five drinks will raise the BAC to approximately 100 to 150 mg/dL.

D. **Distribution.** Ethanol is mildly polar and is water and to some extent lipid soluble. It distributes in the total body water with a volume of distribution (V_d) of approximately 0.6 L/kg.

E. **Metabolism and elimination.** Eighty percent to 90% of an ethanol dose is metabolized in the liver; a small amount is excreted unchanged by the kidneys and the lungs. Metabolism generally follows zero-order kinetics; a fixed milligram amount is metabolized per unit time. A typical nontolerant adult metabolizes approximately 7 to 10 g of ethanol (one drink) per hour with a subsequent decrease in BAC of approximately 15 to 20 mg/dL/h. Tolerant individuals may metabolize ethanol faster and BAC may decrease at a rate of up to 30 to 40 mg/dL/h. The metabolic rates for both nontolerant and tolerant drinkers has significant individual variation. Ethanol is primarily metabolized by the alcohol dehydrogenase pathway found in the cytoplasm of hepatocytes:

$$\text{Ethanol} + NAD^+ \rightleftharpoons \text{Acetaldehyde} + NADH + H^+$$
Alcohol Dehydrogenase

$$\text{Acetaldehyde} + H_2O + NAD^+ \rightleftharpoons \text{Acetate} + NADH + H^+$$
Alcohol Dehydrogenase

$$\text{Acetate} \rightleftharpoons \text{Acetyl CoA} \rightleftharpoons CO_2 + H_2O$$
Krebs Cycle   Krebs Cycle

In chronic alcoholics, this pathway increases the NADH/NAD$^+$ ratio, changes the redox potential of the hepatocyte, and contributes to the development of lactic acidosis and alcoholic ketoacidosis. The microsomal ethanol oxidizing system (MEOS) is a secondary pathway that accounts for about 10% of ethanol metabolism but which becomes increasingly active at higher ethanol concentrations.

F. **Drug-drug interactions**

1. **Acute intoxication** may block the metabolism of and lead to increased levels of drugs such as aspirin, benzodiazepines, barbiturates, phenytoin, and tricyclic antidepressant agents. Ethanol may also have synergistic effects with other sedative-hypnotic agents.

2. **Chronic intoxication** stimulates microsomal enzymes and increases the metabolism of drugs such as isoniazid, phenytoin, tolbutamide, and warfarin.

3. **Disulfiram effects.** Disulfiram is a pharmaceutical agent used to prevent ethanol abuse. By blocking alcohol dehydrogenase, disulfiram causes the accumulation of acetaldehyde, and nausea, vomiting, abdominal pain, flushing, headache, and chest pain. Other agents have disulfiram-like effects in the presence of ethanol, for example: cephalosporins, coprinus-containing mushrooms, griseofulvin, metronidazole, and sulfonamides (for more on disulfiram, see Chapter 43).

VI. **Clinical presentation**

A. **GI.** Nausea, vomiting, and abdominal pain are commonly associated with acute intoxication. In the chronic alcoholic, abdominal pain may be related to esophagitis, gastritis, ulcer disease, pancreatitis, hepatitis, or cirrhosis.

B. **CNS**

1. **Acute intoxication/altered mental status (AMS).** Ethanol acts as a sedative hypnotic agent. Low BACs are associated with exhilirated and euphoric feelings and disinhibited actions. At higher serum levels, there is increasing CNS depression with slurred speech, altered perception of the environment, impaired judgement, ataxia, incoordination, nystagmus, and increased combativeness. The patient may experience blackouts. At very high serum levels, the patient may develop coma and respiratory depression. It is difficult to accurately predict which symptoms will be associated with a particular serum ethanol level in a particular patient, especially one who may be tolerant following chronic exposure. A rough guide to the acute neurologic effects of intoxication in the nontolerant patient is found in Table 66-2. Significant effects on judgement and motor control may occur with BACs of 25 to 50 mg/dL. Hypoglycemia is another manifestation of acute intoxication and may contribute to AMS, particularly in children, and may be associated with malnutrition in the chronic alcoholic. Other causes of AMS should be con-

TABLE 66-2. *Clinical signs in the intolerant ethanol drinker*

Ethanol level (mg/dl)	Clinical manifestations
30	Mild euphoria and disinhibition
50	Mild incoordination
100	Ataxia
200	Drowsiness and confusion
300	Stupor
400+	Possible hypoglycemia, hypothermia, respiratory failure, coma, and death

sidered in the patient with acute intoxication or chronic alcoholism, particularly when there is no resolution of symptoms after an appropriate period of observation. The differential diagnosis of altered mental staus in the alcohol intoxicated patient includes hypoglycemia, electrolyte and acid-base disturbances, coingested toxins, intracranial hemorrhage or mass lesion, intracranial infections, postictal phenomenon, withdrawal phenomenon, and Wernicke-Korsakoff syndrome.

2. Wernicke-Korsakoff syndrome

    a. Etiology. Ethanol interferes with thiamine (vitamin B1) absorption and ethanol-induced hepatic disease leads to decreased thiamine storage and decreased activation to coenzyme thiamine pyrophosphate. Although structural lesions have been identified, the exact mechanism for how thiamine deficiency leads to these lesions is unknown. Administration of glucose may deplete thiamine stores, precipitating Wernicke s disease. Thiamine deficiency may also lead to wet beriberi cardiomyopathy.

    b. Wernicke's encephalopathy. Ocular disturbances (diplopia, blurred vision, bidirectional nystagmus, lateral gaze palsy), gait ataxia, and confusion. These disturbances are amenable to thiamine therapy.

    c. Korsakoff psychosis. Permanent state of cognitive dysfunction characterized by the inability to remember recent events or learn new information (retrograde/anterograde amnesia) and confabulation. This may be a chronic form of Wernicke's encephalopathy and may not be amenable to thiamine replacement.

C. Alcohol withdrawal. A constellation of signs and symptoms associated with the cessation or reduction of alcohol intake in a tolerant individual, generally characterized by a hyperadrenergic state (for more on withdrawal, see Chapter 70).

    1. Minor. Minimal sympathetic symptoms including tremor, anxiety, sleep disturbance, nausea, vomiting, flushed skin, sweating, tachycardia or hypertension.Symptoms begin 6 to 8 h after alcohol intake is reduced and may last for several days.

    2. Moderate. Increased sympathetic symptoms and visual, auditory, tactile or olfactory hallucinations which occur 24 to 36 h after reduced ethanol intake. Despite hallucinations, the patient is usally oriented.

    3. Severe. Increased sympathetic symptoms with fever, altered mental status, or convulsions ("rum fits").

a. **Seizures.** One or more generalized tonic-clonic convulsions which occur 7 to 48 h after cessation of alcohol intake. A seizure may be the first manifestation of withdrawal before other symptoms. One third of patients with alcohol withdrawal seizures will develop delirium tremens. Patients with idiopathic or posttraumatic epilepsy may have seizures 6 to 24 h following even moderate doses of ethanol.

b. **Delerium tremens (DTs).** Autonomic hyperactivity with fever, tachycardia, tachypnea, hypertension, sweating, restlessness, agitation, confusion, disorientation, and hallucinations. DTs do not usually occur before 3 days of abstinence and are associated with a mortality rate of up to 15%, which may be related to concomitant medical problems.

4. **Other neurologic manifestations.** Cerebellar degeneration, peripheral neuropathy

D. **Alcoholic ketoacidosis**

1. **Etiology.** The patient with chronic alcoholism stops eating and drinking because of significant abdominal pain. Hormonal and metabolic derangements on top of depleted hepatic glycogen stores lead to increased lipolysis and oxidation of free fatty acids to the ketoacids B-hydroxybutyrate and acetoacetate.

2. **Clinical.** Symptoms may include nausea, vomiting, abdominal pain, anorexia, hypothermia, hypotension, tachycardia, Kussmaul (hyperpneic) respirations, fruity breath odor. Metabolic derangements generally resolve in 12 to 24 h with therapy.

3. **Laboratory.** There is a positive anion-gap metabolic acidosis with positive urine and serum ketones. Mixed acid-base disorders due to concomitant medical illness may complicate the evaluation. Acidosis is frequently accompanied by hypokalemia (for more on anion-gap acidoses, see Chapter 12).

E. Other clinical effects of chronic alcoholism

1. **Cardiovascular.** Cardiomyopathy, arrhythmias.

2. **Hematologic.** Bone marrow depression, thrombocytopenia, anemia, leukopenia.

3. **Infectious.** Cellulitis, meningitis, peritonitis, pneumonia, sepsis.

4. **Metabolic.** Hyperuricemia, hypoalbuminemia, hypocalcemia, hypoglycemia, hypokalemia, hypomagnesemia, hypophosphatemia, lactic acidosis, hyperthermia, hypothermia.

5. **Nutritional.** Pellagra, beriberi.

6. **Psychiatric.** Alcoholic hallucinosis, depression, bipolar disorder, personality disorders, suicide.

7. **Teratogenic.** Fetal alcohol syndrome.

VII. **Laboratory**

A. **Serum ethanol concentration.** Following acute intoxication in nontolerant individuals, a higher BAC is associated with more significant neurologic impairment (Table 66-1). Individual variation in pharmacokinetics and tolerance make it difficult to associate specific clinical findings with a particular BAC. Many states have adopted the level of 80 to 100 mg/dL as a legal definition of intoxication. Fatalities have been associated with ethanol doses of approximately 3 g/kg in children and 5 to 8 g/kg in adults; fatalities are generally associated with BACs greater than 500 mg/dl.

B. **Serum osmolality** may be a helpful surrogate if BACs are unavailable. If there is a significant difference between the measured and calculated (estimated) serum osmolalities, some of the difference may be attributable to ethanol. Serum osmolality increases approximately 0.22 mOsm/L for each 1 mg/dL in serum ethanol. Serum osmolality may also be increased by methanol and ethylene glycol (see Chapter 15).

C. **Exhaled air ethanol analyzers ("breathalyzers")** give relatively accurate approximations of BAC as long as the patient is cooperative and has not ingested any ethanol-containing products, belched, or vomited within 15 to 30 min of the assay. At equilibrium, the alveolar air/blood ratio of ethanol is 1:2,100.

D. **Saliva ethanol assays** can give a qualitative estimate of the serum ethanol concentration as long as the patient has not ingested any ethanol-containing substance near the time of the assay.

E. **Serum glucose.** Hypoglycemia may be observed, especially in children or malnourished adults.

F. In order to evaluate the **differential diagnosis** of intoxication or chronic health effects, other diagnostic studies may be useful, such as the following.

   1. Arterial blood gas
   2. Electrocardiogram
   3. Serum electrolytes, blood urea nitrogen, creatinine, calcium, phosphorus, and magnesium
   4. Complete blood count
   5. Urinalysis
   6. Stool guaiac
   7. Cervical spine x-rays
   8. Computed tomography (CT)
   9. Lumbar puncture
   10. Serum ketones
   11. Amylase
   12. Urine or serum toxicologic screen

VIII. **Management**

A. **Airway/breathing.** Insure a patent airway in the patient with altered mental status and significant CNS depression. For patients who cannot maintain their own airway, endotracheal or nasotracheal intubation is indicated.

B. **Circulation.** Hypovolemia or shock should be treated with fluid resuscitation. Initial resuscitation may be performed with isotonic saline solutions. In the setting of ethanol intoxication, dextrose containing fluids may also be appropriate, particularly as a maintenance fluid.

   1. Adults: 1 to 2 L initial fluid bolus
   2. Children: 20 mL/kg initial fluid bolus

C. Altered mental status

   1. A patient with a depressed level of consciousness with depressed respirations may be opioid intoxicated and should receive naloxone, 1 to 2 mg i.v. as an initial bolus.
   2. An accurate fingerstick glucose level may be determined by glucometer. If there is evidence of hypoglycemia or if a rapid glucose measurement is

unavailable, glucose should be administered at a starting dose of 0.5 to 1.0 g/kg.

    a.   Adults—$D_{50}W$: 50 to 100 mL i.v. (1 to 2 mL/kg)

    b.   Children—$D_{25}W$: 2 to 4 mL/kg. A 20 mL/kg bolus of i.v. fluid containing 5% dextrose (i.e., D_5W) will also deliver 1 g/kg dextrose.

   3.   Thiamine 100 mg i.v. will treat and may prevent Wernicke's encephalopathy. Thiamine, folate 1 mg, and a multivitamin solution can be added to the i.v. fluid solution.

D.   **Gastric decontamination.** Gastric decontamination is generally not indicated for acute ethanol intoxication because ethanol is rapidly absorbed and is unlikely to be recovered at the time a patient arrives to a health care facility. Ethanol is poorly adsorbed to activated charcoal. If ethanol intoxication is a complicating factor of another significant toxic ingestion, gastric decontamination and the administration of activated charcoal may be indicated. If gastric lavage is considered in the comatose or lethargic patient, the patient should be intubated to protect the airway during the procedure. Syrup of ipecac is rarely indicated in the acutely intoxicated adult, especially in the setting of depressed mental status or depressed levels of consciousness.

E.   **Hemodialysis** will increase the elimination of ethanol and can be considered for a patient with an extremely high BAC, and severe acid-base and electrolyte abnormalities which do not respond to more general therapeutic strategies.

F.   **Withdrawal.** In order to treat withdrawal, a sedative-hypnotic agent to which the patient is cross-tolerant, such as a benzodiazepine or a barbiturate is preferred. Occasionally, exceedingly large doses are necessary to sedate the withdrawing patient and in these cases, the patient may need to be intubated. Butyrophenones and phenothiazines have the disadvantage of lowering the seizure threshold and interfering with thermoregulation (for more on withdrawal, see Chapter 70).

   1.   Diazepam 5 to 20 mg i.v./p.o. q4h p.r.n. mild symptoms

   2.   Diazepam 10 to 20 mg i.v. every 20 min until moderate symptoms resolve and then prn recurrence of symptoms

   3.   Diazepam 10 to 40 mg i.v. every 20 min until severe symptoms resolve, up to 200 mg total dose. If the clinical response is still inadequate, then intubate the patient and start pentobarbital 3 to 5 mg/kg i.v. bolus followed by 100 mg/h (1 to 3 mg/kg/h) as a continuous infusion, titrated to clinical effect. Pentobarbital may cause hypotension.

   4.   Other therapeutic regimens utilizing lorazepam or chlordiazepoxide can also be utilized.

G.   **Metabolic derangements.** Alcoholic ketoacidosis is managed with volume resuscitation and dextrose administration as described above. Other fluid and electrolyte abnormalities such as hypokalemia or hypomagnesemia should be corrected if identified.

H.   **Psychiatric evaluation.** Following necessary medical therapy, patients with acute psychiatric illness such as suicidal ideation require immediate evaluation. Patients seeking alcohol detoxification may also benefit from urgent evaluation. Any patient with an apparent drinking problem should be referred for counseling.

IX. **Disposition**

A. Mild/moderate acute ethanol intoxication can generally be managed with hydration and observation. When the patient is awake, thinking clearly, and able to ambulate without assistance, he/she may be discharged, preferably in the company of a family member or friend. Outpatient followup should be arranged.

B. Admission is indicated for the following:

1. Significant respiratory depression or altered mental status.
2. Moderate or severe withdrawal.
3. Any significant metabolic derangement requiring medical management.
4. Any significant medical complication of alcoholism.
5. Significant mixed overdose.
6. Significant trauma.
7. Suicidal ideation.
8. Any child and most adolescents.
9. Patients without appropriate home-care settings.

Acknowledgement: The author would like to acknowledge the work of J. Albert Avila, Eric W. Schmidt, and Constance G. Nichols, who contributed to this chapter in an earlier edition.

Selected Readings

Harwood-Nuss A, ed. Emergency aspects of alcoholism. *Emerg Med Clin North Am* 1990;8:731–956.

Mendelson JH, Mello NK, eds. *Medical diagnosis and treatment of alcoholism.* New York: McGraw-Hill, 1992.

Seventh special report to the U.S. Congress on alcohol and health. Rockville, MD: U.S. Department of Health and Human Services, 1990.

Valenzuela CF, Harris RA. Alcohol: neurobiology. In: Lowinson JH, Ruiz P, Millman RB, Langrod JG, eds. *Substance abuse: a comprehensive textbook.* 3rd ed. Baltimore: Williams & Wilkins, 1997.

Emergency Toxicology, Second Edition,
edited by Peter Viccellio.
Lippincott–Raven Publishers, Philadelphia © 1998.

67

Nicotine

Jeffrey R. Brubacher

*Department of Emergency Medicine, Vancouver General Hospital and Health Sciences
Medicine, Vancouver, British Columbia, Canada V6N2G7*

I. **Introduction.** Nicotine use in the form of cigarette smoking is widespread. In the United States, an estimated 28% of adults are smokers (1). Nicotine is highly addictive; between one-third and one-half of occasional users become regular smokers. Ninety percent of smokers have tried to quit, but only 2% to 3% succeed in any given year. Adolescents are a major target of tobacco company advertising dollars, and an estimated 3,000 adolescents start smoking regularly every day. Seventy-five percent of adult smokers become "addicted" before age 21. The chronic health effects of tobacco are well known. An estimated 400,000 Americans will die from tobacco-related diseases such as coronary artery disease, COPD, and lung cancer (1–3). The potential for acute toxicity from nicotine is less appreciated. Most cases of acute nicotine toxicity occur in children who ingest cigarette butts, nicotine patches, or nicotine chewing gum. Toxicity in these cases is usually mild (4). Severe toxicity and death has occurred however following ingestion of concentrated liquid nicotine (5,6).

II. **Sources of nicotine.** Cigarettes are the most common source of nicotine and are responsible for chronic toxicity, but rarely cause acute toxicity. The most common sources of ingested nicotine are nicotine gum, discarded cigarette butts, and nicotine patches. There is a considerable amount of nicotine remaining in cigarettes and used nicotine patches. Tobacco workers who absorb nicotine from green tobacco leaves may suffer from green tobacco sickness (7,8). People have become ill from ingesting salad made of tobacco (9). Concentrated nicotine was formerly used as a pesticide. Enemas made from boiling tobacco in water have been used for treating intestinal parasites and constipation (6,10). Table 67-1 lists the nicotine content of various sources of nicotine.

III. **Pharmacology**

    A. **Mechanism of action and toxicity.** Nicotine binds to specific acetylcholine receptors known as nicotinic receptors. These receptors are found at autonomic ganglia, at neuromuscular junctions, in the adrenal medulla, and in the CNS. In the brain, the highest concentrations of nicotine receptors are in the limbic system, the brain stem, and the midbrain. Low doses of nicotine will stimulate these receptors, whereas high doses will depress them. Postganglionic muscarinic acetylcholine receptors are found in parasympathetic nerves and in the sympathetic nerves that mediate sweating. While muscarinic receptors are not directly affected by nicotine, they will be stimulated indirectly due to increased firing of preganglionic fibers. Thus, in the autonomic

TABLE 67-1. *Sources of nicotine*

Source	Concentration of nicotine
Cigarettes	13–30 mg total nicotine per cigarette (delivered nicotine is much less)
	5–7 mg nicotine in a discarded cigarette butt
	3–8 mg total nicotine in a "low-nicotine" cigarette
Cigars	15–40 mg total nicotine
Chewing tobacco	~7.8 mg nicotine/gram
Snuff	~14 mg nicotine/gram tobacco
Nicotine resin gum	2 or 4 mg/piece
Nicotine patches	8.3–114 mg/patch
Green tobacco leaves	1.5–5.4% nicotine by dry weight
Tobacco enemas	Cigarettes or tobacco soaked in water, administered as enema; treatment for intestinal parasites or constipation; high (variable) concentrations of nicotine
Nicotine-containing pesticides	Nicotine sulfate and other salts, discontinued by 1950; ~40% nicotine

nervous system, stimulation of preganglionic nerves results in combined sympathetic and parasympathetic stimulation. Stimulation of nicotinic receptors at the neuromuscular junction results in fasciculations, muscle weakness, and paralysis. At the adrenal glands, nicotine causes catecholamine release. Central nicotine receptor stimulation is responsible for the addicting properties of nicotine. Low doses of nicotine may have beneficial effects such as increased alertness, improved memory, and improved mood. In overdose, nicotine acts centrally to cause headache, agitation, seizures, confusion, and coma. Acute nicotine toxicity is the net result of stimulation followed by depression of all these receptors (11).

B.   Pharmacokinetics. Nicotine is a water and lipid soluble tertiary amine, composed of a pyridine and a pyrrolidine ring. Inhaled nicotine in cigarette smoke is rapidly absorbed through pulmonary capillaries and delivered in high concentrations to the brain. The average cigarette will deliver 1 to 3 mg of nicotine when smoked. Nicotine in chewing tobacco, cigars, and pipe smoke is readily absorbed across the buccal mucosa. Nicotine in liquid pesticides or dissolved in the dew on moist tobacco leaves is readily absorbed percutaneously. Ingested nicotine is well absorbed in the gastrointestinal tract (GI) but has a significant first-pass effect. This first-pass effect is avoided by smokers or by those who chew tobacco. Once absorbed, the half-life of nicotine is 1 to 4 h. About 80% of absorbed nicotine is metabolized to cotinine in the liver and the remainder is excreted unchanged in the urine. Cigarette smoking induces the hepatic enzymes responsible for nicotine metabolism such that chronic smokers metabolize the drug more rapidly. The "therapeutic" level of nicotine in the average pack per day smoker is 25 to 35 ng/mL. Smokers will usually adjust their smoking habits to maintain this level even when using low-nicotine cigarettes. This can be attained by inhaling more deeply, inhaling more frequently, or smoking more cigarettes. The volume of distribution of nicotine is about 1 L/kg (10–12). Cigarette smoke induces hepatic microsomal enzymes. This results in enhanced metabolism of many drugs including theophylline, warfarin, propranolol, lidocaine, caffeine, and nicotine. Ethanol appears to enhance the cardiovascular response to nicotine causing increased heart rate and blood pressure. Thus smokers may be at greater risk of dysrhythmias and sudden death when they consume ethanol (13).

IV. **Clinical presentation.** The chronic effects of cigarette smoking are well known and will not be discussed here. The majority of acute exposures to nicotine occur in children who ingest cigarettes, cigarette butts, nicotine patches or nicotine gum. These ingestions are usually benign. In the past four years, there were 38,295 ingestions of tobacco products reported to the American association of poison control centers toxic exposure surveillance system. Of these, there were no fatalities and only 22 cases of major toxicity (14–17). The most common findings are minor GI complaints such as nausea, vomiting, and diarrhea (4,18). More severe symptoms such as pallor, salivation, tachycardia, hypertension, lethargy, unresponsiveness, apnea, and seizures have been reported following ingestions of these products but are clearly uncommon (5,19–21). Symptoms correlate with amount ingested: ingestion of fewer than three cigarette butts, one pinch of snuff or part of a cigarette typically result in minimal or no symptoms. On the other hand, most children who ingest an entire cigarette, nicotine chewing gum, or more than 7.5 g of snuff will develop symptoms (4). Nicotine patches contain large amounts of nicotine even after use and severe toxicity might be anticipated after ingestion of these patches. Adults who chew the product often develop severe toxicity that may include seizures and coma (22,23). The majority of pediatric exposures to nicotine patches reported to date have been inconsequential (23,24). Toxicity may also develop from dermal application of these patches. Concentrated nicotine in liquid form causes a rapid onset of severe toxicity. Seizures, coma, respiratory muscle weakness, and cardiovascular arrest may occur within minutes of ingestion or rectal administration of these products (6,25,26). Initial hypertension and tachycardia is followed by hypotension and bradycardia. Patients will have muscle fasciculations followed by weakness or paralysis. Intercostal muscle weakness may result in respiratory failure (25). Severe nicotine poisoning will often resemble organophosphate poisoning with diaphoresis, salivation, diarrhea, vomiting, bronchospasm, increased respiratory secretions, and muscle weakness. Persons who work in the tobacco industry may develop symptoms of mild nicotine toxicity. Dew collected on wet tobacco leaves contains nicotine that can be absorbed through the skin. Affected workers develop "green tobacco illness," a syndrome of nausea, vomiting, dizziness, headache, and weakness. Dust in tobacco processing factories contains nicotine that can be inhaled and absorbed through the lungs resulting in similar symptoms (7,8,27).

V. **Laboratory findings.** Laboratory abnormalities in nicotine poisoning are reflective of end-organ involvement. Severe toxicity may cause acidosis or hypoxia. Electrocardiographic abnormalities should be sought in severely symptomatic persons. Serum and urine nicotine levels can be determined and may rarely be helpful in diagnosis if history is unavailable. Nicotine levels will not affect acute management, however, and should not be sent routinely in patients with known ingestion of nicotine containing products.

VI. **Management.** GI decontamination decisions should be made with awareness of the following facts: most ingestions of tobacco products result in minimal toxicity, vomiting is an early manifestation of nicotine toxicity, and severe nicotine toxicity is characterized by rapid development of seizures, coma, or respiratory failure. For these reasons, induction of emesis is contraindicated and orogastric lavage should be reserved for persons with severe toxicity who have not vomited or for those with massive ingestions who present prior to emesis. The majority of persons who seek medical care after nicotine ingestion require activated charcoal only. Asymptomatic children who have ingested only part of a cigarette, a few cigarette butts, or a small amount of snuff (one pinch or less) can be managed without GI decontamination. Skin decontamination is important in toxicity from nicotine patches or liquid nicotine preparations. There is no specific antidote for nicotine toxicity and medical care is supportive. Patients who are hypertensive and a tachycardic following nicotine ingestion should be managed expectantly since these findings are transient and typically followed by hypotension and bradycardia. Nicotine induced seizures should be treated with benzodiazepines followed by barbiturates. Other causes of seizures, particularly hypoxia, should be sought and corrected. Respiratory failure is common in severe nicotine poisoning both because of muscle weakness and from parasympathetic stimulation resulting in bronchospasm and increased bronchial secretions. The patient's respiratory status must be carefully and repeatedly assessed. Endotracheal intubation and mechanical ventilation decisions should be made according to the usual criteria. Atropine should be given to patients with severe muscarinic symptoms, particularly bradycardia or hypoxia from respiratory secretions and bronchospasm. The endpoint of atropine administration in patients with hypoxia from muscarinic excess is correction of the hypoxia. Tachycardia is not a contraindication to atropine in this setting and may resolve with correction of hypoxia. Hypotension is first treated with fluids. Pressors may be required if this is not successful. If the history is unreliable, the clinician should consider poisoning with other agents. Caustic ingestion should be considered in the child with salivation and vomiting after an unknown ingestion. Management in this case may include endoscopy. Persons who develop vomiting, diarrhea, respiratory secretions, hypoxia, and other muscarinic symptoms after an unknown ingestion should be considered to have taken an organophosphate or a carbamate. In addition to atropine, these patients should receive pralidoxime. Early nicotine toxicity may cause dilated pupils, diaphoresis, hypertension, tachycardia, and agitation and mimic poisoning with cocaine or amphetamines. Cooling and benzodiazepines are important in the management as in patients with cocaine toxicity. Determination of acetaminophen levels, assessment of acid-base status with either arterial blood gas or measurement of anion gap, and an electrocardiogram to screen for tricyclic toxicity are essential in the evaluation of every patient following an intentional overdose.

VII. **Disposition.** Children who are asymptomatic after ingestion of part of a cigarette, a cigarette butt, or a small amount of snuff may often be managed at home. GI complaints such as vomiting may herald more severe symptoms and mandate hospital evaluation. Ingestions of an entire cigarette, of more than three cigarette butts, or of nicotine gum are usually followed by symptoms, and all such children should have a medical evaluation. There are limited data concerning outcome after ingestion of nicotine patches by a child. Most of these ingestions appear to be benign (28) unless the patch was chewed, but there is still a concern about possible delayed toxicity. For this reason, we recommend that all children who have ingested a nicotine patch receive activated charcoal and a medical evaluation. All adults who have ingested any form of nicotine with suicidal intent require medical and psychiatric evaluation. Symptoms following nicotine ingestions occur rapidly. A person who remains asymptomatic or whose symptoms have resolved after a 4-h observation period may be safely cleared medically. Nicotine patches may have the potential for delayed toxicity. We recommend a 6-h observation period for children who have ingested a nicotine patch. In addition parents should observe for vomiting, excess salivation, and other signs of nicotine toxicity and return to the emergency department should these occur. Persons with persistent symptoms should be admitted to hospital. Patients with protracted vomiting, seizures, muscle fasciculations or weakness, hypoxia, unstable vital signs, or other significant findings require admission to an intensive care setting where cardiac monitoring and cardio-respiratory support is available.

References

1. Anderson Y. Tobacco ingestions in children. *Clin Pediatr* 1989;28:592–593.
2. Benowitz NL, Jones RT, Jacob P. Additive cardiovascular effects of nicotine and ethanol. *Clin Pharmacol Ther* 1986;40: 420–424.
3. Borys DJ, Setzer SC, Ling L. CNS depression in an infant after the ingestion of tobacco: a case report. *Vet Hum Toxicol* 1988;30:20–22.
4. Boylan B, Brandt V, Muehlbauer J, et al. Green tobacco sickness in tobacco harvesters—Kentucky, 1992. *MMWR* 1993;42: 237–240.
5. Califano JA. The wrong way to stay slim. *N Engl J Med* 1995;333:1214–1216.
6. Caraccio T, Litovitz T. Toxicity from transdermal nicotine patch exposures [Abstract]. *Vet Hum Toxicol* 1993;35:349.
7. Fiore MC. Trends in cigarette smoking in the United States: the epidemiology of tobacco use. *Med Clin North Am* 1992;76:289–303.
8. Garcia-Estrada H, Fishman CM. An unusual case of nicotine poisoning. *Clin Toxicol* 1977;10:391–393.
9. Ghosh SK, Parikh JR, Gokani VN, et al. Occupational health problems among tobacco processing workers: a preliminary study. *Arch Environ Health* 1985;40:318–321.
10. Harchelroad F, Potts K, Burdick J, et al. Oral absorption of nicotine from transdermal therapeutic systems [Abstract]. *Vet Hum Toxicol* 1992;34:332.
11. Henningfield JE. Nicotine medications for smoking cessation. *N Engl J Med* 1995;333:1196–1203.
12. Lavoic FW, Harris TM. Fatal nicotine ingestion. *J Emerg Med* 1991;9:133–136.
13. Le Houzec J, Benowitz NL. Basic and clinical psychopharmacology of nicotine. *Clin Chest Med* 1991;12:681–699.
14. Litovitz TL, Holm KC, Bailey KM, et al. 1991 Annual report of the American Association of Poison Control Centers national data collecting system. *Am J Emerg Med* 1992;10:452–505.
15. Litovitz TL, Holm KC, Bailey KM, et al. 1992 Annual report of the American Association of Poison Control Centers toxic exposure surveillance system. *Am J Emerg Med* 1993;11:494–555.
16. Litovitz TL, Holm KC, Bailey KM, et al. 1993 Annual report of the American Association of Poison Control Centers toxic exposure surveillance system. *Am J Emerg Med* 1994;12:546–584.
17. Litovitz TL, Holm KC, Bailey KM, et al. 1994 Annual report of the American Association of Poison Control Centers toxic exposure surveillance system. *Am J Emerg Med* 1995;13:551–597.
18. Malizia E, Andreucci F, Alfani F. Acute intoxication with nicotine alkaloids and cannabinoids in children from ingestion of cigarettes. *Hum Toxicol* 1983;2:315–316.
19. Manoguerra AS, Freeman D. Acute poisoning from the ingestion of nicotiana glauca. *J Toxicol Clin Toxicol* 1983;19: 861–864.
20. McGinnis JM, Foege WH. Actual causes of death in the United States. *JAMA* 1993;270:2207–2212.
21. McKnight RH, Levine EJ. Detection of green tobacco illness by a regional poison center. *Vet Human Toxicol* 1994;36: 505–510.
22. Oberst BB, McIntyre RA. Acute nicotine poisoning: case report. *Pediatrics* 1953;11:338–340.
23. Salomon M. Nicotine. In: Goldfrank LG, Flomembaum NE, Lewin NA, et al., eds. *Goldfrank's toxicologic emergencies.* 5th ed. Norwalk, CT: Appleton & Lange, 1994:997–1008.
24. Saxena K, Scheman A. Suicide plan by nicotine poisoning: a review of nicotine toxicity. *Vet Hum Toxicol* 1985; 27:495–497.
25. Singer J, Janz T. Apnea and seizures caused by nicotine ingestion. *Pediatr Emerg Care* 1990;6:135–137.
26. Smolinske SC, Spoerke DG, Wruk KM, et al. Cigarette and nicotine chewing gum toxicity in children. *Hum Toxicol* 1988;7:27–31.
27. Woolf AD, Burkhart K, Caraccio T, et al. Toxicity from transdermal nicotine patch exposure [Abstract]. *Vet Hum Toxicol* 1993;35:349.
28. Yuen JA, Ashbourne JF, Croteau DR. Review of transdermal nicotine exposures [Abstract]. *Vet Hum Toxicol* 1993;35:349.

Emergency Toxicology, Second Edition,
edited by Peter Viccellio.
Lippincott–Raven Publishers, Philadelphia © 1998.

68

Abuse of Volatile Substances

Francis J. DeRoos

Department of Emergency Medicine, University of Pennsylvania, Philadelphia, Pennsylvania 19104

I. **Introduction.** The deliberate inhalation of volatile compounds for their intoxicating effects is best termed volatile substance abuse (VSA). Other terms used to describe this practice include glue sniffing, solvent abuse, and inhalant misuse. The vast majority of these abused substances are hydrocarbons although any volatile compound (defined as a substance that is gaseous or readily evaporates at room temperature, that produces a desirable alteration in cognitive function and is minimally irritating to the mucous membranes and lungs) can be used. In addition, these products tend to be inexpensive, legally obtained, and readily available such as common household products. The typical volatile substance user is a young adolescent male living in an impoverished environment (1). They are more likely to use other drugs, particularly ethanol, their families tend to be broken and dysfunctional, and they adjust and perform poorly in school. Some studies have reported anywhere from a 3% to 13% prevalence of solvent abuse in high school students. This is probably an underestimation because solvent abusers tend to drop out of school, which is where most of these data are collected (2). Although the majority of use is limited to a brief period of social experimentation, over one fifth of the deaths are in first-time users (3). In addition, some patients progress to become chronic volatile substance users into adulthood or possibly move on to "harder" drugs such as opioids (4). Other unique demographic groups associated with VSA include Native Americans, polydrug users in which VSA are only used occasionally when their "drug of choice" is not available, and industrial workers with access to solvents at the worksite (5,6). Many different terms are associated with VSA. Sniffing refers to directly inhaling vapors from a container, such as a typewriter correction fluid bottle. Huffing refers to inhaling vapors from a cloth that is saturated with the volatile substance and held over or near the nose and mouth. Bagging refers to inhaling and exhaling into a bag that has been filled with a small amount of a volatile substance. Initial solvent abuse involves sniffing, but as experience and possibly tolerance increases, abusers progress to huffing and ultimately bagging. This progression of methods corresponds to the increase in inspired solvent concentration.

II. **Sources of agents.** Most volatile substances are hydrocarbons that are readily available as common household products and can be divided into six structural classes. Table 68–1 highlights these six structural classes, and lists common sources and typical examples for each. Many common sources contain several different volatile agents so the toxicity may be difficult to ascribe to one particular compound. In addition, many studies have demonstrated that various populations have "favorite" agents of abuse. This selectivity is often dictated by avail-

TABLE 68-1. *Chemical classes, common sources, and typical examples of volatile substances*

General chemical class	Common sources	Typical examples
Aliphatic hydrocarbons	Motor fuel	Gasoline
	Stove and lamp fuel	Kerosine
	Lighter fuel	Butane, isopropane
	Plastic, rubber cement	*n*-Hexane
	Hair spray	Butane, propane
Halogenated hydrocarbons	Solvent	Carbon tetrachloride (rare now)
	Typewriter correction fluid	Trichloroethylene (TCE)
	Paint, varnish remover	Methylene chloride
	Spot remover	1,1,1-Trichloroethane (TCA), TCE
	Dry cleaning agents	Tetrachloroethylene (perchloroethylene)
	Aerosol propellant	Chlorofluorocarbons (Freons)
	Refrigerant	Chlorofluorocarbons (Freons)
Aromatic hydrocarbons	Solvent	Benzene, dimethylbenzene (xylene)
	Airplane glue	Toluene
	Spray paints	Toluene
Aliphatic nitrites	Room "odorizers"	Isobutyl nitrite, butyl nitrite
	Cyanide antidote kit	Amyl nitrite
Ketones	Solvent	Most ketones
	Nail polish remover	Acetone
Ethers	Solvent	Many ethers
	Computer cleaner	Dimethyl ether

ability and not necessarily potency (7). Aliphatic hydrocarbons are straight chain molecules containing one to 16 saturated carbons. As their length increases so does their viscosity. Examples include butane, hexane, gasoline, and kerosene. They are used primarily as fuels and lubricants. Halogenated hydrocarbons are aliphatic chains with one or several halogen substitutions including F, Cl, Br, and I. These are highly volatile and frequently abused. Examples include methylene chloride, chloroform, carbon tetrachloride, trichloroethylene, 1,1,1-trichloroethane, the chlorofluorocarbons (trade name Freon compounds), and halothane. Common sources include many solvents and spot removers, refrigerant fluid, and aerosol propellants. Several brands of typewriter correction fluid, traditionally containing 1,1,1-trichloroethane, have eliminated this halogenated compound in favor of a less toxic aliphatic hydrocarbon, naphtha. Aromatic hydrocarbons are all based upon benzene which is a six carbon ringed structure with alternating single and double bonds. Examples include benzene, toluene (methylbenzene), and xylene (dimethylbenzene). These chemicals can be found in many solvents particularly those for paint (in spray paint), glues, and plastics. Because of their abundance and rapid CNS penetration these are frequently abused. Alkyl nitrites are aliphatic chains containing a nitrite group ($R-NO_2$). These are unique because they are abused as sexual enhancers in young males particularly in the homosexual community. Two common examples include amyl nitrite and isobutyl nitrite. Amyl nitrite is a medicinal found in pearls in the cyanide antidote kit and as a vasodilator. Isobutyl nitrite is widely available as a room odorizer. Common brandnames include "Black Jack," "Hardware," "Locker Room," "Rush," and "Satan's Scent" (8). Ethers are compounds in which two aliphatic groups are joined by an oxygen molecule (general formula R-O-R′). The carbon side chains can have alkyl substitutions. Chemical examples include "ether" (which is actually diethyl ether), dibutyl ether, and methyl propyl ether. These can also be found in various solvents particularly for dyes, gums, paints, and oils and as a high-energy fuel source to prime engines or as rocket fuel (9). Ketones are compounds in which two aliphatic or aromatic groups are joined by a carbon that is double-bonded to an oxygen molecule. General formula R-(C=O)-R'. The smaller the side groups, the more volatile, and the more frequently abused, the substance. Examples include acetone, methylethyl ketone (MEK), and methyl isobutyl ketone. Sources of abuse include nail polish remover and other solvents for varnishes, gums, and adhesives.

III. **Pharmacokinetics.** Although VSA encompasses a vast group of compounds they all tend to be highly lipophilic. This allows them to be easily absorbed through the lungs, and obtain rapid serum levels with subsequent distribution to the brain and other highly fatty organs. Although the data is limited, protein binding appears to be small while the volumes of distribution are relatively great for most of these compounds. Thus while serum levels may peak within 15 to 30 min after a hit of a particular substance, its half-life may be hours or days. Elimination is determined by the substance's primary chemical classification. In general, aliphatics, halogenated hydrocarbons, ethers, and ketones leave the serum the way they entered; via pulmonary ventilation. In contrast the aromatics tend to undergo oxidation via the hepatic mixed function oxidases (P-450's) and subsequent conjugation with glycine and sometimes glucuronic acid. For example, toluene is first oxidized into benzoic acid and subsequently conjugated with glycine forming hippuric acid (10). These conjugated metabolites are then eliminated in the urine. Alkyl nitrites may undergo direct hydrolysis into free nitrite and an alcohol. Several halogenated hydrocarbons undergo complex oxidative metabolism within the liver. This varies for each particular agent.

IV. **Clinical presentation and pathophysiology.** While all of these compounds are abused for their CNS effects, several classes of compounds also have significant toxicity to other organ systems. This discussion of the clinical presentation and mechanisms of toxicity will be organized by organ system rather than each structural class to avoid redundancy. Please refer to Table 68-2 for a general overview of the toxic manifestations of each structural class.

  A. **CNS**

      1. **Acute.** The most prominent physiologic manifestation of VSA is the acute alteration in cognitive function sought by abusers. Clinically the acute central depressive effects are nonspecific and similar to ethanol intoxication. Initially they include euphoria, disinhibition, and excitation. As the intoxication increases drowsiness, incoordination of speech and gait, hallucinations, and disorientation develop. The most potent agents, notoriously the halogenated hydrocarbons, can also induce profound obtundation and coma (7). The disinhibitive effects place abusers at high risk for trauma and unlawful activity. These agents are felt to act by altering neural membrane function rather than effecting neurotransmitters directly (11). The effects typically last for 0.5 to 2 h but may last much longer depending upon each substance's rate of elimination as well as whether the abuser was repetitively dosing or "stacking" his doses while still inebriated. The signs and symptoms of acute intoxication appear to follow a dose-related progression so the greater the blood level, the more profound the intoxication (12,13). While there is no evidence of physical addiction developing, this inebriated state can be psychologically craved (7).

TABLE 68-2. *Clinical manifestations of each chemical classification*

General chemical class	Clinical manifestations
Aliphatic hydrocarbons General, *n*-hexane	Acute and chronic encephalopathy Myocardial sensitization to catecholamines Peripheral neuropathy
Halogenated hydrocarbons General, methylene chloride, halothane, carbon tetrachloride	Acute and chronic encephalopathy Myocardial sensitization to catecholamines Carbon monoxide Hepatic failure
Aromatic hydrocarbons General, benzene, toluene	Acute and chronic encephalopathy Myocardial sensitization to catecholamines Multiple myeloma Aplastic anemia Acute myelocytic leukemia Type I (distal) renal tubular acidosis
Aliphatic nitrites	Acute encephalopathy Methemoglobinemia Hemolytic anemia
Ketones General, methyl n-butyl ketone (MBK)	Acute and chronic encephalopathy Peripheral neuropathy
Ethers General	Acute and chronic encephalopathy

2. **Chronic.** Long-term abuse of these agents can also produce permanent cerebral encephalopathy. These abnormalities can vary from mild cognitive deficits to profound dementia (14,15). The mildest effects, often termed an organic affective syndrome, involve reversible mood changes such as irritability, depression, and apathy (16). With longer periods of abuse, signs may progress to short term memory and psychomotor deficits. The most severe chronic encephalopathy develops as a result of long term abuse, usually years, and is often associated with demonstrable structural CNS damage such as cortical atrophy (15). This dementia manifests with significant impairment in judgment, personality, and cognitive abilities. Other well-described syndromes often associated with this dementia include Parkinsonism, cerebellar dysfunction, and optic neuropathy, and other cranial neuropathies, particularly V and VII (17,18). In general as the severity of the encephalopathy increases, the reversibility becomes less likely and the prevalence of structural abnormalities progressively greater (16). While the pathophysiology of this chronic encephalopathy is not well characterized, it is not hard to imagine how these organic solvents may slowly "dissolve" the highly lipid brain away over time. Typical pathologic findings include gliosis of the long tracts with cerebral and cerebellar atrophy (19). Before 1976 when tetraethyl lead was still present in U.S. gasoline, lead encephalopathy was an additional hazard reported in gasoline sniffers (20,21).

B. Peripheral nervous system. Two volatile substances have been definitively associated with peripheral neuropathies namely *N*-hexane (an aliphatic) and methyl butyl ketone (a ketone). Both of these compounds are metabolized to a neurotoxin, 2,5-hexadione, which is responsible for the peripheral neuropathy (22). This neuropathy is an insidious and painless sensorimotor polyneuropathy which follows a glove and stocking distribution. The small fibers (i.e., those involved in light touch and temperature) are affected initially and symptoms progress from distal to proximal. It is classified as distal axonopathy or "dying back" neuropathy which is the typically caused by most neurotoxins (23). Interestingly, a similar compound methyl ethyl ketone does not produce a peripheral neuropathy alone but significantly potentiates *n*-hexanes and methyl butyl ketones toxic effects (24). This synergistic effect of a nontoxic compound illustrates the difficulty in determining causal agents for clinical effects. Trichloroethylene has been associated with a slowly reversible trigeminal neuropathy since the 1940s when it was used as an anesthetic agent (25). It is postulated that its metabolites, including dichloroacetylene are the actual neurotoxic agents (26).

C. Cardiovascular. Perhaps the most common cause of death from VSA is from its cardiotoxic effects. This event was first labelled "sudden sniffing death" after a nationwide epidemic where adolescents acutely died from dysrhythmias in the setting of solvent abuse (27,28). The mechanism of toxicity is by potentiation of endogenous catecholamine effects upon the myocardium (29,30). This results in spontaneous ventricular tachycardia or fibrillation upon any stimulation. Aliphatic and halogenated hydrocarbons appear to be the most potent myocardial sensitizers although aromatic hydrocarbons have also been implicated (31,32). As with most anesthetic agents, direct myocardial depression can also occur during severe intoxications (33).

D. Hepatic. Several of the halogenated hydrocarbons, including halothane, chloroform, and carbon tetrachloride, have been associated with a central lobular hepatitis (34,35). This may present with signs and symptoms typical for any hepatitis such as jaundice, right upper quadrant pain, nausea and vomiting, malaise, and dark urine. The classic example is carbon tetrachloride, which was previously used as a spot remover. This agent which is metabolized via the mixed function oxidase system (P450) into a free radical (CCl_3) which peroxidizes membrane lipids thus destroying the hepatocyte (36).

E. Renal. Toluene, found in glues, spray paints, and varnishes and is a "favorite" volatile substance of abuse, can cause a type I (distal) renal tubular acidosis. This manifests with significant electrolyte disturbances including a hyperchloremic metabolic acidosis, profound hypokalemia (1.5 to 2.0 meq/dL), and hypophosphatemia (37). As a consequence of the severe hypokalemia and hypophosphatemia rhabdomyolysis may ensue with subsequent acute tubular necrosis. Weakness, fatigue, and abdominal pain are common complaints. On physical examination, the weakness is diffuse, symmetric, and can be as severe as quadraparesis. The mechanism for the cause of the renal tubular acidosis may involve interference with hydrogen ion transport or cell membrane permeability (38).

F. Hematologic. There are three distinct effects of abused solvents upon the hematopoietic system. The first two have the same clinical features as hypoxia including headache, fatigue, lightheadedness, and dyspnea. Methylene chloride, a common paint and varnish stripper, is metabolized in the liver into carbon monoxide (39). Carboxyhemoglobin levels can rise to toxic levels (as high as 50%) and may require therapy with 100%, or possibly hyperbaric, oxygen to avoid permanent cerebral injury (40,41). Alkyl nitrites, such as amyl nitrite and isobutyl nitrite, are potent oxidizing agents and can convert hemoglobin (Fe^{2+}) to methemoglobin (Fe^{3+}) (42). This impairs oxygen transport and the patient develops cyanosis, dyspnea, and fatigue. In addition, these agents can rarely produce a hemolytic anemia in patients susceptible to oxidizing stressors, such as those with G-6-P-D deficiency (43). Cyanosis is usually noted with methemoglobin levels over 15% of the total hemoglobin (42). Chronic exposure to benzene, an aromatic hydrocarbon which historically was used extensively in shoe manufacturing and currently as a general solvent, is associated with multiple myeloma and acute myelocytic leukemia (44). Benzene's toxicity is the result of its metabolites concentrating within the bone marrow and forming several cytotoxic compounds (45).

V.   Laboratory findings. Most patients who present acutely intoxicated with solvents or with a significant history of abuse should receive general laboratory studies including electrolytes, blood urea nitrogen, creatinine, urinalysis, ECG, and pulse oximetry. Consider measuring transaminases, bilirubin, alkaline phosphatase, and coagulation studies as markers of hepatic insult in halogenated hydrocarbon exposures. A complete blood count is indicated to screen for anemia, leukopenia, leukocytosis, and thrombocytopenia in aromatic exposures. If clinically suspected either by the contents of the product being abuse (high risk of methylene chloride exposure with a paint stripper) or the clinical presentation, carboxyhemoglobin and methemeglobin levels can be determined. An electrocardiogram should be obtained to evaluate for any dysrhythmias. In border states where patients have access to lead containing gasoline, blood lead levels should be sent. The diagnosis of sovent intoxication is based solely on clinical presentation. Although many of these agents can be identified in serum using gas chromatography and mass spectrometry, these techniques are not widely available, they are expensive and often time consuming, the substances in question may be present at very low levels in the serum (very lipophilic with large volume of distribution) and the results are seldom important (46). If quantitative results are obtained, however, they appear to correlate with the degree of toxicity (47,13). Qualitative screening of the urine for the metabolites of aromatic hydrocarbons. is used to monitor both workers at high risk of job site exposures and former volatile substance abusers during treatment programs.

VI.   Management. Treatment of acute solvent intoxication is primarily supportive. Initial evaluation and stabilization should focus on the patients ability to protect his airway and for dysrhythmias. Initial preparation includes cardiac monitoring, i.v. access, and, possibly, supplemental oxygen. Identification of all the products used is essential after patient stabilization. A poison information center or the manufacturer should be utilized to determine every ingredient. If any electrolyte abnormalities are present they should be corrected and rhabdomyolysis should be aggressively treated. Patients with evidence of a toxic hepatitis, typically from halogenated hydrocarbons, may benefit from n-acetylcysteine therapy (48). Patients with elevated carboxyhemoglobin levels after methylene chloride exposure should be treated using standard therapies. Patients with methemoglobin levels greater than 20% or those with symptoms or evidence of hypoxia should receive 1 to 2 mg/kg of methylene blue. The methylene blue enhances the enzymatic conversion of methemoglobin back to hemoglobin (42). If dysrhythmias occur, the strict adherence to standard resuscitation protocols may be detrimental.

Because these agents sensitize the myocardium to catecholamines, epinephrine, which is a first-line agent in ventricular tachycardia or fibrillation, may precipitate or worsen dysrhythmias. A more rational approach is the use of β receptor antagonists to blunt the myocardial response to catecholamines. Clinically, propranolol has been efficacious in stopping and suppressing dysrhythmias induced by another halogenated hydrocarbon and myocardial sensitizer, chloral hydrate (49). As with ethanol intoxication, patients with acute solvent intoxication should slowly return to their premorbid state within a few hours. If the patient worsens or does not improve cognitively over time, the patient should be reevaluated for other potential causes of altered mental status including intracranial injuries, infections (including sepsis and meningitis), and other intoxicants.

VII. **Disposition.** Patients who present clinically ill with dysrhythmias, profound CNS depression or seizures, those who have persistent cognitive dysfunction despite 4 to 6 h of observation, and those with electrolyte abnormalities, hepatitis, or rhabdomyolysis should all be admitted to the hospital for more intensive monitoring and therapy. Patients whose acute symptoms resolve over 4 to 6 h of observation and who are not chronic abusers may be discharged to a community primary care provider with a referral for substance abuse counseling. Those patients who clinically improve but who are significant abusers may benefit from intensive inpatient detoxification therapy.

References

1. Beauvais F. Volatile solvent abuse: trends and patterns. *NIDA Res Monogr* 1992;129:13–41.
2. Barnes GE. Solvent abuse: a review. *Int J Addict* 1979;14:1–26.
3. Johns A. Volatile solvent abuse and 963 deaths. *Br J Addict* 1991;86:1053–1056.
4. Dinwiddie SH, Reich T, Cloninger CR. The relationship of solvent use to other substance use. *Am J Drug Alcohol Abuse* 1991;17:173–186.
5. Coulehan JL, Hirsch W, Brillman J, et al. Gasoline sniffing and lead toxicity in Navaho adolescents. *Pediatrics* 1983;71:113–117.
6. Parker SE. Use and abuse of volatile substances in industry. *Hum Toxicol* 1989;8:271–275.
7. Rosenberg NL, Sharp CW. Solvent toxicity: a neurological focus. *NIDA Res Monogr* 1992;129:117–169.
8. Fisher AA. "Poppers" or "snappers" dermatitis in homosexual men. *Cutis* 1994;34:118–122.
9. Linden CH. Volatile substances of abuse. *Emerg Med Clin North Am* 1990;8:559–578.
10. von Oettingen F, Neal PA, Donahue DD. The toxicity and potential dangers of toluene: preliminary report. *JAMA* 1942;118:579–584.
11. Kalf G, Post G, Snyder R. Solvent toxicology: Recent advances in the toxicology of benzene, the glycol ethers, and carbon tetrachloride. *Ann Rev Phamacol Toxicol* 1987;27:399–427.
12. Benignus VA. Health effects of toluene: a review. *Neurotoxicology* 1981;2:567–588.
13. Mackay CJ, Campbell L, Samuel AM, et al. Behavioral changes during exposure to 1,1,1-trichloroethane: time-course and relationship to blood solvent levels. *Am J Ind Med* 1987;11:223–239.
14. Fornazzari L, Wilkinson DA, Kapur BM, Carlen PL. Cerebellar, cortical and functional impairment in toluene abusers. *Acta Neurol Scand* 1983;67:319–329.
15. Lazar RB, Ho SU, Melen O, Daghestani AN. Multifocal central nervous system damage caused by toluene abuse. *Neurology* 1983;33:1337–1340.
16. Baker EL, Fine LJ. Solvent neurotoxicity: the current evidence. *J Occup Med* 1986;28:126–129.
17. Uitti RJ, Snow BJ, Shinotoh H, et al. Parkinsonism induced by solvent abuse. *Ann Neurol* 1994;35:617–619.
18. Hormes JT, Filley CM, Rosenberg JL. Neurologic sequelae of chronic solvent vapor abuse. *Neurology* 1986;36:698–702.
19. Escobar A, Aruffo C. Chronic thinner intoxication: clinico-pathologic report of a human case. *J Neurol Neurosurg Psychiatry* 1980;43:986–994.
20. Boeckx RL, Postl B, Coodin FJ. Gasoline sniffing and tetraethyl lead poisoning in children. *Pediatrics* 1977;60:140–145.

21. Robinson RO. Tetraethyl lead poisoning from gasoline sniffing. *JAMA* 1978;240:1373–1374.
22. Spencer PS, Shaumburg HH. N-hexane and methyl n-butyl ketone. In: Spencer PS, Shaumburg HH, eds. *Experimental and clinical neurotoxicology.* Baltimore: Williams & Wilkins, 1980:456–475.
23. Shaumburg HH, Spencer PS. Recognizing neurotoxic disease. *Neurology* 1987;37:276–278.
24. Saida K, Mendell JR, Weiss HS. Peripheral nerve changes induced by methyl n-butyl ketone and potentiated by methyl ethyl ketone. *J Neuropathol Exp Neurol* 1976;35:207–225.
25. Buxton PH, Hayward M. Polyneuritis cranialis associated with trichloroethylene poisoning. *J Neurol Neurosurg Psychiatry* 1967;30:511–518.
26. Waters EM, Gerstner HB, Huff JE. Trichloroethylene I. An overview. *J Toxicol Environ Health* 1977;2:671–707.
27. Bass M. Sudden sniffing death. *JAMA* 1970;212:2075–2079.
28. King GS, Smialek JE, Troutman WG. Sudden death in adolescents resulting from the inhalation of typewriter correction fluid. *JAMA* 1985;253:1604–1606.
29. Chenoweth MB. Ventricular fibrillation induced by hydrocarbons and epinephrine. *J Ind Hyg Toxicol* 1946;28:151–158.
30. Mullin LS, Azar A, Reinhardt CF, et al. Halogenated hydrocarbon-induced cardiac arrhythmias associated with release of endogenous epinephrine. *Am Ind Hyg Ass J* 1972;389–396.
31. Flowers NC, Horan LG. Nonanoxic aerosol arrhythmias. *JAMA* 1972;219:22–27.
32. Nahum LH. The mechanism of sudden death in experimental acute benzol (benzene) poisoning. *J Pharmacol Exp Ther* 1934;50:336.
33. Harris WS. Toxic effects of aerosol propellants on the heart. *Arch Intern Med* 1973;131:162–166.
34. Neuberger JM. Halothane and hepatitis. *Drug Safety* 1990;5:28–38.
35. Ritt DJ, Whelan G, Werner DJ, et al. Acute hepatic necrosis with stupor and coma. *Medicine* 1969;48:151–172.
36. Recknagel RO. Carbon tetrachloride hepatotoxicity. *Pharm Rev* 1967;19:145–208.
37. Taher SM, Anderson RJ, McCartney R, et al. Renal tubular acidosis associated with toluene "sniffing." *N Engl J Med* 1974;290:765–768.
38. Ramsey J, Anderson HR, Bloor K, Flanagan RJ. An introduction to the practice, prevalence and chemical toxicology of volatile substance abuse. *Hum Toxicol* 1989;8:261–269.
39. Langehennig PL, Seeler RA, Berman E. Paint removers and carboxyhemoglobin. *N Engl J Med* 1976;295:1137–1140.
40. Kaufman D, Lipscomb JW, Leikin JB, et al. Methylene chloride report of five exposures and two deaths. *Vet Hum Toxicol* 1989;31:352–356.
41. Rioux JP, Myers RAM. Hyperbaric oxygen for methylene chloride poisoning: report on two cases. *Ann Emerg Med* 1989;18:691–695.
42. Curry S. Methemoglobinemia. *Ann Emerg Med* 1982;11:214–221.
43. Brandes JC, Bufill JA, Pisciotta AV. Amyl nitrite-induced hemolytic anemia. *Am J Med* 1989;86:252–254.
44. Austin H, Denzell E, Cole P. Benzene and leukemia. A review of the literature and risk assessment. *Am J Epidemiol* 1988;127:419–439.
45. Greenlee WF, Sun JD, Bus JS. A proposed mechansim of benzene toxicity. Formation of reactive intermediates from poyphenol metabolites. *Toxicol Appl Pharmacol* 1981;59:87–195.
46. Patel R, Benjamin J. Renal disease associated with toluene inhalation. *J Toxicol Clin Toxicol* 1986;24:213–223.
47. Charbonneau M. Brodeur J, du Souich P, Plaa GL. Correlation between acetone potentiated CCl^-_4-induced liver injury and blood concentrations after inhalation or oral administration. *Toxicol Appl Pharm* 1986;84:286–294.
48. DeFerreyra EC, Castro JA, Gomez MID, et al. Prevention and treatment of carbon tetrachloride hepatotoxicity by cysteine. Studies about its mechanism. *Toxicol Appl Pharmacol* 1974;27:558–568.
49. Graham SR, Day RI, Lee R, et al. Overdose with chloral hydrate: a pharmacological and therapeutic review. *Med J Aust* 1988;149:686–690.

Emergency Toxicology, Second Edition,
edited by Peter Viccellio.
Lippincott–Raven Publishers, Philadelphia © 1998.

69

Sports Drugs of Abuse

Cathleen Clancy

*Maryland Poison Center; University of Maryland Baltimore, School of Pharmacy,
Baltimore, Maryland 21201-1180; Department of Emergency Medicine, Georgetown University
Medical Center, Washington, D.C. 20007; National Capital Poison Center; Department of
Emergency Medicine, George Washington University Medical Center, Washington, D.C. 20016*

Performance-enhancing, or ergogenic, drugs have been used for as long as competitive sports have been practiced. The ancient Greek Olympic athletes consumed herbs and mushrooms to improve their performance. French athletes used a mixture of coca leaves and wine in the 19th century, and the Aztecs ingested myocardium from sacrificed human beings (1). Drug testing at the Olympic Games began in 1968. There are now three major regulatory organizations governing amateur athletic competitions: the International Olympic Committee (IOC), the U.S. Olympic Committee (USOC), and the National Collegiate Athletic Association (NCAA) (2). The goal of these organizations is not only to insure fairness but to protect the athletes' health. The general categories of drugs and activities that are banned by the International Olympic Committee are anabolic agents, peptide and glycoprotein hormones and analogues, stimulants, diuretics, and narcotics. Prohibited methods include agents that physically manipulate the urine (i.e., probenecid, diuretics) and blood doping. Specific agents are banned for specific sports (e.g., beta-blockers in rifle sports, sedatives in the pentathlon). Numerous other agents are restricted to use by athletes with specific approval. These restricted agents include alcohol, marijuana, corticosteroids, β_2 agonists, beta-blockers, and local anesthetics (3). More information may be obtained by writing the U.S. Olympic Committee Drug Education and Doping Control Program (One Olympic Plaza, Bldg. 32, South End, Colorado Springs, CO 80909). In addition to the numerous hormonal agents and medications, there are a vast array of nutritional supplements available over-the-counter (OTC) that are avidly consumed.

ANABOLIC-ANDROGENIC STEROIDS

I. **Introduction.** Androgens clearly increase lean body mass and body weight in athletes who are involved in a systematic program involving weight training and diet modification. These nitrogen-retaining, anabolic, qualities cannot be separated from the often less desirable, androgenic properties which stimulate male phenotype and male secondary sexual characteristics. The profound health risks associated with chronic abuse of androgens prompted the introduction of drug testing in the 1968 Olympic Games. Surprisingly, the vast majority of abusers are not competitive athletes but rather young people seeking cosmetic improvement. In a 1993 survey of 30,000 people, 0.9% of males over the age of 12 had taken anabolic steroids at some time (4). A more recent questionnaire administered to 16,000 Canadian students (sixth grade and above) revealed that 2.8% of the respondents had used anabolic-androgenic steroids in the previous year. Of those taking steroids, 29.4% reported that they injected them; and of these, 29.2% reported sharing needles. Another study found that 6.6% of high school seniors had abused androgens, and that 35% of these were not even engaged in organized athletics (5).

II.   Sources of agent. The term anabolic-androgenic steroids includes a wide variety of natural and synthetic derivatives of testosterone. The clinical indications for androgen therapy include hypogonadism, hereditary angioedema, endometriosis, and some chronic anemias. Androgens are marketed for human and veterinary use, and illegally imported from other countries. Both oral and parenteral preparations are abused. Most preparations are synthetic but some contain hormones extracted directly from animal gonads. Among athletes, the most commonly used oral agents are methandrostenolone, oxandrolone, stanozolol, oxymetholone, and methyltestosterone. The common parenteral agents are esters of nandrolone, testosterone, and methenolone. Veterinary products include boldenone, mibolerone, and injectable stanozolol.

III.   Pharmacology and properties of agents

    A.   Mechanism of action and toxicity

        1.   Physiology. The Leydig cells of the human testes produce testosterone. Testosterone acts directly on the androgen receptor and is converted to dihydrotestosterone or estradiol. The 5α-reductase enzymes (see **VIII.H**) convert testosterone to the more potent dihydrotestosterone which binds avidly to the androgen receptor. The aromatase enzyme complex transforms testosterone into estradiol which binds to the estrogen receptors producing female characteristics. A number of other hormone preparations effecting these metabolic pathways are also used and abused in the athletic community (see **VIII**).

        2.   Doses. The doses of anabolic-androgenic steroids used by athletes are 10 to 100 times higher than those recommended for replacement therapy. Often multiple steroids and other drugs are used at the same time.

    B.   Pharmacokinetics. Testosterone hormone is degraded quickly by the liver rendering oral preparations inactive. The metabolites and parent compound are then excreted in the urine. Synthetic oral preparations are alkylated at the 17α-hydroxy position rendering them resistant to first pass metabolism. Intramuscular preparations are esterified at the 17β-hydroxy position and often marketed in an oil-based vehicle which allows for a depot injection lasting about 2 weeks (Fig. 69-1). Patches deliver a decreasing amount of testosterone over a 24-h period. Implantable pellets containing trenbolone (Finaplix) are also available. Following subcutaneous implantation the pellets must be replaced every 4 months. Some athletes extract the trenbolone with methanol and administer the dried product parenterally. Neither patches or pellets are commonly abused by athletes.

IV.   Clinical presentation

    A.   Who gets it. Athletes use a number of patterns of androgen administration to try and maximize performance. Typically users take two to four drugs at a time ("stacking") at escalating doses that peak either in the middle ("pyramid") or at the end of a 12 week cycle. The timing of the cycle is related to upcoming athletic events and testing requirements. Commonly users will begin with oral preparations, then advance to the use of parenteral agents. Eventually the serious user will add antiestrogen agents (see **VIII.A**) to inhibit gynecomastia and human chorionic gonadotrophin (hCG) to decrease testicular atrophy. The gynecomastia and other female traits are stimulated by the estrogens formed by the aromatization of testosterone. Habituation to these drugs is common since the desired changes in body physique are lost when the androgens are discontinued. Most adverse effects only become apparent after chronic abuse, however some manifestations may be seen in the first cycle.

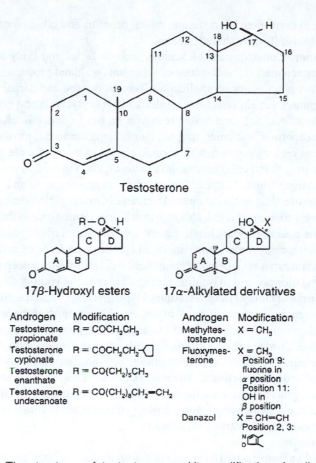

Fig. 69-1. The structures of testosterone and its modifications for clinical use.

B. Manifestations of toxicity. Clinical manifestations are related to androgen or estrogen effects on the hormone receptors, nonsterile injection technique, and transmission of blood borne diseases by shared needles.

    1. Major. Cardiovascular abnormalities include hypertension, cardiomyopathy, reduced glucose tolerance, atherosclerosis, and a marked increase in the LDL/HDL ratio. High density lipoprotein levels are decreased without significant alterations in the low density lipoprotein levels. These effects appear to be reversible after discontinuation of the drugs. Myocardial infarction and strokes in young athletes are often a result of anabolic-androgenic steroid abuse. Erythrocytosis and increased thrombogenesis may also contribute to cardiovascular morbidity (6). The oral, alkylated androgens often cause a reversible elevation of the liver enzymes. However, prolonged abuse may result in peliosis hepatis (rare hemorrhagic cystic degeneration of the liver), hepatitis, and hepatocellular carcinoma. Behavioral effects include mood instability, increased aggression ("roid rage"), major depression, and even psychosis (7). Adolescent abusers may have premature closure of the epiphysial plates resulting in permanent short stature. AIDS, hepatitis and other blood borne diseases may be transmitted by shared needles.

2. **Minor.** Cutaneous manifestations include facial and body acne, alopecia, striae ("stretch marks"), and increased sebaceous oil gland production. Musculotendinous injury is a frequent complication. Tendon rupture and carpal tunnel syndrome are common. Insulin resistance resulting in hyperglycemia and glycosuria is a frequent side effect. Salt and water retention causing edema is also common. In men, azoospermia, testicular atrophy, painful gynecomastia, prostatic hypertrophy, and lactation are common with chronic abuse. In women, male pattern baldness, hirsutism, clitoral enlargement, hoarse voice, and virilization are permanent effects of androgen abuse. However amenorrhea, aggressiveness, and acne seem to resolve when the drug is discontinued. Decreases in immunoglobulins and thyroid hormones have also been reported, although the clinical significance of these changes is unclear.

3. **Sine qua non.** The classic patient would be an athletic, well-muscled male with acne, increased mammary tissue, and perhaps evidence of parenteral drug abuse. A female patient might have pronounced virilization with a deep voice, acne, male pattern baldness, and masculine changes in her facial contours.

C. **Time course of clinical manifestations.** Hyperglycemia, fluid retention and mood changes may be seen within the first week of abuse, whereas most of the androgen and estrogen mediated complications take months to appear. The physical changes associated with the androgen or estrogen effects, primarily virilization or feminization, tend to be permanent; while the anabolic effects, increased muscle bulk and decreased body fat, are transient.

D. **Effect of drug interactions.** Anabolic steroids increase the metabolism of oral hypoglycemic agents and decrease the metabolism of carbamazapine. The 17-alkylated androgens may cause hemorrhages and a prolonged prothrombin time in patients receiving oral anticoagulation with warfarin-type agents.

V. **Laboratory findings**

A. **Utility of various tests.** Urine testing for androgens utilizes gas chromatography/mass spectrometry to compare the ratio of testosterone to epitestosterone. Epitestosterone is an inactive metabolite of testosterone that is secreted from the testes, but is not derived from the metabolism of testosterone. A ratio of more than 6 : 1 indicates androgen abuse. Both men and women normally have ratios of 1 : 1.

B. **Time course for abnormalities.** The increased frequency of drug testing at athletic events has encouraged the use of agents that are rapidly metabolized and excreted, like stanazol and testosterone. These agents may be completely eliminated within a few days (8). Most athletes discontinue oral preparations 2 to 4 weeks before competition and injectable preparations 3 to 6 weeks before competition to ensure a negative test. Long lasting preparations like nandrolone decanoate which may be detected in the urine up to 6 months after injection, are no longer used. False positives may occur in athletes who ingest the meat of animals who have been fed or injected with anabolic steroids (9).

VI. **Management.** The management of an acute overdose involves psychiatric assessment and evaluation for coingestants. The treatment of a chronic abuser, however, is a complex psychosocial undertaking. The most specific therapeutic intervention is discontinuation of the drugs. No decontamination or enhanced elimination is required. Over time, many clinical manifestations will resolve while others are permanent.

VII. Disposition. Patients should be admitted if they are suicidal or violent or if the androgen abuse has lead to severe complications (i.e., stroke, myocardial infarction, depression).

VIII. Other related hormones

A. Antiestrogen agents. These agents are used to decrease the aromatization of testosterone or to decrease the estrogen binding at the receptor. They are available in table form and are abused by chronic androgen abusers to decrease gynecomastia and lactation. Tamoxifen (Nolvadex) is a competitive antagonist at the estrogen receptor, and testolactone (Teslac) is a tablet that inhibits steroid aromatase activity. Mesterolone (Pro-viron), a 1-methyl testosterone derivative, is used in Great Britain.

B. Clenbuterol. Clenbuterol is a β_2 agonist that is banned by the IOC, USOC and the NCAA as an anabolic steroid because of its anabolic and lipolytic activity (see below).

C. Gonadotrophin releasing hormones (GnRHs). Luteinizing hormone stimulates the testes to produce testosterone. Gonadotrophin releasing hormones initially increase circulating luteinizing hormone although chronic administration may actually decrease circulating gonadotropins. These drugs are used by some athletes to increase circulating testosterone as a substitute for androgenic-anabolic steroids. Drugs in this class include gonadorelin acetate (Lutrepulse, Factrel), goserelin (Zoladex), histrelin (Supprelin), leuprolide (Lupron Depot), nafarelin (Synarel), and the synthetic steroid analogue, danazol (Danocrine). Gonadorelin is structurally identical to endogenous GnRH, is clinically available for intravenous use, and recommended for use in patients with primary hypothalamic amenorrhea. Histrelin and leuprolide are synthetic nonpeptide agonists of naturally occurring GnRH. Nafarelin is a synthetic analog and agonist of naturally occurring GnRH, is available in a nasal spray, and is clinically indicated for the treatment of central precocious puberty. While many GnRH agonists do increase circulating testosterone after acute administration, chronic exposure may actually decrease circulating testosterone.

D. Growth hormone. See below.

E. Human chorionic gonadotrophin (hCG). This is a polypeptide produced by the human placenta. The commercially available preparation is derived from the urine of pregnant women. The alpha subunit is identical in structure to the alpha subunits of LH and FSH. The action of hCG is virtually identical to that of LH. It causes stimulation of the Leydig cells of the testes to produce testosterone and stimulates the ovaries to produce progesterone. The perception in the muscle building community is that hCG should be taken during a steroid "cycle" to prevent testicular atrophy. HCG produces precocious puberty when used therapeutically for children with cryptorchism and hypogonadotrophic hypogonadism. HCG is only available for IM injection (Pregnyl, Profasi).

F. Insulin. Insulin is also used by body builders in varying combinations with growth hormone, steroids, clenbuterol, thyroid hormone, or insulin-like growth factor (IGF-1). By increasing the quantity of glucose and amino acids that enter cells, insulin is thought to decrease body fat and increase muscle size especially in combination with other anabolic agents. The doses range from 20 to 40 units/day of a regular plus NPH in divided doses. High carbohydrate meals or glucose snacks are eaten just prior or just after insulin administration to prevent hypoglycemia (10).

G. Insulin-like growth factor (IGF-1). Cell-culture grade IGF-1 is only available on the black market and is administered parenterally. There are no clinically accepted indications for use. The mechanism for the anticatabolic action touted in the muscle building community involves an IGF receptor and increased insulin responsiveness. The increased insulin responsiveness decreases the hyperglycemia caused by GH and anabolic steroids and increases muscle growth. This is the same mechanism that has lead to abuse of other insulin mimickers (see below).

   H. 5-α reductase inhibitors. 5-α reductase is the enzyme that converts testosterone to dihydrotestosterone. Inhibition of this enzyme is thought to decrease some of the androgenic side effects (male pattern baldness, hirsutism, voice changes) without affecting the anabolic qualities. These drugs are popular in women who are chronic abusers of anabolic androgenic steroids. Finasteride (Proscar) is the prototype 5-α reductase inhibitor. It is available by prescription in tablet form and usually prescribed for prostatic hypertrophy. A number of OTC products are used as a substitute. An extract from the plant, *Serenoa repens* (saw palmetto, American dwarf palm tree) is marketed as Permixon and putatively blocks the binding of dihydrotestosterone and testosterone at the receptor and may also have estrogenic activity. Other "natural compounds" having similar activity include gamma linolenic acid, which is found in evening primrose oil, borage seed oil (Barlean's Borage Seed Oil), and hydroxycitric acid (Citrimax). Hydroxycitric acid is reported to interfere with liver conversion of glucose into fatty acids by interfering with NADPH, which is required for the activation of 5-α reductase.

GROWTH HORMONE

   I. Introduction. Growth hormone (GH) is a naturally occurring polypeptide hormone produced by the pituitary gland and manufactured synthetically. Pituitary gland deficiency of this hormone results in dwarfism. Excess quantities of GH prior to adolescence leads to gigantism, whereas after closure of the epiphyseal plates, acromegaly results.

   II. Sources of agent. Prior to 1985 dwarfism was treated with GH extracted from human pituitary glands (Asellacrin, Crescormon, Grorm). The use of cadaveric pituitary glands resulted in the transmission of Creutzfeldt-Jakob Disease and presumably other blood borne diseases. In 1985 a synthetic recombinant GH became commercially available and is marketed as Humatrope, Nutropin, and Protropin. Since then, abuse by athletes has increased dramatically.

   III. Pharmacology and properties of agents
   A. Mechanism of action and toxicity
   1. **Physiology.** Growth hormone is actually a family of structurally related proteins produced by the anterior pituitary cells. These polypeptide hormones maintain the normal linear growth from birth to the attainment of adult height. Growth is promoted by the generation of somatomedins, specifically insulin-like growth factor (IGF-1), which promotes anabolism, facilitating the growth of muscle, bone, and cartilage. IGF-1 can also be obtained on the black market and methods of administration are described in numerous body building magazines (see above). When excessive quantities of GH are present prior to the closure of the epiphyseal plates children grow significantly taller and seem to have a prolonged period of growth. After the closure of the epiphyseal plate, GH causes minimal increase in height but progressive enlargement of the hands, feet, skull and jaw resulting in progressive facial distortion. GH also causes muscles growth and the enlargement of the internal organs; heart, liver, spleen, and kidneys.
   2. **Doses.** Athletes have been reported to take as much as 20 times the clinically recommended dosages. Since GH levels are regulated by negative feedback loops it is

unclear whether exogenous administration can cause significant serum elevations. In addition to down-regulating endogenous production, the available receptors also seem to decline. Other drugs and amino acids are often used to increase the endogenous release of GH, including propranolol, vasopressin, clonidine, cyproheptadine (Periactin), levodopa, arginine, ornithine, and lysine. A combination of arginine and lysine seems particularly popular (11).

B. **Pharmacokinetics.** GH has a very short half-life and less than 1% is excreted in the urine. Administration is usually every 1 to 2 days by intramuscular injection. GH is often taken in combination with other agents.

IV. **Clinical presentation**

A. **Who gets it.** Body builders and athletes use growth hormone as a replacement for anabolic-androgenic steroids, since urine testing does not reveal GH. In one survey, 5% of 224 males reported past or present use of GH (12). Nonathletic adolescents use GH in an attempt to artificially increase their height. The estimated cost for ergogenic quantities of recombinant GH is in the range of $1,000 to $1,500 for an 8-week supply (13). Clinical manifestations are seen with chronic abuse. Few complications of acute exposure to GH have been reported, although sharing needles and unsterile injection techniques may lead to infection.

B. **Manifestations of toxicity**

1. **Major.** Cardiomegaly, hyperlipidemia, hypertension, and cardiomyopathy are frequent complications of chronic abuse. Cardiomyopathy is the most common cause of death (14). Diabetes, osteoporosis, impotence in men, and amenorrhea in women are common. Prior to 1985, or even now, if human cadaveric extracts are used slow viruses and other blood borne pathogens may infect the abuser (i.e., Creutzfeldt-Jakob disease). Sharing needles and syringes imposes the risk of AIDS and hepatitis.

2. **Minor.** Carpal tunnel syndrome and increases in the size of muscles is common although muscle strength is not increased. Over time progressive myopathy and peripheral neuropathy develops and abusers may develop diffuse weakness. Gigantism may occur in prepubescent athletes. Antibodies to endogenous GH may impair future response to endogenous GH.

3. **Sine qua non.** A classic patient would be a body builder with a bloated abdomen, coarse features and evidence of parenteral drug abuse.

V. **Laboratory findings.** Currently, there is no reliable method of urine testing for GH or any of the other peptide hormones including adrenocorticotrophic hormone (ACTH), human chorionic gonadotrophin (hCG), erythropoietin, and gonadotropin releasing factors.

VI. **Management.** The management of an acute overdose involves psychiatric assessment and evaluation for coingestants. The treatment of a chronic abuser, however, is a complex psychosocial undertaking. The most specific therapeutic intervention is discontinuation of the drugs. No decontamination or enhanced elimination is required. Over time some clinical manifestations will resolve but most of the bone growth is permanent.

VII. **Disposition.** Patients should be admitted if they are suicidal or violent or if they manifest severe complications of GH abuse (i.e., cardiomyopathy, diabetes, infections, etc.).

ERYTHROPOIETIN

I. **Introduction.** Recombinant erythropoietin administration is the latest method of induced erythrocythemia, "blood doping." Historically, numerous methods to increase the number of oxygen-carrying red cells have been employed. Homologous blood transfusion, autologous blood transfusion, and endurance training at high altitudes have been used to increase the endurance athletes hematocrit. More recently even hyperbaric oxygen therapy has been used to enhance performance.

II. **Sources of agent.** Erythropoietin is a glycoprotein that is produced by the kidney and regulates red blood cell production. In 1977 erythropoietin was isolated and purified from human urine but the available quantities limited clinical use. The gene that codes for erythropoietin was cloned in 1985 and recombinant erythropoietin became available in Europe in 1987. A series of deaths in cyclists and orienteers from Europe around that time has been postulated to have been related to this new drug. Recombinant erythropoietin (Epogen) is produced commercially by recombinant DNA techniques from chinese hamster ovary cells and has been available in the United States since 1989. Abuse has been reported in athletes competing in endurance events. Unfortunately, conclusive laboratory confirmation of abuse is not usually available.

III. **Pharmacology and properties of agents**
    A. **Mechanism of action and toxicity**
        1. **Physiology.** Studies suggest that when an athlete's total hemoglobin increases by 10% to 20% there is an improvement in endurance performance. One study reported a 23% increase in the time required to reach exhaustion on a submaximal running test following the reinfusion of 800 mL of an athlete's blood that had been withdrawn 3 months earlier (15). Clinically significant elevations in hematocrit are usually seen 2 weeks after erythropoietin administration and may peak as long as 6 weeks later.
        2. **Doses.** Clinically recommended doses of erythropoietin 7 to 450 U/kg in divided doses, three times a week. The erythrocythemia is dose dependant.
    B. **Pharmacokinetics.** Recombinant erythropoietin can be administered intravenously or subcutaneously. The half-life is 3 to 5 h following the intravenous route and approximately 20 h after subcutaneous administration. Metabolism is by the erythroid precursors and also occurs in the liver. Less than 5% is excreted in the urine.

IV. **Clinical presentation**
    A. **Who gets it.** Endurance athletes show the greatest benefit from the increased oxygen carrying capacity conferred by abuse of erythropoietin. There is a considerable delay in the onset of clinical effect and extreme variability in the rate and level of erythrocythemia. The athlete may use erythropoietin 2 weeks before competition and develop symptoms 5 weeks later as the hematocrit continues to rise.
    B. **Manifestations of toxicity.** Adverse effects are dose dependant. Manifestations include complications from the increased number of red blood cells, from unsterile injection techniques, and needle sharing. Hyperviscosity syndrome and hypertension are the most common life-threatening complications. Manifestations may include congestive heart failure, seizures and thrombotic events (i.e., myocardial infarction, stroke).

V. **Laboratory findings.** Urine testing for recombinant erythropoietin is of limited value since such small quantities are excreted. Other testing methods are limited by the drugs short half-life and the prolonged clinical effects. Measurement of hemoglobin and hematocrit values has been proposed as a surrogate for direct detection of blood doping and erythropoietin abuse.

VI. Management. The management of an acute overdose requires psychiatric assessment and evaluation for coingestants. The effects of erythropoietin will not become evident for at least 1 to 2 weeks following administration. Phlebotomy and hydration may be required in the management of severe polycythemia. The treatment of a chronic abuser is a complex psychosocial undertaking. The most specific therapeutic intervention is discontinuation of the drugs. No decontamination or enhanced elimination would be efficacious since the half-life of erythropoietin is short.

VII. Disposition. Patients should be admitted if they are suicidal or violent or if follow-up is unreliable. Clearly admission is also warranted if significant polycythemia is evident or has led to severe complications (i.e., myocardial infarction, seizures).

VIII. Other related techniques

   1. **Homologous transfusions.** Homologous transfusions are clearly the least safe method of blood doping and are now rarely used in the athletic community. Complications include severe hemolytic reactions, anaphylaxis, fever, urticaria, and the transmission of blood borne infections (16).

   2. **Autologous transfusions.** The procedure for autologous blood transfusions involves phlebotomy of 2 units of blood approximately 1 to 2 months before competition. The blood is then separated from the plasma and appropriately frozen. Freezing is the preferred method of storage since blood that is refrigerated will last only 3 weeks. The athlete continues a normal training regimen and then reinfuses the blood 1 to 7 days before competition. Autologous transfusions are relatively safe as long as the infusion and the storage of blood are performed by licensed and trained personnel. Complications of polycythemia, and infections from poorly stored blood or unsterile infusion techniques may occur (16).

   3. **Hyperbaric oxygen (HBO).** In the past, HBO has been used in an extraordinarily wide variety of illnesses. Traditionally the indications for HBO involved diseases or injuries associated with anoxia (i.e., nonhealing ulcers, crush injury, reperfusion injury, carbon monoxide intoxication, etc.). The use of HBO in sports medicine is growing. HBO is recommended by some authorities early in the course of rehabilitation for musculoskeletal injuries to reduce pain, speed up recovery, and hasten the return to active training (17). One study of football players with minor injuries documents a 70% decrease in the amount of time injured (18). Another study found significantly improved performance on a treadmill test up to 3 h after HBO therapy (19). Although not yet mainstream this method of "blood doping" is on the rise.

STIMULANTS

Stimulant drugs include a broad range of agents including amphetamines, β_2 adrenergic agonists (clenbuterol, albuterol), caffeine, cocaine, ephedrine, methylphenidate (Ritalin), phenylephrine, pseudoephedrine, phenylpropanolamine, and strychnine. Stimulants increase alertness, reduce fatigue, and enhance performance in athletic events. Amphetamines have a particularly notorious reputation for causing morbidity and mortality in the athletic community. These agents are also used in combination ("stacked"). Ephedrine (20 mg), caffeine (200 mg), and aspirin (300 mg) is currently a popular combination. β_2 adrenergic agonists are commonly prescribed for asthma but are also classified as stimulants, some agents possess anabolic qualities especially when they are administered orally or by injection. Most β_2 adrenergic agonists are prohibited by the IOC, except the following which are restricted to athletes with written permission: salbutamol (Albuterol), salmeterol

(Serevent), and terbutaline (Brethair). The β_2 agonist clenbuterol has become increasingly popular in recent years. In addition to its stimulating properties clenbuterol, seems to exhibit "anabolic qualities" and increases muscle mass while decreasing lipogenesis. The clinical manifestations of toxicity for all the stimulant agents are quite similar and may be found in individual chapters. Clenbuterol is discussed in more detail below.

CLENBUTEROL

I. **Introduction.** Clenbuterol is a β_2 adrenergic agonist that has gained popularity over recent years because of anabolic and lipolytic effects. These qualities have been utilized for years by veterinarians and breeders of livestock. In the 1992 Olympics abuse by athletes became evident.

II. **Sources of agent.** Clenbuterol is one of a group of drugs known as nutrient partitioning agents because of their ability to decrease the amount of fat produced per pound of feed in the cattle industry. Clenbuterol is marketed for asthma in other countries under a variety of trade names including Clembumar, Novegam, Clenasma, Broncoterol, and Spiropent. In the United States, only veterinary preparations are commercially available and they are approved for use only as tocolytics or bronchodilators. Human poisoning from the ingestion of beef liver from animals illegally fed clenbuterol has been reported (20,21).

III. **Pharmacology and properties of agents**

A. **Mechanism of action and toxicity**

1. **Physiology.** Stimulation of the β_2 adrenergic receptors causes dilation of the blood vessels perfusing skeletal muscle, and relaxation of the smooth muscle in the uterus and bronchi. These actions are mediated by the stimulation of adenyl cyclase, which catalyzes the formation of cyclic-3,5 adenosine monophosphate from adenosine triphosphate. Additionally, clenbuterol seems to induce hypertrophy of skeletal muscle cells, shifts fiber type from Type I (slow twitch) to Type II (fast twitch), and increase the glycolytic capacity of muscle. Presumably these effects are mediated by the β_2 adrenergic receptors, although the precise mechanism has not been elucidated. The β_2 adrenergic receptor is also involved in the flux of sodium and potassium at the cell membrane. Stimulation of the β_2 receptor results in elevated intracellular potassium and decreases serum potassium.

2. **Doses.** The doses used by athletes are 3 to 4 times the dose used therapeutically in the treatment of asthma.

B. **Pharmacokinetics.** The half-life of clenbuterol is 27 h and absorption from oral ingestion is almost 100%. Large amounts are excreted in the urine unchanged. Clenbuterol is cleared from the body in less than 5 days.

IV. **Clinical presentation**

A. **Manifestations of toxicity.** The major clinical manifestations are similar to those seen following overdose with sympathomimetics or other β_2 adrenergic agonists. Cardiovascular effects of overdose include tachycardia, palpitations, supraventricular arrhythmias, hypertension, angina, and myocardial infarctions. In patients with premorbid atherosclerosis myocardial infarctions or stroke are more likely to develop. Neurological finding may include muscle tremor, headaches, anxiety, and drowsiness even at therapeutic doses. In the overdose setting seizures, cerebral hemorrhage, and cerebral infarction may occur. Nausea, vomiting, and diarrhea are common, especially in supratherapeutic dosages. Metabolic abnormalities, including hyperglycemia, and hypokalemia, are common in a true overdose.

V. Laboratory findings

    A. Utility of various tests. Monitor the serum glucose and potassium. Evidence of ischemia or hypokalemia may be found on an electrocardiogram. Urine testing will reveal exposure to β_2 adrenergic agonists. The Food Safety and Inspection Service of the U.S. Drug Administration conducts specific tissue testing for clenbuterol in show animals and condemns the meat from these animals if clenbuterol is found (21).

    B. Time course for abnormalities. The onset of clinical manifestations in sympathomimetic overdose is variable and dependent on the agent and route of administration. In general, symptoms develop soon after therapeutic blood levels are reached and subside as the levels decline. Chronic administration of salbutemol (Alupent) in rats has been associated with benign smooth muscle tumors although no chronic effects in man have been reported.

VI. Management. Specific therapeutic intervention is required only in severely symptomatic patients (i.e., myocardial infarction, hypertensive crisis, seizures). There is no specific antidotal therapy. Symptomatic and supportive care is recommended. Aggressive potassium replacement is rarely warranted since the serum potassium will usually return to normal within 24 to 36 h. However, if the serum potassium falls below 3.0 mEq/L or there are electrocardiographic changes consistent with hypokalemia, replacement is advisable.

VII. Disposition

    A. Admission criteria. Patients should be admitted if they are suicidal or violent or if follow-up is unreliable. Admission is also warranted if signs of significant toxicity are evident (i.e., myocardial infarction, hypertensive crisis, and seizures).

    B. Discharge criteria. Patients may be discharged from the emergency department (ED) if they are asymptomatic after 4 to 6 h of observation and there is no possibility of suicidal intention or coingestants.

NUTRITIONAL SUPPLEMENTS

Nutritional supplements have become an increasingly important part of the American diet. Athletes and muscle builders are particularly responsive to aggressive advertising claims of improvement in health and strength. A recent survey of 12 issues of popular health and bodybuilding magazines revealed 89 brands, 311 products, and 235 unique ingredients. Of a total of 914 ingredients, the most frequently mentioned were; amino acids—type not specified (40%), chromium (30%), branched—chain amino acids (27%), minerals—type not specified (26%), vitamins—type not specified (26%), boron, inosine, smilax, carnitine, dibencozide, gamma-oryzanol, and ginseng. The most frequently promoted health benefit was muscle growth (22). Most adverse reactions from abuse and overdose are never reported or published. Occasionally serious toxicity is recognized by the medical community as in the case of gamma-hydroxybutyrate and L-tryptophan.

GAMMA-HYDROXYBUTYRATE

I. Introduction. Gamma-hydroxybutyrate (GHB) was aggressively marketed as an agent that increases the release of growth hormone, relieves insomnia and enhances weight loss. In the Spring of 1990, use of GHB in the athletic community increased dramatically. GHB was being used as a replacement for L-tryptophan, another nutritional supplement. L-tryptophan banned in November 1989 by the Department of Health and Human Services following linkage to a series of patients diagnosed with of Eosinophilia Myalgia Syndrome (23). By November 30, 1990 there were 22 cases of GHB-related illness reported to poison centers and the Department of Health and Human Services recommended that all sales of this agent be discontinued (24,25).

II. **Sources of agent.** GHB was originally synthesized in 1960 and was found to effectively cross the blood brain barrier and to induce a sleep-like state. Early uses as an anesthetic agent were aborted when lack of analgesia and seizures were reported. In 1963 GHB was found to occur naturally in the human brain, and because of its structural similarity to gamma-aminobutyric acid (GABA) action as a neurotransmitter was postulated. This agent was marketed under a variety of trade names and sold OTC. Currently the structurally similar agent beta-hydroxy, beta-methylbutyrate is touted as nutritional aid that increases lean body mass and strength.

III. **Pharmacology and properties of agents**

   A. **Mechanism of action and toxicity**

   1. **Physiology.** GHB ($HOOC\text{-}CH_2\text{-}CH_2\text{-}CH_2\,OH$) is structurally similar to GABA ($NH_2\text{-}CH_2\text{-}CH_2\text{-}CH_2\text{-}COOH$) and glutamate ($HOOC\text{-}CHNH_2\text{-}CH_2\text{-}CH_2\text{-}COOH$). Some evidence suggests that a presynaptic GHB/$GABA_B$ receptors located in the ventrobasal nucleus of the thalamus mediate the absence-like seizures induced by GHB (26). GHB is used therapeutically in the treatment of narcolepsy, sleep paralysis, hypnagogic hallucinations, and automatic behavior.

   2. **Doses.** Doses of 10 mg/kg produce short term amnesia, 20 to 30 mg/kg produce drowsiness and sleep, and higher doses, 50 to 70 mg/kg result in hypnosis and hypotonia, but little analgesia. The actual quantity of active drug available in one teaspoon, which is the recommended "dose," is extremely variable. Doses producing symptoms range from 1 to 6 teaspoons.

   B. **Pharmacokinetics.** Absorption from the gastrointestinal (GI) tract is rapid and the onset of systemic effects occurs within 15 min. GHB is metabolized to carbon dioxide and eliminated in expired air. Less than 2% to 5% is excreted in the urine (27).

IV. **Clinical presentation**

   A. **Who gets it.** This agent is currently banned by the U.S. Food and Drug Administration, although it is still available on the black market. Other nutritional agents have largely replaced GHB, including glutamate, beta-hydroxy, and beta-methylbutyrate. No clinical data on poisoning by the newer agents is currently available.

   B. **Manifestations of toxicity.** Neurologic manifestations predominate, ranging from somnolence and delirium to coma. Seizures, both grand mal and petite mal, are common. Hallucinations and extrapyramidal effects may also occur. Respiratory depression progressing to apnea is also common at higher doses. Bradycardia, vomiting, and hypothermia have also been reported.

V. **Laboratory findings.** There are no specific diagnostic tests available for GHB. Symptomatic patients should undergo cardiac monitoring, arterial blood gases, and frequent oximetry.

VI. **Management.** The management of an acute overdose requires psychiatric assessment and evaluation for coingestants. The sedative effects of GHB should become apparent with the first few hours. Gastric decontamination should include activated charcoal and a cathartic. Ipecac is contraindicated. There is no specific antidote and therapy is primarily supportive.

VII. **Disposition**

   A. **Admission criteria.** Patients should be admitted if they are suicidal or violent or if follow-up is unreliable. Admission is also warranted if signs of significant toxicity are evident (i.e., respiratory depression, coma, and seizures).

B. **Discharge criteria.** Patients may be discharged from the ED if they are asymptomatic after 4 to 6 h of observation and there is no possibility of suicidal intention or coingestants.

VIII. **Other related agents**

A. **Bicarbonate and phosphate supplements. Sodium bicarbonate** supplements are reported to enhance the uptake of creatine into muscles and prolong anaerobic capacity. Lactic acid is produced in muscles following intense activity and ingestion of baking soda does produce elevations in serum pH. One study showed that baking soda (300 mg/kg) enhanced isokinetic leg extension/flexion exercises (28). In another study, racing times improved 2.8 seconds in trained runners competing in an 800-m race (29). Immediate effects include nausea, vomiting, bloating, burping, and stomach pain. Chronic or excessive ingestion may result in hypernatremia, hypokalemia, alkalosis, volume overload, and lethargy progressing to coma. There is no specific test to detect bicarbonate ingestion. **Phosphates** are ingested prior to competition in order to increase serum 2,3-diphosphoglyceride, shift the hemoglobin-oxygen dissociation curve, and improve oxygen delivery to tissues (30).

B. **Other agents.** Other agents that have recently become popular include **creatine monohydrate** and the insulin mimickers, **chromium picolinate** and **vanadyl sulfate.** Reports of serious toxicity have not been published. **Creatine monohydrate** is a newer nutritional supplement and claims to have cell-volumizing effects, to produce a positive nitrogen balance, increase lean muscle mass, and increase strength. No toxicity data has been published. **Chromium picolinate** is a combination of picolinic acid, an amino acid metabolite, and trivalent chromium, a mineral found in the human body in trace amounts. The side effects include nausea and hypoglycemia in susceptible individuals. The risk of hypoglycemia is minimal in well-fed athletes but is a concern in patients with diabetes. There have been no reported cases of chromium toxicity resulting from this agent. Recent studies have suggested that chronic use of chromium picolinate may cause chromosomal damage in chinese hamster ovary cells (31), but otherwise there have been few serious cases of toxicity reported. **Vanadyl sulfate** is a form of vanadium that improves insulin sensitivity and may enhance glucose and amino acid entry into cells. Advertisements claim that it increases muscle hardness and fullness, and helps prevent protein breakdown. The side effects include nausea and hypoglycemia in susceptible individuals. If large amounts are ingested chronically, symptoms of vanadium poisoning may develop. Symptoms of vanadium poisoning include mania, tremor, mental status changes, epistaxis, arrhythmias, bronchoconstriction, and a green coloration of the tongue.

References

1. Thein LA, Thein JM, Landry GL. Ergogenic aids. *Phys Ther* 1995;75:426–439.
2. Goldwire MA, Price KO. Sports pharmacy: counseling athletes about banned drugs. *Am Pharm* 1995;NS35:24–30.
3. Woolley BH, Birrer RB. Drugs and sports. In: Editor, Richard B. Birrer: *Sports medicine for the primary care physician.* 2nd ed. CRC Press, Inc., Boca Raton, Florida 1994:443–444.
4. Yesalis CE, Kennedy NK, Kopstein AN, Bahrke MS. Anabolic-androgenic steroid use in the United States. *JAMA* 1993;270:1217–1221.
5. Buckley WE, Yesalis CE, Friedl KE, Anderson WA, Streit AS, Wright JE. Estimated prevalence of anabolic steroid use among male high school seniors. *JAMA* 1988;260:3441–3445.

6. Ferenchick GS, Hirokawa S, Mammen EF, Schwartz DA. Anabolic-androgenic steroid abuse in weight lifters: evidence for activation of the hemostatic system. *Am J Hematol* 1995;49:282–288.

7. Pope HG, Katz DL. Psychiatric and medical effects of anabolic-androgenic steroid use: a controlled study of 160 athletes. *Arch Gen Psychiatry* 1994;51:375–382.

8. Bagatell CJ, Bremner WJ. Androgens and men—uses and abuses. *N Engl J Med* 1996;334:707–714.

9. Kicman AT, Cowan DA, Myhre L, Nilsson S, Tomten S, Oftebro H. Effect on sports drug tests of ingesting meat from steroid (methenolone)—treated livestock. *Clin Chem* 1994;40:2084–2087.

10. Phillips B. *Muscle Magazine 2000* 1996;50:32.

11. Catlin DH, Hatton CK. Use and abuse of anabolic and other drugs for athletic enhancement. *Adv Intern Med* 1991;36:399–424.

12. Rickert VI, Pawlak-Morello C, Sheppard V, et al. Human growth hormone; a new substance of abuse among adolescents? *Clin Pediatr* 1992;31:723–726.

13. Haupt HA. Anabolic steroids and growth hormone. *Am J Sports Med* 1993;21:468–474.

14. Wadler GI. Drug abuse update. *Med Clin North Am Sports Med* 1994;78:439–455.

15. Ekblom B, Goldbard A, Gullbring B. Response to exercise after blood loss and reinfusion. *J Appl Physiol* 1972;33:175–180.

16. Wadler GI, Hainline B. Blood doping and erythropoietin. In: Ryan AJ, ed. *Drugs and the athlete*. Philadelphia: F A Davis Co, 1989, pgs 172–177.

17. Jain SC, et al. Effect of phosphate supplementation on oxygen delivery at high altitude. *Int J Biometeor* 1987;31:249.

18. James PB, Scott B, Allen MW. Hyperbaric oxygen therapy in sports injuries. *Physiotherapy* 1993;79:571–572.

19. Cabric M, Mecved R, Denoble P, Zivkovic M, Kovacevic H. Effect of hyperbaric oxygenation on maximal aerobic performance in a normobaric environment. *J Sports Med Phys Fitness* 1991;31:362–366.

20. Pulce C, Lamaison D, Keck G, Bostvironnois C, Nicolas J, Descotes J. Collective human food poisonings by clenbuterol residues in veal liver. *Vet Hum Toxicol* 1991;33:480–481.

21. Aikman B. *United States Department of Health and Human Services press release: Clenbuterol*. FDA, April 9, 1991.

22. Philen RM, Ortiz DI, Auerbach SB, Falk H. Survey of advertising for nutritional supplements in health and bodybuilding magazines. *JAMA* 1992;268:1008–1011.

23. Belongia EA, Hedberg CW, Gleich GJ, et al. An investigation of the cause of the eosinophilia-myalgia syndrome associated with tryptophan use. *N Engl J Med* 1990;323:357–365.

24. German GE. *United States Department of Health and Human Services press release: gamma hydroxybutyrate*. FDA, November 9, 1990.

25. *MMWR* 1990;39:47. Vol 39, No 47, pages 861–863.

26. Banerjee PK. Presynaptic gamma-hydroxybutyric acid (GHB) and gamma-aminobutyric acid$_B$ (GABA$_B$) receptor-mediated release of GABA and glutamate (GLU) in rat thalamic ventrobasal nucleus (VB): a possible mechanism for the generation of absence-like seizures induced by GHB. *J Pharmacol Exp Ther* 1995;273:1534–1543.

27. Dyer J. Gamma-hydroxybutyrate: a health-food product producing coma and seizure-like activity. *Am J Emerg Med* 1991;9:321–324.

28. Coombes J, McNaughton LR. Effects of bicarbonate ingestion on leg strength and power during isokinetic knee flexion and extension. *J Strength Cond Res* 1993;7:241–249.

29. Wilkes K, Gledhill N, Smyth R. Effect of acute induced metabolic alkalosis on 800-, racing time. *Med Sci Sports Exerc* 1983;15:277–280.

30. Jain KK. *Textbook of hyperbaric medicine*. 2nd rev. ed. Seattle, Toronto, Bern: Hogrefe and Huber Publishers, 1996.

31. Sterns DM, Wise JP, Patierno SR, Wetterhahn KE. Chromium (III) picolinate produces chromosome damage in Chinese hamster ovary cells. *FASEB J* 1995;9:1643–1649.

Selected Readings

Gapherty NA. Performance-enhancing drugs. *Orthop Clin North Am* 1995;26:433–442.

Melia P, Pipe A, Greenberg L. The use of anabolic-androgenic steroids by Canadian students. *Clin J Sports* 1996;6:9–14.

Woolley BH. The latest fads to increase muscle mass and energy. *Postgrad Med* 1991;89:195–205.

Emergency Toxicology, Second Edition,
edited by Peter Viccellio.
Lippincott–Raven Publishers, Philadelphia © 1998.

70

Drug Withdrawal Syndromes

Richard J. Hamilton

Allegheny University Hospital, Philadelphia, Pennsylvania 19129-1121

I. **Introduction.** Every withdrawal syndrome has two characteristics: a preexisting physiologic habituation to a substance, the continuous presence of which prevents physiologic derangement, and decreasing concentrations of that substance. The condition should not be confused with simple tolerance. A patient is tolerant to a drug when higher doses are required to produce a given response. For example, while many people are tolerant of ethanol, opioids, or sedative-hypnotic, not all patients exhibit a withdrawal syndrome when these agents are discontinued. The circumstance in which tolerance develops without a subsequent withdrawal syndrome probably depends on the pharmacology of the agent and the physiologic characteristic of the patient. Animal models suggest that withdrawal symptoms can be demonstrated even after short courses of opioids. Even if this situation applies to humans, however, it is probably subclinical. It is also important to differentiate withdrawal syndromes (where reinstatement of an agent with similar pharmacologic activity is therapeutic) from what may be better described as postintoxication syndromes. Individuals who develop tolerance to cocaine require larger, repetitive doses to achieve the sympathomimetic effects of the first single dose. Many of these patients present to emergency departments (EDs) many hours later (after the resolution of the sympathomimetic phase) with hypersomnia, restlessness, and movement disorders. While these symptoms occur as drug levels decrease, reinstatement of the drug or merely continuing use of the drug will not return the patient to physiologic "normal." This discussion may appear merely semantic at first; however, proper understanding of the physiology of withdrawal clarifies therapy. Patients in opioid withdrawal should be treated with agents with opioid receptor activity, patients in ethanol withdrawal should be treated with pharamcologic agents with GABA-minergic activity; patients with clonidine withdrawal should be treated with central alpha-adrenergic agonists. However, patients with hypersomnia and akathisia after a cocaine binge should not be treated with sympathomimetics. These patients require benzodiazepines until the postintoxication syndrome (thought to be from dopaminergic depletion) resolves. This syndrome has been labeled the "cocaine washed-out" syndrome.

II. **Neuropharmacology**

   A. **GABA receptor**

      1. $GABA_A$ receptors are postsynaptic receptors which, when activated, hyperpolarize the postsynaptic neuron by an inward chloride current. Note that these receptors do not act through G protein messengers. These receptors have separate binding sites for GABA, barbiturates, benzodiazepines, and picrotoxin. Many drugs have GABA

receptor activity without a clearly identified binding site (e.g., ethanol, etomidate). Only high-dose barbiturates can open the GABA chloride channel without concomitant binding of a GABA molecule. Ethanol, benzodiazepines, etomidate, and propofol are examples of drugs that merely enhance the affinity of GABA to its receptor and are classified as indirect GABA agonists.

2. GABA$_B$ receptors mediate presynaptic inhibition (by preventing Ca^{2+} influx) and postsynaptic inhibition (by increasing K$^+$ efflux). In addition these presynaptic receptors provide feedback inhibition of GABA release. Unlike GABA$_A$ receptors, they function through G protein messengers. Baclofen is the only clinically important GABA$_B$ agonist.

B. Opioid receptor

1. There are three classes of opioid receptors mu, kappa, and delta. Each of these receptors has three subtypes. Each subtype is responsible for a broad range of opioid effects which often overlap with other subtypes. Stimulation of either kappa$_1$ or kappa$_3$ receptors results in analgesia and miosis; only stimulation of the mu$_2$ receptor results in analgesia and respiratory depression. However, large doses can overcome a drug's low affinity for a particular receptor subtype. Agonist-antagonist opioids (pentazocine, butorphine, and nalbuphine) attempt to exploit this subtle difference and provide analgesia (kappa agonist) while preventing respiratory depression (mu antagonist). Fentanyl, morphine, and heroin (diacetyl morphine) are mu and kappa agonists. Nalmefine and naloxone are mu, kappa, and delta antagonists. Naltrexone is a kappa and mu antagonist. Opioids inhibit neurons by activating a rectifying K$^+$ efflux current and reducing the activity of adenyl cyclase through the G protein. Adenyl cyclase activates inward Na$^+$ current and this enhances the intrinsic excitability of the neuron.

C. Alpha$_2$ receptor

1. Alpha$_2$ receptors are located in the CNS and peripheral nervous system. Stimulation of peripheral postsynaptic alpha$_2$ receptors results in vasoconstriction, hypertension, and bradycardia and prevents acetylcholine release. This results in some anticholinergic symptoms, especially dry mouth. Stimulation of central presynaptic alpha$_2$ receptors inhibits sympathomimetic output and results in bradycardia, hypotension. Clonidine is a central and peripheral alpha$_2$ agent. It exhibits the peripheral effects only in the initial period after a toxic dose.

D. Adenosine receptor

1. Adenosine$_1$ receptors are located in the CNS and autonomic nervous system and function as pre- and postsynaptic inhibitory neurotransmitters. They act on the presynapse to decrease release of neurotransmitters, and on the postsynapse to terminate neuronal transmission. Adenosine$_2$ receptors are found on the cerebral vasculature and promote vasodilation. They are also found in the peripheral vasculature and serve a similar function.

E. Nicotine receptors

1. Nicotinic receptors are a type of acetylcholine receptors located in the autonomic ganglia, adrenal medulla, CNS, spinal cord, neuromuscular junction, and carotid and aortic bodies. Nicotinic receptors are fast-response cation channels that are not

coupled to G proteins. This distinguishes them from muscarinic receptors, which are coupled to G proteins. The ubiquitous nature of these receptors underscores nicotine's systemic effects.

III. **Neuropharmacology and physiology of withdrawal**
    1. **GABA agonists**
        a. **Ethanol and GABA$_A$ agonists.** Acute exposure to ethanol and GABA$_A$ agonists results in enhanced binding of GABA to the GABA receptor by increasing receptor affinity for GABA. Ethanol and other solvents may achieve this effect by acting on the cell membrane to change conformation of the GABA receptor protein complex. Indirect acting GABA agonists (benzodiazepines, low dose barbiturates, etomidate, propofol) do this by binding to other locations on the GABA receptor complex. Chronic exposure results in decreased GABA production as well as enhanced expression of GABA$_A$ receptors. This may be an adaptation to the increased affinity that these receptors have for GABA from chronic exposure to GABA enhancing agents. During withdrawal, receptor affinity returns to its less sensitive, native state. Since GABA production has been suppressed and GABA$_A$ receptors have increased in number, inhibitory control of excitatory neurotransmitters and pathways such as glutamate, NMDA, norepinephrine, and dopamine is lost. This results in the clinical syndrome of withdrawal—CNS excitation (seizures, tremor, hallucinations), and autonomic stimulation (tachycardia, hypertension hyperthermia, diaphoresis). Restoration of inhibitory control by administration of GABA$_A$ agonists is essential for resolution of this life threatening syndrome. Blockade of particular effects of withdrawal may be achieved with agents that antagonize dopaminergic and sympathomimetic amines (beta-blockers, haloperidol) but use of these agents result in additional risks such as hypotension, decreased seizure threshold, and hyperthermia, all of which ultimately exacerbate the syndrome. Long-acting GABA$_A$ agonists that can be administered in a loading dose are the ideal agents for the treatment of withdrawal. Diazepam is the benzodiazepine with the best profile. Phenobarbital has been used successfully because of its long half-life. Since benzodiazepines only enhance GABA binding, and maximum receptor occupancy is lowered in withdrawal because of decreased GABA production and increased receptor numbers, the indirect acting agents must be used at higher doses than normal. In fact, they can be ineffective even at doses that are so high (e.g., gram quantities of diazepam) that excipients such as propylene glycol may approach toxicity. For this reason, high-dose i.v. barbiturates are advantageous in refractory cases because they can open GABA chloride channels without GABA binding.

        b. **Baclofen (GABA$_B$ agonist).** The pre- and postsynaptic inhibitory properties of baclofen allow it to paradoxically cause CNS excitation in acute overdose and withdrawal. In large overdoses, baclofen stimulates presynaptic GABA$_B$ auto receptors which results in a decreased release of GABA$_A$ and subsequent loss of inhibitory tone. Therapeutic use of baclofen results in an increased inhibitory tone and it is useful for CNS-mediated muscle spasticity. When the drug is withdrawn, a disinhibition similar to $GABA_A$ withdrawal occurs. Many case reports of baclofen withdrawal describe hallucinations and psychosis as prominent symptoms, and these may be no different than the withdrawal symptoms of $GABA_A$ agonists. Interestingly, many patients complain of double vision.

2. **Opiates and opioids.** Chronic exposure to opiates (only drugs directly derived from opium) and opioids (all drugs with opioid receptor efficacy) results in a decreased efficacy of this receptor to open potassium channels. The mechanism is unclear, but chronic exposure does not appear to result in alterations in opioid peptides or receptors that adequately explain withdrawal. However, alterations in postreceptor, intracellular pathways may explain dependence and withdrawal. Chronic exposure to opioids increases the expression of adenyl cyclase through activation of the transcription factor cAMP response element-binding protein (CREB). This results in an up regulation of cAMP pathway proteins such as inward Na^+ channels. The enhanced excitability and an increased firing rate can only be blocked by higher levels of opioids. Without them, the patient experiences withdrawal symptoms, largely because of uninhibited activity at the locus coeruleus.

3. **Clonidine.** Clonidine lowers blood pressure by reducing the sympathetic outflow from the CNS. Twenty-four hours after discontinuation of clonidine, norepinephrine levels rise as a result of enhanced efferent sympathetic activity. Clonidine elimination half-life is 14 h, and most patients in withdrawal still have a clonidine level for a period of time. Simultaneous use of beta-blockers will exacerbate withdrawal, as alpha receptor stimulation rises in the face of beta-blockade.

4. **Caffeine.** Caffeine antagonizes the inhibitory effect of adenosine binding. Acute exposure results in increases in heart rate, ventilation, gastrointestinal (GI) motility, and gastric acid secretion, and motor activity. Chronic exposure results in tolerance to the effects of large acute administrations of the drug. This appears to be associated with adenosine$_1$ receptor occupancy by caffeine. Studies seem to suggest that chronic caffeine exposure regulates adenosine$_1$ receptors by various possible mechanisms, such as increases in receptor number, increases in receptor affinity, or enhancing receptor coupling to the G protein. However, many studies offer conflicting data. One well done in vivo animal study demonstrates that the adenosine receptor has a threefold increase in affinity for adenosine at the height of withdrawal symptoms. This model suggests that chronic adenosine$_1$ receptor occupancy by caffeine results in increase in receptor affinity for adenosine, thus restoring state of physiologic balance (normal motor inhibitory tone). When caffeine is withdrawn, the enhanced receptor affinity results in a strong adenosine effect and clinical symptoms of withdrawal—headache (cerebral vasodilation), fatigue, and hypersomnia (motor inhibition).

5. **Nicotine.** Nicotine provides it pleasurable reward through the dopaminergic neurons of the mesocortical and mesolimbic systems. These systems connect the ventral tegmental area with the frontal cortex and the limbic system. Nicotine increases dopamine release in the nucleus accumbens (a mesolimbic structure). It is believed that this is the area in which drugs of abuse (similar effects have been demonstrated for opioids, ethanol, amphetamines, and cocaine) have their self-reward effect.

IV.   **Clinical withdrawal syndromes and treatment**
  A.   **GABA agonists**
    1.   **GABA$_A$ agonists**
      a.   **Ethanol.** GABA$_A$ withdrawal syndromes should be suspected in any patient who uses a GABA$_A$ agent and develops any combination CNS excitation (seizures, tremor, hallucinations) and autonomic stimulation (tachycardia, hypertension hyperthermia, and diaphoresis). Ethanol withdrawal is easily diagnosed in patients with the social and physical stigma of alcoholism, but should also be considered in any patient who develops these symptoms after a period of abstinence (such as a hospital admission or imprisonment). Ethanol withdrawal often manifests as a brief generalized seizure. Many ethanol withdrawal patients are mistakenly given the diagnosis of seizure disorder because this seizure can occur prior to typical withdrawal manifestations and their is often evidence of prior CNS trauma on CT scan or EEG. Autonomic symptoms usually develop within a few hours. The patient becomes increasingly more agitated, diaphoretic, febrile, tachycardic, and hypertensive, and finally develops intractable seizures. Alcohol addicted patients may exhibit withdrawal symptoms anytime their ethanol level drops, even though the ethanol level is still elevated. Untreated mortality arises from hyperthermia, intractable seizures, and aspiration pneumonia. Care must be taken to differentiate withdrawal patients from those exhibiting alcoholic hallucinosis. The latter patients have normal vital signs and exhibit formed, persecutory auditory hallucinations which dissipate when ethanol levels drop. Withdrawal patients more typically have a progression from loose visual hallucinations to frank delirium. Treatment, like withdrawal, should be considered along a continuum. Patients who exhibit only minimal withdrawal symptoms such as mild anxiety or tremor can be treated with oral agents. These mild withdrawal syndromes should be treated because evidence exists to support the theory of "kindling," in which each successive withdrawal is worse than the prior. Long-term potentiation by NMDA neurons appears to be the mechanism. Intravenous therapy should be considered if the patient develops cardiovascular or CNS symptoms. Table 70-1 lists suggested therapeutic approaches. The goal of therapy should be to rapidly load patients with diazepam to a resolution of clinical manifestations and rebolus periodically as needed. In contrast, chlordiazepoxide has also been used, but offers no unique benefits over diazepam. Lorazepam is considered inferior to diazepam because it is short-acting and must be redosed at frequent intervals. Large boluses of diazepam are metabolized to active metabolites (desmethyldiazepam) over the withdrawal period (48 to 72 h) and, subsequently, management is greatly simplified. Studies have demonstrated that bolus therapy to a clinical endpoint is more efficacious than scheduled dosing and actually requires smaller total doses. There are occasional withdrawal syndromes so severe that even aggressive diazepam therapy is ineffective, and high-dose i.v. barbiturates with airway protection are the next line of therapy. The comorbidity from concomitant medical illness cannot be overestimated in

TABLE 70-1. *Treatment regimens for ethanol withdrawal*

Clinical manifestations	Drugs	Additional therapeutic modalities
Anxiety, tremor	Diazepam 10 to 20 mg i.v. or p.o., repeat q4h until patient calm and then p.r.n. reoccurrence of symptoms	
Tachycardia, hypertension, agitation	Diazepam 10 to 20 mg i.v., repeat every 20 min until symptoms resolve, and then p.r.n.	Multivitamin, thiamine i.v. infusion; 50% dextrose bolus; volume repletion
Hyperthermia (rectal temperature less than 104°F),	Diazepam 10 to 20 mg i.v., repeat every 20 min until symptoms resolve, and then p.r.n.	Multivitamin, thiamine i.v. infusion; 50% dextrose bolus; volume repletion; cooling blanket
Seizures, uncontrollable agitation	Diazepam 40 mg i.v. every 20 min until symptoms resolve, and consider airway protection; if symptoms not resolved after 200 mg diazepam total and no partial response to 40-mg boluses of diazepam, intubate patient and use pentobarbital 3 to 5-mg/kg bolus followed by 100 mg/h drip titrated to effect and blood pressure	Multivitamin, thiamine i.v. infusion; 50% dextrose bolus; volume repletion; cooling blanket
Rectal temperature greater than 104°F		Multivitamin, thiamine i.v. infusion; 50% dextrose bolus; volume repletion; cooling blanket; rapid ice immersion until rectal temperature falls to 102°F and then remove and dry

ethanol withdrawal patients. Indeed, it may have been pneumonia, meningitis, or sepsis which prevented the usual alcohol consumption. Thus, consider CSF, urine and blood cultures, as well as empiric antibiotic therapy for all patients with fever or altered mental status. In addition, the high metabolic needs and the poor nutritional state of the withdrawing alcoholic require special therapy. Thiamine (100 mg i.v.) assists in cerebral carbohydrate metabolism, supplemental dextrose reduces the need for fatty acid metabolism, and multivitamins address the many cofactor deficiencies that accompany alcoholism.

b.   **Benzodiazepines and barbiturates.** Benzodiazepine and barbiturate withdrawal symptoms are similar to alcohol withdrawal symptoms except that they may develop as late as 14 days after cessation of drug administration. Severe benzodiazepine withdrawal should be treated no differently than severe ethanol withdrawal, except the expected time course for resolution of withdrawal symptoms is much longer. Although no studies have been done addressing treatment regimens, most practitioners advise administration of boluses of diazepam or phenobarbital until resolution of symptoms, followed by a decrease of 10% of that total dose each day for 10 days. Patients without withdrawal symptoms who are being detoxified electively can be started on half the equivalent diazepam or phenobarbital daily dose and subsequently decreased by 10% each day. Flumazenil is a short-acting benzodiazepine receptor antagonist that is used to reverse benzodiazepine induced conscious sedation. It is capable of rapidly inducing a withdrawal syndrome in patients who are habituated to benzodiazepines. Seizures are the immediate sign of withdrawal and can occur without the return to consciousness. Higher than normal doses of benzodiazepines may be required to treat seizure activity and benzodiazepine receptor antagonism can be expected to last from 1 to 2 h depending on the dose of flumazenil used.

2. **GABA$_B$ agonists (baclofen).** Suspect this withdrawal syndrome in patients being treated for muscle spasticity in spinal cord diseases who suddenly develop an altered mental status. In particular, case reports highlight the development of seizures, hallucinations, psychosis, dyskinesia and visual disturbances. It seems most common for this to occur 24 for 48 h after discontinuation of baclofen during an admission to the hospital for an unrelated medical problem. Intrathecal baclofen pumps have become an effective replacement for oral dosing, and withdrawal can occur from this modality as well. Reinstatement of the prior baclofen dosing schedule appears to resolve these symptoms within 24 to 48 h. Benzodiazepines and GABA$_A$ agonists, not phenytoin, are the appropriate treatment for seizures induced by baclofen withdrawal.

B. **Opioid withdrawal.** Symptoms progress from drug craving, yawning, rhinorrhea, and piloerection to nausea, vomiting, diarrhea, diaphoresis, and mild tachycardia. Chronicity relates to pharmacology of the opiate of abuse. Methadone withdrawal starts 24 h after the last dose and lasts over 72 h. Heroin withdrawal will begin 6 h after the last dose and is usually fully manifest at 24 h. Withdrawal is physically and emotionally painful, but not life threatening as long as adequate hydration and nutritional support are maintained and morbidity from emesis can be minimized. Treatment with methadone (10 mg of i.m. or 20 mg p.o.) is enough to blunt withdrawal symptoms without providing euphoria, although it may not eliminate drug craving. Maintenance programs often use higher daily doses to achieve this effect. Very high doses (greater than 100 mg of methadone per day) are used to flood opioid receptors so that intercurrent heroin abuse will not result in euphoria and drug seeking behaviors is deterred. Clonidine is an effective adjuvant in opioid withdrawal. It acts on the locus coeruleus to open the same potassium channels that opiates open, and corrects many aspects of the withdrawal syndrome. However, acute dosing regimens are not well defined. Clonidine is most useful in conjunction with methadone maintenance and a structured detoxification program. It can be considered in situations where hospital policy does not permit methadone administration. Opioid withdrawal can be induced by the use of opioid receptor antagonists or mixed agonist-antagonists in opioid habituated patients. Often, this is the result of administering large doses of naloxone to opioid addicted patients who present with an opioid toxidrome. The frequency of this problem can be decreased by using a low initial starting dose, supporting oxygenation, gauging the therapeutic effect, and redosing based on clinical grounds. If acute withdrawal makes the patient a behavioral problem, diazepam can be administered for sedation. Withdrawal symptoms should resolve in 2 or 3 h as the naloxone is eliminated.

C. **Clonidine withdrawal.** Twenty-four hours after discontinuation of clonidine, the patient begins to experience headache, flushing, sweating, and anxiety. Hypertensive encephalopathy and death have been reported in rare cases. Blood pressure rises to near or above pretreatment levels by 48 h. The clonidine elimination half-life is 14 h, and most patients in withdrawal still have a measurable clonidine level for a period of time. There appears to be an association with high-dose therapy (greater than 1.2 mg/day) or concomitant beta-blocker therapy and an increased likelihood and severity of withdrawal. The clonidine patch is less likely to result in withdrawal after removal because drug remains in the subcutaneous tissues and declines over several days. Reinstitution of clonidine is therapeutic. Severe symptoms may be immediately reversed with i.v. phentolamine. Beta-blockers are absolutely contraindicated.

D. Caffeine withdrawal. Caffeine dependence and withdrawal has been demonstrated in patients who take as little as 129 mg/day of caffeine—the equivalent of an average 5-oz cup of coffee. Symptoms of anxiety, depression, headaches, sleepiness, and decreased alertness and activity peak on at 24 to 48 h and decrease over 1 week. Most patients will correctly identify the source of their symptoms and medicate with the appropriate dose and preferred form of caffeine. Clinicians should consider this entity in the patient who is being evaluated for headache symptoms.

E. Nicotine withdrawal. Smoking cessation is the primary cause for nicotine for withdrawal, although discontinuation of any tobacco product can lead to this syndrome. Cigarette craving is an important problem for hospitalized patients who are not permitted to smoke as well as office visits for smoking cessation. Nicotine withdrawal manifests largely as cigarette craving and subjective dysphoric symptoms. There are some symptoms of irritability, restlessness, and a decrease in heart rate and blood pressure. Cardiac symptoms resolve over 3 to 4 weeks, but cigarette craving may persist for months to years. The nicotine transdermal system (patch) and nicotine polacrilex (gum) can be used to provide nicotine without the additional health risks of tobacco. The dose of nicotine is then reduced over several weeks by lowering the dose of the patch or by decreasing the number of gum tablets chewed per day. Acute therapy is most easily achieved with use of the gum, as rapid chewing releases an immediate dose of nicotine

V. Neonatal withdrawal syndromes

A. GABA agonists. Maternal addiction to alcohol can result in a neonatal withdrawal syndrome that is characterized by varying degrees of tremor, nystagmus, clonus, opisthotonus, hypertonia, seizures, sleeplessness, crying, asymmetric or hyperactive reflexes, abnormal Moro reflex, excessive mouthing or rooting, diarrhea, vomiting, inability to feed, startle, sweating, and inability to thermoregulate. Symptoms usually begin within three days after birth. This syndrome can develop in children who do not have the fetal alcohol syndrome. In addition, mothers who are alcohol addicted but abstained from alcohol sometime during the third trimester do not have children with alcohol withdrawal symptoms. It is reasonable to expect similar symptoms in children of mothers with perinatal benzodiazepine and barbiturate addiction. Treat with phenobarbital at a loading dose of 16 mg/kg/24 h to produce a 24-h serum level of 20 to 30 µg/mL. This can be maintained with a dose of 2 to 8 mg/kg/24 h. Once withdrawal symptoms are controlled for 72 h, begin to taper the phenobarbital dose at 10% per day. Elixirs of phenobarbital contain 14 to 25% ethyl alcohol; parenteral forms contain 67.8% propylene glycol, 10% ethyl alcohol, and 1.5% benzyl alcohol.

B. **Opioids.** The neonatal opioid withdrawal syndrome occurs within 2 weeks of birth. It shares characteristics of the adult opiate withdrawal syndrome—GI distress (vomiting and diarrhea), irritability, yawning, sneezing, hypertonicity, hyperacusis, diaphoresis, lacrimation, and tremulousness. In neonates, these symptoms are accompanied by mottling, fever, myoclonic jerks, and seizures. This latter symptom is only characteristic of opioid withdrawal in neonates and occurs in roughly 8% of children born to mothers on methadone maintenance and only 1% of those born to mothers who use heroin. Paregoric appears to be more effective than diazepam in controlling and preventing these seizures while preserving the suck reflex. Paregoric is a combination of anyhydrous morphine (0.4 mg/mL), camphor, alcohol 46%, and benzoic acid (4 mg/mL). Some clinicians prefer a 1:25 dilution of opium tincture because it contains only 0.7% alcohol and no camphor or benzoic acid. Dosage for either drug is 0.2 mL every 3 h, increased by 0.05 mL at each dose until withdrawal symptoms are controlled up to a maximum of 0.7 mL per dose. Once the patient is stable, therapy is continued for 3 to 5 days and decreased gradually over a 2- to 4-week period. Parenteral morphine should be reserved for short term therapy of only severe withdrawal symptoms because it contains sodium bisulfite and phenol which may cause anaphylactic reactions and hyperbilirubinemia, respectively, when administered chronically. Methadone has been used for neonatal withdrawal, but its long half-life (26 h) makes dosing adjustments difficult in the neonate.

C. **Caffeine.** Caffeine withdrawal should be considered in the evaluation of an infant with irritability, jitteriness, and vomiting. One study detected caffeine in the serum of six of eight infants with these symptoms. All mothers gave a history of heavy caffeine use, and none were drug or alcohol addicted. The symptoms and caffeine levels persisted for a few days and then resolved spontaneously.

Suggested Readings

American Academy of Pediatrics Committee on Drugs. Neonatal drug withdrawal. *Pediatrics* 1983;72:895–902.

Booth BM, Blow FC. The kindling hypothesis: further evidence from a U.S. national study of alcoholic men. *Alcohol Alcoholism* 1993;28:593–598.

Brown M, Salmon D, Rendell M. Clonidine hallucinations. *Ann Intern Med* 1980;93:456–457.

Charness ME, Simon RP, Greenberg DA. Ethanol and the nervous system. *N Engl J Med* 1989;321:442–454.

Christie MJ, Williams JT, North RA. Cellular mechanisms of opioid tolerance: studies in single brain neurons. *Mol Pharmacol* 1987;32:633–638.

Coles CD, Smith IE, Fernhoff PM, et al. Neonatal ethanol withdrawal: characteristics in clinically normal, nondysmorphic neonates. *J Pediatr* 1984;105:445–451.

Glue P, Nutt D. Over-excitement and disinhibiton. Dynamic neurotransmitter interaction in alcohol withdrawal. *Br J Psychiatry* 1990;157:491–499.

Herzlinger RA, Kandall SR, Vaughan HG Jr. Neonatal seizures associated with narcotic withdrawal. *J Pediatr* 1977;91:638–641.

Kaplan GB, Greenblatt DJ, Kent MA, Cotreau-Bibbo MM. Caffeine treatment and withdrawal in mice: relationships between dosage, cocentrations, locomotor activity and A1 adenosine receptor binding. *J Pharm Exp Ther* 1993;266: 1563–1571.

Maldonado R, Blendy JA, Tzavara E, et al. Reduction of morphine abstinence in mice with mutation in the gene encoding CREB. *Science* 1996;273:657–659.

Manikant S, Tripathi BM, Chavan BS. Loading dose diazepam therapy for alcohol withdrawal state. *Indian J Med Res* 1993;98:170–173.

McGowan JD, Altman RE, Kanto WP Jr. Neonatal withdrawal symptoms after chronic maternal ingestion of caffeine. *South Med J* 1988;81:1092–1094.

Nestler EJ. Under siege: the brain on opiates. *Neuron* 1996;16:897–900.

Ochoa EL, Li L, McNamee MG. Densensitization of central cholinergic mechanisms and neuroadptation to nicotine. *Mol Neurobiol* 1990;4:251–287.

Prakash A, Das G. Cocaine and the nervous system. *Int J Clin Pharmacol Ther Toxicol* 1993;31:575–581.

Reid JL, Dargie HJ, Davies DS, Wing LMH, Hamilton CA, Dollery CT. Clonidine withdrawal in hypertension. *Lancet* 1977;1171–1174.

Rivas DA, Chancellor MB, Hill K, Freedman MK. Neurological manifestations of baclofen withdrawal. *J Urol* 1993;150: 1903–1905.

Saitz R, Mayo-Smith M, Roberts MS, et al. Individualized treatment for alcohol withdrawal. *JAMA* 1994;272:519–523.

Siegfried RN, Jacobson L, Chobal C. Development of an acute withdrawal syndrome following the cessation of intrathecal baclofen therapy in a patient with spasticity. *Anesthesiology* 1992;77:1048–1050.

Silverman K, Evans SM, Strain EC, et al. Withdrawal syndrome after the double-blind cessation of caffeine consumption. *N Engl J Med* 1992;327:1109–1114.

Sporer KA, Lesser SH. Cocaine washed-out syndrome. *Ann Emerg Med* 1992;21:112.

Stolerman IP, Shoaib M. The neurobiology of tobacco addiction. *Trends Pharmacol Sci* 1991;12:467–473.

Strain EC, Mumford GK, Silverman K, et al. Caffeine dependence syndrome. *JAMA* 1994;272:1043–1048.

Trabulsy ME. Cocaine washed-out syndrome in a patient with acute myocardial infarction. *Am J Emerg Med* 1995;13: 538–539.

PART VII

Environmental Toxins

Emergency Toxicology, Second Edition,
edited by Peter Viccellio.
Lippincott–Raven Publishers, Philadelphia © 1998.

71

Nitrogen Oxides and Silo-Filler's Disease

Rivka S. Horowitz

Division of Biology and Medicine, Brown University, Providence, Rhode Island 02903

I. **Introduction.** The oxides of nitrogen are a family of labile substances capable of causing pulmonary injury and, less commonly, methemoglobinemia. The nitrogen oxides of toxicological significance include nitrogen dioxide (NO_2), its dimer, nitrogen tetroxide (N_2O_4), and nitric oxide (NO). Nitric oxide is a unique substance: it is both an environmental pollutant and an endogenous cellular mediator. It has earned the designation "molecule of the year" because of the critical role it plays in the regulation of normal physiological functions (1).

II. **Sources of nitrogen oxides**

   A. **Occupational exposure.** Occupational exposure to nitrogen oxides occurs in a variety of environments. The diversity of occupations in which nitrogen oxide toxicity threatens workers' health underscores the importance of obtaining a thorough occupational history. Examples of populations at risk include the following:

   1. **Farmers** exposed to high concentrations of nitrogen oxides in or near silos (see silo-filler's disease below)

   2. **Firefighters** exposed to potentially lethal concentrations of nitrogen oxides resulting from the combustion of nitrogen-containing materials

   3. Oxyacetylene and electric arc **welders** generating nitrogen dioxide from high temperature reactions between atmospheric nitrogen and oxygen

   4. Military and **aerospace** personnel exposed to the missile fuel oxidizer nitrogen tetroxide

   5. Workers involved in the manufacture and use of **nitric acid** and **explosives**

   B. **Nonoccupational exposure**

   1. **Ice skating arenas.** Inadequate ventilation of nitrogen oxides produced from ice-resurfacing machines may result in clinically significant exposure amongst skaters and spectators in indoor ice skating arenas.

   2. **Air pollutants.** Nitrogen dioxide and nitric oxide are also atmospheric pollutants released from automobile exhaust and industrial smokestack emissions, especially from electrical power plants. In urban areas, peak nitrogen dioxide concentrations occur twice daily, corresponding to rush-hour traffic patterns to and from work. The importance of atmospheric release of nitrogen oxides is twofold: they are direct pulmonary toxicants, and they participate in the formation of ozone, a substance with known pulmonary toxicity. The Clean Air Act and its subsequent amendments require the Environmental Protection Agency to set air quality standards to protect

public health and welfare and which place environmental limits on air pollutants, including nitrogen dioxide, ozone, and other hazardous pollutants. While the bulk of regulatory action is aimed at atmospheric control of nitrogen oxides, there are actually higher ambient levels measured inside the home than outdoors. The sources of indoor nitrogen dioxide include gas stoves, space heaters, cigarette smoke, and exchange from outdoor air.

III. **Mechanism of action and toxicity**

A. **Pulmonary toxicity.** The lung is the primary target of nitrogen dioxide toxicity. The mild irritant, warning properties of nitrogen dioxide, however, may produce only minimal symptoms despite prolonged exposure. Its poor solubility in water results in negligible interaction with the proximal airway and permits its continued inhalation and deposition at the terminal and respiratory bronchioles (2). Nitrogen dioxide induces pulmonary injury in at least three ways: it is converted to nitric and nitrous acids in the distal airway where it exerts direct toxic effects on Type I pneumocytes and ciliated airway cells (3); it initiates free radical generation in the terminal bronchioles resulting in protein oxidation (4), lipid peroxidation (5) and consequent cell membrane damage; and it alters macrophage and immune function causing impaired resistance to infection (6). The nature of these changes are complex and varies depending on the concentration, chronicity and temporal pattern of exposure.

B. **Methemoglobinemia and hypoxemia.** Inhalation of nitrogen dioxide may result in methemoglobinemia, although this complication is reported less often than the pulmonary toxicity. Nitric oxide is absorbed through the lungs and rapidly binds to hemoglobin forming nitrosylhemoglobin (NOHb). This complex is readily oxidized to methemoglobin. In addition, the nitrosylhemoglobin complex preferentially binds nitric acid instead of oxygen (7) and causes a "left shift" of the oxygen-hemoglobin dissociation curve (8) further impairing tissue oxygenation.

C. **Therapeutic potential of nitric oxide.** In contrast to its potential toxicity, the potent vasodilatory effect of nitric oxide has been exploited as a promising therapeutic agent. Inhaled nitric oxide has been administered to adults with high-altitude pulmonary edema (9) and neonates with persistent pulmonary hypertension of the newborn (10). Oxygenation improved in the majority of these patients without adverse systemic effects. Interestingly, methemoglobin levels in the neonates treated did not exceed 2.3% (10). These preliminary studies show promise for the use of inhaled nitric oxide as an effective therapeutic agent.

IV. **Pharmacokinetics and properties of nitrogen oxides**

A. **Absorption, distribution, metabolism, and elimination.** The primary route of exposure to the oxides of nitrogen is via the lungs, although the potent oxidizing property of nitrogen tetroxide results in severe burns upon dermal contact. Nitric oxide is readily absorbed into the blood from the lungs and complexes with hemoglobin to form nitrosylhemoglobin, which in turn forms methemoglobin. Residual inhaled nitric oxide is excreted as nitrate in the urine (11).

B. **Physical properties.** Nitrogen dioxide is heavier than air, a fact which makes human and animal exposure more likely since the gas tends to collect in layers at the surface of the ground or just above silage, rather that diffusing and escaping into the atmosphere (see silo-filler's disease). It is reddish-brown to yellow in color, poorly soluble in water, and has an acrid odor resembling household bleach. Nitric oxide and nitrogen tetroxide are colorless gases, although nitrogen tetroxide retains its brown-yellow color when in liquid form. Liquid nitrogen tetroxide spontaneously oxidizes to nitrogen dioxide once exposed to air.

V. **Clinical presentation.** The first reported death from nitrogen dioxide fumes was colorfully described in 1804 and retold 170 years later in a descriptive narrative published in the *Journal of the American Medical Association*. The article describes in vivid detail the clinical sequelae and deaths of a nitric acid salesman and his dog accidentally exposed to nitrogen dioxide gas from a leaking nitric acid vial (12).

A. **Who is at risk?**

1. **Occupational exposures**

a. **Farmers working in or around silos—silo-filler's disease.** Immediate life-threatening or insidious respiratory disease may occur in farm workers who have been exposed to nitrogen oxides (principally nitrogen dioxide) while working in or near silos. Crops stored in silos rapidly undergo denitrification and fermentation under anaerobic conditions. These complex biochemical reactions result in the generation of gaseous mixtures consisting of high concentrations of nitrogen oxides and carbon dioxide, and depletion of oxygen. This process begins within hours of ensilage so that farmers entering a silo to level out the surface crops may be exposed to high concentrations of nitrogen dioxide. Furthermore, because nitrogen dioxide has only mild irritative properties, an exposed worker may continue to work in the silo, noting no or minimal symptoms. Concentrations in silos may exceed 2,000 ppm, far in excess of lethal doses. The characteristic odor or brown-red cloud need not be present for significant pulmonary injury to occur. Furthermore, because nitrogen dioxide is heavier than air, it flows down and accumulates in the chutes on the outsides of silos and at ground level. Thus, one need not enter the silo to be exposed to toxic concentrations of nitrogen dioxide. Safety guidelines dictate that workers not enter a silo for two weeks from the time crops are stored, at which time the active biochemical processes resulting in nitrogen dioxide generation have ceased. Upon re-entry, farm workers must ventilate the silos with powerful fans usually built into the silo for this purpose.

b. **Military personnel working with missile fuel.** Military personnel working with the liquid missile fuel oxidizer nitrogen tetroxide and civilians living in close proximity to missile silos are at risk should spillage occur. Accidental spillage of nitrogen tetroxide at a missile silo complex has occurred and resulted in death and serious injury (13).

c. **Welders.** High-temperature reactions between atmospheric nitrogen and oxygen from oxyacetylene and electric arc welding, results in the generation of high concentrations of nitrogen dioxide.

d. **Firefighters.** Burning nitrogen-containing materials release nitrogen oxides, putting firefighters at risk if adequate personal protective equipment is not used.

e. **Manufacturers of nitric acid and explosives**

    2. Nonoccupational exposure

        a. Exposure in **indoor ice skating arenas.** Release of nitrogen dioxide from ice-resurfacing machines in indoor ice skating rinks has resulted in clinically significant disease in skaters and spectators (14). Faulty ventilation from the same apparatus has also been responsible for carbon monoxide release.

B. Clinical syndromes. Illness caused by inhalation of nitrogen dioxide may result in a spectrum of disease (15). Factors influencing symptom development include concentration of nitrogen dioxide and duration of exposure.

    1. Acute exposure. Workers exposed to nitrogen dioxide may have symptoms ranging from mild cough and mucous membrane irritation to immediate collapse and death. Unfortunately, the absence of initial symptoms or the development of transient or mild manifestations following exposure to nitrogen dioxide does not preclude later development of clinically significant disease.

    2. Latency period. Following a latency period ranging from a 2 to 48 h, exposed patients may develop progressive dyspnea, bronchospasm, fever, cough, cyanosis and a clinical and radiographic picture of non-cardiogenic pulmonary edema. Patients who survive this, may go on to develop further pulmonary disease weeks to months later.

    3. Late sequelae. Approximately 2 to 8 weeks after nitrogen dioxide exposure, some patients develop progressive dyspnea, cough, fever and diffuse reticulonodular pattern on chest x-ray, consistent with bronchiolitis obliterans (16). Lung biopsy confirms the diagnosis. Patients who had minimal symptoms after initial exposure, may present for the first time with bronchiolitis obliterans.

    4. Methemoglobinemia. Methemoglobinemia should be suspected in dyspneic or cyanotic patients exposed to nitrogen oxides.

C. Clinical clues in the diagnosis of nitrogen oxide–induced pulmonary disease. There are no pathognomonic signs to aid in the diagnosis of nitrogen oxide–induced pulmonary disease. A thorough work history focusing on possible exposure to respiratory toxicants, should be obtained from all patients presenting with acute respiratory symptoms, non-cardiogenic pulmonary edema or bronchiolitis obliterans, for whom a clear etiology is unknown. Similarly, there are no clinical features distinguishing nitrogen oxide-associated bronchiolitis obliterans from the same syndrome caused by other toxicants.

D. Differential diagnosis. The differential diagnosis for dyspnea, non-cardiogenic pulmonary edema and bronchiolitis obliterans is immense. Specific occupations, such as farming, however, expose workers to a number of hazardous materials capable of causing respiratory disease. These include **moldy hay,** which may result in farmer's lung, a type of extrinsic allergic alveolitis; **grain dust,** implicated in the etiology of asthma in farmers; and **organophosphate** or **carbamate** poisoning resulting in cholinergic crisis. Welders may develop respiratory symptoms associated with **metal fume fever** from inhalation of zinc oxide fumes.

VI. Laboratory. There are no laboratory tests specific to nitrogen oxide–induced illness. Pulmonary function tests reveal both obstructive and restrictive disease (17). Patients who develop immediate or delayed respiratory symptoms after exposure to nitrogen dioxide present with a variety of chest x-ray findings ranging from normal to that of non-cardiogenic pulmonary edema. The chest x-rays of patients with bronchiolitis obliterans typically reveal a diffuse reticulonodular pattern similar to miliary tuberculosis (18), although patchy infiltrates may occasionally be seen. A lung biopsy confirms the diagnosis of bronchiolitis obliterans.

VII. Management

  A. General guidelines. Supportive management is the mainstay of therapy for all phases of nitrogen oxide–induced respiratory illness. Patients should be advised that a latency period exists following resolution of initial symptoms, and that delayed, life-threatening pulmonary edema and/or dyspnea due to bronchiolitis obliterans may occur. Although no controlled trials have documented the efficacy of high-dose steroid treatment in nitrogen oxide–induced pulmonary disease, most authors recommend its use in symptomatic patients. The data on the early use of steroids is anecdotal and controversy exists as to whether the early use of steroids prevents late sequelae, such as bronchiolitis obliterans. It is generally well accepted, however, that patients who develop bronchiolitis obliterans should be maintained on steroids until resolution of their symptoms. The long-term prognosis for nitrogen dioxide–induced pulmonary disease is good if the patient survives the acute exposure. In general, bronchiolitis obliterans resolves without chronic sequelae in patients treated with steroids. Patients with methemoglobinemia and cardiopulmonary compromise should be treated with methylene blue.

VIII. Disposition. Patients with a history of shortness of breath or loss of consciousness due to nitrogen dioxide exposure should be admitted to the hospital and observed for a minimum of 24 h. Overall clinical improvement and resolution of hypoxia or methemoglobinemia dictate appropriate time of discharge. Patients should be followed in an out-patient setting for a minimum of 2 to 3 months following exposure to rule out development of bronchiolitis obliterans.

References

1. Culotta E, Koshland DE. NO news is good news. *Science* 1992;18:258:1862–1865.
2. Goldstein E, Goldstein F, Peek N, Parks NJ. Absorption and transport of nitrogen oxides. In: Lee SD, ed. *Nitrogen oxides and their effects on health.* Ann Arbor, MI: Ann Arbor Science Publishers, 1983:143–160.
3. Evans MJ, Stephens RJ, Cabral LJ, Freeman G. Cell renewal in the lungs of rats exposed to low levels of NO_2. *Arch Environ Health* 1972;24:180–188.
4. Prutz WA, Monig H, Butler J, Land EJ. Reactions of nitrogen dioxide in aqueous model systems: oxidation of tyrosine units in peptides and proteins. *Arch Biochem Biophys* 1985;243:125–134.
5. Sagai M, Ichinose T. Lipid peroxidation and antioxidative protection mechanism in rat lungs upon acute and chronic exposure to nitrogen oxide. *Environ Health Perspect* 1987;73:179–189.
6. Jakab JJ. Modulation of pulmonary defense mechanisms by acute exposures to nitrogen dioxide. *Environ Res* 1987;42:215–228.
7. Gibson QH, Roughton FJW. The kinetics and equilibria of the reactions of nitric acid with sheep hemoglobin. *J Physiol* 1957;136:507–526.
8. Kon K, Maeda N, Shiga T. Effect of nitric oxide on the oxygen transport of human erythrocytes. *J Toxicol Environ Health* 1977;2:1109–1113.
9. Scherrer U, Vollenweider L, Delabays A, et al. Inhaled nitric oxide for high-altitude pulmonary edema. *N Engl J Med* 1996;334:624–629.
10. Roberts JD, Polaner DM, Lang P, Zapol WM. Inhaled nitric oxide in persistent pulmonary hypertension of the newborn. *Lancet* 1992;340:818–819.

11. Yoshida K, Kasama K. Biotransformation of nitric oxide. *Environ Health Perspect* 1987;73:201–206.
12. Ramirez R. The first death from nitrogen dioxide fumes: the story of a man and his dog. *JAMA* 1974;229:1181–1182.
13. Yockey CC, Eden BM, Byrd RB. The McConnell Missile Accident: clinical spectrum of nitrogen dioxide exposure. *JAMA* 1980;244:1221–1223.
14. Karlson-Stiber C, Hijer J, Sjoholm A, Bluhm G, Salmonson H. Nitrogen dioxide pneumonitis in ice hockey players. *J Intern Med* 1996;239:241–256.
15. Douglas WW, Hepper NG, Colby TV. silo-filler's disease. *Mayo Clin Proc* 1989;64:291–304.
16. Lowry T, Schuman LM. "silo-filler's disease"—a syndrome caused by nitrogen dioxide. *JAMA* 1956;162:153–160.
17. Jones GR, Proudfoot AT, Hall JI. Pulmonary effects of acute exposure to nitrous fumes. *Thorax* 1973;28:61–65.
18. Delaney LT, Schmidt HW, Stroebel CF. silo-filler's disease. *Mayo Clin Proc* 1956;31:189–198.

Selected Readings

Elsayed NM. Toxicity of nitrogen dioxide: an introduction. *Toxicology* 1994;89:161–174.
Epler GR. Editorial. silo-filler's disease: a new perspective. *Mayo Clin Proc* 1989;64:368–370.
Hayhurst ER, Scott E. Four cases of sudden death in a silo. *JAMA* 1914;63:1570–1572.
Mayorga MA. Overview of nitrogen dioxide effects on the lung with emphasis on military relevance. *Toxicology* 1994;89:175–192.

Emergency Toxicology, Second Edition,
edited by Peter Viccellio.
Lippincott–Raven Publishers, Philadelphia © 1998.

72

Hydrogen Sulfide

Kenneth A. Hirsch

Department of Emergency Medicine, J. T. Mather Memorial Hospital, Port Jefferson, New York 11777; State University of New York at Stony Brook, University Hospital, Stony Brook, New York 11794-7400

A. **Properties of hydrogen sulfide (H_2S)**
1. **Sources.** It may be released from decomposing organic matter (e.g., sewage, manure) and from mixtures involving sulfuric acid or other sulphur acids. H_2S is used in farming, brewing, tanning, glue making, metal recovery, rubber vulcanizing, heavy water production, and oil and gas exploration, and processing. It is also found in natural sulphur springs and mines running through sulphurous rock ("stink damp"). Ingested soluble inorganic sulfide salts may release H_2S in vivo.
2. **Physical and chemical properties.** It is a highly toxic, colorless gas heavier than air. At low concentrations (0 to 25 ppm), it possesses the odor of rotten eggs; higher concentrations (50 to 150 ppm) lead to rapid paralysis of the olfactory nerve with resultant loss of sense of smell.
3. **Mechanism of action and pathophysiology.** It is believed to act as a cytochrome oxidase poison, blocking the terminal element of the electron transport chain, which catalyzes the reduction of molecular oxygen to water, thereby resulting in intracellular hypoxia. This blockage of cellular respiration is similar to the actions of cyanide and possibly carbon monoxide. Recognition of this similarity has resulted in toxin-specific treatment possibilities.
4. **Pharmacology and pharmacokinetics.** H_2S gas is rapidly absorbed and acts as a local irritant at low concentrations. Vapor concentrations as low as 50 ppm may cause toxicity, while high concentrations (over 1,000 ppm) lead to collapse within seconds and may be rapidly fatal. It may have a direct effect on the carotid body, to briefly cause hyperpnea; subsequent respiratory depression and apnea occur from action on the brain stem. H_2S is normally detoxified by undergoing spontaneous oxidation to sulfate of thiosulfate. H_2S binds to methemoglobin to form sulfmethemoglobin, which undergoes autoxidation. The half-life of sulfmethemoglobin is 2 h at 24°C. Some H_2S is excreted, unchanged, by the lungs. The body has a large capacity to detoxify sulfide, so toxicity is mostly related to concentration of exposure and less related to duration.

B. **Clinical presentation**
1. **History.** At exposure to low concentrations (0 to 25 ppm), the odor of rotten eggs is detected. At higher concentrations (over 50 to 150 ppm), the sense of smell is rapidly paralyzed. Symptoms of acute poisoning progress from local irritation of

mucous membranes, headache, nausea, cough, dizziness, and dyspnea, to pulmonary edema, seizures, coma, and death. Exposure to high concentrations (over 1,000 ppm) leads to collapse within seconds ("knockdown"). If exposure is brief (e.g., the wind shifts, or the subject is rapidly removed to fresh air), recovery may be equally rapid; otherwise, death may occur in minutes. Chronic low level exposure may be associated with reduced lung function as measured by FEV1/FVC; neurophysiological abnormalities such as headaches, depression, and personality changes; chronic eye irritation; and abnormalities of fetal/neonatal brain tissue development.

2. **Physical examination**
   a. **Eyes.** Keratoconjunctivitis with tearing, burning, pain, and redness.
   b. **Cardiovascular.** Hypotension, tachycardia, bradycardia, and arrhythmia.
   c. **Respiratory.** Respiratory depression, marked cyanosis, and pulmonary edema. Apnea is a grave sign often followed by hypoxic seizures, cardiovascular collapse, and death.
   d. **Neurologic.** Confusion, disorientation, seizures, coma, and death.
   e. **Gastrointestinal.** Nausea and vomiting.
   f. **Dermatologic.** Erythema and cyanosis.

3. **Course.** Eye complications from prolonged exposure to low concentrations almost always resolve completely. Symptoms from nonfatal exposures will sometimes resolve in hours, although prolonged recoveries are common. Neurologic sequelae have been known to occur. Very brief exposure to even extremely high concentrations may reverse rapidly, with return to normalcy in minutes; however, more prolonged exposure to high concentrations leads rapidly to death.

C. **Differential diagnosis.** Acute H_2S poisoning most closely resembles cyanide and carbon monoxide poisoning. A history of the odor of "rotten eggs" points to H_2S, although this may be absent due to olfactory nerve paralysis. History of the nature of exposure (e.g., industrial exposure) is of great use. Sudden collapse ("knockdown") is characteristic of exposure to high concentrations of H_2S. As H_2S poisonings are often industrial, there is frequently more than one person overcome; the sudden collapse of several coworkers should raise suspicion of H_2S.

   1. **Keratoconjunctivitis.** Prolonged exposure to low concentrations of H_2S may result in eye symptoms alone. History of the characteristic "rotten egg" odor points to H_2S as the etiology.

D. **Laboratory analysis**
   1. **General**
      a. **Arterial blood gases.** Acidosis is often present due to anaerobic metabolism. Hypoxia results from pulmonary edema.
      b. **Electrocardiogram.** May show tachycardia, bradycardia, or cardiac arrhythmias.
      c. **Chest x-ray.** May show pulmonary edema. This may be due to the direct irritant effect of H_2S on the pulmonary epithelium.
      d. **Medication levels.** If indicated (e.g., theophyllin, digoxin).
      e. **Urinalysis.** May show albumin, casts, and/or red blood cells.
      f. **Electrolyte balance.** Should be watched closely as severe metabolic acidosis may develop due to anaerobic metabolism.

2. **Toxin-specific laboratory.** Very limited.
   a. Monitor methemoglobin levels.
   b. Lead acetate test paper detects presence of H_2S in the air.
   c. Quantitative hydrogensulfide ion in blood is not readily available.
E. **Management**
   1. **General.** Remove from exposure, with rescuer safety a must. Protect the airway, and intubate if necessary. Administer 100% oxygen. Aggressive supportive therapy is essential. Naloxone 2.0 mg and dextrose 25 g, if there is altered mental status.
      a. **Hypotension.** Treat with i.v. fluids, Trendelenburg position, and dopamine or norepinephrine if necessary.
      b. **Pulmonary edema.** Suction upper airway as necessary. Furosemide, nitrates, aminophyllin, and bicarbonate if necessary. Monitor ABGs and consider CPAP in the nonintubated patient, PEEP in the intubated patient if Po_2 cannot be maintained above 50 with high concentrations of oxygen alone. Monitor fluids with Swan-Ganz catheter.
      c. **Eyes.** Irrigate copiously. Local anesthetic may be necessary for initial evaluation, and for pain control. Consider an ophthalmologic consultation if irrigation does not relieve symptoms. Olive oil drops have been suggested for symptomatic relief of burning sensation.
      d. **Skin.** Wash thoroughly all exposed areas.
      e. **Seizures.** Treat with i.v. diazepam. May require phenytoin.
      f. **Aspiration pneumonia.** A common complication leading to superimposed bacterial infection. Start antibiotics at the first sign of pulmonary infection.
   2. **Toxin-specific therapy**
      a. **Nitrites.** Cyanide Antidote Kit (Lilly). Amyl nitrate inhalation and i.v. sodium nitrite in the same dose as for cyanide (amyl nitrate inhaled for 30 s/min until sodium nitrite can be given i.v., 300 mg in adults). The sodium thiosulfate from the cyanide kit is felt to be unnecessary. Nitrite-induced methemoglobin is believed to bind sulfide ions, removing them from the cytochrome oxidase system.
      b. **Hyperbaric oxygen.** Recent reports are encouraging. If supportive treatments and nitrites have failed, hyperbaric treatment should be attempted. This may be particularly helpful when pulmonary edema is present and may be of use even hours after exposure.
   3. **Management controversies.** Mainly center around the use of nitrites. Some research indicates that nitrites take too long to work and do not function well in the presence of the high doses of oxygen being used in the treatment of H_2S poisoning. Numerous reports of improvement after treatment with nitrites make it prudent to administer the nitrites in the cyanide antidote kit in cases of H_2S poisoning. In addition, since cyanide poisoning may present in a similar fashion to H_2S poisoning, use of the antidote kit would be effective if cyanide was the actual culprit.
F. **Disposition and follow-up**
   1. **Minor exposure.** Keratoconjunctivitis only—may be discharged home to follow-up with ophthalmologist. Skin irritation only—may be discharged after cleansing.

2. **Significant exposures.** Patients who have been unconscious or who are exhibiting respiratory, cardiac, or neurologic signs should be admitted for monitoring and close observation. Although coma may disappear rapidly, full recovery is usually slow. Watch for pulmonary edema or for aspiration pneumonia.

3. **Long-term follow-up.** Sequelae are generally neurologic, possibly due to changes in brain neurotransmitter content. These sequelae may resolve completely; however, there are reported cases of prolonged or possibly permanent sequelae. Baseline and annual neurological and neuropsychological testing for at least 5 years has been suggested for those patient presenting in coma or with evidence of neurotoxicity.

4. **Hyperbaric treatment.** Candidates should be transferred to the nearest appropriate facility if a hyperbaric chamber is not readily available.

Selected Readings

Beck JF, Bradbury CM, Connors AJ, et al. Nitrite as an antidote for acute hydrogen sulfide intoxication? *Am Ind Hyg Assoc J* 1981;42:805.

Burnett WW, King EG, Grace M, et al. Hydrogen sulfide poisoning: review of 5 years' experience. *Can Med Assoc J* 1977;117:1277.

Gosselin RE, Smith RP, Hodge HC. *Clinical toxicology of commercial products.* 5th ed. Baltimore: Williams & Wilkins, 1984.

Gregorakos L, et al. Hydrogen sulfide poisoning: management and complications. *Angiology* 1995;46:1123–1131.

Guidotti TL. Occupational exposure to hydrogen sulfide in the sour gas industry: some unresolved issues. *Int Arch Occup Environ Health* 1994;66:153–160.

Hoidal CR, Hall AH, Robinson MD, et al. Hydrogen sulfide poisoning from toxic inhalations of roofing asphalt fumes. *Ann Emerg Med* 1986;15:826.

Kilburn KH. Case report: profound neurobehavioral deficits in an oil field worker overcome by hydrogen sulfide. *Am J Med Sci* 1993;306:301–305.

Kilburn KH, Warshaw RH. Hydrogen sulfide and reduced-sulfur gases adversely affect neurophysiological functions. *Toxicol Ind Health* 1995;11:185–197.

Reiffenstein RJ, et al. Toxicology of hydrogen sulfide. *Annu Rev Pharmacol Toxicol* 1992;32:109–134.

Richardson DB. Respiratory effects of chronic hydrogen sulfide exposure. *Am J Ind Med* 1995;28:99–108.

Smilkstein MJ, Bronstein AC, Pickett HM, et al. Hyperbaric oxygen therapy for severe hydrogen sulfide poisoning. *J Emerg Med* 1985;3:37.

Smith RP, Gosselin RE. Hydrogen sulfide poisoning. *J Occup Med* 1979;21:93–97.

Smith RP, Kruszyna R, Kruszyna H. Management of acute sulfide poisoning. *Arch Environ Health* 1976;176.

Snyder JW, et al. Occupational fatality and persistent neurological sequelae after mass exposure to hydrogen sulfide. *Am J Emerg Med* 1995;13:199–203.

Stine RJ, Slosberg B, Beacham BE. Hydrogen sulfide intoxication. *Ann Intern Med* 1976;85:756.

Tvedt B, et al. Brain damage caused by hydrogen sulfide: a follow-up study of six patients. *Am J Indust Med* 1991;20: 91–101.

Warenycia MW, et al. Monoamine oxidase inhibition as a sequel of hydrogen sulfide intoxication: increases in brain catecholamine and 5-hydroxytryptamine levels. *Arch Toxicol* 1989;63:131–136.

Whitcraft DD, Baily TD, Hart GB. Hydrogen sulfide poisoning treated with hyperbaric oxygen. *J Emerg Med* 1985;3:23.

Emergency Toxicology, Second Edition,
edited by Peter Viccellio.
Lippincott–Raven Publishers, Philadelphia © 1998.

73

Cyanide

James G. Ryan

Department of Emergency Medicine, North Shore University Hospital, Manhasset, New York 11030

I. Properties

    A. Sources and forms of toxin

        1. Naturally occurring forms

            a. Certain plants contain high quantities of amygdalin, which is converted to cyanide in the small intestine by bacteria in the presence of the enzyme emulsin.

            b. These plants may contain hundreds to thousands of milligrams of amygdalin per kilogram. Amygdalin when broken down is approximately 6% cyanide, and the lethal dose of cyanide is approximately 0.5 to 1.0 mg/kg, or about 70 mg for an adult man.

            c. Prunus species

                (1) Amygdalin is present in the leaves, flowers, bark, and seeds.

                (2) Chokecherry, wild black cherry, peach, plum, apricot, bitter almond, cherry laurel, mountain mahogany.

            d. Sorghum species

                (1) Johnson grass

                (2) Sorghum

                (3) Sudan grass

                (4) Arrow grass

            e. Linum species

                (1) Flax

                (2) Yellow pine flax

            f. Pear, apple, crabapple seeds

            g. Jetberry bush (jet beads)

            h. Elderberry

            i. Hydrangea

            j. Bamboo

            k. Cassava

            l. Cycad nut

            m. Lima beans

            n. Linseed

    2. Other sources

        a. Cyanide gas

           (1) Fumigation of insects and rodents

           (2) Cigarette smoke

           (3) Used for capital punishment

           (4) Product of combustion of petrochemicals

           (5) Product of combustion in fires, especially involving plastics, wool, and silk

           (6) By-products of industries such as petroleum refining, ore extraction, electroplating, metal heat treating

        b. Liquid and solid forms. Cyanide salts and solutions containing these salts are used in metal cleaning, electroplating, organic synthesis, extraction of metals, photographic chemicals, and mining.

        c. Medicines that liberate cyanide

           (1) Nitroprusside

           (2) Laetrile contains amygdalin that is converted to cyanide in the GI tract (nontoxic i.v.).

           (3) Succinonitrile, an antidepressant

        d. Nitriles are substances that liberate cyanide when metabolized in vivo

           (1) Some nitriles may also liberate hydrogen cyanide gas, which may cause inhalation exposure.

           (2) Nitriles are absorbed readily through the skin.

           (3) Symptoms may be delayed up to 12 h owing to a time lapse in the conversion to cyanide.

           (4) These substances are generally found in chemical industries. Recently, they have been used in household artificial nail removers.

        e. Exposure in fires

            (1) Cyanide gas is known to be released by combustion of various substances, such as wool, silk, nylon, synthetic rubber, polyurethanes, and asphalt.

           (2) Studies have yielded marked disparity in the frequency of elevated cyanide levels in patients exposed to fires.

           (3) Some studies have shown elevated levels in as many as 90% of fire victims.

B. Mechanism of action

    1. Cyanide is a cellular poison that can readily bind to many enzymes, having a metallic component. The enzyme considered responsible for most of the toxic effects of cyanide is cytochrome oxidase, which is the terminal enzyme involved in aerobic metabolism. Inhibition of this enzyme results in a histotoxic anoxia due to paralysis of aerobic metabolism. Cyanide has been shown to initially bind to the protein portion of this enzyme and to later attach to the iron component (1). This reaction is reversible but forms a relatively stable complex.

    2. Cyanide has been shown to bind to many other proteins, such as nitrate reductase, myoglobin, ribulose diphosphate carboxylase, and catalase (1). Lipid metabolism and calcium transport have also been shown to be altered. The significance of these effects in the toxicology of cyanide is not yet determined.

3. The organ systems most susceptible to the cellular anoxia caused by cyanide are the CNS and cardiovascular system, as would be expected from anoxia from any cause. In animal studies, the first symptoms were attributable to CNS disturbances, with death resulting from seizures or inhibition of the central respiratory centers (2). At high blood concentrations (if subjects received artificial ventilation) cardiac arrest occurred, but respiratory arrest was seen consistently at lower blood cyanide levels than were cardiac events.

C. **Pharmacology and pharmacokinetics**

1. **Absorption**

   a. Oral absorption of cyanide is rapid, and the toxic effects can present within minutes. Animal studies (2,3) using large doses have shown respiratory arrest to occur as soon as 3 min after ingestion. Although absorption may not be as rapid with smaller doses, human overdoses generally involve doses far above the minimally lethal dose.

   b. Patients who ingest cyanogenic plants, laetrile, or a nitrile compound frequently have a prolonged delay before the development of symptoms. Laetrile and cyanogenic plants require that amygdalin be converted to cyanide in the GI tract before absorption can occur. Nitriles are metabolized to cyanide after absorption. Either of these processes may take as long as 12 h, thereby delaying evidence of toxicity for many hours.

   c. Respiratory absorption is almost immediate, with rapid onset of symptoms. Patients with a severe exposure often become unresponsive within seconds and succumb rapidly without supportive care.

   d. Dermal exposure is rare but has been reported with large surface area exposures. Nitrile compounds are more readily absorbed through the skin, and their toxicity would likewise be delayed.

2. **Distribution.** After absorption, cyanide distributes to a volume of approximately 40% total body weight. This distribution is rapid and is completed within 5 min after a single i.v. dose (4). The cyanide is transported to its ultimate site by the blood, with approximately 60% bound to plasma proteins, a small amount present in RBCs, and the remainder present as free cyanide.

3. **Elimination.** Cyanide is eliminated from the body by several mechanisms.

   a. It is excreted in small amounts in the urine and via the lungs as well as being incorporated into cyanocobalamin (vitamin B_{12}), oxidized to formate and carbon dioxide, and incorporated with cystine.

   b. The most important mechanism of elimination, accounting for 80%, is its conversion to **thiocyanate.** The exact in vivo mechanism for this reaction has not been elucidated, but two enzymes, rhodanese and mercaptopyruvate sulfur transferase, have been implicated. The conversion to thiocyanate also requires a sulfur donor, such as thiosulfate, to allow the reaction to proceed. This reaction is practically irreversible; and once thiocyanate is formed, it is eliminated via the kidneys. The rate-limiting factor in this reaction appears to be the presence of a sulfur donor. It may be enhanced by the addition of additional sulfur donors.

    c. At 3 h, approximately 90% of injected cyanide has been shown to be eliminated in the dog model (4).

II. Clinical presentation

A. History

1. Clues to the diagnosis of cyanide poisoning are often easier to evaluate if related to the setting of the poisoning. Cyanide is a relatively uncommon ingredient in household items but may be present in metal cleaning solutions and photographic chemicals, and it has been described in the nitrile form in artificial nail removers. As well as these home sources, patients, especially children, may be exposed to cyanide by ingesting cyanogenic plants (see **I.A.1**)

2. Cyanide and nitrile compounds are used or are **by-products of many industries,** especially chemical synthesis, metal extraction, fumigation, photography, jewelry making, and the petrochemical industry. Any patient who presents with signs or symptoms suggestive of cyanide poisoning in this setting should be evaluated. Such patients frequently present with a sudden loss of consciousness or respiratory arrest, but it should be remembered that nitrile compounds produce a more protracted course.

3. With the increasing inclusion of cyanogenic substances in household products, the risk of **fire-induced** cyanide toxicity would be expected to increase. The risk of cyanide from fires varies greatly among studies, but those treating patients exposed to toxic gases from a fire must clearly include cyanide poisoning in the differential diagnosis.

4. Cyanogenic substances are also used for **medical treatment.** Nitroprusside use may lead to cyanide toxicity, but this fact should be recognized and monitored by the clinician administering the medication. Patients with a malignancy who develop symptoms attributable to cyanide should be evaluated for the surreptitious use of laetrile. As with nitriles, laetrile may take a while for conversion to cyanide and may produce a less acute picture.

B. Physical examination is usually not helpful except for a couple of findings.

1. Classically, cyanide has been said to produce an odor of bitter almonds. This finding, although helpful if present, cannot be relied on. Studies have shown that 20% to 40% of the population are not capable of recognizing this odor. This finding is not only true for untrained people but for trained personnel as well, such as chemists.

2. The other finding is the **funduscopic appearance** of the arteries and veins. With cyanide poisoning, the veins have a red color, in contrast to the usual blue tint, and are difficult to distinguish from the arteries. This change is due to the decreased tissue extraction of oxygen, resulting in high venous oxygen saturation. The reliability of this finding has not been evaluated in clinical studies.

3. The remainder of the examination is nonspecific and not helpful.

C. Course

1. The course of **acute cyanide poisoning** depends on the route of ingestion, the dose of cyanide, and whether cyanide itself or a precursor that requires conversion was

ingested. Respiratory exposure to high levels of cyanide gas (more than 270 to 300 ppm) usually results in immediate onset of symptoms and may be fatal in less than 1 min. Lower concentrations (100 to 200 ppm) may be fatal with longer exposures, and levels of more than 100 ppm may produce mild symptoms or death with exposures lasting 1 h (5).

2. Oral ingestion may also produce rapid onset of symptoms. Because many human overdoses involve doses far greater than the minimal lethal dose, the onset of symptoms is frequently rapid. Animal studies have shown that absorption of cyanide decreases with a more alkaline stomach and that normally most cyanide is absorbed within 2 to 3 h of ingestion, suggesting that the time course of an oral ingestion should be fairly rapid and should peak within several hours.

3. Substances such as nitrile compounds and amygdalin from plants require **conversion** to cyanide before they can produce symptoms. This conversion occurs in the GI tract in the case of amygdalin and nitriles, and it may take 12 h or longer before toxicity becomes evident. Because of this delay, patients suspected of ingesting these substances require longer periods of observation in order to monitor for peak absorption and symptoms.

III. **Laboratory analysis**
  A. **General tests**
    1. **Hematology.** Cyanide has not been shown to have any specific effects on the WBC count, hemoglobin, hematocrit, or platelet count.
    2. **Chemistries.** Because of the blockade of aerobic metabolism, cyanide produces an anion gap metabolic acidosis secondary to the production of lactic acid. Glucose catabolism is also altered, and the blood glucose level may be elevated (1,6). The remainder of the chemistries show no specific abnormality.
    3. **Blood gas analyses**
      a. PaO_2 and oxygen **saturation** are unaltered by cyanide except in severe cases where respiratory failure occurs.
      b. pH and $PaCO_2$ are altered in different ways, depending on the severity of poisoning. Initially, patients may exhibit a respiratory alkalosis due to hyperventilation in response to tissue hypoxia. As toxicity worsens, a metabolic acidosis develops, also caused by the inability of the tissues to extract and utilize oxygen. As the patient's status worsens, respiratory depression occurs, and respiratory acidosis and respiratory failure may occur.
      c. Mixed venous oxygen sampling reveals an increased level of oxygen owing to the decreased tissue extraction (7). This finding can be helpful, as critically ill patients would be expected to have normal if not increased oxygen extraction. A decreased arteriovenous (AV) oxygen difference has few causes: a physiological AV shunt, hydrogen sulfide poisoning, sodium azide poisoning, and cyanide poisoning.
  B. **Toxin-specific tests**
    1. Specific cyanide levels can be measured, but the assays require several hours to perform and are therefore not useful for acute management. The **Lee-Jones test** is a quick bedside test that can qualitatively detect the presence of cyanide using gastric

aspirate (8). To perform this test, a few crystals of ferrous sulfate are added to 5 to 10 mL of gastric aspirate. To this mixture, five drops of 20% NaOH are added; and the solution is boiled and then cooled. After cooling, 10 drops of 10% HCl are added. The development of a greenish-blue color indicates the presence of cyanide. This test is not specific for cyanide, as other substances such as salicylates, barbiturates, antidepressants, phenothiazines, and benzodiazepines, may also produce a green-blue discoloration.

2. The specific **cyanide level** is the gold standard test and should be done even though the results may not be readily available. These levels are usually performed on whole blood, but some laboratories use serum or plasma. There is a good correlation between these levels, and the preference for whole blood is more historical than practical. These results, once obtained, must be evaluated with consideration to the 1- to 3-h biologic half-life of cyanide in vivo and the rapid disappearance of cyanide in improperly stored specimens.

3. Range of toxicity. The data presented below are adapted from Rumack (5) and Nassau County Poison Control protocols.

IV. Management

A. General measures

1. **ABCs**
   a. Evaluate adequacy of airway.
   b. Assess adequacy of oxygenation and ventilate.
      (1) Do not give mouth-to-mouth resuscitation without a barrier.
      (2) Administer high-concentration oxygen.
      (3) Intubate if necessary.
   c. Maintain blood pressure via fluids and pressor agents as necessary.

2. **Seizures.** Administer diazepam and phenytoin as per standard seizure protocol.

3. **Arrhythmias**
   a. Supraventricular
      (1) Sinus tachycardia is expected.
      (2) Other arrhythmias are treated as per standard protocols.
   b. Ventricular. Malignant ventricular arrhythmias are treated as per standard protocols.

4. **Detoxification**
   a. Respiratory. Remove patient from site, using precautions to avoid exposure of rescuers.
   b. Dermal. Wash skin thoroughly with water, wearing gloves to protect rescue personnel.
   c. Oral
      (1) Emesis may be dangerous, as the patient may become rapidly obtunded and aspirate.
      (2) Nasogastric lavage may be useful for removing toxin remaining in the stomach.
      (3) Charcoal, especially in the superactivated form, has been shown to bind cyanide and should be administered in patients with cynaide toxic-

ity. Greater benefit would be expected in patients with a recent ingestion or in patients who have ingested compounds that undergo degradation to cyanide and have a delayed onset of toxicity. Since superactivated charcoal is no longer commercially available activated charcoal
should be given.

(4)   Cathartic. One dose may be given with charcoal.

B.   Toxin-specific measures. Many forms of therapy have been proposed to treat cyanide
poisoning, all of which have some inherent problems. The current treatment in the United
States is a combination of nitrite and thiosulfate. Other agents have been used, but no clear
advantage has been shown with alternative therapies. This section focuses on the use of
the nitrite-thiosulfate combination and then briefly discusses alternative therapies.
Hydroxycobalamin has now been studied as an effective antidote with minimal adverse
effects and in fact may replace the current therapy.

1.   **Nitrite-thiosulfate**

   a.   For many years, nitrites were thought to cause removal of cyanide from tissues
   by the preferential binding of cyanide to the methemoglobin induced by these
   agents. This hypothesis has come into question owing to the observation that
   the cyanide antagonism is rapid and occurs faster than methemoglobin formation (1). The cyanide antagonism of nitrites has also been shown to persist
   despite the administration of methylene blue to prevent formation of methemoglobin (9). These findings have led to the proposals that cyanide may act
   by vasodilation or another unknown mechanism, and the issue remains unresolved.

   b.   Thiosulfate provides a sulfur donor to promote the conversion of cyanide to
   thiocyanate, which is nontoxic and can be excreted by the kidneys. The exact
   site of action of thiosulfate and involvement of rhodanese in this reaction
   remains controversial, as rhodanese is a mitochondrial enzyme and thiosulfate has difficulty getting into the mitochondria. Some researchers have
   suggested that the transformation to thiocyanate may involve albumin and a
   sulfur donor, with minimal involvement of rhodanese. The injection of thiosulfate has been estimated to increase cyanide elimination by 13-fold and has
   been shown to restore respiration to dogs poisoned with cyanide within
   3 min.

   c.   Administration of the **nitrite-thiosulfate kit** must be carefully monitored to
   prevent adverse reactions, which may be severe and life-threatening because
   of the toxicity of the nitrites. Sodium nitrite causes **methemoglobinemia,**
   which if severe can be fatal. The dose of nitrites must be corrected for weight
   and hemoglobin content. The other adverse effect of nitrites is **hypotension.**
   The currently available kit contains amyl nitrite for rapid inhalation, sodium
   nitrite for i.v. injection, and sodium thiosulfate for i.v. injection. The amyl
   nitrite is estimated to give a methemoglobin level of 5% when inhaled for
   30 s. Since amyl nitrite is not as effective as i.v. sodium nitrite it should only
   be used if i.v. access cannot be obtained. Sodium nitrite is given at a dose of
   0.9 mg/kg/g Hgb i.v. to a maximum of 300 mg (10 mL of 3% solution) for

adults, which should yield a methemoglobin level of 10% to 12%. Methemoglobin levels should be monitored if multiple doses of sodium nitrite are administered. Sodium nitrite should be administered slowly at a rate of 2 to 5 mL/min to prevent hypotension. Sodium thiosulfate can be given at a dose of 12.5 g i.v., or 50 mL of a 25% solution, for adults or calculated as per the chart below for children. If an inadequate response occurs, half of these doses may be repeated in 0.5 h.

2. Hydroxycobalamin (vitamin B$_{12}$) has been studied as a potential cyanide antidote; it has few if any adverse effects. Hydroxycobalamin binds cyanide with a greater affinity than cytochrome oxidase to form cyanocobalamin, or vitamin B$_{12}$, which can then be excreted in the urine.

    a. In Europe, thiosulfate has been combined with hydroxycobalamin in a kit and has resulted in successful treatment.

    b. The main advantage of hydroxycobalamin over the nitrites is its lack of adverse effects, such as methemoglobin formation and hypotension. This agent can be administered safely to critically ill patients without the fear of impairing oxygen-carrying capacity.

    c. The current dose in Europe is about 4 g.

    d. Currently, the only preparation of hydroxycobalamin available in the United States is an i.m. dose of 1 mg/mL for the treatment of pernicious anemia. To give the 4-g dose used in cyanide toxixity, 4,000 vials or 4 L of this preparation would be required.

3. Other methemoglobin forming agents, most notably DMAP (dimethyl-4-aninophenol) have been shown to rapidly produce methemoglobinemia and attenuate cyanide toxicity. A recent study in rats showed a beneficial effect of treating with both DMAP and sodium nitrite and that thiosulfate increased the degree of protection from cyanide toxicity, when added to this regimen (10). Whether the use of these two methemoglobin forming agents together will be beneficial or will produce clinically toxic methemoglobinemia requires further investigation. No clear benefit has been shown with other methemoglobin producing agents as compared to nitrites.

4. Agents that have alpha-adrenergic properties have been found to antagonize the toxic effects of cyanide. Both chlorpromazine and phenoxybenzamine have been shown (1,11) to protect against cyanide toxicity but only in the presence of thiosulfate. This effect can not be demonstrated when these agents are given alone or with sodium nitrite and it is blocked by the administration of methoxamine (an alpha-blocking agent). The mechanism for this has not been elucidated and their role in human ingestions is unclear.

5. Oxygen has been shown to augment the action of the nitrite-thiosulfate treatment regimen and should be administered. No advantage has been shown with hyperbaric oxygen over normobaric oxygen.

6. Other agents, such as protein kinase C inhibitors, inhibitors of lipid peroxidation, and cobalt porphyrins have shown promising results in animal studies but

these products have not been studied are not available for use in humans at the present time.

C. **Controversies—whom to treat?** Because the diagnosis of cyanide poisoning is usually clinical and without prompt laboratory confirmation and because the current treatment is associated with potentially severe toxicities, the decision as to which patients with suspected cyanide poisoning should be treated is difficult. It can usually be based on the particular form of cyanide ingested and the clinical status of the patient.

1. Patients with a **respiratory exposure** manifest their symptoms immediately. If these patients have a clear exposure history and develop significant toxicity (neurologic, respiratory, cardiac, and metabolic acidosis) treatment should be given. Patients with no or only mild symptoms do not require treatment, as no further absorption occurs once the patient is removed from the environment. Patients without a clear history of cyanide exposure, such as fire victims, provide a more difficult situation. Other toxic gases may explain the symptomatology, and there is often a combined intoxication, most notably with carbon monoxide. Some studies have found an increased risk of toxic cyanide levels in patients with carbon monoxide levels of more than 15%. Giving nitrites to these patients has the theoretical risk of further impairing oxygen transport by methemoglobin formation. The antidote kit, however, only produces methemoglobin levels of 10% to 12% in single doses. Such low methemoglobin levels are unlikely to cause significant clinical deterioration and may be life saving in the case of cyanide toxicity. Since the cyanide level is rarely available in a clinically useful time, the cyanide kit should empirically be administered to these patients.

2. Patients with an oral exposure should also be treated if they have significant symptoms. Asymptomatic patients should be observed for several hours and do not require treatment unless symptoms develop. Efforts to prevent further absorption (lavage, superactivated charcoal) may prevent or diminish toxicity. If patients have ingested a substance that requires conversion to cyanide, observation should be extended to at least 12 h. These patients may also benefit from GI decontamination procedures.

3. Patients who present with no history of **exposure** and with lactic acidosis of unknown etiology should have cyanide poisoning in their differential diagnosis. As discussed above, the methemoglobin levels produced by a single dose of the cyanide kit is unlikely to cause significant clinical deterioration and should be administered if cyanide toxicity is strongly suspected.

V. **Disposition and follow-up**

A. Because of the rapid onset of cyanide toxicity, patients who develop no symptoms immediately after a respiratory exposure or within 3 to 4 h after an oral exposure can probably be discharged following a brief period of observation. If the patient has ingested a substance that requires conversion to cyanide, observation should be extended to at least 12 h.

B. Many patients who recover from cyanide poisoning have no sequelae, but cases of **encephalopathy**, as seen with anoxia, have been reported. Whether it is the result of cyanide itself or of a hypoxic insult due to respiratory insufficiency is unclear.

References

1. Way J. Cyanide intoxication and its mechanism of antagonism. *Annu Rev Pharmacol Toxicol* 1984;24:451.
2. Christel D, et al. Pharmokinetics of cyanide in poisoning in dogs and the effect of 4-dimethylaminophenol or thiosulfate. *Arch Toxicol* 1977;38:177.
3. Klimmek R, Fladerer H, and Weger N. Circulation, respiration, and blood homeostasis in cyanide poisoned dogs after treatment with 4-dimethylaminophenol or cobalt compounds. *Arch Toxicol* 1979;43:121.
4. Sylvester D, et al. Effects of thiosulfate on cyanide pharmacokinetics in dogs. *Toxicol Appl Pharmacol* 1983;69:265.
5. Rumack B. Cyanide poisoning. Presented at the Symposium on Respiratory Care of Chemical Casualties, U.S. Army Research and Development Command, 1983.
6. Way J, et al. The mechanism of cyanide intoxication and its antagonism: cyanide compounds in biology. *Ciba Found Symp* 1988;232.
7. Michenfelder J, Tinker J. Cyanide toxicity and thiosulfate protection during chronic administration of sodium nitroprusside in the dog. *Anesthesiology* 1977;47:441.
8. Hall A, Rumack B. Hydroxycobalamin/sodium thiosulfate as a cyanide antidote. *J Emerg Med* 1987;5:115.
9. Way J, et al. Recent perspectives on the toxicodynamic basis of cyanide antagonism. *Fundam Appl Toxicol* 1984;239.
10. Bhattacharya R. Therapeutic efficacy of sodium nitrite and 4-dimethylaminophenol or hydroxylamine co-administration against cyanide poisoning in rats. *Hum Exp Toxicol* 1995;14:29.
11. Kong A, et al. Effect of chlorpromazine on cyanide intoxication. *Toxicol Appl Pharmacol* 1983;71:407.

Selected Readings

Anderson, R, et al. Cyanide exposure in fires. *Lancet* 1978;91.
Beamer W, Shealy R, Prough D. Acute cyanide poisoning from laetrile ingestion. *Ann Emerg Med* 1983;112:449.
Bismuth C, et al. Cyanide poisoning from propionitrile exposure. *J Emerg Med* 1987;5:191.
Brivet F, et al. Acute cyanide poisoning: recovery with non-specific supportive therapy. *Intensive Care Med* 1983;9:33.
Clark C, Campbell D, Reid W. Blood carboxyhaemoglobin and cyanide levels in fire survivors. *Lancet* 1981;1332.
Cottrell J, et al. Prevention of nitroprusside-induced cyanide toxicity with hydroxycobalamin. *N Engl J Med* 1978;298:809.
Graham D, et al. Acute cyanide poisoning complicated by lactic acidosis and pulmonary edema. *Arch Intern Med* 1977; 137:1051.
Hall A, and Rumack B. Clinical toxicology of cyanide. *Ann Emerg Med* 1986;15:1067.
Kong A, et al. Effect of chlorpromazine on cyanide intoxication. *Toxicol Appl Pharmacol* 1983;71:407.
Lambert R, et al. The efficacy of superactivated charcoal in treating rats exposed to a lethal oral dose of potassium cyanide. *Ann Emerg Med* 1988;17:595.
Litovitz T. An unexpected source of poisoning. *Emerg Med* 1989;May:45.
Litovitz T, Larkin R, Myers R. Cyanide poisoning treated with hyperbaric oxygen. *Am J Emerg Med* 1983;1:94.
Pechacek T, et al. Smoke exposure in pipe and cigar smokers. *JAMA* 1985;254:3330.
Shragg T, Albertson T, Fisher C. Cyanide poisoning after bitter almond ingestion. *West J Med* 1982;136:65.
Silverman S, et al. Cyanide toxicity in burned patients. *J Trauma* 1988;28:171.
Ten Eyeck R, Schaerdel A, Ottinger W. Stroma-free methemoglobin solution. *Am J Emerg Med* 1985;3:519.
Way J, et al. Effect of oxygen on cyanide intoxication. *Toxicol Appl Pharmacol* 1972;22:415.

Emergency Toxicology, Second Edition,
edited by Peter Viccellio.
Lippincott–Raven Publishers, Philadelphia © 1998.

74

Carbon Monoxide Poisoning

Stuart N. Chale

Department of Emergency Medicine, State University of New York at Stony Brook, University Hospital, Stony Brook, New York 11794-7400

The dangers of carbon monoxide have been known since Claude Bernard reported that the gas causes death by hypoxia. Today, carbon monoxide is the leading cause of mortality by poisoning in the United States, responsible for approximately 3,500 deaths per year (1). Carbon monoxide is a tasteless, colorless, odorless gas produced by the incomplete combustion of carbon compounds. Clinically, exposure produces signs and symptoms that are varied and nonspecific, which along with the fact that the patient cannot simply detect it, makes for a very difficult diagnosis. The possibility of carbon monoxide poisoning is obvious for the victim of fire and smoke inhalation. The diagnosis can be easily missed, however, in patients presenting from home or work with headache, nausea, or flu-like symptoms. Some of these patients may have been exposed to carbon monoxide produced from heaters, furnaces, or internal combustion engines in improperly vented areas. The diagnosis for many of these patients is missed if carbon monoxide poisoning is not considered in the differential diagnosis.

I. **Sources of carbon monoxide**

    A. **Endogenous sources.** The human body continuously produces a small amount of endogenous carbon monoxide, originating from the catabolism of the protoporphyrin ring of hemoglobin and to a small extent non-hemoglobin heme. In a normal subject this concentration may account for a carboxyhemoglobin saturation of 0.4% to 0.7%. In females the endogenous production of carbon monoxide is twice as great during the progesterone phase of the menstrual cycle as during the estrogen phase (2). In patients with hemolytic anemia, where there is a much greater breakdown of red blood cells and hemoglobin, the endogenous carbon monoxide production can produce carboxyhemoglobin levels as high as 4% to 6%. In general, the endogenous production of carbon monoxide does not produce any symptoms or toxicity in the normal subject.

    B. **Exogenous sources.** Carbon monoxide is produced by the incomplete combustion of carbonaceous material. The major source in developed countries is the **internal combustion engine.** In the United States automobiles account for approximately 60% of the carbon monoxide produced. The carbon monoxide concentrations on a congested highway during peak periods can reach 100 parts per million (ppm). As a reference point, the industrial standard is a maximum of 50 ppm for a standard 8-h workday as set by the Occupational Safety and Health Administration (OSHA). Carbon monoxide toxicity can occur in any building or stadium where internal combustion engines are used when ventilation is inadequate. This has occurred in ice hockey rinks from the ice resurfacing machine (3), at truck and tractor pulls (4), and in warehouses from propane powered fork-lifts (5). **Industry** accounts for approximately another 20% of the total carbon monoxide production. In the **home,** carbon monoxide can be produced from poorly vented water heaters, furnaces, fireplaces, and space heaters. During the winter months when space heaters are used, the diagnosis of carbon monoxide poisoning is often missed when patients present with flu-like symptoms. Even a properly operating gas stove can produce a significant concentration of carbon monoxide owing to incomplete combustion of the gas. **Tobacco** smokers are heavily exposed to carbon monoxide. Cigarette smoke averages about 400 ppm carbon monoxide. For a person smoking one pack of cigarettes per day, the average daytime carboxyhemoglobin levels approach 5% to 6%. A two- to three-pack per day smoker has a level of 7% to 9% saturation, and a heavy cigar smoker may reach a saturation of 20% (6). **Second-hand cigarette smoke** in homes of heavy smokers has also been shown to produce elevated levels of carboxyhemoglobin in the nonsmokers (7). **Firefighters** and **fire victims** are exposed to the greatest carbon monoxide concentrations. Carbon monoxide levels can reach 10% (100,000 ppm) in a major fire. Because of the increase in minute ventilation that occurs with the strenuous work of firefighting, lethal carboxyhemoglobin levels can be reached in less than 1 min (8). An unusual source of carbon monoxide has been found in **paint removers** that contain methylene chloride. Methylene chloride can be absorbed through the respiratory or GI system and is metabolized to carbon monoxide. Methylene chloride is only slowly released from the body, so carbon monoxide toxicity can be delayed and carboxyhemoglobin levels may continue to rise even after the source is removed.

II. **Mechanism of action.** Carbon monoxide is felt to have several mechanisms of toxicity.

    A. The gas is readily absorbed across the alveolus and **combines with hemoglobin** with an affinity of 210 to 270 times greater than oxygen (9). This displacement of oxygen from hemoglobin leads to a decrease in oxygen transport and causes tissue hypoxia. Normal blood contains 20 volumes percent (vol. %) of oxygen, with 18 vol. % bound to hemoglobin and 2 vol. % dissolved in plasma. Normal cellular metabolism results in an average extraction of approximately 5 vol. %. The brain and heart extract the greatest percentage of oxygen, 6.1 and 11.0 vol. %, respectively. Therefore, these tissues are the earliest and most greatly affected by a reduction in oxygen delivery.

    B. Hemoglobin tetramers to which carbon monoxide is bound hold onto its oxygen molecules with high affinity. This **Haldane effect** shifts the oxyhemoglobin dissociation curve to the left. Therefore oxygen unloading occurs only at a much lower tissue oxygen tension in the presence of carboxyhemoglobin, worsening tissue hypoxia. To put this information in perspective, a healthy person releases 5 vol. % of oxygen at a tissue Po_2 of 40 mm Hg. A person with a hematocrit that is 50% of normal releases the same amount of oxygen at a tissue Po_2 of 27 mm Hg, and a person with a carboxyhemoglobin level of 50% requires a tissue Po_2 of 14 mm Hg to release the same amount of oxygen. This level of hypoxemia is highly dangerous.

    C. An additional 10% to 15% of carbon monoxide is located in the **extravascular tissues,** bound to myoglobin, cytochrome oxidases, and hydroperoxidases. Carbon monoxide binds to myoglobin with an affinity approximately 40 times greater than oxygen, which may cause direct myocardial depression leading to hypotension, ventricular arrhythmias, and cardiac arrest. Neurologic injury due to carbon monoxide poisoning has been shown to correlate with the degree of hypotension. Areas of the brain with the poorest blood supply, such as watershed areas, are the most severely affected (10).

D. The most controversial mechanism of toxicity is carbon monoxide's **effects on cellular respiration.** Carbon monoxide has been shown to reversibly bind cytochrome oxidases a3 and P450. In vitro studies have shown that carbon monoxide inhibits the respiratory function of mitochondria (11).

    1. In support of a tissue toxicity of carbon monoxide, Goldbaum and associates performed experiments in dogs comparing the effects of inhaled carbon monoxide with transfusion of erythrocytes containing carbon monoxide. Dogs inhaling carbon monoxide died, whereas dogs transfused to a similar level of carboxyhemoglobin remained asymptomatic. The explanation given was that inhaled carbon monoxide produces significant carbon monoxide tension in the blood that may be transferred to cellular sites. There it causes toxicity by its effects on cytochrome oxidases (12).

    2. Other authors (13,14) have disputed the effects of carbon monoxide on cytochrome oxidases. Carbon monoxide binds to cytochromes with an affinity similar to that of oxygen. Evidence suggests that the in vivo concentration of carbon monoxide at the level of the cytochromes is not great enough to affect oxygen utilization (14).

    3. Goldbaum's experimental results may be explained by carbon monoxide's effect on myoglobin and the resulting hypotension and ischemic anoxia (13). Still, effects other than reduced oxygen transport by hemoglobin poisoned by carbon monoxide cannot be ignored, and the clinical presentation of the patient may be much worse than the measured blood carboxyhemoglobin suggests (15).

III. Absorption and elimination

A. Carbon monoxide is readily **absorbed** through the lungs and rapidly bound to hemoglobin. Absorption is dependent and proportional to the duration of exposure, the concentration of carbon monoxide in the environment, and the alveolar ventilation rate. The partial pressure of oxygen is also important. In environments where the oxygen content is low, as in a burning building, higher levels of carboxyhemoglobin result (8).

B. Elimination of carbon monoxide is predominantly respiratory; only about 1% is metabolized to carbon dioxide. The **half-life** of carbon monoxide in a healthy adult breathing 21% oxygen (room air) is 4 to 5 h. This time is reduced to 80 to 90 min when breathing 100% oxygen. Breathing 100% oxygen at 3 atmospheres pressure (hyperbaric oxygen) reduces the half life to less than 30 min. This is the basis for treating carbon monoxide poisoning with 100% oxygen or hyperbaric oxygen therapy. The half-life may vary considerably among individuals, and recurrent measurements are needed to guide therapy (16).

IV. Clinical presentation

A. Acute toxicity. The presenting signs and symptoms of a patient acutely intoxicated by carbon monoxide are highly variable and depend on the degree of exposure and physical activity of the patient at the time of exposure. The central nervous system and heart extract the greatest amount of oxygen from the blood; therefore these organs are responsible for most of the presenting features.

1. The clinical manifestations of carbon monoxide poisoning are only approximately correlated to the measured carboxyhemoglobin level (Table 74-1). It must be noted that the absolute level does not always correlate with the patient's presentation. Severe reactions and death have been reported with a measured carboxyhemoglobin level of only 10%. Common presentations are as follows:

   a. Levels of 10% to 20%: Headache, dyspnea on exertion, and weakness predominate.

   b. Levels of 20% to 30%: Severe headache and nausea may appear.

   c. Levels of 30% to 40%: Severe headache, nausea and vomiting, and impaired judgment may be seen.

   d. Levels of 50% to 60%: Confusion, syncope, seizures, and coma predominate.

2. With none of the signs and symptoms diagnostic for carbon monoxide poisoning, patients with low-level poisoning are often misdiagnosed. During winter months several studies have shown that up to 5% of patients presenting to the emergency department with complaints of headache, dizziness, and weakness had a carboxyhemoglobin level higher than 10%. Most of these patients were found to be using space heaters or fireplaces with improper venting (17). These patients would have been misdiagnosed as having a flu-like syndrome if carbon monoxide toxicity was not considered. Multiple household members presenting with the simultaneous onset of a flu-like syndrome suggests carbon monoxide poisoning.

B. **Neurologic complications.** Many of the initial symptoms and physical findings are directly related to the level of hypoxia in the CNS produced by carbon monoxide.

1. Headache, lightheadedness, and nausea are some of the most common symptoms of **mild intoxication.** The headache is typically throbbing in nature or described as "different" from usual headaches; it is presumably due to reflex vasodilatation secondary to CNS tissue hypoxia (18). The cerebral vasodilatation that occurs is proportional to the levels of carboxyhemoglobin, however there is great variability in this increase in brain blood flow between patients (19). **More significant intoxications** result in cognitive impairment, ataxia, visual and auditory abnormalities,

TABLE 74-1. *Approximate correlation of carboxyhemoglobin level and symptoms*

Carboxyhemoglobin level (%)	Symptoms[a]
0–5	None
5–10	None; or slight headache, decreased exercise tolerance, and increased angina pectoris in patients with coronary artery disease
10–20	Mild dyspnea on exertion, mild headache
20–30	Throbbing headache, mild nausea
30–40	Severe headache, dizziness, nausea and vomiting; impaired judgment and manual dexterity
40–50	Confusion, syncope
50–60	Syncope, coma, seizures
60–70	Coma, seizures, cardiorespiratory depression; death
>70	Failing hemodynamic status; death

[a]Symptoms listed for each level are in addition to those already listed for lesser levels.

seizures, and coma. Symptoms are directly related to the level of cerebral hypoxia and hypoperfusion and not necessarily the level of carboxyhemoglobin, particularly if measurement is delayed.

2. In patients who die from carbon monoxide poisoning acutely, the **brain is diffusely edematous.** In patients who survive but die shortly thereafter, findings of **ischemic anoxia** are found. The areas most affected are those with the poorest blood supply: white matter; hippocampus; globus pallidus; and, in gray matter, the watershed areas. This damage correlates with the degree of hypotension induced by carbon monoxide poisoning more than the degree of hypoxemia produced. It is likely that injury is induced by a combination of hypotension, hypoxia, vasodilatation, and cerebral edema, which leads to a decreased supply and utilization of glucose and localized acidosis.

C. **Cardiovascular complications**

1. Carbon monoxide has **direct cardiac toxicity.** Atrial and ventricular arrhythmias, including ventricular fibrillation, may be seen with severe intoxications. Angina or myocardial infarction may be induced. In patients with preexisting coronary artery disease, even low levels of carboxyhemoglobin may lead to angina and reduced exercise tolerance (18). However low levels of 3% to 5% carboxyhemoglobin has been shown not to increase ventricular ectopic beats in patients with coronary artery disease (20).

2. Hemodynamic effects are variable and inconsistent. Tachycardia is frequently seen, but bradycardia may occur in severely intoxicated patients, presumably due to severe myocardial or CNS hypoxia. In animal models, hypotension is frequent and severe. In humans, however, only mild hypotension is usually seen, and hypertension has been reported. Left ventricular dysfunction may also occur in the severely intoxicated patient (21).

3. Increasing levels of **ambient carbon monoxide** has been shown to be the only major gaseous pollutant associated with increased hospital admissions for congestive heart failure in the elderly. This was independent of season, temperature and other measured gaseous pollutants (22).

D. **Pulmonary complications**

1. Shortness of breath and dyspnea on exertion are characteristic.

2. Tachypnea is a common finding, but the lung examination is often normal unless other chemical toxins are involved or the poisoning is severe.

3. With severe poisoning, pulmonary edema and pulmonary hemorrhage may be seen. Pulmonary edema may be secondary to left ventricular dysfunction or to the direct effects of carbon monoxide and hypoxia on the lung parenchyma. In fire victims and patients with smoke inhalation, pulmonary findings may also be due to heat injury or chemical toxins.

E. **Dermatologic manifestations.** The classic cherry red appearance of the skin and mucous membranes is actually uncommon, occurring in fewer than 15% to 20% of patients and usually associated with carboxyhemoglobin levels of 30% to 40% or more. Pale or cyanotic skin is encountered more frequently. Occasionally one sees areas of erythema, edema, and blister formation resembling second-degree burns with severe carbon monoxide poisoning. These lesions are often found in areas of pressure necrosis but may occur in any area of skin (23).

F. Ophthalmologic manifestations. Patients may complain of blurred vision, decreased light sensitivity, and decreased dark adaptation. With severe poisoning, frank blindness may occur. These symptoms are usually related to the effects of carbon monoxide on the CNS, although abnormal retinal findings have been reported. One may see venous engorgement and tortuosity, disk edema, and flame-shaped hemorrhages. Although not common, retinal findings may increase one's suspicion for carbon monoxide poisoning (24).

G. Miscellaneous findings. Patients with severe toxicity who are found unconscious may suffer from rhabdomyolysis, falling into a position that may compromise muscular blood supply and lead to pressure myonecrosis. The resulting myoglobinuria may lead to acute tubular necrosis and renal failure. Disseminated intravascular coagulation and hemolytic anemia have also been reported with carbon monoxide poisoning.

V. Laboratory analysis

A. Carboxyhemoglobin levels should be measured as early as possible to establish the diagnosis of carbon monoxide poisoning. If some time has elapsed since exposure, especially if the patient has been treated with 100% oxygen, the carboxyhemoglobin level underestimates the degree of initial toxicity. In fact, a low carboxyhemoglobin level may be a poor predictor of the degree of poisoning. Carboxyhemoglobin should be measured from an arterial or venous blood sample using spectrophotometric methods (co-oximeter). Although not as accurate, carboxyhemoglobin levels can be estimated from expired air using a breath analyzer for carbon monoxide. This method can be most helpful in the field, especially to screen firemen who are potentially poisoned.

B. Arterial blood gas assays are poor indicators of carbon monoxide poisoning (25). The PaO_2 is often normal, as it is a measure of oxygen dissolved in plasma, not a measure of oxygen bound to hemoglobin. It therefore does not reflect an elevated carboxyhemoglobin level. Because the oxygen saturation is usually determined from a nomogram based on pH and PaO_2 it too often is normal despite an elevated carboxyhemoglobin level; determination of oxygen saturation should be by direct measurement, not by nomogram. The $PaCO_2$ may be slightly lowered owing to the tachypnea and hyperventilation. Metabolic acidosis usually correlates with severe poisoning and a poor prognosis. Metabolic acidosis may also signify coexisting cyanide toxicity. In patients with mild carbon monoxide toxicity and no respiratory distress, an arterial blood gas should be unnecessary (25). Serum electrolytes need only be obtained in the moderate to severely poisoned patient, and may reveal an anion gap metabolic acidosis due to elevated levels of lactic acid. They provide baseline renal function values if rhabdomyolysis is suspected, and may reveal hyperglycemia, which is occasionally seen.

C. In severely poisoned patients, CBC, platelets, fibrinogen, and fibrin split products should be obtained to rule out the rare occurrences of hemolytic anemia and disseminated intravascular coagulation.

D. Chest roentgenogram should be obtained in all symptomatic patients. Up to 30% of carbon monoxide poisoned patients have an abnormal chest film. Alveolar infiltrates, perivascular and peribronchial cuffing, and a diffuse ground-glass appearance may be seen. In severely poisoned patients, there may be pulmonary edema and hemorrhage (26).

E. ECG should be obtained in all patients with significant or symptomatic poisoning, chest pain, or history of coronary artery disease.

Carbon monoxide can produce ischemic changes, conduction disturbances, and dysrhythmias. Patients who are admitted for carbon monoxide poisoning should be admitted to a monitored unit to watch for dysrhythmias. Serial cardiac enzymes should be assayed in all patients with new ECG changes or chest pain, and in all severely poisoned patients to detect myocardial injury.

VI. **Long-term sequelae**

A. Neurologic and psychiatric disturbances have been observed in the patient poisoned by carbon monoxide. They may occur at the outset of intoxication or days to weeks later after a period of apparent total recovery. The incidence of major sequelae is estimated to be as high as 10% (10,27) but may be lower with more prudent use of hyperbaric oxygen therapy (28).

B. Almost every known neurologic and psychiatric syndrome has been reported from carbon monoxide poisoning. Complications can be **dramatic,** such as parkinsonian syndromes, cortical blindness, dementia, peripheral neuropathies, seizure disorders, Wernicke's aphasia, psychosis, and manic depression; or they may be more **subtle,** such as apathy, fatigue, irritability, minor memory disturbances, or difficulty with decisions. Often the subtle changes are picked up by the family members and brought to the attention of the physician.

C. It has been recommended that all patients with carbon monoxide poisoning undergo **careful neuropsychiatric screening** after being treated, and then again approximately 3 weeks later (29). Patients with delayed neuropsychiatric sequela have shown improvement when treated with hyperbaric oxygen therapy, even after this time period.

VII. **Treatment**

A. Initial treatment of carbon monoxide poisoning begins in the prehospital setting. Patients must be removed from the source of the carbon monoxide and have their respiratory function maintained.

1. The most widely accepted treatment for carbon monoxide poisoning is **100% oxygen** provided by a tight-fitting mask preferably with rubber seals, and endotracheal intubation for patients with a depressed mental status. This therapy should be started in the prehospital setting if possible or as soon as carbon monoxide poisoning is suspected. Therapy should not be delayed while awaiting confirmatory carboxyhemoglobin levels.

a. Oxygen therapy works by mass action effects, diluting carbon monoxide attached to hemoglobin, myoglobin, and cytochromes. The half-life of carboxyhemoglobin is reduced from 4 to 5 h to about 80 min when 100% oxygen is substituted for room air. There is great individual variation in carboxyhemoglobin half-lives, however, and follow-up levels are recommended to guide treatment.

b. One can also estimate the highest carbon monoxide level reached if the length of time and treatment modality prior to carboxyhemoglobin measurement are known.

2. A blood sample for carboxyhemoglobin assay should be obtained as early as possible and oxygen therapy continued while awaiting results. All patients who are symptomatic after carbon monoxide exposure should be treated with 100% oxygen despite a low carboxyhemoglobin level.

3. In cases of smoke inhalation, one must always be alert for the possibility of toxicity from poisonous gases other than carbon monoxide. Cyanide poisoning is a likely candidate. In fact cyanide poisoning may be responsible for more of the clinical findings than carbon monoxide (30). Treating indiscriminately for cyanide however is not advised. The standard treatment for cyanide including, amyl nitrite, sodium nitrite, and sodium thiosulfate produces up to 30% methemoglobinemia which would worsen the hypoxemia already produced by carbon monoxide poisoning. If the patient does not respond to normal treatment with 100% oxygen or has signs and symptoms more severe than the carboxyhemoglobin level would suggest, then cyanide poisoning should be considered and treated accordingly.

4. Hyperbaric oxygen at 3 atmospheres pressure further reduces the half-life of carboxyhemoglobin to approximately 23 min. The amount of dissolved oxygen in the plasma increases to about 6.6 vol. % at 3 atmospheres, enough to meet the demand of most tissues, independent of hemoglobin.

B. **Hyperbaric oxygen therapy**

1. Indications for hyperbaric oxygen therapy are controversial. There have been no prospective randomized double blind studies on humans comparing hyperbaric oxygen with 100% normobaric oxygen therapy. Most of the data for hyperbaric oxygen is based on isolated case reports and small case series showing that patients treated with hyperbaric oxygen did better, including the reduction of the many neuropsychiatric sequelae discussed earlier.

2. There are reports of patients improving with hyperbaric oxygen after not responding to treatment with normobaric 100% oxygen (15). Patients who initially improved with 100% oxygen but then returned with neurologic complaints have also been shown to benefit from hyperbaric oxygen therapy (28). It has been suggested that the late sequelae of neuropsychiatric changes due to carbon monoxide toxicity can be avoided with the use of hyperbaric oxygen therapy. Most investigators have referred to a study by Smith and Brandon (27), who found a 10.8% incidence of delayed neuropsychiatric sequelae from carbon monoxide poisoning when not treated with hyperbaric oxygen. Unfortunately, the mode of therapy for many of these patients was not noted, and apparently 100% oxygen was not used routinely.

3. Hyperbaric oxygen therapy has several **disadvantages** that should be factored into any decision regarding therapy. Most hospitals do not have a hyperbaric chamber, thereby necessitating transfer of the patient to another facility. The stability and suitability for transport must be considered in this decision. Moreover, there are a number of complications of hyperbaric oxygen therapy, including emesis, seizures, agitation, rupture of tympanic membranes, blocked sinuses, worsening of a pneumothorax, and loss of hypoxic drive in patients with chronic obstructive pulmonary disease (31).

4. The decision to send a patient for hyperbaric oxygen therapy must be individualized on a patient-by-patient basis, depending on the severity of symptoms, the patient's stability, and time from the nearest compression chamber. There are no absolute guidelines for the use of hyperbaric oxygen. The following criteria, however, have been assembled from several sources to help guide in the decision to institute hyperbaric oxygen therapy (15,32,34).

    a. Any patient with a carboxyhemoglobin level higher than 25%.
    b. Any acute or chronic neurologic symptoms.
    c. Myocardial ischemia or dysrhythmia.
    d. Methylene chloride intoxication, depending on symptoms and carboxyhemoglobin levels.
    e. Unconsciousness or history of unconsciousness for more than 5 min.
    f. Pregnant patients with a carboxyhemoglobin level of 10% or more or with any symptoms.
    g. Metabolic acidosis with pH less than 7.20.

5. Cardiac dysrhythmias should be treated with the appropriate antiarrhythmics in addition to oxygen therapy. Any patient with dysrhythmias should be admitted and monitored for at least 24 h.

6. Acidemia shifts the oxyhemoglobin dissociation curve to the right, counteracting to some extent the left shift caused by carbon monoxide. Bicarbonate therapy may worsen the left shift and further worsen tissue hypoxemia. Therefore treatment of a metabolic acidosis should rely on oxygen therapy and improvement of the hemodynamic status (35).

VIII. **Special considerations**

A. **Pediatric patients.** There is essentially no difference in the treatment of carbon monoxide toxicity when dealing with the pediatric population. They may present with the same signs and symptoms as adults, and the same neuropsychiatric sequelae have been reported after exposure (36). Hyperbaric oxygen therapy should be instituted under the same circumstance as for the adult. It should be noted, however, that infants, because of their higher respiratory rate, may be more severely intoxicated than older children and adults under otherwise identical conditions (37).

B. **Pregnant patients.** Carbon monoxide poisoning in the pregnant patient represents a more complicated situation. Fetal hemoglobin has a greater affinity for carbon monoxide than does adult hemoglobin. Therefore the fetal carboxyhemoglobin concentration may be higher than the maternal concentration. Placental transfer of carbon monoxide is slow, however, and it takes longer to reach these levels. It also takes longer for the carboxyhemoglobin level in the fetus to fall, requiring longer oxygen therapy. Therapy with 100% oxygen at normobaric pressures should probably be continued for five times the length of time it takes to normalize the maternal carboxyhemoglobin level (16,38). Experience with hyperbaric oxygen therapy in the pregnant woman is limited. In animal studies, hyperbaric oxygen has been shown to be teratogenic and causes fetal resorption. Although there are few reported cases of pregnant patients treated with hyperbaric oxygen, no adverse effects in the fetus have been documented. Treatment with hyperbaric oxygen has been recommended by some authorities for all symptomatic pregnant women (16) or pregnant patients with a carboxyhemoglobin level higher than 10% (32).

C. Altitude. Experimentally it has been shown that baseline carboxyhemoglobin levels increase in a linear fashion with increasing altitude in animals. This increase was noted when both clean air or low levels of carbon monoxide were inhaled. Although not studied in humans, this may suggest that patients living at high altitudes would have higher than expected carboxyhemoglobin levels as a baseline, prior to any exposure (33).

IX. Disposition

A. Criteria for hospital admission for carbon monoxide intoxication are essentially the same as those for hyperbaric oxygen therapy:

Any history of loss of consciousness.

Minor neurologic complaints or deficits that fail to clear with 100% oxygen.

Major neurologic deficits, seizures, ataxia, confusion, or neuropathy.

Clinical or ECG evidence of ischemia or dysrhythmias.

Metabolic acidosis.

Abnormal chest radiograph.

Pregnant patients with any symptoms or a carboxyhemoglobin level higher than 10%.

Carbon monoxide intoxication due to a suicide attempt.

Carboxyhemoglobin level higher than 25%.

With carboxyhemoglobin levels of 25% to 39%, clinical judgment must be exercised.

B. All patients admitted to the hospital should be observed and monitored for arrhythmias.

C. Patients with less severe intoxications whose symptoms clear with 100% oxygen therapy may be discharged directly from the emergency department. Patients should receive instructions to return if there is a recurrence of any symptom. Routine follow-up at approximately 3 weeks is mandatory to assess for subtle neuropsychiatric sequelae.

References

1. Public Health Service. *Vital statistics of the United States.* Washington, DC: Government Printing Office, 1976.
2. Coburn RF. Endogenous carbon monoxide production. *N Engl J Med* 1970;282:207.
3. Kwok PW. Evaluation and control of carbon monoxide exposure in indoor skating arenas. *Can J Public Health* 1983; 74:261.
4. Carbon monoxide levels during indoor sporting events. *MMWR* 1994;43:21–23.
5. Fawcett TA, Moon RE, Fracica PJ, Mebane GY, Theil DR, Piantadosi CA. Warehouse workers' headache: carbon monoxide poisoning from propane-fueled forklifts. *J Occup Med* 1992;34:12–15.
6. Stewart RD. The effect of carbon monoxide on humans. *Annu Rev Pharmacol* 1975;15:409.
7. Kachulis CJ. Second-hand cigarette smoke as a cause of chronic carbon monoxide poisoning. *Postgrad Med* 1981;70:77.
8. Stewart RD, et al. Rapid estimation of carboxyhemoglobin level in firefighters. *JAMA* 1976;235:390.
9. Roughton FJW, Darling RC. The effect of carbon monoxide on the oxygen hemoglobin dissociation curve. *Am J Physiol* 1943;141:17.
10. Garland H, Pearce J. Neurological complications of carbon monoxide poisoning. *Q J Med* 1967;36:445.
11. Chance B, Erecinska M, Wagner M. Mitochondrial responses to carbon monoxide toxicity. *Ann NY Acad Sci* 1976; 174:193.
12. Goldbaum LR, Orellano T, Dergal E. Mechanism of the toxic action of carbon monoxide. *Ann Clin Lab Sci* 1976;6:372.
13. Olson KR. Carbon monoxide poisoning: mechanisms, presentations, and controversies in management. *J Emerg Med* 1984;1:233.
14. Coburn RF. Mechanisms of carbon monoxide toxicity. *Prev Med* 1979;8:310.
15. Myers RAM, et al. Value of hyperbaric oxygen in suspected carbon monoxide poisoning. *JAMA* 1981;246:2478.
16. Pierce EC, chairperson. A registry for carbon monoxide poisoning in New York City: Hyperbaric Center Advisory Committee, Emergency Medicine Service, City of New York. *J Toxicol Clin Toxicol* 1988;26:419.

17. Heckerling PS. Occult carbon monoxide poisoning: a cause of winter headache. *Am J Emerg Med* 1987;5:201.
18. Grace TW, Platt FW. Subacute carbon monoxide poisoning: another great imitator. *JAMA* 1981;246:1698.
19. Benignus VA, Petrovick MK, Newlin-Clapp L, Prah JD. Carboxyhemoglobin and brain blood flow in humans. *Neurotoxicol Teratol* 1992;14:285–290.
20. Dahms TE, et al. Effects of carbon monoxide exposure in patients with documented cardiac arrhythmias. *J Am Coll Cardiol* 1993;21:442–450.
21. Penney DG. A review: hemodynamic response to carbon monoxide. *Environ Health Perspect* 1988;77:121.
22. Morris RD, Naumova EN, Munasinghe RL. Ambient air pollution and hospitalization for congestive heart failure among elderly people in seven large U.S. cities. *Am J Public Health* 1995;85:1361–1365.
23. Myers RAM, Synder SK, Majerius TE. Cutaneous blisters and carbon monoxide poisoning. *Ann Emerg Med* 1985; 14:603.
24. Ferguson LS, Burke MI, Choromokos ER. Carbon monoxide retinopathy. *Arch Ophthalmol* 1985;10:66.
25. Lebby TI, et al. The usefulness of the arterial blood gas in pure carbon monoxide poisoning. *Vet Hum Toxicol* 1989; 31:138.
26. Sone S, et al. Pulmonary manifestations in acute carbon monoxide poisoning. *AJR* 1974;120:865.
27. Smith JS, Brandon S. Morbidity from acute carbon monoxide poisoning at three-year follow-up. *BMJ* 1973;1:318.
28. Myers RAM, Synder SK, Emhoff TA. Subacute sequelae of carbon monoxide poisoning. *Ann Emerg Med* 1985; 14:1163.
29. Myers RAM, Messier LD, Jones DW. New directions in the research and treatment of carbon monoxide exposure. *Am J Emerg Med* 1983;2:226.
30. Breen PH, et al. Combined carbon monoxide and cyanide poisoning: a place for treatment. *Anesth Analg* 1995;80: 671–677.
31. Sloan EP, et al. Complications and protocol considerations in carbon monoxide poisoned patients who require hyperbaric oxygen therapy: report from ten-year experience. *Ann Emerg Med* 1989;18:629.
32. Van Meter K. Syllabus for hyperbaric medicine in emergency medicine. Presentation for the ACEP Scientific Assembly, Washington, DC, September 1989.
33. McGrath JJ. Effects of altitude on endogenous carboxyhemoglobin levels. *J Toxicol Environ Health* 1992;35:127–133.
34. Mathieu D, et al. Acute carbon monoxide poisoning: risk of late sequelae and treatment by hyperbaric oxygen. *Clin Toxicol* 1985;23:315.
35. Peirce CE. Treating acidemia in carbon monoxide poisoning may be dangerous. *J Hyperbaric Med* 1986;1:87.
36. Lacey DJ. Neurologic sequelae of carbon monoxide intoxication. *Am J Dis Child* 1981;135:195.
37. Gozal D, et al. Accidental carbon monoxide poisoning: emphasis on hyperbaric treatment. *Clin Pediatr* 1985;24:132.
38. Longo LD. The biological effects of carbon monoxide on the pregnant woman, fetus and newborn infant. *Am J Obstet Gynecol* 1977;129:69.

Emergency Toxicology, Second Edition,
edited by Peter Viccellio.
Lippincott–Raven Publishers, Philadelphia © 1998.

75

Ionizing Radiation

Jonathan L. Burstein

Division of Emergency Medicine, Harvard Medical School; Department of Emergency Medicine,
Beth Israel Deaconess Medical Center, Boston, Massachusetts 02215

Exposure to ionizing radiation, while rare, evokes great fear and apprehension in most medical personnel. Medical response to radiation accidents and exposures requires specific technical knowledge as well as a general grasp of radiation biology. Ionizing radiation produces its effects by ionizing biological chemicals and producing free radicals in tissue. This damages cellular components such as nucleic acids and proteins, thereby disrupting cellular function and reproduction and causing cell death. Large-scale exposures such as occurred near the Chernobyl nuclear reactor are unusual, but smaller scale accidents can be expected due to the widespread use of radioactive materials in medicine, science, and industry (1–3). The possibility of nuclear terrorism, whether via contamination or an explosive device, casts a grim shadow over the future. Medical personnel may be required to deal with multiple casualties suffering from radiologic injury as well as traumatic injury. This discussion will focus on the issues directly related to acute radiation poisoning rather than the trauma-related problems peculiar to an atomic explosion, or the long-term effects, such as carcinogenesis, of radiation exposure.

I. **Sources of radioactive materials**
    A. **Nuclear power plants.** There are approximately 100 nuclear power plants in the United States and about 500 worldwide (4). These are all fission plants, most operating with light-water coolant systems. This coolant water is radioactive and represents a hazard if released into the environment (such as through a breach of the reactor's piping system, not just the reactor containment vessel). Some reactors, such as at Chernobyl, do not have containment buildings, greatly increasing the risk of radioisotope spread in the event of a breakdown (3). Reactor accidents may release various isotopes with different spectra of risks and effects, and may affect large areas and numbers of people.
    B. **Medical radiation.** Both therapeutic radiation sources and roentgenographic equipment may be sources of radiation exposure. Radiotherapy, of course, is predicated on the toxic effects of radiation on mammalian cells. Accidental overexposure can lead to acute radiation toxicity (5). Medically useful isotopes such as technetium can also be sources of radiation poisoning, via accidental release or spillage or overdose. Medical devices containing radioactive material have also occasionally caused radiation exposure through improper disposal (6).
    C. **Industry and science.** Radioisotopes and devices have widespread uses in industry and scientific investigations, for uses ranging from materials analysis to manufacturing to food processing to chemical engineering. Any major industrial area or scientific facility may

have quantitities of radioisotopes sufficient to pose a toxic threat if improperly handled. In addition, transport of isotopes (and waste) may present a threat even in communities without local sources of radioisotopes.

D. **Environmental sources.** These include naturally occurring radon gas, fallout products from atmospheric nuclear tests, and naturally occurring isotopes in atmosphere, rock, and seawater. In general, except under specific circumstances (e.g., radon accumulating in a closed space) the exposure from such sources is low (7,8).

II. **Types of radioisotopes and dosimetry**

A. **Dosimetry.** Radiation is usually measured in rads, standing for *r*adiation *a*bsorbed *d*ose. One rad represents 100 ergs/g of absorbed energy of any type of radiation. The Gray (Gy) is defined as 100 rads. For biological exposures, the rem (*r*adiation *e*quivalent *m*an) is often used, with one Sievert (Sv) equalling 100 rem. The unit rem takes into account the amount of damage caused to human tissue by the radiation. In general, one rad is approximately equal to one rem, except for radiation sources such as neutrons or heavy nuclei which can cause greater damage to human tissue than other forms of radiation, and which therefore will have a higher number of rem than rads for a given amount of radiation energy. Actual determination of exposure in a radiation accident may be difficult unless the exposed individual was wearing a personal dosimeter, but calculations and estimates may be made using various measuring devices and theoretical models.

B. **Measurement devices** (9,10). The Geiger-Mueller counter is a versatile detector for beta and gamma (see below) surveys of areas, objects, or people. It is based on a vacuum tube which produces a measurable electric current when exposed to ionizing radiation. It is quite useful for monitoring scene safety and the progress of decontamination. Personal dosimeters, based on film or electronics, provide a cumulative record of the amount of radiation exposure at the site of the dosimeter. Dosimeters are available in various sensitivities, and should be mandatory equipment for all personnel working in a radiation environment. Neutron detectors will detect neutron beam emissions; they are rarely useful to medical or health physics personnel, since neutron sources are rare.

C. **Alpha radiation.** The alpha particle is a helium nucleus accelerated to high speed. Natural sources include uranium, thorium, polonium, and radium. Although most alpha particles will be stopped by skin, they pose a significant risk if inhaled or ingested, as their great mass (and hence energy) allows them to produce significant tissue damage if in direct contact with vulnerable tissue (10).

D. **Beta radiation.** The beta particle is a high energy electron. Common sources of beta particles include carbon 14, phosphorus 32, strontium 90, and cathode ray tubes such as are found in televisions and video monitors. Beta particles are usually blocked by a thin light metal shield or several layers of cloth, such as normal clothing (10).

E. **Gamma radiation.** These emissions are photons. Iodine 125, iodine 131, and cobalt 60 are typical gamma-emitters, as are x-ray and radiotherapy machines. Gamma-rays have high energy, and therefore great penetration This gives them the ability to cause toxic effects at great distances from the emitter. They will only be blocked by heavy shielding (inches of lead or feet of concrete) (10).

F. **Neutrons and heavy ions.** These particles can cause immense cellular damage due to their mass and speed. Neutrons are created in the fission chain reactions found in power reactors and atomic explosions, accounting for the great radiotoxicity seen in those directly exposed to such sources. These particles are also produced in many experimental particle accelerators. Neutron exposure can *create* radioisotopes in biological material, which can then decay and produce further damage (10).

G. **Background radiation.** Annual yearly background radiation is about 360 millirem (mrem). This is due to exposure to radon, cosmic rays, and the radiation sources of everyday life (e.g., a color television exposes a viewer to about 1 mrem/year). A standard AP chest x-ray accounts for 10 mrem of exposure (3,11).

III. **Kinetics and routes of toxicity**

A. **Kinetics.** The effect of whole-body radiation exposure depends on the total dose received. This quantity is dependent on rate of emission from the source, total time of exposure, quantity of interposed shielding, and distance from the source (since radiation dose drops off according to an inverse-square law with respect to distance, i.e., doubling the distance quarters the dose). Effects given below (see **IV**) are based on a single exposure. The calculation of expected effects for multiple exposures is more complex (3,10,11).

B. **Irradiation.** This type of exposure does not produce continuing damage once the patient is removed from the source, nor does the patient pose a radiation risk to rescuers unless the source was a neutron emitter, in which case the patient's own tissues may actually become radioactive.

C. **Surface contamination.** In this case, the patient is actually physically contaminated with radioactive materials. They will continue to produce exposure until removed, and pose a continuing hazard to both patient and rescuers.

D. **Inhalation, ingestion, and wound contamination.** In these types of exposure, substances such as alpha-emitters may wreak tremendous damage by directly irradiating internal body structures with their massive particles. The patient may suffer incorporation of radioisotopes into body structures, producing continuing exposure. These patients may pose a continuing risk to rescuers. Certain specific treatments are available to block absorption of ingested or inhaled radioactive substances, or to remove them once absorbed. Some of these therapies are discussed below (see **VI**).

IV. **Clinical effects as a function of dose**

A. **Acute radiation syndrome** (1–3,9,11–13). Whole body radiation dosage produces a characteristic clinical syndrome known as the acute radiation syndrome. Especially radiosensitive tissues include the gastrointestinal (GI), reproductive, and hematopoietic systems (especially lymphocytes). The syndrome typically has three phases. These are the prodrome, latent, and manifest-illness phases. The LD_{50} for acute radiation exposure for humans is about 400 rem, while the LD_{90} is about 1,000 rem. A direct dose of over 5,000 rem will be lethal within 1 h, primarily due to CNS effects. During the prodrome, the patient may exhibit nausea and vomiting, diarrhea, salivation, fever, fatigue, abdominal pain, and dehydration. This phase will typically only occur if the total dose was over 100 rem. If the dose was over 600 rem, the syndrome may become evident within 2 h; otherwise it can take up to 6 h to appear. If vomiting occurs within 1 h, or is accompanied by obvious CNS dysfunction (confusion, stupor, coma), the absorbed dose was most likely lethal. The latent phase typically is present in doses below the lethal dose. It may last up to several weeks. In general, the higher the dose the shorter the latent phase. In high-dose exposures (over 400 rem), it may be entirely absent. The manifest-illness phase is characterized by hematopoietic and GI dysfunction and failure, as well as alopecia. The components of the blood decrease in the following order: lymphocytes within 24 to 48 h, then granulocytes (days), platelets (1 to 2 weeks), and finally erythrocytes. Pancytopenia eventually occurs if the exposure was over 400 to 600 rem. Recovery, if it occurs, may take up to a month. Vomiting, diarrhea, intestinal sloughing and hemorrhage can lead to severe dehydration and electrolyte disturbances. Death will usually occur in 2 weeks if the total dose was 1,000 rem or more.

B. Extremity injury. This pattern of injury is similar to that of thermal burns, and may be managed in much the same way, although radiation injury tends to heal more slowly than thermal injury, and is complicated by an obliterating endarteritis which is specific to radiation damage. Early involvement of surgeons trained in plastic or burn surgery is recommended (11).

V. Laboratory findings

A. Absolute lymphocyte count. This is probably the single most useful screening measurement of total dose and prognosis. An absolute lymphocyte count of over 1,500 cells/mL^3 at 48 h postexposure essentially rules out significant whole-body exposure. A count below 1,000 cells/mL^3 at 24 h, or below 500 at 48 h, indicates severe exposure (11,13,14).

B. Platelet count, erythrocyte count, and granulocyte count. These are normal initially but will drop according to the time course given above (see **IV.A**).

VI. Management

A. Decontamination. Meticulous decontamination is necessary to prevent further exposure of the patient or rescue and medical personnel. This should be done in an isolation area, and all materials leaving the area should be assayed for radioactivity. Soap and water is usually sufficient for skin and hair decontamination; shaving hair should be avoided so as not to cut the skin. Eyes and mucous membranes may be irrigated with normal saline. If wound incorporation has occurred, chelation or surgical debridement may be necessary. Inhalation contamination may be treated by pulmonary lavage through a double-lumen endotracheal tube, under general anesthesia. For ingestion contamination, gastric lavage, whole bowel irrigation, or chelation therapy may be used. All lavage fluids must be assayed for radioactivity and disposed of properly. More elaborate protocols have been developed for specific radioactive agents (11–14). The dose exposure of the decontamination team must be monitored, and personnel rotated as needed. A radiation expert must be actively involved to assure team safety and effective decontamination.

B. Supportive care. Meticulous attention to fluid and electrolyte management and infection control procedures is mandatory in all victims of radiation exposure. Specific non–radiation-related injuries and illnesses should receive appropriate management, which may begin simultaneously with decontamination. Bone marrow transplantation may be necessary in those with initial exposure over 400 rem (2,11).

C. Specific antidotes

1. Preventing absorption. For some radionuclides, administering blocking agents will reduce absorption, especially for ingested material. Examples include potassium iodide given orally to block thyroid uptake of radioactive iodine, and nonradioactive forms of calcium, zinc, strontium, and potassium to block uptake of radioactive forms of these elements (1–3,11,13,14). Specific assistance may be obtained from REAC/TS (see **VII**).

2. **Chelation** (11,13,14). Once ingested, inhaled, absorbed from an open wound, or otherwise incorporated into body tissues, some radioisotopes can only be removed by chelation therapy. The most useful chelating agent, especially for actinides (plutonium, americium, and neptunium) and rare earths, is diethylenetriaminepentaacetic acid (DTPA), which is available from REAC/TS in both zinc-DTPA and calcium-DTPA forms. The zinc form appears to be less toxic but also less effective than the calcium form. The initial dose in cases of such contamination should be 1 g of calcium-DTPA diluted in 250 mL of D5W and given over 90 min. Follow-up doses of the calcium form may be given daily over 5 days. DTPA-bound radionuclides are excreted in the urine; monitoring of the urine, patient secretions, blood, and whole body radiation must be continued during therapy. REAC/TS should always be involved in the treatment of such a patient (and in fact in all radiation-exposed patients), and will be able to recommend specific chelators for particular radionuclides.

D. **Disposition.** Most patients suspected or known to have sustained a radiation exposure should be decontaminated, admitted to an acute-care hospital, placed on reverse isolation for infectious-disease control, receive meticulous supportive care, and be monitored until it is clear they are not ill. Baseline laboratory studies, including complete blood count, platelet count, and electrolytes should be obtained. The absolute lymphocyte count, as discussed above, is usually the most useful test to follow, and the 48-h value may be sufficient to establish that the patient is not at further risk. Specific problems such as radiation burns or injuries may require the involvement of particular subspecialists. A completely asymptomatic, decontaminated patient who is not leukopenic or thrombocytopenic may be discharged from the emergency department only if the patient will reliably follow up at 48 h for repeat lymphocyte and platelet counts.

VII. **Resources.** Local Poison Control Centers can provide some assistance in cases of radiation exposure. In addition, in the United States, the Federal Government has a network of offices run by the Department of Energy which can provide aid in the case of a radiation accident. The appropriate Department of Energy Regional Coordinating Office should be notified immediately in case of any radiation exposure. Medical advice and assistance can be obtained 24 h a day from the Radiation Emergency Assistance Center/Training Site (REAC/TS) (Oak Ridge, TN, 615-576-1004).

References

1. Conklin JJ, Walker RI, Hirsch FF. Current concepts in the management of radiation injuries and associated trauma. *Surg Gynecol Obstet* 1983;156:809–829.
2. Champlin RE, Kastenberg WE, Gale RP. Radiation accidents and nuclear energy: medical consequences and therapy. *Ann Intern Med* 1988;109:730–732.
3. Vyas DR, Dick RM, Crawford J. Management of radiation accidents and exposures. *Pediatr Emerg Care* 1994;10: 232–237.
4. World list of nuclear power plants. *Nucl News* 1993;36:43–62.
5. Saenger EL, Silberstein EB, Aron B, et al. Whole and partial radiotherapy of advanced cancer. *Am J Roentgen Radiat Ther Nucl Med* 1973;117:670–685.

6. Andrews G. Mexican Co-60 radiation accident. *Isotopes Radiat Technol* 1963;1:200–201.
7. ACGIH 1994–1995 threshold limit values for chemical substances and physical agents and biological exposure indices. Presented at the American Conference of Governmental Industrial Hygiene, Cincinnati, 1994.
8. Diffre P. Radionuclides in the environment. *J Environ Pathol Toxicol Oncol* 1990;10:276–280.
9. Saenger EL. Radiation accidents. *Am J Roentgenol* 1960;84:715–728.
10. Shapiro J. *Radiation protection*. Cambridge, MA: Harvard University Press, 1990.
11. Saenger EL. Radiation accidents. *Ann Emerg Med* 1986;15:1061–1066.
12. Leonard RB, Ricks RC. Emergency department radiation accident protocol. *Ann Emerg Med* 1980;9:462–470.
13. Pons P, Sullivan Jr JB. Radiation and radioactive emergencies. In: Sullivan JB and Krieger GR, eds. *Hazardous materials toxicology*. St. Louis: CV Mosby, 1992, 441–450.
14. NCRP. *Management of persons accidentally contaminated with radionuclides*. Report no. 65. Bethesda, MD: National Council on Radiation Protection and Measurements, 1979.

Emergency Toxicology, Second Edition,
edited by Peter Viccellio.
Lippincott–Raven Publishers, Philadelphia © 1998.

76

Foodborne Toxins

Patricia L. VanDevander

Department of Emergency Medicine, Lutheran Medical Center, Wheat Ridge, Colorado 80033

Foodborne illness is a frequent complaint of persons seeking medical attention due to the gastrointestinal (GI) distress and systemic symptoms that may result. However, only estimates can be made about the total number of people with "food poisoning" since the illnesses are often self-limited. There are numerous causes of foodborne illness and even a greater variety of food sources implicated in the etiology of illness (see Chapters 82 and 84). Increased public awareness about safe food handling and preparation techniques probably accounts for a decreased incidence of some types of foodborne illnesses. However, there has been an increase in the *variety* of foodborne illnesses. These patterns are probably a result of a change in the techniques used for food production and preparation, more food being imported, and the diversification of eating habits (1).

I. Properties of the agent

A. Sources of the toxin

1. Bacteria may produce enterotoxins either in food prior to its ingestion (preformed) or after contaminated food has been ingested. In this second method, the bacteria attach themselves to the intestinal epithelium and then produce toxin.

2. In suspected food poisoning cases, it is helpful to identify the incubation period (time from food ingestion to onset of illness) so as to narrow down the etiologic agent. Cases where illness begins within 1 h of food ingestion are probably due to chemical poisoning. With an incubation period between 1 h and 7 h, preformed toxin is often the culprit. In comparison, cases in which toxin must be elaborated in the gut have incubation periods greater than 8 h (2).

3. The bacteria and preformed toxin must be able to withstand the acidic environment and digestive enzymes of the upper GI tract to cause their deleterious effects. These seemingly less than optimal conditions for microorganisms and proteins are partially bypassed because the ingested food buffers the acid in the stomach, thus creating a safe passage (3).

B. Mechanism of action of toxin

1. With a few exceptions, there are two basic mechanisms by which enterotoxins cause illness. Enterotoxins can cause the increased production of intracellular cyclic adenosine monophosphate (cAMP), which then induces active secretion of chloride ions by the intestinal cells and inhibits absorption of sodium chloride. Thus, a large chloride gradient occurs across the intestinal membrane and one loses large amounts of fluids and electrolytes (i.e., cholera toxin).

2. Enterotoxins can have a direct cytotoxic effect on the intestinal cells. In this scenario, the enterotoxin causes the small intestine absorptive cells to die by shutting down their protein synthesis. The cells then slough off, exposing the lamina propria that then bleeds. As a result of this cellular damage the intestine is unable to absorb fluids and electrolytes (i.e., Shiga toxin).

II.   Sources of the agent

A.   *Bacillus cereus* is capable of producing two different enterotoxins; thus, two separate forms of illness may result from the ingestion of its spores. The spores formed from this rod-shaped, gram-positive, aerobic organism are widely spread in the environment. Specifically with regard to foodstuffs, they are found in grains, spices, and raw foods. Outbreaks of illness (which occur year-round) have been reported with the ingestion of boiled or fried rice (4) and noodles, vegetable and meat soups, poultry (5), sauces, and desserts (6–8).

1. Emetic toxin is heat-stable and causes a milder form of illness, with nausea, vomiting, and abdominal cramps. There may or may not be any associated diarrhea. The incubation period is from 1 to 6 h, with symptoms lasting from 6 to 24 h (6).

2. Diarrheal toxin is heat-labile and causes significant abdominal pain and tenesmus with profuse diarrhea. Nausea and vomiting may or may not be reported during this illness. The incubation period is longer than with the milder form of illness. Symptom onset is usually 8 to 16 h after ingestion, with a duration of 12 to 24 h (6).

3. Mechanism of action of the toxin is unknown.

4. Diagnosis can be made by isolation of organisms from the stool or vomitus plus isolation of a minimum of 10^5 organisms in 1 g of the implicated food.

5. Treatment is supportive with fluid replacement.

6. Prevention of this illness is achieved by cooling cooked foods rapidly to less than 7°C (44.6°F) or keeping them above 55°C to 60°C (131°F to 140°F). Also, cooled foods should be reheated thoroughly before consuming (7).

B.   *Clostridium botulinum* produces heat-resistant spores that germinate under anaerobic conditions and produce a very potent neurotoxin. It is thought that as little as 1 μg of toxin could be lethal for a human. Unlike infants, adults who ingest food containing only the spores do not usually get neurotoxic effects. This organism is a gram-positive bacillus that is widely distributed, especially in soil. The two forms of food-related botulism in humans are classic and infant.

1. Mechanism of action by this heat-labile neurotoxin, called "botulin," is through irreversible binding with the nerve endplates. Seven specific toxins designated A through G are produced by the spores; however, only three (A, B, and E) are commonly implicated in human botulism. Each molecule of botulin consists of one heavy chain and one light chain. The irreversible binding occurs when the heavy chain attaches to the presynaptic membrane of the motor nerve endplate. Endocytosis of the toxin then occurs, coupling through an enzymatic process takes place, and the light chain blocks the calcium-mediated release of acetylcholine from the presynaptic membrane. Thus, there is no transmitter release. This all takes place at the cholinergic nerve junctions (9,10).

2. Clinical presentation of classic botulism (which is the most common in adults) occurs when one ingests food contaminated with the preformed toxin. The toxin is

absorbed in the duodenum and jejunum, where it then passes into the bloodstream (11). Often, the toxin is produced by spores in food that was inadequately prepared during the home canning process. Food sources implicated include beef stew (12), green beans and other vegetables, commercial pot pies, and seafood in Alaska (10). The incubation period is from 12 h to several days. Illness often begins with influenza-like symptoms and is soon followed by cranial nerve palsies and a symmetrical, descending weakness or paralysis. The person does not develop a fever or any sensory deficits from the toxin. Eventually, large muscle groups become involved, and if respiratory support is not instituted, the person dies due to respiratory failure (13).

3. Clinical presentation of infant botulism was first described in 1976 and is most common in children from 3 weeks to 6 months of age (14). Illness occurs after the child ingests food contaminated with spores, which then germinate in the bowel and produce the toxin. Signs of toxicity may be evident within hours or delayed up to 24 days (mean, 11 days) after ingesting the spores. Food sources have included honey and corn syrup. Constipation is often the initial sign, followed by hypotonia, generalized weakness, poor sucking, and a weak cry (15). The lack of fever and descending paralysis are similar to that previously noted with adults in the classic form of botulism. The overall mortality is 3% to 5% in hospitalized patients (14).

4. Diagnosis is mainly by an accurate history and physical examination. Confirmation laboratory studies include demonstration of the organism or the toxin in the stool (100% and 86%, respectively), serum, or suspected contaminated food (14). EMG results are characteristic, but not specific, for botulism (11).

5. Treatment is supportive. Decision to intubate is based on physical assessment and changes in vital capacity (less than 12 mL/kg). The trivalent antitoxin made from horse serum will bind any unbound toxin; however, this only stops progression of the neurologic compromise and does not resolve the existing deficits. The dose of antitoxin, which may be repeated in 4 h with severe cases, is one vial i.v. plus one vial i.m. Hypersensitivity to the antitoxin occurs in 9% to 20% of patients. Therefore, skin testing should be done before antitoxin administration. Recovery of function takes place over 2 to 3 months as new axons, axon terminals, and motor endplates are formed. Immunity does not develop to the toxin after acquiring the disease (11).

6. Prevention is by proper food handling and preparation. Bulging food containers and spoiled food should be avoided.

C. *Clostridium perfringens* is a common cause of food-related illness but is also normal flora of the human intestinal tract. This gram-positive, anaerobic, nonmotile rod that produces heat-stable spores is widespread in soil, thus making it easier for foodstuffs to become contaminated. The majority of food poisoning outbreaks are due to type A strains, although the rare type C strains have been implicated historically in illness associated with the ingestion of undercooked pork. The endospores are heat resistant, while the endotoxin is heat labile. This is a very common foodborne toxin that contaminates meat, poultry, and spices (16,17). Illness occurs after ingestion of the infected due to elaboration of toxin during sporulation of the organism within the intestine. Type C produces the same toxin as Type A but also produces large amounts of alpha toxin and the lethal, necrotizing beta toxin (which causes severe hemorrhagic enteritis) (18).

1. Mechanism of action of the heat-labile enterotoxin is mostly unknown, although it is thought that it induces a calcium ion-dependent breakdown of the small bowel brush border causing secretion of fluid into the bowel lumen (19). It is also similar to the enterotoxin produced by enterotoxigenic *Escherichia coli* (18).

2. Clinical presentation is with watery diarrhea and abdominal cramping after an incubation period of 6 to 24 h (median 12 h) after ingestion of infected food. Fever, nausea, and vomiting are much less common. The illness then resolves over the next 24 to 36 h (19).

3. Treatment is supportive care with fluids for dehydration.

4. Prevention is by eating the hot foods soon after cooking, cooling prepared foods as quickly as possible to less than 7°C (45°F) and thoroughly reheating food before consumption to 71°C to 100°C (160°F to 212°F) (18).

D. *E. coli* is part of the normal bowel flora and most strains are harmless. However, when this gram-negative rod has at least one virulence factor, it becomes a pathogenic strain able to produce disease. Most of the public focus recently has been on *E. coli* O157:H7. However, there are four forms of *E. coli* that are capable of causing human disease through contaminated food: enterotoxigenic (ETEC); enterohemorrhagic (EHEC); enteroinvasive (EIEC); and enteropathogenic (EPEC) (20). Only ETEC and EHEC will be discussed here, as they are the two most frequently identified forms of *E. coli* in foodborne outbreaks in the United States.

1. ETEC: This group is most commonly associated with "traveler's diarrhea." However, it has also been reported in the United States as the etiologic agent in outbreaks of foodborne illness. This has included food from a Mexican-style restaurant in Wisconsin, French Brie cheese on a cruise ship, drinking water at Crater Lake National Park (20), and from airline food and a buffet dinner (21).

a. Mechanism of action is by two toxins, known as heat-labile (LT) and heat-stable (ST), which are produced by these organisms within the small bowel. Each organism will produce one or both of these toxins. The LT toxin, which is inactivated in 30 min at 60°C, is similar to cholera toxin produced by *Vibrio cholerae*. It affects directly on cAMP within the epithelial cells to increase chloride secretion from the crypt epithelial cells and inhibits sodium absorption from the villous tip epithelial cells. An outpouring of water thus causing the loss of large amounts of fluid follows this increased osmolarity load into the lumen. The ST is able to withstand 100°C for 30 min (20).

b. Clinical presentation of infection with this strain of *E. coli* are symptoms most similar to that of cholera with watery diarrhea and dehydration. In contrast to cholera, mild abdominal cramps are present, and vomiting may or may not be present. The infectious dose is thought to be between 10^8 to 10^{10} organisms with an incubation period of 8 to 44 h (average 26 h) and an illness duration of 24 to 30 h (20).

c. Diagnosis is by clinical history and the presence of fecal leukocytes or a positive stool culture. Methods for laboratory identification are not widely available but can be done at the Center for Disease Control if needed.

d. Treatment is focused on rehydration. Antibiotics and antimotility medication may help the symptoms but they may also prolong the time the bacteria is in the intestinal tract. If antibiotics are used the choice is a fluoroquinolone like ciprofloxacin 500 mg p.o. b.i.d. $\times$ 3 to 5 days or TMP 160 mg plus SMX 800 mg p.o. b.i.d. $\times$ 3 days. Antibiotic prophylaxis is controversial. Loperamide 4 mg followed by 2 mg after each stool with a maximum dose of 16 mg/day added to the antibiotic regimen is thought to be of benefit as well (22).

2. EHEC: This type of *E. coli* has received the most publicity recently because of the large outbreaks and severity of illness associated with it (23). It was first described in the United States in 1982 as **O**157:**H**7 (24). Several of the implicated sources have included: undercooked ground beef (25–31), apple cider (32), contaminated water (33–35), and dry-cured salami. It is not invasive but it has an antigen that adheres to the intestinal epithelium while the toxin is elaborated.

   a. Mechanism of action is by one or both Shiga-like toxins: Shiga-like toxin I (SLT-I) or Shiga-like toxin II (SLT-II).

   b. Clinical presentation of infection with this form of *E. coli* begins after an incubation period of 3 to 4 days with a watery, profuse diarrhea. The diarrhea may progress to being bloody within 2 to 3 days of onset along with severe abdominal cramping or pain, nausea, and vomiting. Fever is uncommon. Most patients' illness resolves over 1 week, although 2% to 7% (especially children) will develop hemolytic uremic syndrome (HUS) after the diarrhea resolves (30,32). HUS has a classic triad of hemolytic anemia, thrombocytopenia and acute renal failure. The patients must be hospitalized to monitor their renal function and for development of other complications including intussusception and toxic megacolon.

   c. Diagnosis is by clinical history and presentation initially. Identification of fecal leukocytes may only be present in one-third of patients and rectal bleeding may be so profuse that this organism is not suspected (31). Stool culture for the organism must be done using sorbitol-MacConkey media.

   d. Treatment is supportive. Antimotility medication is not recommended and antibiotics are not thought to be helpful and may even be harmful.

   e. Prevention of transmission of this organism includes thoroughly cooking beef, pasteurization of milk, and good hygiene prior to handling food (26).

E. *Shigella sonnei* is one of four Shigella species capable of producing human illness known as bacillary dysentery or shigellosis. The serogroup D form of Shigella is the most common cause of shigellosis reported in the United States, accounting for 70% to 80% of cases (36,37). Foodborne transmission of this bacteria occurs when an infected food handler, who has used poor hygiene, directly contaminates the food which is then ingested by an unsuspecting person. Shigella may also be spread by ingesting contaminated water or from person to person by the fecal-oral route. Only a small number of organisms, 10 to 100, need be ingested to cause illness, as Shigella is a very infectious organism. *S. sonnei* is a nonmotile, facultative anaerobic, gram-negative rod. The food items most often linked to Shigella outbreaks included salads, particularly when they are "made with potatoes, chicken, tuna or shrimp" (37). Other implicated foods include raw oysters, apple cider, beans, cream puffs, and hamburger (38) and other cold meats (39).

1. Mechanism of action for Shigella to cause illness is by either of two methods.
   a. The organism infects the absorptive cells of the terminal ileum and proximal colon causing a cytotoxic effect with shut down of cell protein synthesis. This leads to cell death and sloughing with exposure of the lamina propria, ulceration, and bleeding from the denuded areas.
   b. The production of an enterotoxin (Shiga toxin) by the organism within the intestine causes a local inflammatory reaction responsible for the watery diarrhea seen early in the illness. There is also associated cell sloughing, ulceration and bleeding. Different species of Shigella produce different amounts of toxin, with *S. dysenteriae* being the most potent with the production of 1,000 times more toxin than *S. sonnei* (37).

2. Clinical manifestations of shigellosis begin to occur from 24 h to 7 days after ingestion of the contaminated food. Watery diarrhea is present from the beginning of the illness but within 24 h it tends to become bloody with mucous and lasts from a few days to 2 weeks. Fever, chills, dehydration, vomiting and tenesmus are also commonly part of this illness. In infants it is not uncommon for high fevers to cause seizures. Rarely, *S. sonnei* may cross the lamina propria and cause bacteremia or HUS (36,37). Infection with this organism has also been associated with Reiter's syndrome and reactive arthritis. Once the signs and symptoms have subsided some individuals will continue to shed *S. sonnei* in their stool for up to 5 months thus making them potential organism transmitters (38).

3. Diagnosis of shigellosis can be confirmed using stool or food samples for culture of the organism. Examination of the stool will show many polymorphonuclear cells (37).

4. Treatment includes rehydration, especially infants and the elderly. Without antibiotics, illness generally resolves within 1 day to 4 weeks (average 7 days). Antimotility drugs are not recommended due to the potential development of toxic megacolon. If the stool culture is positive for the organism antibiotics are recommended. For adults trimethoprim (TMP) 160 mg plus sulfamethoxazole (SMX) 800 mg p.o. q12h for 3 to 5 days and for pediatrics TMP 10 mg/kg/day plus SMX 50 mg/kg/day in two equal doses p.o. q12h for 3 to 5 days are the current first choice recommendations. Alternate therapy for adults would include either ciprofloxacin 500 mg p.o. b.i.d. or ofloxacin 300 mg p.o. b.i.d. for 3 to 5 days; for pediatrics, it is nalidixic acid 55 mg/kg/day p.o. in four equally divided doses for 3 to 5 days (38). Shigella acquired by travelers to the Far East, India, Brazil, or Latin America have shown resistance to TMP-SMX and ampicillin (36).

5. Prevention is by insisting that food handlers practice good personal hygiene, ensuring that a safe chlorinated water supply is available in areas with substandard sanitation and proper refrigeration and cooking of food.

F. *Staphylococcus aureus* is one of 23 Staphylococcal species and one of the most common causes of foodborne illness. It is also the most common cause of noninfectious food poisoning. *S. aureus* is found in humans on the skin and in the nasopharynx; it is not uncommon for a food handler to be the source for the food contamination. This organism is a gram-positive, facultative anaerobe that occurs worldwide and produces its toxin optimally at 37°C with pH 6.5 to 7.5. Foods that have been implicated in illness as a result of the exotoxin produced by this organism include cheese, chocolate milk, butter, ice cream, rice balls, baked ham, fermented sausage, canned corned beef, potato and meat salads, custard and cream-filled bakery goods, and Easter eggs (40).

1. Mechanism of action by the preformed toxin is initiated in the intestinal tract but the site of action has not been defined.
2. Clinical manifestations of the toxin are GI in origin and include nausea, vomiting, diarrhea, and abdominal cramps. The incubation period is 1 to 7 h with symptoms lasting 24 to 48 h. There are no sequelae of the illness and it is only rarely fatal in the pediatric and geriatric populations.
3. Diagnosis is based on history and clinical presentation but the enterotoxin can be isolated from the implicated food if necessary.
4. Treatment is symptomatic with rehydration being the most often required therapy.
5. Prevention of illness is possible by having food handlers use good hygiene and using clean equipment in food preparation. Additionally, cooked food that is not being immediately served should be stored in small lots below 10°C or above 45°C. The organism is destroyed in food by cooking the food for 30 min at more than 60°C (40).

G. *Vibrio cholerae* is a small, curved gram-negative organism that is transmitted via fecal-oral route with the ingestion of fecally contaminated water or food. An infectious dose is considered to be 10^8 organisms (41). This organism is the cause of "cholera." In the United States there have been reported cases in Texas and Louisiana coastal areas from raw or undercooked shellfish and crustaceans. In addition there continues to be an increase in cases reported in travelers who have acquired the organism during international travel (42). Cholera is still endemic in parts of Asia or India (43), with 70% of persons being asymptomatic, 15% to 23% with mild or moderate nonbloody diarrhea and 2% to 5% of adults with severe diarrhea causing dehydration (41).

1. Mechanism of action for the illness is by the enterotoxin called "choleragen." The organism multiplies within the bowel but it does not spread beyond the intestinal tract. The choleragen is similar to *E. coli* LT.
2. Clinical presentation begins with vomiting quickly followed by an increase in bowel peristalsis and loose stools. The incubation period is from 12 to 72 h. The diarrhea may be mild but typically it is profuse (8 to 15 liters of fluid/day) and causes severe dehydration which leads to death if fluid and electrolyte replacement are not maintained (41). When the diarrhea is significant the stool becomes "rice water-like" in appearance due to the mucous, epithelial cells and large number of vibrios in the stool. It also loses most of its odor. Abdominal pain is usually not one of the significant associated symptoms, nor is fever a predominant sign. Children may become hypoglycemic for unknown reasons, but this may account for a change in mental status along with the changes expected from the electrolyte and water depletion. When antibiotics are used the duration of the diarrhea is shortened. The illness has a duration of 4 to 7 days (41).
3. Diagnosis should be made on clinical suspicion initially (watery diarrhea, lack of fever and minimal abdominal pain) so as to not delay fluid replacement therapy.

Examination of the stool may show a few fecal leukocytes but rarely red blood cells. The quickest way to identify *V. cholerae* is by darkfield or phase microscopy. In addition, both stool and rectal swabs can be cultured for the organism (44).

4. Treatment is directed at aggressive fluid and electrolyte replacement. If replacement is adequate (fluid in = fluid out) throughout the illness, there is less than 1% mortality with cholera. Without treatment, there is a 60% mortality rate due to dehydration and electrolyte loss (43). Fluid replacement may be achieved orally (1 tsp table salt plus 4 tsp. sugar added to 1 liter of water) or intravenously using WHO solution (4 g NaCl plus 1 g KCl plus 5.4 g Na lactate plus 8 g glucose/L of water). The current antibiotic recommendation for adults is doxycycline 100 mg p.o. q12h or a fluoroquinolone with TMP-SMX as an alternative. For pediatrics TMP 5 mg/kg and SMX 25 mg/kg p.o. b.i.d. for 3 to 5 days is suggested (44). Antimotility agents (loperamide) and bismuth subsalicylate have been used as adjuncts with good results.

5. Prevention of acquiring cholera is possible by purifying water sources, washing and cooking foods thoroughly and using good hygiene and sanitation. The general rule "boil it, cook it, peel it, or forget it" does apply here.

H. *Yersinia enterocolitica* as the infectious source of foodborne illness is not as common in the United States as it is in Europe and Canada. This gram-negative rod is acquired by humans through the ingestion of contaminated food (45). The virulent forms of this organism have a surface protein which help it adhere to and invade the intestinal epithelial cells. Not only does this organism produce a heat-stable enterotoxin (similar to *E. coli* ST) causing human illness, but due to its invasive ability hematogenous spread of the organism may also occur rarely. Foods that have been identified as sources of this organism causing illness include beef, oysters, chocolate milk and pasteurized milk, tofu, bean sprouts, and raw pork intestines (46,47).

1. Mechanism of action of the enterotoxin (which may or may not be produced by the virulent organism) is by the stimulation and increased production of epithelial cell guanosine monophosphate (GMP). However, it is thought that illness is primarily due to the invasiveness of the organism. The organism causes intestinal mucosal ulcerations as well as lesions in the Peyer's patches and enlargement of the mesenteric lymph nodes (46).

2. Clinical illness caused by this organism and its toxin is called "yersiniosis." After the ingestion of an inoculum of 10^9 organisms, the incubation period is from 24 h to 7 days. The duration of illness is then 1 to 3 days if complications do not occur. Presenting symptoms include fever, diarrhea, headache and severe abdominal pain that may mimic appendicitis (fever, right lower quadrant pain and leukocytosis). The abdominal pain is due to swelling of the mesenteric lymph nodes. Blood or mucous may be seen in the stool. Children are more often infected than adults and have more severe symptoms (45,46). Complications of this infection include rectal bleeding, ileal perforation, erythema nodosum, exudative pharyngitis, septicemia and a reactive polyarthritis (46). The arthritis begins 1 to 14 days after the acute enteritis and has an unknown mechanism. However, it is observed that these patients have high IgA serum antibodies to *Y. enterocolitica* not found in patients without arthritis

development (47). Symptoms have been noted to last for more than one month but less than 12 months in most patients (46). Septicemia is less common as a complication than arthritis and tends to occur in adults with preinfectious chronic disease. Patients who receive iron chelation are at a particular risk as this enhances the growth of *Y. enterocolitica*. Septicemic patients have developed endocarditis, osteomyelitis, hepatic or splenic abscesses, meningitis or wound infections (46).

3. Diagnosis can be made by isolation of organisms from feces, blood, mesenteric lymph node tissue, pharyngeal exudate or cerebrospinal fluid depending on the clinical scenario.

4. Treatment with antibiotics for the GI symptoms or mesenteric adenitis is undefined in terms of shortening the illness duration as it is usually self-limited (45,46). Kihlstrom (47) found that antibiotics did not influence intestinal or reactive arthritis symptoms. On the other hand, *Y. enterocolitica* septicemia (which causes mortality in 50% of cases) should be aggressively treated with gentamicin, chloramphenicol, TMP-SMX, doxycycline or ciprofloxacin (45,46).

5. Prevention is focused on public health measures such as public education about not consuming uncooked meats and encouraging dairies to be more diligent in preventing the contamination of pasteurized milk.

References

1. CDC. Acute hepatitis and renal failure following ingestion of raw carp gallbladders—Maryland and Pennsylvania, 1991 and 1994 [Editor's note]. *MMWR* 1995;44:565–566.
2. Bean NH, et al. Foodborne disease outbreaks, 5-year summary, 1983–1987. *MMWR* 1990;39:15–54.
3. Taylor SL. Disease processes in foodborne illness. In: Cliver DO, ed. *Foodborne diseases*. San Diego: Academic Press, 1990:17–43.
4. CDC. *Bacillus cereus* food poisoning associated with fried rice at two child day care centers—Virginia 1993. *MMWR* 1994;43:177–178.
5. Slaten DD, et al. An outbreak of *Bacillus cereus* food poisoning—are caterers supervised sufficiently? *Public Health Rep* 1992;107:477–480.
6. Tauten CU. Other bacillus species. In: Mandell GL, ed. *Principles and practice of infectious disease*. 4th ed. New York: Churchill Livingstone, 1995:1890–1894.
7. Tauxe RV, Hughes IM. Food-borne disease. In: Mandell GL, ed. *Principles and practice of infectious disease*. 4th ed. New York: Churchill Livingstone, 1995:1012–1024.
8. Johnson EA. *Bacillus cereus* food poisoning. In: Cliver DO, ed. *Foodborne diseases*. San Diego: Academic Press, 1990:127–135.
9. Hambleton P. *Clostridium botulinum* toxins: a general review of involvement in disease, structure, mode of action, and preparation for clinical use. *J Neurol* 1992;239:16–20.
10. Simcock PR, et al. Neuro-ophthalmic findings in botulism type B. *Eye* 1994;8:646–648.
11. Bleck TP. *Clostridium botulinum*. In: Mandell GL, ed. *Principles and practice of infectious disease*. 4th ed. New York: Churchill Livingstone, 1995:2178–2182.
12. CDC. *MMWR* 1995;44:200–202. Foodborne botulism—Oklahoma, 1994. *JAMA* 1995;273:1167.
13. Sugiyama H. Botulism. In: Cliver DO, ed. *Foodborne diseases*. San Diego: Academic Press, 1990:107–125.
14. Wigginton JM, Thill P. Infant botulism: a review of the literature. *Clin Pediatr* 1993;Nov:669–674.
15. Kothare SV, Kassner EG. Infant botulism: a rare cause of colonic ileus. *Pediatr Radiol* 1995;25:24–26.
16. CDC. *Clostridium perfringens* gastroenteritis associated with corned beef served at St. Patrick's day meals—Ohio and Virginia, 1993. *MMWR* 1994;43:137,143–144.
17. Roach RL, Sienko DG. *Clostridium perfringens* outbreak associated with minestrone soup. *Am J Epidemiol* 1992;136:1288–1291.
18. Johnson EA. *Clostridium perfringens* food poisoning. In: Cliver DO, ed. *Foodborne diseases*. San Diego: Academic Press, 1990:229–240.

19. Lorber B. Gas gangrene and other clostridium-associated diseases. In: Mandell GL, ed. *Principles and practice of infectious disease.* 4th ed. New York: Churchill Livingstone, 1995:2182–2195.

20. Doyle MP, Cliver DO. *Escherichia coli.* In: Cliver DO, ed. *Foodborne diseases.* San Diego: Academic Press, 1990:209–215.

21. CDC. Foodborne outbreaks of enterotoxigenic *Escherichia coli*—Rhode Island and New Hampshire, 1993. *MMWR* 1994;43:81,87–89.

22. Sanford JP, et al., eds. *The Sanford guide to antimicrobial therapy.* 27th ed. Vienna, VA: Antimicrobial Therapy, Inc., 1997.

23. Ostroff SM, et al. Surveillance of *Escherichia coli* O157 isolation and confirmation United States, 1988. *MMWR* 1991;40:1–5.

24. Ostroff SM, et al. Infections with *Escherichia coli* O157:H7 in Washington State. *JAMA* 1989;262:355–359.

25. Bell BP, et al. A multistate outbreak of *Escherichia coli* O157:H7–associated bloody diarrhea and hemolytic uremic syndrome from hamburgers: the Washington experience. *JAMA* 1994;272:1349–1353.

26. CDC. Preliminary report: foodborne outbreak of *Escherichia coli* O157:H7 infections from hamburgers—Western United States, 1993. *MMWR* 1993;42:85–86.

27. CDC. Outbreak of *Escherichia coli* O157:H7 infection—Georgia and Tennessee, June 1995. *MMWR* 1996;45:249–251.

28. Le Saux N, et al. Ground beef consumption in noncommercial settings is a risk factor for sporadic *Escherichia coli* O157:H7 infection in Canada. *J Infect Dis* 1993;167:500–502.

29. MacDonald KL, Osterholm MT. The emergence of *Escherichia coli* O157:H7 infection in the United States: the changing epidemiology of foodborne disease. *JAMA* 1993;269:2264–2266.

30. CDC. Update: multistate outbreak of *Escherichia coli* O157:H7 infections from hamburgers—Western United States, 1992–1993. *MMWR* 1993;42:258–263.

31. Berkelman RL. Emerging infectious diseases in the United States, 1993. *J Infect Dis* 1994;170:272–277.

32. Besser RE, et al. An outbreak of diarrhea and hemolytic uremic syndrome from *Escherichia coli* O157:H7 in fresh-pressed apple cider. *JAMA* 1993;269:2217–2220.

33. Keene WE, et al. A swimming-associated outbreak of hemorrhagic colitis caused by *Escherichia coli* O157:H7 and *Shigella sonnei. N Engl J Med* 1994;331:579–584.

34. CDC. Lake-associated outbreak of *Escherichia coli* O157:H7—Illinois, 1995. *MMWR* 1996;45:437–439.

35. Swerdlow DL, et al. A waterborne outbreak in Missouri of *Escherichia coli* O157:H7 associated with bloody diarrhea and death. *Ann Intern Med* 1992;117:812–819.

36. CDC. *Shigella sonnei* outbreak associated with contaminated drinking water—Island Park, Idaho, August 1995. *MMWR* 1996;45:229–231.

37. Doyle MP. Shigella. In: Cliver DO, ed. *Foodborne diseases.* San Diego: Academic Press, 1990:205–208.

38. DuPont HL. Shigella species (bacillary dysentery). In: Mandell GL, ed. *Principles and practice of infectious disease.* 4th ed. New York: Churchill Livingstone, 1995:2033–2038.

39. Hedberg CW, et al. An international foodborne outbreak of shigellosis associated with a commercial airline. *JAMA* 1992;268:3208–3212.

40. Bergdoll MS. Staphylococcal food poisoning. In: Cliver DO, ed. *Foodborne diseases.* San Diego: Academic Press, 1990:85–106.

41. Vugia DJ, et al. Surveillance for epidemic cholera in the Americas: an assessment. *MMWR* 1992;41:27–33.

42. CDC. Cholera associated with international travel, 1992. *MMWR* 1992;41:664–668.

43. Doyle MP, Cliver DO. Vibrio. In: Cliver DO, ed. *Foodborne diseases.* San Diego: Academic Press, 1990:241–245.

44. Greenough WB. *Vibrio cholerae* and cholera. In: Mandell GL, ed. *Principles and practice of infectious disease.* 4th ed. New York: Churchill Livingstone, 1995:1934–1944.

45. Doyle MP, Cliver DO. *Yersinia enterocolitica.* In: Cliver DO, ed. *Foodborne diseases.* San Diego: Academic Press, 1990:223–228.

46. Butler T. Yersinia species (including plague). In: Mandell GL, ed. *Principles and practice of infectious disease.* 4th ed. New York: Churchill Livingstone, 1995:2070–2078.

47. Kihlstrom E, et al. Intestinal symptoms and serological response in patients with complicated and uncomplicated *Yersinia enterocolitica* infections. *Scand J Infect Dis* 1992;24:57–63.

Emergency Toxicology, Second Edition,
edited by Peter Viccellio.
Lippincott–Raven Publishers, Philadelphia © 1998.

77

Foreign Bodies

†Philip I. Hubel and °David Barlas

†*Department of Emergency Medicine, North Shore Long Island Jewish Health System, Great Neck, New York 11021; °Department of Emergency Medicine, New York University School of Medicine; North Shore University Hospital, Manhasset, New York 11030*

Any patient presenting to the emergency department (ED) with a foreign body comes with the expectation of having the extraneous object immediately removed. The physician must approach the problem judiciously, positively identify the location of the foreign body, and, according to its life-threatening potential, formulate a timely response.

I. **Airway foreign bodies**

   A. **Nose**

   1. The nose is probably the most common site of foreign bodies in small children, who have a proclivity for inserting small, brightly colored objects, foodstuffs, and jelly beans into one or both nostrils. If the children do not present quickly after nasal insertion, they can present with a unilateral, foul-smelling discharge (1). **Complications** resulting from nasal foreign bodies and their removal include mucosal trauma and aspiration. Presence of septal hematoma, uncontrolled epistaxis, or cerebrospinal fluid (CSF) are emergencies and should prompt specialist intervention. Button batteries are particularly injurious, causing superficial burns of the nasal mucosa and nasal septal perforation secondary to tissue necrosis (2–5).

   2. Removal is usually not difficult when the practitioner is well prepared. A small child should be in a papoose or swaddled, and a good light source or headlamp should be available. **Repeat examination** should be performed after successful removal to exclude the presence of more foreign bodies. Specialist intervention is necessary if removal attempts fail.

      a. Forceps in conjunction with a nasal speculum of appropriate size are often successful at removing most nasal foreign bodies.

      b. Suction with a rigid, narrow catheter (i.e., tonsil adapter) can help extract smooth, round objects that are difficult to grasp with forceps.

      c. Cyanoacrylate adhesive (Super Glue) has been successfully used for removing nasal foreign bodies. A small amount of glue is placed on the blunt end of a cotton swab, which is then carefully introduced into the canal to make contact with the object. Both swab and object are removed after 60 s (6).

      d. Positive pressure is an interesting technique that has been found to be well tolerated and effective. Under supervision, a parent gives the child a "kiss." The child's patent nostril is occluded, and a sharp puff of air is introduced during the kiss, expelling the object onto the parent's cheek (7).

B. Ears

1. Any and all types of objects—organic, inorganic, and living—have been retrieved from human ears. The items most commonly removed from children's external auditory canals are cockroaches, paper wads, toy parts, earring parts, hair beads, eraser tips, and food (8). Button batteries lodged in the ear can produce severe tissue destruction (2). **Complications** include tympanic membrane perforation, ossicle damage, epithelial necrosis, chondritis, facial nerve paralysis, and hearing impairment.

2. Removal, as with nasal foreign bodies, begins with preparation. The practitioner must use good tools (preferably an operating otoscope), good light, good restraint, and good sense. Straightening the ear canal is accomplished by posterosuperior traction on the pinna. The patient should be advised of the extreme sensitivity of the auditory canal and to expect some discomfort. Sedation or analgesia such as nitrous oxide should be offered. Following successful removal, a **repeat examination** should be performed to detect complications or retained foreign body fragments.

   a. Forceps extraction is the simplest method of removing a foreign body in the canal, and is the preferred method for removing insects and vegetable matter. Insects should first be killed with mineral oil, alcohol, or topical lidocaine.

   b. Irrigation of the canal is another effective method to remove foreign bodies. Water is directed past the object, against the tympanic membrane, and against the back side of the foreign body through a small-gauge plastic i.v. catheter, driving it out. *Contraindications* to this method are a history of tympanic membrane perforation or a tendency of the object (e.g., insects and vegetable matter) to absorb water and swell.

   c. Tightly wedged, smooth, round foreign bodies in the ear canal remain the most difficult to remove. A rigid, narrow suction device (e.g., tonsil adapter) may be able to adhere to the object, permitting removal under direct visualization. A new method using cyanoacrylate adhesive (Super Glue) has used successfully to remove a soybean from a 16-year-old boy (9). The glue was placed on the blunt end of a cotton swab, which was then introduced into the canal to make contact with the bean. Removal was easy, safe, and effective.

3. A specialist should be called if the object cannot be removed quickly or atraumatically.

C. Tracheobronchial

1. Eighty percent of tracheobronchial foreign bodies occur in children less than 3 years old, and only 10% occur in persons older than 15 years old. Aspiration of foreign objects accounts for 2,000 deaths per year, with an incidence of 0.8 per 100,000 children 0 to 9 years old, in a male/female ratio of 2:1. Of all deaths from foreign body aspiration, 61% occur in children less than 1 year old, and 94% in children under 5 years.

2. **Etiology.** Food is the predominant foreign body (10); and although it occurs more commonly in children, everyone can be subjected to the "cafe coronary" and its potentially lethal results. Risk factors for food aspiration include inadequate dentition (your mother always said to chew your food), intoxication, food inappropriate for age, and stuffing the mouth. The most commonly recovered foods are meat (hot dogs), seeds (peanuts), raw carrots, hard candy, grapes, and raisins. Peanuts are the

most commonly aspirated foreign body in children (11,12), as many parents are still unaware that peanut ingestion can be hazardous in young children. Inorganic objects have included earrings, toys, and pacifiers that can pull apart into pieces. About 80% to 90% of airway foreign bodies are located in the bronchial tree.

3. Symptoms can range from none to life-threatening depending on location and size of the object relative to the airway lumen. In up to 80% of patients there is a history of witnessed choking (13). Hoarseness and stridor are significantly more common in upper airway entrapment (10), whereas subglottic obstruction can produce a clinical picture simulating croup or asthma (14). The triad of wheezing, coughing, and decreased breath sounds is diagnostic of a lower airway foreign body in as many as one-half of cases. Other findings may include labored respiration, retractions, tachypnea, and asymmetry of ventilation secondary to air trapping. Foreign body aspiration must be considered in all children with new or unexplained wheezing or stridor.

4. There are four basic **obstructive mechanisms** by which foreign bodies lead to lower airway pathology.
   a. Check valve, where inhaled air cannot be expelled past obstruction, resulting in hyperinflation.
   b. Stop valve, where the foreign body creates a total obstruction with atelectasis distally.
   c. Ball valve, where the foreign body dislodges during expiration and reimpacts during inspiration leading to atelectasis.
   d. Bypass valve, when the foreign object causes a partial obstruction, resulting in decreased aeration.

5. Diagnosis may be facilitated by radiographs if the patient is stable.
   a. Soft-tissue neck radiographs may demonstrate subglottic narrowing of the upper airway with a homogeneous, poorly defined radiodensity within the narrowed segment (14). There may also be hyperextension of the neck with dilatation of the hypopharynx on the lateral radiograph.
   b. Chest radiographs most commonly displayed unilateral hyperlucency (38%) or atelectasis (25%), a radiopaque object (15%), or no abnormality (19%) in a review of 155 children with bronchoscopy-proven foreign bodies (12). Children with tracheal foreign bodies had a normal chest radiograph 50% of the time. If the initial radiograph is normal but there is a strong suspicion of a radiolucent foreign body, a chest radiograph taken during inspiration may accentuate emphysema ipsilateral to a bronchial foreign body. A radiograph taken during expiration may reveal a mediastinal shift away from the object because of air trapping. If available, fluoroscopy may reveal similar findings. In the uncooperative infant or developmentally delayed patient, decubitus radiographs cause a unilateral chest compression comparable to expiration in the lung on the side against the table. Air trapping is evident when the lung containing the foreign body is against the table.

6. **Treatment**
   a. Immediate treatment of **upper airway obstruction** is indicated only when there is a completely obstructed airway. Attempts to assist someone who is moving air past the foreign body can produce complete obstruction.

(1) Prehospital treatment consists of the abdominal thrust and well-known **Heimlich maneuver.** In children under 1 year of age, repetitions of four back blows and four chest thrusts are the accepted maneuvers, because vigorous abdominal compression can produce traumatic asphyxia and injury to thoracic and abdominal structures.

(2) In the hospital, completely obstructing foreign bodies should be removed with the aid of **direct laryngoscopy.** If the object is beyond reach, creation of an artificial airway is the next step. **Cricothyrotomy** is the accepted procedure. If the foreign body is at the cricoid it can be pushed into the right mainstem bronchus, allowing aeration through the left lung. If a specialist is available, a **tracheostomy** can be performed.

b. Treatment of **lower airway obstruction** can be performed by a specialist using a rigid bronchoscope under controlled conditions in the operating suite.

II. GI tract foreign bodies

A. Foodstuffs are the most frequent impacted GI tract foreign body in **adults.** The elderly patient with dentures or the intoxicated patient may swallow an incompletely chewed bolus of meat owing to altered sensation in the mouth. Psychotic or demented patients are also at risk for foreign body ingestion (15–17).

B. Children put everything in their mouths, and coins are the most commonly impacted foreign body. Toys and batteries are also found with regularity. Ingestions tend to occur during nonschool months or in high-risk situations, and repeat ingestions are not uncommon (17–20).

C. Foreign bodies usually lodge at points of **physiologic narrowing.** Most are located in the esophagus at the level of the cricopharyngeus muscle, aortic arch, or gastroesophageal junction. Patients of any age with motility disorders or pathologic strictures are also at higher risk for impaction. Sharp or pointed objects such as fish bones also have a tendency to lodge in the esophageal mucosa.

D. Complications of esophageal foreign bodies depend on the nature of the object and duration of impaction. A sharp, pointed object, impaction for more than 24 h, and poor removal technique all may lead to esophageal perforation and mediastinitis. Lesser trauma may result in laceration and delayed stricture formation. Prolonged impaction can lead to inflammation, tracheal compression, and respiratory symptoms. Button batteries are especially troublesome and can severely injure the esophagus by several mechanisms.

E. Diagnosis can usually be made by history. Adults can usually localize the foreign body by symptoms of pain, pressure, or dysphagia. Uncooperative or preverbal children can be more problematic. Clues to the diagnosis include refusal to eat, increased salivation, drooling, and vomiting. However, anywhere from 16% to 44% of children have been found to be asymptomatic after esophageal foreign body impaction (18,21,22). It is therefore recommended that all children with a history of possible foreign body ingestion undergo radiographic evaluation. Expedient diagnosis is essential because the risk of complications increases and the success of removal declines with prolonged impaction.

1. Soft-tissue radiographs of the neck and chest can locate radiopaque foreign bodies. Unfortunately, in one study only 24% of endoscopically proven esophageal fish bone impactions were identified by plain film (23).

   2. Contrast radiography should be attempted if plain films do not identify the object (15,17). After verifying that the patient can swallow, administer a water-soluble agent (Gastrografin) alone or on a small cotton pledget. Gastrografin is safe in the mediastinum but causes pulmonary edema if aspirated. Barium leaves a better coating, is safe if aspirated, but forms granulomas in the mediastinum.

   3. CT scanning, with its excellent soft-tissue detail, can accurately localize esophageal foreign bodies that are not seen with either plain or contrast radiography but still suspected (24).

   4. External metal detectors have been able to accurately localize metallic GI tract foreign bodies in small studies (25,26).

F. Treatment of esophageal foreign bodies entails prompt removal, particularly when there is a chance of perforation. Several techniques are described.

   1. Endoscopy is the standard method for removing any esophageal foreign body, and is the method of choice for patients with esophageal pathology, objects that have been impacted for a prolonged period (greater then 24 h), and sharp objects. Endoscopy is the definitive method to search for foreign bodies that are still suspected despite a negative radiographic evaluation or when other modes of retrieval have failed (15,17,22,27).

   2. A **Foley catheter** can be used under fluoroscopic guidance by an experienced physician to draw out blunt objects such as coins that have been lodged in the esophagus for a short period of time. In a survey of 2,500 cases, there was a 95% success rate and one serious complication (28). One center treated 421 children over an 11-year span and achieved success in 91%. Major complications occurred in 1% (19).

   3. **Glucagon** at a dose of 0.5 to 2.0 mg i.v. (may be repeated twice) is a lower esophageal muscle relaxant that can facilitate egress of smooth foreign objects out the lower end of the esophagus. It is noninvasive, but contraindicated if esophageal stricture is suspected. There was a 69% success rate in a series of 48 patients in which an effervescent agent and water were also utilized (29).

   4. Papain, an enzymatic meat tenderizer, is no longer recommended because of the risk of esophageal perforation (15).

G. Once in the **stomach,** most foreign bodies pass unimpeded (17,22). One should beware, however, of large objects lodged in the stomach. More than 50% of patients who had swallowed objects that were more than 6.5 cm in length required surgery for their removal (30). Other areas where foreign objects can lodge are the cecum, appendix, hepatic and splenic flexures, and a Meckel's diverticulum. A foreign body's progress through the GI tract can monitored with stool inspections and/or serial radiographs. Surgical removal is indicated if symptoms occur.

H. Ingestions of cocaine packets by the "body packer" drug smuggler presents the physician with a formidable GI decontamination. Packets usually contain 3 to 7 g of cocaine; 1 to 3 g of cocaine powder can be lethal if the packet ruptures (31). In such cases an abdominal radiograph may demonstrate multiple, well-defined, homogeneous oval or oblong densities, especially if surrounded by a crescent of air (double-condom sign) (32). The standard methods of GI decontamination (ipecac, lavage, enema, cathartics) should be avoided because of the high risk of packet rupture.

I. Button batteries are being used with increasing frequency in a variety of devices including hearing aids, watches, and calculators. Most contain a heavy metal such as mercury and an alkaline electrolyte. Esophageal impaction can result in injury may occur by four mechanisms: electrolyte leakage; alkali produced from external currents; mercury toxicity; and pressure necrosis (33).

    1. Early removal of ingested disk batteries is indicated for esophageal impaction, large diameter (more than 21 to 23 mm in diameter), signs and symptoms of abdominal pain, tenderness, and guarding, or prolonged contact with a specific site. Complications from disk batteries that have traversed the esophagus are rare. Most batteries (68.8%) pass through the GI tract within 48 h, 85.4% within 72 h, and 98.8% within 4 days (34).

    2. When viewed in an anterior projection, disk batteries demonstrate a double-density shadow due to the bilaminar structure of the battery. On lateral view, the edges of most disk batteries are round and present a step-off at the junction of the cathode and anode. These findings are differentiated from coins, which do not have a double density on frontal projection, have a much sharper edge, and have no visible step-off (35).

J. Appropriate **discharge instructions** to all patients with an intestinal tract foreign body would be to return to the ED if the foreign body is not observed to pass within 4 days (2 days if it is a battery) or if any symptoms occur.

K. Rectal foreign bodies present a slightly different problem for the physician. Adults are at risk for objects inserted during sexual activity. On the other hand, children most often present with misplaced thermometers. Patients are often embarrassed and reluctant to give the history. The diagnosis should be made by digital examination, and only on occasion are radiographs necessary (36). If possible, removal of the foreign body should be done transanally, occasionally with local anesthesia and sedation. Rarely, when the object is not palpable, removal should be performed in the operating room under general anesthesia. All rectal removal of foreign bodies must be followed by sigmoidoscopy to look for damage.

References

1. Werman HA. Removal of foreign bodies of the nose. *Emerg Med Clin North Am* 1987;5:253.
2. Kavanagh KT, Litovitz T. Miniature battery foreign bodies in auditory and nasal cavities. *JAMA* 1986;255:1470.
3. Skinner DW, Chui P. The hazards of "button-sized" batteries as foreign bodies in the nose and ear. *J Laryngol Otol* 1986;100:1315.
4. Capo JM, Lucente FE. Alkaline battery foreign bodies of the ear and nose. *Arch Otolaryngol Head Neck Surg* 1986;112:562.
5. Fosarelli P, Feigelman S, Pearson E, Calimano-Diaz A. An unusual intranasal foreign body. *Pediatr Emerg Care* 1988;4:117.
6. Hanson RM, Stephens M. Cyanoacrylate-assisted foreign body removal from the ear and nose in children. *J Pediatr Child Health* 1994;30:77.
7. Baklin SA. Positive-pressure technique for nasal foreign body removal in children. *Ann Emerg Med* 1995;26:658.
8. Baker MD. Foreign bodies of the ears and nose in childhood. *Pediatr Emerg Care* 1987;3:67.
9. Pride H, Schwab R. A new technique for removing foreign bodies of the external auditory canal. *Pediatr Emerg Care* 1989;5:135.
10. Laks Y, Barzilay Z. Foreign body aspiration in childhood. *Pediatr Emerg Care* 1988;4:102.
11. Brown TC, Clark CM. Inhaled foreign bodies in children. *Med J Aust* 1983;2:322.

12. Burton EM, Brick WG, Hall JD, Riggs W Jr, Houston CS. Tracheobronchial foreign body aspiration in children. *South Med J* 1996;89:195.
13. Wiseman NE. The diagnosis of foreign body aspiration in childhood. *J Pediatr Surg* 1984;19:531.
14. Gay BB Jr, Atkinson GO, Vanderzalm T, Harmon JD, Porubsky ES. Subglottic foreign bodies in pediatric patients. *Am J Dis Child* 1986;140:165.
15. Ginsberg GG. Management of ingested foreign objects and food bolus impactions. *Gastrointest Endosc* 1995;41:33.
16. Roark GD, Subramanyam K, Patterson M. Ingested foreign material in mentally disturbed patients. *South Med J* 1983;76:1125.
17. Webb WA. Management of foreign bodies of the upper gastrointestinal tract: update. *Gastrointest Endosc* 1995;41:39.
18. Hodge D III, Tecklenburg F, Fleisher G. Coin ingestion: does every child need a radiograph? *Ann Emerg Med* 1985;14:443.
19. Shunk JE, Harrison AM, Corneli HM, Nixon GW. Fluoroscopic foley catheter removal of esophageal foreign bodies in children: experience with 415 episodes. *Pediatrics* 1995;96:791.
20. Taylor RB. Esophageal foreign bodies. *Emerg Med Clin North Am* 1987;5:301.
21. MacPherson RI, Hill JG, Othersen HB, Tagge EP, Smith CD. Esophageal foreign bodies in children: diagnosis, treatment, and complications. *Am J Roentgenol* 1996;166:919.
22. Schweich PJ. Management of coin ingestions: any change? *Pediatr Emerg Care* 1995;11:37.
23. Evans RM, Ahuja A, Rhys Williams S, Van Hasselt CA. The lateral neck radiograph in suspected impacted fish bones: does it have a role? *Clin Radiol* 1992;46:121.
24. Braverman I, Gomori JM, Polv O, Saah D. The role of CT imaging in the evaluation of cervical esophageal foreign bodies. *J Otolaryngol* 1993;22:344.
25. Biehler JL, Tuggle D, Stacy T. Use of the transmitter-receiver metal detector in the evaluation of pediatric coin ingestions. *Pediatr Emerg Care* 1993;9:208.
26. Ros SP, Cetta F. Metal detectors: an alternative approach to the evaluation of coin ingestions in children. *Pediatr Emerg Care* 1992;8:134.
27. Sundgren PC, Burnett A, Maly PV. Value of radiography in the management of possible fishbone ingestion. *Ann Otol Rhinol Laryngol* 1995;104:501.
28. Campbell JB, Condon VR. Catheter removal of blunt esophageal foreign bodies in children. *Pediatr Radiol* 1989;19:361.
29. Robbins MI, Shortsleeve MJ. Treatment of acute esophageal food impaction with glucagon, an effervescent agent, and water. *Am J Roentgenol* 1994;162:325.
30. Gracia C, Frey CF, Bodai BI. Diagnosis and management of ingested foreign bodies: a ten-year experience. *Ann Emerg Med* 1984;13:30.
31. Boehnert MT, Lewander WJ, Gaudreault P, Lovejoy FH Jr. Advances in clinical toxicology. *Pediatr Clin North Am* 1985;32:193.
32. Beerman R, Nunez D Jr, Wetli CV. Radiographic evaluation of the cocaine smuggler. *Gastrointest Radiol* 1986;11:351.
33. Kost KM, Shapiro RS. Button battery ingestion: a case report and review of the literature. *J Otolaryngol* 1987;16:252.
34. Litovitz TL. Battery ingestions: product accessibility and clinical course. *Pediatrics* 1985;5:469.
35. Maves MD, Lloyd TV, Carithers JS. Radiographic identification of ingested disc batteries. *Pediatr Radiol* 1986;16:154.
36. Busch DB, Starling JR. Rectal foreign bodies: case reports and a comprehensive review of the world's literature. *Surgery* 1986;100;512.

Emergency Toxicology, Second Edition,
edited by Peter Viccellio.
Lippincott–Raven Publishers, Philadelphia © 1998.

78

PCBs and Dioxins

Raquel L. Gibly

Division of Emergency Medicine, University Medical Center, Tucson, Arizona 85724

I. **Introduction.** There are many types of halogenated aromatic compounds. These compounds are typified by polychlorinated biphenyls (PCBs), polybrominated biphenyls (PBBs), polychlorinated dibenzo-*p*-dioxins (PCDDs), polychlorinated diphenylethers (PCDEs), polychlorinated dibenzofurans (PCDFs), and polychlorinated naphthalenes (PCNs) (Fig. 78-1). These compounds are not found naturally. They are synthesized and used diversely in commercial and industrial applications.

II. **Sources.** PCBs have been widely used as hydraulic fluids, heat transfer fluids, organic diluents, plasticizers, lubricants, flame retardants, adhesives, laminating agents, dusting agents, and dielectric fluids for capacitors and transformers. PCNs and PBBs were primarily used as flame retardants. PCDDs, PCDEs, PCDFs and many other halogenated aromatics are formed as byproducts during the synthesis or combustion of other industrial halogenated aromatics.

PCBs are ubiquitous in the environment, and all humans have been and will continue to be exposed to them. The primary source of exposure is ingestion of contaminated food or fish. Small amounts are inhaled through the air. Dairy products contain PCBs, and breastfed infants may be exposed through breast milk. High risk of occupational exposure occurs in the following professions: electric cable repair, electroplating, emergency response teams, firefighting, hazardous waste handling or site operation, heat-exchange equipment repair, metal finishing, paving, roofing, pipefitting, plumbing, manufacture of timber products, transformer/capacitor repair, waste-oil processing. PBBs are not used as diversely, and are not found freely in the environment. PBB contamination is restricted to Michigan's lower peninsula. Production of PBBs was stopped in 1974, and U.S. production of PCBs was stopped in 1977. Significant quantities of these products as well as their byproducts can still be found in older transformers and capacitors, and as global contaminants in our ecosystem (1,2).

Major incidents of poisoning from halogenated aromatic products include the following (3):

1949—Nitro, West Virginia—Monsanto plant contamination by intermediary product in trichlorophenol production (Tetrachloredibenzo-p-dioxin (TCDD)).

1962–1970—Vietnam—Agent Orange defoliant (TCDD) exposure.

1968—Yusho, Japan—Contamination of rice-oil with PCBs and PCDFs.

1971—Times Beach, Missouri—Spraying of TCDD contaminated sludge oil for dust control.

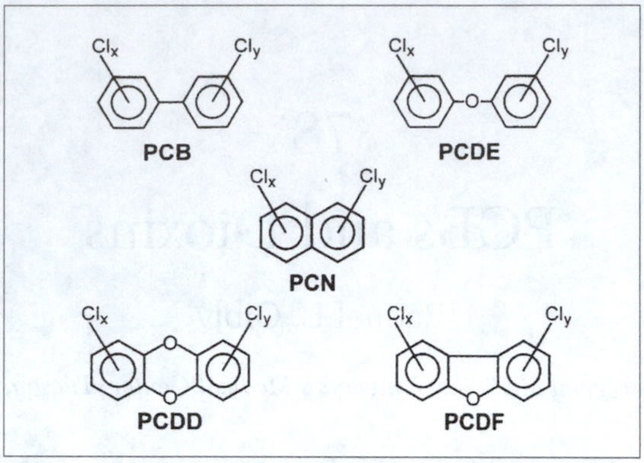

FIG. 78-1. Physical structures of selected polyhalogenated aromatic hydrocarbons

1973—Michigan—Firemaster flame retardant accidentally introduced to cattle feed (PBB and polybromodibenzofuran (PBDF) exposures).

1976—Seveso, Italy—ICMESA plant runaway reaction at trichlorophenol plant causing TCDD exposure

1979—Taichung county, Taiwan—Contamination of rice-oil with PCBs and PCDFs (Yucheng disease).

III. Polychlorinated biphenyls (PCBs)

A. Properties of agent

1. **Sources and forms of toxins.** PCBs are very versatile secondary to their wide range of physical properties, chemical stability and miscibility with organic compounds. For the most common sources of these products, see **II.** Due to detection of PCBs in the environment, a ban was placed on the use of PCBs, and in the late 1970s, use and production of this product in the United States was stopped. Significant quantities still exist in dielectric fluids of older transformers and capacitors (2).

2. **Physical and chemical properties.** The polycyclic halogenated aromatics have multiple sites for halogen substitution allowing many different isomers and congeners to be formed. PCBs have 1 to 10 chlorine atoms attached to a biphenyl structure with the empirical chemical formula $C_{12}H_{10-n}Cl_n$, where $n = 1$–10. There are 209 different PCB congeners. Some of the commercial names for PCBs include Aroclor (USA), Phenoclor (France), Kanechlor (Japan), Fenclor (Italy), Soval (USSR), Clophen (Germany), and Delor (Czechoslovakia). The IUPAC numbering system has arranged the PCBs in ascending order based on number of substituted chlorine molecules from 1 to 209. Aroclors, the major PCBs used in the United States, are identified by a four digit numbering system in which the last two digits represent the chlorine content by weight percent (i.e., Aroclor 1242 = 42% chlorine by weight) (2,4). Most products are mixtures of many congeners and isomers, and the same products exact congeneric composition may vary from lot to lot (4).

PCBs are inert chemicals with a high degree of lipophilicity. They are fairly resistant to degradation and hydrolysis. They are relatively water insoluble, but are very soluble in nonpolar organic solvents and biological lipids. The higher the amount of halogenation, the greater the toxicity of the product. Fires and other sources of high temperature can greatly increase the toxicity of PCBs by the formation of byproducts such as PCDFs and PCDDs (1,3).

3. **Mechanism of action/pathophysiology.** PCBs and other similar halogenated aromatic hydrocarbons are thought to share similar mechanisms of action. A few congeners bind to a cellular Aromatic hydrocarbon receptor (Ah receptor) which regulates the synthesis of a variety of proteins. Others induce a variety of microsomal systems including the cytochrome P-450–dependent monooxygenases in the liver. Some induce toxicity directly by their physical structure, with the congeners substituted in both para, at least two meta, and no ortho positions, representing the most potent class of these physical toxins (4).

4. **Pharmacology and pharmakokinetics**

   a. **Absorption.** PCBs are highly lipophilic and are readily absorbed from the GI tract via a passive process across cell membranes. They are also readily absorbed through the dermal and inhalational routes. Absorption efficacy increases with the degree of ring chlorination, up to a point. Increased protein binding also occurs with increased halogenation (4).

   b. **Distribution.** PCBs are rapidly cleared from the blood (minutes-hours) and deposited in tissues, especially liver and muscle. They are stored mostly in skin and adipose tissue due to their highly lipophilic nature. PCBs are excreted into milk and also undergo transplacental transfer (4).

   c. **Metabolism.** PCBs are metabolized in the liver by the cytochrome P-450 microsomal system to polar metabolites that undergo conjugation with glutathione or glucuronic acid. They also undergo sulfation reactions. Different enzymes are induced depending on the number and position of the chlorine atoms within the PCB isomer (5). Rate of metabolism is dependent upon the ring substitution pattern, degree of ring chlorination, and levels of enzymes in the target tissue. The higher the degree of chlorination the slower metabolism. It is important to note that different species metabolize PCBs in different ways.

   d. **Elimination.** Elimination follows first-order kinetics with elimination half-lives 0.5 to 2.6 years (4). The main routes of excretion are fecal and urinary. More highly chlorinated congeners are predominantly excreted in the feces (up to 60%). For less chlorinated compounds, urinary excretion predominates. Small amounts of parent compound may be excreted unchanged in the feces, but only metabolites are found in the urine and bile. Breast milk is also an important route of elimination of PCBs.

B. **Clinical presentation**

   1. **History.** PCBs themselves are found to cause very few systemic symptoms. Nonspecific and vague subjective symptoms such as general malaise, weight loss, anorexia, oral mucous pigmentation, and palmar sweating have been reported with PCB exposure (6). Subjective complaints of tiredness, depression, dizziness, head-

ache, equilibrium problems, blurred vision, joint pains and muscle weakness have been reported, but these symptoms were not correlated with body burdens (3,5). Skin is the most sensitive organ to show toxicity to the PCBs. Chloracne, a refractory follicular skin eruption resembling acne, is the "hallmark" of poisoning by polychlorinated and polybromated cyclic aromatic compounds (i.e., PCBs, PCNs, PCDFs, PCDDs), and is the most commonly reported toxic effect (3,7,8). PBBs have not been causally linked to any human clinical illness (5), although neurologic symptoms have been noted after exposure. Because these products are often mixtures, it is difficult to assign the cause of symptomatology to exactly one product. Symptoms & signs related to other polyhalogenated benzenes include weight loss, hyperhidrosis, unusual body odor, nausea, vomiting, diarrhea, neuropathies with documented demyelination, persistent bronchitis, unspecified joint problems, and porphyria of the hepatic type as characterized by hyperpigmentation, hypertrichosis, traumatic and actinic bullae, milia, and scars, with evidence of liver damage (3,4). Inhalation exposure can cause upper respiratory irritation, cough, chest pain/tightness, and changes in pulmonary functions (decrease FEV_1 and FVC). Ocular effects include edema of the eyelid, congestion/hyperemia of the conjunctivae, eye discharge (PCDFs), and enlargement of the Meibomian glands (4,8–10) (Table 78-1).

2. **Physical examination.** The basic chloracne lesions are comedones and yellow cysts. Unlike juvenile acne, chloracne has a predilection for malar crescents, periauricular and retroauricular skin, axillae, and scrotum, and causes little local inflammation (7,8). It is frequently accompanied by hyperpigmentation of the face, nails, lips, axillae and mouth. Meibomian gland involvement and conjunctivitis can be present with ophthalmic chloracne (8).

3. **Clinical course.** Chloracne can occur as a result of chronic or acute exposure by any route. Lesions usually appear within 2 to 4 weeks of exposure but can appear as late

TABLE 78-1. *Signs and symptoms reported with polyhalogenated hydrocarbon exposure*

Cutaneous	Respiratory
Chloracne	Chronic bronchitis
Comedones, hyperkeratosis, follicle enlargement	Persistent cough
Hyperpigmentation	Hepatic
Skin, nails, mucous membranes	Liver enlargement
Hyperhidrosis	Porphyria
Hirsutism	Gastrointestinal
Elastosis	Digestive disorders
Ocular	Anorexia/weight loss
Hypersecretion of the Meibomian glands	Nonspecific
Conjunctivitis	Muscle aches/pains
Discharge	Hemorrhagic cystitis
Neurologic	Sleep disturbances
Headaches	Depression
Numbness	Loss of energy
Weakness	Decreased libido
Fatigue	
Cold intolerance	
Memory loss	
Neuropathy/neuritis	

Data from refs. 2, 8–10.

as 2 or more months after the exposure. Lesions usually regress over a 4 to 6 month period, assuming no additional exposure, although some dermal lesions have been known to persist for over 30 years (8). A grading system has been suggested to assess the severity of chloracne lesions (Table 78-2) (11). There is no evidence for increased rates of mortality, teratogenesis, carcinogenesis, fetotoxicity, genetic mutations, or immunologic deficiencies in humans with exposure to PCBs or TCDDs (3). It should be noted that animal studies linking these parameters to PCB exposure have been done, but the relevance of extrapolating this data to humans is questionable (3,12).

C. **Differential diagnosis.** Evaluation of the dermal lesions should include acne vulgaris and porphyria cutanea tarda. Exposure to one polychlorinated hydrocarbon should raise suspicion about exposure to multiple compounds in this family since these are usually mixtures of products and contaminants.

D. **Laboratory analysis.** Serum PCB levels may be measured by gas chromatography-mass spectrometry or gas chromatography-hydrogen flame ionization detection. A nonfasting blood sample should be used. Mean serum levels in nonoccupationally exposed adults are 7 to 30 ppb (5). Levels can be 2.5 times higher in people who regularly eat fish (4). PCB levels in human adipose are generally less than 3 ppm, but levels up to 33 ppm have been reported (5). Human milk levels range from 40 to 100 ppb (9). In newborns, PCBs can be measured from umbilical cord blood, and are expected to be 10% of the maternal level (9). Liver enzymes should be checked. Various studies have shown increases in SGOT, SGPT, GGT, alkaline phosphatase, and LDH, that correlate to increased PCB levels. However, there is no evidence for long term hepatotoxicity, and increased liver function tests, as well as fatty infiltration of the liver and hepatomegaly were noted to be reversible, therefore, the clinical significance of these findings remains in question (4,5). PCBs do induce the hepatic microsomal system. This can be monitored using the Caffeine Breath Test (CBT) which indirectly measures hepatic cytochrome activity by measuring the amount of exhaled radiolabeled CO_2 produced by the liver microsomal system from ingested radiolabeled caffeine (4). Depressed levels of T_4 have been found in rats after PCB exposures but not in humans. No significant changes in T_3, T_3 uptake, thyroxine, or free thyroxine index have been noted (4). No significant changes in hematologic or renal parameters have been noted. For diagnosis of chloracne, histology is helpful in acute cases, although in chronic cases, histopathology is nonspecific (7). PBB exposure has not revealed any hematologic abnormalities.

TABLE 78-2. *Choracne grading system*

Grade	Description
1	No change
2	Few comedones in specific sites only
3	More comedones in specific sites/No cysts
4	Numerous comedones in specific sites with cysts
5	Numerous comedones and cysts in specific and other sites
6	As above with inflammatory changes

    E. Management
        1. General. General decontamination should include immediate removal of the patient from sources of contamination such as clothing, food, water, and air. Gloves should be used to avoid contact with contaminated clothing and substances. For dermal exposure, the skin and hair should undergo multiple washes with soapy water. For inhalational exposures, basic airway and breathing management including oxygen therapy with the use of 100% humidified oxygen and bronchodilators as clinically indicated. For ocular exposure, irrigate the eyes with copious amounts of water for at least 15 min. Eye exam is warranted if irritation persists. For oral exposure, emesis is not any value in chronic or remote exposures. In the unlikely event of an acute ingestion, induction of emesis is not recommended secondary to the high risks of aspiration. Benefits of administering activated charcoal in an acute ingestion are unknown; nonetheless, due to its relatively benign effects, charcoal is frequently recommended at a dose of 1 g/kg orally (50 to 75 g for an average adult) (9). Treatment of chloracne is not very successful. Topical retinoic acid, oral 13-cis-retinoic acid (isotretinoin), oral antibiotics, peeling agents, and dermabrasion, have all been reported with varying effectiveness (7,8).
        2. Toxin-specific measures. There are no specific treatments, antidotes, or chelating agents available.
  F. Disposition and follow-up. Since most exposures are occupationally related, or accidental environmental exposures, removal, containment, and disposal of the offending agent should be performed to prevent further exposure. Depending on the patient's symptoms, long term follow-up can be arranged, and the patient monitored for abnormalities, resolution of symptoms, and laboratory abnormalities. Dermatologic consultation should be obtained in the presence of dermal lesions as these may be extremely hard to deal with, and may require very long term follow-up.

IV. Dioxins and furans
  A. Properties of agent
    1. Sources and forms of toxins. Polychlorinated dibenzodioxins (PCDDs or "dioxins") and polychlorinated dibenzofurans (PCDFs or "furans") usually coexist as unwanted contaminants produced during combustion or incineration of polychlorinated compounds. They are formed from the incomplete burning of waste products containing chlorine such as PVC and plastic, chemical manufacturing processes, recirculation of environmental reservoirs, and processes involving chlorine bleaching or municipal sludge. They are also formed in coal-burning power plants, exhaust from diesel engines, the making of white paper products, home fireplaces, and cigarette smoke (11,13,14). They are produced naturally in small amounts by volcanoes and forest fires (13). Dioxins are also formed during the production of many chlorinated organic solvents, hexachlorophene, and the herbicide 2,4,5-T, which was removed from the market but which was a component of the defoliant Agent Orange. Agent orange, agent pink, agent purple and agent green were all herbicides used in Vietnam, and were all contaminated with varying amounts of dioxins (11). Occupational exposure occurs primarily during the production of trichlorophenol (TCP). Since 1983, dioxins are no longer manufactured

in the United States. Other occupations with the greatest risk of exposure include firefighters, environmental and hazardous waste clean-up crews, municipal waste incinerator workers and people involved with the manufacture of chlorinated herbicides, germicides and organic solvents.

Dioxins are ubiquitous in the environment (13). Food accounts for over 90% of human exposure, with the major sources being meat, fish, and dairy products. Only 1% comes from breathing contaminated air (10). Only a minor amount ($\simeq 0.01\%$) comes from drinking contaminated water. The present exposure of the general population to environmental levels of TCDD and related compounds present in milk, fish, other consumer products, and other media, should not be of concern. There are no known cases of human fatalities from acute exposure to dioxins (15).

2. **Physical and chemical properties.** There are 75 congeners of the polychlorinated dibenzo-*p*-dioxins, also known as "dioxins." The most studied isomer is the most toxic, 2,3,7,8-Tetrachlorodibenzo-*p*-dioxin (TCDD). Because dioxins have similar effects and modes of action, the phrases "TCDD" and "dioxins" are often used interchangeably. TCDD is colorless, odorless, lipid-soluble, and only slightly soluble in water (13). It is solid at room temperature (16). There are 135 different congeners of polychlorinated dibenzofurans (PCDFs).

3. **Mechanism of action/pathophysiology.** Dioxins work by binding to the cellular Ah receptor to form an Ah-ligand complex. Binding affinities of the various PCDDs and related compounds are dependent upon the shape and electronic configuration of the molecules. This complex then induces the cytochrome P-450 systems in liver and other tissues (10). The Ah-ligand complex is transported into the nucleus where it binds to DNA recognition sites and alters the expression of specific genes and may act as a promoter for initiation of somatic mutation (17).

4. **Pharmacology and pharmacokinetics**
   a. **Absorption.** The mechanisms of absorption are poorly understood (10).
   b. **Distribution.** Due to the high lipophilicity of these products, the greatest concentrations are found associated with lipids and in adipose tissue. High concentrations are also found in liver, pancreas, skin, and muscle. TCDD crosses the placenta and accumulates in breast milk, allowing fetuses and newborns to have an increased risk of exposure, although no cases of dioxin toxicity has been reported by these routes.
   c. **Metabolism.** TCDD undergoes monohydroxylation, dihydroxylation, and monomethoxylation, but the exact mechanisms are not well established (16).
   d. **Elimination.** Elimination is by the fecal route for 80% to 100% of these products. Both parent compound and metabolites are found fecally. Only minor amounts of metabolites are found in the urine (11).

B. **Clinical presentation**
   1. **History.** No syndromes in humans have been associated with exposure to these polychlorinated compounds except chloracne (see PCBs) (16). People acutely exposed have exhibited symptoms such as chemical burns to skin and mucous mem-

branes, eye irritation, headache, muscle pains, nausea and vomiting. "Wasting away syndrome," characterized by anorexia, listlessness, weakness, and emaciation, has been seen in animals, but not humans, after exposure to lethal doses of dioxins (16). After a latent period of as little as 2 weeks or as long as years, chloracne, porphyria cutanea tarda, hirsutism, hyperpigmentation, polyneuritis, hand dystonias, and hepatomegaly have been noted. As with PCBs, the most specific indicator of this type of exposure is the presence of chloracne (11,16).

2. **Physical examination.** See PCBs.

3. **Clinical course and long-term effects.** Chloracne can be a long term problem and may be progressive regardless of limited exposure. Teratogenicity, carcinogenicity and reproductive effects in humans have been greatly studied and much debate and controversy exists as to whether conclusive conclusions can be drawn (14). There is an association between the development of soft tissue sarcomas and dioxin exposure, but this is inconclusive and some studies dispute this association (11). Many confounding factors exist including exposure to multiple products mixed with the dioxins, differing social factors and associated risk factors of exposed workers. There is suggestive evidence for relationships to other cancers in humans, but currently there is insufficient data to draw conclusions (11). No structural malformations in newborns have been conclusively linked to dioxin exposure (11,16).

C. **Differential diagnosis.** See PCBs.

D. **Laboratory analysis.** Serum analysis for dioxins is very expensive to perform (more than $1,000.00), and requires a large amount of serum (more than 250 cc) (11,16). Tissue levels are also very difficult and expensive to perform. When ordered, these levels are measured by gas chromatography and mass spectrometry, with a margin of error being 20% to 50% on samples measuring less than 100 ppt (parts-per-trillion) (11). The dioxin levels in the average human population are as follows: serum, 5 ppt; adipose tissue, 4 to 130 ppt; human milk, 2 ppt; background levels, 3 to 10 ppt for TCDD, and 250 to 1000 ppt for octachloro-benzo-*p*-dioxins (10,11). Blood levels are reflective of tissue levels. TCDD concentrations in body lipids of greater than 50,000 ppt have been tolerated in humans with no or only minor side effects with the exception of chloracne (15). Furan levels are considerably lower (10). Liver function tests, CBC, PT, serum lipids, and uroporphyrins should be obtained in an acute exposure. An increase in T_4 and TSH in infants has been associated with high dioxin levels in the milk fat of nursing mothers (11). Hyperlipidemia may persist for as long as 10 years after an acute exposure, but the clinical significance of this is yet unknown (11). Formal neurologic testing should be done in patients suffering from neuropathy or neuritis.

E. **Management.** See PCBs.

F. **Disposition and follow-up.** See PCBs.

References

1. Safe S. Polchlorinated biphenyls, dibenzo-*p*-dioxins, dibenzofurans, and related compounds: environmental and mechanistic considerations of toxic equivalency factors. *Toxicology* 1990;21:51–88.
2. Safe S. Polychlorinated biphenyls (PCBs) and polybrominated biphenyls (PBBs): biochemistry, toxicology and mechanism of action. *Crit Rev Toxicol* 13(4)319–95, 1984.

3. Tindall JP. Chloracne and chloracnegens. *J Am Acad Dermatol* 1985;13:539–558.

4. U.S. Department of Health and Human Services. *Toxicology profile for polychlorinated biphenyls*. Washington, DC: USDHHS, August 1995.

5. Shields PG, Whysner A, Chase KH. Polychlorinated biphenyls and other polyhalogenated aromatic hydrocarbons. In: Sullivan JB, Kreiger GR, eds. *Hazardous materials toxicology*. Baltimore: Williams & Wilkins, 1992:748–755.

6. Takamatsu M, Oki M, Maeda K, et al. PCBs in blood of workers exposed to PCBs and their health status. *Am J Ind Med* 1984;5:59–68.

7. Coenraads PJ, Brouwer A, Olie K, et al. Chloracne, some recent issues. *Dermatol Clin* 1994;12:569–576.

8. Zugerman C. Chloracne, clinical manifestations and etiology. *Dermatol Clin* 1990;8:209–213.

9. Poisondex. *Toxicologic managements: PCB-PBB. Volume 90*. Micromedix, Inc. Englewood, Colorado. 1974–1996.

10. Dickson LC, Buzik SC. Health risks of "dioxins": a review of environmental and toxicological considerations. *Vet Hum Toxicol* 1993;35:68–77.

11. Poisondex. *Toxicologic managements: dioxins. Volume 90*. Micromedix, Inc. Englewood, Colorado. 1974–1996.

12. Golub MS, Donald JM, Reyes JA. Reproductive toxicity of commercial PCB mixtures: LOAELs and NOAELs from animal studies. *Environ Health Perspect* 1991;94:245–253.

13. Agency for Toxic Substances and Disease Registry. U.S. Department of Health and Human Services, Public Health Service, Atlanta, Georgia. Dioxin toxicity. *Am Fam Phys* 1993;47:855–861.

14. Kociba RJ, Schwetz BA. Toxicity of 2,3,7,8-tetrachlorodibenzo-*p*-dioxin (TCDD). *Drug Metab Rev* 1982;13:387–406.

15. Kimbrough RD. How toxic is 2,3,7,8-tetrachlorodibenzodioxin to humans? *J Toxicol Environ Health* 1990;30:261–271.

16. Andrews JS. Polychlorodibenzodioxins and polchlorodibenzofurans. In: Sullivan JB, Kreiger GR, (eds). *Hazardous materials toxicology*. Baltimore: Williams & Wilkins, 1992:756–761.

17. Skene SA, Dewhurst IC, Greenberg M. Polychlorinated dibenzo-*p*-dioxins and polychlorinated dibenzofurans: the risks to human health. A review. *Hum Toxicol* 1989;8:173–203.

PART VIII

Animal Toxicology

Emergency Toxicology, Second Edition,
edited by Peter Viccellio.
Lippincott–Raven Publishers, Philadelphia © 1998.

79

Arthropod Envenomation

Karl A. Sporer

Department of Surgery, University of California, San Francisco, Department of Emergency Services, San Francisco General Hospital, San Francisco, California 94110

The phyla Arthropoda is the largest division of the animal kingdom and includes the class Insecta (bees, wasps, caterpillars, ants) and class Arachnida (spiders, scorpions). This group of animals collectively accounts for a huge number of envenomations in clinical practice.

I. **Brown recluse spider.** Spiders from the family Loxoscelidae are responsible for essentially all of the documented cases of spider bites associated with serious skin necrosis. *Loxosceles reclusa* is the most clinically significant in the United States because of its high prevalence, but other species exist as well: *L. refuscens, L. unicolor (deserta), L. arizonica, L. devia,* and *L. laeta. L. laeta* was imported from South America and is potent, but no human bites have been reported in the United States, and *L. unicolor* and *L. arizonica* rarely come into contact with humans (1).

   A. **Location.** The brown recluse spider is widely distributed throughout the southern and central United States. The spider has been reported as far west as California and as far east as New Jersey but is especially concentrated in Oklahoma, Missouri, Kansas, Tennessee, and Arkansas; it is seen in lesser concentrations in Kentucky, Louisiana, Texas, Nebraska, Iowa, Alabama, Georgia, and Ohio. The incidence of bites increase from April through October and occur most commonly in the morning (2).

   B. **Description**

      1. The brown recluse spider ranges from 1 to 3 cm in length (from rostral to caudal leg tip) and is light to dark brown. These spiders have a characteristic violin- or fiddle-shaped dark brown to yellow marking on the dorsal cephalothorax. They have long, slender legs relative to the body and have three pairs of eyes, in contrast to the usual four noted in most spiders. This point may be helpful for identifying partially demolished spiders (3).

      2. The recluse is a passive spider that lives in dark places; it is rarely seen because of its nocturnal hunting habits. It prefers a warm, dry climate, and its natural habitat is outdoors in wood piles, among debris, under stones, or in any spot that can afford it a dry, protected location. In the colder habitats, the recluse spider tends to live indoors in basements or storage areas and is more likely to come into contact with humans. Brown recluse spiders are not aggressive and bite only when they are inadvertently crushed against the skin of an unsuspecting human. The most common contact occurs when someone puts on some old clothes, lies on a sheet or blanket without shaking it out, or steps into a shoe without checking (2).

C. **Venom**

1. Spiders have a pair of horny fangs called chelicerae. Their venom is injected from modified salivary glands through these hollow chelicerae. The brown recluse venom is composed of sphyngomyelinase D, the primary dermonecrotic and hemolysis factor, along with other enzymes, including hyaluronidase, proteases, collagenase, esterases, phospholipase, deoxyribonuclease, ribonuclease, and alkaline phosphatase, which help promote local spread of the venom and have some role in chemotaxis, necrosis, and platelet aggregation.

2. Sphyngomyelinase D has been shown to be the active agent in dermonecrosis (4,5). The intradermal injection of this toxin produces the characteristic necrotic lesions with systemic symptoms. The toxin is capable of producing direct cell death and hemolysis, activating the complement cascade, and chemotactically attracting polymorphonuclear (PMN) leukocytes (6).

3. There is a subsequent brisk coagulation of platelets and occlusion within small capillaries that sparks the complement cascade and attracts a pronounced infiltration of PMNs (7). A neutrophilic dermatosis similar to pyoderma gangrenosa has been described and is a likely explanation for the lengthy healing period of these lesions (8).

D. **Cutaneous manifestations**

1. Bites from the brown recluse spider can range from insignificant irritation to full-thickness ulceration with severe systemic symptoms. The patient's size, the spider's size, and the amount of envenomation probably add to the variable nature of these bites. In addition, it has been suggested that natural immunity acquired from prior spider bites can produce an amelioration of symptomatology. Multiple injections of venom in animals leads to the development of serum antibodies and immune protection (9). Patients with repeat spider bites have been noted to have less reactive subsequent lesions.

2. Berger (10) described two carefully documented cases of brown recluse bites that resolved after days of expectant therapy. These patients had no evidence of former immunity as determined by the lymphocyte transformation test. He concluded that many (maybe most) brown recluse bites resolve with minimal symptoms, and only a small percentage develop the characteristic lesions (10).

3. The brown recluse spider bite may be relatively painless, or it can produce a mild sting and go unnoticed initially. Necrosis may develop rapidly over a matter of hours or slowly over days. Pain secondary to ischemia usually peaks within 2 to 18 h. In most cases the lesion is diagnostic within 6 to 8 h.

4. Classically, there is initial erythema, edema, and tenderness that progresses to a blue-gray vasoconstrictive halo that spreads around the puncture site. After 12 to 18 h, a bleb or dull gray macule forms at the site and is accompanied by a surrounding zone of erythema and edema. The erythema is replaced by a characteristic violaceous discoloration of the skin. Gradually, this necrotizing lesion widens, and the edge becomes uneven. The necrotic center eventually sinks below the normal level of the skin. The violaceous color and skin depression help differentiate this bite from other arthropods' bites.

5. The central ischemic lesion may cause necrosis within 3 to 4 days and later forms an eschar within 4 to 7 days. The ulcerated lesion heals slowly over 4 to 6 weeks (occasionally as long as 4 months). The wound may leave extensive residual scarring and may require eventual reconstructive surgery. Lesions have been noted to be more severe in areas of fatty tissue, such as the thighs or buttocks (2,11).

E. **Systemic manifestations**

1. Only a fraction of patients with diagnostic brown recluse spider bites develop systemic symptoms, but they can be severe and are responsible for all the reported deaths. These reactions have no correlation with the severity of the cutaneous lesion. One study of 18 bites reported two patients with hemolysis and five others with symptoms of nausea, vomiting, rash, abdominal pain, and headache (12).

2. Systemic symptoms usually occur within 24 to 48 h. Typically, they include fever, chills, malaise, nausea, vomiting, myalgias, hemolysis, and disseminated intravascular coagulation (DIC). Renal failure, coma, hypotension, and seizures have been noted in some rare patients. The hemolytic anemia can be difficult to diagnose because it can occur rapidly or take 2 to 3 days to appear. Systemic loxoscelism with little or no skin involvement has been described. It usually occurred in children and presented with massive hemolysis (13).

F. **Laboratory analysis.** There are no readily available laboratory tests to confirm brown recluse spider bites. The lymphocyte transformation test and various immunoassays are being studied but none of these are currently available (14,15,15a,15b). Most laboratory work is needed to exclude or confirm the presence of hemolysis and hemoglobinuria or hematuria. Thus a baseline urinalysis, CBC with platelets, and creatinine assay are useful in all but the most trivial bites. Daily monitoring of these parameters is indicated for serious wounds.

G. **Treatment of cutaneous lesions**

1. Local wound care, ice, and delayed debridement are the mainstays of therapy of the brown recluse spider bite. Attention to local wound care, rest, elevation, and tetanus status are equally important. Much of the literature concerning treatment is replete with anecdotal cases and no controlled human studies. Many of the wounds studied are presumptive necrotic arachnidism and further cloud the picture. Most recommendations concerning treatment come from some authors' experience and a small group of animal experiments.

2. Early excision has not been shown to be effective. The venom spreads quickly through the tissues, and it is impossible to determine which bite will progress to a significant lesion. One prospective study of presumptive spider bites found that individuals fared better with medical treatment and delayed closure than did the group with early surgical excision (16). A successful regimen usually requires allowing the necrotic area to demarcate with subsequent excision with wide margins.

3. Ice packs are thought to be useful because sphyngomyelinase D is more active at higher temperatures. It also correlates with the clinical experience of several authors (2,17). Intermittent ice bags are probably soothing and useful so long as care is taken not to inflict a cold injury on susceptible patients.

4. **Dapsone.** Use of the PMN inhibitor dapsone has been suggested for large lesions (18). A prospective study of 31 patients demonstrated that wound healing was

significantly better in the dapsone-treated group than in the group without dapsone (16). Dapsone is used in doses of 50 to 100 mg divided into twice-a-day doses after ruling out glucose-6-phosphate dehydrogenase (G6PD) deficiency. Despite the relatively few studies confirming efficacy, the complication rate of hemolysis and methemoglobinemia is low enough to warrant therapy with this drug (19,20).

5. Prophylactic antibiotics (2) and steroids (21,22) are not useful. Antivenom, hyperbaric oxygen, and electroshock therapy have been tried with variable degrees of success (19,20,23).

6. Treatment of the systemic effects of the brown recluse spider bite includes steroid therapy and meticulous supportive care. Systemic corticosteroids have not been proved effective in controlled studies, but most investigators recommend them (2). Prednisone 1 to 2 mg/kg/day or its equivalent may be given and quickly tapered by day 7.

7. Transfusions of packed red blood cells and fresh frozen plasma are given as indicated for hemolysis, and urine alkalinization is useful for preventing renal failure.

8. For patients with necrotic lesions, baseline CBC, urinalysis, and platelet count should be performed and monitored for several days. Patients with systemic symptoms should be admitted.

II. **Black widow spider,** or *Latrodectus mactans,* is found throughout the United States but is most common in the Southeast, Southwest, and California. It is characteristically shiny black with a red hourglass shape in its bulbous abdomen. The spider grows to a body size of 15 mm and a leg spread of 30 mm. The male of the species is too small to penetrate the dermis of humans and is of no clinical concern. The black widow makes coarse, irregular webs in dimly lit places both indoors and out and is not aggressive toward humans.

A. **Venom.** Latrodectus venom is a novel and potent toxin. The venom causes an indiscriminate release of neurotransmitters and accounts for most of the symptoms of latrodectism. This venom works to depolarize synaptic membranes by opening nonspecific ionic channels that allow the ingress of calcium intracellularly (24,25). This depolarization promotes calcium-independent release of neurotransmitters and inhibits reuptake. High serum concentrations of calcium antagonize the neurotransmitter-releasing effect of the venom and allows the normal release via nerve stimulation (26).

B. **Clinical syndrome**

1. Latrodectism produces a characteristic clinical syndrome that can be explained on the basis of uncontrolled discharge of acetylcholine and norepinephrine. It is rarely fatal. The bite itself commonly goes unnoticed, or a small needle-like prick may be noted. Within 10 to 20 min, however, localized pain and throbbing begin. The pain quickly spreads to the rest of the extremity, followed by generalized symptoms of chest pain with tightness and dyspnea, abdominal cramping, and the characteristic facies latrodectismica (a flushed, sweating face contorted in a painful grimace with conjunctivitis and trismus of the masseters) (27,27a). General restlessness, localized sweating, and hypertension have been universally noted. The board-like rigid abdomen has been often confused with an acute abdomen and has caused unnecessary surgery. The bite site may develop mild redness or urticaria.

2. In one series of patients, onset of symptoms ranged from 30 min to 6 h (median 2 h). All of the patients had muscular pain, 64% had abdominal pain, 36% had nau-

sea and vomiting, and 27% had headache. Recovery time ranged from 8 to 32 h, with a mean of 18 h (28). Laboratory studies are normal except for an occasional leukocytosis.

C. Treatment consists in calcium gluconate, adequate analgesia, and muscle relaxants.

1. Calcium gluconate 1 to 2 mL/kg i.v. (up to 10 mL) may be given slowly. This treatment is often efficacious in relieving the muscle spasms but must commonly be repeated in several hours. It has proved to be more effective than methocarbamol (29).

2. There is extensive experience with the use of black widow antivenom in Australia. A report of 2,144 cases, most treated with antivenom, had only a 0.54% rate of anaphylactic reactions (30). Antivenom is undoubtedly the most specific and most permanent relief; series in the United States, however, revealed a high complication rate, and many believe that the risk of serum sickness and anaphylaxis is statistically greater than the risk of death from the black widow spider bite (31). Latrodectus antivenom is usually reserved for the patients at greatest risk, the extremes of age, those with hypertensive cardiovascular disease, pregnancy, and serious envenomation (31a,31b).

3. All patients who require calcium gluconate or muscle relaxers to relieve their pain should be admitted to the hospital to observe for recurrence of symptoms.

III. **Scorpion stings**

A. In the United States, the only scorpion whose sting is dangerous to humans is *Centruroides sculpturatus*. It is found mainly in Arizona and some contiguous parts of Texas, New Mexico, northern Mexico, and small areas of California.

B. *C. sculpturatus* can range from 1 to 7 cm in length and carries its venom and stinging apparatus in its tail. It is usually active on warm nights. The species is unusual in that it lives mainly in or near trees. Scorpions are not generally aggressive toward humans, but they do sting repeatedly when threatened or handled (32).

C. **Venom**

1. The venom of *C. sculpturatus* is primarily a neurotoxin. It contains no enzymes to cause local tissue destruction and so characteristically creates no local inflammatory response at the sting site.

2. **Mechanism of action.** Normal depolarization is controlled by the regulation of sodium influx and potassium efflux through the the cell membrane. This neurotoxin causes sodium channels to remain open longer than usual after depolarization and blocks voltage gated potassium channels. This sequence creates a widened action potential and causes repetitive firing of axons (32,33,33a).

D. **Clinical presentation.** Most scorpion stings occur on the extremities.

1. There is an immediate onset of pain without visual signs of inflammation at the site. Over minutes to an hour, the pain travels up the extremity and may become generalized. In severe cases, cranial nerve dysfunction may be noted, as may blurred vision, rotary eye movements, tongue fasciculations, loss of pharyngeal muscle control with attendant difficulty with secretions, stridor, and occasional respiratory arrest. There may also be evidence of excessive somatic neuromuscular activity, which manifests as uncontrollable jerking of the extremities or severe restlessness.

    2. Most patients with *C. sculpturatus* envenomation experience only local or extremity pain that usually resolves within 4 to 6 h and certainly by 24 h. Eight percent of stings produce symptoms of cranial nerve dysfunction or somatic neuromuscular excitation.

    3. As expected, small children are more likely to have severe symptoms because of relatively greater envenomations (32).

E. Treatment of patients with local and extremity pain consists in local ice, attention to wound care, and analgesia. Treatment of severe envenomations consists in specific scorpion antivenom and strict attention to airway management. There have been no controlled studies to assess the various modalities.

    1. A series of 12 children with serious *C. sculpturatus* envenomation were treated with barbiturate sedation. They were all hospitalized in an intensive care unit (ICU) and two patients developed respiratory arrest (34). There are obvious difficulties in sedating a patient with marginal respiratory control.

    2. A series of patients treated with intravenous antivenom prepared from goats was much more successful (35). Administering antivenom intravenously to patients with serious manifestations would reverse the neurologic symptoms within minutes to an hour (35,35a,35b). Two recent series demonstrated antivenin to be reasonably safe with mild immediate hypersensitivity reactions occurring 8% of the time, but were generally mild. This therapy is promising and should be reserved for serious life-threatening envenomations. As yet, Food and Drug Administration (FDA) approval does not exist.

IV. Hymenoptera

A. The order Hymenoptera includes the bee, wasp, and ant. Common characteristics include two pairs of wings, one pair of antennae, and three body segments (head, abdomen, and thorax) (36).

B. Bee venom includes a list of toxins: melittin, dopamine, histamine, phospholipase A2, hyaluronidase, apamin, and a mast cell degranulator. Melittin constitutes 50% of the dry weight of bee venom and is capable of producing histamine release from mast cells, contracting smooth muscle, and producing inflammation (37). Wasp venom is similar.

C. Local reactions begin with a sharp, stabbing pain followed by burning pains for minutes. A local wheal-and-flare reaction forms with central erythema and subsequent edema that may last days. Treatment of local reactions consists in removing any stingers (remember that the bee stinger may still contain uninjected venom and should be removed by scraping with a scalpel to avoid further envenomation), local wound care, and analgesia (38).

D. Anaphylactic reaction is the most common effect of serious, deadly arthropod envenomation.

    1. Any patient with signs of systemic reaction (shock, bronchospasm, generalized urticaria, or angioedema) should be treated with parenteral epinephrine. Those not in shock should receive epinephrine 1:1,000 0.1 mL/kg s.q. up to 0.5 mL. Because the shock state may hinder absorption, these patients should receive epinephrine 1:10,000 0.1 mg i.v. slowly (0.1 mL of epinephrine 1:1,000 in 10 mL normal saline) (39). Sometimes an epinephrine infusion is necessary (1 mL of epinephrine 1:1,000 in 250 mL 5% dextrose).

2. Diphenhydramine 50 to 100 mg i.v. and usteroids parenterally are recommended.

3. All patients with serious reactions to Hymenoptera should be referred to an allergist for desensitization.

E. Fire ants *(Solenopsis richteri* and *S. invicta)* were introduced into the United States in Alabama around 1920. By now they have invaded the Gulf Coast and are expected to infiltrate large parts of California. Fire ants grasp the skin with their jaws and then inflict multiple stings in a circular pattern. There is an immediate wheal-and-flare reaction that lasts several hours. A superficial vesicle with clear fluid and mild surrounding edema appears and after 8 to 10 h develops the characteristic sterile pustule (40). Therapy mostly consists in local wound care. Ice, sodium bicarbonate paste, and papain have been suggested, but none has proved effective (41,42).

V. **Lepidoptera.** Venomous caterpillars and moths are a common problem in the southern United States. The puss caterpillar *(Megalopyge opercularis)* is the most common (43). Envenomation occurs by contact with specialized hollow spines with venom spines at their base. Treatment consists in removing the spines, wound care, and analgesia as required. Systemic reactions do not occur.

References

1. Wilson DC, King LE. Spiders and spider bites. *Dermatol Clin* 1990;8:277.
2. Wasserman GS, Anderson PC. Loxoscelism and necrotic arachnidism. *J Toxicol Clin Toxicol* 1983–1984;21:451.
3. Gertsch WJ. *American spiders.* New York: Van Nostrand Reinhold, 1979.
4. Berger RS, Adelstein EH, Anderson PC. Intravascular coagulation—the cause of necrotic arachnidism. *J Invest Dermatol* 1978;61:142.
5. Kurpiewski G, et al. Platelet aggregation and sphyngomyelinase D activity of a purified toxin from the venom of *Loxosceles reclusa. Biochim Biophys Acta* 1981;687:467.
6. Gebel HM, Campbell BJ, Barrett JT. Chemotactic activity of venom from the brown recluse spider *(Loxosceles reclusa). Toxicon* 1979;17:55.
7. Smith CW, Micks DW. The role of polymorphonuclear leukocytes in the lesion caused by the venom of the brown spider, *Loxosceles reclusa. Lab Invest* 1970;22:90.
8. Rees RS, Fields JP, King LE. Do brown recluse spider bites induce pyoderma gangrenosum? *South Med J* 1985;78:283.
9. Smith CW, Micks DW. A comparative study of venom and other components of three species of Loxosceles. *Am J Trop Med Hyg* 1968;17:651.
10. Berger RS. The unremarkable brown recluse spider bite. *JAMA* 1973;225:1109.
11. Majeski JA, Durst GG. Necrotic arachnidism. *South Med J* 1976;69:887.
12. Hollabaugh RS, Fernandes ET. Management of the brown recluse spider bite. *J Pediatr Surg* 1989;24:126.
13. Taylor EH, Denny WF. Hemolysis, renal failure, and death, presumed secondary to bite of brown recluse spider (necrotic arachnidism). *South Med J* 1966;59:1209.
14. Berger RS, Millikan LE, Conway F. An in vitro test for *Loxosceles reclusa* spider bites. *Toxicon* 1973;11:465.
15. Finke JH, Campbell BJ, Barrett JT. Serodiagnostic test for *Loxosceles reclusa* bites. *Clin Toxicol* 1974;7:375.
15a. Barret SM, Romine-Jenkins M, Blick KE. Passive hemagglutination inhibition test for diagnosis of brown recluse spider bite envenomation. *Clinical Chemistry* 1993;10:2104.
15b. Barbaro KC, Cardoso JL, Eickstedt VR, Mota I. IgG antibodies to Loxosceles sp. spider venom in human envenoming. *Toxicon* 1992;9:1117.
16. Rees RS, et al. Brown recluse spider bites: a comparison of early surgical excision versus dapsone and delayed surgical excision. *Ann Surg* 1985;202:659.
17. King LE. Brown recluse spider bites: stay cool. *JAMA* 1985;254:2895.
18. King LE, Rees RS. Dapsone treatment of a brown recluse bite. *JAMA* 1983;250:648.
19. Rees RS, et al. The diagnosis and treatment of brown recluse spider bites. *Ann Emerg Med* 1987;16:945.
20. Barrett SM, Romine-Jenkins M, Jenkins DE. Dapsone or electric shock therapy of brown recluse spider envenomation. *Ann Emerg Med* 1991;20:459.

21. Jansen GT, et al. The brown recluse spider bite: controlled evaluation of treatment using the white rabbit as an animal model. *South Med J* 1971;64:1194.
22. Fardon DW, et al. The treatment of brown spider bites. *Plast Reconstr Surg* 1967;40:482.
23. Svendson FJ. Treatment of clinically diagnosed brown recluse spider bites with hyperbaric oxygen: a clinical observation. *J Ark Med Soc* 1986;83:199.
24. Finkelstein A, Rubin LL, Tzeng MC. Black widow spider venom: effect of purified toxin on lipid bilayer membranes. *Science* 1976;193:1009.
25. Rauber A. Black widow spider bites. *J Toxicol Clin Toxicol* 1983–1984;21:473.
26. Pardal JF, Granata AR, Barrio A. Influence of calcium on ^{3}H-noradrenaline release by *Latrodectus atheratus* (black widow spider) venom gland extract on arterial tissues of the rat. *Toxicon* 1979;17:455.
27. Maretic Z. Latrodectism: variations in clinical manifestations provoked by Latrodectus species of spiders. *Toxicon* 1983;21:457.
27a. Muller GJ. Black and brown widow spider bites in South Africa. A series of 45 cases. *South African Medical Journal* 1993;83:399.
28. Timms PK, Gibbons RB. Latrodectism—effects of the black widow spider bite. *West J Med* 1986;144:315.
29. Key GF. A comparison of calcium gluconate and methocarbamol (Robaxin) in the treatment of latrodectism (black widow spider envenomation). *Am J Trop Med Hyg* 1981;30:273.
30. Sutherland SK, Tinca JC. Survey of 2144 cases of red-back spider bites. *Med J Aust* 1978;2:620.
31. Moss HS, Binder LS. A retrospective review of black widow spider envenomation. *Ann Emerg Med* 1987;16:188.
31a. Handel CC, Izquierdo LA, Curet LB. Black widow spider (Latrodectus mactans) bite during pregnancy. *Western Journal of Medicine* 1994;160:261.
31b. Scalzone JM, Wells SL. Latrodectus mactans (black widow spider) envenomation: an unusual cause for abdominal pain in pregnancy. *Obstetrics and Gynecology* 1994;83:830.
32. Currey SC, et al. Envenomation by the scorpion *Centuroides sculpuratus. J Toxicol Clin Toxicol* 1983–1984;21:417.
33. Moss J, Thoa NB, Kopin IJ. On the mechanism of scorpion toxin-induced release of norepinephrine from peripheral adrenergic neurons. *J Pharmacol Exp Ther* 1974;190:39.
33a. Martin BM, Ramirez AN, Gurrola GB, Nobile M, Prestipino GM, Possani LD. Novel K(+) channel blocking toxins from the venom of the scorpion Centruroides limpidus limpidus Karsch. *Biochemical Journal* 1994;304:51.
34. Rimsza ME, Zimmerman DR, Bergeson PS. Scorpion envenomation. *Pediatrics* 1980;66:298.
35. Russell FE, Timmerman WF, Meadows PE. Clinical use of antivenin prepared from goat serum. *Toxicon* 1970;8:63.
35a. Gateau R, Bloom M, Clark R. Response to specific *Centruroides sculpturatus* antivenom in 151 cases of scorpion stings. *Journal of Toxicology, Clinical Toxicology,* 1994;32:165.
35b. Bond GR. Antivenin administration for *Centruroides* scorpion sting: risks and benefits. *Annals of Emergency Medicine,* 1992;21:788.
36. Ellenhorn MJ, Barceloux DG. *Medical toxicology.* New York: Elsevier Science, 1988.
37. Habermann E. Bee and wasp venom. *Science* 1972;177:314.
38. Green VA, Siegel CJ. Bites and stings of hymenoptera, caterpillar and beetle. *J Toxicol Clin Toxicol* 1983–1984;21:491.
39. Barach EM, et al. Epinephrine for treatment of anaphylactic shock. *JAMA* 1984;251:2118.
40. DeShazo RD, Butcher BT, Banks WA. Reactions to the stings of the imported fire ant. *N Engl J Med* 1990;323:462.
41. Ginsberg CM. Fire ant envenomation in children. *Pediatrics* 1984;73:689.
42. Ross EV, Badame AJ, Dale SE. Meat tenderizer in the acute treatment of imported fire ant stings. *J Am Acad Dermatol* 1987;16:1189.
43. Pinson RT, Morgan JA. Envenomation by the puss caterpillar *(Megalopyge opercularis). Ann Emerg Med* 1991;20:562.

Selected Readings

Barbaro KC, Cardoso JL, Eickstedt VR, Mota I. IgG antibodies to Loxosceles sp. spider venom in human envenoming. *Toxicon* 1992;9:1117.

Barret SM, Romine-Jenkins M, Blick KE. Passive hemagglutination inhibition test for diagnosis of brown recluse spider bite envenomation. *Clin Chem* 1993;10:2104.

Bond GR. Antivenin administration for *Centruroides* scorpion sting: risks and benefits. *Ann Emerg Med* 1992;21:788.

Gateau R, Bloom M, Clark R. Response to specific *Centruroides sculpturatus* antivenom in 151 cases of scorpion stings. *J Toxicol Clin Toxicol* 1994;32:165.

Martin BM, Ramirez AN, Gurrola, GB, Nobile M, Prestipino GM, Possani LD. Novel K$^+$ channel blocking toxins from the venom of the scorpion *Centruroides limpidus* limpidus Karsch. *Biochem J* 1994;304:51.

Muller GJ. Black and brown widow spider bites in South Africa. A series of 45 cases. *S Afr Med J* 1993;83:399.

Emergency Toxicology, Second Edition,
edited by Peter Viccellio.
Lippincott–Raven Publishers, Philadelphia © 1998.

80

Reptilian Envenomation

Victor M. Garcia-Prats

*Department of Emergency Medicine, Alton Oshner Medical Foundation,
New Orleans, Louisiana 70121*

Reptilian envenomation can be considered a multiple-toxin poisoning (1). The spectrum of patient presentations and the variety of patients' responses to treatment challenge the clinician's knowledge and skill. As suburbia creeps closer to the wilderness, as our society becomes increasingly mobile, and as the number of weekend campers rises, an encounter with a venomous reptile becomes more likely. Considering the increased volume in illegal trade by collectors of exotic reptiles, one can understand the subtleties and complexities involved in snakebite presentation. Approximately 8,000 poisonous snakebites per year are reported in the United States (1). In the past, a variety of treatments were advocated with variable results; even today there are several schools of thought. To choose one method of treatment over another blindly would be foolish because of the ever-evolving schemes of treatment suggested in the literature. As with many other diseases, the treatment of snakebite is controversial. The key is to be aware of the facts and choose treatments accordingly.

I. **Properties of agent**

   A. **Sources of agent**

      1. Snakes and lizards are grouped under the class Reptilia, order Squamata; within this classification are found the venomous snakes and lizards. There are four principal families of snakes: Boidae, Colubridae, Elapidae, and Viperidae. There are no venomous snakes within the family Boidae, so the focus is on snakes in the three other families.

      2. The rear-fanged Colubridae are known for their fixed hind fangs and are represented by dangerous snakes, such as the African boomslang, which is not endemic to the United States; however, most Colubridae have no fangs and are completely harmless. Some colubrids found in the United States, such as ring-necked snakes and hog-nosed snakes, that have been considered to be nonvenomous have been reported to have saliva with toxic effects similar to the effects of venom (2).

      3. Found within the family Elapidae are the well-known and dangerous cobras and mambas. Three kinds are found in the United States. The Eastern coral snake, *Micrurus fulvius fulvius,* is spread throughout the southern states, extending into the Mississippi Basin. The Texas coral snake, *Micrurus fulvius tenere,* appears from eastern Texas into western Louisiana and southern Arkansas; and the Arizona coral snake, *Microides euryxanthus euryxanthus,* is found in Arizona and western New Mexico. These species are known for their brightly colored alternating bands. Because of the increased interest in these snakes by zoos and private collectors, encounters with patients bitten by the exotic Elapidae must be considered possible.

4. Old World and New World vipers and pit vipers are classified in the family Viperidae. The groups that pose the greatest threat within the United States are in three genera: Agkistrodon, Sistrurus, and Crotalus. These snakes can be found throughout the country except for parts of Maine and parts of Wisconsin, Michigan, Minnesota, North Dakota, Oregon, Montana, and Washington. The Eastern diamondback rattlesnake extends throughout the southern portions of Mississippi, Alabama, and Georgia, through the entire state of Florida, and in the eastern portion of South Carolina. The distribution of the Western diamondback rattlesnake extends from the central portion of Arkansas, Oklahoma, and central, northern, and western Texas, through the southern three-quarters of New Mexico and Arizona, touching extreme Southern California (3).

5. The distribution of the other species is too complex to discuss in detail here, and specific textbooks should be consulted for definitive discussions on this subject (1). The genera mentioned here differ from true vipers because **pit vipers** have an advanced neurosensory receptor located between the eye and the nostril. This heat-detecting pit is the reason for these snakes being called pit vipers; it is one of several ways to identify these toxic snakes. In the United States the family Viperidae is represented by three genera and 17 species, including the copperhead, cottonmouth, massasauga, pygmy rattlesnake, and true rattlesnakes (among which the eastern and western diamondbacks are considered to be the most dangerous).

6. The focus of this chapter is on the families Elapidae and Viperidae because they cause most venomous snakebites; coral snakes cause fewer than 2% of these bites.

7. **Venomous lizards** in the United States are classified in the family Helodermatidae, of which there are two species, *Heloderma suspectum* and *Heloderma horridim*. The Gila monster inhabits the Great Sonoran Desert region of Arizona and Mexico, and the beaded lizard has been confirmed in Mexico and Guatemala. Utah and Nevada have also been cited as areas of habitation for the Gila monster. These lizards are prized specimens for collectors throughout the United States; hence encounters outside their natural habitat regions are possible.

B. **Forms of toxin.** A venom is a toxic substance produced by a plant or animal in a highly developed secretory organ or group of cells, and one which the animal can deliver during a biting or stinging act (1).

1. In venomous snakes the toxin is produced within a gland located behind the eye and transmitted, when muscles contract to excrete it, via a duct into the hollow, fixed, short fangs of Elapidae or the curved, elongated fangs of Viperidae. In vipers, the fangs are usually retracted posteriorly and sheathed; during the act of striking, however, the fangs are brought forward.

2. **Snake venom** is a complex mixture of compounds that provide the snake an offensive and defensive armamentarium. Venom functions as part of the snake's food-gathering mechanism, enabling it to immobilize its victim and begin the digestive process prior to ingestion. The defensive function enables the snake to retreat after the initial strike. Defensive doses of venom are somewhat smaller in volume and concentration than the food-gathering dose (3).

   a. Venom components and activity can vary according to the family and species of snake but also by subspecies, geographic area, age of the snake, time of year, and the snake's nutritional status (4). The complex makeup of venom has yet to be completely defined, but it is generally composed of metal ions, enzymes, and low-molecular-weight peptides and polypeptides (molecular weight 6,000 to 30,000 Daltons).

b. In the past, general characteristics were applied to certain venoms because of their predominant effects (e.g., neurotoxin or cardiotoxin); however, these terms should be avoided because an entire spectrum of effects of venom can be observed.

c. Generally speaking, the **enzymatic components** of snake venom cause local and sometimes systemic effects, and the **nonenzymatic components** provide lethality.

   (1) **Enzymes** that have been found in venoms include phospholipase A, venom proteases, hyaluronidase, and amino acid esterases. Their net effect is to cause an increase in cell wall permeability, with hemolysis, disruption, and alteration of connective tissue allowing further spread of the toxin; muscle and subcutaneous tissue damage leading to necrosis; and promotion of intravascular clotting and fibrinolysis resulting in a defibrination syndrome.

   (2) The components of venom that cause systemic effects can be categorized as nonenzymatic, low-molecular-weight peptides and polypeptides. The presence of these **lethal compounds** varies among species of snakes; they can be grouped into hemorrhagins, cardiotoxins, and neurotoxins.

      (a) **Hemorrhagins** exert their main toxic effect on the lung; they disrupt endothelial cell junctions and alveolar septa, which results in increased hemorrhage into the pulmonary arterial and arteriolar walls, intraalveolar movement of blood and transudates, and eventually pulmonary congestion and increased lung weight (3,5). These effects can also occur locally at the bite site, causing hemorrhagic edema and systemic bleeding, leading to shock.

      (b) **Cardiotoxin,** found particularly in cobra venom, is toxic to the heart. It is a depolarizing agent that affects skeletal, cardiac, and smooth muscle membranes as well as the neuromuscular junction (3).

      (c) **Neurotoxins** can be found in elapid, hydrophid, vipirid, and crotalid venoms. They are neuromuscular nondepolarizing blocking agents with different methods of action. The venom of the Mojave rattlesnake is predominantly neurotoxic, and a neurotoxic component has been found in the Eastern diamondback rattlesnake as well.

d. During injection, the snake bypasses the primary barrier, the skin, depositing venom in blood vessels, peritoneum, subcutaneous tissue, or muscle. **Absorption of venom** through these sites is variable, but it takes place most rapidly through the blood vessels. In subcutaneous tissue the venom is transported to other sites via the lymph channels and capillary bed.

e. **Distribution of venom** depends on protein binding, membrane permeability, and pH, with entry into tissue based on the rate of blood flow and tissue mass. Certain components of venom have a high affinity for certain receptor tissues.

Upon reaching these tissues, venom crosses the membrane by four methods of transport: passive diffusion, facilitated diffusion, active transport, and pinocytosis (3).

f.   **Venom is excreted** by the kidney; however, kidney function can be decreased because of the indirect effects of venom on blood cells (hemoglobinuria) and muscle cells (myoglobinuria).

g.   Table 80-1 (6) shows the range of **toxicity** of snake species found in the United States. Other factors lending to variations in toxicity include the age and size of the snake and the amount of venom injected. The age, size, and general health of the victim are also important. For example, a child requires more antivenin than an adult because the ratio of venom concentration to tissue is greater, and less total body fluid is available as a diluent.

II.   **Clinical presentation** of a snakebite may be straightforward and obvious, but not always. The history may be vague and confusing and the physical findings minimal or absent. Thus, the clinician may be challenged by a hypotensive, unconscious adult or a child with acute seizures but no obvious clue to the cause. Therefore, understanding the snake and its habits, the initial signs and symptoms of snakebite, and how it progresses can be lifesaving.

A.   Snakes have no means of internal temperature control; thus, their active times occur when temperatures range from 22°C to 32°C; they hibernate during cold weather. Most snakebites take place during the months of April through October. Snakes generally are relatively nonaggressive unless threatened, but there are times in the life cycle when aggressiveness can increase.

TABLE 80-1. *Comparative toxicity of snake venoms*

Species of rattlesnake (Crotalus)	Average length of adult (in.)	Approximate yield, dry venom (mg)	Intraperitoneal LD_{50} in mice (mg/kg)	Intravenous LD_{50} in mice (mg/kg)
Eastern diamondback (*C. adamanteus*)	32–65	370–700	1.89	1.68
Western diamondback (*C. atrox*)	30–65	175–320	3.71	4.20
Prairie (*C. viridis viridis*)	32–46	35–100	2.25	1.61
Southern Pacific (*C. viridis helleri*)	32–48	75–150	1.60	1.29
Mojave (*C. scutulatus*)	22–40	50–90	0.23	0.21
Sidewinder (*C. cerastes*)	18–30	18–40	4.00	—
Moccasins (*Agkistrodon*)				
Cottonmouth (*A. piscivorus*)	30–50	90–145	5.11	4.00
Copperhead (*A. contortrix*)	24–36	40–70	10.50	10.92
Coral snakes (*Micrurus*): eastern coral (*M. fulvius*)	16–28	2–6	0.97	—

Modified from ref. 6.

B. Snakebites may occur during encounters in "wild" areas, but more frequently the event takes place in the patient's home surroundings and often while snakes are being handled by collectors.

C. Review of cases yields certain facts about the **victims:** They are usually males (4:1) age 10 to 19 years, and the bite site is usually an extremity (65%), predominantly the hands, fingers, ankles, and feet (7). A high incidence of snakebite is associated with alcohol use by the victim.

D. **Identification of the snake** is important but should be left to experts such as the herpetologist at the local zoo. Attempts at exact identification by a lay person can lead to serious errors. However, certain characteristics of poisonous snakes can be noted.

   1. To identify the **Crotaldae subfamily,** look for the heat-detecting organ located in the pit between the eye and the nostril. Other important characteristics are a triangular-shaped head, vertical elliptical pupils, and a single row of subcaudal plates (Fig. 80-1) (8,9).

   2. **The coral snakes** found in the United States have none of these danger signs; however, their sequential bands of color are a distinctive feature. Certain nonpoisonous snakes have mimicked these sequential bands as a defense mechanism, but in these snakes the bands do not completely encircle the body and they follow a different sequence of colors. The fully encircling bands of the black-snouted coral snake are in a consistent pattern of yellow or white, red, and black; thus, remembering the saying, "Red on yellow kill a fellow; red on black, venom lack" can help to identify coral snakes.

E. **On physical examination** of the patient, the earliest signs to look for are **bite marks** made by the anteriorly oriented fangs.

   1. The usual number of punctures is two; however, there can be one to three marks present because a fang could have been lost or a replacement fang may be present without the older one having been shed.

   2. Because of its efficient venom transport mechanism, the **crotalid** bite is a quick event; however, the **coral snake** has shorter, fixed fangs, so a longer "chewing" action is necessary to inject venom. This is an important point about which to question the patient.

   3. The **coral snake's** puncture marks are usually separated by a distance of 2 to 8 mm; however, to complicate matters, sometimes no visible marks can be found.

F. **Symptoms**

   1. **With crotalid envenomation,** local pain and swelling are noted most frequently and progress rapidly up the extremity, particularly within the first hour, then more slowly over the next several hours. Within the first 30 min, the patient may complain of weakness or numbness and tingling of the face and lips. Skin discoloration can be noted early with associated regional lymph node pain and swelling. With a severe envenomation or with inadequate treatment, the signs and symptoms can progress rapidly with petechiae, ecchymoses, bleb formation, and subsequent necrosis. Further worsening signs are hypotension with development of a shock-like state and cardiac dysfunction. Nausea and vomiting can occur with hematemesis and associated bloody diarrhea and hematuria as coagulopathy evolves.

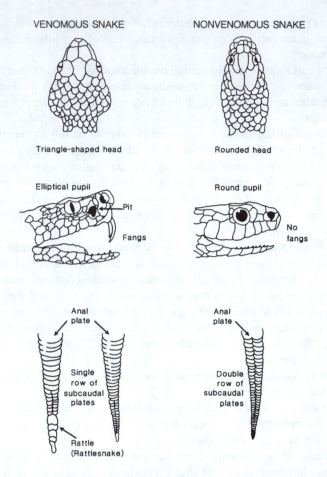

FIG. 80-1. Left: Head of a poisonous pit viper. **Right:** Head of a harmless snake. (Adapted from Keiser, E.D. *The Poisonous Snakes of Louisiana and the Emergency Treatment of Their Bites.* New Orleans: Louisiana Wild Life and Fisheries Commission; Lafayette Natural History Museum, 1971, p. 5; and from Otten, E.J. Venomous Animal Injuries. In P. Rosen, F.J. Baker, and G.R. Braen (eds.), *Emergency Medicine.* St. Louis: C.V. Mosby Company, 1983, p. 679. With permission.)

2. With the **Eastern diamondback rattlesnake,** fasciculations and seizure activity may occur, particularly in children. Subsequent multiple organ failure, especially of the heart, lung, and kidney, results from the direct effect of the venom and secondarily from fluid shifts and losses, hemoglobin loss, and myoglobulin excretion.

3. A patient sustaining a **coral snake bite** may show no early signs of envenomation, although subsequent progression may be rapid. Pain, swelling, and local skin changes may be minimal. This stage may soon be followed by numbness, weakness of the extremity, and, after several hours, euphoria, drowsiness, tremors, and salivation. After 5 to 10 h, patients may have slurred speech and diplopia with the development

of dysphagia, dyspnea, progressive flaccid paralysis, and eventually death from respiratory paralysis and cardiac failure.

III. **Differential diagnosis.** A key to the diagnosis of envenomation is awareness of all possibilities that can produce the presenting signs and symptoms. The spectrum of potential causes ranges from a simple thorn puncture to the complexity of sepsis with disseminated intravascular coagulation.

   A. One must consider **toxins** from a black widow spider or venomous marine animal or a **hypersensitivity reaction** to various insect stings or bites, primarily from Hymenoptera.

   B. **Acute neurologic syndromes,** rapidly progressing ascending **paralyses** from any cause, and **chemical toxins** resulting in salivation, pupillary changes, confusion, and seizures must be considered as possible etiologies.

   C. A localized **crush injury** with swelling, tissue injury, and muscle necrosis involving renal failure secondary to myoglobulin release must be part of the differential diagnosis.

   D. **Other causes of hemolytic anemia,** whether an intrinsic defect or an intracorpuscular abnormality, must be reviewed, as well as causes of thrombocytopenia, such as decreased bone marrow production or increased peripheral destruction of platelets.

   E. The diagnosis is pinpointed by combining the history, physical findings, and laboratory results and gradually eliminating possibilities from the diagnostician's list.

IV. Laboratory analysis provides the treating physician with a looking-glass into the evolution of envenomation. These studies should be followed closely throughout the patient's stay in the emergency room or intensive care unit (ICU). Combining the clinical appearance with the laboratory results can guide the physician through treatment dilemmas.

   A. While examining a newly presented envenomated patient, one should develop a baseline of the signs and symptoms as well as of cardiac, neurologic, renal, pulmonary, and hematologic function. As the patient's symptoms evolve, the clinician can focus attention on particular studies.

   B. When the patient arrives in the emergency room, the following **basic studies** should be performed: CBC; platelet count; coagulation studies (including prothrombin time, fibrinogen level, and fibrin split products); electrolytes, creatinine, and BUN levels; and blood type and crossmatch. With these parameters, the clinician can follow the patient's renal function, volume status, and coagulation system.

   C. **Pulmonary status** should be monitored with repeated chest roentgenograms and arterial blood gas measurements (ABGs), because with fluid shifts, increased endothelial permeability, and the direct effects of the venom, the development of adult respiratory distress syndrome (ARDS) is a possibility.

   D. **ECGs** can monitor cardiac function.

   E. **Urinalysis** initially and with subsequent bedside checks using a dipstick can signal developing hematuria or myoglobinuria.

   F. Attempts to develop assays that identify the presence of venom at the puncture site or within the patient's serum have met with little success. A **radioimmunoassay** was developed for this purpose in Australia during the 1970s, but it has never become a practical methodology and is useful only as a research tool. The **enzyme-linked immunosorbent assay** bridges the gap because it can detect small amounts of antigen and antibody. Unlike the radioimmunoassay, the reagents are inexpensive, stable, and have a short performance time. A field device was developed in Australia to identify the venoms of five dangerous snakes; however, in the United States no tests are commercially available and no laboratories provide clinical detection of snake venom. Testing would yield only a positive result for pit viper envenomation without species specificity because of cross-reactivity of the antigens. As techniques and venom antigens are refined, this method may be of practical use in the future (10).

V. Management of a snakebite can be fraught with excitement, fear, and confusion if it is not handled in an organized, controlled manner. One should view the situation as having a realistic endpoint and proceed toward it in methodical steps. The overall concern is controlling the situation by understanding the challenge and the complications that can be expected.

   A. **At the scene.** The key to treatment of a snakebite at the scene is to proceed with first aid steps and move to the nearest medical facility. Delaying definitive treatment can cause further injury.

   1. The person bitten always experiences fear and possibly panic, so the initial effort should be to **calm the patient.** Do not allow him or her to exert himself or herself by running. The patient should be removed from the area and be made to sit or lie down with the affected extremity in a neutral position.

   2. Attempts to **locate the snake** are important for later identification; however, be sure that the search is done safely so others are not bitten. The snake should be killed with a long tree limb or stick, is possible. Note that the reflex biting action of a dead snake, even with a severed head, can persist for up to 60 min.

   3. Once these steps have been taken, the patient's bitten **extremity is immobilized** as a fracture would be, using whatever methods are available. It has been suggested that, in an attempt to delay lymphatic flow, two methods can be utilized: the lymphatic constricting band and the elastic wrap. The key to placement of either is the amount of pressure with which it is applied; thus, the bands should be maintained at less than venous pressure.

      a. The **lymphatic constricting band** should be placed proximal to the bite, testing the band so that one or two fingers can be placed easily underneath it. This band should be repositioned proximal to the evolving edema every 10 to 15 min.

      b. It has been suggested that in cases of an **elapid snakebite,** an **elastic-type** wrap should be placed over the affected extremity beginning over the bite marks and continuing along the length of the extremity. A splint can then be applied for immobilization (11).

   4. The method of **incision and suction** advocated in the past has been a source of controversy because of the damage to tissue caused by this technique. A product developed recently may resolve this controversy and should be seriously considered as care on the scene. The Sawyer Extractor **vacuum pump** with different-sized mouthpieces for maximum suction is described as a spring-loaded, two-chambered suction device that can generate 1 atmosphere of negative pressure and can be placed using only one hand (Fig. 80-2). No incision is advocated prior to placement of this suction device over the puncture site (12). The function of the device is to draw out venom through the path left by the fangs. Experimentally, with placement of suction after a 3-min delay, 23% of labeled venom was removed after 3 min and 34% was removed after 30 min (13). The scientific jury is still out on this device, but it is promising.

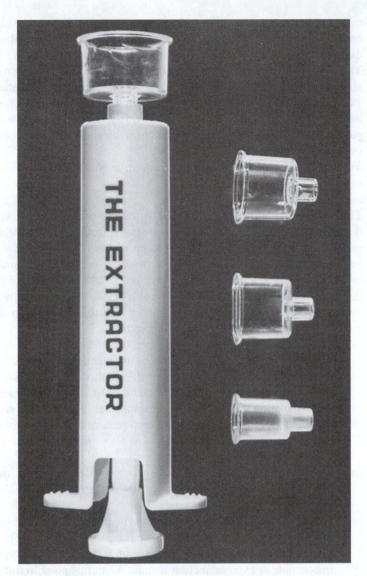

FIG. 80-2. Sawyer Extractor with mouthpieces of various sizes for maximum removal of venom.

B. At the hospital

1. Once a poisonous snakebite is diagnosed, **initial evaluation** entails monitoring **vital signs** and a thorough, rapid general examination, with the understanding that, if indicated, appropriate **advanced cardiac life support** measures should be taken. The subsequent focused examination should emphasize the bitten area, noting the amount of swelling by the measured circumference of the extremity. The level to which this swelling extends and any loss of vascular and neurologic function should also be noted. A baseline **physical examination** of the cardiac, neurologic, respira-

tory, and hematologic systems should be documented. The patient should be placed on a **cardiac monitor** and vital signs measured frequently. The **laboratory studies** discussed previously (see **IV**) should be performed.

2. Throughout the next 24 h (longer if the patient's condition warrants it), vital signs should be monitored frequently, fluid intake and output documented, and physical examination repeated. Progression of swelling, discoloration, necrosis, or bleb formation should be noted. The purpose of this process is to follow continually the patient's overall condition because the aggressiveness of treatment depends on the evolution of these signs and symptoms.

3. Two large-bore **i.v. lines** should be started, avoiding the affected extremity, and **crystalloid fluids** begun.

C. **Toxin-specific measures**

1. The definitive treatment for snakebite is the use of **antivenins,** which have been developed through much research and are being further refined. Delaying this treatment enhances the risk of subsequent complications. Antivenins are suspensions of venom-neutralizing antibodies derived from the sera of hyperimmunized animals using simple ammonium sulfate fractionation (14). Most suspensions are polyvalent, that is, derived from the venom of several species. The two most widely used antivenins in the United States are the crotalid polyvalent antivenin and coral snake antivenin, both produced by Wyeth Laboratories.

    a. One of the greatest difficulties when treating snakebite is determining **how much** antivenin to use. There have been several attempts in the past to provide clinicians with a grading system. As this method evolves, it is becoming understood that this is not a cold, hard, factual definition of treatment but, rather, a fluid gradation. One should understand that this time is a starting point for treatment and that the patient's overall presentation determines the amount of antivenin to use. (Of course, one must take into account the species of snake and its size to help refine this method.)

    b. For **crotalid** antivenin use, Wingert (15) described the method used at Los Angeles County, University of Southern California Medical Center (Table 80-2).

    c. For **elapid** bites, different tactics must be used because the venom is a neurotoxin, and signs of envenomation are not present initially. This false sense of security can lead one to complacence until the sometimes rapid evolution of irreversible or even fatal clinical signs. With this point in mind, three to four vials of antivenin should be given to patients showing no signs of envenomation and five to six vials to patients with symptoms of pain or numbness or with neurologic signs. The antivenin is given in increments of three vials up to a maximum total dose in the range of 10 vials (16).

    d. North American coral snake antivenin (Wyeth) can counter the effects of bites by the **Eastern coral snake** and the **Texas coral snake.** However, it has no effect against bites of the Arizona coral snake. Fortunately, there have been no reported deaths from these bites, and supportive therapy has been sufficient.

TABLE 80-2. *System for grading envenomation*

Envenomation	Reaction	Dosage
None	No local or systemic reactions	No antivenin
Minimal	Local swelling but no systemic reactions	5 vials
Moderate	Swelling that progresses beyond the site of the bite together with a systemic reaction, laboratory changes, or both	10 vials
Severe	Marked local reaction, severe symptoms, and laboratory abnormalities	10–15 vials

Adapted from ref. 15.

    e. Because antivenin is derived from horse serum, the recipient should be tested for **sensitivity.** This testing should take place only when one is committed to giving antivenin because the testing itself can sensitize the patient. Instructions for sensitivity testing can always be found in the package insert. Beginning with a 1:10 dilution of antivenin, 0.02 mL is given intradermally, noting during the next 15 min any signs of reactivity. As a control, normal saline is also given in the same amount.

    f. During this period, drugs should be made available to counter any major reaction that occurs during sensitization testing and venom administration. It has been suggested that **diphenydramine** be given in a dose of 50 to 100 mg i.v. prior to the antivenin dose. **Epinephrine** may also be considered.

    g. Antivenin is reconstituted and diluted in 500 mL normal saline and is given over 1 h, with readministration of more antivenin as the patient's condition warrants it. The rate of administration can be increased if the patient's condition deteriorates. Antivenin can be given up to 24 h after the bite, but treatment is most efficacious within 4 h. It has been shown that for patients with coagulopathy continued antivenin use for up to 72 h is beneficial (15).

    h. An envenomated **child** requires more antivenin than an adult because children have less tissue mass to delay venom spread, less extracellular fluid for dilution, and less protein for binding; a child also receives a greater dose of venom per kilogram of body weight than an adult (16).

  2. In addition to antivenin administration, the clinician should consider **prophylactic antibiotics** to cover the gram-negative pathogens found in snakes' mouths (15). The patient's **tetanus** status should be determined and tetanus toxoid given if needed; additionally, 250 U of tetanus immunoglobulin should be given.

  3. The wound should be cleansed and a padded splint applied. Observation for bleb formation and tissue necrosis should continue, with debridement beginning after days 3 to 5. The use of fasciotomy has fallen into question, with the primary method of delaying tissue destruction being the adequate use of antivenin.

D. Treatment of specific effects. Venom has **multiple sites of action** locally and systemically, resulting in several main effects. In addition, the factors released by the patient in response to the venom further complicate the picture. The direction of treatment after baseline evaluation is toward stabilizing the patient's condition and lessening the untoward effects of the venom. The cornerstone of treatment is antivenin therapy, which counters local (e.g., tissue damage) and multisystem effects (e.g., coagulopathy).

1. Movement of fluid due to changes in membrane permeability into affected tissues can lead to **hypovolemia.** Intravenous fluids should be given using plasma or albumin as the primary resuscitative fluid; crystalloids are not indicated. Dramatic shifts have been seen, and management may require central venous pressure or Swan-Ganz catheter placement. The use of vasopressors should be avoided.

2. **Hemolysis** can be monitored and hematocrit and red blood cell mass maintained by the infusion of packed red blood cells or whole blood. The resulting hemoglobinuria and myoglobinuria due to muscle damage can lead to renal failure. Therefore, adequate urine flow is mandated to prevent this occurrence.

3. The hematologic system is the target for various components of venom, and a spectrum of **coagulopathies** may be seen. Platelet aggregation can occur, resulting in thrombocytopenia. In this case, platelet packs can be given to maintain adequate levels. Thrombin-like enzymes can mediate fibrinogen into ineffectual fibrin, leading to hypofibrinogenemia and defibrination syndrome. Antivenin is the treatment of choice. The serum fibrinogen level can be monitored; and when this level begins to rise, an adequate amount of antivenin may be given (5). Supportive treatment for bleeding with fresh frozen plasma, cryoprecipitate, platelets, or packed or whole blood is indicated.

4. As mentioned, the lung is affected directly, resulting in increased lung weight and congestion. **ARDS** has been described as a worst-case scenario (5); therefore, ABGs should be monitored, and if the patient's condition deteriorates, intubation and respiratory control are necessary.

5. Two types of **hypersensitivity reactions** can be seen in response to horse serum-derived antivenin.

    a. **Type I anaphylactic reaction** has been alluded to previously. The difficulty arises when the patient has a known sensitivity to horse serum or reacts significantly during testing. The clinician must decide whether the treatment is absolutely necessary. In a life-threatening situation, when antivenin must be given, i.v. antihistamine (diphenhydramine 50 to 100 mg) and titrated epinephrine (1 mg in 100 mL saline) have been shown to control the severe manifestations (17). Slowing antivenin administration also can provide better control. Close monitoring by the physician is essential.

    b. **Serum sickness** (type II complex–mediated reaction) is a well-documented complication that can occur up to 3 weeks after antivenin administration. This reaction can occur in any patient receiving any amount of antivenin, but it is seen most frequently with increasing doses of antivenin. Symptoms include fever, enlarged lymph nodes, urticarial rash, and painful joints. Treatment consists in antihistamines, steroids, or both; hospitalization is not always necessary. It has been suggested that to prevent this sequela a tapering dose of steroids should be considered in patients receiving eight vials or more of antivenin (18).

6. **Envenomation by an exotic species** can occur because of increasing interest in collecting these rare specimens. Sources of antivenin for these species may be difficult to find, but they should be considered. Consulting with the herpetologist at the local zoo is helpful for identifying the species involved. In addition, a supply of a variety of antivenins is usually available to the zoo. Local poison control officials should be contacted. Note that the University of Arizona College of Pharmacy coordinates a clearinghouse for snakebite information and can be contacted by telephone at (520) 626-6016.

VI. **Heloderm poisoning.** The **Gila monster,** a representative species of the heloderms known for its tenacious bite, is a large (300 cm) reptile with a round, thick tail. This lizard has few enemies other than humans, and its venom apparatus is used as a defense mechanism rather than for food gathering.

A. The **venom,** released from glands located in the lower jaw, has been known to cause local pain, anaphylactic reactions, hypotension, and coagulopathy. It is absorbed by capillary action during the bite. The lizard's teeth are solid, sharp, grooved, and recurved; and the grooved surface is the conduit by which venom is injected into the victim. Similar to snake venom, heloderm venom is a complex mixture of proteins, including amine oxidase, hyaluronidase, serotonin, and phospholipase A.

B. Because of these similar enzymes, **presentation** after a bite may involve local pain with edema and cyanosis surrounding the bite. There is capillary leakage and third spacing of fluid with resultant hypotension and diaphoresis. Coagulopathy with elevated prothrombin time and partial thromboplastin time, the appearance of fibrin split products, and a decrease in serum fibrin and platelets have been described (19).

C. **Treatment** initially is oriented toward **removing the lizard** from the affected extremity. Various methods have been attempted, including prying the jaw open with a stick, cutting the strong masseter muscles, or immersing the bitten part (with lizard attached) into cold water. Further treatment consists in immobilizing the affected extremity, cleansing the wound, and removing any broken teeth left in the area of the bite. Intense local pain, which may last upt to 8 h, can be treated with **local anesthetics** or **parenteral analgesics**. The patient's **tetanus injections** should be brought up to date. Hypotension can be treated with crystalloid infusion or colloids if necessary. Vasopressors have also been required. The coagulopathy usually resolves with time, and stabilization with appropriate blood products is all that is required. Antibiotics usually are not required. Continued wound care and possible physical therapy round out the treatment regimen.

References

1. Russell FE. Snake venom poisoning in the United States. *JAMA* 1975;233:341.
2. McKinstry DM. Evidence of toxic saliva in some colubrid snakes of the United States. *Toxicon* 1978;16:523.
3. Russell FE. *Snake venom poisoning*. Philadelphia: Lippincott, 1980.
4. Van Mierop LHS. Poisonous snakebite: a review. Part 1. Snakes and their venom. Part 2. Symptomatology and treatment. *J Fla Med Assoc* 1976;63:191.
5. Curry SC, Kunkel DB. Death from a rattlesnake bite. *Am J Emerg Med* 1985;300:227.
6. Russell FE, Puffer HW. Pharmacology of snake venoms. *Clin Toxicol* 1970;3:433.

7. Wingert WA, Wainschel J. A quick handbook on snake bites. *Med Times* 1977;105:68.
8. Keiser ED. *The poisonous snakes of Louisiana and the emergency treatment of their bites*. New Orleans: Louisiana Wild Life and Fisheries Commission, Lafayette Natural History Museum, 1971.
9. Otten EJ. Venomous animal injuries. In: Rosen P, Baker FJ, Braen GR, eds. *Emergency medicine*. St. Louis: Mosby, 1983:677–694.
10. Minton SA. Present tests for detection of snake venom: clinical applications. *Ann Emerg Med* 1987;16:932.
11. Sutherland SK, Coulter AR, Harris RD. Rationalisation of first-aid measures for elapid snakebite. *Lancet* 1979;1:183.
12. Hardy DL. First aid for snakebite: the Extractor vacuum pump. *Tucson Herpetol Soc Newslett* 1989;2:3.
13. Bronstein AC, Russell FE, Sullivan JB. Negative pressure suction in the field treatment of rattlesnake bite victims. *Vet Hum Toxicol* 1986;28:485.
14. Sullivan JB. Past, present, and future immunotherapy of snake venom poisoning. *Ann Emerg Med* 1987;16:938.
15. Wingert WA. Venomous snake bites. In: Auerbach PS, Geehr EC, eds. *Management of wilderness and environmental emergencies*. 1st ed. New York: Macmillan, 1983:352–378.
16. Otten EJ. Antivenin therapy in the emergency department. *Am J Emerg Med* 1983;1:83.
17. Loprinzi CL, et al. Snake antivenin administration in a patient allergic to horse serum. *South Med J* 1983;76:501.
18. Jurkovich GJ, et al. Complications of Crotalidae antivenin therapy. *J Trauma* 1988;28:1032.
19. Preston CA. Hypotension, myocardial infarction, and coagulopathy following Gila monster bite. *J Emerg Med* 1989; 7:37.

Selected Readings

Kunkel DB. Bites of venomous reptiles. *Emerg Med Clin North Am* 1984;2:563.

Emergency Toxicology, Second Edition,
edited by Peter Viccellio.
Lippincott–Raven Publishers, Philadelphia © 1998.

81

Amphibian Toxins

Phillip L. Rice

Brooklyn, New York 11215

All the amphibia—toads, frogs, salamanders, and newts—have secretory glands that produce several classes of substances, which in turn have multiple functions. The most important actions of these substances are to prevent desiccation, control the growth of microorganisms and infections, and discourage predators. Infection and death follow ablation of these secretory glands.

I. **Classification and location.** There are more than 2,600 species of amphibians, the most important toxicologically being the **toads** of the family Bufonidae and **frogs** of the families Atelopodidae, Dendrobatidae, Discoglossidae, Hyliade, Phyllomeduses, Pipidae, and Ranidae. Poisonous **newts** include those of the genera *Taricha* and *Triturus*. *Salamander* toxins are mainly found in the species of the genus *Salamandra*. The Bufonidae can be found in the southwestern part of the United States, particularly along the Colorado River. The most poisonous groups are found in the tropical regions of the world. Salamanders and newts are located mostly in the Southwest.

II. **Toxins**

   A. The amphibia have elaborated a remarkable diversity of **secondary metabolites,** including more than a dozen classes of alkaloids, peptides, biogenic amines, bufodienolides (bufogenins), and proteins (Table 81-1). Each secondary metabolite may exist with one or more of the others, giving rise to a mixed clinical picture. On the whole, there are no specific antidotes, and treatment is supportive, with removal of the unabsorbed toxin being a key component of therapy.

   B. **Sites of toxins.** Although some of the toxic compounds occur in eggs or larva, most have been found in the skin of adult amphibians. These skin secretions have been used as deadly arrow poison for centuries by the Cholo Indians of Columbia and others in South America (1).

   C. **Route of toxicity.** Amphibians do not inject their venom; rather, it is absorbed after ingesting the animals, their eggs, or their larva. Most poisonings occur in dogs, cats, and children. When attacked, the amphibians secrete a milky substance on their skin from their glands, and children handling them contaminate their fingers with the secretions. Occasionally, there are reports of ingestions by adults, but hand to mouth spread is the commonest form of poisoning. Dart poisoning has yet to become a major problem.

   D. **Specific toxins.** Many of the toxins are newly identified, with little known about them, although there are some major toxins about which much is known.

TABLE 81-1. *Amphibian toxins*

Main categories	Sample compounds
Peptides	Angiotensin
	Bombesins
	Bradykinins
	Demorphins
	Granuluiberin
	Tryptophyllins
	Thyroid-releasing hormone
	Vasoactive intestinal peptide
	Xenospin
Bufodienolides (bufogenins)	
Biogenic amines	Dopamine
	Epinephrine
	Histamine
	Norepinephrine
	Serotonin
	Tryptamine
	Tyramine
Alkaloids	
N-Methylated or cyclicized	*N*-Methylhistamine
	Spinace amine
Water-soluble	Ephippootoxin
	Chiriquitoxin
	Saxitoxins
	Tetrodotoxins
	Zetekitoxins A, B, C
Lipophilic	Dentrobatid
	Batrachotoxins
	Decahydroquinolones
	Histrionocotoxins
	Indolizidines
	Pumilotoxins
	Calycanthine
	Chimonanthine
	Morphine
	Noranabasamine
	Samandarine

1. The alkaloids, defined as cyclic nitrogen-containing compounds with a limited distribution in nature, comprise a wide variety of substances with much structural diversity. They are divided into three categories.

   a. *N*-Methylated or cyclized congeners of the various biogenic amines (e.g., *N*-methylhistamine and spinace amine).

   b. Highly water-soluble compounds comprised mainly of the tetrodotoxins found in a wide variety of animals. Others in this group are the saxitoxins; ephippootoxin; zetekitoxins A, B, and C; and chiriquitoxin (1). These compounds have primarily cardiotoxic as well as hypotensive effects, which appear to be due to the combination of blockage of vasomotor nerve impulses and relaxation of vascular smooth muscle. They specifically block the sodium channels in the membranes of excitable cells. As a result, the sodium currents are inhibited and the action potential is blocked (2).

(1) Ingestion of these toxins results in tingling of the oral cavity with salivation, muscle weakness and motor incoordination, skin numbness, vomiting, and diarrhea, and a generalized paralysis with ensuing convulsions and death in severe cases. Death results invariably from respiratory paralysis.

(2) Respiratory support is a key component of treatment of severe intoxications. Generally, treatment is supportive with early gut decontamination. Oral cavity lavage, stomach emptying via ipecac or lavage, activated charcoal, and cathartics should be used along with vascular support (3).

c. Variety of **lipophilic compounds** including the samandarin and dedrobatid alkaloids, frog chimonanthine, frog calycanthine, noranabasamine, and morphine.

(1) Samandarin is a potent toxin that is said to act on the CNS and has hypertensive and anesthetic properties. Investigation continues with respect to its toxicologic properties (4).

(2) Dentrobatid alkaloids include the batrachotoxins, histrionocotoxins, indolizidines, pumilotoxins, and decahydroquinolines (1). Of these substances, batrachotoxin is the most well studied. Batrachotoxin does not affect the action potential–generating system of either nerve or muscle; moreover, the acetylcholine sensitivity of the muscle and end-plate is unaffected, suggesting blockade of transmission in the presynaptic terminal. It does not inhibit sodium and potassium ATPase as does ouabain. Instead, it appears to cause a specific and irreversible increase in the permeability of excitable membranes, especially the presynaptic terminal, to sodium ions. This increase in sodium permeability results in depolarization of the presynaptic terminal and a concomitant calcium-dependent increase in acetylcholine release. The subsequent transmitter release appears to be due to complete depolarization of the nerve terminal (5). The effects of batrachotoxin can be prevented by tetrodotoxin and saxitoxin compounds, which block passive diffusion of sodium ions through excitable membranes (2). The extreme toxicity of batrachotoxin is related to its effects on cardiac conduction, which results in extrasystoles, ventricular tachycardia, and ventricular fibrillation. It causes slowing of respirations as well as increased tidal volume. It has been suggested that batrachotoxin also has a CNS effect (5). The other compounds in this class, such as the pumiliotoxins, can produce ataxia, clonic convulsions, and death with 20 min. Pumiliotoxins act through facilitation of release of calcium from the sarcoplasmic reticulum (3).

(3) A puzzling occurrence for which there is no immediate explanation is that morphine, a well-known plant alkaloid, has been detected in trace amounts in the skin of *Bufo marinus* (1).

2. Biologically active peptides include bradykinins, physaelaemins (also termed tachykinins), caeruleins, bombesins, sauvagine, dermorphin, thyroid-releasing hormone (TRH), vasoactive intestinal peptide (VIP), angiotensins, hemolytic or toxic peptides, enzymes, and tryptophyllins. Many of these peptides have human analogues with similar activity: bradykinins, TRH, VIP, and angiotensins.

   a. Tachykinins or physaelaemins have potent hypotensive actions as well as being potent stimulators of smooth muscle.

   b. Caeruleins have the peptide structure and activity of cholecystokinin.

   c. Bombesins are found in the GI tract as well as in the CNS, where they act as typical neuropeptides, interfering in thermoregulation, glucoregulation, and food intake.

   d. The activity spectrum of **sauvagine** is essentially similar to that of corticotropin-releasing factor (CRF) with some important differences. Unlike CRF, the amphibian peptide inhibits prolactin, thyroid-stimulating hormone, and growth hormone release from the anterior pituitary.

   e. Dermorphin possesses an extraordinary potent opioid activity both peripherally and centrally. It inhibits the peristaltic reflex and is unsurpassed in its analgesic action on the CNS. The potency of demorphin is 1000 times greater than that of dynorphin, the enkephalins, and morphine, and 15 times greater than that of beta-endorphin.

   f. The pharmacologic activity of other peptides (e.g., carnosine, granuliberin, xenospin, and tryptophyllins) continues to be investigated (6).

3. Biogenic amines found in amphibian skin include serotonin (5-hydroxytryptamine), histamine, tyramine, tryptamine, epinephrine, norepinephrine, and dopamine. Serotonin is by far the most common and in the highest concentration in many amphibians (7). Most of the biogenic amines act in a stimulatory fashion; but, depending on exposure, amount absorbed, and amount of each biogenic amine present, the response varies.

4. The last important group of toxins are the **bufodienolides** (bufogenins), which are cardioactive agents similar to digitalis compounds. These toxic glycosides are sufficiently potent to cause death within 10 to 15 min in children and small animals.

   a. Clinical syndrome develops within a few minutes after children place their fingers coated with the glandular secretions in the mouth. The initial sign is profuse salivation, with pulmonary edema, cardiac dysrhythmias, hypertension, and prostration developing within minutes. Convulsions develop rapidly; and death due to cardiac arrest may be observed as early as 15 min after initial contact with the toxic secretions.

   b. Treatment is largely aimed at removing as much of the unabsorbed secretions as possible from the mouth and controlling the clinical signs. Washing the victim's mouth with abundant water, frequently from a garden hose or a similar supply of vast quantities of water, and administering stropine to control salivation are early treatments that should be promptly implemented (3).

      (1) Barbiturates or **benzodiazapines** should also be administered to control convulsions.

(2) Maintenance **phenytoin** therapy is recommended because of its anti-dysrhythmic properties for glycoside-induced cardiac dysrhythmias.

(3) Calcium gluconate may be useful for combating some of the physiologic effects. **Artificial respiration** to maintain respiratory function may be needed. **Phenoxybenzamine** is recommended to block the alpha-adrenergic receptors.

(4) Propranolol is used to block the beta-adrenergic receptors. It also has an antifibrillatory action against the cardiac glycosides. This therapy has proven effective in **experimental cases,** apparently because the cardiac syndrome produced by the *Bufo* toxin is similar to the synergistic effect of cardioactive glycosides and ephedrine (3).

References

1. Daly JW, et al. Further classification of skin alkaloids from neotropical poison frogs (Dendrobatidae) with a general survey of toxic/noxious substances in amphibia. *Toxicon* 1987;25:1023–1095.
2. Goodman LS, Gilman A. *The pharmacological basis of therapeutics*. New York: Macmillan, 1985.
3. Casarett LJ, et al. *Toxicology—the basic science of poisons*. New York: Macmillan, 1986.
4. Casarett LJ. *Toxicology. The basic science of poisons*. New York: Macmillan, 1975.
5. Sebben A, et al. A tetrodotoxin-like substance found in the Brazilian frog: *Brachycephalus ephippium. Toxicon* 1986;24:799–806.
6. Erspamer V. Half a century of comparative research on biogenic amines and active peptides in amphibian skin and molluscan tissues. *Comp Biochem Physiol* 1984;79C:1.
7. Rosegmini M, et al. Indole, imidazode and phenyl-acylamines in the skin of one hundred and forty American amphibian species other than bufonids. *Comp Biochem Physiol* 1986;85C;139.

Emergency Toxicology, Second Edition,
edited by Peter Viccellio.
Lippincott–Raven Publishers, Philadelphia © 1998.

82

Marine Toxins

Paul Krochmal

Guilford, Connecticut 06437

Exposures to marine toxins are increasingly frequent. They are seen primarily in two settings, ingestions and through envenomation or contact. Since virtually all exposures to marine toxins are associated with preformed toxins, there is a relatively short lag between exposure and the development of symptoms.

I. Ingested toxins

A. Scombroid poisoning

1. **Source.** Scombroid poisoning is named for the family Scombroidea, which includes tuna and mackerel, although this syndrome can occur after ingestion of any red (dark-fleshed) species containing high levels of histidine. Mahi mahi (dolphinfish), a nonscombroid fish, is implicated more often than any other source. If the fish are improperly handled, they undergo bacterial decomposition, which converts histidine to histamine. Histamine is both heat and cold stable and is thought to be responsible for the symptoms of this illness (1). Normally, the histamine concentration is less than 1 mg/100 g of fish. In toxic fish the level exceeds 20 to 50 mg/100 mg of fish and may be much higher.

2. Symptoms begin rapidly, usually within less than 1 h, and resolve in about 12 h. The most frequent symptoms are dizziness, headache, diarrhea, and a burning or peppery feeling in the mouth. Flushing of the face and chest, nausea and vomiting, abdominal cramps, tachycardia, pruritus, and bronchospasm may occur. Scromboid poisoning may be confused with a monosodium glutamate (MSG) reaction. Since urticaria may occur, victims may mistakenly believe they are allergic to fish.

3. Diagnosis rests on the history and clinical symptoms. Some patients report a peppery ("Cajun") or even metallic taste.

4. Laboratory analysis is useful only for looking at histamine levels in the fish suspected to be the source of the outbreak. The U.S. Food and Drug Administration (FDA) has established 50 mg/100 g as a hazardous level of histamine in tuna. Levels measured in outbreaks have been much higher (more than 500 mg/100 g).

5. **Course and therapy.** Scombroid poisoning is usually mild and self-limited. More severe cases have been managed according to symptoms. Various antihistamines including hydroxyzine, which is also an antiemetic, have been used. Bronchodilators are appropriate if the patient is wheezing. Cimetidine has been used, but the use of

all therapy has been anecdotal and symptom-directed. There is a theoretical danger to patients on INH, which blocks histaminase.

6. Prevention of scombroid poisoning is important. A fish should be continually iced or refrigerated from the time it is caught until it is cooked. Cooking does not eliminate histamine once it has formed. Freezing once the histamine is present also does not prevent the illness. All improperly handled fish should be discarded.

B. Ciguatera poisoning

1. **Pathophysiology.** Ciguatera is the most common form of poisoning from ingesting fish. There are more than five toxins implicated. They are colorless, odorless, tasteless, and heat-stable. They are not affected by freeze-drying or gastric acid. These toxins include ciguatoxin, a fat-soluble compound, and maitotoxin, a water-soluble component. The mode of action is still controversial. The water-soluble component has anticholinesterase activity, which may not be a factor in vivo. The ciguatoxin may interfere with calcium receptor sites, which affect the sodium channels of neural, muscle, and myocardial cell membranes. Toxin-induced hypertension and tachycardia have been suppressed in animal models with phentolamine. Ciguatoxin may increase heart rate and contraction, whereas, maitotoxin appears to be a cardiac depressant. The toxin is potent, and 2 to 5 g of fish is enough to kill 50% of mice. The LD_{50} is 0.45 µg/kg.

2. **Source.** Ciguatera poisoning originates in bottom-dwelling algae in tropical waters around coral reefs. These algae are consumed by herbivorous fishes, which are then eaten by carnivorous fishes. Ciguatoxic fish feed on the food chain of bottom dwellers. Fish feeding on plankton are not thought to be ciguatoxic. Ciguatera poisoning usually occurs between latitudes 35 degrees N and 35 degrees S. There can be great variation within a region, and there is no way to predict which fish are safe. Many species have been implicated. The best known is the barracuda, but the illness actually takes its name from the "cigua," or turban shellfish. Larger fish are thought to be at more risk than smaller members of the same species, but it is a relative risk. Moray eels are particularly dangerous to eat. The viscera, including liver, are likely to be the most toxic. There is no way to detect a ciguatoxic fish by appearance or smell. It is not associated with the freshness of the fish or bacterial food poisoning. Interestingly, some investigators believe that these toxins are elaborated in areas where the reef has been recently disturbed and may represent a biologic defense of the reef ecosystem. Ciguatera poisoning may be seen in nonendemic areas (2). While cold-water fish are thought not to be associated with ciguatera poisoning, the syndrome has been reported after ingestion of farm-raised salmon possibly fed contaminated food (3).

3. **Clinical presentation.** The onset of symptoms is consistently rapid but shows great variation, which may reflect the different toxins, local conditions, and ethnic responses to the illness; even gender differences have been described. Symptoms may occur within 30 min of ingestion and generally develop within 3 h. The early symptoms are usually gastrointestinal (GI): abdominal pain, nausea, vomiting, and diarrhea. There may be an increase in severity and the beginning of non-GI symptoms, which may be delayed by hours or even days and may persist for weeks.

Muscle pains, weakness, exhaustion, and cardiovascular and neurologic symptoms may be seen, as may hypotension, paresthesias, pruritus, headache, and ataxia. Nightmares and hallucinations are reported. Diaphoresis, visual disturbances, and a maculopapular desquamating rash can occur. A possibly pathognomonic symptom is the reversal of hot and cold perception, which occasionally develops 3 to 5 days after onset. Interestingly, some symptoms such as pruritus may last weeks. Apparently, the toxin can accumulate in humans as well as fish. Prior ciguatera poisoning affects immunity and may place the patient at greater risk for a severe reaction. Alcohol ingestion may cause exacerbation of the syndrome, especially the pruritus. Symptoms may wax and wane. Fatalities have been reported. Deaths may be more common with severe intoxications.

4. Diagnosis is made on clinical grounds. Any patient who presents with acute gastroenteritis associated with unusual cardiovascular or neurologic symptoms should have a dietary history pursued. However, even GI symptoms, which comprise the most common presentations, occur in only 75% to 85% of poisonings. The diagnosis can be substantiated only by testing the fish itself.

5. There is no generally available **laboratory test** that identifies ciguatoxin in humans; and routine laboratory tests yield only nonspecific abnormalities, such as an elevated white blood cell count. Assays for ciguatoxin can be performed on fish. There is also a field test, the "stick test," which is an immunoassay and works well for screening fish.

6. Treatment is supportive.

   a. Induced **emesis** or gastric **lavage** may be of use if the patient presents early and is not vomiting spontaneously. Magnesium-containing cathartics are theoretically contraindicated because they could exacerbate the calcium channel blockade, which is thought to be one of the mechanisms of toxicity. Antiemetics such as **hydroxyzine** are recommended; and hydroxyzine may also help with pruritus. **Crystalloid** infusion is recommended for volume replacement and control of hypotension. **Atropine** has been used successfully for bradyarrhythmias and hypotension. Intravenous **calcium gluconate** has been used successfully but not consistently for cardiac and neurologic symptoms. Its use is based on the pharmacology of ciguatoxin and not on the treatment of hypocalcemia, which is not a diagnostic standard. **Mannitol** as an intravenous infusion has been reported as a possible therapy (4). Alcohol should be avoided, as should fish-based foods.

   b. The best treatment is **prevention.** Despite the cost to the fishing industry, the **stick test** offers the best hope of avoiding this potentially lethal problem. A field bamboo stick test is a colorimetric immunoassay and is currently being used to test fish in some areas.

C. **Clupeotoxin fish poisoning**

1. The **pharmacology** of clupeotoxin fish poisoning is basically unknown. This group of fish includes herring, sardines, and anchovies. These fish feed on plankton. There is no way to recognize a clupeotoxic fish by its appearance, and freshness is not related to toxicity.

2. **Clinical presentation.** This syndrome is characterized by a violent onset of symptoms, rapid death, and a high mortality. The symptoms begin within 30 to 60 min of ingestion. There is a sharp metallic taste, abdominal pain, vomiting, and diarrhea. Further manifestations include headache, tachycardia, hypotension, respiratory distress, progressive muscular paralysis, and death, which can occur within 15 min of the onset of symptoms. The fatality rate has been reported as high as 45%.

3. **Treatment** is not well studied. The disease is rare, and the only recommendations are supportive intensive care and prevention, which means avoiding these fish during the summer months.

D. **Tetrodotoxin fish poisoning**

1. **Source.** Tetrodotoxin is best known as the highly potent, lethal toxin that is associated with fugu, a delicacy in Japan now also allowed on a limited basis in the United States. Tetrodotoxin is aminoperhydroquinazolone, a heat-stable, water-soluble compound. Tetrodotoxin is concentrated in the skin and viscera, especially the liver and the gonads. Lesser amounts of the toxin may be found in the muscles. This poison interferes with sodium channels and affects the central and peripheral nervous systems as well as the myocardium and skeletal muscle. Interestingly, although thought of as a pufferfish or fugu toxin, this chemical has been isolated from other species, including the blue-ringed octopus, some crabs, bivalves, and a variety of amphibians. The **lethal dose** is 10 µg/kg.

2. **Clinical presentation.** Tetrodotoxin is well studied, as Japan considers fugu a delicacy. The case fatality rate is approximately 60%, with death usually occurring within the first 24 h. Apparently, the symptoms of mild paresthesias and flushing are thought to be an exhilarating experience. When symptoms do develop, they are rapid, seen most frequently within 10 to 45 min, although they have been delayed for several hours. Oral paresthesias are usually the first symptom, followed by lightheadedness, generalized paresthesias, or a sense of numbness that makes the victim feel as if he or she is "floating." Hypersalivation, diaphoresis, and GI symptoms may develop. Neurologic symptoms include weakness, ataxia, paralysis, and gross muscular coordination. Mentation can be maintained with respiratory support to avoid anoxia. Victims may also develop desquamation as well as extensive subcutaneous hemorrhage thought to be due to a disseminated intravascular coagulation-like syndrome. Hematemesis may be present. Most deaths are early.

3. **Diagnosis** is clinical, based on the history and the timely association with a suspicious meal. The constellation of GI, neurologic, and possibly hematologic symptoms, perhaps followed by cardiovascular collapse, in the setting of ingesting a tetrodotoxic fish suggests the diagnosis.

4. **Treatment** is entirely symptomatic and supportive. Removal of the toxin from the GI tract has been suggested, as these victims present early after the ingestion. Gastric lavage with a 2% sodium bicarbonate solution has been suggested. (One can also inactivate the toxin—and the taste of the fish—by cooking with baking soda for a long time.) Removal may be followed by charcoal and perhaps sorbitol. There is a theoretic objection to magnesium-containing cathartics in that they may augment a calcium channel blockade. Beyond basic cardiovascular and respiratory support, it has been suggested that anticholinesterase inhibitors may help the theoretic prob-

lem of reduced release of acetylcholine at the neuromuscular junction. Remember that these patients may be wide awake despite life-threatening problems. **Patients with minor symptoms** should be simply observed. Nothing should be given orally to patients with dysphagia. Eight hours of observation are recommended.

5. Prevention is easily achieved by following the biblical admonition against eating all scaleless fish. Unfortunately, the culturally dependent demand for these fish as a delicacy means we will gain more experience managing this problem.

E. **Paralytic shellfish poisoning (PSP)**

1. **Source.** PSP occurs after ingesting filter-feeding shellfish and sometimes the carnivorous mollusks that feed on them. The toxin originates in the dinoflagellates on which they feed. Dinoflagellates and other phytoplankton are important as the primary producers of the food supply in the sea. These organisms use photosynthesis but also have some animal-like feeding characteristics. In the correct setting these organisms can "bloom," increasing their concentration 1,000-fold. These blooms discolor the water, resulting in the infamous red tide or another color depending on the organism. The blooms are common during the summer months and can kill birds and fish. Shellfish can become toxic even in the absence of such a bloom. Several toxins are elaborated, the best known being saxitoxin, an alkaloid neurotoxin. This compound is water-soluble and heat-stable. Hence it may become concentrated in a broth. Saxitoxin appears to block neuromuscular conduction by interfering with sodium movement. The maximum safe level is 80 μg/100 mg of shellfish.

2. **Clinical presentation.** Symptoms begin within minutes to hours. Oral paresthesias occur first and spread to the extremities. Victims rapidly show a constellation of GI and neurologic symptoms including vomiting and diarrhea, dysphagia, incoordination, and weakness. They may progress to flaccid paralysis and respiratory failure. If there is no paralysis, the syndrome is sometimes described as neurotoxic shellfish poisoning. Nevertheless, the greatest danger is respiratory paralysis, and these patients should be observed for this complication. Without respiratory support there is significant mortality.

3. Diagnosis is usually made by the history.

4. There are no direct **laboratory tests** available to the clinician to confirm the diagnosis. The toxin can be measured, and a level of 75 to 80 μg/100 g of shellfish is considered hazardous. During particularly toxic blooms, the level may be 100 times as high.

5. Treatment includes gastric emptying and irrigation with 2% sodium bicarbonate. Like tetrodotoxin, saxitoxin may be inactivated in an alkaline medium. Charcoal is recommended. Magnesium-containing cathartics are theoretically contraindicated because they may contribute to decreased nerve conduction. Respiratory support, when indicated, is life-saving.

6. Prevention is still the most important approach. In the Northern Hemisphere the danger period is May to October. Even if a bloom has passed, the shellfish may remain toxic. There is variation from area to area, and local governments quarantine areas when they are suspicious.

F. **Fish botulism.** Foodborne botulism associated with fish is thought to represent approximately 13% of foodborne outbreaks of this disease in the United States (5). *C. botulinum* produces a neurotoxin which is responsible for the illness. Botulism is discussed in Chapter 76.

G. **Pelagic paralysis.** This designation was suggested as a common name for puffer fish poisoning and ciguatera and paralytic shellfish poisoning. These conditions are difficult to distinguish clinically, and symptoms result from interference with sodium channels in conducting cell membranes. "Pelagic," a term that basically means pertaining to the sea, has not been widely adopted.

II. **Envenomation and contact toxins**

A. **Invertebrate porifera (sponges)**

1. **Pathophysiology.** Sponges produce poisonings in three ways. First, contact with certain sponges can produce a localized dermatitis similar to *Rhus*-induced dermatitis (e.g., poison ivy). Second, toxin may be introduced by the spicules, which are the framework of sponges and which may cause microtrauma to the skin. Third, there are some envenomations attributed to handling sponges that are really due to the stinging tentacles of small coelenterates that have taken up residence with the sponges.

2. **Clinical presentation.** Some sponges produce crinotoxins, which can be direct dermal irritants. Most victims have a limited local dermatitis that subsides in a week. A few victims have systemic reactions such as erythema multiforme or an anaphylactoid reaction. In cases where the toxins are introduced by spicules, there may be increased systemic symptoms such as arthralgias.

3. Treatment consists in cleaning the area. Adhesive tape can be used to remove any remaining spicules. Vinegar (dilute acetic acid) or alcohol has been suggested for cleaning the skin. If inflammation appears topically, steroids may be of use. Systemic steroids and antihistamines may be required if the reaction is severe.

4. Gloves are the best **prevention.** One should also not crush an unidentified sponge.

B. **Coelenterates**

1. **Source.** Coelenterates are primitive animals with simple cellular differentiation. There are three main groups: hydrozoa, including the Portuguese man-of-war, scyphozoa or jellyfish, and anthozoa or sea anemones and corals. Most coelenterates are innocuous, but there is at least one species that can kill an adult human in minutes. There are two primary forms of coelenterates: the sessile polyp and the free-swimming medusae. Coelenterates are predators and feed on fish and shellfish.

2. **Toxin.** The poison apparatus is the nematocyst, which is a specialized cell that when touched or chemically stimulated ejects a sharp tube-like thread that injects venom. There are a number of types of nematocysts and many toxins. The primary effects of all the toxins are pain, paralysis, and an urticaria-like reaction. These toxins are potent marine toxins with an LD_{50} in mice as low as 50 µg/kg. They are thought to act by hemolysis, which begins as massive cellular potassium loss.

3. **Hydrozoa.** This group consists in both sedentary and free-floating animals. Coming in contact with the tentacles of the hydroids or the branches of fine coral may result in a stinging or burning sensation that becomes a rash. The skin should be cleaned with sea water and dried gently. Fresh water or brisk rubbing of the area may result in any remaining nematocysts joining in the envenomation. Dilute acetic acid

(vinegar) or isopropyl alcohol can be applied. The skin reaction may require topical steroids. In the group hydrozoa there is the Portuguese man-of-war *(Physalia physalis),* which is a floating animal up to one-third of a meter in length and with tentacles that may stretch 30 m underneath the surface. Each tentacle may have hundreds of thousands of nematocysts. Detached tentacles on a beach can still discharge the nematocysts.

4. **Scyphozoa.** This group contains the larger jellyfish, such as the deadly **box-jellyfish** *(Chironex fleckeri),* which is usually found off Australia. The box-jellyfish can cause death within minutes, with a mortality rate of 15% to 20%. The sting is intensely painful. There is a toxic skin reaction that includes wheals, discoloration, and perhaps blisters. With severe stings, collapse and death may occur in minutes. Adherent tentacles should be removed from the victim with 5% acetic acid (vinegar). Care should be taken to be sure the rescuer does not become a victim. *Chironex* antivenin is available and can be lifesaving if administered early; it carries the risk of serum sickness, however, as do other antivenins. Skin reactions to the sting may persist for months. Other scyphozoa, such as **sea nettles,** may be found in more temperate waters. Sea nettles may cause moderately severe stings but are not as dangerous as the box-jellyfish.

5. **Anthozoa.** Anemones are the members of this class that concern us. Often found in shallow water, they may appear to be undersea flowers, attracting the unwary or accidental contact. They cause, via their nematocysts, a severe dermatitis and, rarely, systemic reactions. The dermatitis may be persistent and cause local necrosis, and there may be secondary infection. It is an anemone that attaches itself to the base of some sponges and may cause a reaction that can be confused with that from the sponge itself.

6. Management of coelenterate envenomations can be approached in a general way. Special attention to this possibility is necessary whenever someone collapses while in the water.

   a. Mild envenomations usually are confined to dermatitis. There may be pruritus and paresthesias as well as local pain. The skin may show the track of the tentacle. There may be wheals, blistering, and discoloration due to petechiae. One such dermatitis, erroneously attributed to sea lice, occurs when larval forms are trapped under the swim suits of bathers (7).

   b. With more **severe envenomation** the skin manifestations may be more severe, and a systemic reaction may be seen. These systemic reactions may be neurologic, cardiovascular, or GI. The man-of-war and anemone stings are the most painful, and that of the box-jellyfish is the most deadly.

   c. Systemic reactions must be managed first. Any remaining tentacles or nematocysts must be removed or detoxified with 5% acetic acid. Hypotension should be managed with crystalloid. Patients with systemic reactions should be observed and monitored (including renal function). *Chironex fleckeri* is the only species with a specific antivenin. Pain control is often necessary and can be improved by treating the dermatitis. Rinse victims with sea water, not fresh water. Do not rub with a towel or clothing to remove tentacles, as these practices may release more nematocysts; use forceps or a glove. The toxins are best inactivated by 5% acetic acid (vinegar). There is also a commercial preparation called "Stingose" (aluminum sulfate and surfactant), which may be beneficial. Systemic drugs are of value only for allergic manifestations. Local steroids may be useful after removing the nematocysts.

C. **Mollusks.** Two groups of mollusks are hazardous.

1. The first is a small group of gastropods called **"cone shells,"** which have a venom apparatus as part of their feeding apparatus. In humans the sting can vary from the sting sensation with local symptoms to death. The toxin is a neuromuscular blocker and can cause muscular paralysis and respiratory failure. Rare and found mostly in the Indo-Pacific area, these animals should be handled with respect and with gloves. Prevention is superior to the supportive care otherwise available. Interestingly, an experimental pain medication has been isolated from this venom (6).

2. Cephalods are often harmless, although some small octopus species can paralyze or kill adult humans. This group includes the Australian blue-ringed octopus. These species frequent shallow waters. The toxin is secreted in the salivary gland and is transmitted when the animal bites. The venom may be injected deep into the tissues. The toxin, called "maculotoxin" or "cephalotoxin," contains a number of components, but the most significant is identical to tetrodotoxin, which blocks peripheral nerve conduction and is most often associated with fugu (see **I.D**). The course of these envenomations is much like that associated with fugu except for the local wound. These bites may be lethal and are best treated supportively. Unless hypoxic, the victims often remain conscious. Respiratory support is essential. Prevention is the best available approach. All of these animals should be treated with respect and handled with gloves.

D. **Echinoderms.** This phylum includes starfish, sea urchins, and sea cucumbers, which are potentially dangerous. In this group the venom is associated with spines. Retained fragments of these spines may provoke chronic local problems. All retained fragments should be carefully removed.

1. Starfish produce a toxic slimy secretion that is carried into the victim on the animal's spines. Multiple punctures with the most venomous starfish can cause major systemic reactions, but most result in a contact dermatitis.

2. Sea urchins have specialized venom delivery systems. Some sea urchins have hollow, venom-filled spines and others triple-jawed pedicellariae (a specialized stalk that seizes whatever it contacts and injects venom). Careless divers and curious children who come in contact may be envenomated. These stings are painful and may be associated with systemic reactions. Immersion of the wound in hot, nonscalding water for 1 h is recommended as treatment of local pain.

3. Sea cucumbers produce a toxin called "holothurin," which produces a contact dermatitis. This substance is concentrated in tentacles, which the animal uses to defend itself.

E. **Vertebrates.** There are a number of venomous marine vertebrates.

1. Stingrays, found along the warmer shorelines of the United States, come in various sizes. They are bottom-dwelling, often lying in the mud or sand. Their venom appa-

ratus is a spine on the tail, and the usual envenomation is to a human lower extremity after someone accidentally steps on the stingray. The toxin is a combination of enzymes that can cause major systemic reactions including cardiac arrhythmias. Treatment consists in irrigation of the wound that always accompanies the envenomation. Soaking in warm, nonscalding water may affect heat-sensitive components of the toxin. Prevention means caution in high-risk waters, as the spine can go through a boot.

2. Weeverfish are among the most dangerous poisonous fish, with painful and potentially fatal stings. They are a sedentary fish, are found in temperate waters, and bury themselves in shallow bottoms. The most common injury is to the lower extremity of fishermen and other waders by the spines, which are located with the forward dorsal fin and with the operculum. Not only can these fish survive hours out of water, but the venom remains active after death. The venom, called a "ichthyoacanthotoxin" (fish venom), has several components and is at least partially heat-labile. Envenomation results in pain and local discoloration and edema. Healing may take months. Major systemic symptoms can also occur. Immersing the wound in hot, nonscalding water may inactivate parts of the venom.

3. Catfish have many species equipped with spines associated with the introduction of venom. The toxin has multiple components that produce an injury after being introduced by the spines. There are both local and systemic reactions. Hot, nonscalding water to the wound may help with heat-sensitive components. Catfish should not be handled by the dorsal or pectoral fins, where the spines are found.

4. Scorpion fish include a variety of fish with venoms that range in severity from mild to life-threatening. The most famous is the stonefish, which lives a sedentary life in shallow water in tropical areas. The venom apparatus in multiple species is associated with venom glands. The venom of a stonefish can be lethal. Some of the tropical scorpion fish that appear in aquariums may also be dangerous. Handling dead fish can be hazardous as well. Treatment consists in wound care and immersion in hot, nonscalding water to destroy heat-labile components of the venom. A stonefish antivenin is available.

5. Sea snakes are reminiscent of venomous terrestrial snakes with poisonous fangs. Sea snake bites are most common in fishermen who inadvertently trap these snakes in their nets. The bite is painless but leaves tiny puncture marks. The venom can cause hemolysis, rhabdomyolysis, myoglobinuria, and renal failure. Symptoms usually occur early if there is envenomation. Care parallels the care of poisonous snake bites on land. A polyvalent sea snake antivenin is available.

References

1. Morrow JD, et al. Evidence that histamine is the causative toxin of scombroid-fish poisoning. *N Engl J Med* 1991; 324:716.
2. DeFusco DJ, et al. Coma due to ciguatera poisoning in Rhode Island. *Am J Med* 1993;95:240.
3. DiNubile MJ, Hokama Y. The ciguatera poisoning syndrome from farm-raised salmon. *Ann Intern Med* 1995;122:113.
4. Palafox NA, et al. Successful treatment of ciguatera fish poisoning with intravenous mannitol. *JAMA* 1988;259:2740.
5. Centers for Disease Control. Fish botulism—Hawaii, 1990. *MMWR* 1991;40:412.
6. Gibbs WW. A new way to spell relief: v-e-n-o-m. *Sci Am* 1996;274:28.
7. Freudenthal AR, Joseph PR. Seabather's eruption. *N Engl J Med* 1993;329:542.

Selected Readings

Auerbach PS. *Wilderness medicine*. 3rd ed. St. Louis: Mosby, 1995.

Bengston K, et al. Sudden death in a child following jellyfish envenomation by *Chiropsalmus quadrumanus*. *JAMA* 1991;266:1404.

Burnett JW. Jellyfish envenomation syndromes updated. *Ann Emerg Med* 1987;16:1000.

Centers for Disease Control. Scromboid fish poisoning—Illinois, South Carolina. *MMWR* 1989;38:140.

Halstead BW. *Poisonous and venomous marine animals of the world*. 2nd ed. rev. Princeton, NJ: Darwin Press, 1988.

Mills AR, Passmore R. Pelagic paralysis. *Lancet* 1988;333:161.

Sanders W Jr. Intoxications from the seas: ciguatera, scombroid, and paralytic shellfish poisoning. *Infect Dis Clin North Am* 1987;1:665.

Sims JK. A theoretical discourse on the pharmacology of toxic marine ingestions. *Ann Emerg Med* 1987;16:1006.

Tu AT. Biotoxicology of sea snake venoms. *Ann Emerg Med* 1987;16:1000.

PART IX

Plant Toxicology

Emergency Toxicology, Second Edition,
edited by Peter Viccellio.
Lippincott–Raven Publishers, Philadelphia © 1998.

83

Systemic Poisonous Plant Intoxication

†Mark S. DeManuelle and °R. Scott Orava

† Metairie, Louisiana 70005-3342; °Department of Emergency Medicine, Valley Lutheran Hospital, Mesa, Arizona 85206

Many plants produce GI irritation alone, but space limitations prevent discussion of each of them.

I. **Management.** In general, GI tract decontamination is indicated for patients who present within 1 to 2 h following substantial ingestions of potentially toxic plants. If a patient is already vomiting during the initial evaluation, the stomach may already be empty; in this case, GI evacuation is unnecessary. If a patient is already experiencing catharsis, a cathartic is usually not needed. Activated charcoal is indicated in all potentially serious ingestions, and whole bowel irrigation (WBI) may also be considered. Symptomatic patients after 6-h observation should be considered for admission.

   A. If a patient is **markedly ill** from the ingestion, monitor the fluid and electrolyte balance to avoid dehydration and hypotension. Positive identification of the ingested plant material is essential in these cases. Beware of using the common names of plants, as they vary regionally and the genus and species names may overlap. Pesticides may also cause symptoms of intoxication after plant ingestion and may cloud the clinical picture.

   B. Whenever there is any question that plant toxicity may be involved, call the nearest poison control center.

   C. Ideally, every emergency department (ED) should have an atlas of poisonous plants for easy identification. Despite the hundreds of photographs and drawings of poisonous plants available, they are clearly insufficient for even the experienced physician frantically trying to identify an ingested plant. Hence, each ED must have someone available for plant identification; depending on the community, it may be a botanist, horticulturist, or nursery owner.

II. **Specific plants**

   A. *Abrus precatorius* (rosary pea, jequirity bean). This vine produces pods that contain red seeds 1 cm in length. Each seed has a small black area. Others are black with a white center or white with a black center. This plant is commonly found in southern Florida, Hawaii, and the Caribbean.

      1. **Toxic part.** The entire plant is toxic. The seeds are used in jewelry and as an abortifacient.

      2. **Toxin.** Abrin is a toxaalbumin that inhibits protein synthesis and causes cell death.

      3. **Presentation.** Severe irritation of the upper GI tract occurs more than 2 h after ingestion. Delayed cytotoxic effects occur in the liver, CNS, kidney, and adrenal glands 2 to 5 days after exposure. Severe toxicity has occurred with one-half to two chewed

beans. Tachycardia and hypotension result from fluid loss, and severe dehydration and bloody diarrhea occur. Liver function tests are abnormal. Fever, meiosis, leukocytosis, hypoglycemia or hyperglycemia, seizures, and CNS depression may occur.

4. **Management**
   a. Aggressive decontamination using GI lavage or WBI for any exposure is imperative, as is attention to the patient's fluid and electrolyte balance.
   b. Administer activated charcoal and a cathartic (in the absence of diarrhea). Maintain adequate fluid volume to prevent acute renal failure. Monitor liver function tests and hematocrit.

B. *Aconitum* **species** (e.g., monkshood). This tall perennial has blue or pink helmet-shaped flowers and lobed leaves.
   1. **Toxic part.** The entire plant is toxic, although the toxin is most highly concentrated in the roots and seeds. Recreational ingestions and medicinal extracts cause many of the poisonings. A few grams of plant material contains a lethal adult dose.
   2. **Toxin.** Aconitine, a norditerpene alkaloid. Interference with the sodium-potassium pump occurs, causing high-grade heart block. When *intracellular* potassium levels drop, myocardial cells lose electrical function, with asystole as the terminal event.
   3. Laboratory analysis. Radioimmunoassay for digoxin is helpful with plant glycoside intoxication, although toxicity is not directly related to measurable serum levels. With poisonings involving monkshood and other plants any measurable digoxin level in a patient not on digoxin should suggest a significant ingestion.
   4. **Presentation**
      a. Burning of the oral mucosa is followed by a sensation of tightness in the throat. Salivation and mydriasis with visual blurring occur; patients may see yellow halos around objects(xanthopsia). GI symptoms may be severe. Paresthesias, ataxia, and slurred speech occur; and respiratory paralysis, convulsions, and hypotension are possible. Lethal bradycardia with varying degrees of atrioventricular (AV) block, as well as ventricular tachycardia, may occur.
      b. Hyperkalemia may be present and cause inactivity of the myocardium due to loss of excitability. In this state the heart may not respond to a pacemaker, and death may occur within 1 to 2 h of ingestion.
   5. **Management**
      a. Lavage the stomach (inducing emesis with ipecac may cause a vagal reflex), and administer multiple-dose activated charcoal and a cathartic.
      b. Treat bradycardia with atropine; if the bradycardia is refractory, consider inserting a pacemaker. Treat hypotension with fluids followed by vasopressors. Support respiration by mechanical means if necessary.
      c. Monitor potassium levels frequently. Observe the cardiac monitor for T-wave changes. Do not give potassium unless hypokalemia is documented. For hyperkalemia, give glucose and insulin or Kayexalate as indicated.
      d. Most patients who show signs of toxicity should have a pacemaker inserted if they do not respond to initial pharmacologic therapy.
      e. Digibind (Fab fragments) should be used in the presence of life-threatening arrhythmias although some patients have died despite its use. If serum digitalis concentrations are unavailable or are thought to be inaccurate, give 10 vials

(400 mg) over 30 min initially. If cardiac arrest is imminent, a bolus may be given. Monitor the potassium carefully because it may drop rapidly. Because of incomplete cross reactivity with plant glycosides, higher doses may be needed.

    f. Patients should be observed for symptomatology. An estimation of the amount ingested is not an accurate parameter for the level of toxicity present.

C. *Actaea* **species** (e.g., baneberry, cohosh). All members of this genus produce similar toxicity and require the same management. The plant is a perennial with brightly colored berries (red, white, blue, or purple) and feather-like leaves.

    1. **Toxic part.** The roots, sap, and berries are toxic. A few berries can cause severe symptoms.

    2. **Toxin.** Glycoside, a strong purgative (or possibly another unknown toxin, possibly protoanemonin).

    3. **Presentation.** Severe GI irritation occurs with bloody emesis and diarrhea. The toxin has a vesicant action on mucous membranes and skin that causes intense pain. Profuse salivation, tachycardia, delirium, visual hallucinations, and circulatory collapse occur, as may dysuria, polyuria, hematuria, and renal damage. Seizures and paralysis have been seen in large animal ingestions.

    4. **Management.** Empty the stomach, then give demulcents (cold milk or ice cream for GI, cold compresses for skin). Administer i.v. fluids if the patient becomes dehydrated or acidotic. Monitor renal function. Treat other symptoms as they occur.

D. *Arisaema triphyllum* (jack-in-the-pulpit). All members of the genus *Arisaema* are potentially toxic. This herb has red berries and a "flower" (spathe) that is green, brown, or purple and pulpit-shaped, with a pointed hood. The root is tuberous.

    1. **Toxic part.** All parts of the plant are toxic, although the roots are most toxic.

    2. **Toxin.** Consists of needle-like insoluble calcium oxalate crystals (raphides) that can pierce the mucous membranes and proteolytic enzymes in idioblasts which ultimately cause the release of histamine and bradykinin.

    3. **Presentation.** The major symptoms of intoxication are pain and edema of the oropharynx with bullae, increased salivation, and loss of speech lasting up to several days. Necrosis of the mucous membranes may occur, as may respiratory distress if airway edema is severe. Gastric irritation with hemorrhage may occur. Eye exposure may cause corneal damage. Handling the plant may cause dermatitis.

    4. **Management.** Empty the stomach, give demulcents, and apply cold compresses for pain. Analgesics may also help to relieve pain. Steroids and i.v. fluids may be used for severe reactions. For eye exposures copious irrigation, analgesia, and ophthalmologic consultation should be provided.

E. *Atropa belladonna* (deadly nightshade). This perennial bears a dark berry.

    1. **Toxic part.** The entire plant is toxic.

    2. **Toxins.** Atropine and other belladonna alkaloids.

    3. **Presentation.** With the following symptoms: dry mouth, dysphonia, dry skin, hyperthermia, tachycardia, mydriasis, urinary retention, and hallucinations.

    4. **Management.** Empty the stomach. If severe intoxication occurs, give i.v. physostigmine slowly, 0.5 mg for children and 2.0 mg for adults. The dose may be repeated in 30 to 45 min. if necessary.

F. ***Brugmansia*** **species** (angels' trumpet). This small tree has large white conical flowers. As for deadly nightshade.

G. ***Caladium*** **species**. This large, multicolored plant (white, green, and red) has heart-shaped leaves and tuberous roots. As for jack-in-the-pulpit.

H. ***Caltha palustris*** (marsh marigold, cowslip). This perennial, found in wetland regions, has bright yellow flowers and heart-shaped leaves.

    1. Toxic part. All parts of the plant are toxic.

    2. Toxin. Protoanemonin.

    3. Presentation. The first sign of intoxication is inflammation or ulceration of the oropharynx, with blistering of the skin after dermal exposure. Bloody emesis and diarrhea, respiratory depression, hypotension, and convulsions may occur.

    4. Management. Empty the stomach. Support respiration and monitor fluid and electrolyte status carefully.

I. ***Cicuta*** **species** (e.g., water hemlock). Found only near water, this plant grows to a height of 6 to 8 ft. The leaves are compound, and the flowers are small and white or green. The roots are large, white, chambered, and tuberous. When cut they exude a yellow sap. Water hemlock is frequently mistaken for wild parsnips or wild artichokes.

    1. Toxin. Cicutoxin, a long-chain alcohol, is found in all parts of the plant. A single bite of the root can kill an adult in 15 min.

    2. Presentation. Rapid onset of salivation, GI irritation, and severe abdominal pain are followed by trismus, dilated pupils, delirium, and convulsions. Death may occur rapidly. If the patient survives, prolonged defects in cognition have been seen. Hallucinations and nightmares may occur much later.

    3. Management. Maintain an adequate airway because convulsions may occur. Empty the stomach with gastric lavage. Assist ventilation. Administer activated charcoal and cathartics. Control seizures with anticonvulsants. Correct acidosis and establish an adequate urine flow to reduce myoglobinuria secondary to convulsions.

J. ***Colchicum autumnale*** (autumn crocus). This bulbous member of the lily family has long, narrow basal leaves. The flowers are tubular and white to purple; and they bloom in the fall. Distinguishing the autumn crocus from the nontoxic blooming crocus is important. Native to Europe and North Africa but used as a garden plant in North America.

    1. Toxic part. The entire plant is toxic.

    2. Toxin. Colchicine, an antimitotic agent.

    3. Presentation. Following plant ingestion, the latent period may last as long as 12 h. Oropharyngeal pain followed by GI irritation develops, with profuse diarrhea that may lead to fatal hypovolemic shock. Hallucinations, convulsions, and coma may occur; and there may be bone marrow depression and ascending paralysis. Renal involvement with hematuria and oliguria can occur, and liver damage has been seen in some patients. Ingestion during pregnancy may induce genetic changes in humans.

    4. Management

        a. Empty the stomach if vomiting has not already occurred. Administer activated charcoal no matter how late the symptoms occur. Intoxication has a prolonged course because of the slow excretion of colchicine. Fluid resuscitation is usually necessary; analgesics and atropine may alleviate colic and diarrhea, which may last for more than 1 week.

    b. Monitor blood counts daily for leukopenia and thrombocytopenia. Also monitor hepatic function and electrolyte levels closely and give appropriate replacement fluids.

K. *Convallaria majalis* (lily of the valley). This small perennial has bell-shaped white flowers. The few leaves are broad, stiff, and 6 to 8 in. long. Naturalized in Eastern North America but cultivated throughout the United States.

    1. Toxic parts. Essentially all parts of this plant are poisonous.

    2. Toxin. Convallarin, a cardiac glycoside.

    3. Presentation and management. As for monkshood.

L. *Datura stramonium* (jimsonweed, thornapple, locoweed). This annual grows to about 4 ft tall, with tubular white flowers and green fruit covered with thorns. The leaf edges are serrated, and the plant has a foul odor. Native throughout North America.

    1. Toxic part. The entire plant, including the nectar (honey), is toxic. The pollen can cause unilateral mydriasis ("cornpicker's pupil").

    2. Toxins. Belladonna alkaloids (hyoscyamine, atropine, and scopolamine) are present.

    3. Presentation. This plant is used as a deliriant, with potentially disastrous results. The symptoms of intoxication constitute the anticholinergic toxidrome which includes: warm, dry, red skin; mydriasis; dry mouth; tachycardia; hallucinations; hypotension or hypertension; urinary retention; delirium; convulsions; coma; and death. Hyperthermia can occur in children. Four grams of plant material can be lethal to a child.

    4. Management. Empty the stomach and give activated charcoal and a cathartic, even if the patient is treated 24 h after ingestion (because intestinal motility is decreased). Monitor and regulate the patient's temperature. For severe symptoms (hyperthermia, delirium, seizures, hypertension, and arrhythmias), i.v. physostigmine should be given slowly over 5 to 10 min (2.0 mg for adults; 0.5 mg for children). A repeat dose may be required in 20 min.

M. *Delphinium* species (e.g., larkspur). This tall herb has lobed leaves and flowers of many colors, each with a "spur."

    1. Toxic part. The young plants and seeds are especially toxic.

    2. Toxins. Ajacine, delphinoidine, and delphinine are all most highly concentrated in seeds and young plants.

    3. Presentation. GI irritation occurs, as do anxiety or depression, hypotension, and respiratory depression. Intoxication may also present as skin paresthesias, numbness.

    4. Management. Empty the stomach by emesis or lavage. Administer activated charcoal and a cathartic. Maintain blood pressure with fluids and vasopressors if needed. Respiratory support may be necessary.

N. Dieffenbachia (dumbcane, mother-in-law's tongue). This plant has leaves that are large, smooth, and green on the periphery and mottled white in the center. As for jack-in-the-pulpit.

O. **_Digitalis purpurea_** (foxglove). This tall flowering herb has large leaves and tubular, multi-colored flowers. Native to Europe but found throughout the United States, including Hawaii. As for monkshood.

P. **_Gelsemium sempervirens_** (yellow/carolina jessamine). This perennial evergreen vine has yellow tubular flowers and lanceolate leaves. Native to the Southern United States, Mexico, and Guatemala. Cultivated in the United States as an ornamental.

    1. **Toxic part.** All parts of the plant are toxic, as is the nectar (honey). The roots are a source of medicinal drugs and contain the highest concentration of toxin.

    2. **Toxins.** Gelsemine, gelseminine, and gelsemiodine cause either atropine-like symptoms or solanine-like symptoms, depending on the maturity of the plant.

    3. **Presentation.** Headache, difficulty speaking, and dysphagia may be present; and ptosis, diaphoresis motor weakness, respiratory paralysis and failure, tetany, and convulsions may occur.

    4. **Management.** Empty the stomach, and administer activated charcoal. Give i.v. fluids, support respiration, and administer anticonvulsants as needed.

Q. **_Kalmia latifolia_** (mountain laurel). This evergreen shrub has leathery leaves and flowers of variable colors, usually white, pink, or red. Native to the Eastern United States in mountainous wooded areas.

    1. **Toxic part.** All parts of the plant and the nectar (honey) are poisonous. This plant has been used by Native Americans for suicide.

    2. **Toxins.** The plant contains adromedotoxin and grayanotoxins, which hold the sodium channels open in cardiac cells, increasing sodium permeability.

    3. **Presentation.** After a latent period, salivation and lacrimation occur, with GI irritation, diaphoresis, headache, muscular weakness, blurred vision, respiratory depression, ataxia, bradycardia, conduction disturbances including Wolff-Parkinson-White syndrome, and complete AV block. Progressive paralysis, severe hypotension, seizures, coma, and death are possible.

    4. **Management**

        a. Gastric emptying is best performed by lavage; induction of vomiting may stimulate vagal reflexes and worsen arrhythmias. Give charcoal in repeated doses.

        b. Replace fluids as indicated and support respiration. Monitor cardiac rhythm. Give atropine for bradycardia; if it is refractory, a pacemaker may be needed. Administer fluids and vasopressors (dopamine, norepinephrine) for hypotension.

R. **_Karwinski humboldtiana_** (buckthorn). This shrub has elliptical leaves; the mature fruit is black. It grows in the southwestern United States.

    1. **Toxic part.** The fruit is poisonous.

    2. **Toxins.** The plant contains anthracinones and a polyphenol, which cause demyelination.

    3. **Presentation.** After a latent period of several weeks, progressive ascending paralysis may progress for more than 1 month. Respiratory paralysis may also occur.

    4. **Management.** There is no antidote, so all treatment is supportive. If the victim survives, slow improvement results in near-complete recovery.

S. **_Laburnum anagyroides_** (golden chain tree). This tree bears masses of small yellow flowers. The seeds are produced in pods. Native to southern Europe, cultivated in the United States.

1. **Toxic part.** All parts of the tree are poisonous.
2. **Toxin.** Cytisine, an alkaloid related to nicotine.
3. **Presentation.** Rapid onset of emesis occurs with salivation, headache, hallucinations, incoordination, mydriasis, diaphoresis, bradycardia or tachycardia, hypotension, convulsions, and coma. Respiratory paralysis may lead to death.
4. **Management.** When vomiting stops, give activated charcoal and a cathartic. If vomiting has not occurred, perform gastric lavage and protect the airway. Respiratory support may be needed. Treat seizures with anticonvulsants. Treat hypotension with i.v. fluids and administer vasopressors as needed.

T. *Lantana camara.* This sprawling shrub has square stems. The flowers are yellow, orange, or red and occur in flat clusters. The leaves are serrated. Native to tropical America. Naturalized from Florida to Texas.
1. **Toxic part.** The entire plant is toxic, but the unripe berries are the most toxic part.
2. **Toxin.** Lantanidine A. This toxin antagonizes acetylcholine at neuroreceptors. This effect is seen especially in heart and smooth muscle, brain, and exocrine glands.
3. **Presentation.** The symptoms may be delayed for several hours and are similar to those of atropine poisoning: mydriasis, blurred vision, dry mouth, tachycardia, changes in blood pressure, urinary retention, gastroenteritis, lethargy, slowing of respiration, abnormal reflexes, delirium, seizures, coma, circulatory collapse, and death.
4. **Management**
   a. Empty the stomach, since symptoms may be delayed. Treat hypotension with i.v. fluids and vasopressors. Support respiration mechanically if necessary.
   b. For **serious symptoms,** especially severe hypertension, arrhythmias, and hallucinations, give physostigmine 2 mg i.v. over 5 to 10 min (for children: 0.5 mg i.v. over 5 to 10 min).
   c. If the patient is in a **coma,** one dose of physostigmine may be given as a diagnostic tool. If the drug does not work for arrhythmias, alkalinize the patient to pH 7.5.

U. *Narcissus* **species, family amaryllidaceae** (e.g., daffodil, jonquil). This plant is similar to an onion in appearance, with a flowering stalk and white or yellow flowers. Native to Spain.
1. **Toxic part.** The bulbs are toxic and have been mistaken for onions.
2. **Toxins.** Lycorine and other alkaloids are present. Daffodils also contain oxalates.
3. **Presentation.** GI irritation occurs. Skin and eye irritation may occur on contact with plant material.
4. **Management.** The stomach should be emptied unless the patient has already vomited. When vomiting stops, give activated charcoal and a cathartic. Replace fluids as needed to prevent dehydration. Wash the skin thoroughly and irrigate the eyes for 15 min if contact with plant material has occurred. Even though systemic toxicity is uncommon, convulsions and death have been reported.

V. *Nerium oleander.* This evergreen shrub has long, narrow leaves and cone-shaped flowers of varied colors (red, pink, and white). The fruit is borne in pods. Native to Mediterranean region, cultivated in the southern United States, Hawaii, and Japan.

1. **Toxic part.** All parts, including the nectar (honey), are toxic except the roots. The smoke from the burning plant is toxic, as is the vase water. When plant material is used to roast food over a fire, the poisonous sap transferred to the food may be lethal.
2. **Toxins.** Nerioside and oleandrin are cardiac glycosides that act like digitalis but are *much more toxic*.
3. **Presentation and management.** As for monkshood.

W. **Nicotiana tabacum and Nicotiana glauca** (tobacco). This annual or perennial has tubular flowers. Native to South Bolivia, and Northern Argentina. Naturalized in the United States.
   1. **Toxic part.** The whole plant is poisonous when ingested or with cutaneous absorption.
   2. **Toxins.** Nicotine, anabasine, and other chemically related alkaloids.
   3. **Presentation.** Salivation, nausea, and vomiting occur, with convulsions, respiratory paralysis, and circulatory collapse.
   4. **Management.** Provide respiratory support as indicated; empty the stomach, administer activated charcoal, and give anticonvulsants and vasopressors as needed.

X. *Phytolacca americana* (pokeweed). This large shrub grows up to 8 ft tall, with purple branches and dark berries on a vertical stalk. The leaves are oval and pointed. Naturalized in fields and damp woods from Maine to Minnesota, south to the Gulf of Mexico.
   1. **Toxic part.** The roots, uncooked stems, and leaves are toxic. The fruit is the least toxic part. Ten or more uncooked berries can cause serious poisoning in an adult, although only a few can cause toxicity in infants. Leaves that have been boiled twice are still toxic.
   2. **Toxins.** Saponins, glycoproteins, and triterpenes (phytolaccatoxin, phytoloaccinic acid, and phytolaccagenin). This plant also contains oxalic acid, asparagine, and several mitogens.
   3. **Presentation.** Headache and oropharyngeal irritation occur, accompanied by GI irritation within 0.5 to 6 h, which may last up to 48 h. Visual disturbances, diaphoresis, dyspnea, convulsions, coma, and death may ensue. In addition, there may be immunosuppressive effects; and mitogenic cell changes have been seen after exposure (ingestion or contact of toxin with wounds). Examination of blood smears from exposed children has revealed cells resembling proplasmacytes and plasmablasts. Intoxicated patients frequently have lymphoblastoid cells on peripheral blood smears. The lymphocytosis is usually seen 2 to 4 days following an ingestion.
   4. Management. Empty the stomach; give activated charcoal and cathartics if the patient has not already experienced catharsis. Treat hypotension with fluids; then use dopamine if necessary. Control pain and monitor fluid and electrolyte status. Treat seizures with anticonvulsants. Wash exposed skin thoroughly.

Y. *Pieris floribunda and Pieris japonica* (lily of the valley bush). This evergreen shrub has leathery leaves and clusters of white flowers. Native to Japan, cultivated throughout the United States.
   1. **Toxic part.** The leaves and nectar are poisonous.
   2. **Toxins.** Grayanotoxins (andromedotoxins).
   3. **Presentation and management.** As for mountain laurel.

Z. *Podophyllum peltatum* (May apple). This herb has large umbellate leaves, a single white flower, and egg-shaped fruit. Found throughout the United States and southern Canada in moist woods and meadows.

  1. **Toxic part.** The entire plant is toxic, including the green fruit.
  2. **Toxins.** Podophyloresin, a purgative, and alpha- and beta-peltatin, which are antimitotic agents that arrest cellular mitosis. Oral ingestion or dermal exposure may result in toxicity.
  3. **Presentation.** Toxicity usually develops within 4 to 8 h in oral ingestion and 12 to 24 h in dermal exposures. GI irritation occurs with severe purging, hypotension, and dyspnea. Repeated topical exposures or large ingestions can result in an elevated uric acid level with (delayed) renal failure, elevated hepatic enzymes, leukocytosis or leukopenia, thrombocytopenia, lethargy, areflexia, confusion, and coma lasting up to 10 days. If death does not occur, polyneuropathy may progress for 2 to 3 months, and orthostatic hypotension may persist for 6 to 9 months. *Podophyllum* may be teratogenic.
  4. **Management.** Empty the stomach if vomiting has not occurred. Resuscitate the patient with fluids, and give vasopressors if necessary. Administer activated charcoal and antiemetics. Blood component transfusion may be needed. Monitor renal and liver function tests, CBC, electrolytes, and calcium levels. Consider hemodialysis for renal failure. If eye exposure occurs, irrigate the eyes for at least 15 min. If skin exposure occurs, wash thoroughly.

AA. *Prunus* **species** (e.g., apricot, cherry, peach, plum, choke cherry). This species includes several well-known fruits of the family Rosaceae. The fruit is characterized by a fleshy outer layer over a stone or pit.

  1. **Toxic part.** The kernel in the pit is poisonous. Apricot pits cause most of the fatalities in this group. With the exception of the fruit pulp, the rest of the tree is toxic.
  2. **Toxins.** Cyanogenic glycosides (amygdalen), which cause cellular hypoxia.
  3. **Presentation.** Most intoxications involve a delayed onset of abdominal pain and vomiting, changes in respiratory and heart rate, lethargy, severe hypotension, diaphoresis, muscle flaccidity, incontinence, coma, and tetanic convulsions. Acidosis results from the accumulation of lactic acid. Cyanosis may not occur.
  4. **Management.** Determine arterial blood gases, and monitor methemoglobin levels; in pediatric patients, monitor the hemoglobin level in order to gauge the correct dose of sodium nitrite. Empty the patient's stomach, and administer a cathartic. Charcoal is of questionable effectiveness with cyanide poisoning but should be given. A 25% solution of sodium thiosulfate should be instilled into the stomach (300 mL for an adult). Administer anticonvulsants for seizures. Support respiration, correct acidosis, and treat shock with volume expanders. If the patient has an altered level of consciousness or other serious symptoms, administer a cyanide antidote (kit by Eli Lilly Company), starting with amyl nitrite inhalants, then sodium nitrite, then sodium thiosulfate. If marked methemoglobinemia occurs, treat with exchange transfusion. Giving methylene blue to treat the methemaglobinemia causes an increase of free cyanide and worsens intoxication.

BB. *Rheum rhabarbarum* (rhubarb). Rhubarb is a perennial with large, oval leaves on long stalks that become red at maturity. **Boston ivy** (*Parthenocissus tricuspidata*) and **Virginia creeper** (*P. quinquefolia*) each cause similar symptoms that should be treated the same way; they are deciduous woody vines with blue-black fruit. These plants all contain soluble salts of oxalic acid. The symptoms and treatment differ from those of other oxalate-containing plants.

    1. **Toxic part.** The leaf blades are toxic. Ingestion of a small amount of plant material does not usually cause symptomatology.

    2. **Toxins.** Oxalic acid (soluble salts) and anthraquinone glycosides are present.

    3. **Presentation and management.** As for jack-in-the-pulpit.

CC. *Rhododendron* **species** (e.g., azalea, rhododendron). There are more than 750 species in the genus. The leaves are oblong, and the flowers vary in color and are bell-shaped.

    1. **Toxic part.** The entire plant, including the nectar (honey), is toxic.

    2. **Toxins.** Grayanotoxins and andomedotoxins bind to sodium channels in the cell membrane; nerve and muscle cells remain in a state of depolarization.

    3. **Presentation and management.** As for mountain laurel.

DD. *Ricinus communis* (castor bean). This tall shrub has large leaves. The seeds are brown or black, mottled, and encapsulated. Cultivated commercially and as an ornamental.

    1. **Toxic part.** Essentially the entire plant is toxic, although the seeds are the most poisonous part. Chewing one seed may prove fatal to a child, and four seeds may be lethal to an adult. Anaphylaxis may also occur with exposure.

    2. **Toxin.** Ricin, a toxalbumin like abrin, is a phytotoxin that inhibits intestinal protein synthesis. It is a poorly absorbed substance, with its full effect taking up to 5 days.

    3. **Presentation.** After a delay of several hours, severe burning of the oral mucosa appears, similar to an alkali burn; and there may be severe abdominal pain with hemorrhagic gastritis. CNS toxicity is delayed, especially involving the cranial nerves. There is also delayed toxicity of the adrenal glands, liver (resulting in abnormal glucose metabolism), and kidneys (causing uremia leading to death). Tachycardia and hypotension are secondary to fluid loss, which may be fatal. Marked fluid and electrolyte changes occur frequently.

    4. Laboratory analysis. Monitor liver enzymes, serum glucose, renal function, and serum chemistries.

    5. Management

        a. Immediate emptying of the stomach is essential because of the extreme toxicity of the seeds. Activated charcoal is helpful. Cathartics may be indicated if the patient has not already undergone catharsis.

        b. Hypovolemia and electrolyte abnormalities must be corrected. Parenteral hyperalimentation may be required.

        c. A latent period for CNS organ toxicity lasts up to 5 days.

EE. *Robinia pseudoacacia* (black locust). This large tree with compound leaves has a thorned trunk and branches. The white flowers bloom in clusters, and the seeds are produced in pods. Found throughout the United States.

    1. **Toxic part.** The bark, leaves, and seeds are toxic.

    2. **Toxins.** Robitin is a glucosin, and robin is a toxalbumin.

    3. **Presentation and management.** As for rosary pea.

FF. ***Sanguinaria canadensis*** (bloodroot). This plant is a white wildflower with red sap. Found throughout the United States and Southern Canada.

    1. **Toxic part.** All parts of the plant are toxic; the highest concentration of toxin is in the roots.

    2. **Toxin.** Sanguinarine, an alkaloid.

    3. **Presentation.** GI irritation occurs, with bradycardia, hypotension, syncope, coma, paralysis, and death.

    4. **Management.** Empty the stomach. Give activated charcoal and a cathartic. Treat hypotension with fluids; if there is no response, give vasopressors. Support respiration.

GG. **Family Solanaceae**

    1. ***Solanum nigrum*** (black nightshade) and ***Solanum dulcamara*** (deadly nightshade). These plants are herbs or shrubs with spiny or hairy leaves. They have five-toothed flowers, usually white or blue, and berries of several colors, usually black. Native to Europe but has become metropolitan.

        a. **Toxic part.** The entire plant is toxic, with the highest concentrations found in the unripened fruit. Ingestion of small amounts of plant material usually produces toxicity. Fatal intoxications have occurred, more commonly in children.

        b. **Toxin.** Solanine, a glycoalkaloid, which is absorbed slowly.

    2. ***Solanum pseudocapsicum*** (Jerusalem cherry). *Solanum* is a genus with more than 1,700 species. *S. pseudocapsicum* is a shrub with waxy leaves. The flowers are white, and the fruit consists of round orange-red berries. Naturalized in the tropics and the subtropics.

        a. **Toxic part.** The entire plant is toxic, especially the leaves and the unripe berries.

        b. **Toxins.** Solanine, solanidine, and solanocapsine, all of which are glyco-alkaloids.

    3. ***Solanum tuberosum*** (potato plant). The tomato plant and the eggplant are also in this group, and their symptomatology and treatment are similar. Widely cultivated in temperate regions.

        a. **Toxic part.** All parts of the plant except the tuberous root (or fruit, in the case of the tomato and eggplant) are toxic. The tubers, when unripe or overripe, and the sprouts have caused severe poisoning.

        b. **Toxin.** Solanine, a glycoalkaloid, is present throughout the plant, with the highest concentration in the unripe tuber. Fatal intoxication has occurred in children.

        c. **Presentation.** After a latent period of 12 to 24 h, GI irritation, mydriasis, hypothermia or hyperpyrexia, motor paralysis, respiratory depression, convulsions, and circulatory collapse may occur.

        d. **Management.** Empty the stomach, even if the symptoms are delayed. Administer activated charcoal and a cathartic and replace fluids as needed. Support respiration; give anticonvulsants as needed. Monitor and control temperature.

HH. ***Taxus cuspidata*** (Japanese yew) and ***Taxus canadensis*** (American yew). These evergreen shrubs have dark green foliage. The seeds are produced in an aril, a soft red, cup-shaped structure. The leaves are 1 in. long, which distinguishes plants of the *Taxus* species from the *Podocarpus* (also called Japanese yew). *Podocarpus,* which can cause severe gastroenteritis, has leaves 2 to 5 in. long.

1. **Toxic part.** The aril is nontoxic. The remainder of the plant, including the seeds within the aril, is toxic.
2. **Toxin.** Taxine, a potent, rapidly absorbed alkaloid that appears to block conduction in the heart.
3. **Presentation.** Symptoms occur within 1 to 3 h. Gastric irritation occurs, with mydriasis, dyspnea, and cardiac arrhythmias including third-degree AV block and ventricular tachycardia and fibrillation. Hyperkalemia, hypotension, convulsions, coma, and respiratory failure occur. Death may ensue within 30 min of ingestion. Chewing the leaves may produce anaphylactoid reactions.
4. **Management.** Perform gastric lavage with a large-bore tube. Administer activated charcoal and a cathartic. Monitor cardiac rhythm carefully. Treat hypotension with fluids followed by dopamine. Consider inserting a pacemaker in the presence of third-degree block. Support respiration and treat anaphylactoid reactions with epinephrine, steroids, fluids, and respiratory support. Monitor electrolytes and replace fluid losses. Ventricular fibrillation may be refractory to all modes of therapy.

II. *Veratrum viride* (false hellebore, corn lily). This tall perennial has pleated leaves.
1. **Toxic part.** All parts of the plant are poisonous.
2. **Toxins.** Veratrine and more than five other veratrum alkaloids depolarize cellular membranes, especially the vagus nerve endings.
3. **Presentation.** The following symptoms may occur: salivation and diplopia, severe GI irritation, diaphoresis, confusion, paralysis, blurred vision, bradycardia, hypotension, hypertension, hypothermia, respiratory depression, syncope, seizures, coma, and death (from asphyxiation).
4. **Management.** Empty the stomach and administer activated charcoal. Give atropine for bradycardia, and replace fluids as needed. Monitor blood pressure closely, and give atropine and vasopressors for hypotension. Support respiration. Administer nifedipine or nitroprusside for severe hypertension.

JJ. *Wisteria sininsis.* This vine or shrub bears flower clusters of varied colors. The seeds are produced in pods.
1. **Toxic part.** The seed pods are the most dangerous part of the plant, but all parts are toxic. Ingestion of two seeds can cause serious illness.
2. **Toxin.** Wisterin, a glycoside.
3. **Presentation.** GI irritation is followed by lethargy, convulsions, paralysis, hypovolemic shock, and respiratory failure.
4. **Management.** Empty the stomach if vomiting has not occurred, and then give activated charcoal; administer a cathartic if catharsis has not occurred. Perform fluid resuscitation, and give antiemetics as needed. Treat convulsions with anticonvulsants, and support respiration as needed.

KK. *Zygadenus paniculatis* and *Zygadenus venenosus* (e.g., death camas). This perennial bulbous herb of the lily family resembles the wild onion, but the odor is lacking. The pale flowers bloom in clusters on stalks.
1. **Toxic part.** All parts of the plant are poisonous, including the pollen and honey.
2. **Toxins.** Zygadenine, protoveratridine, veratrine, and neogermitrine.

3. **Presentation.** The main symptoms are oropharyngeal and gastric irritation, with bradycardia, hypothermia, hypotension, and convulsions.
4. **Management.** The stomach should be emptied. Resuscitate the patient and administer i.v. fluids. Give atropine for bradycardia and hypotension, and vasopressors as needed.

Selected Readings

Frohne D, Pfander HJ. Trans. Bisset NG. *A color atlas of poisonous plants: a handbook for pharmacists, doctors, toxicologists and biologists*. London: Wolfe, 1984.

Hardin JW, Arena JM. *Human poisoning from native and cultivated plants*. Durham, NC: Duke University Press, 1977.

Lampe KF, McCann M. *AMA handbook of poisonous and injurious plants*. Chicago: American Medical Association, 1985.

Poisindex. Denver: Micromedex, 1996.

Schmutz EM, Breazeale L. *Plants that poison*. Flagstaff, AZ: Hamilton/Northland Press, 1988.

Emergency Toxicology, Second Edition,
edited by Peter Viccellio.
Lippincott–Raven Publishers, Philadelphia © 1998.

84

Mushroom Poisoning

Richard D. Shih

*Department of Emergency Medicine, Morristown Memorial Hospital,
Morristown, New Jersey 07962*

I. **Introduction.** Mushrooms are the aboveground fruit of certain fleshy fungi. Approximately 5,000 different species exist in the United States, of which about 100 are poisonous and 10 potentially fatal if ingested (Table 84-1). The incidence of poisoning has been increasing due to the rising popularity of mushroom foraging ("Mother Earth" movement) and natural products. More than 9,000 mushroom exposures were reported to the American Association of Poison Control Centers in 1995. Eighty percent of these exposures involved children younger than 6 years of age, and more than 90% resulted in minimal or no toxicity. Most poisonings occur in the spring and fall when the temperature and wet conditions favor mushroom growth. Many edible mushrooms resemble poisonous ones and are often difficult to differentiate by visual inspection even by experts. Common myths about differentiating poisonous mushrooms are unreliable. Examples of these include the following: "animal bite marks are only found on edible mushrooms"; "edible mushrooms do not tarnish silver spoons"; "boiling, drying, or salting mushrooms can detoxify them"; "if the skin from the cap of a mushroom can be peeled then it is edible"; and "poisonous mushrooms will turn vinegar milky." The majority of United States mushroom-related deaths involve ingestions of Amanita species (especially *A. phalloides* and *A. virosa*). The most important aspect of clinical management is to differentiate exposure to mushrooms with respect to low versus high risk of toxicity. This is achieved by definitive identification of the mushroom involved if possible and/or assessing the clinical presentation with special attention to the time of symptom onset. Late onset of symptoms, greater than 6 h after exposure, is more likely due to exposure from mushrooms with the potential for severe toxicity.

II. **Mechanism of action and pharmacokinetics.** The poisonous mushrooms are classified into eight different groups based on the primary toxin and/or the clinical toxicity.

   A. **Cyclopeptides.** Prototypical mushroom—*Amanita phalloides*. Although many of the mushroom families contain cyclopeptides in low concentrations, Amanita and Galerina mushrooms have the highest concentrations and are the most dangerous. The main types of cyclopeptide toxins are the phallotoxins and amatoxins. The phallotoxins interrupt actin polymerization and impair cell membrane function. They are poorly absorbed and are felt to be responsible for the severe gastrointestinal (GI) effects which occur early. Amatoxins are rapidly absorbed, have significant enterohepatic circulation, and are excreted in urine. They inhibit RNA polymerase II, interfering with protein synthesis. These toxins are felt to be responsible for the hepatic, renal and CNS effects.

TABLE 84-1. *Some potentially lethal mushrooms*

Cyclopeptides
    Aminita phalloides, Aminita virosa
    Conocybe filaris
    Galerina autumnalis
    Lepiota helveola, Lepiota josserandii
Gyromitrin, *Gyromitra esculenta*
Orellanine/orelline, *Cortinarius orellanus*

B. **Gyromitrin.** Prototypical mushroom—*Gyrometra esculenta.* Gyromitrin is hydrolyzed to monomethylhydrazine. The exact mechanism of this toxin is not entirely understood but may involve inhibition of pyridoxine and pryridoxal phosphate leading to decreased concentrations of gamma-aminobutyric acid (GABA, an inhibitory neurotransmitter). GABA depletion is responsible for the CNS symptoms associated with toxicity. These toxins are also hemoglobin oxidizers capable of causing hemolysis and methemoglobinemia. Gyromitrins are predominantly hepatic metabolized, with small amounts excreted by the lungs and kidneys.

C. **Orellanine and orelline.** Prototypical mushroom—*Cortinarius orellanus.* These toxins are bypyridyl in structure resembling the herbicides paraquat and diquat. They inhibit renal alkaline phosphatase, effecting adenosine triphosphate production and causing renal tubulointerstitial effects.

D. **Muscarine.** Prototypical mushroom—*Clitocybe delbata.* Although this toxin was originally discovered in *Amanita muscaria,* this mushroom contains only small amounts of this toxin. Muscarine is an alkaloid acting as an agonist at peripheral parasympathetic neurons causing cholinergic effects. This toxin is predominantly metabolized in the liver, with some renal elimination.

E. **Coprine.** Prototypical mushroom—*Coprinus atramentarius.* Coprine is a glutamine derivative that inhibits acetaldehyde dehydrogenase and dopamine decarboxylase (similar to the effects of disulfuram). It is metabolized in the liver and renally excreted.

F. **Ibotenic acid and muscimol.** Prototypical mushroom—*Amanita muscaria.* These toxins resemble GABA and interact with multiple CNS neurotransmitters to produce their effects. Effects from antagonism of parasympathetic neurons may predominate leading to different central and autonomic nervous system effects especially anticholinergic symptoms. These toxins are predominately metabolized by the liver, with some renal excretion.

G. **Psilocybin and psilocin.** Prototypical mushroom—*Psilocybe cubensis.* These indole toxins resemble serotonin structurally. They interact with CNS neurotransmitters to produce their LSD-like CNS effects. Psilocybin is hepatically converted to the more potent psilocin and predominantly hepatically eliminated.

H. **Multiple gastrointestinal toxins.** Many different mushrooms contain toxins that are strong gastrointestinal irritants. Most of the toxins have yet to be isolated and individually identified.

III. **Clinical presentation.** The clinical features of toxicity depend on the specific mushroom and amount of toxin involved in the exposure. The maturity and the growing conditions of the mushroom can effect toxin concentration. Eight general groups of poisonous mushrooms have been classified based on the toxin that is present (Table 84-1).

A. Cyclopeptides. Prototypical mushroom—*Amanita phalloides*. This mushroom causes four stages of poisoning. The initial asymptomatic phase lasts from 6 to 24 h, with most patients presenting between 8 and 10 h after consumption. This leads to the gastrointestinal (GI) phase, which is characterized by the sudden development of severe nausea, vomiting, and diarrhea often described as cholera-like. The GI symptoms are typically more severe than caused by other poisonous mushrooms and may lead to dehydration and hypotension perfusion. The GI phase lasts between 12 and 24 h and leads to another relative asymptomatic phase. This stage is characterized by a general clinical improvement, which may be interpreted incorrectly as recovery. Patients often develop mild clinical and laboratory evidence of hepatic dysfunction. This relative asymptomatic phase lasts several hours to several days and may progress rapidly to the hepatic phase, which is characterized by severe hepatic failure and other end organ dysfunction. Most patients who die do so from hepatic failure 7 to 10 days after ingestion. The mortality rate with modern supportive care is between 10% and 30%. Patients that recover do so over several weeks, with 10% to 20% going on to develop a picture of chronic active hepatitis.

B. Gyromitrin. Prototypical mushroom—*Gyrometra esculenta*. Gyromitrin intoxication is also associated with a delayed onset of symptoms. Patients typically develop mild to moderate GI symptoms 6 to 12 h after ingestion. CNS symptoms of weakness, headache, seizures, and ataxia may also occur. Hemolysis, methemoglobinemia, and hepatic effects may occur in severe cases. The mortality rate has been reported as high as 14%. However, most cases result in minor symptoms and mushroom-related deaths rarely involve this toxin.

C. Orellanine and orelline. Prototypical mushroom—*Cortinarius orellanus*. Mushrooms containing this toxin are found very rarely in North America, and, thus, poisoning is uncommon in the United States. This toxin is associated with a delay in symptom onset, beginning with constipation and gastritis 24 to 48 h after ingestion. Symptoms of progressive renal dysfunction are often the presenting complaints up to 3 weeks after initial ingestion. Associated findings include oliguria, fever, chills, myalgias, anorexia, and headaches. Renal toxicity often requires hemodialysis. Partial or full recovery may occur over weeks to months.

D. Muscarine. Prototypical mushroom—*Clitocybe delbata*. Ingestion is quickly followed by symptoms within 15 to 60 min. Signs and symptoms of cholinergic excess predominate. This cholinergic toxidrome includes salivation, lacrimation, nausea, vomiting, abdominal pain, defecation, diaphoresis, and miosis. Symptoms are usually mild and improve over the next several hours. Severe cases may be associated with seizures, bradycardia, and wheezing. Mortality is unlikely with good supportive care.

E. Coprine. Prototypical mushroom—*Coprinus atramentarius*. The symptom onset for this toxin is variable depending on if and when ethanol is consumed by the patient. A reaction is visible if alcohol is consumed up to 72 h after ingestion. The disulfiram-like syndrome occurs 0.5 to 2 h after alcohol ingestion and is characterized by flushing, headache, parasthesias, nausea, vomiting, diaphoresis, chest pain, and tachycardia. Mortality is unlikely, with symptoms resolving after 4 to 6 h.

F. Ibotenic acid and muscimol. Prototypical mushroom—*Amanita muscaria*. Poisoning from these toxins are more commonly due to recreational abuse for their hallucinogenic effects. Symptoms begin soon after ingestion, with CNS effects predominating. Mental status alteration, hallucinations, visual complaints, agitation, ataxia, seizures, muscle fasciculations and psychosis can occur. Anticholinergic symptoms of flushing, mydriasis, dry skin, decreased bowel sounds, and urinary retention may be very prominent.

G. Psilocybin and psilocin. Prototypical mushroom—*Psilocybe cubensis*. Exposure from these toxins are usually in the setting of recreational drug abuse. Symptoms begin shortly after exposure. Hallucinations, weakness, anxiety, and dysphoria may occur. Symptoms typically resolve within several hours without chronic sequelae.

H. Multiple GI toxins. A large number of potential mushrooms produce a similar clinical picture characterized by rapid onset of GI symptoms. The nausea, vomiting, abdominal pain, and diarrhea begin 30 min to several hours after ingestion. Symptoms can be severe and last several days but more typically are mild to moderate and resolve after 12 to 24 h.

IV. Diagnostic tests

A. A number of tests can be performed on a mushroom sample if available. Results from these tests may help in identification of the mushroom involved in an unknown exposure. These tests should be performed by a trained expert such as a mycologist (located by contacting a botanical garden, poison center, mushroom club, or university).

B. If a sample is brought with the patient, try not to bruise or damage the mushroom and place it in a paper bag rather than a plastic container to prevent decomposition. If a sample is not available, gastric contents can be aspirated to obtain a specimen and/or filtered to obtain mushroom spores.

C. Tests performed on mushroom samples include spore printing, spore examination, testing with Meltzer's reagent, and the Meixner's test (see textbooks cited for the performance and interpretation of these tests).

D. Serum, gastric, urine and fecal specimens from the exposed patient can be assayed for specific toxins and may help to diagnose the specific mushroom involved. Techniques include radio-immunoassay, high-pressure liquid chromatography, gas chromatography-mass spectroscopy and infrared spectroscopy.

V. Management

A. The main clinical issue involves determining the lethality of the mushroom involved. This is accomplished by either identifying the mushroom or by clinical assessment.

B. The clinical assessment of poisonous mushrooms is based on the signs and symptoms seen and their time of onset (early versus late) relative to mushroom ingestion.

1. Late onset of symptoms, greater than 6 h after mushroom exposure, is consistent with potentially lethal mushrooms: cyclopeptides, gyromitrin, and orellanine/orelline-containing mushrooms.

2. Early onset of symptoms, less than 2 h after mushroom exposure, is consistent with poisonous mushrooms that have limited toxicity: muscarine, coprine, ibotenic acid/muscimol, psilocybin/psilocin, or diverse GI toxin–containing mushrooms.

C. If a sample of the mushroom is available, identification of the specific mushroom involved is the most helpful piece of information in determining the patient's potential for serious illness and guides subsequent treatment. If a sample is available, a trained expert (mycologist) should be involved to help identify the mushroom.

D. Implementation of general measures such as gastric lavage, activated charcoal, induced emesis, and cathartics depends on the likelihood that a potentially lethal mushroom is involved. These forms of gastric decontamination should be aggressively utilized if there is a strong clinical suspicion of a potentially lethal mushroom.

E. Specific toxin/mushroom therapy. A number of specific toxin antidotes and methods of enhanced elimination have been utilized. However, there is little evidence that these modalities are useful. Consideration for their use should be made in consultation with a medical toxicologist or poison center.

  1. Cyclopeptides. Prototypical mushroom—*Amanita phalloides*

    a. Antidotes. Many antidotes have been suggested for this mushroom poisoning. Good controlled studies are lacking to support efficacy for any of these agents. Silibinin (20 to 50 mg/kg/day i.v.) and penicillin (300,000 to 1,000,000 U/kg/day i.v.) have shown the most promise in animal and clinical studies. Other agents with less scientific support include thiocytic acid, dexamethasone, vitamin C, cytochrome C, cimetidine, *N*-acetylcysteine, kutkin, and aucubin.

    b. Enhanced elimination. Forced diuresis, continuous gastroduodenal aspiration, common bile duct cannulation and drainage, hemodialysis, and charcoal hemoperfusion have been utilized but none of these modalities are accepted as standard therapy. Multidose oral activated charcoal adsorbs amatoxins and may be beneficial. It should be routinely offered with this poisoning.

    c. Other. Liver transplantation has been performed in several cases and may be life-saving. Patient selection criteria are not clear and remain the most controversial aspect of this therapeutic modality. Early consultation with a liver transplant team should occur for any patient that manifests progressive hepatic dysfunction.

  2. Gyromitrin. Prototypical mushroom—*Gyrometra esculenta*. This toxin may partially exert its effects by inhibiting pyridoxine metabolism. Pyridoxine administration (25 mg/kg i.v.) may reverse these effects. Methylene blue can be administered to patients that develop symptomatic methemoglobinemia.

  3. Orellanine and orelline. Prototypical mushroom—*Cortinarius orellanus*. No specific antidotes are available for this mushroom. Charcoal hemoperfusion may enhance toxin elimination and should be considered especially in patients who are already receiving hemodialysis.

  4. Muscarine. Prototypical mushroom—*Clitocybe delbata*. Atropine (1.0 mg i.v. every 5 min until secretions are controlled) administration is useful for patients with cholinergic effects. Bronchodilators may be useful for patients manifesting bronchospasm.

  5. Coprine. Prototypical mushroom—*Coprinus atramentarius*. There is no specific antidote for this toxin and supportive care is generally all that is required. Patients rarely manifest serious problems.

  6. Ibotenic acid and muscimol. Prototypical mushroom—*Amanita muscaria*. Although anticholinergic features may predominate, physostigmine is not generally needed or recommended. Sedation with benzodiazepines is an effective and pre-ferred therapy for agitated patients.

7. **Psilocybin and psilocin.** Prototypical mushroom—*Psilocybe cubensis*. Patients should be offered a quiet room and reassurance. Sedation with benzodiazepines may rarely be needed for very agitated patients.

8. **Diverse GI toxins.** No specific antidotes exist for this diverse group of toxins. Fluid therapy, antiemetics and antimotility agents may be useful.

F. **Pitfalls in management**

1. Not considering that different species of poisonous mushrooms may grow in the same area and be harvested and ingested together. This could make clinical assess-ment based on time to onset of symptoms difficult and misleading.

2. Interpreting the relative asymptomatic phase of cyclopeptide poisoning (the improvement in initial GI symptoms prior to the development of hepatic dysfunc-tion) as patient recovery.

3. Not having a high degree of suspicion to rule-out life-threatening mushroom exposures.

4. Attempting to identify a sample using a photo atlas or textbook can lead to mis-labeling a poisonous mushroom as benign.

5. Not utilizing consultants (mycologist or a poison control center) to help manage suspicious cases.

VI. **Conclusions.** Mushroom exposures occur frequently. Most cases involve young children. Although outcome is favorable in the majority of cases, severe toxicity and death does occur. A high vigilance to assess possible exposure to potentially lethal mushrooms is the key to the successful diagnosis and management of these cases.

Selected Readings

Ammirati JF, Traquair JA, Horgen PA. *Poisonous mushrooms of the Northern United States and Canada.* Minneapolis: University of Minnesota Press, 1986.

Floersheim GL. Treatment of human amatoxin mushroom poisoning: myths and advances in therapy. *Med Toxicol* 1987; 2:1–9.

Galler GW, Weisenberg E, Brasitus TA. Mushroom poisoning: the role of orthotopic liver transplantation. *J Clin Gastroenterol* 1992;15:229–232.

Hanrahan JP, Gordon MA. Mushroom poisoning: case reports and a review of therapy. *JAMA* 1984;251:1057–1061.

O'Brien BL. A fatal Sunday brunch: Amanita mushroom poisoning in a Gulf Coast family. *Am J Gastroenterol* 1996;91: 581–583.

Pinson CW, Daya MR, Benner KG, et al. Liver transplantation for severe Amanita phalloides mushroom poisoning. *Am J Surg* 1990;159:493–499.

Rumack BH, Salzman E, eds. *Mushroom poisoning: diagnosis and treatment.* Boca Raton, FL: CRC Press, 1979.

Emergency Toxicology, Second Edition,
edited by Peter Viccellio.
Lippincott–Raven Publishers, Philadelphia © 1998.

85

Poisoning from Herbs and Related Products

†William S. Pearl and °Lewis S. Nelson

*†Department of Emergency Medicine, Emory University School of Medicine,
Atlanta, Georgia 30303; °Department of Emergency Services, New York University,
Bellevue Hospital, New York, New York 10016*

The consumption of botanical products for healing, rejuvenating, or mind-altering properties has been practiced throughout recorded history. The ancient Chinese recorded empirical data on materia medica several thousand years ago. Other cultures, such as the Assyrians, Greeks, Romans, and Egyptians, also catalogued herbal remedies. The advent of modern allopathic medicine has not eliminated the use of traditional herbal therapies. Their use remains prevalent, constituting a rapidly expanding, multimillion dollar industry. Patterns of herb and alternative therapy use relate to ethnic, cultural, and societal custom. Thus, an appreciation of ethnopharmacology is not solely of interest to the medical anthropologist: the subject is quite relevant to Western practitioners, particularly those practicing in ethnically diverse urban centers. In current vernacular, "herbal" implies any botanical medicinal product harvested or marketed for consumption in an unprocessed form, or as an extract or decoction of the raw material. There is no logic supporting the popular conception that herbal products are safer, more natural, or more holistic than pharmaceutical medications. On the other hand, the discovery, purification, and characterization of naturally occurring products, many well known to traditional healers, continues to contribute to the modern formulary. According to a recent survey, 3% of the U.S. population acknowledged using herbal therapy within the preceding year. A survey in rural Mississippi found a 71% incidence of herbal remedy use during the prior year. Twenty-two percent of HIV-infected patients attending an AIDS clinic had used herbal remedies in the preceding 3 months. Prevalence of nontraditional therapy use is also high among those closely tied to the Asian, African, or Latino communities, food fadists, patients with eating disorders, and health food enthusiasts. Patients with chronic diseases or cancer are likely to use alternative therapies. Of concern, 72% of those using alternative therapies did not inform their physicians. Therefore, physicians should specifically inquire about the use of herbal products. Some herbal toxicities are predictable, based on known botanical content (Tables 85-1 and 85-2). Many other adverse effects are idiosyncratic. Most commonly, however, herbal toxicity is secondary to product contamination, accidental or intentional substitution, or adulteration of otherwise safe products. The manufacture, importation, and sale of herbal products are exempt from most governmental regulation. Thus, product content frequently varies by manufacturer or batch. The wide spectrum of herbal toxicity prevents discussion of all reported and possible adverse reactions. This chapter contains examples selected based on their recent, historic, or epidemiological importance. Because natural product content is often unknown to the acute care physician, and because their adverse effects are not commonly appreciated, the information presented is based upon the most likely clinical picture.

TABLE 85-1. *Herbs and their toxicities*

Botanical name	Common names	Distribution, source, or most likely setting for exposure	Clinical toxicity, based on recent case reports (1966–1995) or historical association with clinical toxicity, which is supported by known toxic constituents	Anticholinergic	Hepatotoxicity	Digoxin activity	Hematologic	Hemodynamic effect	GI symptoms	CNS effects	Nephrotoxicity	Hypoglycemia	Allergy
Acillea milefoleum	Yarrow	WHM	Coagulopathy/bleeding				y						y
Acontium spp.	Monkshood, Wolfsbane, Chanwu, Caowu	CM, WHM	Ventricular arrhythmias, paresthesias					d	y	d			
Actaea sp.	Baneberry, Cohosh	WHM	—										
Aesculus spp.	Horse chestnut	WHM	—				y		y		y		y
Allium spp.	Garlic, Dasuan	WHM, CM, AYM	—				y		y				
Aloe sp.	Aloe	WHM, CM, AYM, LA, AP	Diarrhea						y				y
Angelica spp.	Tang-kuei, Du-huo, Bai-zhi	CM	—				y						
Anthemis nobilis	Chamomile	WHM	Anaphylaxis/allergy						y				y
Arnica spp.	Arnica, Arniflor	WHM, American Indian	Dermatitis						y				y
Arctium lappa	Burdock	WHM	Anticholinergic syndrome							dl,sx		y	y
Aristolochia spp.	Snakeroot (virginian), Fangchi	WHM, CM	Renal failure							y	y	y	
Artemisia spp.	Wormwood, Absinthe, Mugwort, Qinghaosu	CM, WHM	Seizures, euphoria, hallucinations							s,sx			y
Asclepias tuberosa	Pleurisy root	WHM	—			y							
Atractylis Gummifera	White chameleon	Mediterranean, N. Africa	Multiorgan		y		y		y	d	y	y	
Atractylodes sp.	Bai-zu, Pai-chu	CM	—										
Atropa Belladona	Deadly nightshade	AC	Anticholinergic syndrome	y	y					d		y	
Azadirachta indica	Margosa oil, Chinaberry	CM, AYM	Multiorgan		y				y	dl,sx	y		
Berberis Vulgaris	Barberry, Cheunlin	CM, WHM	Bilirubin elevation							d,sx			
Calendula officinalis	Calandula, Marigold	WHM	Dermatitis, Allergy										y
Callipesis laureola	Impilia	South Africa	Multiorgan		y		y		y	d	y	y	
Carissa acokanthera	Bushmans poison	Africa, AP, O, AC, IP	—			y							
Carissa spectabilis	Wintersweet	South Africa; Australia: OM, AC	—			y							
Cassia spp.	Senna	WHM, CM	Diarrhea		y				y				
Catha edulis	Khat	Middle East, N. Africa	Sympathomimetic effect					h		s			
Caulophyllum sp.	Blue cohosh	WHM	—						y				
Cerbera manhas	Sea mango	AP, O, AC, IP	—			y							
Chrysanthemum spp.	Chrysanthemum	CM, WHM	Allergy						y				
Commiphora molmol	Myrrh	CM	Dermatitis										
Convallaria majalis	Lilly of the valley	WHM, O, AC, IP	—			y			y				y

Botanical name	Common name(s)	Availability	Potential toxicity							
Corynanthe yohimbe	Yohimbine	WHM, Africa	Hypertension, anxiety							
Crotalaria spp.	Bush tea	Jamaica, Equador	Veno-occlusive liver dx				h		s	
Cytisus spp.	Broom	WHM, O	—	y		y				
Datura spp.	Jimson weed, Thorn apple, Locoweed, Yangjinhua	WHM, CM, AC, IP	Anticholinergic syndrome	y	y			y	dl, sx	y
Dictamnus dasycarpus	CM for skin disorders	CM								
Digitalis spp.	Foxglove	O, AC, IP	Digitalis poisoning	y	y			y		
Dipterix odorata	Tonka bean	WHM	Anticoagulant, bleeding	y		y		y		
Echinacea spp.	Coneflower	WHM	—							y
Ephedra spp.	Ephedra, Mormon tea, Ma-huang	WHM, CM, substance of abuse	Hypertension, euphoria, mania				h		s	
Galega officinalis	Galega, Goats rue	WHM	Dermatitis		y					
Gaultheria procumbens	Wintergreen, oil of	commonly available	Antiplatelet activity, salicylate poisoning		y				y	y
Glycyrrhiza glabra	Licorice	CM, WHM	Hypertension, Hypokalemia, Myopathy		y		h			
Gynura segetum	Tu-san'chi	CM	Veno-occlusive liver dx	y						
Heliotropium spp.	Hathisunda	AY, CM	Veno-occlusive liver dx	y						
Hydrastis candadensis	Goldenseal, Yellow puccoon	WHM	—		y			y	s	y
Hyoscyamus niger	Black henbane	CM, Asia, AC	Anticholinergic syndrome	y		y			dl, sx	y
Hypericum perforatum	St. John's wort, Klamath	WHM, CM	—							
Ilex paraguayensis	Paraguayan tea	LA	—		y				s	
Isatis tinctoria	Dyers wood root, Pan-lan-ken	WHM, CM	—							
Juniperus communis	Juniper	WHM	—						s	y
Lactuca virosa	Wild lettuce	WHM	—						d	y
Larrea tridentata	Chapparal, Creosote bush	WHM, American Indian	Hepatitis	y						
Liliacea family	Autumn crocus, Glory lily	WHM, CM	Colchicine poisoning	y	y				d	y
Lobelia spp.	Lobelia, Indian tobacco	WHM	Nicotine-like effects		y				s	
Lycium chinensis	Wolfberry, gougizi, kuo-chi-tzu	CM	—					y		y
Mandragora officinarum	Mandrake (European)	WHM, CM, IP	Anticholinergic syndrome	y	y			y	dl, sx	y
Mentha pulegium, Hedeoma pulegiodes	Pennyroyal	WHM, IP	Multiorgan		y				d	y
Mormodica sp.	Bitter gourd, Kerla	AYM	—		y					
Nepeta cataraia	Catnip	WHM	—							
Nerium oleander	Oleander (common)	O, AC, IP	Digitalis poisoning	y		y		y	s	
Panax spp.	Poke, Pokeweed, Inkberry, Crowberry, Garget, Jalap	CM	HTN, diarrhea, dermatitis				h	y		y
Phytolacca americana		WHM	Diarrhea, GI bleeding					y	d, sx	y
Podophyllum spp.	May apple, Mandrake (American)	WHM, CM, AC	Multiorgan		y			y	d	y
Prunella vulgares	Prunella, Woundwort	CM, WHM	—		y		d		d	
Rauwolfia spp.	Snakeroot, Serpentwood, Chotchand	AYM, WHM	Somnolence, gynecomastia				d		d	y
Rehmenia glutionsa	Shent-ti-huang, Rhemenia	CM	—							y

(continued)

TABLE 85-1. *Continued*

Botanical name	Common names	Distribution, source, or most likely setting for exposure	Clinical toxicity, based on recent case reports (1966–1995) or historical association with clinical toxicity, which is supported by known toxic constituents	Potential toxicity, including reported effects of unclear clinical significance, in vitro effects									
				Anticholinergic	Hepatotoxicity	Digoxin activity	Hematologic	Hemodynamic effect	GI symptoms	CNS effects	Nephrotoxicity	Hypoglycemia	Allergy
Rhamnus catharticus	Buck thorn	WHM	—						y				
Rumex spp.	Dock root	WHM	—						y				
Salvia miltiorrhiza	Salvia, Tan-shen	CM	Inhibits warfarin excretion				y			d		y	
Salix caprea	Linn	AYM	G6PD-related hemolysis					d	y				
Sanguinara candensis	Red puccone, Bloodroot	WHM, NAI								d			
Scutellara sp.	Skullcap	CM, WHM	Hepatitis		y								
Senecio sp.	Ragwprt, Gordolobo, Bush tea	WHM, LA, Jamaica	Veno-occlusive liver dx		y			d		d			
Stephania sp.	Jin Bu Huan	CM, AC	Hepatitis, bradycardia		y			d		d			
Strychnos nux-vomica	Strychnine	Hawaii, AC, CM	Hyperreflexia, opisthotonis							s,sx	y		
Symphytum spp.	Comfrey	WHM	Veno-occlusive liver dx		y								
Tanacetum parthenium	Feverfew	WHM	Oral ulcers				y		y				y
Taxacarum officinalis	Dandelion	WHM, CM											y
Teucrium spp.	Germander	WHM, Mediterranean	Hepatitis		y								
Thevetia peruviana	Oleander (yellow)	O, AC, IP	Digitalis poisoning			Y			y	d, sx			
Trichosanthes kirilowii	Chinese cucumber, Compound Q, Gualogen	CM	—						y			y	
Trifolium pratense	Red clover	WHM	—				y						
Tussilago farfara	Coltsfoot, Horsefoot, Coughwort	WHM, CM	Venoclusive liver dx		y								
Urginea maritima	Squill, Sea onion	Mediterranean	Digitalis toxicity			Y							
Valariana officinalis	Valerian	CM, WHM	Hepatitis		y					d			
Veratrum spp.	False Hellebore	WHM, CM, AC	Bradycardia, hypotension					d	y	d			
Viscum album	Mistletoe (European)	WHM, CM	—		y				y	d			

y, yes; d, decrease (BP or CNS); h, hypertension; s, stimulant or euphoriant; dl, delerium; sx, seizure; WHM, Western herbal medicine; CM, Chinese medicine; AYM, Aruvdic (India); AP, Asia-Pacific; LA, Latin America; IP, intentional poisoning; O, ornamental plant; AC, accidental or intentional substitute.

TABLE 85-2. *Nonplant toxins or adulterants found in alternative medications*

Constituent	Common names	Distribution, source, or most likely setting for exposure	Clinical toxicity, based on recent case reports (1966–1995) or historical association with clinical toxicity, which is supported by known toxic constituents	Anticholinergic	Hepatotoxicity	Digoxin activity	Hematologic	Hemodynamic effect	GI symptoms	CNS effects	Nephrotoxicity	Hypoglycemia	Allergy
Antibiotics	Chloramphenicol, Sulfa	CM	—				y				y		
Auricularia polytricha	Black tree fungus, Mo-er	CM	Antiplatelet/bleeding				y				y		
Bacteria/yeast aggregate	Kombucha	WHM	Hepatitis		y								
Benzodiazepine	Diazepam	CM								d			
Cantharis vesicatora	Spanish fly, Ban-Mao	CM, WHM, homeopathy	Cutaneous blisters, multiorgan failure		y		y	d	y	d	y		
Diuretic	Hydrochlorathiazide	CM											
Heavy Metals	Pb, As, Hg, Cu, Cd	CM, AYM, WHM, LA	Multiple organs		y		y		y		y		
L-Tryptophan	L-Tryptophan	—	Eosinophilic myalgia						y	d			
NSAID's	Phenylbutazone, Aminopyrone, Mefenemate, Indocin	CM, AYM, LA	Aplastic anemia, renal failure				y		y		y		
Skin of *Bufo* spp. frogs	Bufalin	CM	Digitalis poisoning			y							
Steroids	Hydrocortisone and others	CM	Cushing syndrome					h		s			
Warfarin	Coumadin	LA, CM, WHM	Coagulopathy				y				y		y

Potential toxicity, including reported effects of unclear clinical significance, in vitro effects.

y, yes; d, decrease (BP or CNS); h, hypertension; s, stimulant or euphoriant; dl, delerium; sx, seizure; WHM, Western herbal medicine; CM, Chinese medicine; AYM, Aruvdic (India); AP, Asia-Pacific; LA, Latin America; IP, intentional poisoning; O, ornamental plant; AC: accidental or intentional substitute.

I. **Multiorgan toxicity**
   A. **May apple (Podophyllotoxin) and Autumn crocus (Colchicine).** Podophylotoxin is produced by plants of the genus Podophyllum, of which Mayapple (*P. peltatum*) is indigenous to North America. Accidental consumption of the immature and use of Podophyllum species in herbal medications has resulted in severe toxicity. Podophyllotoxin interferes with several metabolic processes, including mitotic spindle formation, purine synthesis, and the tricarboxylic acid cycle. Clinical manifestations begin within hours and include vomiting, diarrhea, and altered consciousness. Coma ensues and may last for several days. Marked leukocytosis and progressive thrombocytopenia are characteristic. A severe sensory-motor neuropathy can develop over several weeks and resolve over months. Minor elevations of liver enzymes are common. Renal insufficiency and hepatitis have occurred. Management is supportive. Anecdotal reports suggest hemoperfusion is efficacious, and its use should be considered in severe or refractory cases. The autumn crocus (*Colchicum autumnale*) contains colchicine. Fortunately, most responsible herbal guides for laypersons identify this as a potential deadly toxin, and there are no recent reports of clinical toxicity. Colchicine, a multiorgan toxin, is discussed elsewhere.
   B. **Pennyroyal.** Pennyroyal oil is derived from leaves of *Mentha pulegium* and *Hedeoma pulegiodes*. The active constituent is a ketone, pulegone. Pennyroyal has a long history of use as an abortifacient. It is available as leaves for brewing in tea or as an oil. Abdominal pain, vomiting, and diarrhea occur progressively over the first day after ingestion. DIC and hepatic necrosis also develop early. Renal insufficiency, gastrointestinal (GI) bleeding, vaginal bleeding, seizures, and coma follow.
   C. ***Callipesis laureola* and *Atractylis gummifera*.** *Callipesis laureola* (Impilia) is indigenous to Southern Africa. A center in South Africa claimed 50 fatal cases of herbal toxicity from Impilia over an 8-year period. The clinical presentation resembles Reye's syndrome, including vomiting, hypoglycemia, and altered mental status. Renal failure is common. Liver biopsy demonstrates centrilobular necrosis, without fatty changes. *Atractylis gummifera* is indigenous to the Mediterranean region. Exposure is through use as a medicinal herbal or by accidental consumption, particularly in North Africa. Toxicity is characterized by hepatitis, abnormal mental status, seizures, vomiting, diarrhea, acidosis, leukocytosis, and renal insufficiency. The full spectrum of toxicity develops over 6 to 12 h. Toxicity may be due to compounds similar to potassium atractylate. Poisoning is frequently fatal.

II. **Cardiovascular toxicity**
   A. **Aconite.** In Hong Kong, aconitine poisoning accounts for nearly 70% of severe poisoning caused by Chinese medicines, totaling over 600 known cases by 1993. Aconitine, derived from several species, including *Acontium napellus* (monkshood or wolfsbane), is composed of C-19 diterpenoid alkaloids. Clinical toxicity results from improper preparation. Before use, the roots must be soaked or boiled in water to hydrolyze the alkaloids to less toxic forms. The alkaloids activate sodium channels, producing prolonged depolarization and impaired repolarization of excitable membranes. Symptoms of toxicity often begin within 30 min and include GI upset and perioral paresthesias followed by progressive skeletal muscle weakness. Cardiac arrhythmias begin within the first hours after ingestion. Ventricular tachycardia is characteristic. Sinus bradycardia, supraventricular

tachycardia, and Torsades de pointes are reported. Hypotension and bradycardia may respond to fluids and atropine, although vasoactive agents are frequently required. The ventricular arrhythmias are often refractory to cardioversion or lidocaine. Bretrylium, procainamide, amiodarone, and flecanide are not uniformly effective. The arrhythmias usually resolve within 24 h.

B. **Cardiac glycosides: Oleander, Foxglove, and Bufalin.** Many common teas and herbal preparations contain chemical constituents that produce digoxin cross-reactivity in vitro. Despite their ubiquity, clinical toxicity from most cardiac glycosides is unusual due to their poor absorption or low potency. Most human toxicity occurs through accident inclusion in herbal preparations or by suicidal or homicidal intent. Foxglove and Oleander species are common ornamental plants. Foxglove, *Digitalis purpurea* (North America) and *Digitalis lanata* (Europe), contains digoxin and digitoxin, respectively. Poisoning from species of the Dogbane family, Common Oleander *(Nerium oleander)* and Yellow Oleander *(Thevetia peruviana),* is more common, particularly in India. These exposures are usually accidental or suicidal, although they are also used as medicinal agents. As few as eight Oleander seeds or one leaf may produce fatal toxicity. Poisoning is possible from cooking with Oleander twigs as skewers or inhalation of burning leaves. Medicinal products made from the skin or secretions of the toad *Bufo bufo gargarazans* contain bufalin, a cardiac glycoside. Recently, several deaths occurred from the oral use of aphrodisiac products containing Bufalin. These were intended for topical use. Symptoms of glycoside poisoning are similar to pharmaceutical digoxin poisoning. Interpretation of the serum digoxin concentration is difficult, since the assay used and the degree of structural similarity of the cardiac glycoside present to digoxin will affect the result. The serum concentration should not be used to determine toxicity, but is helpful if positive. There are reports of therapeutic response to digoxin-specific antibody fragments in patients with Foxglove or Oleander poisoning. The affinity of the Fab fragment for the toxin is unpredictable. Thus, if there is no response to the initial dose, additional Fab fragments are indicated.

III. **Hepatotoxicity**. Herbal hepatotoxicity typically presents after several weeks or months of continuous herbal use. Most cases resolve after several months of abstinence. However, the pathologic features of hepatotoxic injury vary. Hepatocyte necrosis ranging from focal to extensive, chronic hepatitis, steatosis, cirrhosis, and veno-occlusive liver disease (VOD) are reported.

A. **Pyrrolizidine alkaloids: comfrey and others.** Plants containing pyrrolizidine alkaloids (PZA's) exist worldwide. VOD, similar to Budd-Chiari syndrome, is characteristic of pyrrolizidine hepatotoxicity. Endemic VOD in humans was recognized in Jamaica and Barbados after consumption of bush teas containing Crotalaria and Senecio spp. Epidemic poisoning has occurred. A recent outbreak in Tadjikistan resulted in nearly 4,000 hepatotoxic patients from Heliotropium contamination of the grain supply. Many traditional Asian and Western remedies contain PZA's and have caused hepatotoxicity. Occurrence is sporadic, probably due to variation in PZA content between specimens or variable human susceptibility. Comfrey (*Symphytum officinale*), an herb commonly used in North America, was responsible for several recent cases of VOD. The mechanism of pyrrolizidine liver injury is not fully understood. Metabolism to toxic intermediates by

P-450 enzymes may be responsible. The clinical presentation is variable. Jaundice is typically minimal or absent. Liver biopsy reveals nonthrombotic occlusion of small centrilobular veins, hepatic congestion, centrilobular necrosis and in some cases, cirrhosis. Although fatalities occur, most recover.

B. **Germander, chapparal, valerian root, and sculliteria.** In 1986, an herbal tea containing Germander (*Teucrium chamydres*) was marketed in France as a weight loss adjunct. Subsequently, more than 30 cases of liver injury occurred. Germander containing herbals are now banned in France. It is unclear why germander hepatitis was not previously recognized. The mechanism of toxicity is believed to be activation of a furano compound, neoclerodane, to a toxic intermediate by P-450 enzymes. Massive hepatic necrosis and fatalities have been reported. Approximately 500 million capsules containing Chaparral were marketed in the past 20 years. However, Chaparral (*Larrea tridentata*) hepatotoxicity was not recognized until 1990. Chaparral comes from the leaves of the Creosote bush, native to the deserts of the southwest United States and Mexico. It is marketed as a nutritional supplement, antioxidant and free radical scavenger. Creosote leaves contain a high concentration of nordihydroguiaretic acid (NGDA), believed to be the toxic constituent. NDGA inhibits cylooxygenase and lipoxygenase pathways. Toxicity appears to be idiosyncratic. Numerous cases from Europe and Asia link products containing Scutellaria and Valeriana officinalis, often in combination, with acute hepatitis. These roots, used in Chinese and Western herbal mixtures, are marketed as natural anxiolytics and sleep aids. However many of the products associated with hepatitis contained a mixture of several herbs and the causal relationship between Scutellaria or Valeriana and hepatitis is not firmly established.

C. *Jin Bu Huan.* *Jin Bu Huan* is a traditional Chinese medication used for over 1000 years. Recently, 7 cases of hepatitis occurred in patients using *Jin Bu Huan*. Analysis indicated that toxicity resulted from substitution for a levo-alkaloid herb, Polygala chinensis by levo-terahydropalmatine containing plants, Stephania or Cordalis. It is unclear if the product misrepresentation was accidental or intentional. The average duration of use before symptoms was 20 weeks with resolution over months. A syndrome of CNS depression, respiratory depression and bradycardia occurred in 3 children after accidental overdose on *Jin Bu Huan*. These symptoms resolved completely within 10 h in each case.

D. **Other herbs, nonbotanical therapies, and contaminants.** *Viscum album* (Mistletoe), based on a few case reports, is reported to be hepatotoxic. The strength of this association is dubious. There are numerous reports of hepatitis associated with consumption of Chinese herbal mixtures for eczema, atopic dermatitis, and psoriasis. These mixtures have been prescribed in Europe by Chinese and Western practitioners, and *Radix cortex dam-nimni* is implicated. Nonherbal constituents of alternative "herbal" therapies also produce liver injury. These include Spanish fly (*Cantharis vesicatoria*) and *kochumbu* (a bacteria-yeast aggregate currently popular in the United States). Poisoning from lead contamination may present with elevated liver enzymes; however other organ systems involvement is usually apparent first.

IV. **GI toxicity.** Many plants are GI irritants and produce oral mucosal irritation, nausea vomiting, and diarrhea. Senna and Physellia seed are the active component of commonly prescribed laxatives. Aloe is a potent cathartic and is a favored herbal constituent. Diarrhea is a prominent early feature in Podophyllum species poisoning, as discussed above.

A. **Pokeweed.** Pokeweed (*Phytolacca americana*) leaves are eaten as a salad and the dried root has been used in herbal preparations. Parboiling (boiling, discard the water then reboiling) usually destroys the toxin, but clinical symptoms have still occurred. All parts of the plant are toxic, including the berries that stain contacting surfaces a telltale purple. Pokeweed mitogen, a glycoside saponin, causes severe diarrhea and vomiting. This is frequently accompanied by GI bleeding and hypotension. Lethargy, transient blindness, amblyopia, and convulsions are occasionally associated. Symptoms begin within several hours of exposure and resolve within 24 to 48 h. Therapy is supportive.

V. **CNS toxicity**
   A. **Stimulants and euphoriants: caffeine, ephedra, and essential oils.** Herb-based stimulants are widely available and often contain familiar substances. Many are advertised as legal alternatives to illicit substances in counterculture magazines such as High Times. Most of these contain *Ma-Huang,* also known as Mormon tea (*Ephedra nevadensis*), which contains ephedrine. The chemical structure of ephedrine is markedly similar to amphetamine. Not surprisingly, street samples of cocaine have revealed ephedrine upon analysis. Caffeine, a methylxanthine typically available as coffee (*Coffee arabica*), is also the active ingredient in mate, or Paraguay tea (*Ilex paraguayensis*). The caffeine content of paraguay tea is higher than coffee. Substitution of *Datura stramonium* for mate resulted in an epidemic of anticholinergic poisoning in New York City. Ginseng, claimed to have antifatigue and ergometric properties, is discussed below. Its combination with the MAO inhibitor phenylzine induced mania. Some street samples of Ginseng contain ephedra. Essential oils euphoriants have a rich history of use. Europe in the 18th century enthusiastically used absinthe, containing thujone, the distillation product of wormwood (*Artemesia absinthum*). It has been postulated that Van Gogh was under the influence of absinthe at the time of his infamous delusional states. Catnip (*Nepeta cataria*) has been reported to have mildly hallucinogenic effect in humans, presumably due to the essential oil nepetalactone. The most common euphoriant available today is the cannabinol containing marijuana (*Cannibis satiiva*).
   B. **CNS depression: valerian, rauwolfia, and L-tryptophan.** Twenty three cases of overdose of soporific products containing Valerian root (Valeriana officinalis), passionflower (Passiflora spp.), hops (*Humulus lupulus*), or gentian (Gentiana spp.) were reported to the National Poisons Unit in London in 1991. Most of these patients suffered from drowsiness without serious sequelae. Valerian root (*Valeriana officinalis*), a widely used soporific, has been reported to produce coma in overdose. Snakeroot (*Rauwofia serpentina*), which contains reserpine, may have the longest history of use as a tranquilizer, and is associated with hypotension in overdose due to depletion of catecholamines. L-Tryptophan was marketed in the 1980's as a natural sedative. Its sale is now prohibited because of its association with eosinophilic myalgia syndrome.
   C. **Anticholinergic syndrome.** Substitution or intentional use of medicinal herbs containing tropane alkaloids is frequently reported in the medical literature. Anticholinergic Datura species are used in Chinese, Western, and Native American medicine. However, recent cases of Dautura toxicity are often due to "recreational misadventure." Seven cases of severe anticholinergic poisoning occurred in New York in 1994 from ingestion of "Paraguay tea," a product imported from South America. Analysis revealed scopalamine and hyoscyamine. These are not constituents of *Ilex paraguariensis,* the proported constituent of this tea. Several common Chinese medications contain belladonna alkaloids. In a recent series, 15% of adverse effects to Chinese medications in Hong Kong were attributable to anticholinergic poisoning.

VI.   **Endocrine disturbances**

A.   **Hypertension and mineralocorticoid excess: Ginseng, Yohimbine, and Licorice.** The invigorating, restorative, and curative properties of Ginseng are a paradigm of Chinese medicine. Ginseng, in various forms, is sold in most pharmacies and supermarkets in the United States. Several plant species are used in "Ginseng" preparations. *Panax ginseng* is indigenous to China, Japan, and Korea. American Ginseng, *Panax quinequefolius,* grows in the Eastern United States and is cultivated for local use and export. Ginseng species contain a family of glycosylated steroids, ginsenosides. Siberian Ginseng, *Eleutherococccus senticosus,* is an unrelated species that does not contain ginsenosides. Reported in vitro and animal effects include hypertension, hypotension, antithrombotic, thrombogenic, improved memory, improved psychomotor effect, adrenocortical stimulation, alterations in glucose metabolism, as well as androgenic and estrogen effects. Other studies indicate no effect on the same systems. These inconsistent findings may be explained by variation in gensenoside composition and content between species and samples. Many studies and clinical reports include the chemically distinct Siberian Ginseng extract. Some "street" samples of commercial Ginseng products contain no Ginseng at all or a substitute, Chinese silk vine (*Periploca sepium*). The Ginseng abuse syndrome, a constellation of hypertension, nervousness, diarrhea, and dermatitis occurred in 10% of users in an uncontrolled, self-reported case series. Isolated hypertension is also reported. Other reported adverse effects include mastalgia and postmenopausal vaginal bleeding. Neonatal androgenization from maternal use of Siberian Ginseng has been reported. However subsequent lot analysis suggest the product may have in fact contained Chinese silk vine. Yohimbine, derived from the African *Pausinystalia yohimbe* tree, is an alpha-2 blocker that is efficacious in some forms of impotence. It is marketed as a natural aphrodisiac and vitalizing agent. Overdose produces hypertension and anxiety. The hypertensive response may be greater in combination with tricyclic antidepressants. Atrial fibrillation has been reported. Licorice root, derived from Glycerrhiza spp, is widely used in herbal preparations. Glycyrrhezenic acid, contained in licorice root, is a potent inhibitor of renal 11-beta-hydroxysteroid dehydrogenase. Inhibition of this enzyme blocks conversion of cortisol to cortisone; Cortisol, a more potent mineralocorticoid, accumulates. Clinical effects include sodium and water retention, hypoglycemia and hypertension. Hypokalemic myopathy with weakness or paralysis may occur in chronic users.

B.   **Hypoglycemia, hyperthyroidism, and glucocorticoid excess.** Many Asians use Karela (*Momordica charantia*) for its hypoglycemic effect. Hypoglycemia is possible when used in combination with an oral hypoglycmic agent. Kelp, a food stable in the orient, is an herbal constituent touted to promote weight loss. However, the large iodine content of kelp has resulted in thyrotoxicosis. Individuals with underlying thyroid dysfunction should use kelp products with caution. Herbal products used for arthritis or asthma are commonly adulterated with corticosteroids. Typically, patients have a dramatic clinical response prior to the onset of adverse symptoms related to the steroids.

VII.   **Renal insufficiency.** Herb-induced nephrotoxicity generally occurs in the setting of multi-organ system failure or volume depletion. Adulteration with NSAIDs is common and has produced renal failure. Rhabdomyolysis and renal failure occur after ingestion of hemlock, usually consumed by the uninitiated herb forager.

A. **Chinese herbs nephropathy.** Between 1990 and 1992, more than 80 cases of herb-induced renal failure occurred in Belgium. Most patients attended a single weight loss clinic which was distributing pills containing a mixture of Chinese herbs. Prior to the epidemic, the manufacturer altered the pill content, allegedly by adding *Stephania tetrandra* and *Magnolia officinalis*. However, analysis of toxic specimens did not reveal alkaloids characteristic of Stephania tetrandra. Aristolochic acid, a nephrotoxin found in Fangchi (*Aristolochia clematis*) but not in Fangji (Stephania spp.) was isolated from herbal products. Thus, the accidental or intentional use of *Aristolochia clematis* is believed to be responsible for these cases of renal failure. The course of renal failure from Chinese herbs nephropathy is progressive, resulting in end stage disease over a period of months. The histological pattern resembles Balkan nephropathy. Interestingly, aristolochic acid had been implicated as a possible cause of Balkan nephropathy.

VIII. **Hematological abnormalities.** Many herbs contain natural coumarins or exert antiplatelet effects in vitro or in vivo. Indeed, the anticoagulant effect of coumarin was discovered when cattle developed a hemorrhagic illness from consumption of spoiled sweet clover. A clinical bleeding diathesis from herb use is rare but is reported. *Salvia miltiorrhiza* (Danshen), used in Chinese medicines, inhibits warfarin elimination, prolonging prothrombin times. Many topical preparations contain methyl salicylate (oil of wintergreen), which is absorbed through the skin and inhibits platelet function. Most serious hematological toxicity is a result of product contamination or adulteration. Chinese medications used for arthritis or pain relief, are frequently adulterated with NSAIDs. Sporadic cases of agranulocytosis from phenylbutazone and aminopyrine are reported. Warfarin contamination has also been reported. Unexplained anemia, especially in the presence of GI or neurological symptoms should raise suspicion of lead poisoning.

IX. **Allergic reactions.** Plant allergens in topical and oral herbal medications are responsible for contact dermatitis and systemic allergic reactions. Reports of anaphylaxis to plants in the Compososatea family, including Chamomile, dandelion, and Artemisa, are widely cited. Any herb of the Compositea family is potentially sensitizing. Bonesetters' disease, a contact dermatitis, is caused by application of an herbal mixture near fracture sites. It may be caused by Myrrh, a component in many Chinese medications.

X. **Heavy metal poisoning associated with herbal products.** Lead, mercury and arsenic contamination and toxicity have frequently been associated with herbal or alternative remedies. In many cases the metal is considered an integral component of the product; contamination of otherwise nontoxic products also occurs. A recent investigation of the metal content of traditional Asian remedies noted that 64% contained lead or mercury and 41% contained arsenic. Surma, a paste predominantly of lead sulfide (85%) has been used in India to preserve and enhance eyesight and for cosmetic purposes. Many cases of toxicity have occurred. Azarcon (lead tetroxide) and Greta (lead oxide) are Mexican remedies for diarrhea. Hmong refugees from Laos use a lead containing traditional remedy (paylooah) for fever in children.

XI. **General management.** Initial steps should follow the standard approach of airway management, stabilization, and GI decontamination. Activated charcoal is indicated for most ingestions, unless the product is known to be nontoxic or unresponsive to charcoal. Consider whole bowel irrigation when consumption of a product containing heavy metal is suspected. Also consider skin decontamination for those harvesting or handling herbal products and those who present with dermal manifestations of poisoning. The possibility of pesticide contamination should likewise be considered. Evaluating a patient with suspected or known herbal poisoning can be daunting. Thousands of potential toxins exist. Above all, a high index of suspicion must be maintained. Identifying the organ systems most affected may help to narrow the list of possible agents. Obtain an electrocardiogram in those exhibiting any systemic toxicity or hemodynamic instability, or after potentially toxic ingestion of known cardiotixic products. Cardiac glycosides are present in many plants. Obtain a digoxin level when signs or symptoms of glycoside toxicity are present. Obtain serum electrolytes, a CBC, liver enzyme tests, coagulation studies, and an arterial blood gas (ABG) for signs of systemic toxicity. The use of toxicology screens should be directed by the clinical toxidrome. Do not dismiss the possibility of coingestion or contamination toxicity from more traditional substances of abuse or misuse. Serum, urine, or product screening for a potential toxin after asymptomatic ingestion of an unknown herbal product is probably unwarranted. Likewise, known specimens producing expected toxicity will not generally require body fluid analysis. For suspected toxicity from an unidentified product, or when the degree of toxicity is out of proportion to the quantity of toxin ingested, qualitative and quantitative analysis should be conducted. Consider heavy metal analysis for patients with suggestive symptomatology, particularly those who chronically ingest Asian herbal preparations. The local poison control center and public health authorities should be informed whenever product contamination, adulteration, or heavy metal poisoning is considered.

References

1. Eisenberg DM, Kessler RC, Foster C. Unconventional medicine in the United States: prevalence, cost and patterns of use. *N Engl J Med* 1993;328:246–252.
2. Frate DA, Croom EM, Frate JB. Self treatment with herbal and other plant-derived remedies: rural Mississippi 1993. *MMWR* 1995;44:204–207.
3. Kestin M, Miller L, Littlejohn G. The use of unproven remedies for rheumatoid arthritis in Australia. *Med J Aust* 1985; 143:516–518.
4. Verhoef MJ, Sutherland LR, Brkich L. Use of alternative medicine by patients attending a gastroenterology clinic. *Can Med Assoc J* 1990;142:121–125.
5. Pearl WS, Leo P, Tsang WO. Use of Chinese therapies among Chinese patients seeking emergency department care. *Ann Emerg Med* 1995;26:735–738.
6. Cassidy DE, Drewry J, Fanning JP. Podophyllum toxicity: a report of a fatal case and a review of the literature. *J Toxicol Clin Toxicol* 1982;19:35–44.
7. Wei-Fong Kao, Dong-Zong Hung, Wei-Jen Tsai. Podophyllotoxin intoxication: toxic effect of bajiaolian in herbal therapeutics. *Hum Exp Toxicol* 1992;11:480–487.
8. Kowalchik C, Hylton WH, eds. *Rodale's Illustrated encyclopedia of herbs.* Emmaus, PA: Rodale Press, 1987.
9. Keys JD. *Chinese herbs: their botany, chemistry and pharmacodynamics.* Rutland, Vermont: Charles E Tuttle Co., 1976.
10. Pui-Hay P. Herbal poisoning caused by adulterants or erroneous substitutes. *J Trop Med Hyg* 1994;1997:371–374.
11. Sullivan JB, Rumack BH, Thomas H. Pennyroyal oil poisoning and hepatotoxicity. *JAMA* 1979;242:2873–2874.
12. Watson AR, Coovadia HM, Boola KD. The clinical syndrdome of Impila *(Callipelis laureola)* poisoning in children. *S Afr Med J* 1979;55:290–292.
13. Gold CH. Acute renal failure from herbal and patent remedies in blacks. *Clin Nephrol* 14;1980:129–134.
14. Larrey D, Pageux GP. Hepatotoxicity of herbal remedies and mushrooms. *Semin Liver Dis* 1995;15:183–188.
15. Chan TY, Tomlinson B, Tse LK, Chan JC. Aconite poisoning due to Chinese herbal medicines: a review. *Vet Hum Toxicol* 1994;36:452–455.
16. Tai YT, But PP, Young. Adverse effects from traditional Chinese medicine. *Lancet* 1993;341:892.

17. Kapoor S. Cardiovascular aspects of aconite poisoning in human beings. *Indian Heart J* 1969;21:329–338.

18. Tai Y, But P, Young K. Cardiotoxicity aftter accidental herb-induced aconite poisoning. *Lancet* 1992;340:1254–1256.

19. Clark RF, Selden BS, Curry SC, Digoxin-specific Fab fragments in the treatment of oleander toxicity in a canine model. *Ann Emerg Med* 1991;20:1073–1077.

20. Safadi R, Levy I, Amitai Y, Caraco Y. Beneficial effect of digoxin-specific Fab antibody fragments in Oleander intoxication. *Arch Intern Med* 1995;155:2121–2125.

21. Rich SA, Libera JM, Locke RJ. Treatment of foxglove extract poisoning with digoxin-specific Fab fragments. *Ann Emerg Med* 1993;22:1904–1907.

22. Brubacher J, Hoffman RS, Bania T. Deaths associated with a purported aphrodisiac—New York City, February 1993 to May 1995. *MMWR* 1995;44:853–855,861.

23. Radford DJ, Gillies AD, Hinds JA. Naturally occurring cardiac glycosides. *Med J Aust* 1986;144:540–543.

24. Longrich L, Johnson E, Gault MH. Digoxin-like factors in herbal teas. *Clin Invest Med* 1993;16:210–218.

25. Huxtable RJ. The harmful potential of herbal and other plant products. *Drug Safety* 1990;5:126–136.

26. Datta DV, Khuroo MS. Mattocks AR. Herbal medicines and veno-occlusive disease in India. *Postgrad Med J* 1978; 54:511–515.

27. Lyford CL, Vergara CG, Moeller DD. Hepatic veno-occlusive disease originating in Ecuador. *Gastroenterology* 1976; 70:105–108.

28. Bach N, Thung SN, Schaffer F. Comfrey herb tea–induced hepatic veno-occlusive disease. *Am J Med* 1989;87:97–99.

29. Koumana CR, Ng M, Lin HJ. Hepatic veno-occlusive disease due to toxic alkaloid in herbal tea. *Lancet* 1982;2: 1360–1361.

30. Huxtable RJ, Awang DVC, Ridker PM. Pyrrolizidine poisoning. *Am J Med* 1990;89:547–548.

31. Anonymous. Chaparral-induced toxic hepatitis—California and Texas, 1992. *MMWR* 1992;41:812–814.

32. Larrey D, Vial T, Pauwels A. Hepititis after Germander *(Teucrium chamaedrys)* administration—another instance of herbal medicine hepatotoxicity. *Ann Intern Med* 1992;117:129–132.

33. Itoh S. Marutani K. Nishijima T. Matsuo S. Liver injuries induced by herbal medicine, *syo-saiko-to (xiao-chai-hu-tang).* *Dig Dis Sci* 1995;40:1845–1848.

34. Kane JA, Kane SP, Jain S. Hepatitis induced by traditional Chinese herbs: possible toxic components. *Gut* 1995;36: 146–147.

35. Miskelly FG, Goodyer LI. Hepatic and pulmonary complications of herbal medicines. *Postgrad Med J* 1992;68:935–936.

36. MacGregor FB, Abernethy VE, Dahabra S. Hepatotoxicity of herbal remedies. *BMJ* 1989;299:1156–1157.

37. Graham-Brown R. Toxicity of Chinese herbal remedies. *Lancet* 1992;340:673.

38. Perharic-Walton L, Murray V. Toxicity of Chinese herbal remedies. *Lancet* 1992;340:674.

39. Pillans PI, Eade MN, Massey RJ. Herbal medicine and toxic hepatitis. *NZ Med J* 1994;107:432–433.

40. Cheng KC, Lee HM, Shum SF, Yip CP. A fatality due to the use of cantharides from *Mylabris phalerata* as an abortifacient. *Med Sci Law* 1990;30:336–340.

41. Perron AD, Patterson JA, Yanofsky NN. Kombucha "mushroom" hepatotoxicity. *Ann Emerg Med* 1995;26:660–661.

42. Keen RW, Deacon AC, Delves HT. Indian herbal remedies for diabetes as a cause of lead poisoning. *Postgrad Med J* 1994;70:113–114.

43. Woolf GM, Petrovic LM, Rojter SE. Acute hepatitis associated with the Chinese herbal product *Jin Bu Huan. Ann Intern Med* 1994;121:729–735.

44. CDC. *Jin Bu Huan* toxicity in children—Colorado 1993. *MMWR* 1993;42:633–636.

45. Harvey J, Colin-Jones DG. Mistletoe hepatitis. *BMJ* 1981;282:186–187.

46. Saxe TG. Toxicity of medicinal herbal preparations. *Am Fam Physician* 1987;35:135–142.

47. Kassler WJ, Blanc P, Greenblatt R. The use of medicinal herbs by human immunodeficiency virus-infected patients. *Arch Intern Med* 1991;151:2281–2288.

48. Roberge R, Brader E, Martin M. The root of evil—pokeweed intoxication. *Ann Emerg Med* 1986;15:470–473.

49. Meggs WJ, Weisman R, Hoffman RS. Anticholinergic poisoning associated with an herbal tea—New York City 1994. *JAMA* 1995;273:1166–1167.

50. Chan TYK. Anticholinergic poisoning due to Chinese herbal medicines. *Vet Hum Toxicol* 1995;37:156–157.

51. Siegel RK. Ginseng abuse syndrome: problems with the panacea. *JAMA* 1979;241:1614–1615.

52. Greenspan EM. Ginseng and vaginal bleeding. *JAMA* 1983;249:2018.

53. Jones BD, Runkings AM. Interaction of ginseng with phenelzine. *J Clin Psychopharmacol* 1987;7:201–202.

54. Perharic L, Shaw D, Murray V. An appeal to pharmacists to report adverse effects of herbal and vitamin products. *Pharm J* 1994;252:479.

55. Koren G, Randor S, Margin S. Maternal ginseng use associated with neonatal androgenization. *JAMA* 1990;264:2866.

56. Awang DV. Maternal use of ginseng and neonatal androgenization. *JAMA* 1991;265:1828.

57. Awang DV. Maternal use of ginseng and neonatal androgenization. *JAMA* 1991;266:363.

58. Bahrke MS, Morgan WP. Evaluation of the ergogenic properties of ginseng [Review]. *Sports Med* 1994;18:229–248.

59. Caradonna P, Gentilon N, Servidei S. Acute myopathy associated with chronic licorice ingestion: reversible loss of myoadenylate deaminase activity. *Ultrastruct Pathol* 1992;16:529–535.

60. Farese R, Biglieri E, Shackleton C. Licorice-induced hypermineralocorticoidism. *N Engl J Med* 1991;325:1223–1227.
61. Cumming AA, Boddy K, Brown JJ. Severe hypokalemia with paralysis induced by small doses of liquorice. *Postgrad Med J* 1980;56:526–529.
62. DeSmet P, Smeets O. Potential risks of health food products containing yohimbine extracts. *BMJ* 1994;309:958.
63. Anonymous. Drug points: overdose of yohimbine. *BMJ* 1992;304:548.
64. Capobianco DJ, Brazis PW, Fox TP. Proxmial-muscle weakness induced by herbs. *N Engl J Med* 1993;329:1430.
65. Aslam MO, Stockley IH. Interaction between curry ingredient (kerla) and drug (chlorpropramide). *Lancet* 1979;1:607.
66. Leatherdale BA, Panesan RK, Singh G. Improvement in glucose tolerance due to *Mormordica charantia* (Kerla). *BMJ* 1981;282:1823–1824.
67. Skare S, Hirsch HJ. Iodine-induced thyrotoxicity in apparently normal thyroid glands. *Acta Endocrinol* 1980:94:332–336.
68. Shilo S, Hirsch HJ. Iodine-induced hyperthyroidism in a patient with a normal thyroid gland. *Postgrad Med J* 1986;62:661–662.
69. Joseph AM, Bitts T, Garr M. Stealth steroids. *N Engl J Med* 1991;324:62.
70. Forster PJ, Calverley M, Hubball S. *Chuei-Fong-Tou-Geu-Wan* in rheumatoid arthritis. *BMJ* 1979;2:308.
71. Rubin BK, Legatt DF, Audette RJ. The Mexican asthma cure: systemic steroids for gullible gringos. *Chest* 1990;97:959–961.
72. Abt AB, Oh JY, Huntington RA. Chinese herbal medicine induces acute renal failure. *Arch Intern Med* 1995;155:211–212.
73. Van Ypersele de Strihou C, Vanherwghem JL. The tragic paradigm of Chinese herbs nephropathy. *Nephrol Dial Transplant* 1995;10:157–160.
74. Vanherweghem JL, Depierreux CT, Abramowicz D. Rapidly progressive interstital renal fibrosis in young women: association with slimming regimen including Chinese herbs. *Lancet* 1993;341:387–391.
75. Rizzi D, Basile C, DiMaggio A, Sebastio A, Introna F, Rizzi R, Scatizzi A, DeMarco S, Smialek JE. Clinical spectrum of accidental hemlock poisoning—neurotoxic manifestations, rhabdomyolyis and acute tubular-necrosis. *Nephrol Dial Transplant* 1991;6:939–943.
76. Hogan RP. Hemorrhagic diathesis caused by drinking and herbal tea. *JAMA* 1983;249:2679–2680.
77. Tam LS, Chan TY, Leung WK. Warfarin interactions with Chinese traditional medicines: danshen and methyl salicylate medicated oil. *Aust NZ J Med* 1995;25:258.
78. Nelson L, Shih R, Hoffman R. Aplastic anemia induced by an adulterated herbal medication. *J Toxicol Clin Toxicol* 1995;33:467–470.
79. Ries CA, Sahud MA. Agranulocytosis caused by Chinese herbal medicines. *JAMA* 1975;231:352–355.
80. Lightfoot J, Blair HJ, Cohen JR. Lead intoxication in an adult caused by Chinese herbal medication. *JAMA* 1977;238:1539.
81. Bruynzeel DP, van Ketel WG, Young E. Contact sensitization by alternative topical medicaments containing plant extracts. *Contact Dermatitis* 1992;27:278.
82. Lee TY, Ham TH. Myrrh is the putative allergen in bonesetters herbs dermatitis. *Contact Dermatitis* 1993;29:279.
83. Arnold WN. Vincent Van Gough and the thujone connection. *JAMA* 1988;260:3042–3044.
84. Edison M, Philen RM, Sewell CM. L-Tryptohan and the eosinophillia-myalgia syndrome in New Mexico. *Lancet* 1990;335:645–648.
85. Jackson B, Reed A. Catnip and the alteration of consciousness. *JAMA* 1969;207:1349–1350.
86. FDA. Warning issued about street drugs containing botanical sources of ephedrine. *JAMA* 1996;275:1534.
87. Levitt C, Paulson D, Duval K, Folk remedy–associated lead poisoning in Hmong children—Minnesota. *MMWR* 1983;32:555–556.
88. Holtan N, Hall S, Knight F. Nonfatal arsenic poisoning in three Hmong patients—Minnesota. *MMWR* 1984;33:347–349.
89. Baker D, Brender J, Davis KC. Cadmium and lead exposure associated with pharmaceuticals imported from Asia—Texas. *MMWR* 1989;38:612–614.
90. Smitherman J, Harber P. A case of mistaken identity: herbal medicine as a cause of lead toxicity. *Am J Ind Med* 1991;20:795–798.
91. Perharic L, Shaw D, Colbridge M. Toxicologic problems resulting from exposure to traditional remedies and food supplements. *Drug Safety* 1994;11:284–294.
92. Tse CY, Chin DKF, Teoh R. Poisoning by Chinese herbs. *J Hong Kong Med Assoc* 1989;41:177–178.
93. Baker S, Thomas PS. Herbal medicine precipitating massive haemolysis. *Lancet* 1987;1:1039–1040.
94. Capwell RR. Ephedrine-induced mania from an herbal diet supplement. *Am J Psychiatry* 1995;152:647.
95. Jaffe AM, Gephardt D, Courtemanche L. Poisoning due to ingestion of *Veratrum viride* (false hellebore). *J Emerg Med* 1990;8:161–167.
96. Hammerschmidt DE. Szechwan purpura. *N Engl J Med* 1980;302:1191–1193.
97. Norcross WA, Ganiats TG, Ralph LP. Accidental poisoning by warfarin-containing herbal tea. *West J Med* 1993;159:80–82.

 98. Gorey JD, Wahlquist ML, Boyce NW. Adverse reaction to a Chinese herbal remedy. *Med J Aust* 1992;157:484–486.
 99. Siegel RK. Herbal intoxication: psychoactive effects from herbal cigarettes, tea and capsules. *JAMA* 1976;236:473–476.
100. Ridker PM. Health hazard of unusual herbal teas. *Am Fam Physician* 1989;39:153–156.
101. D'Arcy PF. Adverse reactions and interactions with herbal medicines. Part 1. Adverse reactions. *Adverse Drug React Toxicol Rev* 1991;10:189–208.
102. D'Arcy PF. Adverse reactions and interactions with herbal medicines. Part 2. Drug interactions. *Adverse Drug React Toxicol Rev* 1993;12:147–162.

Emergency Toxicology, Second Edition,
edited by Peter Viccellio.
Lippincott–Raven Publishers, Philadelphia © 1998.

86

Differential Diagnosis of Poisonings

Howard C. Mofenson

*Department of Emergency Medicine, Long Island Regional Poison Control Center, Winthrop
University Hospital, Mineola, New York 11501*

The manifestations of poisonings are listed by systems in this chapter. The inspection portion of the physical examination (skin changes and odors) and vital functions are presented first because they are the first encountered. The manner of presentation is to briefly describe the pathophysiology, medical conditions that produce the manifestations, and the toxic substances, usually in an alphabetical list, that have been reported to produce the manifestation. An asterisk indicates that the substance is more frequently involved in producing the manifestation.

INSPECTION OF THE PATIENT

   I.   **Odor** (1–7). The sense of smell functions as a warning of environmental hazards, but it is not a reliable early warning in most instances. The odor on the patient's breath, from the gastric contents and other body excretions, may give an **important clue to the identity of the substance.** The odor may be the same as the substance itself or indicate a metabolite. On the other hand, **the odor does not indicate that that substance is the cause of the patient's condition.** For example, the odor of ethanol on the breath may be noted in a comatose patient, when a head injury is the etiology of the coma. Odors may also be obscured and not detected by certain genetic inabilities to detect certain odors. About 45% to 50% of the general population cannot detect the odor of cyanide.

   A.   **Medical conditions** that cause disorders of smell include chronic diseases, endocrinopathies (Addison's disease, Cushing's syndrome, diabetes mellitus, hypothyroidism, pseudohyperparathyroidism, Turner's syndrome, and Kallmann's syndrome—anosmia and hypogonadism), infections (hepatitis, influenza, meningitis), local lesions (adenoid hypertrophy, allergic rhinitis, cocaine insufflation, nasal polyposis (cystic fibrosis, aspirin), neurosis and psychosis, sinusitis, Sjogren-Larsen's syndrome, multiple sclerosis, nutritional deficiencies (vitamin B_{12} deficiency, zinc deficiency), and temporal lobe epilepsy. Androsterone in underarm secretion has a woody smell of urine. Some of the medical conditions with specific aromas are listed in Table 86-1. The inborn errors of metabolism that produce specific odors are listed in Table 86-2.

   B.   **Odors as clues to intoxications.** The following are different odors and their potential agents or conditions.

   1.   *Acetone.* Acetone, chloral hydrate, isopropanol, metabolic acidosis (salicylate, diabetic and alcoholic ketoacidosis, and other causes).

   2.   *Airplane glue* (aromatic). Ethchlorvynol, toluene, aromatic hydrocarbon inhalation.

TABLE 86-1. *Common medical conditions and aromas*

Medical condition	Aroma
Ammonia-like	Uremia
Beer-like	Scrofula (tuberculosis)
Fruity	Diabetic and alcoholic ketoacidosis
Fresh-baked brown bread	Typhoid fever
Putrid	Scurvy, anaerobic infections
Sweetish	Diphtheria

3. *Alcohol.* Ethanol (no alcohol odor with ethylene glycol or vodka). The odor of ethanol may be a red herring; exclude other causes of coma.

4. *Ammonia.* Ammonia or uremia.

5. *Bitter almonds* (the odor of silver polish, not detectable by 50% of population). Cyanide cyanogenic plants.

6. *Bleach* (hypochlorite). Hypochlorite.

7. *Carrots.* Cicutoxin of water hemlock.

8. *Coal gas.* Carbon monoxide is odorless but mixed with illuminating gas for detection.

9. *Disinfectants.* Creosote, phenol.

10. *Formaldehyde.* Formaldehyde, methanol.

11. *Foul* (**unpleasant**). Bromides, foreign body in orifice, lithium.

12. *Hay (newly mown).* Low-level phosgene.

13. *Hemp (burnt rope).* Marijuana.

14. *Garlic.* Arsenic, dimethylsulfoxide (DMSO), malathion, parathion, yellow phosphorous, selenium, tellurium, zinc phosphide.

15. *Mothballs.* Camphor, naphthalene, paradichlorobenzene.

16. *Peanuts.* Rodenticide: Vacor (now banned).

17. *Pears.* Chloral hydrate, paraldehyde.

18. *Rotten eggs.* Disulfiram, hydrogen sulfide, hepatic failure, mercaptans, *N*-acetylcysteine.

19. *Shoe polish.* Nitrobenzene.

20. *Violets (urine specimen).* Turpentine.

21. *Vinegar.* Acetic acid (some photograph film developer fluid is glacial acetic acid).

TABLE 86-2. *Inborn errors of metabolism with abnormal odor*

Inborn error	Urine and body odor
β-Methycrotonyl glycemia	Tomcat urine
Glutaric acidemia type II	Sweaty feet
Isovaleric acidemia	Sweaty feet
Maple syrup urine disease	Maple syrup
Methionine malabsorption	Cabbage
Phenylketonuria	Mousy or musty
Trimethylaminuria	Rotting fish
Tyrosinemia	Rancid
Oasthouse disease	Hoplike (beer)
Hawkinsinuria	Swimming pool

Data from *Nelson's textbook of pediatrics.* 1992.

22. ***Vinyl shower curtain.*** Ethchlorvynol.
23. ***Wintergreen.*** Methylsalicylate.
24. ***White paste.*** Phenol.

II. **Dermatology** (8–21)

A. **The appearance** of the skin may be a clue to the nature of the exposure. In California, which has the most comprehensive reporting of occupational diseases, skin diseases accounted for 40% of reported occupational diseases, and 70% of these diseases was due to external contact.

B. **Percutaneous absorption** occurs readily by lipophilic substances, including some organophosphates and polychlorinated biphenyls, but is much slower by hydrophilic substances. **Substances are absorbed 40 times faster from the scrotum than from the forearm.** Solubility and pH do influence absorption. Plastic occlusive dressing enhances absorption. Solubility and pH influence absorption. Examples of intoxications caused by topical applications include the following:

1. Boric acid absorbed through inflamed and denuded skin has caused seizures, renal impairment, and epidermolysis in infants (13).
2. Lidocaine as Xylocaine 2% is absorbed through mucosa, resulting in seizures, dysrhythmias, and death.
3. Lindane (Kwell) improperly applied has caused seizures (10,11).
4. Potent corticosteroid topical preparations have suppressed adrenal function.
5. Glycol in gauze pads has led to metabolic acidosis.
6. Promethazine (Phenergan 2% Cream) caused neurologic manifestations.
7. Diphenhydramine (Caladryl) has produced toxic encephalopathy (8,9).
8. TAC (Cocaine 11%) misapplied to mucosa has produced seizures and death.
9. Aniline dyes stamps on diapers caused methemoglobinemia (19).
10. Hexachlorophene skin application caused vacuolization of the brain in premature neonates (14,15).
11. Pentachlorophenol caused toxic syndrome of profuse diaphoresis, fever, tachycardia, and tachypnea (16,17), and hyperbilirubinemia (18).
12. Isopropyl alcohol caused intoxication in alcohol sponging (12).
13. DEET, diethyltoluamide, misused on the skin of children, can produce encephalopathy and death (20,21).

C. **Toxic skin reactions** (22–25)

1. **Contact dermatitis irritative.** Local reversible inflammation to a single application without immunologic response. It is not as severe as allergic dermatitis. When contact is discontinued, rash resolves spontaneously in 1 to 3 weeks. Children under 8 years of age are more susceptible. Irritant dermatitis is insidious in onset.

   a. **Common irritants in the home and workplace**

      (1) **Home products.** Bleaches, copper and metal brighteners, detergents, drain cleaners, fertilizers, furniture polishes, oven cleaners, pesticides, pet shampoos, rug shampoos, scouring pads and powders; soaps, toilet bowl and window cleaners.

      (2) **Workplace substances.** Acids and alkali, benzoic acid, cleaning products, epoxy resins, foams (insulation foams), non–carbon-required paper, powders (aluminum, carbon silicate, cement, cleaning agents, metallic

oxides), particles (ore particles in mining, plant particles, plastics, sawdust, wool), volatile substances (ammonia, formaldehyde, organic solvents).

2. **Corrosion—direct chemical action ulceration and necrosis.** Acids coagulate skin proteins, and alkali remove surface lipids. Causes include hydrofluoric acid, ethylene oxide, cement, and alkyl mercury products.

3. **Phototoxicity—occurs on sun-exposed areas.** The skin lesions are macular and nonpruritic. *Ultraviolet light (UV-A) light* of the wave length of 315 to 400 nanometers is involved.

   a. Phototoxicity may be induced by molecular changes in the skin, and the **inducers** include 6-methylcoumarin (methoxypsorben), polyaromatic, hydrocarbons (anthracene, acridine, phenanthrene) after shave lotions with musk ambrette; medications (chlorpromazine, coumarin derivatives; nalidixic acid, phenothiazines, sulfonamides, sulfonylureas, tetracycline and thiazide diuretics); sunscreen compounds (*p*-aminobenzoic acid).

   b. **Phototoxic dermatitis** must be **differentiated** from xeroderma pigmentosum, porphyria, systemic lupus erythematosus, pellagra, dermatomyositis, and allergic contact dermatitis.

4. **Allergic contact responses.** About 30% of occupational skin disease is allergic. Allergens are haptens of less than 500 Daltons. Irritative and allergic dermatitis may coexist. In a sensitized person, inflammation begins about 12 h after exposure and peaks in about 50 h and may last 4 days to several weeks (usually about 14 to 21 days). If the entire skin is involved, it is called **exfoliative dermatitis.** Cross-reactivity with similar substances may occur. Common allergens include the following:

   a. Metals, including nickel, chromium, cobalt, and organomercurials, but other metals are not sensitizers.

   b. Plant sensitizers, including toxidendron genus, composite family, and *Primula obvconia.*

   c. Rubber additives, antioxidants, and polymerization accelerators—mercaptobenzthiazide, thiuram, *p*-phenylenediamine (used in rubber industry), resorcinol.

   d. Epoxy oligomer.

   e. Methyl methacrylate and other acrylics.

   f. Formaldehyde.

   g. Topical medications—neomycin, benzocaine.

   h. *p*-Aminophenol and hydroquinone in photographic film developers.

   i. Germicides—formaldehyde-releasing compounds, paraben, quaternary ammonium compounds.

   j. Grains—barley, oat, rye, wheat.

   k. Fragrances and perfumes—balsam of Peru, Benzyl alcohol, cinnamic acid, citronella derivatives.

   l. Plastic resins epoxide, formaldehyde-based acrylics, phenolic compounds.

D. **Differences between irritant dermatitis and allergic dermatitis** are listed in Table 86-3. Common allergic dermatitis groups are listed in Table 86-4.

TABLE 86-3. *Irritant and allergic dermatitis*

Irritant dermatitis	Allergic dermatitis
Less pruritus	Extensive pruritus
Insidious onset	Abrupt onset
Exposed areas	Unexposed and exposed areas
More erythema	More vesiculation

E. **Cutaneous reaction patterns**
   1. **Chemical acne or chloracne.** There are about 4,000 cases worldwide. Onset is typically *delayed 2 to 4 weeks* after exposure. The pathology is involves replacement of atrophic sebaceous glands with keratin filled cysts. The morphology consists of dry skin with comedones, straw-colored cysts, milia, papules and, if all follicles involved, bizarre "**pebbled appearance.**" Chloracne usually regresses over 4 to 6 months, but a few cases have lasted 30 years. Table 86-5 indicates its distinction from acne.
      a. Compounds that **can cause chloracne** include polyhalogenated dibenzofurans, polychlorinated dibenzodioxins (2,3,7,8-tetrachlorodibenzo-*p*-dioxin) associated with elevated porphyrin excretion, hyperpigmentation, hypertrichosis changes in lipid metabolism, and hepatic effects. Epidemic occurred in Japan "rice-oil disease," in Taiwan, and in Seveso, Italy. Other compounds that cause chloracne include polychlornaphthalene, polychlorobiphenyls (PCBs), polybrominated biphenyls (PBBs), pentachlorophenol, azobenzenes, azoxybenenes.
   2. **Fiberglass physical dermatitis** associated with fibers of more than 4.5 μm and extensive pruritis. Microscopic examination of the skin may reveal the fibers.
   3. **Urticarial reactions.** Urticaria occurs in 15% to 23% of the general population (38). Contact urticarial reactions are wheal and flare (hives) reactions that occurs immediately to 30 to 60 min after direct exposure and disappear within 24 h. The causes include animal products (danders, hair, saliva), chemicals (ammonia, alcohol, paraben, polyethylene glycol), cosmetics (hair products, nail polish, perfumes), foods, medications (bacitracin, cephalosporins, chloramphenicol, gentamicin, neomycin, salicylic acid)
      a. **Chronic urticaria** is daily or almost daily for 6 weeks (38). For features of chronic urticaria, see Table 86-6.
      b. **Immunologic.** IgE-mediated mainly by histamines released by the mast cells in persons previously sensitized and activation of the complement cascade and systemic effects may occur.

TABLE 86-4. *Common allergic dermatitis groups*

Irritant dermatitis	Allergic dermatitis
Aromatic amines	Hydroxyquinoline
Benzothiazides	Phenolic compounds
Caine-type anesthetics	Phenothiazines
Ethylenediamine compounds	Streptomycin group of antibiotics
Halogenated genocides	Thiurans

TABLE 86-5. *Differential of chloracne and acne vulgaris*

Chloracne		Acne vulgaris
Age not specific	age	13–26 years
face (crow's feet and malar crescent below and outside eyes), neck, earlobes, shoulders, abdomen, legs, buttocks and genitalia	Site	central-face, chest, back and chest
dry skin with comedones, straw colored cysts, milia, papules and if all follicles involved bizarre "pebbled appearance"	Morphology	oily skin, comadones, papules, pustules and scars

    c. **Nonimmunologic** (release of vasoactive substances bradykinins, histamines and other inflammatory mediators) produced by acids (acetic, benzoic, cinnamic, sorbic), alcohols (ethyl, butyl), balsam of peru, benzocaine, cold temperatures, cobalt chloride, dimethylsulfoxide (DMSO), formaldehyde, witch hazel, sodium benzoate, esters of nicotinic acid.

4. **Cutaneous granulomas** are a foreign body reaction to talc, silica, beryllium (which is immunologic), zirconium, and chromium salts in tattoos.

5. **Pigmentary changes**

    a. **Hypopigmentation** is usually due to damage to melanocyte or interference with melanin synthesis by compounds that contain tyrosine (a building block of melanin). It takes 2 to 4 weeks and may take up to 6 months to become visible. Loss of skin melanin is detected by failure to fluoresce under Wood's light. It is indistinguishable from **vitiligo** clinically, which affects 1% of the general population and may be associated with autoimmune and endocrine abnormalities. **The common compounds** include the following:

        (1) **Phenols.** Benzylchlorphenol (antiseptic, butylphenol (varnish, lacquers, antioxidant, in soaps), creosol (disinfectant), hydroxyconiine (photo-processing, skin lighteners, antioxidants in synthetic rubber industry), phenylphenol (fungicide, disinfectant, rubber industry).

TABLE 86-6. *Features of commonest types of chronic urticaria*

Type of urticaria	Age (years)	Sites and lesions	Angio edema	Diagnostic tests
Idiopathic	20–50	Generalized pink-pale	Yes	—
Symptomatic dermatographism	20–50	Linear wheal, red flare	No	Light stroking of skin, immediate wheal
Physical				
Cold	10–40	Pale or red contact site	Yes	10-min ice pack causes wheal 5 min after removal
Pressure	20–50	Palms, soles,	No	Perpendicular pressure waist lasts 24 h; causes after 1–4 h
Solar site	20–50	Exposure to UV for 290–690 μm	Yes	Irradiation by a 2.5-kW 30–120 causes wheal 30 min
Cholinergic	10–50	Pink wheals on trunk	Yes	Exercise or hot shower

Data from ref. 18.

(2) **Catecholic compounds.** Pyrocatechol (antiseptic), butylcatechol (astringent).

(3) **Burns** (chemical and thermal).

(4) **Arsenic.**

b. **Hyperpigmentation** (melanosis) follows episode of dermatitis or inflammation. UV radiation, causing melanin synthesis, is a frequent cause.

(1) **Hyperpigmentation** can be produced by barbiturates, phenolphthalein (fixed drug reaction), heavy metals (arsenic, silver argyria, bismuth and mercury), 4-aminoquinolones in antimalarial, phenothiazines, tetracycline, busulfan. Topically, it can be caused by creosote and aromatic chlorinated hydrocarbons.

(2) **Differential diagnosis** is birth marks and staining by heavy metals (silver salts), nitrosylated compounds (nitric acid ordinitrophenol), or derivatives of coal distillation.

6. **Cancer.** There are more than 500,000 new nonmelanoma neoplasms (squamous cell, basal cell carcinoma) annually in the United States and 28,000 melanomas. The **incidence of melanoma has increased more than 700% in the past 60 years.** The reasons for this increase may be associated with depletion of the ozone layer. If this rate of cancer continues the risk in a decade for a lifetime could be 1%.

a. **The wave length of skin cancer** is 280 to 315 nanometer of UV-B. The first association between occupational malignancy and environmental chemical was made by Percival Pott in 1775, when he reported scrotal cancer among London chimney sweeps; later the cancer was discovered to be caused by exposure to polycyclic aromatic hydrocarbons.

b. **Other causes of skin cancer** include UV light, ionizing radiation, phenolic compounds, physical trauma and burns, aliphatic hydrocarbons and inorganic arsenic compounds (arsenic in water at 0.05 mg/L). The latent period for skin cancer may be 20 years.

(1) **Inorganic arsenic compounds** initially cause mild erythema and hyperhydrosis of the palms and soles followed by firm symmetrical punctate keratoses. White hyperkeratoses develop on ankles, shins, and dorsum of hands. A diffuse hyperpigmentation with white atrophic macules ("rain drops on a dusty road") may be seen and basal cell or squamous cell carcinoma secondary to arsenic may develop.

(2) **A sunscreen (*p*-aminobenzoic acid derivatives) of 15** allows the person to remain outdoors for 5 h before minimal erythema. Persons of Celtic origin (Scotch, Welsh, or Irish) and those with certain **conditions (albinism, xeroderma pigmentosum, and porphyria)** are at risk for developing skin cancer (Table 86-7).

F. **Skin appearance** (26–45). Asterisk indicates most frequently encountered.

1. **Acneform lesions.** Bromides, corticosteroids, dactinomycin, exposure to greases and oils, heavy cosmetic use, iodides (in kelp tablets), isoniazid, lithium, phenytoin, mechanical (from friction and pressure), polychlorinated or polybrominated biphenyls, TCCD ("dioxin"). Acne medicamentosa from medications (see **E.2**).

TABLE 86-7. *Toxic skin reactions and causes*

Skin toxic reaction	Common causes
Contact dermatitis	
Irritative	Fiberglass, corrosive, soaps
Allergic	Nickel, chromates
Chemical burns	Corrosives acids, alkali, phenols, hydrofluoric acid, phosphorous
Acne	Oils, fats, tars
Chloracne	Dibenzofurans, PCB, dioxin
Pigmentary	Aniline, arsenic, phenol
Cancer	UVL, radiation, arsenic
Hair loss	Thallium, arsenic, radiation

2. **Alopecia hair** (30–34).
    a. **Alopecia** (30–33). Onset and pattern of loss can indicate etiology, e.g., androgenic pattern baldness. Scaring alopecia is caused by physical agents, infection, some dermatologic conditions, and skin neoplasms. Nonscarring by drugs, febrile illness, traction, endocrine, and nutritional.
        (1) **Toxins/drugs.** Alkylating chemotherapeutic agents*, allopurinol*, amiodarone, androgens*, anticoagulants (coumarin, warfarin), antithyroid, arsenic*, beta-adrenergic blockers, bismuth, boric acid, burns, caustics, chloroquine, chloral hydrate, cimetidine, colchicine and autumn crocus*, contraceptives* (oral), coumarin anticoagulants, cytotoxic*, (cyclophosphamide, doxorubicin), melphalan, methotrexate, vinblastine, vincristine), didanosine*, ergot, ethambutol, heavy metals* (especially arsenic, gold, lead, lithium, mercury, thallium*), heparin, hydroxyurea, imipramine, L-dopa, metoprolol (48), paclitaxel, pesticides, phenol, NSAIDs, radiation*, salicylates*, selenium and selenious acid (gun bluing), thallium*, thiouracil, thioglycolates, valproic acid, excess vitamin A* (30–33).
        (2) **Medical illness.** Alopecia areata, ectodermal dysplasia, endocrine (hyperthyroidism, hypopituitarism), lichen planus, lupus erythematosus (systemic and discoid), mechanical, nutritional deficiencies, scleroderma, sarcoidosis, theologian defluvium (psychic stress, rapid weight loss, high fever, parturition and shedding of hair 2 to 4 months later), tinea capitis, trichomania, tumor (basal cell, metastatic).
    b. **Discoloration of hair.** Green from copper, blue from cobalt, yellow from picric acid.
3. **Local skin stains**
    a. **Black.** Chloramphenicol, osmium trioxide, silver salts.
    b. **Brown-yellow local skin stains.** Bromine (yellow), bromides (yellow), chlorine (yellow), chromate (yellow-brown), creosol (brown), dinitrobenzene (yellow), formaldehyde (brown), iodine (brown), nitric acid (yellow-brown), nitrogen oxide (yellow-red), phenol (brown), picric acid (yellow), testryl (yellow), trinitrotoluene (yellow).

    c. **Blue local skin stain.** Methylene blue, oxalic acid.

    d. **Bronze.** Arsenic, arsine.

    e. **Green local skin stain.** Copper salts

4. **Bulla.** Acetylcarbromal (coma), allergic contact dermatitis, barbiturates*, caustics and corrosives, carbon monoxide* (coma), coma (sweat gland necrosis) from neurologic and overdose conditions, dihydrocodeine (coma), epidermolysis bullosa, erythema multiforme bullosa, glutethimide (coma), heroin (coma), imipramine (coma), impetigo (bullous), insect bites, marine injuries, methadone (coma), methaqualone (coma), morphine (coma), nitrazepam (coma), phenobarbital* (coma), phenolphthalein, (fixed drug reaction), snake envenomation, scromboid fish poisoning, sedative-hypnotics* (coma and barbiturates; 6.5% of 200 patients had bulla), thermal burns (35,37).

    a. **Medical bullous skin diseases** include pemphigus (vulgaris, foliaveus, paraneoplastica, pemphgoid), herpes gestationis, epidermolysis bullosa acquistra, dermatitis herpetiformis, chronic bullous dermatosis of childhood, linear IgA dermatosis of adulthood, erythema multiforme minor, erythema multiforme major (Steven-Johnson syndrome; SJS), toxic epidermal necrolysis (secondary to medications especially sulfonamides, antibiotics, phenytoin, and other anticonvulsants) (27).

    b. **Pemphigus-induced injury** is diagnosed by the following:

        (1) Evidence that the onset of the lesions is related to the intake of a certain drug.

        (2) Acanthocytosis of epidermal cells detected on histopathologic examination.

        (3) Positive direct immunofluorescence staining of intercellular substance with either IgG or C3 (29).

        (4) Drugs implicated in inducing pemphigus include the following:

            (a) **Antibiotics.** Cephalexin, ceftriaxone, ethambutol, isoniazid, penicillin, rifampin.

            (b) **Thiols.** Captopril, gold sodium, thiomalate, mercaptopropyllglycine, methimazole, penicillamine piroxicam, thiopronine, tyritinol.

            (c) **Parazolone derivatives.** Aminopyrine, aminophenazone, azopropyrine, oxyphenylbutazone, phenylbutazone).

            (d) **Miscellaneous.** Digoxin, enalapril, heroin, interleukin-2 and interferon-beta, L-dopa, lysine acetylsalicylate, nifedipine, phenobarbital, propranol (29).

5. **Burns.** Caustic/corrosive, detergents (electric dishwasher machine type), fluorides, formaldehyde, heavy metal salts (copper, mercury, zinc), hydrofluoric acid (rust removers), iodine, oxalic acid (rust removers), permanganate, phenols, phosphorous, pine oil, silver nitrate, sodium bisulfite, thioglycolate.

6. **Cyanosis.** The concentration of reduced hemoglobin in capillary blood is increased to 5 g/dL by lack of atmospheric oxygen, hypoventilation, inadequate absorption of oxygen, impaired respiratory movements, or increase in metabolism and oxygen demand or 1.5 g/dL of methemoglobin or 0.5 g/dL of sulfhemoglobin.

    a. **Methemoglobinemia and sulfhemoglobinemia are oxygen resistant.** Acetanilid, carbon monoxide, CNS depressants, CNS stimulants, dinitrophenol, hypoxia and hypoxemia from any cause, methemoglobinemia (aniline and azo dyes, dinitrobenzene, local anesthetics (benzocaine), nitrates, nitrites, nitrobenzene, nitrophenol, phenacetin, trinitrotoluene), salicylates, sulfhemoglobin (hydrogen sulfide) produces green tint to cyanosis.

  7. **Dark skin.** Argyria produced by chronic silver absorption, chrysiasis produced by chronic gold absorption, chronic bismuth poisoning.

  8. **Desquamation.** Arsenic, boric acid ("boiled lobster appearance"), acrodynia (chronic mercury), causes of toxic epidermal necrolysis.

  9. **Diaphoresis. Diaphoretic** is organic and the most frequent medical causes are hypoglycemia, sepsis, withdrawal, or heat stroke. The toxicologic causes include arsenic, carbamates, ciguatera fish poisoning, CNS stimulants* (amphetamines, cocaine), cholinergic mushrooms*, cholinergic medications* (physostigmine, neostigmine), cimetidine, herbicides (dinitrophenol, pentachlorophenol) fluorides, hypoglycemia* from any cause, iodides, insulin*, mercurials, nicotine, nitrites, opioids, organophosphate insecticides*, salicylates*, serotonin (5-HT) syndrome*, sulfonylurea hypoglycemics*, withdrawal from ethanol*, opioids, and sedative-hypnotics. An asterisk indicates most frequent. Oriented times three but acting strange is functional illness. The **most perfuse diaphoresis** occurs with heat exhaustion, hypoglycemia, myocardial infarction, pulmonary embolus, sepsis, organophosphate insecticide intoxication and pentachlorophenol intoxication.

 10. *Dry and flushed.* Anticholinergics, antihistamines, ethanol.

 11. *Erythema multiforme.* Anticonvulsants (hydantoins), antihistamines, arsenicals, barbiturate, chlorpropamide, codeine, corticosteroids, cimetidine, dapsone, griseofulvin, hydralazine, mercurials, penicillin, phenothiazines, phenolphthalein, phenytoin, salicylates, sulfonamides, thiazides. Physical factors, such as cold, radiation, sunlight.

 12. **Erythema nodosum.** Contraceptives (oral hormonal), halides, penicillins, sulfonamides, tetracyclines.

 13. **Flushed.** See flushing syndromes.

    a. **Flushing** due to sympathomimetic or hypotension (associated with perspiration); or if due to vasoactive chemicals such as histamine, kinins, prostaglandins (not associated with perspiration). **Medical causes** may be autonomic epilepsy, carcinoid tumors, insulinoma, mastocytosis, pheochromocytoma, and urticaria pigmentosa (localized mastocytosis) (38–40).

    b. **Flushed skin** may be due to the presence of excessive oxyhemoglobin as in cyanide or carbon monoxide intoxication (rarely found in living patient), dilation of the cutaneous vasculature by anticholinergics, or release of histamine or a pigment produced by a medication such as rifampin (38–40).

    c. **Other causes of flushing** are anticholinergics*, antihistamines*, boric acid*, carbamazepine, carbon monoxide (rarely), cyanide (rarely), dinitrophenol, disulfiram reaction*, ethanol*, monosodium glutamate*, monoamine oxidase inhibitors (MAOI) with tyramine reaction, niacin (nicotinic acid)*, nicotinamide, nitrites*, rifampin (overdose)*, sympathomimetics, scromboid fish poisoning*, toxic shock syndrome, vancomycin by rapid infusion* (38–40).

    d.   **Flushing syndromes** (38–40)

        (1)   **With ethanol.** Antabuse-type reaction, genetic predisposition (Asians, American Indians), chloral hydrate, tyramine, MAOI.

        (2)   **Without ethanol.** Excess niacin, nicotinic acid, nitrates, carcinoid syndrome, Zollinger-Ellison syndrome, **pheochromocytoma, carcinoid** syndrome, cluster headache, migraine headache.

14.   **Hirsutism.** Androgens, corticosteroids, diazoxide, minoxidil, phenytoin, progestins.

15.   **Jaundice.** See yellow.

16.   **Keratinization.** Arsenic, thallium.

17.   **Lupus-like reactions.** Beta-blockers, ethosuximide, flecainide, hydralazine*, isoniazid*, labetalol, methyldopa, minoxidil, nitrofurantoin, penicillamine*, phenothiazines, phenytoin, procainamide*, quinidine, sulfonamides, tocainide, tetracycline, trimethadione.

18.   **Pallor.** Arsenic trioxide, benzene (chronic), carbon monoxide (acute), chlorates, clonidine, colchicine (acute), epinephrine (Epi) (acute), ergot, hemolysis (aniline, fava beans, naphthalene, others), insulin (acute), lead (chronic), mercury (chronic), phenols, phosphorous (chronic), solanine, trinitrotoluene, vanadium.

19.   **Pruritic.** Anticholinergic, boric acid, ciguatera fish poisoning, cobalt, *Datura stramonium,* phenytoin, rifampin, scombroid fish poisoning.

20.   **Purpura.** Anticoagulants (medical or in rodenticides), benzene (chronic), disseminated intravascular coagulation, ergot, envenomations (insects, spiders, snakes), quinine, sulfonamides, salicylates

    a.   **Mechanical purpura.** Glass cup suction (chin), suck on arms, rubber arrowhead suction (forehead), ECG suction cups (chest) (28).

21.   **Scleroderma.** Associated with organic solvent exposures.

22.   **SJS,** or erythema multiforme bullosa, described in 1922. In 1956, Lydell introduced the term **"toxic epidermal necrolysis."** It leaves the surface looking scalded.

    a.   SJS and TEN have similar histopathologic features. SJS is also a synonym for erythema multiforme bullosa or major and has target lesions predominantly on the extremities. Erythema multiforme occurs after infections with herpes simplex and mycoplasma and has a benign course. Patients with widely disseminated purpuric macules and blisters are likely to have drug-induced SJS. SJS resolves into more toxic epidermal necrolysis within a few days. Substances that produce SJS are listed in Table 86-8.

    b.   **Clinical and laboratory findings** that alert to drug-induced SJS include the following:

        (1)   **Cutaneous findings.** Confluent erythema, facial edema, central facial involvement, skin pain, palpable purpura, skin necrosis, blisters or epidermal detachment, positive Nikcolsky's sign, mucous membrane erosions, urticaria, swelling of the tongue.

        (2)   **General findings.** High fever, of more than 40°C, enlarged lymph nodes, arthralgia or arthritis, dyspnea, wheezing or hypotension.

TABLE 86-8. *Drugs with Serum Johnson Syndrome (SJS)*

Allopurinol[a]	Vasculitis
Amithiozone	Allopurinol
Aminopenicillins[a]	Penicillins and aminopenicillins[a]
Barbiturates[a]	Phenytoin[a]
Benzodiazepines	Propylthiouracil
Carbamazepine[a]	Pyrazolone
Cephalosporins[a]	Sulfonamides[a]
Chlormezanone	Raynaud's disease or digital necrosis
Co-trimethoprim[a]	Beta-adrenergic blockers (propranolol)
Ethambutol	Bleomycin
Isoxicam	Ergot alkaloids
NSAID[a,b]	Serum sickness (SS)
Phenytoin	Serum preparations
Rifampin	Vaccines
Sulfonamides[a]	Resemble SS (fever, rash, arthralgias)
Sulfonylureas	Beta-adrenergic blockers
Tetracycline[a]	Streptokinase
Tetracycline[a]	β-Lactam antibiotics (cefachlor 1:2,000)[a]
Trimethoprim[a]	
Trioxsalen	
Vancomycin	

[a]= more common.
[b]NSAID, nonsteroid antiinflammatory drugs, especially phenylbutazone.
Modified from ref. 1 and Strom BL, et al. *Arch Dermatol* 1991;127:831.

    (3) Laboratory. Eosinophil count of more than 1,000/mm³, lymphocytosis with atypical lymphocytes, abnormal liver function tests. Neutropenia suggests poor prognosis. **Other texts include** additional causes of SJS/TEN: acetaminophen, chloramphenicol, colchicine, dapsone, gold salts, nitrofurantoin, phenolphthalein, and salicylates.

  23. Yellow skin

    a. *Jaundice.* See hepatic system.

      (1) Hepatocellular and cholestatic damage. Acetaminophen (late), amanita phalloides and related mushrooms, anesthetic agents (halothane), cephalosporin (ceftriaxone), chlorinated hydrocarbons (chloroform, carbon tetrachloride, trichloroethylene), chloral hydrate, chlorpromazine, erythromycin, ethanol, heavy metals (arsenic, gold, iron), phenothiazines (chlorpromazine), phosphorous, solvents.

      (2) Hemolytic substances. Aniline, antimalarial agents (especially in G-6-PD deficiency), arsine gas, benzene, cephalosporins, castor beans (ricin), copper, fava beans, jequirity bean, naphthalene especially with G-6-PD deficiency, nitrites, salicylates, snake venom and sulfonamides.

    b. *Systemic staining.* Atabrine, carotenemia* (clear sclera), epoxy resins, quinacrine, picric acid, rifampin, vitamin A.

  F. *Fixed drug reaction.* Fixed drug eruption is a cutaneous inflammatory reaction that manifests by solitary or multiple well-defined macules, which may become bullous. The lesions occur within a few hours of ingesting the drug and characteristically recur in the same location with each subsequent dose. They heal in 10 to 14 days and leave residual hyper-pigmentation. Systemic symptoms are uncommon. The time to sensitization is weeks to years. **Agents causing a drug fixed reaction** include analgesia (acetaminophen, acetyl-salicylic acid, codeine, ibuprofen); antimicrobials (ampicillin, griseofulvin, metronidazole, nystatin, sulfonamides, tetracycline, trimethoprim); sedative-hypnotics (barbiturates, chloral hydrate); sympathomimetics (pseudoephedrine, tetrahydrozolamine); miscellaneous (digitalis, diphenhydramine, emetine, phenolphthalein, phenothiazine) (35).

G. *Dating of injuries to the skin.* The color changes that take place in bruises over time allow approximating of dating of injuries. Skin changes to temporary red or pink due to capillary dilation resulting from mild trauma. If the capillaries are broken, red cells extrude and the reddened skin will not blanch with pressure. After 0 to 2 days, the contusion becomes swollen and tender blue-purple, and at 1 to 3 days becomes blue to bluish brown. As the hemoglobin is changed to biliverdin, bilirubin, and hemosiderin, the skin changes to green at approximately 6 (range 5–7) days, and yellow-brown at 8 to 9 (range 8–14) days. The skin returns to normal in 2 to 4 weeks (Fig. 86-1) (41).

H. **Fingernails.** The average growth of the thumb nail is 0.10 mm/day, and it is possible to assess the approximate time of the insult that has marked the nails. The length of the furrow correlates with the duration of the condition that has affected the nail matrix. An abrupt limit to the furrow indicates an acute attack, whereas a slope indicates more protracted disease (46). In 1846, Beau described transverse lines and depressions in the nails following severe acute disease (47). **Medical conditions associated with Beau's lines** are acrodermatitis enteropathica, acute illness, (severe), alopecia areata, carpal tunnel syndrome, epidermolysis bullosa, epileptic convulsions (severe), eczema (chronic), fungal infections, hypocalcemia, Hodgkin's disease, hypopituitarism, malaria, menstrual cycle, manicuring (overzealous), measles, paronychia, psoriasis, Raynaud's disease, trauma (washboard), zinc deficiency. **Substances associated with Beau's lines** include cancer chemotherapy, dapsone (47), fluorosis, heavy metals* (arsenic, thallium), metoprolol (47), phenytoin exposure in utero, and retinoids (49). **Substances associated with softening of the nail** include formaldehyde, alkali, acids, paraquat.

I. **Pruritus** (51,52). Pruritus is the itch. It is the commonest symptom of a rash, but patients may have pruritus without a rash.

   1. **Systemic diseases** associated with pruritus without diagnostic skin lesions.
      a. **Definite association** with pruritus with systemic diseases, including chronic renal failure, hepatobiliary disease, Hodgkin's disease (15%), hyperthyroidism (5%), polycythemia vera (14% to 25%), and psychogenic state.
      b. **Possible association** with diabetes mellitus, hypothyroidism, internal malignancy, iron deficiency anemia. Case and anecdotal reports of association with

```
Day 1    2    3    4    5    6    7    8    9    10    13    21    28
Red-blue|  Blue-purple|  Green  Yellow-brown--->|resolved
```

FIG. 86–1. Dating of injuries to skin

AIDS, carcinoid syndrome, dumping syndrome, mastocytosis, multiple myeloma, neurologic disorders, and Sjogren syndrome.

c. **Medication reaction** with or without a rash. The agents most involved include
allopurinol, aconite, carbamazepine, nitrofurantoin, penicillins, phenylbutazone,
streptomycin, and sulfonamides. Drugs that **affect the mast cells** and cause
histamine release by nonallergic mechanisms are codeine, estrogens, meperidine, morphine, salicylates, radiocontrast media and vancomycin. Cocaine and
aconite have sensation of insects under the skin. "Magnan's sign" in cocaine
addiction.

d. **Pruritus produced by hepatic cholestasis** include anabolic steroids, captopril, chlorpropamide, erythromycin estolate, oral contraceptives, phenothiazines, tolbutamide, and trimethoprimsulfamethoxazole.

2. **Dermatologic disorders** occur with diagnostic skin lesions and include atopic dermatitis, contact dermatitis, dermatitis herpetiformis, insect bites, lichen planus,
miliaria, pediculosis, psoriasis, ringworm, and scabies.

3. **Bite reactions** to *Sarcoptes scabiei,* flea bites, other insects. Dry skin and fiberglass
are other causes.

4. **Workup. History** of gradual or acute, nature (continuous, burning, prickly), time
occurs, location, relationship to hobbies and occupation and provoking factors such
as air, water, exercise, atopy, bathing habits, pets, sexual history, travel history, prior
treatment. **Laboratory tests** includes CBC, BUN, creatinine, alkaline phosphatase,
bilirubin, T4 and TSH, blood glucose, chest x-ray. Skin biopsy if etiology obscure
after workup. **Treatment** is ice pack to localized pruritus. Sedating antihistamine
1 h before bedtime (hydroxyzine, cyproheptadine). Nonsedating antihistamines are
not effective.

III. **Cardiovascular system** (53,54). The effects of poisoning and overdose on the cardiovascular
(CV) system are disturbances in: **conductivity** (chronotropy)—rhythm and rate; **contractility**
(inotropy)/cardiac pump function; and **vascular tone, including preload or intravascular
volume and afterload or vascular resistance.** The pattern of the pulse, blood pressure (BP),
cardiac conduction, and type of dysrhythmia may aid in the recognition of the toxic agent.
However, hypoxia, shock, hypothermia, and other superimposed complications may distort the
typical pattern. **The heart and vasculature are affected directly or by alterations in autonomic function. Direct membrane depression** delays impulse conduction and is referred to
as the "quinidine-like" action. The **sympathetic response** increases the automaticity, conduction velocity, contractility of the heart, lengthens the refractory period and produces constriction of most vascular beds. The **parasympathetic response** delays conduction velocity
through the AV node (vagotonic block) and the ventricular tissue, diminishes contractility,
shortens the refractory period and generally produces vasodilation. There are **two type of
parasympathetic receptors:** the nicotinic receptor, which may produce tachycardia and
hypertension, and the muscarinic receptor, which produces bradycardia and hypotension. The
table shows classes of alpha- and beta-adrenergic agents, the syndromes they produce and their
antagonists, and the specific receptor, action, agonist, syndrome and antagonist are summarized (Table 86-9).

TABLE 86-9. *Classes of alpha- and beta-adrenergic agents*

Receptor	Action	Agonist	Syndrome	Overdose antagonist
Alpha-1	Vasoconstriction Postsynaptic Signal pathway: Phospholipid C activation[a]	Phenylephrine Methoxamine Metaraminol Phenylpropanol-amine (PPA)	Hypertension, mydriasis, sweating, reflex bradycardia	Prazosin
Alpha-2	Vasodilation Decreased CNS sympathetic outflow Feedback inhibition of NE release. Signal pathway: Inhibition adenyl-cyclase[b]	Clonidine Guanabenz Guanfacine Imidazoline	Hypotension, miosis, dry skin, bradycardia	Yohimbine
Alpha-1 and -2		Norepinephrine Epinephrine Phenylpropanol-amine		Phentolamine Phenoxybenz-amine
Beta-1	Inotropic Chronotropic Signal pathway: adenylcyclase activation[c]	Epinephrine Norepinephrine Isoproterenol	Hypertension, mydriasis, sweating, tachycardia	Acebutolol Atenolol Esmolol Metoprolol
Beta-2	Vasodilation Bronchial dilation Signal pathway: adenylcyclase activation[d] Hypokalemia	Isoproterenol Terbutaline Albuterol Isoetarine	Normotensive miosis, wide pulse, tremor, hyperglycemia	Propranolol Nadolol Pindolol Timolol Epinephrine
Beta-1 and -2	Usually produces beta-1 effects	Isoproterenol Metaproterenol	Normo/hypotensive miosis, tachycardia, and beta-2 effects	Propranolol Nadolol Pindolol Sotalol
Alpha and beta	—	Labetalol Acebutolol	—	—
Dopamine[e]	—	Dopamine	—	—

[a]Alpha-1 receptors are located in blood vessels; phospholipid C results in cleavage of phosphoinositol into inositol phosphate and diacylglycerol; this action leads to increase in intracellular calcium and vasoconstriction.

[b]Alpha-2 receptors are located on neurons where they inhibit norepinephrine release from postganglionic fibers and decrease sympathetic outflow from the brain stem regulatory areas, and on blood vessels where they produce vasoconstriction by inhibiting adenyl cyclase, reducing intracellular cyclic AMP levels.

[c]Beta-1 receptors are located in the heart where they mediate increases in heart rate, contractility, and conduction velocity, which increases adenyl cyclase activity.

[d]Beta-2 receptors are located in smooth muscle and blood vessels and produce bronchial dilation and vasodilation by increases in adenyl cyclase activity.

[e]Dopamine receptors are present on renal and splanchnic blood vessels and postganglionic sympathetic nerves; they produce vasodilation and inhibition of norepinephrine secretion.

A.   **Sudden cardiac arrest** (sudden CV collapse). About 3% to 9% of ventricular fibrillation (VF) remains unexplained even after postmortem examination.

1.   **Medical conditions** associated with cardiac arrest include severe acidosis and alkalosis, Addison's disease, aortic dissection, atherosclerotic coronary heart disease (most common), anaphylaxis, congenital heart disease (aberrant coronary blood vessel, medial sclerosis of the coronary vessels, endocardial fibroelastosis, glycogen storage disease), cardiac tamponade, cardiomyopathy (hypertrophic, viral, bacterial), dysrhythmias and prolonged QT syndromes, drugs illegal (cocaine, amphetamines, phenylpropanolamine), electric shock, electrolyte abnormalities (calcium, magnesium, potassium, magnesium), hypoglycemia, hypoxia form any cause (carbon monoxide poisoning), hypo- and hyperthermia, insect bites and stings, medications (allergy, adverse reaction or overdose), myocardial infarction, neurologic disorders (cerebrovascular accident, convulsions, brain stem compression, infection), pulmonary embolism, respiratory failure (RF) with hypoxia and/or hypercapnia, shock from any etiology), sepsis, substances (chlorinated hydrocarbons, i.e., 1,1, 1-trichloroethane), sudden infant death syndrome (SIDS), tension pneumothorax, upper airway obstruction, valvular heart disease (mitral valve prolapse).

2.   **Medications most likely to cause cardiac arrest** from allergy, adverse reaction or overdose include antihypertensive agents, insulin, nitrates, opioids, penicillin, propranolol, quinidine, sedative-hypnotics, sulfonamides, theophylline, Torsades de pointes (TDP) from interaction of ketoconazole and terfenadine or hismanal, erythromycin and terfenadine or hismanal, and warfarin.

3.   **Complications of cardiorespiratory resuscitation** include hypoxic encephalopathy, endotracheal tube injury (laceration, fractured teeth, epistaxis), spinal cord injury, pneumothorax, pneumomediastinum, subcutaneous emphysema, hemothorax, atelectasis, foreign body, aspiration, hemopericardium and cardiac tamponade, lacerated coronary or ruptured ventricle, acute gastric dilation, gastroesophageal reflux, liver or splenic laceration, acute renal failure, fat embolism, volume over load, metabolic alkalosis (excess sodium bicarbonate or posthypercapnic).

B.   **Sinus rate and AV nodal conduction** (55–57)

1.   **Sinus rate.** Autonomic input: sympathetic beta stimulation increases conduction, cholinegic stimulation decreases conduction.

2.   **Beta-1 agonists** increase the rate, including albuterol, amphetamine, Epi, cocaine, theophylline/caffeine.

3.   **Beta-1 antagonists** (beta-blockers) decrease the heart rate.

4.   **Alpha-2 agonists** decrease the central sympathetic output and decrease the rate, including clonidine, guanabenz, methyldopa, oxymetazoline, and tetrahydrozoline.

5.   **Cholinergic stimulation** decreases the rate including cholinesterase inhibitors, digitalis glycosides, and centrally increased vagal tone from many causes. Cholinergic inhibition increases rate, including anticholinergic agents and cyclic antidepressants.

6.   **AV nodal conduction.** Decreased conduction (AV blocks) are produced by adenosine, digitalis glycosides, calcium channel blockers, antidysrhythmic class 1c and III (bretylium.)

B. **Bradycardia** mechanism may be produced by excess cholinergic activity or depressed sympathomimetic activity such as cholinergic medications (carbamates), organophosphate insecticides; vagotonic cardiac glycosides); interference with release or depletion of the catecholamines (beta-adrenergic blockers); damage or membrane depression of the myocardium including chloroquine, cyclic antidepressants, antidepressants, 1a antidysrhythmic (quinidine, procainamide, disopyramide) and 1c (encainide, flecainide); increased intracranial pressure (ICP) (lead encephalopathy and vitamin A toxicity producing Cushing's reflex bradycardia and hypertension; CNS depressants (opioids, sedative-hypnotics); initial reflex bradycardia alpha-adrenergic agonists (clonidine and phenylpropanolamine); electrolytes (potassium and magnesium); heavy metals; and lithium.

1. **Bradycardia** in an adult of less than 60 bpm may occur with sleep, sedation, vagal stimulation such as bowel movement, hypothyroidism, and athletic heart. Bradycardia under 1 year of age is less than 80 bpm.

2. The **common intoxications** that produce bradycardia include alpha-1 adrenergic antagonists, alpha-2 adrenergic agonists, amantadine, antidysrhythmic agents (especially disopyramide, lidocaine, phenytoin, procainamide, quinidine), arsenic, astemizole, beta-adrenergic blockers, calcium channel blockers, cardiac glycosides, cholinergic agents (physostigmine, neostigmine), CNS depressants (barbiturates-late), chloroquine, clonidine (AV block), cyclobenzaprine, ipecac (emetine), lead, lithium, nonbarbiturate sedative-hypnotics (late), opioids, organophosphate insecticides, phenytoin, quinidine (wide QRS), pentamidine, phenothiazines, sympathomimetics, terfenidine, tricyclic and cyclic antidepressants (preterminal).

C. **Tachycardia** mechanisms may be due to excess anticholinergic activity, including *Amanita muscaria,* antihistamines, anticholinergic phenothiazines, tricyclic antidepressants (TCA); stimulation of release of catecholamines amphetamines, caffeine, cocaine, ephedrine, phencyclidine, theophylline; inadequate venous return due to vasodilation (nitrites, disulfiram, antihypertensives) or inadequate volume; hypoxia due to carbon monoxide, cyanide, hydrogen sulfide and methemoglobinemia (oxidizing agents); direct injury to myocardium or increased metabolism; and withdrawal from ethanol or sedative-hypnotics.

1. **Tachycardia** is produced by fever (increases of 10 beats for each degree of temperature above 38°C), hypovolemia, sepsis, hyperthyroidism, and congestive heart failure.

2. The **common intoxications** that produce tachycardia include alcohols and glycols (early), *A. muscaria,* anticholinergic agents, antidysrhythmic agents (but not calcium channel blockers), antihistamines, cardiac glycosides, CNS stimulants (amphetamine, cocaine, carbon monoxide, cyanide, methylphenidate, phenylpropanol-amine), Epi, ethanol withdrawal, hallucinogens, hypoglycemic agents, hypokalemia (diuretics, theophylline, salicylates) nicotine, nitrates and nitrites, phencyclidine, phenothiazines, salicylates, sedative-hypnotics (early), sympathomimetics (theophylline), thyroid, tricyclic and cyclic antidepressants (early), withdrawal states.

D. **Dysrhythmia** mechanisms include spontaneous depolarization (automaticity) due to theophylline or digitalis; abnormal impulse conduction (reentry) such as nodal reentry with digitalis intoxication and hyperkalemia; and "triggered" responses such with TDP.

1. They may be caused by direct or indirect sympathomimetic effects, anticholinergic effects, CNS-altered regulation of peripheral autonomic activity, direct effects on the myocardial membrane, secondary to hypotension, hypoxia, disturbances in acid-base balance and electrolyte, and myocardial ischemia.

2. Correction of hypoxia and metabolic derangements (electrolytes, hypoglycemia, acid-base disturbances) will spontaneously rectify many dysrhythmias.

3. The **common intoxications likely to produce dysrhythmias** are amphetamines, anticholinergics, antidysrhythmics, beta-blockers, calcium channel blockers, carbon disulfide (occupational), carbon monoxide, cardiac glycosides, chloral hydrate, chloroquine, clonidine, cocaine, fluorocarbons, lithium, nicotine, phenothiazines, quinidine, solvents, sympathomimetics, theophylline, tricyclic and cyclic antidepressants.

4. **Any antidysrhythmic medication** can also produce a dysrhythmia. The antidysrhythmic agents are Class 1a—quinidine, procainamide, disopyramide; Class 1b—lidocaine, phenytoin, tocainide, mexiletine; Class 1c—flecainide, encainide; Class 2—beta-adrenergic blockers; Class 3—amiodarone, bretylium, sotalol; Class 4—calcium channel blockers; and Class 5—digoxin.

5. **Prolongation of the QRS wave and QT interval** is seen with TCA intoxication, quinidine, phenothiazine overdose, or hypocalcemia as occurs in ethylene glycol poisoning.

   a. **Substances causing QRS prolongation** include amantadine, *antidysrhythmic agents 1a (quinidine, procainamide, disopyramide) and 1c (encainide, flecainide), beta-adrenergic blockers, *chloroquine, digitalis glycosides (complete heart block), diphenhydramine, fluoride, heavy metals, hyperkalemia, hypocalcemia (as occurs in ethylene glycol), hypomagnesemia, lithium, phenothiazine (thioridazine), propoxyphene, quinine, thallium, *TCA (slowing of the inward fast Na^+ conductance of the action potential in the heart).

   b. **QRS widening of more than 0.12 s in the limb leads.** This is highly suggestive of serious poisoning with any cyclic antidepressants, and other membrane depressant drugs, which reflects **inhibition of the fast sodium-dependent channel and depolarization of the cardiac tissue.** It is usually accompanied by QT interval prolongation, AV block, and depressed cardiac contractility. The QRS interval prolongation may also be due to ventricular escape rhythm in a patient with complete heart block (digitalis or calcium channel antagonist poisoning).

   c. The **differential of wide QRS** includes intrinsic disease of the myocardium associated with myocardial infarction, **hyperkalemia** with large undulating "sine wave" pattern and markedly widened QRS with peaked T waves and eventually asystole, and **hypothermia** core temperature of less than 32°C (90°F) causes extraterminal QRS deflection (**J wave or Osborne wave**, which is the end of the QRS and the beginning of the S-T segment), resulting in widened QRS.

   d. **Ventricular tachycardia** (VT) may be seen with drugs that prolong the QT and QRS, including anticholinergics, digitalis, Epi, ethanol withdrawal, hypokalemia (diuretics, theophylline, salicylates), isoproterenol, procainamide, TCA.

4. **QT prolongation.** The QT interval is measured from the onset of the QRS to the **end** of the T wave and represents ventricular repolarization. The QT interval is rate dependent. The corrected QT interval (QTc) is generally used for interpretation. The QTc equals QT divided by the square root of the previous R-R interval in seconds. In the first 6 months of life, the QTc should not exceed 0.46, and in older children should not exceed 0.44.

   a. **A prolonged QT interval** can predispose to VT, TDP, and VF.

   b. **Prolonged QT interval syndromes** include congenital heredity Jervell-Lange-Nielsen syndrome, which is less frequent, autosomal recessive triad of prolonged QT interval, syncope, and congenital deafness. The Romano-Ward, which is more frequent, autosomal dominant prolonged QT, and syncope without deafness. Other causes of prolonged QT interval include metabolic/electrolyte, central or autonomic nervous system, coronary artery disease, mitral valve prolapse

   c. **Torsades de pointes** (TDP), or "twisting of the points," was discovered by Dessertenne in 1960. This dangerous dysrhythmia is a polymorphic VT with varying QRS amplitudes that can degenerate into VF. The peaks of the QRS shift from one side to the other of the isoelectric baseline. TDP has noted to be produced by drugs and toxins that prolong the QT interval (56,57).

      (1) The **commonly reported intoxications that produce TDP** are amantadine, arsenic, anticholinergics (especially atropine), antidysrhythmic agents (Ia *quinidine, disopyramide, *procainamide, Ib lidocaine, mexiletine, tocainide; Ic encainide, flecainide; III amiodarone), chloral hydrate, corticosteroids, diuretics, flouride, *hyperkalemia, hypocalcemia*, hypomagnesemia, lithium, *phenothiazines (especially thioridazine), organophosphate, maprotiline, thallium, TCA, and liquid protein diet (56,57).

E. **Cardiomyopathy.** The true incidence of **idiopathic cardiomyopathy (IDC)** is estimated at about 5 to 8 per 100,000 population, and accounts for 10,000 deaths annually. Blacks and males have a 2.5-fold increase in risk as compared to whites and females. Convincing associations have been reported between beta-adrenergic agonists and moderate alcohol consumption.

   1. **Known causes of dilated cardiomyopathy**

      a. **Toxins.** Acetaminophen, alcoholism, antiretroviral agents (zidovudine, didanosine), antimony, arsenic, chloroquine, cancer chemotherapeutic agents (cyclophosphamide, daunorubicin, doxorubin, bleomycin), carbon monoxide, cobalt, cocaine, emetine, ethanol, hydrocarbons, lead, lithium, mercury, phenothiazines.

      b. **Metabolic abnormalities.** Nutritional (thiamine, selenium, carnathine), endocrinopathies (acromegaly, Cushing's syndrome, diabetes mellitus, hypothyroidism, pheochromocytoma, thyrotoxicosis), electrolyte abnormalities (hypocalcemia, hypophosphatemia)

      c. **Inflammation and infectious**

         (1) **Infectious.** Bacterial (diphtheria), fungal, mycoplasma, parasitic (trichinosis, toxoplasmosis, Chagas' disease) Rickettsia, viral (Coxsackie, cytomegalic, human immunodeficiency).

      (2) Noninfectious. Collagen vascular disorders (scleroderma, lupus erythematosus), dermatomyositis), hypersensitivity myocarditis, sarcoidosis, and peripartum dysfunction.

    d. Neuromuscular causes. Duchenne muscular dystrophy, fascioscapulohumeral muscular dystrophy, Erb's limb-girdle dystrophy, myotonic dystrophy, Friedreich ataxia.

    e. Familial myocardiopathies.

F. Vascular tone (59–69). **Transient hypertension** may be produced by substances acting indirectly to increase the release of norepinephrine (NE) from storage granules or, decreasing the reuptake of NE. Substances may also act directly to decrease the degradation of NE or interact with the alpha receptors. The vascular tone may be reduced by agents that produce myocardial depression and a decrease in cardiac output or dysrhythmias that interfere with cardiac filling. Vascular tone may also be influenced by the agents affecting the autonomic CNS or peripheral effector sites. The cause may be hypoxia, volume depletion, and anaphylaxis. Both hypertension and hypotension may be seen in a single substance poisoning. **Hypertension due to intoxications rarely requires vigorous therapy** (except in cocaine, monamine oxidase inhibitor interaction hypertensive crisis), since it is usually only seen initially, is transient and is often followed by life-threatening hypotension.

    1. Hypertension. Systemic hypertension affects 20% of white and 30% of Black Americans 18 years or older. Adult systolic-diastolic hypertension is defined as a BP of 140/90 or greater. Over 90% of hypertension is **essential hypertension** defined as **diastolic BP** (DBP) mild (90 to 104 mm Hg), moderate DBP (105 to 114 mm Hg), or severe DBP (more than 115 mm Hg). A DBP of more than 90 mm Hg is a risk factor for cerebrovascular and ischemic disease. The presence of papilloedema defines malignant BP regardless of the absolute level of the BP. Less than 10% of hypertensive patients have an identifiable cause.

      a. Medical causes of secondary hypertension are acute porphyria, primary aldosteronism, coarctation of the aorta, oral hormonal contraceptives, congenital adrenal hyperplasia, corticosteroids, Cushing's syndrome, diencephalic syndrome, extrarenal chromaffin tumors, familial dysautonomia, hypercalcemia, lupus erythematosus, pheochromocytoma, renal disease, toxemia of pregnancy.

      (1) Isolated systolic hypertension is defined as SBP of more than 160 mm Hg and indicates increased cardiac output and/or stroke volume. The causes include anxiety, anemia, arteriovenous fistula, aortic rigidity, beriberi, complete heart block, patent ductus arteriosus, thyrotoxicosis.

      (2) Raised ICP can produce hypertension.

      (3) Malignant hypertension is accompanied by retinopathy, and some of its causes are acute glomerulonephritis and hemolytic uremic syndrome.

      b. Drug and toxins that commonly cause hypertension can be classified. The drugs that commonly cause hypertension in overdose are sympathomimetics (agitation), TCA (lethargic, transient hypertension), or beta-adrenergic agonists (agitation).

(1) **Mediated by alpha-adrenergic receptors.** Direct alpha-binding: catecholamines, Epi, NE, phenylephrine, ergotamines, methoxamine.

   (a) Indirect acting. Sympathomimetics, amphetamines, bretylium, cocaine, monoamine oxidase, phencyclidine, cyclic antidepressants, yohimbine, rarely anticholinergic from *Datura stramonium* and *A. muscaria.*

   (b) Direct and indirect acting. Dopamine (DA), ephedrine, metaraminol, naphazoline, oxymetazoline, phenylpropanolamine, pseudoephedrine.

(2) **Not mediated by alpha-adrenergic receptors**

   (a) Angiotensin.

   (b) Beta-adrenergic agonist receptors. Catecholamine release nonselective: isoproterenol, isoxsuprine (Vasodilan), nylidrin (Arlidrin).

   (c) Mediated by beta-2 selective receptors. Albuterol, metaproterenol, terbutaline cause hypertension because 10% to 50% of cardiac beta receptors are beta-2.

   (d) Nicotine (in early stage).

   (e) Nephrotoxic agents.

   (f) Steroids. Glucocorticoids, mineralcorticoids, e.g., licorice.

   (g) Thromoxane A-2.

   (h) Vasopressin.

(3) **Intoxications associated with hypertension with tachycardia** are often noted from anticholinergic agents; CNS stimulants and sympathomimetics (amphetamines, cocaine, ephedrine, and pseudoephedrine, monoamine oxidase [early in overdose and in interactions], phencyclidine, phenylpropanolamine); heavy metals (barium, cadmium, thallium); hallucinogens (mild); nicotine (early stage) thyroid; and withdrawal from antihypertensive agents, from ethanol, and from sedative-hypnotics.

(4) **Intoxications associated with hypertension with reflex bradycardia or AV block** has been reported from intoxications from agents that increase the ICP such as hypervitaminosis A, nalidixic acid, tetracycline, chronic lead poisoning with encephalopathy, and corticosteroids.

(5) **Hypertension may initially be associated with bradycardia** from clonidine, ergot, methoxamine, NE, phenylpropanolamine, and phenylephrine.

f. **Malignant hypertension.** Intoxications or food drug interactions include MAOI interaction, neuroleptic malignant syndrome (NMS), 5-HT syndrome, and stimulants.

2. **Hypotension**

   a. **Medical conditions** that cause severe acidosis and alkalosis, burns, hyperthermia, hypothermia, hypovolemia, hypoxia, external losses (from the GI tract, hemorrhage, kidneys, and skin burns, perspiration and exudation), internal losses (ascites, peritonitis and pancreatitis), infection (septicemia, toxic shock syndrome), anaphylaxis, endocrine disease (adrenal insufficiency, thyroid storm, pheochromocytoma), cardiac causes (dysrhythmias, myopathies), pericarditis, coarctation of aorta, ruptured aortic aneurysm, pulmonary diseases (pneumothorax, thromboembolism).

b. **Intoxications that causes hypotension with tachycardia** include the following:

  (1) **True vascular volume loss**

    (a) **GI losses and hemorrhage.** Antibiotics, heavy metals (arsenic, iron, mercury*), iron, iodides, laxatives, caustic injuries*, lithium, nonsteroidal antiinflammatory agents*, opioid withdrawal, organophosphates and carbamates, plants and mushrooms (castor bean, colchicine, podophyllin, saponin, rosary pea), theophylline, zinc phosphate.

    (b) **Insensible losses.** Amphetamines, cocaine, chlorphenoxy herbicides, dinitrophenols, organophosphates and carbamates, salicylates.

    (c) **Urinary losses.** Diabetes insipidus, diuretics, ethanol, lithium, mercury, salicylates, tetracycline, theophylline.

    (d) **Redistribution** or "third spacing." caustics, snake envenomation, heavy metals, phenol, salicylates.

  (2) **An apparent hypovolemia from vasodilation** due to loss of vascular tone (peripheral venous and arteriolar dilation) such as occurs with particularly some antihypertensive agents*, beta-2–stimulating agents, caffeine, disulfiram reactions*, hydralazine, hyperthermia, nitrites*, sodium nitroprusside, phenothiazines*, theophylline and other methylxanthines.

  (3) **Others.** Alcohols, antihypertensive, anticholinergics, angiotensin converting enzyme inhibitor, calcium channel blockers, cyclic antidepressants, furosemide, opioids, sedative-hypnotics.

  (4) **Depression of cardiac output.** Barbiturates, beta-blockers, Class 1a, 1b antidysrhythmics especially quinidine, calcium channel blockers, sodium channel blockers antihistamines, phenothiazines, and TCA.

  (5) **Dysrhythmias** that interfere with cardiac filling. See dysrhythmias.

  (6) **Plants.** Autumn crocus, azalea, Christmas cherry, corn lily, daffodil, delphinium, foxglove, lily of the valley, mayapple, mistletoe, monkshood, morning glory, mountain laurel, some mushrooms, nutmeg, oleander, podophyllum, *Rauwolfia serpentina,* rhododendrum, star of Bethlehem, tobacco, and yew.

  (7) **Marine food or injury.** Box jellyfish, ciguatera, jellyfish, lionfish, shellfish poisoning, stonefish, and turkeyfish.

  (8) **Common intoxications** that cause this pattern of **hypotension and tachycardia** initially include amanita phalloides, anithypertensive agents, antidysrhythmic agents, arsenic, barbiturates (early), beta-blockers, calcium channel blockers, carbon monoxide (rarely), caustics, clonidine, cyanide, cholinergics, colchicine, copper sulfate, disulfiram with ethanol, hyperthermia, iron, nitrites, MAOI (late in overdose), opioids, organophosphate insecticides (rarely), phenothiazines, rattlesnake envenoma-

tion, sedative-hypnotics, shock from any cause, theophylline, tricyclic and cyclic antidepressants. **Later bradycardia develops in severe intoxications.**

(9) **Common intoxications** that may cause early **hypotension with bradycardia** are sympatholytic agents* (beta-blockers*, bretylium, clonidine, hypothermia, opioids, reserpine, tetrahydrozoline); membrane depressant drugs (beta-blockers*, class 1a, 1b antidysrhythmics*); others— calcium channel blockers*, cardiac glycosides (digitalis), cyanide, flouride, lithium, magnesium, neuroleptics (phenothiazines) organophosphates, sedative-hypnotics; and shock from any cause (late).

c. **Orthostatic hypotension. The test:** after the patient is supine for 2 min, determine BP and pulse rate. After standing 1 min or sitting 2 min recheck the BP, pulse and observe for orthostatic signs such as dizziness, syncope, or lightheaded. A positive test is if the SBP falls more than 20 mm Hg, DBP falls more than 10 mm Hg, pulse increases >10 bpm or signs and indicates 10 to 15 mL/kg volume loss. There is some controversy about this test since it has not been standardized.

(1) **The drugs** associated with orthostatic hypotension include the following:

(a) **Antihypertensive agents** include adrenergic antagonists (guanethidine, bretylium), angiotensin converting enzyme inhibitors, central alpha-2 adrenergic receptor antagonists (clonidine), alpha-methyldopa, guanabenz), ganglionic blockers (Trimethapan), peripheral alpha-1 adrenergic receptor antagonists Prazocin, phenoxybenzamine).

(b) **Vasodilators** (disulfiram, hydralazine, nitrites).

(c) **Calcium channel blockers.**

(d) **Beta-adrenergic blockers.**

(e) **Antianginal agents** (beta-adrenergic blockers, calcium channel blockers, nitrites).

(f) **Antidepressants** (TCA, MAOI).

(g) **Antiparkinson agents** (bromocriptine, L-dopa, pergolide mesylate).

(h) **Diuretics.**

(i) **CNS depressants** (ethanol, opioids, sedative-hypnotics).

(j) **Neuroleptics** (phenothiazines, butyrophenones).

G. **Chest pain** (66)

1. **Medical conditions**

a. **Cardiac conditions. Angina pectoris** (substernal pressure, not severe, lasts only a few minutes and is precipitated by exertion), **coronary artery disease** (myocardial infarction, hypertrophic cardiomyopathy, in pediatric patients Kawasaki's disease, aberrant coronary artery (type IA hyperlipidemia); **myocarditis associated with virus** diseases [Coxsackie, ECHO], **pericarditis** (pain is sharp, pleuritic, retro-sternal with cardiomegaly, intermittent rub heard over sternum in expiration, diffuse ST-T segment elevation changes or downward sloping of the PR on ECG, patients prefer to sit forward); **tuberculosis,**

connective tissue disease, uremia, malignancy, dissecting aneurysm of thoracic aorta (tearing, sudden onset radiating to anterior neck, back, flank and legs); **mitral valve prolapse** (usually female sex, mid-systolic click, pain is brief, stabbing); **aortic stenosis** (pain in 5th to 7th decade of life).

b. **Pulmonary. Pneumonia with pleurisy** (sharp pleuritic chest pain related to respiration or rub), **pulmonary embolus** (birth control pills or estrogen intake, pregnancy, recent pelvic or lower extremity trauma or surgery, burns, deep venous thrombosis, obesity, prolonged immobilization, polycythemia, **hypercoagulation state** [with protein C and S deficiency or antithrombin III deficiency or malignancy], **wide A-a gradient** [$A - aQ2 = 150 - (Pa_{O_2} + [P_{CO_2}/0.8])$ normal is 3 to 4 in patients younger than 20 and age/10 + 10 in patients older than 20 and abnormal PQ ratio, pain is pleuritic, sudden onset, lightheaded, syncope), **pneumothorax** (acute), **acute bronchospasm** (wheezing); **pleurodynia** (epidemic pleurodynia due to Coxsackie B).

c. **Musculoskeletal injury** (dull aching pain with sharp stabbing exacerbations typically occurs after exertion, lasts only 30 to 120 min and exaggerated by motion particularly of the left arm but does not radiate), **costochondritis or, Tietze's disease** or chest wall syndrome (painful point tenderness or one or more costal cartilages with swelling over costochondral or sternocostal junction, pain at rest but exaggerated by trunk and shoulder motions), slipping rib, precordial catch, myalgia, traumatic muscle pain; **thoracic outlet syndrome** caused by compression of the brachial plexus or artery by first rib, cervical rib or scalene muscle, pain is dull aching with paresthesias in ulnar nerve distribution, **traumatic** (bruised or fractured rib).

d. **GI. Esophageal reflux and esophagitis** (35% of normal population have "heartburn" at least once a month, if pregnant daily; **hiatal hernia** (pain is often nocturnal burning substernal resolve with viscous xylocaine and antiacid, treat with H-2 blockers) and **peptic ulcer disease** (relief with food or antacid) or referred from abdomen with peritonitis, pancreatitis)

e. **Psychological. "Panic attack"** (recurrent episodes of sympathetic stimulation causing patient to feel uneasy, pain in left mammary area, stabbing and fleeting, some patients express feeling of imminent death (*"angor animi"*) associated with dyspnea, dizziness, palpitations, abdominal pain. ECG normal except of tachycardia, nitroglycerin relieves in 30 min, often no precipitating stress), and **"hyperventilation syndrome"** (in patients under 40 years of age, tachypnea, substernal chest heaviness, palpitations, paresthesias, dizziness, carpopedal; spasm common, voluntary hyperventilation replicates symptoms, often precipitated by stress event, reduced P_{CO_2} alkalosis, relieve using a rebreathing mask or simple paper bag).

f. **Herpes zoster**

2. **Chest pain.** This may be caused from the **cardiotoxic effects** of drugs and chemicals.

a. Myocardial infarction associated with **vasoconstrictive action** and other factors of the toxic substance such as cocaine.

b. It may be due to an **irritative effect** of the agent on the myocardium such as petroleum distillates or Stoddard's solvent.

    c.   Associated with **pericarditis**, e.g., procainamide, hydralazine, methyldopa.

    d.   Related to **other organs** such as the burning pain of caustic/corrosives on the esophagus.

    e.   Chest pain has been reported from the following **intoxicants** arsenic, carbon monoxide* (CO), caustics/corrosives, CNS stimulants (cocaine, amphetamines), digitalis, heavy metal salts producing esophageal caustic action (copper sulfate, mercuric chloride, zinc sulfate), hydralazine*, ipecac (emetine), irritant gases, marijuana (panic attack), methyldopa*, methylene chloride* (in vivo releases CO), monosodium glutamate*, nicotine, nitroglycerin (medication or working with explosives), and procainamide*.

H.   **Pericarditis.** Pericarditis has been divided into **accumulation of excessive fluid; tamponade** or squeezing of the heart that may prevent diastolic filling; and **hypotensive or obstructive shock.** On ECG S-T segment elevation, usually with an indention in anterior and inferior leads, suggests pericarditis while myocarditis infarction causes S-T segment elevation in only one anatomical location.

    1.   **Medical causes** are as follows: infectious—viral, mycoplasma, bacteria, and *M. tuberculosis;* postmyocardial infarction; trauma and surgery; neoplasms (lung, breast, lymphoma, and leukemia).

    2.   **Pericarditis** has been reported with the following medications even in therapeutic doses: cromolyn sodium, dantrolene, doxorubicin, oral hydralazine, isoniazid, methyldopa, methysergide, minoxidil, penicillin, procainamide, phenytoin, reserpine.

IV.   **Edema** can be generalized and localized (70).

  A.   **Localized edema** can be due to lymphatic or venous obstruction (thrombosis, tumor, radiation, surgery, filariasis), inflammatory disease, allergic processes, physical or chemical trauma, insect stings and bites, immobilized limb or congenital lymphedema, or Milroy's disease.

  B.   **Generalized edema** is associated with right ventricular congestive heart failure, cor pulmonale, pericardial disease, hepatic cirrhosis, hypoalbuminemic states (nephrotic syndrome, protein losing enteropathy, malnutrition, severe chronic disease), acute and chronic renal disease with fluid overload, inferior vena cava obstruction, myxedema, iatrogenic salt overload (enteral feedings, i.v. fluid administration, poisoning), trichinosis, idiopathic cyclic edema, hereditary angioneurotic edema, and parenteral feeding.

  C.   **Drugs and toxins causing generalized edema** are bromocriptine, carbenicillin, corticosteroids, diazoxide, guanethidine, hydralazine, indomethacin, minoxidil, phenylbutazone.

V.   **Respiratory system** (71–82)

  A.   The **effects of overdose and poisoning** on the respiratory system include the following:

    1.   **Depression of the CNS**

    2.   **Obstruction of the upper and lower airways** by a foreign body, aspiration, or bronchospasm.

    3.   **Lung parenchyma.** Involvement by aspiration and/or chemical pneumonitis, fibrosis, interstitial diseases, atelectasis, and pulmonary edema.

    4.   **Pleural disease** with long-term exposure to toxic inhalations.

    5.   **Chest wall disturbances** with substances that produce paralysis of diaphragm and intercostal muscles.

6. **Gases and vapors** that may displace oxygen from the atmosphere, produce irritation of airways, parenchymal involvement.

7. **Systemic diseases** that interfere with transport or tissue uptake of oxygen and the oxygen-carrying capacity of hemoglobin.

B. **Respiratory (ventilatory) failure (RF).** RF may be caused by bacterial and viral pneumonia, viral encephalitis, and myelitis, including poliomyelitis, myasthenia gravis, traumatic or ischemic effects on the CNS or spinal cord. Chest wall rigidity of certain toxins, e.g., tetanus. RF is the most common cause of death from poisoning and overdose producing CNS depression or paralysis of the respiratory muscles.

1. **Depression of the CNS and respiratory center**

    a. **Medical diseases** include encephalitis (viral), embolus or thrombus, head injury, intracranial hemorrhage or infarction especially in the brain stem, increased ICP, primary alveolar hypoventilation, status epilepticus.

    b. **Toxic substances** include alcohols, anesthetics, barbiturates, benzodiazepines (rarely) clonidine, cyclic antidepressants, glycols, opioids, nonbarbiturate sedative-hypnotics.

2. **Neuromuscular paralysis of respiration**

    a. **Medical diseases.** Peripheral nerve and anterior horn disorders include Guillain-Barré syndrome, poliomyelitis, Werdnig-Hoffman's disease (infantile progressive spinal muscle atrophy); myoneural junction include myasthenia gravis, tetanus; and muscular disorders include polymyositis, muscular dystrophies, myotonia.

    b. **Toxic substances** include botulin toxin, marine toxins (paralytic shell fish, tetrodotoxin), neuromuscular blockers (anesthetic agents, magnesium, aminoglycoside), organophosphates, plant toxins (curare, coniine), snake envenomation, strychnine, tetanus, tick paralysis, and triorthocresyl phosphate fuel oil.

3. **Chest wall and pleural disorders,** including severe kyphoscoliosis, flail chest, large pleural effusions or hemorrhage, tension pneumothorax.

4. **Bronchopulmonary disorders**

    a. **Medical causes** include adult respiratory distress syndrome (ARDS), airway obstruction (foreign body, epiglottitis, angioneurotic edema) aspiration, bronchospasm, fibrosis (alveolar, interstitial), neoplasm, pneumonia, obliterative vasculitis, pulmonary edema (cardiac and noncardiac), pulmonary embolus, pulmonary hypertension, status asthmaticus, bronchospasm.

    b. **Toxic substances** include antimony, arsenic, asbestos, barium, cadmium, cobalt, paraquat, Pneumoconioses, antimony, asbestosis, barium, berylliosis, silicosis, coal workers, iron oxide, talc, kaolin, fibrous glass, tungsten, and tin.

    c. **Occupational asthma** includes animal allergens, gums, latex, isocyanate, wood dusts, anhydrides, amines, fluxes, chloramine-T, dyes, formaldehyde, acrylate, drugs and metals) (Table 86-10). Also see occupational and hypersensitivity pneumonitis below, under chemically induced pulmonary dysfunction.

5. **R produces** hypoxia, which results in brain death, cardiac dysrhythmias and cardiac arrest. Hypercarbia results in acidosis, which contributes to dysrhythmias (71).

TABLE 86-10. *Common causes of occupational asthma*

Occupation	Cause
Animal handlers	Animal dander and urine, mites, insects
Adhesive industry	Diisocyanate
Carpenters	Wood dust such as red cedar
Chemical petrol industry	Diisocyanate, acid anhydrides
Cleaners	House dust, cleaning products
Cosmetic workers	Dyes, thioglycollate
Detergent industry	Bacterial enzymes
Electricians	Soldering flux
Electroplaters	Platinum salts, nickel salts
Epoxy resin and plastic workers	Anhydrides (phthalic, tetrachlorophthalic, timellitic)
Food industry	Flour dust, mites, castor beans, green coffee beans, tea leaves, vegetable gums, shellfish
Foundry workers	Diisocyanate, complex amines, furan binder
Hospital workers	Ethylene oxide, formalin, hexachlorophene, latex
Meat packers	Fumes from polyvinyl chloride
Metal workers	Nickel, vanadium, chromium, cobalt, tungsten
Oil extractors	Castor beans, linseed oil, cottonseed
Paint industry	Diisocyanate
Pharmaceutical industry	Antibiotics, enzymes, psyllium, dyes
Polyurethane industry	Diisocyanate used in manufacture
Printing	Gum arabic
Rubber industry	Diisocyanate
Textile industry	Cotton fibers, cotton dust, flax, hemp, wool

C. **Sudden apnea** (72,73)
 1. **Inhalations** of high concentrations of ammonia, acid fumes, carbon monoxide, chlorine, cyanide, hydrogen sulfide, nitrogen dioxide, and sulfur dioxide may result in sudden apnea.
 2. **CNS depressant intoxications** such as anesthetics, anticonvulsants, barbiturates (late), benzodiazepines, carbon monoxide (late), clonidine, ethanol, cyanide (late), neuroleptics, opioids, sedative-hypnotics, and TCA.
D. **Dyspnea.** Acute dyspnea is apparent as increased work of breathing. It may be associated with **obstruction** of the airway passages, involvement of the pulmonary parenchyma that **interferes with oxygen exchange,** and **asphyxiant gases.** It may be apparent where the **oxygen demand is increased** beyond the available supply because of metabolic stimulation.
 1. The **medical pleuropulmonary causes** of acute dyspnea include asthma, upper airway obstruction, foreign body pneumothorax, pneumonia, pulmonary edema (cardiac and noncardiac), asthma gastric aspiration, thromboembolism, atelectasis, pleural effusion, bronchiolitis, flail chest.
 2. The **medical nonpulmonary causes** include decreased pressure of inspired oxygen at high altitudes, acute neuromuscular dysfunction, anemia, obesity, ascites, hyperthyroidism, shock, fever, increased ICP, metabolic acidosis, psychogenic.
 3. **Chronic medical causes** include emphysema or chronic obstructive pulmonary disease, asthma, bronchiectasis, diffuse interstitial lung disease, pleural disease, alveolar disease (neoplasm primary or metastatic, proteinosis, lipid pneumonia), pneumoconioses, paralyzed diaphragm.

4. **The following toxic substances** have been noted to produce acute dyspnea: asphyxiant gases* (methane, propane, carbon dioxide, ethylene dibromide), beta-blockers, herbicides* (dinitrocresol, dinitrophenol), gases* that irritate the upper respiratory tract (anhydrous ammonia, chlorine, sulfur dioxide), gases* that irritate the lower respiratory tract (acrolein, nitrogen dioxide), gases* that interfere with oxygen transport and utilization (cyanide, carbon monoxide, hydrogen sulfide, carbon disulfide), mercury vapors, metabolic acidosis (ethylene glycol, ethanol, iron, isoniazid, lactic acidosis, methanol, salicylates, solvents), hydrocarbon aspiration*, methemoglobinemia (aniline, nitrites and others), methyl bromide, methyl chloride, methylene chloride, paraquat (fibrosis later), solvents (chlorinated hydrocarbons such as trichloroethylene) and withdrawal states. **Chronic dyspnea** is associated with many long-term exposures to asbestos, beryllium, silica, and other worker's pneumonoconiosis.

E. **Tachypnea with and without respiratory distress.**
1. **Direct CNS stimulation.** Amphetamines, caffeine, cocaine, dinitrophenol, salicylates, theophylline.
2. **Hypoxia/acidosis.** Acidosis causes, aspiration, carbon monoxide, cyanide, fever, irritation by gases.
3. **Tachypnea without respiratory distress ("quiet tachypnea").** This is usually from nonpulmonary causes such as fever or an effort to maintain a normal pH by **respiratory compensation. Kussmaul breathing,** when the pH is below 7.25 from metabolic acidosis is an example, although sometimes dyspnea may be present.
4. **Toxic situations** that produce tachypnea with respiratory distress include the following:
   a. **Aspiration** pneumonitis such as seen from petroleum distillate aspirations and gastric aspirations in obtunded patients that have lost their airway protective reflexes.
   b. **Inhaled gases** (carbon dioxide, carbon monoxide, cyanide, hydrogen sulfide) or ingested substances (cyanide, methemoglobinemia producers) that interfere with oxygen transport and/or tissue utilization of oxygen.
   c. **Irritant fumes** from mixing household chemicals or liberated in fires and in industrial accidents.
   d. **CNS respiratory stimulant intoxications** such as salicylates, cocaine, amphetamines and phenylpropanolamine.
   e. **Withdrawal states. Tachypnea and ineffective shallow respirations** (decreased tidal volume) can coexist, producing alveolar hypoventilation.

F. **Slow and shallow respirations**
1. **Central effect.** Clonidine, cyclic antidepressants, ethanol, opioids, sedative-hypnotics.
2. **Neuromuscular.** Botulism, elapid envenomation, neuromuscular blockade, organophosphate, strychnine, tedrotoxin.
3. **Bradypnea and apnea may be caused by** CNS depressant intoxications such as anesthetics, anticonvulsants, barbiturates (late), benzodiazepines, carbon monoxide (late), clonidine, ethanol, cyanide (late), neuroleptics, opioids, sedative-hypnotics, and TCA.

4. **Shallow ineffective respirations** are produced by substances that interfere with the muscles of respiration including paralytic neuromuscular blocking anesthetics, paralytic plant toxins (curare, coniine from poison hemlock), botulism, organophosphate insecticides, nicotine, paralytic shell fish poisoning and tick paralysis, triorthocresyl phosphate fuel oil.

G. **Bronchospasm (wheezing respirations).** "Not all that wheezes is asthma." Medically it may be congenital abnormalities, allergic, infectious, CV, or tumor. **Airway foreign bodies may also cause wheezing.**

1. **Intoxicants that may produce wheezing** and bronchospasm include the following:
   a. **Direct irritation** from gases including chlorine and smoke inhalation, or aspiration of gastric contents or petroleum distillates.
   b. **Pharmacologic effects** such as parasympathetic actions as with organophosphates and beta-adrenergic blockers.
   c. **Hypersensitivity** or allergic reactions include the histamine reactions of scromboid fish poisoning. Salicylates (nasal polyps and asthma), sulfites may cause bronchospasm in susceptible individuals with reactive airway disease.
   d. Agents that may produce bronchospasm include beta-blockers, cholinergic medications, clitocybe and inocybe species mushrooms, and organophosphate insecticides that cause **parasympathetic bronchospasm.**

2. **Occupational hypersensitivity asthma has been reported from** anhydrides (epoxy resin workers), B. subtilis enzymes* (detergent manufacturing workers), diisocyanate* (polyurethane foam workers, foundry workers, and auto painters), metal salts and "metal fume fever" (MFF)* (nickel sulfate, potassium chromate*, platinum, vanadium, zinc* in metal plating and refinery workers), soldering fluxes (electronic workers), wood dust (Western red cedar workers). Other hypersensitivity occupational from natural products include bagassosis (bagasse is the dried fibrous residue of sugar cane) in sugar cane workers, byssinosis in cotton industry workers, and farmer's lung workers in moldy hay. Table 86-10 lists the common cause of occupational asthma, and Table 86-11 differentiates between occupational asthma and hypersensitivity pneumonitis.

TABLE 86-11. *Differences in occupational asthma and hypersensitivity pneumonitis*

	Occupational asthma	Hypersensitivity pneumonitis
Symptoms	Dyspnea, cough, chest tightness	Dyspnea, dry cough, fever, chills
Signs	Wheezes, hyperinflation	Crackles
Time	Immediate or delayed several hours	Delayed 4–6 h
Airways	Medium-sized bronchi and bronchioles	Respiratory bronchioles and alveoli
PFT	Obstruction	Restrictive
CXR	Hyperinflation or normal	Parenchymal infiltrates
Serology	Increase in IgE	Precipitins present in 90%
Mechanisms	Type I or III hypersensitivity, nonimmunologic or irritant	Probable type III hypersensitivity, immune complex
Factors	Asthma, atopy	None known

PFT, pulmonary function tests
Modified from Morgan WK, Lapp NL: *Disease of the airway and lungs.*

H.   Chemically induced pulmonary dysfunction
   1.   *Gases that affect the respiratory tract directly.* These gases are classified by their water solubility.
      a.   **Highly water-soluble gases** produce immediate symptoms, irritate primarily the upper respiratory tract (although massive exposure could involve the lower tract and parenchyma) and are self limited. Because of the good warning property of respiratory tract irritation voluntary prolonged exposure is unlikely. *Examples include* Anhydrous ammonia (fertilizers), chlorine (swimming pools, industrial accidents, bleach), fluorine, formaldehyde, hydrogen chloride, hydrogen fluoride, nitric oxide, sulfur dioxide (pollution).
      b.   **Less water-soluble gases** produce little upper respiratory tract irritation and a delayed onset of symptoms, and affect the lower respiratory tract and parenchyma. Because of poor warning properties prolonged voluntary exposure may occur. Examples are acrolein and aldehydes (from the burning of wool and cellulose fibers), carbonyl chloride, nitrogen dioxide and oxides of nitrogen (pollution), ozone (pollution), and phosgene (polyvinyl chloride, hydrocarbons, styrene). These gases have poor warning properties and prolonged exposure to moderate and low concentrations can occur. Therefore, chemical pneumonitis and delayed (12 to 24 h or longer) noncardiac pulmonary edema may occur.
   2.   **Systemic gases** interfere with oxygen transport in the blood or in the utilization of oxygen in the cells or both. Examples are cyanide, carbon monoxide, hydrogen sulfide (sewer gas), carbon disulfide (rubber industry).
   3.   **Inert gases** displace oxygen from the atmosphere. Examples are butane, propane, methane (marsh gas), carbon dioxide, ethylene dibromide (fumigant), nitrous oxide, helium, neon, dibutyl phalate.
   4.   **Clues to the presence of gases**
      a.   **Color.** Chlorine has a greenish color; nitrogen dioxide has a reddish brown color; bromine has red-brown color, flouring has a yellow color.
      b.   **Odor.** Hydrogen sulfide and carbon disulfide have a rotten egg odor; cyanide has the odor of bitter almonds (silver polish); organophosphates, arsenic and phosphorous have a garlic odor; phosgene has the odor of newly mown hay; and carbon monoxide is odorless but has added to it the odor of coal gas. Some other gases have their own specific odor such as acetone, ammonia, petroleum distillates.
   5.   **Gases with good warning properties.** Ammonia, chlorine, hydrochloric acid, nitric oxide, phosphine, ozone, sulfur dioxide. *Specific pulmonary toxins:* Aluminum (TLV 10 mg/m³⁾—long-term inhalation of fine powders or ore (bauxite) causes pneumoconiosis (Shaver's disease), which progresses to interstitial fibrosis. Increased incidence of cancer in workers. **Ammonia (TLV 25 ppm, IDLH 500 ppm)**—corrosive and irritating to the upper respiratory tract, high water solubility. Severe responses associated with anhydrous ammonia in fertilizers. Good warning properties. **Asbestos (proposed 0.2 fibers/cm³)**—asbestos causes pneumoconiosis, interstitial fibrosis, pleural disease, asbestosis, and neoplasms. The TLV vary with the types chrysotile (serpentine) 2 fibers/cm³ and amphiboles amosite 0.5 mg/cm³, crocidosite 0.2 mg/cm³, other form are 2 fibers/cm³. **Bleomycin (antineoplastic**

agent)—produces interstitia; fibrosis by a free radial mechanism. **Beryllium (TLV 0.002 mg/m³)**—produces irritation and acute pneumonitis, and may progress to interstitial fibrosis and bronchiectasis. It can cause granulomatous disease. It is a pulmonary carcinogen in animals and may be a human carcinogen. **Cadmium (TLV 0.05 mg/m³, IDLH 50 mg/m³)**—acute fume inhalation produces symptoms similar to MFF but progresses onto ARDS and death. High fever is a bad prognostic sign. Chronic fume inhalation produces renal and pulmonary damage, changes obstructive pulmonary function tests with bronchodilator response. Cadmium is carcinogenic in test animals but there is limited data in humans. **Chlorine (TLV 0.5 mg/m³ IDLH 30 mg/m⁻³)**—intermediate or low water solubility and extremely irritating to the eyes and respiratory tract. Good warning properties. **Cobalt (TLV 0.05 mg/m³, IDLH 20 mg/m³)**—causes "hard metal disease," wear-resistant mixture of cobalt and tungsten used in manufacture of drills for grinding. Can produce interstitial fibrosis and giant cell pneumonitis. Cardiomyopathy associated with ingestion. **Copper sulfate (TLV 1 mg/m³ dusts and mists, 2 mg/m³ fumes)**—"Bordeaux solution" causes "Vineyard Sprayer's lung" which results in interstitial fibrosis and adenocarcinoma. They are irritating, may produce corneal ulceration and may cause MFF. **Cotton dust (TLV 0.2 mg/m³, IDLH 500 mg/m³)**—chronic exposure, a respiratory syndrome called **byssinosis.** Starts first day of workweek continues all week. Can lead to irreversible airway obstruction. **Hydrochloric acid (TLV 5 ppm IDLH 100 ppm)**—high water solubility. See occupational medicine. Good warning properties. **Isocyanates**—widely used in manufacture of polyurethane, urethane, and spandex. Contain $N \div C \div O$ group which is very reactive upon inhalation and dermal contact.

a. **Toluene 2,4 diisocyanate (TLV 0.005 ppm, IDLH 10 ppm).** A potent respiratory tract sensitizer and irritant, produces pulmonary edema for high exposures. Carcinogen in test animals. Sharp pungent odor serves as **good warning property.**

b. **Methyl isocyanate (MIC, TLV 0.02 ppm, IDLH 20 ppm).** Highly reactive corrosive on direct contact Irritating to eyes, skin, and respiratory tract. Severe burns and pulmonary edema. Toxicity not related to cyanide. Adverse effects on fetal development and a sensitizer. Responsible for Brophal, India tragedy of 2,000 deaths and more than 100,00 people affected. **Ozone—(TLV 0.1 ppm, IDLH 10 ppm).** Ozone is low solubility, potent irritant and involves the lower respiratory airway. Has a very short half-life but causes oxidative damage. Ground ozone has nothing to do with the stratosphere ozone but ground ozone is increasing because of the biochemical smog reaction HC + NO_2-UV light $\rightarrow O_3$. **Sharp distinct odor is adequate warning property. Nickel carbonyl (Ni(CO)₄, TLV 0.05 ppm, IDLH 7 ppm)** causes an immediate syndrome of insomnia and irritability, fever, headache, nausea, vomiting, and extreme weakness that lasts for hours and is followed by an asymptomatic period of 12 h to days, then develops pneumonitis, which could be fatal, or recovery can take months. Based on animal tests, it can produce liver and brain damage. It is a teratogenic and carcinogenic agent in test animals. Exposures are largely limited to nickel refining. **Nitrogen dioxide (NO₂) (PEL 3 ppm,**

IDLH 50 ppm) is the cause of **"silo filler's disease."** It has low water solubility and affects the lower airway and can have a significant delay in symptoms. **Pungent odor and irritation occur slightly above TLV and are adequate warning properties.** It may cause bronchiolitis obliterans and interstitial fibrosis. It is a **photochemical smog agent** HCS + NO_2—UV light → O_3 (ozone). It can cause methemoglobinemia. It forms nitrous and nitric acid on contract with water. The clinical picture is triphasic with acute symptoms irritation of eyes and respiratory tract (cough and dyspnea) occurring within hours then a latency period up to a day and pulmonary edema and the ARDS with bronchiolitis obliterans occurring 2 to 6 weeks later. **Nitric acid (aqua fortis, engraver's acid TLV 2 ppm, DLH 100 ppm).** Concentrated solutions corrosive to eye and skin. Vapors irritating eye. Respiratory tract and pulmonary edema has occurred. Chronic inhalation has produced bronchitis and erosion of teeth. **Nitric oxide (NO, nitrogen monoxide, TLV 25 ppm, IDLH 100 ppm)** is slowly converted into nitrogen dioxide in the air. **Has sharp sweet odor below TLV and good warning properties.** Can cause obstructive pulmonary disease and based on animal studies methemoglobinemia. **Paraquat (TLV 0.5 mg/m³ and IDLH 1.5 mg/m³).** Paraquat concentrates in the lung and causes pulmonary fibrosis by the classic free radial mechanism. One swallow of a 20% solution is fatal. Treatment is multiple dose activated charcoal. Direct contact causes corrosion. Causes pulmonary fibrosis and multiple organ failure. Dithionate test is 1 part of urine, 0.5 parts of sodium dithionate in 1 N sodium hydroxide. A deep blue color indicates the presence of paraquat or diquat. **Phosgene (carbonyl chloride TLV 0.1 ppm, IDLH 2 ppm).** See occupational medicine. Irritating to lower respiratory tract. Insidious because odor is poor warning property. Hay-like odor at low concentrations Sharp, pungent as high concentrations. **Phosphine (hydrogen phosphide, TLV 0.3 ppm, IDLH 200 ppm).** Extremely irritative gas to respiratory tract can cause fatal pulmonary edema. Multisystem poison with early symptoms of diarrhea, nausea, vomiting cough, headache, and dizziness. **Has fishy garlic odor detected below TLV and is good warning property.** Ignites spontaneously with air. Used as aluminum phosphide fumigant. **Radon** is a naturally occurring radioisotope made from decaying uranium and respirable "radon daughters" release alpha particles causing lung carcinoma. Guideline for safety is less than 4 pcu/L. **Silica.** See pneumoconiosis below. **Silicon** is Si, and silica is SiO_2. **Sulfur dioxide (SO_2) (PEL 2 ppm, IDLH 100 ppm)** occurs when there is high sulfur, soft coal burning when there is an air inversion causing high sulfur smog with increased respiratory mortality and morbidity. SO_2 has high water solubility. See occupational medicine. It causes upper airway irritation but in massive doses can cause bronchiolitis obliterans. **Pungent suffocating odor with a "taste" and irritation good warning properties. Vanadium pentoxide (PEL 0.05 mg/m³ IDLH 70 mg/m³)** is highly irritating to the eyes, skin and respiratory tract. Tracheobronchitis, emphysema and pulmonary edema may occur. Low level exposure may cause greenish discoloration of the tongue.

I. *Metal Fume Fever (MFF)*

  1. MFF is a syndrome that occurs on exposure to fresh metal oxide fumes. Metal fumes are **solid particles less than 0.1 μm in diameter.** There is latent period. More than 1000 patients with MFF are reported each year in the United States. It has been called "Monday morning fever," "brass chills," or "Foundry fever" when reexposed at the beginning of each work week. The pathogenesis is unknown but it is unrelated to hypersensitivity or immunologic mechanisms. ***Common settings* are** brass foundries, zinc smelters, welding, soldering, grinding, galvanizing, chrome plating, and metal cutting.

  2. **Sources** include zinc oxide (the most common and the PEL TLV-TWA is 5 mg/m³), brass which is a combination of up to 45% zinc, copper, cadmium. It is important to differentiate MFF from cadmium fume pneumonitis, which is more serious, results from direct pulmonary toxicity, and may result in ARDS and renal failure. Other metals that cause MFF include aluminum, antimony, arsenic, cobalt, copper, iron, manganese, mercury, nickel, platinum, selenium, silver, and tin. It occurs in association with galvanization process which is coated with zinc to prevent corrosion. Welding of galvanized steel typically causes MFF. Beryllium does not cause MFF.

  3. A similar condition called **"polyfume" fever** occurs from heating the fluoropolymers like polytetrafluoroethylene (Teflon) above 300°C which causes thermodegradation. Cigarette smoking is a major risk factor probably secondary to contamination of the cigarettes with polymers. Fluoropolymers are responsible for atmospheric ozone depletion.

  4. **Manifestations.** Acute self-limited illness.

  (1) **Sudden onset** after a delay of a few hours (4 to 8 h) of brief "flu-like" reaction, often when at home, after exposure and unrecognized.

  (2) A sweet **metallic taste** develops first and may herald the onset. Over the next few hours the symptoms may progress to high fever, chills, frontal headache, diaphoresis, malaise, myalgia, cough, chest and back pain, sore throat, hoarseness, and thirst. **Physical findings may reveal moist rales at bases of the lungs with or without wheezing.** The white blood cell count may be elevated to 12,000 to 16,000. The chest radiograph is normal.

  (3) **Maximum symptoms** occur 10 to 12 h postexposure, followed by **resolution** the next day at 12 to 48 h.

  (4) With time, **tolerance** to the symptoms develops but is lost following a few days of nonexposure. Therefore, it recurs after a weekend.

  (5) **There is no specific test to confirm the diagnosis.** Urine samples for metals are not useful because the oxides are poorly absorbed and background excretion of endogenous metals is variable (zinc, copper, manganese). Complete resolution of symptoms and pulmonary functional abnormalities by 24 to 48 h favors the diagnosis. Nonspecific findings include elevation of the LDH, leucocytosis, and occasionally abnormal chest radiograph with increased interstitial markings and vascular engorgement. Broncho-alveolar lavage (BAL) is positive for neutrophils with elevated levels of inflammatory cytokines in the lavage fluid.

Differential diagnosis: Influenza, bronchitis, pneumonia, or pulmonary embolism.
Management:

1. Prevention with appropriate ventilation and protective equipment.
2. MFF usually resolves within 24 to 48 h without treatment.
3. Oxygen should be administered for hypoxemia and bronchodilators if there is bronchospasm.
4. There is no role for chelator unless there is concomitant systemic poisoning.
5. **Exclude direct pulmonary metal toxicity** from cadmium, mercury, and oxides of nitrogen, phosgene which may be generated by heating of other substances. *Laboratory:* Urine screens for heavy metals. Metal levels may be elevated, confirming exposure. Leucocytosis of 12,000 to 16,000 is often present. **Chest radiograph is normal in MFF, and pulmonary infiltrates seen in hypersensitivity pneumonitis are absent. Precipitating antibodies seen in hypersensitivity are absent in MFF.** Arterial blood gases may show hypoxemia if extensive pulmonary involvement.

J. **Interstitial fibrosis** is the end result of many pulmonary pathologic processes resulting in restrictive pulmonary function tests. The etiology includes but is not limited to— aluminum (Shaver's disease), asbestos, beryllium, bleomycin (classic interstitial fibrosis), coal dust lung (anthracosis, "black lung"), cobalt ("hard metal disease"), copper, nitrofurantoin, mercury fumes, paraquat, silica, talc.

K. **Bronchiolitis obliterans** is caused by many pulmonary toxins resulting in restrictive deficit. It develops after 2 to 6 weeks. It may occur after exposure to ammonia, beryllium, chlorine, nitrogen dioxide ("silo filler's disease"), ozone, and phosgene.

L. **Pulmonary granuloma**
   a. Medical causes include **infections** such mycobacteria (tuberculosis, avium, leprosy) bacteria (especially brucella, yersinia), spirochetes, protozoa (toxoplasmosis, toxocara), viral (cat scratch disease, acquired immunodeficiency), chlamydia (lymphogranuloma), fungi; **idiopathic** such as **sarcoid,** systemic lupus, Wegener's granulomatosis, histiocytosis X, chronic granulomatous disease of childhood, neoplasms.
   b. **Extrinsic alveolitis** such as Farmer's lung, Bird fancier's lung, hypersensitivity conditions such as Mushroom worker, Maple bark strippers, Coffee bean workers, Bagassosis.
   c. **Chemicals and radiation** such as **beryllium,** zirconium, mineral oils, silica, starch, talc, cromolyn sodium, methotrexate, cancer chemotherapy. It is classically caused by beryllium and resembles sarcoidosis. A positive lymphocyte transforming test occurs with beryllium.

M. **Pneumoconioses.** Pneumoconioses are the **dust diseases** of the lung caused by occupational exposures to fibrosing dusts. They are demonstrable radiologically and have restrictive pulmonary function tests. Most important are **aluminum** (Shaver's disease), antimony, **asbestosis,** barium (baritosis), berylliosis, **coal workers** (which may cavitate, become necrotic and cough up black sputum called melanoptosis), **cobalt** (hard metal), fibrous glass, Kaolin, iron oxide, silicosis caused by quartz and other forms of crystalline **silica,** silver, talc, tin, titanium, and hard metal disease caused by **cobalt-tungsten** (elemental tungsten is a gray-white heavy high which melts to hard polyvalent metallic element that resembles chromium and molybdenum in many properties and is used for electrical purposes, drilling and grinding), zirconium, and rare earth metals.

N. **Cancer. Occupational Cancer** was first recognized by Percival Pott in chimney sweeps in London. More recently it has been associated with asbestos (lung and mesothelioma), benzene (myelogenous leukemia and lymphoma), vinyl chloride (angiosarcoma of the liver), arsenic (cancer of the skin, lung and liver), bischloromethyl ether (oat cell carcinoma of the lung), ionizing radiation and dioxin is still controversial. Table 86-12 lists the agents associated with lung cancer. Tobacco use, particularly smoking, is linked to more than 430,000 deaths per year in the United States. About 114,000 of these deaths are caused by lung cancer (87). On the basis of 30 epidemiologic studies the EPA has concluded that environmental tobacco smoke is a **human carcinogen.** Research on the hazards of smoking tobacco has recently shown an association between exposure to tobacco smoke by **passive smoking** and adverse health effects, including lung cancer, respiratory diseases, brain tumors, asthma, and asthmatic exacerbations.

O. **Angioedema (angioneurotic edema). The substances** include azithromycin, barium, captopril, enalapril, griseofulvin, iodine, lamtrigine, meprobamate, monosodium glutamate, penicillin G, providine-iodine, quinidine, sulfides, tartrazine dye, thiamine.

P. **Hypoxia.** Hypoxia can be caused by **insufficient oxygen in the ambient air** including displacement by inert gases; **interference with oxygen absorption** by the lung because pneumonia and pulmonary edema; and **cellular hypoxia** which may be present despite normal arterial oxygen tension. The routine measurement of oxygen measures the oxygen dissolved in the plasma but does not measure oxygen content or oxygen saturation. A direct measure of the oxygen content is by co-oximeter will show decreased oxyhemoglobin saturation. The pulse oximeter gives falsely near normal readings. Hypoxia may also be caused medically by bacterial or viral pneumonia, heart failure due to myocardial infarction, shock or other causes. **The other causes for hypoxia** include erroneous venous blood sampling, other infectious causes of pneumonia, and myocardia damage secondary to infarction and trauma. **The toxicologic causes of hypoxia** include the following:

1. **Inert gases** (carbon dioxide, methane, propane, and nitrogen).
2. **Agents causing cardiogenic pulmonary edema** characterized by low cardiac output and elevated pulmonary wedge pressure (antidysrhythmic agents type 1a (quinidine, procainamide, disopyramide), beta-adrenergic blockers, and verapamil and TCA.

TABLE 86-12. *Agents associated with occupational lung cancer*

Acrylonitrile	Production of plastics and petrochemicals
Arsenic	Copper smelting, manufacture of pesticides
Asbestos	Production, construction
Bis(chloromethyl)ether	Manufacture of exchange resins
Beryllium	Metal processing
Cadmium	Smelting and manufacture of batteries
Chromium	Manufacture of pigments, leather products, plating
Cigarette smoke	Asbestos
Mustard gas	Production, warfare
Nickel	Smelting, electrolysis
Radon	Mining
Vinyl chloride	Production of polyvinyl chloride

3. **Agents causing cellular hypoxia** by limiting hemoglobin oxygen binding capacity (carbon monoxide, methemoglobinemia, sulfhemoglobinemia) or interference with cellular oxygen utilization (cyanide, carbon disulfide, hydrogen sulfide).

4. Substances causing increase in pulmonary capillary permeability and **noncardiogenic pulmonary edema** (ARDS) are characterized by low or normal pulmonary wedge pressure and include cocaine, opioids, paraquat, phosgene, salicylates, sedative-hypnotics (ethchlorvynol), smoke inhalation.

5. **Pneumonia** (aspiration of gastric contents, aspiration of petroleum distillates, chlorine and irritant gases, MFF?).

6. **Pulmonary fibrosis** (paraquat).

Q. **Pulmonary edema.** Pulmonary edema, both cardiac and noncardiac, may develop from intoxications. All the substances that can cause chemical pneumonia may cause pulmonary edema.

1. **Noncardiac pulmonary edema** usually involves pulmonary capillary permeability, lacks the signs of congestive heart failure and the pulmonary wedge pressure will be low or normal and the cardiac output increased or normal. The substances that may cause this include opioids (especially i.v. but also inhaled heroin) (76), barbiturates and nonbarbiturate sedative-hypnotics (ethchlorvynol IV), organophosphate insecticides, aspiration (hydrocarbons, gastric contents in coma and convulsions), irritant gases (chlorine, nitrogen dioxide, metal and polyfume fever), paraquat (noncardiogenic as well as fibrosis), cyanide, carbon monoxide and salicylates (25% of adults with chronic salicylate poisoning) (75). They may damage the alveolar-capillary membrane producing increased capillary permeability and pulmonary edema, especially with i.v. fluid overload.

2. **Cardiogenic pulmonary edema** has an elevated pulmonary wedge pressure and low cardiac output. Drugs associated with heart failure may be involved.

3. Other toxins such as cocaine may cause a **massive sympathetic discharge resulting in neurogenic pulmonary edema.** Pulmonary edema may also be produced by **aspiration** of many toxins or the gastric contents and by inhalation of **chemical irritants** such as ammonia, chlorine, phosgene, sulfur dioxide, oxides of nitrogen, ozone, smoke inhalations, and metal fumes. **Fires** liberating carbon monoxide and cyanide may result in pulmonary edema.

R. **ARDS** (77,78)

1. First described by Ashbaugh in 1967 and characterized by dyspnea, hypoxia, decreased pulmonary compliance, and bilateral pulmonary infiltrates. ARDS is a catastrophic insult that leads to extravascular lung fluid. It occurs in individuals with previously healthy lungs. Mortality is usually 50%.

2. **Pathophysiology** starts with noncardiac pulmonary edema as a primary feature of ARDS resulting from increased permeability of the alveolar-capillary interface and the effects of other inflammatory mediators. The excess fluid, usually removed by the lymphatics, can not be adequately managed and accumulates. This allows for the alveoli and interstitium to become flooded with transudate. The end result is pulmonary shunting (lung areas are perfused but underventilated), decreased compliance, pulmonary hypertension, and increased dead space.

3. **ARDS may be caused by** anaphylaxis, burns, postcardioversion, DIC, diabetic ketoacidosis, embolism (air, amniotic, fat), near drowning, pancreatitis, pneumonia (including aspiration pH of less than 2.5, and PCP), sepsis, shock, smoke inhalation, strangulation, trauma, toxic gas inhalation, uremia.

4. **Toxic substances that may produce ARDS** include ammonia, barbiturates, cadmium, chlordiazepoxide, colchicine, Dextran 40, ethchlorvynol, fluorescein, heroin, methadone, nitrous oxide, oxygen, phosgene, propoxyphene, salicylates, thiazides.

S. **Pneumonitis and pulmonary impairment** (79–85). **Parenchymal pulmonary damage has been reported from the following substances:** ammonia, asbestos (brake lining, fireproofing), bagassosis (sugar cane residue—bagasse), beryllium (resembles sarcoid), byssinosis (cotton, flax or hemp, "brown lung disease"), cadmium welding, carbon disulfide, chlorine, chromates, detergent manufacturing (*B. subtilis* proteolytic enzymes), farmer's lung (mold thermophilic actinomyces), halogen gases, hydrocarbon aspiration, hydrogen sulfide, manganese, maple bark disease (mold Alternaria), mercury (inorganic) vapor, nitrofurantoin, nitrous oxide, paraquat, petro chemicals, petroleum distillates, phosgene, silicosis, silo filler's disease due to nitrogen dioxide, toluene diisocyanate (TDI) hypersensitivity (polyurethane, plastic industry), turpentine, zinc chloride.

T. **Pulmonary renal syndrome (PRS, Goodpasture's syndrome)** (86). This syndrome is defined as lung hemorrhage and renal failure. The term "pulmonary renal syndrome" is used synonymously with "acute glomerulonephritis" and "pulmonary hemorrhage." It was discovered by Ernest Goodpasture in studying histopathology of victims of the 1919 influenza epidemic. It is mediated by immune, infectious, and toxic chemical causes. **Most frequent entities producing PRS** include the following:

1. **Immune complex diseases.** Systemic lupus erythematosus, Henock-Schonlein, subacute bacterial endocarditis), Berger's disease, cryoglobulinemia, idiopathic rapidly progressive glomerulonephritis.

2. **Antinuclear circulating antibodies.** Wegener's granulomatosis, periarteritis nodosa, sarcoidosis, D-penicillamine, trimellite anhydrase, used in industry for epoxy resins, and vinyl plastics.

3. **Nonimmune infections.** *Legionella pneumonia.*

U. **Drug-induced bronchopulmonary disorders** (87,88). **Reported reactions to selected drugs** include the following:

1. ACE inhibitors (cough, and mild obstruction).

2. Amiodarone (interstitial pneumonitis/fibrosis, hypersensitivity, noncardiac pulmonary edema, ARDS).

3. Alkylating agents (busulfan, cyclophosphamide, melphalan, chlorambucil give interstitial fibrosis and pneumonitis, alveolar proteinosis).

4. Aminoglycoside (impaired neuromuscular transmission respiratory muscle dysfunction).

5. Beta-blockers (bronchospasm in patients with hyperreactive airway disease).

6. Bleomycin (interstitial fibrosis and pneumonitis), carmustine (BCNU interstitial fibrosis, and pneumonitis).

7. Cocaine (alveolar hemorrhage, noncardiac pulmonary edema, interstitial pneumonitis, bronchiolitis obliterans).

8. Ethchlorvynol (noncardiac pulmonary edema).
9. Gold (bronchiolitis obliterans, hypersensitivity pneumonitis).
10. Methotrexate (hypersensitivity and interstitial pneumonitis, fibrosis, noncardiac pulmonary edema).
11. Nitrofurantoin (hypersensitivity and interstitial pneumonia, vasculitides, pleuritis, fibrosis).
12. Nonsteroidal antiinflammatory drugs (bronchospasm, hypersensitivity pneumonia).
13. Opioids (respiratory depression, noncardiac pulmonary edema, fibrosis, granulomas, and vasculitis in i.v. abusers).
14. Penicillins (pneumonia).
15. Penicillamine (bronchiolitis, Goodpasture-like syndrome, interstitial pneumonia/fibrosis).
16. Pentamidine (bronchospasm).
17. Phenytoin (mediastinal lymphadenopathy, vasculitis).
18. Salicylates (bronchospasm, nasal polyposis, noncardiac pulmonary edema).
19. Sulfonamides (vasculitis, pneumonia, bronchospasm).
20. Vinca alkaloids (vincristine gives interstitial pneumonitis, fibrosis, and bronchospasm).

VII. **Temperature** (89–106). **Temperature readings are often presented in either fahrenheit (F) or centigrade (C) the conversion factors for these are C × 1.8 + 32 = °F or F − 32 × 0.55 = °C.** For each degree of temperature more than 37°C (98.6°F), pH decreases 0.015, P_{CO_2} increases 4.4%, and Pa_{O_2} increases 7.2%. The opposite occurs for each degree less than 37°C. Electrolytes changes are increase or decrease in potassium and sodium, increased BUN and glucose. The ECG shows nonspecific ST segment depression, T wave, PVC, SVT. Nonspecific cerebrospinal fluid (CSF) pleocytosis.

A. **Temperature elevation**

1. **Febrile states are regulated temperature elevations** and develop secondary to a physiologic readjustment of the thermoregulatory set-point to a higher level. The most frequent cause is infection. Antipyretic medications act to inhibit prostaglandin synthesis and reduce the temperature of infections.

2. **Hyperthermia** is unregulated temperature elevation. **The autoregulatory mechanism of fever is not functioning** and the temperature is usually more than 40°C (104°F) and may rise to dangerous levels. These types of temperature elevation are **referred to as hyperthermia or heat illness similar to heat stroke.** Toxicologic temperature elevations require external cooling measures and control of excess muscular activity such as convulsions. Antipyretics are not useful in these cases. A frequent cause of fever **following intoxication** is aspiration pneumonia. Table 86-13 lists the toxicologic causes of temperature elevation, their mechanisms, and a summary of their management. Temperature elevation associated with toxicologic emergencies may be due to the following:

   a. **Direct effect on hypothalamic set-point** by interference with or depletion of DA (phenothiazines, H-2 blockers).

   b. **CNS stimulation, muscular hyperactivity and seizures, increase in metabolic rate** (amoxapine, amphetamines and derivatives, cocaine, lithium, lyser-

TABLE 86-13. *Intoxications that produce temperature elevation*

Agent	Mechanism	Specific therapy
Amphetamines[a]	CNS stimulation, seizures, muscular hyperactivity	Benzodiazepines
Anesthetic agents[a] (halothane, succinylcholine)	Muscle rigidity	Dantrolene
Anticholinergic[a]	Decreased perspiration	—
Antihistamines	Decreased perspiration	—
Boric acid	Seizures	Benzodiazepines
Caffeine	CNS stimulation, seizures	Benzodiazepines
Muscular hyperactivity		
Camphor	CNS stimulation, seizures	Benzodiazepines
Cocaine[a]	CNS stimulation, seizures, muscular hyperactivity	Benzodiazepines
Delirium tremors[a]	Tremors, muscular activity	Benzodiazepines
Ethanol withdrawal	CNS stimulation	Benzodiazepines
Lithium	Tremors, muscle rigidity. Haloperidol interaction?[a]	—
Malignant hyperthermia	Muscle rigidity, increased metabolism	Dantrolene
Metal fume fever	May effect thermoregulation	—
Monoamine oxidase inhibitors	Serotonin	Benzodiazepines
Drug interactions[a]	Muscle rigidity	Dantrolene
	Muscle rigidity	Dantrolene
MNS[a]	May effect thermoregulation	—
Pentachlorophenol	Interferes with oxidative phosphorylation	—
Phencyclidine	CNS stimulation, muscular hyperactivity	—
Phenothiazines	Anticholinergic activity	—
MNS[a]	Muscle rigidity, may effect thermoregulation	Dantrolene
Polymer fume fever	May effect thermoregulation	—
Salicylate	Interferes with oxidative phosphorylation CNS stimulation	—
Sedative-hypnotic withdrawal[a]	CNS stimulation	Benzodiazepines
Thyroid excess	Increase in metabolism	Propylthiouracil
Tricyclic antidepressants	Anticholinergic activity	—

[a]May result in malignant hyperthermia. All malignant hyperthermia requires, in addition to specific agent, external cooling, acid-base, and fluid and electrolyte repair. Antipyretics are not indicated or effective.
MNS, malignant neuroleptic syndrome.

gic acid diethylamide (LSD), maprotiline, MAOI, phencyclidine, strychnine, agents causing dystonia).

   c. **Excess muscle activity** (amphetamines, cocaine, isoniazid, thyroid).

   d. **Impaired thermoregulation** (MFF).

   e. **Hypermetabolic state**. Amphetamines, cocaine, dinitrophenol, salicylates, thyroid).

   f. **Interference with oxidative phosphorylation** (salicylate, dinitrophenol, pentachlorophenol).

   g. **Dehydration** (diuretics).

   h. **Hypersensitivity** (antibiotics).

   i. **Impaired heat dissipation** (anticholinergic agents, antihistamines).

   j. **Peripheral vasoconstriction and conservation** (sympathomimetics).

   k. **Destruction of cell and liberation of cellular contents** and IL-1 (chemotherapeutic agents, trauma).

    l.   Genetic (malignant hyperthermia, NMS, and G6PD deficiency).

    m.   Poikilothermic environmental (heat stroke, MFF, phenothiazines).

  3. Medical differential diagnosis. Infection (especially malaria); dehydration, endocrine (hypothalamic disorder, thyroid storm, pheochromocytoma); heat stroke, and hyperthermic syndromes. Muscular rigidity suggests hyperthermic syndromes.

  4. Complications are hyperthermia, acidosis, dysrhythmias, rhabdomyolysis (RDM) and myoglobinemia, hepatic damage, coma with neurologic sequel, coagulopathy and disseminated intravascular coagulation, cardiac, acute tubular necrosis (ATN), and renal failure.

B. Hyperthermia syndromes (Table 86-13). The hyperthermia syndromes are life-threatening elevation of temperature. The syndromes all have altered mental state, rigidity, acidosis and temperature elevation except the 5-HT syndrome. They may occur as

  1. Malignant hyperthermia, an autosomal dominant **genetic inborn error** of muscle metabolism (incidence 1:15,000) on exposure to certain halogenated anesthetic agents, particularity halothane and succinylcholine.

  2. NMS in patients chronically on antipsychotic agents and associated with muscle rigidity, metabolic acidosis, and altered mental state. It is an idiosyncratic reaction to neuroleptic medication—phenothiazines and butyrophenones. It may be genetic reaction.

  3. Malignant hyperthermia associated with drug interactions such as when synthetic opioids (meperidine, dextromethorphan and possibly others) or TCA are administered to patients receiving MAOI.

  4. Anticholinergic overdose interferes with the dissipation of heat by inhibiting perspiration.

  5. 5-HT syndrome may occur with or without hyperthermia primarily in patients taking MAOI who take serotonergic drugs such as meperidine, 5-HT inhibitors (fluoxetine, sertraline, paroxetine) and is characterized by irritability, rigidity, myoclonus, diaphoresis, and hyperthermia. Parkinson "drug holidays" have cause 5-HT like syndromes.

C. Heat stroke (101,102). Heat dissipation mechanisms of the body (sweating, radiation, and convection) are overwhelmed by the absorption or production of heat. Theoretically exhaustion and heat stroke were differentiated by primary water or salt loss. In reality pure forms are very rare. When body temperature reaches 42°C, oxidative phosphorylation becomes uncoupled. Membranes become more permeable and sodium influx increases, depolarization occurs. The hallmark is neurologic disability.

  1. Underlying causes are the environment, behavioral activities (exertional and nonexertional), chronic and congenital illness (cystic fibrosis loss of chlorides, anhidrotic ectodermal dysplasia), and age (the elderly and the young infant are more susceptible).

  2. Medications in therapeutic doses, in overdoses or by substance abuse that may contribute heat stroke include antihistamines and anticholinergics, beta-blockers, phenothiazines, and TCA by decreased perspiration; amphetamines, hallucinogens, and thyroid increased heat production; and ethanol by increased heat absorption.

3. **Clinical findings**
   a. Nonspecific. Anorexia, nausea, vomiting, headache, fatigue.
   b. CNS. Confusion or disorientation progressing to coma and posturing.
   c. Skin is red, hot, and dry.
   d. High temperatures of more than 40°C accompanied by tachycardia and hypotension.
4. **Differential diagnosis** from heat exhaustion which has normal mentation, temperatures less than 39°C, and moist diaphoretic skin but there is overlapping. It is differentiated from most hyperthermia syndromes by the lack of rigidity.

D. **Hypothermia**
   1. **An average of 770 persons (range 586 in 1991 to 1021 in 1983) or 0.2 deaths per million population die from hypothermia in the United States annually. About 50% of these deaths are in persons over 65 years of age. The elderly** have a increased risk for hypothermia because of impaired shivering, lower levels of protective fat, limited mobility, and lower metabolic rate (104). **Other risk factors,** inadequate housing, outdoor sports and water immersion, hypothyroidism, mental illness, starvation, poverty and any immobilizing illness (104,105). **Toxicologic risk factors** are consumption of alcoholic beverages, neuroleptics, sedative-hypnotics including barbiturates and benzodiazepines.
   2. **Hypothermia exists when the patient's core temperature is below 35°C (95°F).** At this temperature the systems responsible for thermoregulation begin to fail. Nuclei in the preoptic anterior hypothalamus coordinate heat conservation. Hypothermia like hypocapnia and alkalosis, shifts the oxyhemoglobin-dissociation curve to the left resulting in decreased oxygen release from hemoglobin into the tissues. Hypothermia can be clinically overlooked since many clinical thermometers measure only as low as 94°F (34.4°C) and the signs and symptoms are not specific.
   3. Hypothermia may also be associated with following **medical conditions** adrenal insufficiency, anorexia nervosa, CV collapse (hemorrhage, dehydration, and sepsis), cold exposure, cold water immersion, CNS trauma and transection of the spinal cord, hypoglycemia, hypothyroid and myxedema, hypopituitarism, malnutrition, and CV accidents.
   4. **Intoxications.** In obtunded patients with an overdose of sedative-hypnotics, hypothermia is a poor prognostic sign.
      a. Mechanisms of intoxications that may produce hypothermia include the following: any agent decreases the level of consciousness interferes with the physiologic response (vasoconstriction and muscle contraction) when the patient is exposed to a cool environment especially, e.g., ethanol, opioids; hypothalamic effects of the agent, e.g., carbon monoxide; impaired heat conservation, e.g., ethanol.
      b. **Most common cause (more than 80% of hypothermia cases) of substance-induced hypothermia is ethanol. Intoxications associated with hypothermia** are aconite, **alpha-antagonists,** barbiturates*, benzodiazepines, beta-blockers,

carbon monoxide*, CNS depressants, clonidine, ethanol* (most common cause), general anesthetics, hypoglycemia* (insulin, sulfonylureas and from any cause), nitrites, opioids, phenothiazines* (97) (second most common cause), sedative-hypnotics*, and TCA*. An asterisk indicates most frequent causes (99).

5. **Early manifestations** include shivering, numbness, fatigue, slurred speech, confusion, poor coordination and impaired gait, combativeness, blueness or puffiness of the skin, and irrationality. Shivering may be a early clue but hypothermic patients with temperatures lower than 90°F (32.2°C) may not shiver or even feel cold (105). **Below 90°F**, muscle tone increases, heart rate slows, respirations become shallow and slow, pupils dilated and fixed, and the patient may appear dead. Since hypothermia may mimic death, the patients should continue to have resuscitative measures until they are "warm and dead." Table 86-14 summarizes the effects of hypothermia at different temperatures.

   a. **Mild 35°C to 32.2°C (95°F to 90°F).** CNS: decreased metabolism, amnesia, apathy, dysarthria, impaired judgement, maladaptive behavior; CV: tachycardia then progressive bradycardia, prolongation cardiac cycle, increase cardiac output and BP. Respiratory (Res): Tachypnea, progressive decrease minute volume, declining oxygen consumption, bronchorrhea, bronchospasm; renal/endocrine (R/E): cold diuresis, increase catecholamines, adrenal steroids, triiodothyronine, thyroxine, increase metabolism with shivering; Neuromuscular (NM): increased muscle tone preshivering, fatigue, shivering-induced thermogenesis, ataxia.

   b. **Moderate, 32.2°C to 28°C (90°F to 82.4°F).** CNS: EEG abnormalities, progressive decrease in level of consciousness, pupillary dilation, paradoxical undressing, hallucinations; CV: Progressive decrease in pulse and cardiac output, increased atrial and ventricular dysrhythmias, nonspecific and suggestive ECG J waves, prolonged systole; Res: hypoventilation, 50% decreases in CO_2 production per 8°C drop, absence airway protective reflexes, 50% decreased in oxygen consumption; R/E: 50% increase in renal flow, no insulin activity; NM: hyporeflexia, decreased shivering-induced thermogenesis, rigidity.

TABLE 86-14. *Manifestations of hypothermia*

Core temperature physiology	Common manifestations
35°C (95°F)	Slurred speech, memory lapse, ataxia
32°C (89.6°F)	Drowsy, amnesic, confused, disoriented, loss of muscle coordination, muscle rigidity, skin cyanotic and edematous, tachycardia
30°C (86°F)	Hypoxia, stuporous, myocardial irritability, decreased CO, bradycardia, J waves on ECG,[a] hypotension, shivering, decreased minute ventilation, bradypnea, ceases 30°C, pallor and cyanosis
28°C (82.4°F)	Dysrhythmia and ventricular fibrillation and asystole, acidosis
26°C (78°F)	Loss of consciousness, areflexia
25°C (77°F)	Apneic, pulseless, areflexia, fixed dilated pupils
20°C (68°F)	Asystole, EMD

[a]"Camel humped" at QRS-ST junction at about 30°C.
EMD, electromechanical dissociation.

    c. **Severe, less than 28°C (82.4°F).** CNS: loss cerebrovascular autoregulation, decliner in cerebral blood flow (CBF), coma, loss ocular reflex, decrease in EEG and ECG activity, CV: decrease BP, heart rate and cardiac output, re-entrant dysrhythmias, decreased ventricular dysrhythmia threshold, asystole; Res: pulmonary congestion, 75% decrease in oxygen consumption, apnea; R/E: decrease renal blood flow parallels decrease in cardiac output, extreme oliguria, poikilothermic, 80% decrease in basal metabolism; NM: no motion, decreased nerve conduction velocity, peripheral areflexia.

    6. **Laboratory values** change with various degrees of hypothermia. Initially respiratory alkalosis followed by respiratory acidosis due to CO_2 retention. The hematocrit increases 2% per °C decline in temperature. The white blood cell count falls but differential is normal. Potassium should be checked frequently because hypothermia masks potassium-induced changes in the ECG. Potassium of more than 6.8 mEq/L is a good indicator of death during acute hypothermia. Cold-induced renal glycosuria does not suggest normoglycemia. Hypothermia is frequently associated with hypoglycemia. Persistent hyperglycemia suggests diabetes mellitus or pancreatitis. Coagulopathies develop in the presence of normal levels of clotting factors since the PT or PTT are routinely performed at 37°C. Hypercoagulopathy may result in thromboembolism (106). **When the blood cools,** the arterial pH increases and the partial pressure of carbon monoxide (P_{CO_2}) falls. For each degree of temperature less than 37°C (98.6°F), the pH increases 0.015, P_{CO_2} decreases 4.4%, and Pa_2 decreases 7.2%. Thus, a pH of 7.4 and a P_{CO_2} of 40 mm Hg at 37°C is equivalent to a pH of 7.55 and a P_{CO_2} 30 mm Hg at 30°C (106).

VIII. **Nervous system** (107)

    A. **Altered mental state.** This is one of the most common manifestations of intoxications (Fig. 86-2). To alter the mental state there must be cortical or ascending reticular activating (ARAS) dysfunction (Fig. 86-2). It is useful to **categorize these manifestations into** CNS depressants; CNS stimulants; hallucinogens; anticholinergic agents; and cholinergic agents. Such a classification allows the clinician to convey to the toxicologic analyst the type of neurologic manifestations present and to direct the analysis toward the most likely substances on the basis of the clinical evaluation. It is **wise not to assume** that the altered mental state is solely associated with the intoxicant but to exclude other treatable causes. It is important to recognize that some substances may uncover an underlying illness or provoke an underlying psychosis. For instance, some drugs such as the phenothiazines may lower the convulsive threshold resulting in seizures of idiopathic epilepsy. **Classification** below lists the substances on the right and the manifestations of the class (not the specific substance) on the left.

    B. **Classification of toxins to the central and autonomic nervous system**

        1. **CNS depressants.** Hallmarks of CNS depressants are CNS depression and lethargy. Most serious intoxications will produce coma eventually if untreated. The primary CNS depressants are listed below with their major manifestations. "Designer drugs" are synthetic analogs of meperidine and fentanyl that are made to avoid legal sanctions. They are many more times potent than morphine. One analog 3-methyl fentanyl is 3000 times more potent than morphine.

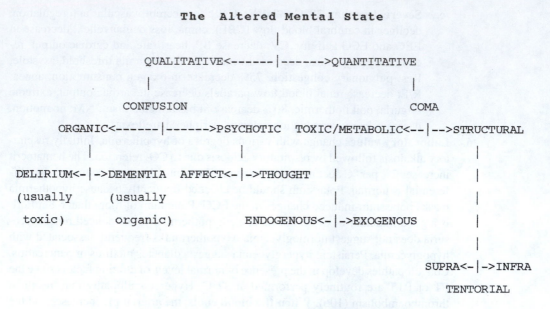

FIG. 86-2. The altered mental state.

a. **CNS depressants:**

Manifestations	CNS Depressants
Bradycardia	Alcohols and glycols
Bradypnea	Anticonvulsants
Shallow respirations	Antidysrhythmics
Hypotension	Antihypertensives
Hypothermia	Barbiturates
Flaccid coma	Benzodiazepines
Miosis	Butyrophenones
Hypoactive bowel sounds	Beta-adrenergic blockers
Frozen addict syndrome	Calcium channel blockers
	Digitalis
	Opioids
	Phenothiazines
	Nonbarbiturate sedative-hypnotics chloral hydrate, glutethimide, methaqualone, methyprylon, ethchlorvynol)
	Tricyclic/cyclic antidepressants

Exceptions to the above manifestations:
1. Barbiturates may produce an initial tachycardia
2. Convulsions are produced by: codeine, propoxyphene, meperidine, glutethimide, phenothiazines, methaqualone, and tricyclic/cyclic anti-depressants
3. Benzodiazepines rarely produce coma that will interfere with cardio-respiratory functions.

4. The "frozen addict syndrome" is due to a neurotoxin from improper synthesis of an analog of meperidine. Its manifestations are similar to permanent type of parkinsonism.

5. Pulmonary edema is common with opioids and sedative-hypnotics.

b. **CNS stimulants.** Hallmarks of CNS stimulants are convulsions and hyperactivity:

Manifestations	CNS Stimulants
Tachycardia	Amphetamines
Tachypnea and dysrhythmias	Anticholinergics
Hypertension	Cocaine
Convulsions	Camphor
Spastic coma	Ergot alkaloids
Toxic psychosis	Isoniazid
Mydriasis (reactive)	Lithium
Agitation and restlessness	LSD
Moist skin	Mescaline and synthetic analogs
Tremors	Metals (arsenic lead, mercury)
	Methylphenidate
	MAOI
	Pemoline (Cylert)
	Phencyclidine
	Salicylates
	Strychnine
	Sympathomimetics (Phenylpropanolamine, Theophylline, caffeine)
	Withdrawal from ethanol, beta-adrenergic blockers, clonidine, opioids, sedative-hypnotics
	Exceptions to the above manifestations are the following: flaccid coma will eventually develop after seizures; anticholinergics produce dry skin and mucosa; and phencyclidine may produce miosis.

c. **Hallucinogens.** There is considerable overlapping in this category; however, the major hallmark manifestation is hallucination:

Manifestations	Hallucinogens
Tachycardia and dysrhythmias	Amphetamines
Tachypnea	Anticholinergics
Hypertension	Carbon monoxide
Hallucinations usually visual	Cardiac glycosides
Disorientation	Cocaine
Panic reaction	Ethanol
Toxic psychosis	Hydrocarbon inhalation (abuse)
Moist skin	Hydrocarbon inhalation (occupation)
Variable bowel sounds	LSD

Mydriasis (reactive)

Marijuana

Hyperthermia

Mescaline (Peyote)

Flashbacks

Mescaline—amphetamine hybrids

Metals (Chronic mercury, arsenic)

Mushrooms (Psilocybin)

Phencyclidine

Plants (Morning glory seeds, nutmeg)

Mescaline-amphetamine hybrids are methylene dioxymethamphetamine (MDMA, ecstacy, "ADAM") and methylene dioxyamphetamine (MDA, "Eve") which have been recently associated with deaths.

d.   Automatic nervous system. Figure 86-3 summarizes the biosynthesis of the catecholamines. Figure 86-4 shows the divisions of the autonomic nervous system. Table 86-15A summarizes the autonomic syndrome effects.

(1)   Anticholinergic. There is overlapping with other categories of drugs particularity the antipsychotic (phenothiazines), antidepressants (tricyclic/cyclic antidepressants) and hallucinogens. The anticholinergic actions of these agents is usually only part of the total action and are not the most important or prominent effect. The modified poem used to recall anticholinergic action is "Blind as a bat, red as beet, hot as a hare, dry as a bone, mad as a hatter, the bowel and bladder lose their tone and the heart runs alone." "Alice in Wonderland" syndrome or Lilliputian type of hallucinations has been frequently reported:

Manifestations	Anticholinergic agents
Tachycardia, dysrhythmias rare	Antihistamines
Tachypnea	Antispasmodic GI preparations
Hypertension (mild)	Antiparkinson preparations
Hyperthermia	Atropine
Hallucinations	Cyclobenzaprine
Mydriasis (unreactive)	Mydriatic ophthalmologic agents
Flushed skin	Over-the-counter sleep agents
Dry skin	Plants (Datura spp.)/mushrooms)
Hypoactive bowel sounds	Phenothiazines
Urinary retention	Scopolamine
	Tricyclic/cyclic antidepressants

(2)   Cholinergic. The mnemonic to remember their major manifestations is **DUMBELS: D**—diarrhea; **U**—urination; **M**—miosis; **B**—bronchospasm and bradycardia; **E**—excess salivation; **L**—lacrimation; **S**—seizures and coma.

Manifestations	Cholinergic agents
Bradycardia-muscarinic effect	Bethanecol
Tachycardia—nicotinic effect	Carbamate insecticides (Carbaryl)
Miosis	Edrophonium
Diarrhea	Organophosphate insecticides

```
           1            2              3                      4
Tyrosine -->Dopa -->dopamine -->norepinephrine -->epinephrine
           5                                 2
Tryptophan --> 5 hydroxytryptophan --> 5 hydroxytryptamine
                                            (serotonin)
```

1. Tyrosine hydroxylase

2. Aromatic L-amino acid decarboxylase also converts 5
-hydroxytryptophan to serotonin

3. Dopamine -B-hydroxylase dopamine to norepinephrine inhibited by
copper reagents such as disulfiram and diethylthiocarbamate.

4. Phenylethanolamine-N-methyltransferase catalyzes the transfer of
methyl group to norepinephrine for formation of epinephrine.

5. Tryptophan hydroxylase

FIG. 86-3. Biosynthesis of catecholamines.

Hypertension (variable)	(Malathion, parathion)
Hyperactive bowel sounds	Parasympathetic agents
Excess urination	(Physostigmine, pyridostigmine)
Excess salivation	Toxic mushrooms (*A. muscaria,*
Lacrimation	Clitocybe spp.)
Bronchospasm	
Muscle fasciculations	
(nicotinic effect)	
Paralysis (nicotinic effect)	

```
1. Parasympathetic
CNS -Preganglionic -<ganglion>-Postganglionic -<neuro junct> effector
      (cholinergic)  Acetyl-  (cholinergic)    acetyl      cell
                     choline                   choline
2. Sympathetic
CNS  Preganglionic -<ganglion>-Postganglionic -<neuro junct> effector
      (cholinergic)  Acetyl-  (adrenergic)     Norepi-     cell
                     choline                   nephrine
                     (ACH)                     (NE)
```

FIG. 86-4. Divisions of the autonomic nervous system.

    e. **Autonomic nervous system tests** include the following:

        (1) **Pupillary function tests.** Response to light in 0.2 to 0.3 s with 2 to 4 mm constriction and accommodation assess the parasympathetic system; dilation to dim light the sympathetic nervous system. Pilocarpine 0.125% eye drops act on end organs affected by acetylcholine and pupil constriction of 0 to 0.5 mm implies parasympathetic action. Epi 0.1% eye drops act directly stimulates the alpha-adrenergic receptors and lack of induction of dilation indicates postganglionic sympathetic lesion. Cocaine 4% to 5% block reuptake NE and indirectly dilate the pupil more than 1.5 mm. Lack of dilation indicates pre- or postganglionic lesion.

        (2) **CV function tests.** Heart response to deep breathing. Pulse rate (6 to 18 bpm) through vagal afferent is reduced with inspiration and increased with expiration.

        (3) **Plasma NE** normal values supine 70 to 750 pg/mL, standing 200 to 1,700 pg/mL: Allow NE with patient supine indicates postganglionic sympathetic lesion, failure of NE to rise when stands suggests either preganglionic or postganglionic disturbance (108).

        (4) **Signs of autonomic insufficiency** are constipation, anhydrosis, postural hypotension, loss of premonitory signs of syncope (diaphoresis and bradycardia), urinary retention, incontinence, night blindness (inability to dilate pupil), nasal congestion (lack of alpha-mediated nasal constriction) and impotence.

        (5) **Substances associated with autonomic insufficiency** include alcoholism, antihypertensive agents, barbiturates, beta-blockers, MAOI, phenothiazines, and TCA.

E. **Neurotransmitters.** Table 86-15B summarizes some of their agonists and antagonists.

    1. **Acetylcholine.** Central fibers project to cerebral cortex and peripheral in the autonomic and somatic motor fibers. **It is released into the synapse by Ca²⁺-dependent exocytosis. It also may involve Na⁺ channels. It has nicotinic and muscarinic receptors.**

TABLE 86-15A. *Autonomic syndromes*

Autonomic syndromes	BP	Pulse	Pupil dilation	Sweat	Peristalsis	Examples
Adrenergic						
Alpha	≫	<	≫	>	<	Phenylpropanolamine
Beta-2	<	≫	0	0	0	Theophylline
Alpha and beta	≫	≫	≫	≫	—	Cocaine, amphetamine, phencyclidine
Sympatholytic	<	>	<	<	<	Clonidine, opioids, phenothiazines
Anticholinergic	>	≫	≫	≪	≪	Atropine
Cholinergic						
Nicotinic	>	>	<	≫	≫	Nicotine
Muscarinic	<	≪	≪	≪	≪	Organophosphates

<,decreased; >, increased; 0, no change.

    a. **Agonist** of muscarinic receptors include the black widow spider bite, guanidine, aminopyrine causes calcium influx and acetylcholine release. Other agents are anticholinesterase physostigmine, pyridostigmine, organophosphate, and carbamate insecticides. Direct agonist of nicotinic receptors are coniine, lobeline, nicotine, succinylcholine, and curare initially.

    b. **Antagonists** are neuromuscular blockers of pancuronium type; anticholinergic agents are amantadine, aminoglycoside, anticholinergics (atropine, antihistamines), botulism toxin, crotalidae venoms, elapidae venoms, hexamethonium (ganglion), cyclic antidepressants, magnesium, phenothiazines, tropicamide and tubocurare (end plate).

2. **Biogenic amines** are **NE, Epi, DA, and 5-HT.** All four types of neurons are affected by cocaine, amphetamines, MAOI, and reserpine. These agents can have several different effects on the same system. Amphetamine releases NE, blocks its reuptake and have metabolites that inhibit monoamine oxidase degradation.

    a. **Sympathomimetic agonist**

        (1) **Direct-acting.** Such as beta-agonist (albuterol and bronchodilators); alpha-agonist (dobutamine, ergot alkaloids, Epi, NE, phenylephrine, tyramine).

        (2) **Indirect-acting stimulants.** amphetamine, amphetamine metabolites, cocaine, MAOI (pargyline, tranylcypromine, phenelzine); alpha-2 antagonist (Yohimbine).

        (3) **Mixed** (DA, ephedrine). Inhibitors of NE uptake (amphetamines, cocaine, cyclic antidepressants).

    b. **Sympathetic antagonists** include the following:

        (1) **Alpha-antagonists.** Cyclic antidepressants, ergot alkaloids, phenothiazines, phenoxybenzamine, quinidine, trazodone.

        (2) **Inhibitors of DA beta-hydroxylase:** Alpha-methyldopa, disulfiram, and MAOI.

        (3) **Beta-antagonists.** Beta-adrenergic blockers, prevent NE release (bretylium, guanethidine, reserpine)

        (4) **Alpha-2 agonist.** Clonidine, guanabenz, and the imidizolines.

3. **Gamma-aminobutyric acid** (GABA) is one of two main inhibitory neurotransmitters mainly in the brain but also in the spinal cord. The other is glycine. GABA is synthesized from glutamate, the main CNS excitatory neurotransmitter, using glutamic acid decarboxylase (GAD) and requiring pyridoxal phosphate from pyridoxine. **Glycine** acts as a postsynaptic inhibitory neurotransmitter in the lower brain stem and the spinal cord. There are **two types of GABA,** receptors **GABA-A** where barbiturates (open channels) and benzodiazepines (open chloride channel in the presence of GABA). **GABA-B** where baclofen, the muscle relaxant acts as an agonist and the benzodiazepines have no effect.

    a. **Agonist** include the muscinol, ethanol, barbiturates, nonbarbiturate sedative-hypnotics, anticonvulsants (phenytoin), and general anesthetic agents enhance its activity. Enhance synthesis of GABA, valproate, baclofen (GABA-B), progabide. Barbiturates and benzodiazepine function if GABA is present and are useful in toxin-induced seizures. These anticonvulsants will cause a

TABLE 86-15B. *Some neurotransmitters and medications that may affect*

Neurotransmitter	Agonist	Antagonist
Acetylcholine	Muscarine	Atropine
	Nicotine	Hexamethonium (ganglion)
	Choline	Tubocurare (endplate)
	Physostigmine	Anticholinergics
	Deanol	Botulism toxin
Norepinephrine	Clonidine	Beta-blockers
Epinephrine	Amphetamine	Phentolamine/phenoxybenamine
	Tyramine	Guanethidine
Dopamine		
Direct	Amantadine	Haloperidol block receptor
	Bromocriptine	Oxiperomide
	Levodopa	Phenothiazine
MAOI	Pargyline	Cyclic antidepressants
	Tranylcypromine	Trazodone
	Phenelzine	Buspirone
Indirect	Amantadine	MPTP → Destroy neurons
	Amphetamines	Reserpine → Block uptake
	Benztropine	Tetrabenazine
	Phencyclidine	—
Inhibit DA reuptake	Amantadine	—
	Cocaine	—
	Diphenhydramine	—
	Methylphenidate	—
	Orphenadrine	—
Serotonin	Clonazepam	Cyproheptadine direct
Enhance synthesis	5-Hydroxytryptophan	Fenfluramine
	L-Tryptophan	Lithium
Block breakdown	MAOI	Methysergide
Direct agonist	Buspirone	Clozapine
Increase release	Amphetamine derivative	Metaclopramide
	Cocaine	Ondansetron
Inhibit reuptake	Amphetamines	Phentolamine
	Cyclic antidepressant	Phenothiazines
	Cocaine	Propranolol
	Dextromethorphan	Trazodone
	Fluoxetine and others	Reserpine
	Meperidine/methadone	—
Gamma-aminobutyric acid	Indirect agonist	Direct antagonist
	Benzodiazepines	Biculline
	Carbamazepine	Cephalosporins
	Ethanol	Fluoroquinolones
	Etomidate	Imipenem
	Phenytoin	Nalidixic acid
Sedative-hypnotics	Penicillin	—
	Barbiturate	Indirect antagonist
	Nonbarbiturates	Cyclic antidepressants
	Steroids	Organochlorines (Lindane)
Enhance synthesis	Valproate	MAOI
GABA site agonist	Baclofen	Picrotoxin
	Progabide	Cyanide→ Inhibit GAD
	—	Domoic acid
	—	Hydrazines (INH)/steroids

response only if GABA is present. Phenytoin is not effective in toxin-induced seizures.

    b. **Antagonists** include the stimulants, picrotoxin, cyanide (inhibits GAD), domoic acid (shell fish poisoning), hydrazides, and isoniazid organochlorine insecticides.

  4. **Glutamate** is the main excitatory neurotransmitter in the CNS, and aspartate is believed to have similar actions. Glutamate is synthesized from alpha-ketoglutamate. **It is released into the synapse by Ca^{2+}-dependent exocytosis. Excess amounts can produce convulsions and neuronal death.**

    a. **Its agonists** are aspartate, glutamate, ibotenic acid, domoic acid (shellfish poisoning).

    b. **Its antagonists** are ethanol, lamotrigine (anticonvulsant), amantadine, bromocriptine, dextromethorphan's metabolite dextrorphan, phencyclidine, ketamine.

  5. **Adenosine,** a purine, lessens oxygen requirements and increase in oxygen and substrate delivery. It is an important inhibitory transmitter and vasodilator. Adenosine triphosphate (ATP) serves as an energy source for substrates for ATP production.

    a. Its **agonists** include inhibitors of uptake (benzodiazepines, papaverine, flumazenil, carbamazepine), and inhibitors of adenosine deaminase (dipyridamole).

    b. Its **antagonists** include A1 and A2 blockade agents (theophylline, caffeine, carbamazepine) (Table 86-15B).

F. **CNS. All patients with altered conscious level must be assumed to have an associated head and neck injury** until these possibilities are excluded. This is especially true with alcoholic patients where trauma is frequently associated. The general medical/surgical causes of altered mental status and coma may be recalled by several mnemonics using the vowels **AEIOU** for metabolic disorders and **TIPS** for other causes. Over 50% of patients presenting with coma at large hospitals had drug ingestions.

  1. **Mnemonic for the causes of altered state of consciousness: Metabolic disorders, AEIOU: A**—Alcohol; **E**—Endocrine (thyroid, blood glucose), Electrolyte disturbances (Ca, Na, Mg), Epilepsy; **I**—Intoxication, insulin; **O**—Oxygen deprivation, opioids, overload fluid; **U**—Uremia and metabolic disorders hepatic, hypertension. **Other causes, TIPS: T**—Trauma, tumor; **I**—Infection (meningitis, encephalitis); **P**—Psychologic, postictal; **S**—Shock, seizures, strokes (CV).

  2. **USC altered mental state scale rating alert** (no evidence of CNS depression): **Euphoria**—feeling of well-being or elation; **Dysphoria**—feeling of discomfort or anxiety; **Drowsy**—all levels between alert and stupor; **Acute organic brain syndrome**—delirium, confusion. disorientation; **Toxic psychosis**—hallucinations, delusions, paranoid ideation, with or without acute organic brain syndrome; **Stupor**—markedly sedated but responsive to verbal or tactile stimuli; **Coma-1**—not responsive to verbal or tactile stimuli but responsive to painful stimuli; **Coma-2**—not responsive to painful stimuli but normal respiration or BP; **Coma-3**—not responsive or abnormally responsive to painful stimuli* but with spontaneous respirations that are slow, shallow or rapid but adequate or with low but adequate BP; **Coma-4**—not responsive or abnormally responsive to painful stimuli* but with apnea, or inadequate reparations or BP, or both. An asterisk indicates decorticate or decerebrate posturing to painful stimuli.

3. **Confusion. Delirium** is acute confusion state with reduced awareness of stimuli and reduced higher level of cortical function. See delirium. **Dementia** is chronic or gradual disturbance in higher cortical function. For differentiating psychiatric (functional disorders) from delirium and dementia, see Table 86–16.

a. **Medical conditions associated with confusion include** Alzheimer's disease (AD) and senile dementia, acute psychosis (postoperative, postpartum), CNS disorders (cerebrovascular disorders, brain tumor, encephalitis, meningitis, following seizures, hepatic failure (alcoholism, drug toxicity, hepatitis), hypercalcemia associated (hyperparathyroidism, osteolytic metastasis, hypervitaminosis D, hypoadrenalism, hyperthyroidism, multiple myeloma), hypocalcemia associated (hypoparathyroidism), hyperglycemia (diabetes mellitus, corticosteroid excess), hypoglycemia (insulin excess, oral sulfonylureas, pancreatic neoplasms, hypoadrenalism, hepatic failure), hypermagnesemia (renal failure exogenous magnesium), hypomagnesemia (malabsorption, pancreatitis, renal disease, alcoholism, diuretics, diabetic ketoacidosis, osteolytic metastasis), hypernatremia associated (dehydration, diabetes insipidius), hyponatremia associated (diuretic use, water intoxication, inappropriate secretion antidiuretic hormone, hypoadrenalism, renal disease), hyperpyrexia and hyperthermia (heat exposure, infection, substance abuse), hypothermia (cold exposure, ethanol, substance abuse, hypothyroidism and myxedema), hyperosmolality (diabetes insipidus, diabetic ketoacidosis, hypernatremia, dehydration), hypoxia, and hypercapnia (CNS

TABLE 86-16. *Characteristics of functional versus organic disorders*

Feature	Functional (psychiatric)		Organic	
	Mood	Schizophrenia	Delirium	Dementia
Focal neurological	No	No	Maybe	No
Asterixis	No	No	Maybe[a]	No
Onset	Gradual	Gradual	Acute	Insidious
Orientation	Normal	Normal	Disoriented	Disoriented
Level of consciousness	Normal	Normal	Fluctuating	Normal (early)
Attention	Normal	Normal	Impaired	Normal (early)
Hallucinations	Rare	Auditory	Visual/tactile	None
Memory deficits				
Short-term	Intact	Intact	Fluctuating	Stable
Long-term	No	No	Impaired	Impaired
Thought process	Grandiose rambling	Complex less	Simple	Disorganized
Delusions	Deprecatory	Elaborate	Incoherent	

[a]Suggestive of toxic-metabolic encephalopathy.

depressant drugs, pulmonary emboli, congestive heart failure, severe anemia, chronic respiratory insufficiency), infections- (febrile illness, sepsis, typhoid fever), metabolic (hepatolenticular degeneration, Huntington, hyperthyroidism, lipid storage diseases), vitamin deficiencies (thiamine [Wernicke Korsakoff], pyridoxine, cyanocobalamin, niacin (dementia, dermatitis, and diarrhea).

  b. **Medications that cause confusion** include the following:

    (1) **Anticholinergic.** Oxybutynin (Ditropan), bowel antispasmodics, antihistamines especially cimetidine.

    (2) **Antidepressants.** Cyclic antidepressants, MAOI, lithium.

    (3) **Antihypertensive.** Clonidine, alpha-methyldopa.

    (4) **Antiparkinson drugs**. L-Dopa (Sinemet), bromocriptine, amantadine (Symmetrel), trihexyphenidyl (Artane), benztropine (Cogentin), biperiden (Akineton), procyclidine (Kemadrin), ethopropazine (Parisol).

    (5) **Bronchodilators.** Aminophylline, theophylline.

    (6) **Beta-blockers**

    (7) **Bromides**

    (8) **Calcium channel blockers**

    (9) **Camphor**

    (10) **Ergot derivatives**

    (11) **Digoxin preparations**

    (12) **Corticosteroid psychosis**

    (13) **Drug withdrawal.** Alcohol (Werniche), barbiturates, opioids, sedative-hypnotics.

    (14) **Hypnotic-sedatives.** Nonbarbiturates (chloral hydrate, ethchlorvynol, glutethimide, meprobamate, methaqualone, methyprylon) and barbiturates

    (15) **Neuroleptics.** Phenothiazines and derivatives.

    (16) **Tranquilizers.** Benzodiazepines.

4. **Acute organic brain syndrome (109–117).** This toxic psychosis presents with disturbed cognition, distorted perception, mood and reality associated with impaired cerebral function. **This includes** delirium, dementia, amnesia, and confusional states. **The most frequently abused substances that produce chemically induced psychosis are** amphetamine derivatives and phencyclidine, although many other psychotropic agents, therapeutic drugs, and occupational chemicals are capable of producing a similar psychosis.

  a. **Acute organic brain syndrome has been observed from:** amphetamines* (lasts longer than cocaine), anticholinergic agents* (hypoactive bowel sounds), antihistamines, barbiturates, carbon monoxide, carbon disulfide (industrial), cardiac glycosides, chloroquine, cocaine*, corticosteroids, dapsone, ergot, ethanol, heavy metals (lead, mercury), inhalants and solvents (industrial and abuse), hallucinogens* (lysergic acid derivatives, marijuana, mescaline), methyl bromide, MAOI (interactions or overdose), phencyclidine* (miosis, rotatory nystagmus), phenytoin, solvents (trichlorethylene), theophylline, withdrawal* particularly from ethanol or sedative-hypnotics.

5. **Delirium** (118–133). **Delirium** is a transient reversible organic mental syndrome characterized by global disturbances in the cognitive processes, and fluctuation in level of consciousness. Classically it is worse at night. The **pathophysiology** is not well understood but the consensus is that delirium results from insufficient cerebral oxidative metabolism and dysregulation or reduced synthesis of the neurotransmitters. It is **clinically** characterized by disturbed arousal (sleep-wake cycle), disorientation, with impaired attention and short memory, slight incoordination, impaired speech, sometimes with anxiety and restlessness. These signs are often accompanied by hallucinations and delusions. **Delirious** patients have clouded sensorium, fluctuating level of consciousness and **visual** hallucinations whereas **psychotic** patients usually have intact sensorium with **auditory** hallucinations, a stable level of consciousness, less confusion, disorientation or autonomic overactivity (Table 86-16).

   a. **Medical conditions** associated with delirium include abscess of brain, severe anemia, CNS circulatory disturbances, encephalitis, high fevers (i.e., sepsis, typhoid), metabolic (hypercapnia, hypoglycemia, electrolyte disturbances, fluid imbalance, hypoxia), hepatic disorders, meningitis, all infections particularly with acquired immune deficiency syndrome (AIDS), porphyria, postconcussion, postconvulsive, postoperative, postpartum, pulmonary embolus, CNS neoplasms, severe fecal impaction, thyrotoxicosis and hypothyroidism, uremia, severe urinary retention, vitamin B deficiency, Wernicke syndrome, and HIV infection.

   b. **Drug-induced delirium** usually has altered sensorium (confusion and disorientation) with **visual** hallucinations. It is caused by the following classes of substances in therapeutic doses and overdoses: alcohols*, anticholinergic*, anticonvulsants * (phenytoin), antihistamines, barbiturates*, benzodiazepines*, digitalis*, ethanol*, ergot derivatives, hallucinogens*, heavy metals (arsenic, lead, mercury, thallium), hydrocarbon inhalation*, opioids*, phencyclidine*, phenothiazines, sedative-hypnotics*, sympathomimetics, CNS stimulants** (amphetamines, cocaine) and tricyclic/cyclic antidepressants*, withdrawal or abstinence from barbiturates, benzodiazepines, ethanol, sedative-hypnotics.

   c. **Mini-mental state examination** (129)

     (1) **Level of awareness.**

     (2) **Attention and calculation.** Count backwards from 100, by 7 for 5 subtractions (for example: 93, 86, 79, 72, 65), or spell "world" backwards (DLROW) Give 7 numbers at one number per second (9185072). Repeat at least 5. More depressed in organic confused state.

     (3) **Orientation.** What is the date, month, day, season, year? Name of hospital, floor, town, county, state? Organically confused patients are typically disoriented as to time and place but **rarely to person.**

(4) Recall. For short-term recall, ask patient to recall previous unrelated three words after the passage of 3 to 5 min. About 80% sensitive and 75% specific. Impairment of memory in organic confusional states, although severe intrusive hallucinations or depression, may appear "pseudo-impaired."

(5) Thought content. Aimed toward delusions of persecution often paranoia or grandiose. "Are you afraid someone will hurt you? Is anyone controlling your mind? Are there thoughts you can't get out of your head? Do you possess any special powers?"

(6) Registration. "Flag, ball, tree," then ask to repeat.

(7) Language. Naming—wrist watch, pencil. Repetition: "No ifs, ands, buts." Command "Take paper in your right hand, fold in half and place on floor. Write a sentence with a subject, a verb and an adjective.

d. Cognitive testing for hyperbaric chamber in carbon monoxide poisoning.

(1) Serial 7's; digit span; forward and backward spelling of three-letter and four-letter words. Functional testing may be more appropriate method for determining the need for HBO among minimally symptomatic patients with carbon monoxide poisoning (131–133).

6. Dementia

a. Dementia (the failing brain) is a clinical state characterized by a decline from a previously attained intellectual level involving the memory, cognitive functions, and adaptive behavior without reduction in arousal so the patient is **otherwise alert.** It is a brain disorder, not the product of normal aging. It differs from mental retardation by higher level of intellectual function and from delirium by its persistence. Beginning at the age of 60 years the frequency of dementia in the population doubles every 5 years. **Pathophysiology** is a dysfunction of cerebrum association areas which integrate perception, thought, and purposeful action. It occurs over months to years. Some varieties can be arrested or reversed. Clinical findings are forgetfulness, repetition of word and/or action, failure at work, getting lost in own neighborhood, reverse sleep cycles, hallucinations, and behavioral change.

b. Commonest form of dementia is **AD,** which may affect as many as 10% over 65 years and 25% to 50% of those over 85% years. There is gradual deterioration and death occurs in about 10 years. Paranoia with persecutory delusion occur in 50%. Early-onset AD is autosomal dominant associated mutations on chromosomes 14 to 21, but majority are sporadic late onset. AD is not a global disorder; it has an identifiable profile of cognitive changes. The second commonest cause of dementia is multiple cerebral infarcts. **Vascular dementia** is intellectual decline produced by ischemic, hypoxic, cardiac disorders, or hemorrhagic brain lesions. **Parkinson disease** is associated overt dementia in 40% and 70% have some degree of cognitive impairment.

c. Arrestable and reversible medical causes of dementia are collagen-vascular (see SLE below), endocrinopathies (thyroid, adrenal, parathyroid disorders), hypoperfusion, intoxications, infections of the CNS (bacterial meningitis, herpes, neurosyphilis, tuberculosis, AIDS encephalopathy), metabolic disorders (hypoxemia, porphyria, Wilson's disease), multiple sclerosis, nutritional disorders (thiamine deficiency, pellagra, folate deficiency, B_{12}), psychiatric (depression) sarcoidosis, space occupying lesions (tumor, subdural hematoma), normal pressure hydrocephalus, and affective disorders. "Pseudodementia" of severe depression must be excluded. **Unusual causes** of dementia are Pick's disease, Huntington's chorea, and Creutsfeldt-Jacob syndrome.

d. **Substances capable of producing dementia** are chronic alcohol* abuse, antibiotics (penicillin and chloramphenicol in elderly), anticholinergic*, anticonvulsants, antidysrhythmic agents, antidepressants, antihistamines*, antihypertensives, antiparkinson drugs, carbon monoxide*, carbon disulfide (sulfur madness), digitalis, hallucinogens, heavy metals* (aluminum, arsenic, copper, lead, manganese, mercury, thallium), hydrocarbon inhalation, insecticides, opioids, lithium, MAOI, neuroleptics, delayed effects of radiation*, organic solvents, major tranquilizers (phenothiazines and butyrophenones), tricyclic/cyclic antidepressants. An asterisk indicates more frequent substances.

e. **Workup for dementia**—CBC, electrolytes, BUN, Creatinine, liver function tests, serum B_{12}, ESR (if evidence decline in health), syphilis serology (history or signs), urinalysis, HIV testing. Chest radiograph and ECG (indicated for exclusion of co-existing medical conditions), serum folate (if have anemia), thyroid function tests. **Dementia-related Information and Resources**—National Alzheimer's Association 1-800-272-3900; Alzheimer's Disease Education and Referral Center (ADEAR) 1-800-438-4380.

7. **Coma and depressed level of consciousness** (134–142). The **pathophysiology** of coma and depressed level of consciousness implies involvement of both cerebral hemispheres or the ascending reticular activating system of the diencephalon, midbrain, pons, and medulla must be involved. **Involvement of the upper brain stem** (diencephalon and mid-brain) produces lighter coma and may be associated with seizure activity. **Lower subtentorial involvement** produces deeper coma and disturbances in circulation and respiration. **Neurostructural** coma has an impaired pupillary light reflex in the early stages and develops respiratory impairment in the late stages, whereas respiratory impairment occurs early and the pupillary light reflex is lost late in **toxic-metabolic coma. Psychiatric disease rarely causes coma.**

a. **Coma may be produced** by the following:

(1) **Substances causing hypoxia** such as agents that interfere with oxygen transport in blood and/or interfere with **tissue utilization of oxygen** (carbon monoxide, cyanide, hydrogen sulfide, and methemoglobin producers) or gases that displace oxygen in atmosphere (carbon dioxide, nitrogen dioxide, butane, propane, methane, aromatic hydrocarbons, solvents).

(2) **CNS depressants** such as alcohols and glycols, anticholinergics, anticonvulsants, antidepressants (lithium, MAOI, and tricyclic/cyclic antidepressants), antihistamines, barbiturates, bromides, neuroleptics (phenothiazines, butyrophenones), opioids, nonbarbiturate sedative-hypnotics (chloral hydrate, ethchlorvynol, methaqualone, glutethimide, and methyprylon), and tranquilizers (benzodiazepines).

        (3) **Hypoglycemia-producing substances** (insulin, oral hypoglycemic agents, ethanol, beta-blockers, and salicylates).

        (4) **Enzyme inhibitors** such as cyanide, heavy metals (arsenic, iron, lead, mercury, thallium), organophosphates, and salicylates.

        (5) **Hallucinogens** such as LSD, mescaline, phencyclidine.

        (6) **Postictal.** See causes of convulsions.

    b. **The most common intoxications that cause coma,** ABCNOT, include **A**—alcohols (mainly ethanol) and glycols (especially ethylene glycol), anticonvulsants; **B**—barbiturates, benzodiazepines, nonbarbiturate sedative-hypnotics; **C**—carbon monoxide; **N**—neuroleptics (phenothiazines); **O**—opioids; **T**—tranquilizers, tricyclic and cyclic antidepressants. Alcoholic patients may be poisoned with ethanol substitutes such as methanol, isopropanol, or ethylene glycol.

    c. **Coma with pulmonary edema** is observed with cholinergic medications, opioids, organophosphate insecticides, and salicylate intoxications.

    d. **Coma with cardiac dysrhythmias** is observed with beta-blockers, CNS stimulants (amphetamines, cocaine, phenylpropanolamine), calcium channel blockers, clonidine, cocaine, digoxin, lead, lithium, phencyclidine, phenothiazines, propranolol, theophylline, TCA.

8. **Coma, seizures, and/or movement disorder** (MD) (143,144). Most of these diseases that include **coma and seizures are of infectious etiology and are characterized by abnormalities in the CSF. Those with persistently normal CSF include** tetanus, cerebral malaria, cat scratch disease, typhoid fever, shigella and can usually be recognized by their extra-cerebral manifestations. Reye's syndrome and hemorrhagic shock by biologic markers. Substances that produce these manifestations include substances of abuse (amphetamine, barbiturates, benzodiazepines, cocaine, opioids, phencyclidine, phenylpropanolamine), and antihistamines, isoniazid, phenothiazines, salicylates, tricyclic and heterocyclic antidepressants. Lead intoxication can be demonstrated by biologic changes and lead levels. **Workup when the etiology is obscure** should include the following:

    a. **CSF** (cell number and type, protein, glucose, protein electrophoresis, interferon alfa titer, viral antibody titers (measles, mumps, rubella, varicella-zoster virus, influenza (A and B), coxsackie, parainfluenza, adenovirus, Epstein-Barr, cytomegalic virus, mycoplasma. Cultures and bacterial cultures and antibody tests).

    b. **Serum tests** should exclude hypoglycemia, electrolyte abnormalities, ionized calcium, calcium, hyperammonemia (urea cycle defects), aminoacidemias, organic acidemias (lactate and pyruvate), ammonia, lead, carbon monoxide, liver function tests and BUN and creatinine, viral antibody titers.

    c. **Urine tests** should include aminoacid chromatography, organic acid chromatography, and toxicologic analysis.

9. **Convulsions** (145–151). Convulsions mandate the exclusion of trauma, a surgical lesions and underlying medical disease before they are attributed solely to toxins. Alcoholic patients may have seizures from hypoglycemia, electrolyte abnormalities, withdrawal, and pontine or subdural hematoma. **Clonic convulsions** may arise from the cerebral cortex and are followed by periods of stupor or coma, i.e., camphor intoxication. **Tonic convulsions** arise from the spinal cord and are accompanied by normal mentation until hypoxia supervenes, i.e., strychnine overdose.

    a. **Classification of seizures and epileptic syndromes.** Convulsions are classified into generalized and partial (focal seizures). Generalized are subclassified on the basis of the presence of absence of various patterns of movement, i.e., tonic, tonic-clonic, atonic, myoclonic. Partial seizures are subclassified according to whether consciousness is maintained (simple partial seizures) or impaired (complex partial seizures formerly called temporal lobe or psychomotor seizures) (Table 86-17).

    b. **Convulsions caused by poisoning or overdose** may be due to the following:

        (1) The **direct effect of the toxin on the inhibiting neurotransmitters,** especially GABA. Isoniazid interferes with the formation of GABA by producing a pyridoxine deficiency and **strychnine** blocks the neurotransmitter inhibitor glycine.

        (2) The **indirect effect of the toxin on metabolic factors** (oxygen, glucose, calcium, electrolytes, magnesium, osmolality).

        (3) The **secondary to toxin-induced organ damage** such as in renal failure, hepatic failure, and CNS hypoxia.

        (4) Secondary to withdrawal of an addicting substance.

        (5) **Lower the convulsive threshold** such as phenothiazines.

        (6) Cerebral edema produced by chronic lead intoxication.

    c. **Hypoxia** is a frequent cause of convulsions. Some toxins suppress respiration through **neuromuscular blockade** and produce hypoxia such as botulism,

---

TABLE 86-17. *International classification of epileptic seizures*

I. Partial (beginning locally) classified as simple or complex on basis of consciousness.
  A. Simple: consciousness preserved.
    1. Motor (Jacksonian contractions of a limb while alert).
    2. Somatosensory (auditory hallucinations, flashing lights, strong taste in mouth or noxious smell).
    3. Autonomic (nausea, vomiting, diaphoresis).
    4. Psychological (Deja' vu or jamais vu, hallucinations).
  B. Complex: impaired consciousness at onset or at onset.
  C. Partial seizures may become secondarily generalized.
II. Generalized—convulsive and nonconvulsive.
  A. Absence (Petit Mal) in children over 3 (usually over 5 years), unresponsive at less than 3 s and have 3 HZ/s spike and wave pattern. Resolves at 18 to 20 years spontaneously. One-third of these patients will have clonic-tonic seizures as adults.
    1. Atypical absence last longer, and children lose train of thought.
  B. Types are myoclonic, clonic, tonic, tonic-clonic, and atonic. Tonic-clonic (Grand Mal) loses consciousness, falls to floor with a cry, becomes stiff and rigid, urinates, defecates, temporary cyanosis, period of clonic jerking followed by limpness and coma. Consciousness returns after 15 min, but fatigue, confusion, and headache last for 1 h.
III. Localized-related (focal): Idiopathic (benign focal of childhood); symptomatic (chronic progressive, temporal lobe, extratemporal) If focal, suggests structural lesion in brain.
IV. Classification of epilepsies and epileptic syndromes— Idiopathic: benign neonatal, childhood absence, juvenile myoclonic, other. Cryptogenic: West syndrome (Infantile spasms), early myoclonic encephalopathy, Lennox-Gastaut syndrome, progressive myoclonic epilepsy.

tedrotoxin (from puffer fish), saxitoxin (from fish ingesting plankton dinoflagellate of the Gonyaulax spp.) and curare-like medications. Others act directly to **suppress the respiratory center** in the CNS and produce hypoxia such as sedative-hypnotics.

d. The **common substances that cause intoxications with convulsions** include alcohol intoxication and withdrawal; amphetamines; amoxapine (act on picrotoxin site) anesthetics (general and local); anticonvulsants (paradoxical effect); antidepressants (newer types especially amoxapine, bupropion, maprotiline); antidysrhythmic agents, antihistamines H-1 blockers (especially in children); beta-blockers; boric acid; butyrophenones (haloperidol); caffeine, camphor; cholinergic blockers, cocaine; cyanide; disopyramide (severe hypoglycemia); ciprofloxacin (block P-450 enzyme and inhibit GABA) essential oils, ethylene glycol; heavy metals particularly lead; insulin; isoniazid; fluoride; insect repellent (*N,N*-diethyl-*M*-toluamide or DEET); insulin, lead (chronic poisoning); lidocaine; lithium; meperidine, MAOI ("serotonin syndrome," act on picrotoxin site), methaqualone; MAOI, nicotine, organochlorine insecticides (Lindane act on picrotoxin site); organophosphate insecticides; opioids (fentanyl, meperidine and propoxyphene toxic metabolites, possible pentazocine); (penicillin in large doses inhibits GABA), phencyclidine; phenothiazines; phenylpropanolamine; phenytoin (overdose); physostigmine; propoxyphene; salicylates; strychnine; sulfonylureas; sympathomimetics; theophylline (adenosine receptor blocker); TCA (act on picrotoxin site); withdrawal of barbiturates, nonbarbiturate sedative-hypnotics, opioids and ethanol. **Refractory seizures:** amoxapine, isoniazid, chronic lead poisoning, strychnine, theophylline.

e. **Specific drug-induced seizures.** Cocaine (15% of 5 to 10 million users), **cyclic antidepressants** especially newer agents, e.g., amoxapine and maprotiline, **isoniazid** seizures begin within 30 to 120 min **theophylline** intractable seizures have a high mortality, **alcohol withdrawal seizures** occur 24 to 48 h after cessation of consumption and lasts 6 h or less. First time alcohol seizures require immediate workup bedside: glucose, electrolytes including calcium and magnesium, BUN, creatinine, liver profile, blood alcohol, CT (6% had mass lesion; therefore, exclude brain infarct, hemorrhage stroke, and subdural hematoma).

f. The **mnemonic** is **WPLASTIC: W**—withdrawal; **P**—PCP*, pesticides, phenothiazines* (chlorpromazine, mesoridazine, thioridazine), propoxyphene; **L**—lead (chronic), lithium*, lindane, lidocaine; **A**—amphetamines*, anticholinergics, antihistamine, alcohol*, antidepressants (cyclic)*, anticonvulsants; **S**—salicylates*, stimulants, strychnine; **T**—theophylline*; **I**—INH*, insulin, Inderal; **C**—CO, cocaine*, camphor*, caffeine.

10. **Spells** (152). These are a sudden onset of symptom or symptoms that are recurrent, self-limited, and stereotypic in nature. An example is facial flushing, which is the most common. Neurogenic (wet flush), is accompanied by perspiration (precipitated by histamines, prostaglandin, polypeptide). Hot flash of postmenopausal women. Direct vasodilatory flush is dry.

a. **History.** Thorough medical, social, family, medication history. Spell history—symptoms characteristic, precipitating and alleviating factors, flush or pallor, BP changes, timing, frequency, and duration. Mental status after spell, list medications prescription, over-the-counter (OTC) products, vitamins.

b. **Physical.** BP, heart rate, orthostatic changes. Skin dermographia, cafe au lait, neurofibroma, body hair distribution. Thyroid function tests hyperthyroidism and hypothyroidism. Left ventricular function. Abdomen mass or bruit. Genitalia testicular atrophy.

c. **Diagnostic tests.** CBC with differential, serum electrolytes, serum glucose, creatinine, calcium, phosphorous, liver function, total protein. Urinalysis, 24-h excretion of metanephrine, 5-hydroxy-indoleacetic acid (5-HIAA), creatinine.

   (1) **Pheochromocytoma** tests false metanephrine and catecholamine false-positives—TCA, labetalol, L-dopa, ethanol, sotolal, amphetamines, methyldopa, benzodiazepines, withdrawal from clonidine and other drugs. False-negatives metyrosine and methylglucamine.

b. **Carcinoid false-positive** for 5-HIAA foods (banana, plantain, pineapple, kiwi, avocados, nuts), cough medicines with guaifenesin, acetaminophen, naproxen, fluororacil. False-negatives for aspirin, L-dopa, phenothiazines.

c. **Mast cell disease.** Interfere with measurements of histamine and metabolites, antihistamines.

d. **Classification of the causes of spells**

   (1) **Pharmacologic.** Withdrawal of adrenergic inhibitor, MAOI treatment and tyramine in foods or sympathomimetic drugs, sympathomimetic ingestion, illegal drugs (cocaine, phencyclidine, LSD), chlorpropamide-alcohol flush, niacin-flush, nitrates-flush, vancomycin "red man syndrome."

   (2) **Endocrine.** Pheochromocytoma*, thyrotoxicosis, primary hypogonadism (menopausal syndrome), pancreatic tumors (insulinoma-hypoglycemia), hypoglycemia, carbohydrate intolerance, "hyperadrenergic spells."

   (3) **CV.** Labile essential hypertension, pulmonary edema, syncope, orthostatic hypotension, baroreflex dysfunction, paroxysmal cardiac dysrhythmias, angina, renovascular disease.

   (4) **Psychologic.** Anxiety attacks, panic attacks (develop abruptly and peak in 10 min, palpitations, sweating, trembling, choking, dyspnea, chest and abdominal pain discomfort, faint, light headed, dizzy, derealization [unreality] or depersonalization [being detached from oneself], hyperventilation), fear of dying and fear of going crazy, paresthesias, chills, and hot flashes.

   (5) **Neurologic.** Autonomic tachycardia syndrome, autonomic neuropathy, migraine, seizure disorder, autonomic seizures, stroke, CV insufficiency.

   (6) **Other.** Mastocytosis*, environmental allergies, carcinoid syndrome*, recurrent idiopathic anaphylaxis, polycythemia vera, POEMS (polyneuropathy, organomegaly, endocrinopathy, M protein, and skin changes). An asterisk indicates syndromes.

11. **Syncope** (153–157). Syncope is transient but complete impairment of consciousness. Syncope is related to transient ischemia of the brain due to hypotension or low cardiac output. It usually starts in the erect position, with a feeling of weakness and unsteadiness, the pulse is weak, the breathing shallow, the face becomes pale or ashen gray, and the skin sweaty. The patient has muscle weakness, loss of postural tone and falls to the floor. The muscles are flaccid but there is no incontinence of urine or feces (in seizures the muscles are rigid and there may be incontinence). Hyperventilation and blurred vision may precede the episode. When the patients falls to the horizontal position the face suffuses pink, the pulse becomes palpable and breathing deepens and immediate awareness of surroundings occurs although muscle weakness remains a short time.

    a.   The **medical etiology of syncope** may be situational, orthostatic, vasovagal, cardiac dysrhythmias, any cause of prolonged Q-T interval (congenital hereditary Romano-Ward and Jervell Nelsen-Lange), CNS diseases (transient ischemic attacks, subclavian steal, migraine), myocardial infarction, and carotid sinus syndrome.

    b.   **Syncope may be associated with the following medications:** anaphylactoid reactions, antidysrhythmic agents (class a), antihypertensive agents, antiparkinsonism agents (L-dopa), beta-blockers, calcium channel blockers, cocaine, digitalis, diuretics, hypoglycemic agents (insulin, sulfonylureas, biquanides), any medication that causes hypotension, nitrites, phenothiazines, any cause of prolonged Q-T interval, and quinidine.

    c.   **Syncope differentiated from seizure.** Recovery is quick, usually no postictal period; postictal creatine kinase (CK) is a nonspecific indicator of recent tonic-clonic seizure.

12. **"Alice in Wonderland" syndrome or Lilliputian type of hallucinations** (158). Intermittent complaints of **bizarre images of the body or objects** such as seeing objects smaller or larger than they are. It is seen in infectious mononucleosis syndrome and anticholinergic poisoning.

13. **ICP** (159)

    a.   **Physiology.** Intracranial volume consists of the brain, vascular blood, CSF, and interstitial water. **Cerebral perfusion** pressure is equal to the mean arterial pressure (MAP) minus the ICP. If the perfusion pressure falls below 40 mm Hg CBF falls to critical pressure levels and ischemia develops. Normal neuronal function requires a CBF of 18 to 20 mL/100 g/min.

    b.   **ICP** causes include mass lesions, brain edema, increased CSF and increased blood volume. **Acute increased ICP** is characterized by changes in personality and mental status, lethargy, headache, and vomiting in the morning, papilloedema, and retinal hemorrhages. The headache may waken the patient at night due to the large vasodilator-related pressure changes that occur in REM sleep. **Chronic pressure changes** can produce decreased upward gaze, and paresis of the VI cranial nerve with diplopia, papilledema, behavioral changes, and weight loss.

        (1)   The **surgical-medical causes** include hydrocephalus, intracranial hemorrhage, and secondary to asphyxia. Other potential causes include

cerebrovascular events, burns, hypertension, infections, pulmonary insufficiency, trauma, tumors.

(2) **Cerebral edema** may be vasogenic (tumors, abscess, trauma contusions, meningitis), interstitial and cytotoxic (intracellular accumulation of water due to hypoxia, Reye's syndrome, and diabetic ketoacidosis (hyperosmolar coma), toxins such as lead).

(3) **Herniation syndromes.** If the pressure increase is rapid or undiagnosed the cranial contents may shift and cause herniation syndromes, which generally follow a rostocaudal progression (Table 86-18). The herniation syndromes are as follows:

(a) **Transtentorial herniation** where the cerebral hemispheres and the deeper nuclear structures are shifted and lead to the displacement of the diencephalon or midbrain.

(b) **Uncal herniation,** a mass in the middle fossa or temporal lobe, produces herniation of the uncus and hippocampal gyrus leading to compression of the oculomotor nerve, posterior cerebral artery, and midbrain.

(c) **Cerebellar herniation** can occur upward through the tentorial notch or downward through the foramen magnum. Upward herniation compresses the dorsal midbrain and downward herniation compresses the medullary structures.

c. **Pseudotumor cerebri (PC) or idiopathic intracranial hypertension (IIH)** (160–164). The diagnosis is made after exclusion of tumors, obstruction of the ventricles, intracranial infection and vascular hypertensive encephalopathy. **The diagnostic criteria** include documented elevation of ICP (more than 250 mm of water or more), no neurologic signs except for papilloedema and occasional abducens nerve paresis and a normal CSF composition, normal ventricles and absence of space-occupying lesion on neuroimaging studies. It was recognized almost a century ago (161). The **exact mechanism** is not known, but some attribute it to cerebral edema, others to abnormal CSF absorption. **PC** occurs with a frequency of 1:100,000 per year in the general population. Its incidence is high in obese women 19 to 21:100,000 and in children 5 to 15 years of age. The major complication is damage to the optic nerve disc as a result of papilledema which may cause permanent visual loss. Clinical find-

TABLE 86-18. *Pattern of herniation syndromes*

	Respiration	Pupils	Eyes	Motor
Transtentorial				
Diencephalon	Cheyne Stokes	Small reaction	Reflexes intact	Decorticate
Midbrain-pons	Hyperventilation	Midposition fixed	Dysconjugate	Decorticate
Medullary	Slow irregularity	Midposition	Absent	Flaccid
Uncal	Increased or normal	Anisocoria fixed	Adductor paresis ptosis	Contralateral hemiplegia[a]
Infratentorial	Compromised	Reactive	Vertical	Asymmetric

[a]Hemiparesis on side opposite the dilated pupil.

ings may include headache, nausea, vomiting, lateral rectus paresis, vertical strabismus, facial paresis, back, and neck pain. Amaurosis fugax, and scotoma have been reported. For the workup of idiopathic ICP, see Fig. 86-5.

(1) Systemic causes include an association with **endocrine disorders** (adrenal insufficiency, female reproductive age group with obesity, rapid weight gain and menstrual irregularities, hypoparathyroid disease, hypothyroid disease and correction of hypothyroidism); malnutrition and renutrition, iron deficiency anemia; pericranial infections in the ear, mastoid and sinuses and lateral sinus thrombosis; lupus erythematosus, head trauma, and renal failure. Questionable etiologies are vitamin A and D deficiencies.

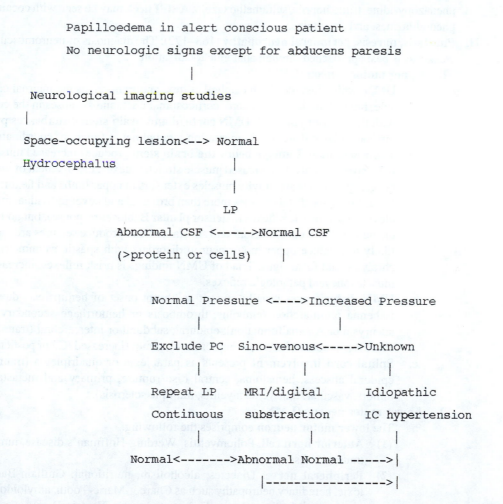

```
Papilloedema in alert conscious patient

No neurologic signs except for abducens paresis

                    |

  Neurological imaging studies

   |

 Space-occupying lesion<--> Normal

 Hydrocephalus                 |

                               |

                        LP

    Abnormal CSF <----->Normal CSF

    (>protein or cells)     |


        Normal Pressure <---->Increased Pressure

             |                        |

        Exclude PC  Sino-venous<----->Unknown

             |           |             |

        Repeat LP   MRI/digital    Idiopathic

        Continuous   substraction   IC hypertension

             |           |             |

        Normal<------->Abnormal Normal ----->|

                 |---------------->|
```

FIG. 86-5. Idiopathic intracranial hypertension (4). Key: PC = Pseudotumor cerebri, LP = Lumbar puncture, CSF = Cerebrospinal fluid, MRI = Magnetic resonance imaging, IC = Intracranial.

(2) **Medications and intoxications** reported to cause PC include corticosteroid therapy and corticosteroid discontinuation withdrawal, cimetidine poisonings, growth hormone (recombinant gene type) therapy (24 case reports) (163), heavy metals (arsenic lead), isotretinoin (Accutane) therapy, L-thyroxine, lithium, minocycline, nalidixic acid therapy, nitrofurantoin, sulfonamides, tamoxifen, tetracycline (outdated) therapy, trimethoprim-sulfamethoxazole, excess vitamin A.

G. **Aseptic chemically induced meningitis** (165–167). **Noninfectious chemically induced meningitis** has a very acute onset and resolves rapidly after discontinuing the medication or exposure. It has been reported from azathioprine, contrast media, cytosine arabinoside, gentamicin (intrathecal with preservatives), isoniazid, nonsteroidal antiinflammatory agents, (ibuprofen associated with and without systemic lupus, sulindac, tolmetin), phenazopyridine, trimethoprim/sulfamethoxazole. **A stiff neck** may be seen with cocaine, phenothiazines, and strychnine.

H. **Paralysis, paresis, peripheral neuropathy** (168–172). The diagnosis of neuromuscular weakness is best approached through anatomic localization.

1. **Upper motor neuron (UMN)**

   a. **UMN,** which includes both cerebral cortex, and transverses the internal capsule, brain stem, and spinal cord, corticospinal tract, and synapses in the cord with the anterior horn cell. **UMN cortical and brain stem** disturbances produce associated disorders in mentation, cranial nerve function, coordination and/or sensation. **Damage below the brain stem** produces increased muscle tone, spastic paralysis, increased muscle stretch reflexes, involvement of muscle groups (affects antigravity muscles extensors in upper limbs and flexors in lower limbs, the distal muscles more than proximal and never individual muscles) and pathologic reflexes (extensor plantar Babinski response), but no fasciculations. Neurologic lesions and substances that produce seizures are more likely to produce upper motor neuron disorders with spastic asymmetrical paralysis, and focal signs. Triad of UMN findings is brisk reflexes, increased muscle tone and pathologic reflexes.

   b. **UMN disturbances** usually present as abrupt onset of hemiparesis due to ischemia or infarction (embolus, thrombosis or hemorrhage secondary to aneurysm or AV malformation); epidural, subdural or intercerebral (trauma); abscess (i.v. abuser, immunocompromised); tumor (increased ICP or postictal).

   c. **Spinal cord involvement** presents as paraplegia or quadriplegia (trauma, epidural abscess, hematoma, central disc rupture, primary and metastatic tumors, vascular, transverse myelitis, multiple sclerosis).

2. **Lower motor neuron (LMN)**

   a. The **lower motor neuron** comprises the following:

      (1) **Anterior horn cell.** Poliomyelitis, Werdnig-Hoffman's disease, tumor, trauma or disc.

      (2) **Peripheral nerve.** Diabetes, alcoholism, nutritional, Guillain-Barré, toxic, hereditary neuropathy such as Charcot-Marie-Tooth, amyloidosis, porphyria, infectious (Lyme disease, diphtheria, Epstein-Barr).

    (3)   **Systemic conditions.** Electrolyte, uremia, collagen, sarcoidosis, tumors.

    (4)   **Myoneural junction.** Myasthenia, gravis, botulism, aminoglycoside toxicity, magnesium overdose, tick paralysis, and Eaton-Lambert syndrome.

    (5)   **Skeletal muscle.** See myopathy in neuromuscular disease.

b.   **The LMN damage results** in distal flaccid paralysis (and with time atrophy), early depressed or absent muscle stretch reflexes, may affect individual muscles or part or all of a limb, and may have fasciculations. **Pathologically** neuropathies are classified into the following:

    (1)   **Axonpathies** with early destruction of cell's axon. Most toxic neuropathies are in this category.

    (2)   **Myelinopathies** or demyelinating disorders with early destruction of myelin sheath.

    (3)   **Neuronal neuropathies** with early destruction of the cell bodies. They can be further divided into type of cell involved motor, sensory, or autonomic system.

c.   The **neuromuscular junction** is affected by a number of disease processes that interfere or destroy acetylcholinesterase causing weakness and fatigability that involves the cranial nerves and may progress to involve the respiratory muscles.

d.   **Myopathies muscle damage** should be differentiated from neuronal. Primary muscle damage is proximal, does not follow root syndromes or nerve distribution, has muscle pain or tenderness, has decreased muscle reflexes late and rarely has complete paralysis and fasciculation. See neuromuscular disease.

e.   The **interruption of nerve impulses** resulting in a lack of muscle contraction has been reported with chemical and toxin-induced disorders including involvement of the **anterior horn and the peripheral nerves** with heavy metals usually arsenic, lead, thallium and alcohol, hydrocarbon exposure, vincristine; **the myoneural junction** (organophosphates, magnesium, botulism, tick paralysis) and **the muscle** (ipecac; see RDM). The **hallmark of toxic neuropathies** is their diffuse and symmetric distribution.

f.   **Specific neuropathies** include the following:

    (1)   **Axonopathies** make up 90% of toxic neuropathies. Long, large fibers are affected preferentially, resulting in diffuse, symmetrical disorders of the extremities. The classic example is the glove and stocking sensory neuropathy which has a distal distribution of arsenic. Lead neuropathy is a typical axonopathy. It is associated with pure motor neuropathy and results in foot or wrist drop. In **Wallerian degeneration,** the toxin may transect the axon with the distal segment dying as often occurs in trauma. Since the nerve cell remains viable it can regenerate and partially recover.

        (a)   **Acrylamide.** Grouting industry gives sensory motor neuropathy.

        (b)   **Hexacarbons** (*n*-hexane, methyl *n*-butyl ketone in glues and varnish) are metabolized to 2,5-hexanedione which damages the cells by forming a pyrrole ring which serves as the toxic compound. *Chronic* exposure produces progressive glove and stocking sensory, motor and autonomic axonopathy. Occurred in shoe industry in 1950s.

(c) **Carbon disulfide.** Rayon industry: sensory motor neuropathy and "sulfur madness."

(d) **Tri-ortho-cresyl phosphate (TOCP)** in single exposure to an organophosphate was responsible for "ginger jake" paralysis producing classic axonopathy with any organophosphate (muscarinic or nicotinic) symptoms. Other organophosphates can produce delayed axonopathies following acute poisonings or with chronic low level exposure.

(e) **Metals** such as arsenic, thallium, mercury, and platinum produce axonopathies. Thallium is painful ascending sensory and later motor axonopathy whereas mercury is largely motor.

   (i) **Arsenic neuropathy** is mainly progressive sensory "glove and stocking" loss with little motor involvement.

   (ii) **Mercury neuropathy** involves sensory nerves and may affect the cerebellum and occipital lobe.

   (iii) **Thallium neuropathy** is progressive, with motor and sensory loss.

(f) **Metabolic toxins** such as colchicine, podophyllin, vincristine, taxol, and other antineoplastic agents, including cisplatin, doxorubicin, taxol, vincristine, and vinblastine, cause toxicity by directly interfering with microtubule function. Other metabolic toxins include disulfiram, Dapsone, ethanol, isoniazid, metronidazole, nitrous oxide, and Vacor, which produce axonopathies.

(2) **Myelinopathies.** Myelin is the insulation of nerves; therefore, its destruction can result in slow and abnormal conduction. Toxins may separate the myelin from the nerve and others may destroy myelin in a segmental distribution. These patients present with generalized weakness and minimal or no sensory problems. The heavily myelinated large motor fibers are more affected than the small diameter myelinated and unmyelinated sensory fibers. Therefore, proprioception, touch, and vibration are impaired, and the small fibers such as pain and temperature and autonomic nervous system are intact. Areflexia is common. The healing is rapid compared to the axonopathies.

(a) **Lead toxicity** is associated with segmental demyelination in animals and a typical axonopathy described in humans. It is classically associated with a pure motor neuropathy—isolated wrist drop and foot drop in adults.

(b) **Buckthorn** (Rhamnus), a plant, chronic ingestion causes ascending paralysis resembling Guillain-Barré. Other plants that may cause paralysis include aconite, azalea, curare, jassamine yellow, lantana, nicotine, poison hemlock, sweat pea.

(c) **Other substances** include **diphtheria toxin** (produces local and distant demyelination syndrome) involves cranial nerves, amidarone, hexachlorophene, and trichloroethylene (involves cranial nerves).

(3) Neuronal neuropathy

    (a) Doxorubin is highly toxic to the dorsal root ganglia and autonomic ganglia. Motor neuron are left intact.

    (b) Pyridoxine neuropathy following large chronic doses of 2 to 3 g per day produced sensory loss with ataxia from impaired proprioception (170).

(4) Toxins causing cranial nerve palsies include amidarone, botulism, diphtheria, carbon disulfide, chloroethylene, ethylene glycol, Guillain-Barré syndrome, hexachlorophene, Lyme disease, organophosphates, and carbamate insecticides.

(5) Toxins affecting the nerve function without causing nerve injury.

    (a) Botulism. Interferes with presynaptic release of acetylcholine leading to motor weakness and autonomic dysfunction. Constipation and dilated pupils.

    (b) Tetanus. Presynaptic inhibition of glycine release. Since glycine has little action above the spinal cord true seizures are uncommon although the motor activity appear like seizures. There is normal mentation and normal EEG if ventilation and hemodynamics are stable. Tetanus has slow onset and recovery.

    (c) Strychnine. It is difficult to distinguish strychnine from tetanus except by its rapid onset and resolution. It interferes with glycine function by *postsynaptic* inhibition of glycine receptors.

    (d) Snake (Elapidae) venom (coral and cobra snakes). It produces significant neuromuscular weakness with death occurring from respiratory compromise. These toxins behave like **curare** in that they bind the *postsynaptic receptors* and render them insensitive to acetylcholine like nondepolarizing neuromuscular blockers such as pancuronium. Examples are cobra and coral.

    (e) Black widow spider venom. This has the ability to produce painful contractions of large muscle groups with the potential of RDM. Venom blocks the synaptic transmission by opening up the without impairing axon conduction. The result is a massive release of acetylcholine resulting in depolarization like succinylcholine.

g. The **drugs and chemicals that may produce paralysis and paresis** include the following: Alcohol (chronic ethanol); aminoglycoside (interfere with release of acetylcholine); botulism, barbiturates (in porphyria); cancer chemotherapeutic agents (cisplatin, doxorubicin, taxol, vincristine, vinblastine); carbon disulfide, carbon monoxide, cyanide; dapsone, disulfiram, dichlorophenoxyacetic acid (2,4 D); ethambutol, ethylene glycol, ethylene oxide, ethyl methyl ketone; **fish food poisoning** (ciguatera, shell fish, tedrodotoxin); fluoride, fluoroacetate, **heavy metals** (arsenic, lead, gold, mercury, thallium, zinc); isoniazid, insects (spiders), ipecac (chronic); magnesium sulfate, manganese, methanol, methyl bromide and chloride, metronidazole; nitrous oxide, *N*-**hexane** (metabolite 2,5-hexanedione), nitrofurantoin; phenytoin; plants (aconite, buckthorn, curare, jassamine, lantana, nicotine, poison hemlock, sweet pea); organophosphate insecticides (delayed "drying back" neuropathy); reptiles (Elapidae species such as coral); solvents (*N*-hexane and methyl ethyl ketone produce the neuropathy by the same toxic metabolite 2,5-hexanedione); thalidomide, trichloroethylene, acrylonitrile, toluene, **triorthocresyl phosphate (fuel);** vitamins (excess pyridoxine); and Vacor produces autonomic neuropathy.

h. **Acute flaccid paralysis** (which develops in minutes, hours, or days) may be observed with food poisonings such as botulism (descending paralysis, cranial nerve involvement, diplopia, dysphagia, dysarthria, dry mouth); carbon monoxide; ciguatera fish (onset within 30 min, temperature reversal, perioral paresthesia); fluoroacetate; insects such as ticks (ascending paralysis, no cranial nerve involvement, no pupil involvement); metabolic disorders such as porphyria if administer barbiturates; organophosphates "intermediate" syndrome usually after treatment of cholinergic crisis; plants (aconite, azalea, curare, jassamine yellow, lantana, nicotine, poison hemlock, sweat pea); shell fish (feels like pepper on tongue, very rapid 15 to 60 min after ingestion) and snakes and spiders.

i. **Subacute or chronic paralysis** (develops in weeks) may be caused by alcoholism (ethanol); carbon disulfide in rayon industry; fuel oil—"Ginger Jake paralysis"—due to triorthocresyl phosphate (TOCP); heavy metals (arsenic, lead, gold, mercury, thallium, zinc); solvents (*n*-hexane, ethyl methyl ketone); pesticides (organophosphate delayed).

I. **Neuromuscular disease** (173,174)

1. **Neuromuscular disorders** are genetic muscular dystrophies; spinal muscular atrophies; neuropathies (Guillain-Barré, autoimmune, diabetes mellitus, and porphyria); myasthenia gravis; Eaton-Lambert; amyotrophic lateral sclerosis; myotonic dystrophy; and familial periodic paralysis.

2. **Endocrine and metabolic disorders** include hyperadrenalism (Cushing's disease) and adrenal insufficiency (Addison's diseases) hyperkalemia, hypokalemia, hypercalcaemia; hypermagnesemia, hypophosphotemia, and hypo- and hyperthyroidism;

3. **Genetic metabolic disorders** are carbohydrate metabolism (McArdle's syndrome, 6-phosphofructokinase deficiency, adult acid maltase deficiency); lipid metabolism (carnitine deficiency); purine metabolism; mitochondrial myopathies.

4. **Infections** include **viral** (influenza, Epstein-Barr, HIV, coxsackie); **bacterial** (staphylococci, streptococci, clostridia); **parasitic** (toxoplasmosis, trichinosis, schistosomiasis, cysticercosis.

5. **Miscellaneous.** Polymyalgia rheumatica, vasculitis, eosinophilia myalgia syndrome, paraneoplastic myopathy.

6. **Myopathies** can be diffuse or focal. Myopathies must be distinguished from neuropathies. Myopathies lack sensory findings, typically involve the proximal muscles, have muscle pain or tenderness, and preserve the deep tendon reflexes until they are very advanced. They do not follow root syndromes or nerve distribution and rarely has complete paralysis and fasciculation. **The medical causes** include dermatomyositis, endocrine disorders, electrolyte disturbances, (hypokalemia associated with anorexia/bulimia) hyperthermia, inherited metabolic myopathies (glycogen

storage disease [Pompe], acid maltase deficiency and phosphorylase deficiency [McArdle's disease], carnitine deficiency [systemic type associated hepatic encephalopathy and cardiomyopathies], muscular dystrophies, nemaline rod disease, periodic paralysis (familial and nonfamilial) polymyositis, RDM, trichinosis, thyroid disorders, and HIV.

7. **Exposure to drugs and chemicals** may account for or contribute to neuromuscular symptoms.

   a. **Peripheral neuropathy** may be caused by anesthetics, anticonvulsants, antimicrobials, botulism, CV agents, cytotoxics, diphtheria toxin, ethanol, fish food (ciguatera), heavy metals, n-hexane metabolite (2,5-hexanedione), organophosphate insecticides, solvents, vitamin B_6, and vaccines. Dimethylaminopropionrile causes bladder neuropathy.

   b. **Neuromuscular junction disorders** may be caused by anticonvulsants, aminoglycoside, CV agents, immunosuppressive agents, organophosphates, tetrodotoxin, tick toxin.

   c. **Toxic myopathy** may be caused by the following:

      (1) Diffuse myopathies can be caused by amidarone, aminocaproic acid, antimalarials, beta-adrenergic antagonists, chloroquine, cimetidine, clofibrate, cocaine, colchicine, corticosteroids, cyclosporin, ethanol, etchlorvynol, heroin, ipecac (chronic use), lovastatin and other lipid lowering agents, penicillin, phencyclidine, propylthiouracil, rifampin, sulfonamides, toluene (chronic inhalation), vincristine, zidovudine. Exposure to barium salts, glycyrrhizic acid may produce muscle weakness. **Inflammatory myopathy** has been produced by D-penicillamine, eosinophilia myalgia syndrome. Toxins from snakes, brown recluse spider, hymenoptera.

J. **Differential diagnosis of generalized weakness in the intensive care unit** (ICU) (175). The mnemonic of generalized muscle weakness is **MUSCLES: M**—medication i.v. administration of corticosteroids—pancuronium, vercuronium, metronidazole, amidarone, zidovudine; **U**—undiagnosed neuromuscular disorder (polymyositis, dermatomyositis, amyotrophic sclerosis, Guillain-Barré, Eaton-Lambert syndrome, myasthenia gravis, acid maltase deficiency, muscular dystrophy; **S**—Spinal Cord damage (ischemic, compressive, hematoma, trauma); **C**—critical illness polyneuropathy; **L**—loss of muscle mass (disuse atrophy, RDM, catabolic state); **E**—Electrolyte disorders (hypokalemia, hypermagnesemia, hypophosphatemia); **S**—Systemic illness (acute porphyria, AIDS, vasculitis neuropathy, endocrine myopathies).

K. **Ataxia** (176–178). **Ataxia or incoordination** of the voluntary muscles resulting in uncertain movements, and a broad based staggering gait has been seen in many intoxications. Ataxia may be sensory (proprioceptive, postural) or cerebellar. If ataxia is due to **sensory loss** its manifestations are increased by closing the eyes. If it is **cerebellar** it is not influenced by loss of visual impulses. Ataxia may be due to impairment of many structures such as the peripheral nerves (see **H.2.g**), posterior columns and spinocerebellar tracts of the spinal cord, cerebellum and cerebello-vestibular spinal cord pathways. **The most common cause of ataxia is an overdose or an intoxication.**

1. **Medical causes**
   a. Epidural hematoma, subdural hematoma, hemorrhage, or stroke.
   b. **Acute cerebellar ataxia** occurs in children, with peak at 3 years of age. It was associated with varicella and other viral illness and with immunizations. CSF pleocytosis occurs in 50%. It has an explosive onset over a few hours with a complete recovery in 8 months in 75% of cases. Other causes include alcoholic cerebellar degeneration, ataxia-telangiectasia, brain abscess, cerebral trauma, dementia (AD), encephalitis (subacute sclerosing panencephalopathy-MRI shows asymmetrical demyelination in subcortical area), Hartnup's disease, hyperthermia, hypoxic encephalopathy, after hepatic encephalopathy, hypoparathyroidism, lipid storage diseases, phenylketonuria, vascular occlusion of the basilar artery.
   c. **Loss of proprioceptive sense or postural tone** occurs with hereditary, polyneuropathy, multiple sclerosis, spinal cord tumor, tabes dorsalis.
   d. **Subacute causes** are posterior fossa neoplasm, indolent posterior fossa abscess, subdural empyema.
   e. **Opisthotonos-myoclonus-ataxia syndrome** may be caused by infections, or toxic-metabolic causes including cocaine, hyperosmolar nonketotic coma, and biotin responsive multiple carboxylase deficiency and in 2% to 3% of cases with occult neuroblastoma.
   f. **Chronic or recurrent** ataxia occur with metabolic disorders (urea cycle disorders, aminoacidopathies), lysosomal storage disorders (metachromatic leukodystrophy presents in second year of life with poor balance, progressing to spasticity and MRI shows periventricular white matter abnormalities) hereditary ataxia, degenerative disease, and paraneoplastic syndromes.
   g. **The most frequent substances** involved are alcohol (ethanol), anticonvulsants (phenytoin, carbamazepine), barbiturates, and benzodiazepines. **Ataxia has also been reported in intoxications** from acrylamide, alcohols (ethanol, isopropyl, methanol), alprazolam, amiodarone, aminoglycoside, anticholinergics, anticonvulsants (carbamazepine, lamotrigine, phenytoin), antihistamines (tripleennamine), baclofen, barbiturates, benzodiazepines, bromides, carbamates, carbon monoxide, carbon disulfide, chloral hydrate, cimetidine, cocaine, dinitrobenzene, ethylene glycol, fish poisoning (ciguatera, shellfish, tedrodotoxin), freon, gabapentin, hallucinogens (mescaline, peyote), hexachlorobenzene, hypoglycemic (insulin and sulfonylureas), hydrocarbon inhalants, glycols (ethylene glycol), isoniazid, L-dopa, lithium, metaclopramide, metals (lead, mercury, thallium), nicotine, opioids (dextromethorphan, diphenoxylate, propoxyphene), organochlorine insecticides (DDT, lindane), organophosphate insecticides, phencyclidine, phenothiazines, phenylbutazone, plants (English ivy, golden chain, lantana, mayapple, mushrooms [groups II, V, VI], Scotch broom), 5-HT inhibitors (fluoxetine, sertraline), sedative-hypnotics (methaqualone), solvents (chlorinated hydrocarbons, trichloroethane, trichloroethylene), toluene inhalation, TCA, turpentine, vincristine, vinyl chloride, zidovudine, zolpidem.

L. MD (179–185). MD are classified as extrapyramidal, usually considered as involving the basal ganglia of the brain and their connections or cerebellum, dystonic reactions, dyskinesia, drug-induced Parkinson rigidity, asterixis, fasciculations, and choreoathetoid movements.

1. **MD have been observed in the following intoxications:** amantadine, anticholinergics, anticonvulsants, antihistamines (diphenhydramine), arsenic, barbiturates, bromocriptine, caffeine, carbon monoxide, carbon disulfide, CNS stimulants (amphetamines, cocaine, phenylpropanolamine), ergot (St. Anthony's Fire), ethanol, lithium, metoclopramide (Reglan), mercury, neuroleptics (phenothiazines, butyrophenones), sedative-hypnotics, and withdrawal states especially ethanol delirium tremens.

2. There are several types of drug-related MD:

   a. **Acute dystonia** is sustained twisting movements and can progress to posturing. They are not dose-related and may occur with single dose, long-term therapeutic doses, or overdose. They may be delayed 5 to 18 h after a single dose but usually occurs within 48 h of starting therapy or after a dose increase. It occurs in 10% to 15% of overdose patients. They are characterized by spasms of the musculature of the head, neck and upper torso, opisthotonos (tetanic contractions of muscles of spine and extremities), torticollis (spasmodic contractions of muscles of the neck), oro-lingual dyskinesia resulting in dysarthria and tongue protrusion, akathisia (desire for motion and unable to sit still) grimacing, and oculogyric crisis (painful upward gaze of the eyes). They may be mistaken for a psychotic episode but the patients have **normal mentation.** The **mechanism** is believed due to **blockade of the dopaminergic receptors** causing a shift in cholinergic-dopaminogenic balance. Predisposing factors appear to be fever and dehydration. Rarely irreversible tardative dyskinesia may occur. The different diagnosis is tetany, tetanus, focal seizures, hypomagnesemia, strychnine and hysteria. **The agents** that cause this as an idiosyncratic reaction include amantadine, antihistamines, bromphenaramine, carbamazepine, L-dopa, loxapine, metaclopramide, orphenadrine, ranitidine, sertraline and the phenothiazines. The high antipsychotic potency, low anticholinergic action phenothiazines like the piperidine group (fluphenazine, perphenazine, prochlorperazine, trifluoperazine) and nonphenothiazine butyrophenones such as haloperidol. It occurs less frequently with medication with high cholinergic blockade such as chlorpromazine and thioridazine. Dystonias should be distinguished from dyskinesia because they can be treated with anticholinergic agents. Dyskinesia should be treated with a sedative muscle relaxant such as diazepam.

   b. **Dyskinesias** are rapid repetitive movements of small local muscle groups such as tongue darting or focal myoclonus but may be generalized The agents that cause this reaction include anticholinergics, anticonvulsants, antihistamines (diphenhydramine), caffeine, CNS stimulants (amphetamines, cocaine, phenylpropanolamine), L-dopa, lithium. These reactions should be treated with a sedative muscle relaxant such as diazepam, not anticholinergics.

c. **Drug-induced parkinsonism** is characterized by pill-rolling resting tremors, rigidity, bradykinesia, postural instability (TRAP), expressionless mask-like face, stooped posture, shuffling gait, and drooling. Prochlorperazine is an important cause of **parkinsonism** in the elderly and late onset side effects such as tardive dyskinesia and dystonia are often permanent. Withdrawal of L-dopa during "Parkinson drug holidays" may produce a bizarre hyperkinetic disorders similar to NMS. It has been seen with alcohol withdrawal and with medications including captopril, carbon disulfide, carbon monoxide*, cyanide, lithium, manganese*, metaclopromide, methanol, methylphenyl-tetrahydropyridine (MPTP—a meperidine analog synthesis by-product that produced the **"frozen addict syndrome,"** neuroleptics, phenytoin, reserpine.

d. **Rigidity of the muscles** is seen with black widow spider bite, lithium intoxication, MAOI, phencyclidine, strychnine poisoning. It is also seen as part of the NMS, 5-HT syndrome, and malignant hyperthermia. The rigidity NMS is caused by DA antagonists such as phenothiazines and butyrophenones.

e. **Asterixis** abnormal muscle tremor consisting of involuntary jerking movements especially of the hands but also seen in the tongue and muscle groups of the foot. When due to hepatic coma is called "liver flap." It is elicited by the patient holding the hand as if stopping traffic. Asterixis implies a toxic-metabolic encephalopathy. **Medical metabolic conditions** causing these movements include hepatic failure, hyperosmolar states, posthypoxia, and renal failure. **Toxins** causing these movements include anticonvulsants, benzodiazepines, bismuth, cyclic antidepressants, ethanol, lead, L-dopa, mercury, methylbromide, sedative-hypnotics.

f. **Fasciculations** are involuntary twitching of muscle fibers seen under the skin. If they occur when a muscle is cold or fatigued it is not pathologic. They are seen in **neurologic diseases** and are attributable to the lower motor neuron damage and deterioration of the anterior horn cells of the spinal cord. They can indicate nicotinic receptor involvement in organophosphate intoxication. **Skeletal muscle** tremors occur with beta-adrenergic agonist drugs. **Other substances** with fasciculations include amphetamines, arsenic, black widow spider bite, caffeine, cocaine, cholinergic agents, ergotamine, fluorides, hypoglycemic agents, lead, lithium, manganese, mercury, nicotine, phencyclidine, scorpion envenomation, shellfish poisoning, snakes, strychnine, tedrodotoxin (pufferfish).

g. **Choreoathetoid movements** are irregular, involuntary spasmodic movements of the limbs and trunk and grimacing of the face. They give the appearance of restlessness and movements flow from one body part to another in an unpredictable fashion. The patients can not maintain a posture for more than a few seconds. Their grip on the examiner's fingers will relax and tighten "milk maid's grasp." **Hemiballismus** type is violent flinging or throwing movements. Chorea movements are exacerbated by action and stress. It must be distinguished from tics, myoclonus, tremor, and dystonia. The **mechanism** is the release of DA in the synaptic connections or deficiency in acetylcholine.

(1) **Medically,** these movements are seen as a major manifestation of rheumatic fever called Sydenham chorea (St. Vitus Dance). It is seen many other conditions including acquired immune deficiency disease, autoimmune disorders (systemic lupus-rare), encephalitis, infectious mononucleosis, Lyme disease, disorders of metabolism (amino acid, carbohydrate, lipid metabolism disorders), cerebral palsy, kernicterus, hyperthyroidism (2%), hepatic encephalopathy, heredodegenerative disorders (Huntington's disease, Wilson's disease—copper deposition in basal ganglia, ataxia telangiectasia, Hallervorden-Spatz, Pelizaeus-Merzbacher) hypocalcemia, hypoglycemia, structural lesions (cerebrovascular accidents, trauma, hemorrhage, tumors). Exclude cervical spine, ocular and neoplastic causes.

(2) **Drug- and toxin-induced movements** that are the result of dysfunction in the basal ganglia may be **observed in idiosyncratic reactions and poisonings** by alcohol, amidarione, anticholinergic, anticonvulsant (phenytoin) antihistamines (chlorphenaramine, meclizine), antiparkinson agents*, contraceptive oral type (with underlying basal ganglia pathology), cyclic antidepressants, diazoxide, droperidol, ergot alkaloids (St. Anthony's Fire), haloperidol, L-dopa, loxapine, phenothiazines* (chlorpromazine, fluphenazine, mesoridazine, molindone, prochlorperazine, promazine, thioridazine, trifluoperazine, triflupromazine, thiothixene), 5-HT reuptake inhibitor (paroxetine), phenytoin, pimozide, phencyclidine, thiethylperazine, theophylline, trimethobenzamide.

h. **Tremors** have been induced by the following substances: acrylamide (acrylic amide used adhesives and grouting), acyclovir, albuterol, aluminum, amidarone, amphetamines, anticholinergic, antihistamines H-1 blockers, antihistamine H-2 blockers (nizatidine, ranitidine) anticonvulsants (carbamazepine, phenytoin, primidone, valproic acid) bromides, caffeine, camphor, chlorambucil, ciprofloxacin, cyclosporin, clonazepam, cocaine, cyclic antidepressants (amitriptyline, nortriptyline), diethyltoluamide (DEET), digitalis, droperidol, ephedrine, ethylene dichloride (soil fumigant and solvent), fenfluramine, flecainide, fluoride, freon, gabapentin, gamma-hydroxybutyric acid (abused as a body builder), glycol ethers, indian tobacco, insulin, lead, L-thyroxine, lidocaine, lithium, marijuana, mescaline, methcathinone (abused stimulant), methylene chloride (paint stripper), mexiletine, organochlorine insecticides, peyote, pimozide, pindolol, piroxicam, propoxyphene, pyrethrins, rauwolfa serpentina (plant), reserpine, risperidone, 5-HT reuptake inhibitors (fluoxetine, sertaline), scorpion fish, selenium, stonefish, thallium, thyroid, trichloroethylene, theophylline, zidovudine.

M. **Trismus (lock jaw)** is tonic contractions of the muscles of mastication, observed with intoxication from aconite, carbon monoxide, nicotine, phenothiazines, strychnine, tetanus (risus sardonicus), and water hemlock. "*Facies lactrodectismica*" is a grimace seen with black widow spider bite.

N. **Slurred speech.** Alcohols (ethyl, methyl, isopropyl), anticonvulsants (carbamazepine, phenytoin, phenobarbital, primidone, prazepam), baclofen, barbiturates (phenobarbital, secobarbital), benzodiazepine (alprazolam, diazepam, triazolam) botulism, bromides, bupropion, cocaine, dantrolene, diethyltoluamide (DEET insecticide), ethylene glycol, fish food poisoning (scromboid fish poisoning, shell fish poisoning, tedrodotoxin poisoning) freon, manganese, marijuana, octopus, phenol, plants (philodendron, poison hemlock), sedative-hypnotics (ethchlorvynol, glutethimide, meprobamate, methaqualone, pyrethrins), risperidone, trichlorethylene, zolpidem.

O. **Behavioral disturbances** (186,187). **The major substances producing behavioral disturbances are** amphetamines, anticholinergic, carbon monoxide, carbon disulfide, cocaine, heavy metals, inhalants, and hallucinogens.

1. **Intoxications associated with behavioral disturbances** (aggression and violence, agitation, anxiety and panic, euphoria, hallucinations, homicidal and suicidal intent, insomnia, hyperexcitability, irritability, paranoia, psychosis) have been reported from amphetamines*, anticholinergics, antidepressants, antihistamines, arsenic, benzodiazepines, bromides, bromocriptine, carbon disulfide, carbon monoxide, cardiac glycosides, cimetidine, cocaine*, corticosteroids, disulfiram, ethanol*, hallucinogens, hypoglycemia from any cause, isoniazid, lead (chronic), L-dopa, lidocaine, lithium, LSD, marijuana, metoclopramide, mescaline, methylphenidate*, methyl bromide (fumigation), morning glory seeds, nutmeg, opioids, phencyclidine*, phenylpropanolamine, phenothiazines, salicylates, scopolamine, solvents, sympathomimetics, theophylline, toluene, triazolam, TCA, vitamins A and D, withdrawal from opioids, sedative-hypnotics and ethanol, yohimbine. Asterisk indicates compounds that are associated with violence.

   a. **Euphoria has been reported to develop** from alcohol, amphetamines, aromatic hydrocarbon inhalation, carbon monoxide, cocaine, opioids, petroleum distillates, trichloroethylene.

   b. **Anxiety and panic** from amphetamine, caffeine, cocaine, ethanol, hallucinogens (especially LSD, marijuana), mercury, phenylpropanolamine, sedative-hypnotics, and stimulants.

   c. **Mania** from amphetamines, anticholinergics, antihistamines, cocaine, methylphenidate, phencyclidine, phenylpropanolamine, salicylates, sympathomimetics, theophylline.

   d. **Paranoia** from amphetamines, anticholinergics, antihistamines, cocaine, ethanol, hallucinogens, methamphetamine, phencyclidine, and TCA.

P. **Violence** (188–191). **Violence** is aggressive assault or combativeness with the use of force. Most people are angry because they feel abandoned, their expectations not met or they haven't been consulted about their treatment. These patients may harm themselves and others. Violence may be psychiatric, situational frustration, or due to organic diseases. **Agitation** is uncontrollable restlessness or excessively excitable. **Psychosis** is a mental derangement which may cause violence or aggression.

1. **Features** of the different causes of violence

   a. **Personality disorder.** Absence of hallucinations, delusions, disorganized thought, intact orientation. History of impulsive behavior, self-mutilation, suicide, sexual promiscuity, drug abuse, shop lifting, frequent physical fights.

    b.   **Schizophrenia or mania** has a gradual onset, hallucinations, delusions (especially persecutory), disorganized thought, orientation intact. History of psychiatric illness.

    c.   **Alcohol and drug intoxication** often have tremor, pupillary changes, hyperreflexia, nystagmus, slurred speech, autonomic hyperactivity, ataxia, history of alcohol or substance abuse.

    d.   **Delirium** has a sudden onset, has disorientation, is waxing and waning, has illusions, and has known medical illness.

  2.   Notice **of potential violence** includes agitation, loud speech, startles easily, tense posture, sits on edge of chair, paces back and forth, clinched fists, tattoos (prison tattoos are black and fuzzy), tattoo says "born to kill." Emergency departments (EDs) should have a code word for trouble "Need Dr. Armstrong here." The prodromal symptoms of violence are increasing anxiety and tension manifest as rigid posturing, verbal abusive and profanity and increasing hyperactivity such as pacing. These signs may indicate the need for immediate intervention. **Note** odors, pupils' size and eye movements, and mental status. Treat violent patients like a king: walk in facing him and back out. For the proposed combativeness score, see Table 86-19.

  3.   **Medical conditions** that have been associated with violent behavior include anemia (severe), AIDS encephalopathy, brain abscess, cerebrovascular accident, chromosomal XXY males, delirium, dementia, electrolyte abnormality, endocrine disorder, hepatic failure, hyperthermia, hypothermia, hyperglycemia, hypertensive encephalopathy, hypoglycemia (hypothermic), hypoxia, infection (fever), neoplasm, porphyria (associated with abdominal pain), seizures, thyrotoxicosis, trauma, vascular malformation, and vitamin deficiency. **Always exclude** hypoxia, hypoglycemia, electrolyte disturbances, metabolic and endocrine disorders. Most patients labeled as violent are schizophrenic, especially of the paranoid type (30% to 40%).

  4.   **Common drugs and substances that cause violent reactions** include ethanol (intoxication, intolerance, and withdrawal), amphetamines, anticholinergics, aromatic hydrocarbons, cocaine, corticosteroids, LSD, opioids (especially after naloxone provoked withdrawal), phencyclidine, sedative-hypnotics (intoxication or withdrawal), and withdrawal from ethanol.

  5.   **Differential diagnosis.** The patient with an **organic etiology** is more confused and disoriented, and has more bizarre behavior. Violence is misdirected and occurs when personal space is invaded. **Violent behavior should be considered to have an**

TABLE 86-19. *Combativeness score*

1	2	3	4	5
Violent	Agitation	Agitation	Less agitation	None
Fully restrained	+	+	Unrestrained	No
Constant attention	+	Intermittent	None	None

Modified from Dublin WR. Overcoming danger with violent patients: guidelines for safe and effective management. *Emerg Med Rep* 1992;13:112.

organic etiology if over 40 years of age without a previous psychiatric history, disorientation, lethargy or stupor, abnormal vital signs, visual hallucinations, or illusions.

Q. Headache. The brain is not a pain-sensitive structure; therefore, **headaches are caused by the following:**

1. **Intracranial irritation** of the pain fibers that innervate the dura, or the vessels of the pia-arachnoid (increased ICP due to meningeal irritation, abscess, tumor, hemorrhage, hypertensive encephalopathy, or edema)

2. **Extracranial pain structures** which include the muscles (trauma, tension, bone disease), blood vessels of the scalp (cluster headaches, migraine, tension), epithelial tissues of the sinus (sinusitis) and structures of the eye and the orbit (eye stain, glaucoma, tumor) or temporomandibular joint.

3. **The toxins that commonly may cause headache** include acetone, anticholinergics, aniline dyes, caffeine, carbon monoxide, corticosteroids, cyanide, digitalis, ergotamine, heavy metals (lead), methemoglobinemia causes, nicotine, nitrites, organophosphate insecticides, quinidine, tetracycline (outdated), sympathomimetics (amphetamines, cocaine, phenylpropanolamine), theophylline, vitamin A (chronic excess).

R. Dizziness and vertigo (192–196). Dizziness means either faintness or vertigo after the elimination of vague terms such as "lightheaded," "faintness," "spinning," "giddiness," and "confusion."

1. **True vertigo** is the sensation of moving in space (subjective) or having objects move around the person (objective). It is a result of a disturbance in the equilibrium apparatus. The maintenance of balance and spatial orientation depend on input from the vestibular labyrinth, visual system and proprioceptive nerves arising from tendons, muscles and joints. Input is received by the vestibular nuclei in the medulla and lower pons via the vestibular branch of the VIII cranial nerve. and from the cerebellum. The vestibular nuclei send efferent fibers to cerebellum, medial longitudinal fasciculus and vestibulospinal tract. Lesions at the inner ear, brain stem, cerebellum may manifest as vertigo. Dizziness when rolling over in bed is vertigo (Table 86-20) for differentiation of central and peripheral vertigo. **Near syncope** (near faint or faintness) due to decreased CBF (perfusion) of the CNS associated with autonomic nervous system compensation (diaphoresis, nausea, tachycardia, cardiac dysrhythmias (rare), hypersensitive carotid, a "vasovagal" reflex (inadequate vasoconstriction or inappropriate vasodilation), orthostatic hypotension (medications rarely cause in patient lying down). **Disequilibrium** is a sensation of imbalance when standing or walking. It reflects a gait disorder. This caused by neurologic disorders, multiple sensory disorders (diabetes mellitus, alcoholism, posterior column diseases), cerebellar-pontine angle disorders (auditory disorders) or posterior fossa tumors, cerebellar degeneration, tertiary syphilis (tabes dorsalis), parkinsonism, transient ischemic attaches and other vascular disorders (CVA, aneurysm and embolism), positive Romberg, and gait disturbances. **Lightheadedness or psychogenic illness** is psychiatric disorders produce unrelenting dizziness throughout the day seen in hyperventilation syndrome, anxiety neurosis, hysterical neurosis, affective disorders, depression. Hyperventilation produces dizziness. **Tests for vertigo** include vision and auditory examination (exclude foreign bodies or impacted wax),

TABLE 86-20. *Differentiation—central and peripheral vertigo*

Feature	Central	Peripheral
Cause	Vascular	Infection labyrinth
	Demyelinating diseases	Meniere, Neuronitis
	Neoplasm	Ischemia, trauma
	Multiple sclerosis	Acoustic neuroma
	Medication or toxin	Medication or toxin
Site	Brain stem or cerebellum	Labyrinth
Onset	Sudden	Insidious
Pattern	Continuous	Intermittent
Severity	Mild	Marked
Duration	Months (may be chronic)	Minutes to days, recurs
Head motion	Little change	Aggravates
Deafness/tinnitus	Usually absent	Often present
Nystagmus	Multiple directions	Unidirectional
Horizontal	Common	Uncommon
Vertical	May be present	Never present
Neurologic	Abnormal	Normal

exclude anemia, BP when erect lying down, Valsalva maneuver, carotid, sinus pressure, hyperventilation (less than Pco_2 causes vasoconstriction), Romberg test, cold caloric test (eye movement slow phase is toward lesion, fast phase nystagmus is away from lesion), the patient falls toward lesion and environment spins away), blood glucose, serologic test for syphilis. **Substances commonly associated with dizziness include** alcohols (ethanol, methanol), aminoglycoside, anticonvulsants (barbiturates, phenytoin, carbamazepine), antihistamines H-1 and H-2, antihypertensive agents (especially ACE inhibitors), benzodiazepines, caffeine, carbon monoxide, drug abuse, environmental toxins, meprobamate, nonsteroidal antiinflammatory agents, quinidine, quinine, salicylates.

IX. **Ocular system** (197,198). The visual apparatus and its muscles are one of the most important tools in the diagnosis of toxicologic problems because they reflects the CNS and the autonomic nervous system response from distant organs. The **pupillary size and response to light** is dependent on a balance between the sympathetic dilation and parasympathetic constriction. **Hypothermia** can produce large, small or midposition fixed pupils. **Anoxia** produces fixed and dilated pupils.

  A. **Eye clues in coma.** Although physiologic pupillary anisocoria (pupils remain same size in dark and light) and congenital microcoria exist, new pupillary signs are used to localize the neurological process.

    1. The **normal eyes** are directed straight ahead with reactive pupils and normal oculocephalic reflexes.

    2. The **oculocephalic reflex** is absent in barbiturates, TCA, and phenytoin poisoning but intact in opioid poisoning.

    3. **Disconjugate deviation** of the eyes verticle or lateral suggests a structural brain stem lesion.

    4. **Conjugate deviation of the eyes.** If ipsilateral indicate cerebral lesion looking away from hemiplegic side. If contralateral pontine lesions look toward hemiplegic side.

5. **Unilateral dilated pupil** suggests supratentorial mass lesion with uncal herniation and compression of third nerve.

6. **Bilateral dilated pupils,** fixed to light suggest irreversible brain damage or anticholinergic poisoning. Also seen with hypothermia and peripheral nerve damage.

7. **Third nerve palsies** (eyes point down and out) and bilateral midpoint fixed pupils suggest thalamic and midbrain lesions.

8. **Irregular pupils** unreactive to light suggest midbrain damage.

B. **Diplopia ("double vision").** Increased ICP, brain tumor, orbital mass, myasthenia gravis, sedative-hypnotics, and botulism.

C. **Mydriasis (dilation of the pupil).** Dilation of the pupil may be due to paralysis of the parasympathetic innervation of the sphincter of the iris (decreased cholinergic action) by anticholinergic agents or stimulation of the sympathetic nerve fibers to the dilator pupillae muscle (increased sympathetic action) by amphetamine or cocaine. Dilated pupil is due to third nerve compression by the expanding supratentorial lesions such as tumor or hematoma (Hutchinson pupil). Mydriasis also occurs in hypoxemia, hypoglycemia, and reflex reaction to pain and vomiting.

1. **Unilateral unresponsive mydriasis,** the ominous sign of uncal brain herniation, CNS infections (meningitis, encephalitis), rarely following seizures, multiple sclerosis may also be seen from glutethimide overdose (200), and with normal mental status from mydriatic drops in one eye or local trauma to the eye. However, it usually requires a CT scan to exclude intracranial pathology.

2. **Blindness produces mydriasis** because the perception of light has been abolished. Dilation of the pupil is produced by the many intoxicants and may be recalled by classifying these by the **mnemonic** of **SHAW: S**—sympathetic agents (amphetamines, cocaine, DA, MAOI); **H**—hallucinogens, pathologic states of hypoglycemia and hypoxia; **A**—anticholinergic agents (atropine, antihistamines, cyclic antidepressants glutethimide); **W**—withdrawal from opioids, sedative-hypnotics, and ethanol.

3. **Mydriasis may be noted in the following intoxications:** anticholinergics*, antihistamine H-1 and H-2 blockers*, barium, benztropine, botulism (delayed)*, bretylium, bromides, caffeine, camphor, carbamazepine, carbon monoxide*, cimetidine, cocaine, curare, cyanide, ergot, ethylene glycol, fluoride, glutethimide (may produce unilateral dilated pupil) (200), hallucinogens (LSD)*, hypoglycemic agents (insulin, oral sulfonylureas), meperidine, methanol (delayed), nicotine, MAOI, mushroom (*A. muscaria,* peyote), plants (box thorn, English ivy, Golden chain, jimson weed, morning glory, nutmeg, Scotch broom, water hemlock, Yew), quinidine, quinine, sertraline, sympathomimetics (cocaine, amphetamines, phenylpropanolamine), thallium, thyroid, toluene, trichloroethylene, TCA*, tyramine food poisoning and withdrawal* from opioids, sedative-hypnotics and ethanol.

   a. **Nonreactive mydriasis** is usually from pure anticholinergic poisoning.

   b. **Delayed mydriasis** occurs from methanol intoxication (formate destruction of the retina) and botulism.

   c. **Opioids that produce mydriasis** are meperidine, diphenoxylate with atropine (Lomotil) and dextromethorphan (paralysis of the iris).

D. **Miosis** (constriction of the pupil or pinpoint pupils) (199). Constriction of the pupil may result from parasympathetic stimulation (increased cholinergic action) such as from organophosphate poisoning, or inhibition of sympathetic stimulation (decreased sympathetic action).

1. **Neurologic causes** include Horner's syndrome (ipsilateral miosis, ptosis and anhidrosis) which result from a lesion in any of the three sympathetic ganglion, small but reactive pupils (oculo-sympathetic paresis) can be seen in hypothalamic lesions, and destructive lesions of the pons disrupt the oculosympathetic pathways and produce pinpoint pupils. **A miotic pupil (1 mm) unresponsive to dim light and naloxone** usually indicates pontine damage of the pupillary centers.

2. **Miosis may be the result of intoxication** from carbamates (medicinal and insecticides), carbamazepine, cholinergic agents, cimetidine, clonidine, edrophonium, guanabenz, methyldopa, miotic eyedrops (pilocarpine), lidocaine, mushrooms (cholinergic clitocybe, inocybe), meprobamate, nicotine, opioids (except dextromethorphan, meperidine and Lomotil), nutmeg, organophosphate insecticides (only 60% of intoxications), phencyclidine, and phenothiazines (almost 80% of cases of overdose), phentolamine, phenoxybenzamine, prazocin, tetrahydrozoline, valproic acid, zolipdem (Ambien).

3. A **simplified method of recalling substances that commonly produce miosis** is **CPOOP: one "C," two "Os"**— organophosphate (and carbamates) and opioids; and **three "Ps"**— phencyclidine, phenothiazines, and pontine lesions.

4. "The flea collar pupil" unilateral constricted pupils occurs when carbamates dust used in flea collars for dogs and cats gets into an eye (1).

E. **Nystagmus** (201–203). **Nystagmus movements are** involuntary rhythmical oscillation of the eyes, with fast movement in one direction and slow in the other. The commonly used mnemonic COWS indicating the eye movements after injecting cold and warm water into the auditory canal (cold opposite and warm same refers only to the fast component). The cerebral cortex is intact if nystagmus is present. Nystagmus may be congenital, frequently present in albinos, seen in amblyopia, occupational in miners, train dispatchers, in labyrinthitis, neurologic diseases and with medications in overdose. The **mechanism for the production of nystagmus** is input passes from the vestibular nuclei to nuclei of the extraocular muscles through the medial longitudinal fasciculus to produce nystagmus. This input may be modified by information from the cerebral cortex and the cerebellum. It may involve the cerebrum, cerebellum, vestibular apparatus, brain stem nuclei for cranial nerves III, IV, VI, VIII, the medial longitudinal fasciculus, and the extraocular muscles. It is normal to have a few beats with extreme lateral gaze. The direction and pattern of the nystagmus may be a clue to the cause or intoxicant.

1. Sustained jerk nystagmus. Impaired vestibular function. Labyrinth disease or its central connection in brain stem.

2. Verticle nystagmus. Brain stem dysfunction or cocaine, diphenhydramine, opioids, phencyclidine, and phenytoin

3. Rotatory nystagmus. Labyrinth disease (fine and maximum in direction of gaze) or central vestibular mechanisms (associated with nausea and vomiting) or intoxication from haloperidol, methanol, and phencyclidine.

4. Horizontal pendular. Seen in albinism, is vestibular origin overdose and from overdose of barbiturate, carbamazepine, ethanol, ethylene glycol, isopropanol, lithium, meprobamate, methanol, phenytoin, phencyclidine

5. Wandering or searching nystagmus is irregular, oscillating searching movements of marked amplitude seen in blind or in persons with poor vision. There is no rapid jerk component.

6. To-and-fro nystagmus. Jelly-like movements seen in congenital nystagmus and spasms nutans. Slow and fast components are not evident.

7. **Drug-induced nystagmus** suggests overdose from anticonvulsants* (but it is present in only 30% of overdoses phenobarbital, clonazepam, diazepam, lamotrigine, phenytoin, primidone, valproic acid), barbiturates, baclofen, cyclic antidepressants (amitriptyline, amoxapine, imipramine), carbon disulfide (rayon, rubber industries) (202,203), clozapine, disulfiram, ethanol*, ethylene glycol*, ethchlorvynol, ethylene oxide, fluoxetine, gabapentin, gamma-hydroxybutyric acid, isoniazid, lithium*, marijuana, nicotine, opioids (vertical), quinine, phencyclidine * (rotatory), phenothiazines (mesoridazine, thioridazine), salicylates, and sedative-hypnotics, ziduvidine. The **mneumonic** for the most common is **LAAP: L**—lithium; **A**—anticonvulsants; **A**—alcohols and glycols; **P**—phencyclidine. The absence of nystagmus does not exclude these substances. For the differentiation of peripheral and brain stem nystagmus, see Table 86-21.

F. **Ophthalmoplegia** is paralysis of all ocular muscles. Externa is paralysis of multiple extraocular muscles has been observed in poisonings from amitriptyline, botulism toxin, carbon monoxide, curare, ergot, ethanol, lead, thallium, vincristine, and Wernicke's encephalopathy (thiamine deficiency).

G. **PC or IIH.** See ICP.

H. **Ptosis.** Drooping of the upper eyelid may be due to paralysis of the levator palpebrae and **is noted from poisonings by** bromides, botulism toxin, curare, lead (chronic), mercury (chronic), phenytoin, thallium, vincristine.

I. **Disturbances of colored vision.** Disturbed color vision, usually all the objects look yellow, may be **observed with intoxications from** amyl nitrite, anticholinergics, arsenic trioxide, barbiturates, bromides, carbon monoxide, chromic acid, digitalis, ethambutol (loss of green), ethanol, hallucinogens (perceptual), iodoform, isoniazid, lead (chronic), methanol, picric acid, quinine, quinidine, salicylates, santonin, solvents, thallium, trichloroethylene.

TABLE 86-21. *Nystagmus*

Feature	Peripheral	Brain stem—posterior fossa
Latent period	2–20 s	None
Duration	<1 min	>1 min
Fatigability	Yes	No
Direction	Unidirectional, never vertical	May change direction: horizontal, vertical, rotatory
Intensity	Severe	Mild or none
Head position	Single vertical	Occur in more than one position

J. **Blindness,** i.e., impaired vision and acute loss of vision (204). Impaired vision and sudden loss of vision has been reported with the following:
1. **Ophthalmologic conditions.** Acute angle-closure glaucoma, optic neuritis, central retinal artery or venous occlusion, internal carotid hemorrhage, posterior uveitis, retinal detachment, retinal/macular hemorrhage, vitreous hemorrhage.
2. **Medical diseases.** Temporal arteritis, increased ICP, migraine, hysteria, arteriovenous malformations, cerebral embolism, multiple sclerosis, and demyelinating encephalopathies.
3. **Traumatic.** Head trauma, lens dislocation, retinal detachment, globe rupture, chemical injury, corneal abrasion.
4. The **following poisoning may produce impaired vision. Acute neurotoxic blindness** is almost exclusively caused by methanol and quinine. Anticoagulants (retinal hemorrhages), amiodarone (keratopathy), anticholinergic (acute/temporary), arsenicals, carbon disulfide (retrobulbar neuritis), carbon monoxide (bilateral)*, caustic/corrosive (direct action; see chemical burns), chloramphenicol (optic neuritis, central scatoma), chloroform, chloroquine (corneal injury, renal damage), cocaine (retinal vessel vasospasm) corticosteroids (emboli, cataracts), deferoxamine, digitalis, (blurred vision disturbed color vision), dinitrobenzene (optic neuritis), dinitrotoluene, ergot derivatives, ethambutol (in therapeutic doses optic neuropathy with central scotoma), hydrogen sulfide, iodoform (optic neuritis), lead encephalopathy, mercury (organic mercury), methanol (formate action on retina)*, naphthalene (retro and optic neuritis), quinine (retro and optic neuritis) and cinchona derivatives, thallium (retrobulbar neuritis), trichloroethylene (retrobulbar neuritis), vitamin A (cerebral edema).

K. **Cataract** (205) is an opacity of the lens of the eye or its capsule or both. Lenticular opacity has been **reported with chronic exposure to** allopurinol, amantadine, amiodarone, busulfan, chloroquine, chloroacetophenone (lacrimator), corticosteroids, dimethyl sulfoxide (in animals), dinitrocresol, dinitrophenol, ergot, naphthalene, phenothiazines especially chlorpromazine, radiation, tamoxifen (used in treating breast cancer), thallium, titanium, excess vitamin D (chronic).

L. **Lacrimation.** Cholinergics, heavy metals, irritant gases, lacrimators (chloroacetophenone), withdrawal states.

M. **Photophobia.** Amiodarone, botulism toxin, chloroquine, Ciguatera fish poisoning, clofibrate, mercury, mydriatics, plants (Boston ivy, caladium, calla, century plant, devil ivy, dieffenbachia, Jack in the pulpit, lantana, rhubarb), digitalis, dimethyl sulfoxide, quinine, scopolamine, sertraline.

N. **Anisocoria** (206). Unequal pupils may be familial or be associated with the following:
1. **Eye disorders.** Iritis, cataracts, glaucoma, blindness, artificial eye, after eye trauma, after mydriatic or miotic eye drops.
2. **Neurologic disorders** such as third nerve compression (cerebral herniation, expanding supratentorial lesion such as a tumor or hematoma), Horner's syndrome, encephalitis, meningitis, and multiple sclerosis.
3. **Drugs** include scopolamine patches, carbamate on flea collar, nose drops inadvertently in the eye. Glutethimide may produce unilateral pupil dilation.

O.   Chemical burns of the eye
   a.   In **alkali injury,** the elevated pH produces saponification of cell-membrane components resulting in cell death. Common causes are cleaning agents (ammonia, drain cleaners), fertilizers, lime products (plaster, mortar), and refrigerants (207,208).
   b.   In **acid injury,** the protein to coagulate in the corneal epithelium and stroma, thus limiting penetration. Common causes are hydrofluoric acid, which has unique penetrating ability and its release of fluoride ions, and sulfuric acid (industrial and battery acid) (208,209).

P.   Intraocular pressure (210–212) is increased by amitriptyline, anticholinrergics (hyoscyamine), desipramine, imipramine, maprotiline, nortriptyline, scopolamine, trimipramine, zietuton.

Q.   Ocular manifestations of some systemic medications and toxins. Most of these manifestations occur on long-term use.
   1.   **Allopurinol.** Cataracts.
   2.   **Amantadine.** Corneal opacities.
   3.   **Amiodarone.** Keratopathy, i.e., small punctate deposits in the basal layer of the cornea.
   4.   **Anticholinergics and antihistamines H-1 blockers.** Mydriasis, photophobia, precipitate narrow angle glaucoma.
   5.   **Beta-adrenergic blockers.** Decrease tear production giving gritty sensation.
   6.   **Bromocriptine.** Myopia, blurred vision.
   7.   **Busulfan.** Cataracts.
   8.   **Chloramphenicol.** Optic neuritis with bilateral blurred vision, central scotoma, and papilledema.
   9.   **Chloroquine.** Cataracts, corneal injury, retinal damage with loss of central vision.
   10.   **Cisplatin.** Blurred vision, altered colored vision.
   11.   **Corticosteroids.** Cataracts and chronic open angle glaucoma.
   12.   **Cyclophosphamide.** Blurred vision, keratoconjunctivitis.
   13.   **Deferoxamine.** Blurred vision, night blindness, blindness, and retinal deposits.
   14.   **Digitalis.** Blurred vision, disturbed color vision, colored halos.
   15.   **Disulfiram.** Retrobulbar neuritis.
   16.   **Ethambutol.** Optic neuropathy with scotoma and reduced vision.
   17.   **Isoniazid.** Optic neuritis.
   18.   **Isotretinoin.** Dry eyes, blepharoconjunctivitis, corneal opacities.
   19.   **Methanol.** Snow-like halos around lights, blindness.
   20.   **Oxygen.** Implicated in retinopathy of prematurity.
   21.   **Phenothiazines.** Deposits on the cornea and lens. Anticholinergic action may precipitate narrow angle glaucoma.
   22.   **Quinine.** Reduction in visual fields, loss of visual acuity, and blindness.
   23.   **Rifampin.** Exudative conjunctivitis, orange-stained tears, and staining of contact lenses.
   24.   **Sympathetic agents.** May precipitate narrow angle glaucoma.
   25.   **Tamoxifen.** Retinal and corneal opacities.

26. **TCA.** Ophthalmoplegia from amitriptyline (211).
27. **Vincristine.** Ptosis due to cranial nerve involvement, blurred vision, night blindness.

X. **Auditory system** (213)

A. **Deafness (hearing loss).** It is estimated that 4% of U.S. population under 45 years of age and 29% of those over 65 years have handicapping loss of hearing. The most common cause is otosclerosis. Human speech is 250 to 3,000 Hz, and the ear can detect sounds from 20 to 20,000 Hz.

1. **Hearing loss from medical diseases** may result from effusions and infections of the middle ear, bacterial infections (meningitis, syphilis, tuberculosis), viral infections in utero (rubella, CMV); genetic and developmental disorders (Jervell- prolonged QT, deafness and sudden death, Waardenburg, Usher, Alport, Hurler's); hyperbilirubinemia (kernicterus); trauma (physical and acoustic environmental excess noise); immune-mediated diseases (lupus erythematosus, polyarteritis nodosa); neoplasms (acoustic neuroma, meningioma), metastatic lesions; Meniere's disease; circulatory insufficiency diseases, otosclerosis, miscellaneous (sarcoidosis, histiocytosis X, Behcet's syndrome, Paget's disease).

2. **Medications and intoxications produce neurosensory type.** It has been reported with aminoglycosides*, anticholinergic, antineoplastic agents* (bleomycin, cisplatin, nitrogen mustard, vincristine, vinblastine) benzene, bromates (hair neutralizers), bupropion, butorphanol, captopril, carbon dioxide, carbon monoxide*, chloroquine, cocaine, cyanide, cyclic antidepressants (doxepin, imipramine, maprotiline, trazadone), dantrolene sodium, dapsone, diflunisal, digitalis, diuretics (ethacrynic acid, furosemide), dinitrobenzene, erythromycin, hallucinogens, heavy metals (arsenic, cobalt, chronic lead), hexane, hydrocarbons (toluene, xylene, styrene) lidocaine, lithium, methanol, minoxidil, nicotine, nitroprusside, nonsteroidal antiinflammatory agents (ibuprofen, ketorolac, mefenamic acid, naproxen, phenylbutazone, piroxicam, sulindac), quinidine, quinine, radiation injury, salicylates, streptomycin, tolbutamide, toluene, trichlorethylene, vancomycin.

   a. **Reversible hearing loss toxins** include nonsteroidal antiinflammatory drugs: ibuprofen, naproxen, indomethacin, piroxicam diuretics (furosemide, ethacrynic acid, acetazolamide, mannitol), antimicrobials (erythromycin, quinine), salicylates, and carbon monoxide.

   b. **Irreversible hearing loss** include antimicrobials, (aminoglycosides, vancomycin), antineoplastic (cisplatin, vincristine, vinblastine, bleomycin, nitrogen mustard), bromates, hydrocarbons (toluene, xylene or styrene), heavy metals (arsenic), and toluene.

B. **Tinnitus** (214–218). Tinnitus is described as ringing or tinkling sound in the ears, is a sensation of sound that does not result from acoustic phenomena, and may result from **medical diseases** (acoustic neuroma, arteriovenous aneurysm, cerumen, fluid, foreign bodies, hypothyroidism, Meniere's disease, otosclerosis, hypertension) or trauma (barotrauma, noise, perforation of the tympanic membrane) and stress. Tinnitus is produced by toxic action on the eight nerve by numerous substances including albuterol*, aminoglycosides*, amphotericin B*, anticonvulsants, antidepressants, antifungal agents, antihistamines antineoplastic agents, bromates*, beta-blockers, caffeine* (tea, coffee), camphor, carbamazepine, carbon disulfide*, carbon monoxide, digitalis, dinitrophenol, diuretics (ethacrynic acid, furosemide), heavy metals, nicotine, nonsteroidal antiinflammatory agents (indomethacin), quinidine (rarely), quinine (tonic water)*, salicylates*, streptomycin, sympathomimetics, turpentine.

XI.   Olfactory system. Nasal perforation etiology includes cocaine insufflation, chromium. For odors, see above.

XII.   GI tract

A.   **Gingivitis, loose teeth, and stomatitis.** Oral damage from poisonings is the result of inflammation and irritation.

1.   It may be **caused by the following substances:** cancer chemotherapeutic agents, caustic/corrosive, ciguatera fish poisoning (tooth pain), heavy metals (arsenic trioxide, mercuric chloride, lead, thallium, zinc chloride), oxalates, phenol, phenytoin phosphorous, and radiation.

B.   **Excessive salivation and drooling. The oral secretions may be increased** by inflammation, irritation, and ulceration such as from caustic/corrosive injuries, by the bitter taste from heavy metals and disulfiram, and from parasympathetic stimulation from organophosphate insecticide poisoning. Also see dysphagia.

1.   The **substances that may cause excessive salivation** are ammonia, baclofen, bethanechol, benzalkonium chloride (Zephiran), butotenine (in skin glands of toads) carbamate insecticides (aldicarb, carbaryl, propoxur), carbamate medication (edrophonium, neostigmine, physostigmine, pyridostigmine), caustics/corrosives, cantharidin (Spanish Fly), clonazepam, clozapine, fluoride, foreign body, gamma-hydroxybutyric acid, heavy metals by irritation and bad taste (arsenic trioxide, copper sulfate, lead, mercuric chloride, thallium), mushrooms (Clitocybe spp., Inocybe spp.), nicotine, organophosphate insecticides (chlorfenvinphos, diazinon, dicrotophos, fenthion, malathion, parathion), plants (Boston ivy, buttercup, calla, century plant, devil's ivy, dieffenbachia, Jack-in-the-pulpit, jonquil, marsh marigold, narcissus, peyote, rhubarb, star of Bethlehem), selenious acid (gun bluing), scorpion bite, substances that paralyze the esophageal mobility, and shellfish poisoning (peppery taste), tetrodotoxin fish food poisoning.

C.   **Decreased salivation and dry mouth. The oral secretions may be diminished resulting in dry mouth by inhibition of salivation** by anticholinergic agents, by parasympathetic paralysis such as in botulism, by hyperventilation and dehydration such as in salicylate intoxication, by hyperthermia such as in cocaine and amphetamine intoxications and by hyperventilation from CNS stimulation.

1.   The **substances that cause dry mouth are** anticholinergic, antihistamines, botulism toxin, CNS stimulants (amphetamines, cocaine), opioids, phenytoin, and salicylates.

D.   **Salivary gland (especially parotid) swelling**

1.   The **medical causes** are allergy, cysts, diabetes mellitus, infections such as mumps and other viruses, infants with HIV, bacterial such as staphylococcal suppurative parotitis, Mikulicz syndrome (associated with lacrimal adenitis and uveitis in patients with TB, leukemia, Hodgkin, lupus), uveoparotid fever of sarcoid or tularemia, cirrhosis of the liver, lactation, pregnancy, Sjogren syndrome (of postmenopausal women), stones, and tumors.

2. **Medications reported to cause enlargement of the salivary glands** are guanethidine, iodine (occasionally from contrast media), phenylbutazone, thiouracil.

E. **Taste (gustation) distortion** is the interpretation of oral ingested material by the taste buds (life-span of 10 days) on tongue, palate, throat, and upper esophagus. The taste sensations are sweet, sour, bitter and salty. Taste is also influenced by aromas.

1. Distortion of taste may occur with **medical conditions** such as local oral conditions (neoplasms, Sjogren syndrome, glossitis, infections, candida); endocrinopathies (Cushing's syndrome, hypothyroidism, diabetes, gonadal dysgenesis, pseudohypoparathyroidism), renal failure, cirrhosis, hepatitis, hysteria, familial autonomic dysfunction, Parkinson disease, and migraine headache.

2. Disorders of taste by substances include amiloride, antithyroid drugs, antineoplastic drugs, biquanides, captopril, carbon monoxide, cocaine, dimethylsulfoxide DMSO (garlic), fish poisoning (Shell fish and ciguetera peppery taste), griseofulvin, heavy metals (metallic taste), lithium, metronidazole, nitroglycerine, penicillamine, phenylbutazone, spirolactone, and rifampin.

F. **Dysphagia** (219,220). **Difficulty in swallowing may be caused by substances that interfere with the swallowing mechanism such as** botulinum toxin, or may be associated with mucosal edema or pain from ulceration such as with alkali or acids.

1. **Dysphagia may occur** from antiseptics (concentrated iodine or quaternary ammonia compounds such as zephiran), caustics/corrosives, diquat, foreign bodies, heavy metals salts (arsenic trioxide, copper sulfate, mercuric chloride, ferrous sulfate, silver nitrate, thallium, zinc chloride), paraquat, phenol, phosphorous, plant irritation or ricin from castor bean, soaps and detergents (anionic, nonionic, cationic), and volatile oils.

2. **Medications associated with dysphagic esophagitis** depend on the physical properties (pH, slow-release formulation) and insufficient quantity of water while in supine position. **Medication implicated** are ascorbic acid, aspirin, chloral hydrate, clindamycin, doxycycline, ibuprofen, indomethacin, lincomycin, minocycline, phenoxymethyl penicillin, potassium chloride, quinidine, theophylline (219).

3. **Water-soluble gums.** Laxatives and antidiarrheal medication labels will say the products contain water-soluble gums and warn to take adequate fluid. The gum could get stuck on the way down, swell up in the throat or esophagus, and cause choking. There have been 199 cases of choking between 1970 and 1992 in products using these gums, including 18 deaths. The FDA has banned all **weight control products using water-soluble gums** in 1992.

G. **Vomiting.** The vomiting center is believed to be the final common pathway that mediates all vomiting. This center does not respond directly to chemical stimuli, but is **activated through the chemoreceptor trigger zone (CTZ).** The CTZ has receptors for various stimuli. NE and acetylcholine receptors mediate impulses responsible for activating the vomiting center. DA and opioid receptors are found in the GI tract and are the mediators of the emetic effect. Afferent impulses carried by the vagus and sympathetic nerves originate in the pharynx and GI tract.

1. **Vomiting is a very common nonspecific manifestation of acute poisoning.** It can be the result of local irritation which occurs within minutes after ingestion of an irritant such as detergents, or syrup of ipecac or it may be due to CNS action on the

vomiting center which occurs after a delay. The list of intoxicants that cause vomiting are too numerous to be of any diagnostic value.

2. **Lack of vomiting** can be an important sign. It may indicate that a toxic dose was not ingested. Most toxic ingestions of nonsteroidal antiinflammatory agents, salicylate, and tobacco vomit as the first sign of toxicity. On the other hand, late vomiting, starting 2 to 6 h, after mushroom ingestion may be an ominous sign that a deadly mushroom has been ingested.

H. **Diarrhea.** Loose, frequent stools may result from increased stimulation of the intestinal musculature such as produced by antibiotics, cathartics, colchicine; stimulation of the parasympathetic nervous system by organophosphate insecticides (diarrhea and miosis); from an inflammatory process after such poisons as heavy metal salts (arsenic, barium, copper, iron, thallium); lithium; opioid withdrawal; and excess vitamins. Diarrhea may be produced by such a great variety of poisons that it lacks significance as a symptomatic diagnostic tool.

I. **Constipation. Failure to have bowel movements resulting in hard difficult passage (221).** Historically, it was defined as fewer than three bowel movements per week, but many patients define it differently. The current working definition for functional constipation is that about two of the following complaints are present for at least 12 months: staining 25% of the time, lumpy or hard 25% of the time, incomplete evacuation 25% of the time, and about two bowel movements per week. Rectal outlet delay is anal blockage of more than 25% of the time, prolonged defecation, or manual disimpaction (when necessary). Constipation may be caused.

a. **Medical conditions,** including mechanical obstruction, metabolic conditions (diabetes mellitus, hypothyroidism, hypercalcemia, hypokalemia, hypomagnesemia, uremia), myopathies (amyloidosis, scleroderma), neuropathies (Parkinson disease, spinal cord injury tumor, multiple sclerosis) or other conditions (depression, degenerative bone disease, autonomic neuropathy, cognitive impairment, immobility and cardiac disease).

b. **Common medications,** including antacids (calcium containing as Tums), anticholinergic drugs* (belladonna which paralyzes the parasympathetic nervous system), antidiarrheal agents (Lopramide, Lomotil), antihistamines* (anticholinergic action), antiparkinson drugs (amantadine anticholinergic action), antipsychotic drugs* (chlorpromazine anticholinergic action), beta-adrenergic blockers (propranolol), calcium channel blockers (verapamil slow transit by effect on autonomic nervous system or smooth muscle), calcium supplements*, clonidine, diuretics* (furosemide dehydrates patient), iron supplements*, opioids* (morphine producing diminished peristaltic waves in large intestine), nonsteroidal antiinflammatory drugs (inhibit normal prostaglandin), sedative-hypnotics, sympathomimetics (ephedrine or terbutaline), tricyclics antidepressants (amitriptyline anticholinergic action) (221).

1. The **following substances may result in constipation:** barium-soluble salts causing spasm of the intestinal musculature, botulism toxin, cicutoxin (water hemlock), heavy metals (lead, thallium and following iron intoxication resulting in residual stricture) (221).

J. Bowel sounds (BS, peristalsis). Bowel sounds are an important physical diagnostic clue.

   1. May be affected by mechanical factors as injury, perforation, peritonitis, or obstruction (adhesions, mass or a foreign body). Distention and ileus may be sign of ischemic infarction secondary to mesenteric arterial spasm (ergot, amphetamine, or cocaine) or extreme hypotension.

   2. Become **hyperactive** by intoxication with cholinergic substances such as organophosphate insecticides, cathartics, CNS stimulants (cocaine and amphetamines), nicotine, and occasional sympathomimetics (theophylline).

   3. May be **hypoactive** or develop ileus from *A. muscaria* mushroom, anticholinergic, antihistamines, soluble barium salts by hypokalemia, botulism toxin, CNS depressants, lead, opioids, phenothiazines, thallium, TCA.

K. Abdominal pain. Abdominal pain may result from ingestions that produce irritation, ulceration, obstruction, or perforation of the intestine. The intoxicant may cause pain by producing hyperactivity or hypoactivity and abdominal distention. If the pain is in the right upper quadrant it could result from hepatotoxic substances, the lumbar area from nephrotoxic agents, the lower abdomen, hypogastrium, from bladder irritants, the epigastrium from damage to the stomach (epigastric pain and hematemesis).

   1. The **common substances that produce severe abdominal pain** are alcohols, particularly isopropanol, antibiotics (especially erythromycin), anticholinergic (distention), antiseptics such as concentrated iodine, bleach above 10% concentration, cantharidin (Spanish fly mythical aphrodisiac), cathartics, caustics/corrosives, cholinergics, corticosteroids (ulcerogenic), colchicine (Autumn crocus plant, medication), food poisonings, fluorides, heavy metals (arsenic, iron, chronic lead, mercuric chloride, copper sulfate, zinc chloride), insect bites (black widow with rigidity, brown recluse), marine bites (jellyfish, Portuguese-man-of-war with rigidity), paraquat, nonsteroidal antiinflammatory agents, opioids (constipation), organophosphate insecticides (hyperactivity), reptile bites, salicylates (ulcerogenic).

L. Abdominal colic. Colic is acute, excruciating, sharp pain indicating spasm or obstruction of the intestine, ureter, or biliary ducts.

   1. **Colic** has been reported in the following intoxications: arsine, black widow spider envenomation, cathartics, caustics/corrosives, colchicine, food poisoning, heavy metals salts (arsenic, soluble barium salts, chronic lead, iron, thallium), marine fish envenomations, methanol, withdrawal states especially from opioids.

M. Hematemesis, hematochezia, melena. See GI bleeding protocol. Blood in vomitus and/or stools may be due to corrosion, ulceration, irritation with capillary injury, substances that affect coagulation, and foreign bodies. **Hematemesis** may not be bright red blood, but is coffee brown because of the formation of acid hematin in acidic stomach. If the source of the bleeding is the stomach or above the upper ileum the blood may undergo transformation and present as a **black stool. Melena** refers to the passage of dark tarry stools. **Hematochexia** the passage of bright red blood. If the source is above the ileum and bleeding briskly or below the upper ileum the stools may be bright red.

   1. **GI bleeding** has been observed from anticoagulants, boric acid, cathartics, caustics/corrosives, ethanol, fluorides, foreign bodies, formaldehyde, heavy metal salts (arsenic, cadmium, chromates, iron, mercury, thallium), isopropanol, nonsteroidal antiinflammatory drugs (especially indomethacin, ibuprofen, phenylbutazone), oxalates, phenol, pine oil, plants (especially castor bean ricin, mushrooms, jequirity bean, pokeweed berries, wisteria), salicylates, and sympathomimetics (theophylline).

N. Colored material
1. **Gastric contents**
   a. **Blue-green.** Boric acid, copper salts, cyanide, iodine with starch, nickel salts.
   b. **Brown.** Iodine, blood as acid hematin.
   c. **Luminous.** Phosphorous.
   d. **Pink.** Ethchlorvynol.
   e. **Red.** Beets, blood, chocolate, Kool-Aid, gelatin (red Jello), mercurochrome, red licorice. May indicate gastric bleeding.
2. **Colored material in bowel movements**
   a. **Black.** Blood from substances that cause hematemesis, or blood in stool, charcoal, nontoxic bismuth salts, fruits (blackberries, huckleberries), iron salts, lead, magnesium dioxide, silver nitrate, spinach.
   b. **Blue.** Boric acid, methylene blue, iodine, and starch.
   c. **Clay.** Alcoholic etiology, barium.
   d. **Green.** Oral antibiotics, bismuth, clofazimine (leprosy medication), indomethacin (from biliverdin), iron, copper sulfate, may indicate bile.
   e. **White.** Aluminum hydroxide antacid.
   f. **Red.** Beets, blood, chocolate, clofazimine, Kool-Aid, gelatin (red Jello), mercurochrome, phenazopyridine, pyrinium pamaote (antihelminth), red licorice, rifampin, senna. May indicate lower intestinal bleeding (anticoagulants, heparin, nonsteroidal antiinflammatory drugs, salicylates).
   g. **Yellow.** Senna.

O. Radiopaque material in GI tract (222–228). **C**—Chlorides including chloral hydrate, carbon tetrachloride, chloroform. **H**—Heavy metals (arsenic, barium, iron, lead, mercury) and halogens. **I**—Iodides, iodine and iodinated substances and iron. **P**—Play-doh, Pepto-Bismol, occasionally phenothiazines. **E**—Enteric coated are not always radiopaque. **S**—Salts—barium, bismuth, calcium, potassium, phosphorous, sodium (salts in tablet form). Solvents of chlorinated hydrocarbons. **S**ome others—Acetazolamide (Diamox), foreign bodies, "body packers" and "body stuffers" (225). Cocaine, heroin, thiamine, some vitamins. **Strongly radiopaque substances are** calcium carbonate, ferrous sulfate, potassium chloride in tablet form. **Substances reported as having varying degrees of radiopacity are** acetazolamide, amitriptyline, antihistamines, chloral hydrate, ferrous gluconate, liothyronine, phenothiazines, phosphorous, sodium chloride, thiamine, tranylcypromine, trifluoperazine, trimeprazine, zinc sulfate and TCA have varying degrees of radiopacity. **A good predictor of radiopacity** is whether it is visible when radiographed through 15 cm or more of water, but placing a tablet directly on an x-ray plate often gives a false-positive radiopacity. **Paradichlorobenzene products are consistently radiopaque** whereas naphthalene products are radiolucent. A third alternative in toilet bowl deodorizers cetrimonitum bromide is also radiopaque (228).

P. GI ulcers (229–235). **Peptic ulcers may be primary or secondary. The mechanisms** that may produce peptic ulcers are increased acid or gastrin secretion (Zollinger-Ellison

syndrome), ischemia, inhibition of prostaglandin synthesis, decreased bicarbonate production (in cystic fibrosis patients), infections with *Heliobacter pylori*. Whether prophylaxis prevents bleeding from **stress ulcers** has been the subject of controversy. A met-
analysis results indicated there was strong evidence for the use of histamine$_2$-receptor
antagonists. Sucralfate may be as effective and is associated with lower pneumonia and
mortality (235).

    1.   The **substances associated with the development of peptic ulcers** are caustics and
corrosives, corticosteroids (controversial), ethanol (damages blood vessels), nonsteroidal antiinflammatory agents (indomethacin, naproxen, piroxicam, sulindac, tolmetin may produce silent perforation), drug-induced life-threatening illness (shock,
dehydration, burns, respiratory distress, renal failure and vasculitis), salicylates.

XIII. **Hepatic system** (236–243). The pharmacologic action of a medication in the body is shown in
Fig. 86-6. The hepatic drug metabolism is mostly by P-450 mixed oxidative function enzymes.
They occur in two phases. **Phase 1** formation of more water-soluble metabolites. Frequently
the metabolite is reactive electrophile. Hydroxylation is the most common reaction. **Phase II**
is conjugation. Glutathione (GSH) a nucleophile commonly detoxifies electrophils (Fig. 86-7).
The liver is affected in many poisonings. After oral ingestion, the most common route of poisoning, the liver is the first organ the toxin encounters after the GI tract. The liver is the major
detoxification unit and excretes many poisons through the bile. Interference with the **blood
supply** to the liver may also interfere with the detoxification of certain chemicals that utilize
the liver as the route of elimination. Chemicals that impair liver function are classified as
intrinsic, which is usually predictable and dose-related, **or idiosyncratic,** which are unpredictable may be associated with hypersensitivity or metabolic idiosyncrasy. The metabolic
enzymes are most concentrated in the centrolobular area of the liver.

    A. **Intrinsic hepatotoxins** are divided into direct and indirect acting toxins.

        1.   The **direct agents,** such as yellow phosphorous and carbon tetrachloride, do physico-
chemical damage to the hepatocyte.

    B. The **indirect hepatotoxins** created by intermediate toxic metabolite or metabolized by
the liver into toxic metabolites include acetaminophen, *Amanita phalloides* mushroom,
anabolic steroids, ethanol, heavy metals, hydrocarbons (halogenated), and methotrexate,
6-mercaptopurine, tetracycline, valproic acid interfere with the hepatocyte metabolic
pathway and secretory mechanisms, or cause hepatic vein thrombosis by pyrrolizidine.

```
DOSE ------------------> BLOOD CONCENTRATION ----------------> EFFECT

    Kinetics                                   Dynamics

    What body does to drug                     What drug does to body
```

Metabolism : by cytochrome C reductase, P450 (mixed function oxidase),
and hydrolyases

FIG. 86–6. Pharmacologic action of medication.

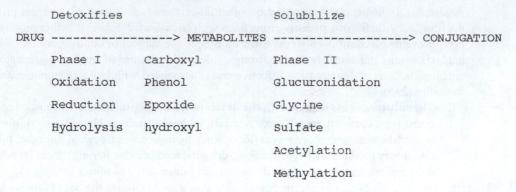

```
        Detoxifies                    Solubilize

DRUG ----------------> METABOLITES -------------------> CONJUGATION

        Phase I      Carboxyl          Phase II

        Oxidation    Phenol            Glucuronidation

        Reduction    Epoxide           Glycine

        Hydrolysis   hydroxyl          Sulfate

                                       Acetylation

                                       Methylation
```

FIG. 86-7. Phases of hepatic metabolism.

C. **Types of hepatic injury**
   1. **Cytotoxic** are the most common type producing injury to hepatocyte. The proto-types are acetaminophen (APAP), carbon tetrachloride.
   2. **Cholestatic** or interference with biliary secretion. Prototypes are erythromycin esto-late and chlorpromazine. It is rarely associated with industrial chemicals and cause elevation in the alkaline phosphatase, 5' nucleotase and gamma-glutamyltranspep-tidase.
   3. **Steatatic** or macrovesicular and microvesicular damage associated with progression fibrosis and cirrhosis. The prototype is chronic ethanol.
   4. **Carcinogenic.** The major carcinogenic lesion is **angiosarcomas of the liver** which may be caused by anabolic steroids, arsenic, copper sulfate used as Bordeau's solu-tion in spraying vineyards (Vine Sprayer's disease), Thiotrast a dye used to delin-eate the coronary vessels that is no longer used, and vinyl chloride plastic workers.
   5. **Idiosyncratic hepatic reactions** are divided into hypersensitivity reaction and metabolic idiosyncratic reactions.
        a. **Hypersensitivity** reactions caused halothane, *p*-aminosalicyclic acid, pheny-toin, and sulfonamides. These reactions are usually associated with systemic symptoms of rash, fever, and eosinophilia. They occur most frequently with phenytoin and are type IV Coombs-Gell immune reaction.
        b. **Idiosyncratic metabolic reactions.** Phenytoin is the prototype. An example is isoniazid, which may account for toxicity in certain susceptible patients by slow clearance or accelerated metabolism. **Idiosyncratic reactions are caused by** allopurinol, chlorpromazine, chlorpropamide, disulfiram, erythro-mycin estolate, halothane, isoniazid, methyldopa (alpha-), nitrofurantoin, phenylbutazone, phenytoin, propylthiouracil.
   6. **Dose-related liver toxicity** where the prototypes are ethanol and acetaminophen. It is generally secondary to electrophilic metabolites. Glutathione is hepatoprotective except in amatoxin which inhibits DNA dependent RNA polymerase. It is made worse by exposure to P-450 **enzyme inducers** including **the mnemonic of POP-PERS: P**—phenobarbital; **O**—organochlorine pesticides; **P**—polycyclic aromatic

hydrocarbons (PAH carcinogenic from fossil fuels and example benzopyrene); **E**—chronic ethanol; **R**—rifampin. **Examples** include acetaminophen metabolite's *N*-acetyl-*p*-benzoquinoneimine (NAPQI), halogenated hydrocarbons of which carbon tetrachloride is the most potent, amatoxins, ethanol, white phosphorous.

7. **Synergistic causes** of liver failure are alcohol and acetaminophen, trimethoprim sulfamethoxazole, rifampin and isoniazid, acetaminophen and isoniazid, amoxicillin and clavulanic acid. The **acetaminophen and alcohol syndrome** which causes extraordinary rises in aminotransferase levels has a case fatality rate of at least 20% and may be the most frequent single cause of acute liver failure in the United States (237,241,242).

8. **Substances that produce hepatic impairment** have been reported in the literature from many chemicals: acetaminophen, aflatoxin (mycotoxin from *Aspergillus flavus*); alcohols (ethanol); allopurinol, analgesics (acetaminophen, salicylates); anesthetics (chloroform, cyclopropane, halothane, methoxyflurane); antibiotics, chloramphenicol, erythromycin estolate (239), nitrofurantoin, sulfonamides (239), tetracycline (239) (i.v. during pregnancy); anticonvulsants (phenytoin, carbamazepine, valproate); antihypertensives (thiazides, chlorthalidone, methyldopa, hydralazine); antithyroid drugs (methimazole, propylthiouracil); antituberculosis drugs (ethionamide, isoniazid, *p*-aminosalicylic acid, pyrazinamide, rifampin); antineoplastic agents (6-mercaptopurine, methotrexate), aromatic hydrocarbons (benzene, toluene, xylene); boric acid; cancer chemotherapeutic agents (azathioprine, chlorambucil, methotrexate, 6-mercaptopurine); chloral hydrate, fluoxatine (240), halogenated hydrocarbons (carbon tetrachloride, trichloroethylene); hormones (androgens, corticosteroids, estrogens); heavy metals salts, (arsenic, antimony, chromates, copper, gold, iron, lead, thallium); herbicides (dinitrophenol, dinitrocresol); hypoglycemic agents (insulin, sulfonylureas); iodoform; MAOI; insecticides (chlorinated), mushrooms—cyclopeptides such as Amanita phalloides, verna, virsosa and Galerina species, and Lopiota species, and monomethylhydralazines, such as Gyromitra and Helvella species); naphthalene; nitrobenzene; 2-nitropropane; nonsteroidal antiinflammatory drugs (indomethacin, phenylbutazone); phenothiazines; pyrrolizidine alkaloids, (in PennyRoyal used as abortion agent); phosphorous (rat poisons); plants (akee, castor bean, fava beans, jequirity bean, Lantana); quinidine; solvents (halogenated hydrocarbons such as trichloroethylene); salicylates, tannic acid, and valproate.

9. **Acute liver impairment**

   (1) **Acetaminophen** (classic dose-dependent hepatotoxin), P-450 metabolized 5% into reactive electrophilic *N*-acetyl-*p*-benzoquinoneimine (NAPQI), which is detoxified by glutathione. It causes centrolobular necrosis.

   (2) **Aflatoxin.** A mycotoxin from *Aspergillus flavus*.

   (3) **Akee plant** (unripe) in Jamaica contains hypoglycin which causes Jamaican vomiting sickness and severe hypoglycemia and steatosis. Hypoglycin is an amino acid found in seed and unripe fruit of the fruit ackee.

   (4) **Amatoxin** is dose-dependent and inhibits DNA dependent RNA polymerase resulting in centrolobular necrosis of the liver.

(5) **Arsenic** produces dose-dependent hepatocellular necrosis and chronically angiosarcoma of the liver.

(6) **Carbon tetrachloride** is the classical dose-dependent hepatotoxin metabolized by the P-450 to free radicals, which are detoxified by glutathione (GSH).

(7) **Copper** in Wilson's hepatolenticular degeneration.

(8) **Halothane** and halogenated hydrocarbon anesthetics cause idiopathic hepatitis.

(9) **Halogenated** hydrocarbons such as carbon tetrachloride, chloroform, and trichloroethylene are dose-dependent hepatotoxic.

(10) **Hexachlorobenzene.** Thousands of Turkish Kurds ingested wheat treated with hexachlorobenzene and developed severe centrolobular necrosis, steatosis, and toxic porphyria.

(11) **Iron salts.**

(12) **Isoniazid** (idiosyncratic hepatitis that resembles viral hepatitis).

(13) **MAOI.**

(14) **Mushrooms** (cyclopeptides such as *Amanita phalloides,* verna, virsosa, Galerina species, Lopiota species, Gyromitra and Helvella species).

(15) **Pyrrolizidine alkaloids** produce damage to the small veins and cause hepatic veno-occlusive disease. Plant genera involved are Crotalaria, Heliotropium, and Senecio. Herbs that contain pyrrolizidine alkaloids and produce toxic hepatitis. Pyrrolizidine alkaloids are esters of the amino-alcohols. They can produce hepatic vaso-occlusive disease of the liver and death (239). They may mimic Reye's disease. They have been implicated in hepatic vaso-occlusive disease. Common names are "Comfrey" (Symphytum spp.) has been linked to liver damage, "Groundsel" (*Senecio longilobus*), "Skullcap" (*Sculltellaria laterifolia*).

(16) **Phosphorous, white or yellow.**

(17) **Solvents** (halogenated hydrocarbon).

(18) **Tetracycline** i.v. during pregnancy.

(19) **Valproate** cytotoxicity and steatosis. Valproate toxicity is unpredictable and non–dose-dependent. Usually occurs under 12 years of age in the first 4 to 6 months of therapy. Risk is 1 in 500 for children under 2 years and 1 in 12,000 for children over 2 years.

j. **Chronic liver impairment.** Chronic liver damage is associated with the following:

(1) **Androgens** (anabolic steroids) are threefold dose-dependent, cholestasis, and carcinogen-producing angiosarcoma of the liver.

(2) **Arsenic chronically.** Angiosarcoma of the liver.

(3) **Aflatoxin.** Same as in acute.

(4) **Beryllium.** Although the main target organs are the lung and the skin it can cause a granulomatous disease of the liver

(5) **Dimethylformamide.** The "universal solvent" can produce hepatocellular necrosis and steatosis.

    (6) **Ethanol** has acute and chronic syndromes. Chronic ethanol is a MBO inducer that causes steatosis (microvesicular)

    (7) **Erythromycin estolate.** Idiosyncratic hepatotoxin causing cholestasis.

    (8) **Isoniazid.** Dose-dependent hepatitis.

    (9) **Nitrofurantoin.**

    (10) **Phenothiazine (chlorpromazine).** Idiosyncratic reaction that produces cholestasis.

    (11) **Phenytoin.** Idiosyncratic reaction, usually hypersensitivity variety with fever, rash, and eosinophilia.

    (12) **Phenol**

    (13) **Phenylbutazone**

    (14) **Rifampin**

    (15) **Salicylates**

    (16) **Sulfonamides**

    (17) **Vinyl chloride** worker in the plastics industry. Angiosarcoma.

    (18) **Vitamin A**

  k. *Clinical and morphologic presentation*

    (1) **Hepatitis acute.** Alpha-methyldopa, isoniazid, phenytoin, nonsteroidal antiinflammatory agents, lovastatin.

    (2) **Cholestatis.** Androgens, oral contraceptives, erythromycin estolate, metronidazole, chlorpropamide, chlorpromazine, nitrofurantoin, rifampin. Increase in alkaline phosphatase and direct bilirubin.

    (3) **Hepatic necrosis.** Acetaminophen, arsenic, carbon tetrachloride, *Amanita phalloides,* disulfiram, ethanol, halothane, iron, isoniazid, methotrexate, methyldopa, phenytoin, procainamide, prophylthiouracil, propylthiouracil, tetracycline, yellow phosphorous.

    (4) **Chronic hepatitis.** Alpha-methyldopa, arsenic, isoniazid, halothane.

    (5) **Fatty change.** Corticosteroids, ethanol, valproate, tetracycline.

    (6) **Neoplasms.** Androgens, oral contraceptives, vinyl chloride.

  l. **Differentiating liver damage** from ethanol from acetaminophen. Ethanol rarely produces LST (SCOT) of more than 300 IU/L and the ALT (SGPT) is greater than the AST (Table 86–22).

  m. **Reye's and Reye's-like syndromes** (244)

    (1) Reye's syndrome is a condition usually occurring in children characterized by a viral syndrome (usually influenza B, or Varicella), vomiting, hepatic encephalopathy, coma and death. About 95% of patients had a history of salicylate ingestion but less than 0.1% of children having a viral illness and treated with aspirin develop Reye's syndrome. **The incidence** was 3.7 per 1 million children less than 17 year of age. The syndrome proceeds from persistent vomiting to encephalopathy by 24 to 48 h.

    (2) **Differential diagnosis of Reye's syndrome** includes the following:

      (a) **Inborn errors** of B-oxidation causing dicarboxylic aciduria (affected usually in neonatal period or early childhood); glutaric

TABLE 86-22. *Clinical features differentiating hepatotoxicity*

	Alcoholic with APAP hepatotoxic	Suicide ingestion of acetaminophen	Alcoholic hepatitis	Viral hepatitis
AST (SGOT) IU/L	Markedly increased, more than ALT	Normal initially, later may be markedly increased	Usually <300, AST 2–3 times greater than ALT	Hundreds to thousands
ALT (SGPT) IU/L	Increased but less than AST	Normal initially, later may be markedly increased	Normal or slight increase	Variable, less than AST
AST/ALT ratio	>2	<2	>2	>1
Prothrombin time	Increased to markedly increased	Normal initially, later may be increased	Increased, usually under 30 s	Increased
Acetaminophen	Normal or slight increase	Increased	Normal	Normal
Acute viral studies[a]	Negative (–)	Negative (–)	Negative (–)	±[b]

[a]Hepatitis B surface antigen, hepatitis B core IgM, hepatitis A IgM.
[b]May be negative with non-A non-B viral hepatitis.
APAP, acetaminophen; AST, aminotransferase (SGOT); ALT, alanine aminotransferase (SGPT).
Adapted from Kumar S, Rex DG. Failure of physicians to recognize acetaminophen hepatotoxicity in chronic alcoholics. *Arch Intern Med* 1991;151:1189–1181. Brent J, Rumack BH. Analgesic, anti-inflammatory, and anti-pyretic agent poisoning. In: Harwood-Nuss A, ed. *The clinical practice of emergency medicine.* Philadelphia: JB Lippincott Co, 1996:450–457.

aciduria type II or multiple acyl CoA dehydrogenase deficiency; systemic carnitine deficiency a rare variant of lipid storage myopathy or carnitine deficiency can be secondary to a variety of inborn errors of metabolism.

(b) **Jamaican vomiting sickness** is an acute intoxication caused by hypoglcin, an amino acid found in seed and unripe fruit of the fruit ackee.

(c) **Pantanoate toxicity.** Synthetic chemical. No cases of human toxicity reported.

(d) **Disorders of urea synthesis and tricarboxylic acid cycle deficiencies.**

(e) **Branched amino acid inborn errors of metabolism** and **valproate toxicity,** which is unpredictable and non–dose-dependent. Usually occurs in under 12 years of age in first 4 to 6 months of therapy. Risk is 1 in 500 for children under 2 years and 1 in 12,000 for children over 2 years.

(f) **Salicylate intoxication and other drugs with carboxylic acid functional group** such as ibuprofen, clofibrate, valproate (described above).

(g) **Other clinical presentations that mimic Reye's syndrome** such as viral hepatitis, viral encephalitis and meningitis, hepatotoxins such as amatoxin or carbon tetrachloride and isopropyl alcohol intoxication.

n.   Clinical syndromes caused by hepatotoxins (245–249)

(1)   Fever, rash, eosinophilia. Idiosyncratic hypersensitivity reaction chlorpromazine, phenylbutazone, anesthetics.

(2)   Acute hepatitis. Carbamazepine, colchine, dantrolene, halothane, iproniazid, isoniazid, indomethacin, papaverine, phenylbutazone, pyrazinamide, salicylates, sulfamethoxazole, sulfisoxazole, tranylcypromine.

(3)   Obstructive jaundice. Chlorpromazine, erythromycin estolate, estrogens, anabolic steroids, terfenadine, ceftriaxone.

(4)   Pseudomononucleosis. Phenytoin.

(5)   Serum sickness. *p*-Aminosalicylic acid, phenytoin, sulfonamides.

(6)   Autoimmune hemolysis. Methyldopa.

(7)   Myalgia, weakness, stiffness, increased CPK. Clofibrate.

(8)   Antinuclear antibodies. Procainamide.

(9)   Associated marrow injury. Anticonvulsants, gold propylthiouracil, chloramphenicol, phenylbutazone.

(10)   Associated pulmonary injury. Amiodarone, sulfonamides.

(11)   Associated renal injury. Gold salts, penicillamine, paraquat, methloxyflurane.

(12)   Fatty liver. Aflatoxin, emetine, ethanol, carbon tetrachloride, chloroform, corticosteroids, tetrachloroethane, trichloroethylene, valproate.

(13)   Fatty liver of pregnancy. Tetracycline.

(14)   Peliosis hepatitis. Anabolic steroids.

(15)   Adenoma and carcinoma. Oral contraceptives, androgens.

(16)   Angiosarcoma. Vinyl chloride monomer, copper sulfate, arsenic, androgens.

(17)   Centrolobular necrosis. Acetaminophen, beryllium, bromobenzene, carbon tetrachloride and other halogenated hydrocarbons, chloroform, furosemide, urethane.

o.   Hepatorenal syndrome. Hepatorenal syndrome is the failure of the liver and the kidneys. **Intoxications causes include** acetaminophen, carbon tetrachloride and other halogenated hydrocarbons (carbon tetrachloride, chloroform, trichloroethylene), glycols (ethylene glycols and others), heavy metals (arsenic antimony, bismuth, boron, cadmium, chromium, copper, gold, lead, lithium, mercury, platinum, thallium, uranium), mushrooms (cyclopeptides such as *Amanita phalloides, verna, virsosa,* Galerina species, Lopiota species, Gyromitra and Helvella species), phosphorous, and tetracycline i.v. during pregnancy.

p.   Pancreatitis (250–260). **Acute pancreatitis** is frequently associated with a number of medications, and **chronic pancreatitis** is associated with chronic alcoholism. In 1987, there were 180,000 hospitalizations in the United States for pancreatitis, with 2,251 deaths. Since the diagnosis usually rests on hyperamylasemia (85% sensitive), but is not specific, other causes of hyperamylasemia must be excluded. The other nonpancreatic causes of hyperamylasemia include marcoamylasemia, diabetic ketoacidosis, ectopic pregnancy, perforated duodenal ulcer, ischemic bowel, and small bowel obstruction. **The serum amylase**

may be normal in as many as 20% of patients with pancreatitis. An elevated serum lipase increases the diagnostic sensitivity to 95% when combined with the serum amylase.

(1) The **medical surgical causes of acute pancreatitis** are obstructive, due to or associated with diseases of the gall bladder or the pancreas itself; traumatic, either accidental or iatrogenic; metabolic associated with hypertriglyceridemia I, IV, V and hypercalcemia associated with hyperparathyroidism, inherited conditions; infection with parasites (*Schistosoma mansoni,* Echinococcus spp., viruses (including cytomegalic virus, Epstein-Barr, HIV, mumps, varicella-zoster), and bacteria; vascular due to ischemia, atherosclerotic emboli and vasculitis; miscellaneous conditions such as penetrating peptic ulcer, Crohn's disease, Reye's syndrome, and hypothermia. Ethanol is the major cause of pancreatitis in the United States, and this is the only common form of pancreatitis that leads to calcification, although the serum amylase rarely exceeds 1,000 IU/L (Table 86-23).

(2) **Pancreatitis has been reported** to be caused by more than 85 drugs (258). Ethanol is the most common toxin causing pancreatitis. These drugs include acetaminophen* intoxication (257), aminosalicyclic acid* (258), amoxapine, azathioprine* (3% to 5%), carbamazepine, cancer chemotherapy (cisplatin, cyclophosphamide, cyclosporine, L-asparaginase, methotrexate, 6-mercaptopurine* 3% to 5%), cimetidine*, cholinergics (spasm of sphincter of oddi), contraceptives (estrogens) (258), corticosteroids*, didanosine+ (23%) (258), diphenoxylate, diuretics (especially thiazides, ethacrynic acid, furosemide), erythromycin* (252,253,254,258), ethanol* (258), isoniazid*, lovastatin, manganese, metronidazole* (258), methanol* (258), methyldopa (258), mushroom (cyclopeptides), nitrofurantoin (258), nonsteroidal antiinflammatory drugs (especially sulindac) (258), opioids (spasm of the sphincter oddi), organophosphate (258), pentamidine+ (258), phenformin, procainamide, rifampin, ranitidine (258), salicylate (258), scorpion venom (258), sulindac, sulfonamides*, tetracycline*, thiazides (especially chlorthalidone), valproic acid+, vitamin D, zinc. An asterisk indicates more frequent cause, and a plus indicates the accumulation of toxic metabolite weeks to months after exposure.

TABLE 86-23. *Ranson's criteria*

On admission	Within 48 h of admission
Age, 55 years	About 6 L volume requirement
Blood glucose >200 mg/dL	BUN increase >5 mg/dL
LDH >350 IU/L	Pao_2 <60 mm Hg
SGOT (AST) >250 IU/L	Hct <10%
WBC >16,000	Serum calcium <8 mg/dL

<3 criteria, 1% mortality; 3–7 criteria, 15% mortality and 50% require ICU admission; >7 criteria, 50% mortality and almost all require ICU admission.
  Data from ref. 7.

XIV. **Renal system** (261–265)

    A. **Renal impairment and failure.** The kidneys are the major excretory organs and, therefore, are exposed directly to the effects of many toxins. As the salt and water is reabsorbed, any substance in the proximal tubular fluid concentrates to many times more than plasma concentration. Examples are **heavy metals** such as chromium and mercury that produce their damage in the proximal convoluted tubules. The **organic compounds** produce their damage in straight portion of the tubules. **Amphotericin B** is nephrotoxic in the loop of Henle. The distal convoluted tubule does not seem to be selectively damaged. In addition active renal secretion into tubular urine is accomplished by the initial accumulation of the substance in proximal renal tubular cells.

        1. The kidney function is also linked to extrarenal factors such as BP, blood volume, sympathetic nervous system, antidiuretic hormone, and the angiotensin-renin system. Any intoxicant producing hemodynamic changes that interfere with renal circulation can impair function, interfere with excretion, and damage the kidneys.

        2. The kidneys commonly suffer **three syndromes with poisoning: ATN** (aminoglycoside), **interstitial nephritis** (most cases are believed to be due to some type of hypersensitivity or toxin), and **postischemic renal failure** (hemodynamic vascular changes).

    B. **Nephrotoxic classification of renal impairment and failure**

        1. **Prerenal extracellular fluid** (ECF) **depletion:** dehydration, shock, hypoalbuminuria (malnutrition, hepatic disease, GI loss, nephrotic syndrome), renal vein thrombosis. In these circumstances, the renal tubules responding vigorously to conserve salt and water to restore ECF.

        2. **Renal**

            a. **ATN.** The commonest cause of renal failure has been reported from the following:

                (1) **Hypoperfusion and postischemia** by prolonged ECF depletion. Heavy metals damage acutely by shock, later by proximal convoluted tubular cells sloughing and obstructing, and vasomotor reaction.

                (2) **Pigments**

                    (a) **Hemoglobinuria** secondary to hemolysis, including aniline, arsine, benzene, cephalosporins, creosol, chlorates, copper, hydralazine, nitrites, nitrofurantoin, phenol, phenazopyridine, sulfonamides, triamterene.

                    (b) **Myoglobinuria** secondary to RDM is often noted in intoxications with amphetamines, cocaine, heroin abuse, phencyclidine, phenylpropanolamine, water hemlock.

                    (c) **Obstruction of tubules by casts** in ethylene and propylene glycol, primidone, sulfonamides intoxications.

                (3) **Drugs and chemicals** produce direct tubular injury by concentration in the tubular epithelium and combination with sulfhydryl groups of proteins resulting in loss of renal tubular function manifest as proteinuria, hematuria, glycosuria urinary casts, oliguria.

                    (a) **Antibiotics.** Amphotericin B, bacitracin, cephaloridine, colistin, gentamicin, kanamycin, neomycin, penicillin) bind to lysosomes and interfere with protein synthesis and cell membranes integrity.

      (b) **Anesthetics.**

      (c) **Diuretics.**

      (d) **Heavy metals.** Arsenic, antimony, bismuth, boron, cadmium, chromium, copper, gold, lead, lithium, mercury, platinum, thallium, uranium.

      (e) **Organic solvents and glycols (with or without hepatic necrosis).** Carbon tetrachloride, trichloroethylene), diethylene glycol, ethylene glycol, glycol ethers.

   (4) Contrast media. Direct cellular toxicity by osmolality or idiosyncrasy. Produces proximal tubular vacuolization, hypercellularity in glomerulus and interstitial hemorrhage.

 b. Acute glomerular injury. Immune complex deposition usually unrelated to nephrotoxins except for some exposure to hydrocarbon fuels, pesticides, and penicillamine.

   (1) Poststreptococcal, systemic lupus erythematosus, periarteritis, malignant hypertension but cases attributed to penicillins, thiazides, phenylbutazone, iodides, i.v. amphetamines.

   (2) Vascular occlusion. Thrombus, embolism, cortical necrosis. Nonsteroidal antiinflammatory agents cause prostaglandin synthesis inhibition, which decreases the renal plasma flow.

 c. Acute interstitial disease

   (1) Infectious pyelonephritis.

   (2) Allergic (usually antibiotics and antirheumatic drugs) thiazides, penicillins, sulfonamides, rifampin, allopurinol, methotrexate (7-OH metabolite).

 d. Postrenal is the obstruction of urine flow.

3. Substances that produce renal impairment. The **three most common nephrotoxins** are aminoglycoside, nonsteroidal antiinflammatory agents, and contrast media. **Renal damage has been reported in poisoning from** acetaminophen (usually reversible), acyclovir, allopurinol, aluminum, aminoglycoside, amphoteric B, antihypertensive agents (angiotensin converting enzyme inhibitors, beta-blockers, calcium channel blockers), anesthetics (Methoxyflurane), aniline, arsenic, ascorbic acid with oxalosis, barbiturates, bacitracin, barium salts (soluble), benzene, bismuth, boric acid, bromates, brown recluse spider, camphor, cancer chemotherapeutic agents (cytoxan, methotrexate), captopril, carbamazepine, cantharidin (Spanish Fly), carbon monoxide, castor bean, cephalosporins, chelating agents, chlorates, chlorinated hydrocarbons, chlordane, chromates, cimetidine, ciprofloxacin, clofibrate, colchicine, copper, clofibrate, cyclophosphamide, contrast media, copper salts, cresol, cyclosporin, deferoxamine, diethylene glycol, dimethyl sulfate, dinitrocresol, dinitrophenol, diphenhydramine, disodium edetate, disopyramide, diuretics (loop diuretics, thiazides), ethylene dichloride, ethylene glycol, gold, glycol ethers, halothane, heavy metal salts, hydralazine, iron salts, iodinated substances, radiocontrast media, isoniazid, isopropanol, labetalol, lead, lithium, marijuana, mannitol, meprobamate, mercurial salts, methanol, methotrexate, methylene chloride, methyl halogens and salicylate, mushrooms (cyclopeptides of Amanita species), myoglobinemia secondary to RDM, nabumetone, nizitidine, nonsteroidal anti-inflammatory agents, oxalates, opioids, paraquat (usually reversible), penicillins, penicillamine, pentamidine, phenol, phosphine, phosphorous, platinum, procainamide, providine-iodine, propylene, quinidine, radiation, ranitidine, rifampin, salicylates, sulfonamides, solvents of chlorinated hydrocarbon variety, thallium, trinitrotoluene, triamterene, trichloroethylene, turpentine, urethane, vitamin D, water hemlock plant, zinc salts.

C. Nephrotic syndrome has been reported with the following: allergens, amphotericin B, aminoglycoside, anticonvulsants, bismuth, captopril, dapsone, doxorubicin, gold, mercury, penicillin, penicillamine, probenecid, rifampin, trimethadione

D. RDM and myoglobinuria (266–274). RDM is a pathologic condition that resulting from the release of the skeletal muscle cell contents—potassium, myoglobin, aldolase, CK, etc.—into the plasma when the muscle is injured. RDM has over 150 causes. **Myoglobin** (MW 17,000 daltons) carries oxygen in the muscle and is filtered by the glomeruli and excreted in the urine. Myoglobinemia and myoglobinuria may occur with or without RDM. Myoglobin may precipitate in the renal tubules resulting in tubular necrosis, and renal failure.

1. Etiologic categories

   a. Toxin- and drug-induced intoxications

      (1) The mechanism and the most frequent of this category include those that produce seizures and muscle hyperactivity (amphetamines, cocaine, malignant hyperthermia, NMS, phencyclidine), hyperthermia (amphetamines, cocaine, malignant hyperthermia, NMS), direct cytotoxic effect on muscle cells (ethanol), or cause prolonged immobilization on a hard surface (CNS depressants, carbon monoxide, ethanol, heroin, sedative-hypnotics).

      (2) RDM/myoglobinuria have been reported with the following: allopurinol, amphetamines*, amphotericin B, amoxapine*, arsenic, barbiturates*, cocaine*, carbon monoxide*, chloral hydrate, clofibrate, codeine, colchicine, cyanide, cyclosporin, dextroamphetamine, diazepam, doxepin, ethchorvynol, ethanol*, ethylene glycol, erythromycin, fish poisoning, fluorouracil, fluoxetine, heroin, insect envenomation (including bee stings), isoniazid*, isopropyl alcohol, lindane, lithium, lovastatin, loxapine*, malignant hyperthermia, mercuric chloride, meperidine, mescaline, methamphetamine, methanol, methcathinone, molindone, MAOI, niacin, orphenadrine, paraquat, pentamidine, phenobarbital, phencyclidine, phenelzine, phenylbutazone, phenytoin, plants and mushrooms (A. phalloides mushroom, poison hemlock, water hemlock), NMS, phenothiazines, propoxyphene, quinidine, quinine, sedative-hypnotics*, 5-HT reuptake inhibitors (fluoxetine, paroxatine, sertraline), 5-HT syndrome, snake envenomation*, spider envenomation (black widow spider, brown recluse)*, terbutaline, toluene, triazolam, verapamil, vitamin A, zidovudine (AZT). glutethimide, heroin, hyperthermia, hypothermia, isopropyl alcohol, lithium, malignant hyperthermia, NMS, methadone, methanol, opioids, phencyclidine, phenylpropanolamine, plants (water hemlock), quinine, salicylates, spider bite* (black widow and brown recluse), snake envenomation*, strychnine, succinylcholine, tetanus, tetany, theophylline, toluene, TCA.

   b.   **Hypoxic** or impaired blood flow and oxygen delivery. From compression in crush injury and coma with pressure ischemia, vasculitis, thrombus or embolus, compartment syndrome, vasoconstriction in cocaine abusers, hypokalemia with severe potassium depletion (diuretics, chronic diarrhea, vomiting, massive black licorice ingestion, amphotericin B, and carbon monoxide poisoning).

   c.   **Direct injury to skeletal muscle.** Trauma, burns, infections (virus—influenza, Coxsackie, hepatitis; bacterial—tetanus, Legionnaire disease, and gram-negative sepsis), and trichinosis.

   d.   **Metabolic due to decreased energy storage or utilization.** Diabetic coma, hyponatremia, hypomagnesemia, hypophosphatemia of less than 1.0 mg/dL, thyroid storm or myxedema, disorders of lipid metabolism (carnitine deficiency, carnitine palmityl transferase deficiency, lovostatin or gemfibrozil with renal failure), cyclosporin, hypothermia.

   e.   **Intrinsic muscle injury** by trauma, polymyositis, dermatomyositis, muscular dystrophies, vigorous exercise, myophosporylase deficiency in McArdle's syndrome. **A syndrome** of muscle pain, weakness, brown urine was described by Meyer-Betz in 1910 and has been linked to strenuous activities as military basic training, weight lifting now known as **"exercise-induced RDM."** It has not been reported to be associated with renal failure (272).

   f.   **Increased energy consumption.** Seizures, delirium tremens, high-voltage shock, tetanus, malignant hyperthermia, heat stroke, drugs (amphetamines, cocaine, NMS, succinylcholine, causing hyperphosphatemia, hyperkalemia, hyperuricemia, metabolic acidosis, and hypocalcemia (268).

2.   **Manifestations of RDM.** The patients are often are agitated, delirious and acutely ill. Myalgia is present in 50%. General findings are muscle pain, cramps, muscle swelling, weakness, and loss of sensation. Sometimes loss of sensation of the overlying skin.

   a.   **Traumatic.** History of crush injury, discolored indurated area with decreased to absent muscle power, signs of volume depletion such as hypotension and tachycardia.

   b.   **Ischemic.** Severe muscle pain, pallor, cyanosis, coldness in affected extremity, agitated, combative behavior in cocaine toxicity.

   c.   **Alcoholic.** Muscle pain, muscle swelling and tenderness and weakness after heavy consumption of alcohol.

   d.   **Metabolic.** Proximal muscle weakness, hypokalemia or hypophosphatemia, history of recurrent muscle cramps, history of taking lovostatin or cyclosporin.

   e.   **Exertional.** Seizures or delirium tremens, stimulants use, hyperthermia, hyperthermia.

   f.   **Complications of muscle damage** are compartment syndrome (10% to 30%), disseminated intravascular coagulation syndrome (DIC), renal failure (33%), and metabolic abnormalities

3. **Laboratory findings**
    a. **Myoglobinuria** is suggested by a reddish brown or smoky urine, clear plasma (excludes hemoglobinuria), and oliguria if renal failure present. The color develops on standing or if in the bladder at acid pH for a period of time. The **urinalysis** in myoglobinuria has an acid pH of less than 5.5, protein positive, pigmented granular casts, renal epithelial cells, uric acid crystals, a positive 3+ or 4+ benzidine or orthotoluidine test (Hematest) but less than 10 red blood cells/HPF. Urine ferroprotein myoglobin of more than 100 mg/dL imparts a brown color. This is the simplest and most practical initial test. **Urine screening tests for myoglobin** may not be completely reliable because of the presence of hypochlorite, microbial peroxidase, ascorbic acid or other oxidizing contaminants. Serum testing is recommended for confirmation. A orthotoluidine dipstick is positive at 0.2 mg/L or 3.1 µmol/L hemoglobin or myoglobin. This is below the level of 3 RBC/HPF, which is considered normal. The method to identify myoglobin is by **radioimmunoassay** which is the most specific and most sensitive and detects myoglobin at a concentration of 0.5 ng/mL (the normal urine contains less than 5 ng/mL). However, this test is not immediately available. There are other immunoassay methods available but they are not as sensitive and specific. A negative ortho-toluidine test for blood (18%) with high CK values indicates that RDM can occur without myoglobinuria.
    b. **Myoglobinemia** in blood is usually below 80 µg/L in males and below 60 µg/L in females. The renal threshold for myoglobin is 2 mg/dL or 20 mg/L. Only the presence of high-concentration myoglobin of more than 1,000 ng/mL is associated with the development of acute renal failure.
    c. **Chemistries.** The creatinine increases faster than blood urea nitrogen (BUN) so the creatinine/BUN ratio is often less than 1:5. If serum creatinine was more than 5 mg/dL, 73% developed renal failure, compared to only 20% if it was less than 3 mg/dL. Other findings are early hyperkalemia (10% to 40% more than 5.5 mEq/L) indicates cellular potassium from injured skeletal muscle, decreased bicarbonate, metabolic acidosis with anion gap, hyperphosphatemia, hypocalcemia (63%) (excess phosphate in the circulation binds with calcium phosphate), hyperuricemia, hypoalbuminemia, and the bilirubin is increased.
    d. **Enzymes.** The **serum CK**/MM isoenzyme (skeletal muscle type) is elevated often over 10,000 IU. The myocardial band will be less than 5% of total CK. The aspartate aminotransferase (AST, formerly SGOT) is elevated.
E. **Hematuria** (275–278). **Microscopic hematuria** is defined as five or more red blood cells per high-power field. Hematuria may have its origin in the kidney, the urinary tract, the bladder or urethra. The gross renal hematuric urine may be grossly brown or red and microscopically show red blood cell casts and proteinuria. Hematuric urine from the upper tract damage may also be associated with edema and hypertension. Hematuric urine from the lower tract, the bladder and urethra is grossly bright red and microscopically shows no red blood cell casts. It is important to exclude organic pathology before attributing hematuria to a chemical intoxication. **Factious hematuria with alleged pain of renal colic is a favorite way for opioid dependent patients to obtain drugs.**

1. **Hematuria has been reported** from acetazolamide, aminoglycoside, anticoagulants, allopurinol, busulfan, chlorates, contraceptives (oral), cyclophosphamide (hemorrhagic cystitis), diphenhydramine, doxorubicin, furosemide, heavy metal salts (gold, lead, mercury), ibuprofen, indomethacin, isoniazid, lithium, methanol, methotrexate, methysergide, mitomycin, naphthalene, nitrofurantoin, nitrates, nonsteroidal antiinflammatory agents, penicillins (especially methicillin interstitial nephritis), phenol, penicillamine, rifampin, sulfonamides, triamterene, turpentine. vitamin D (Table 86-24).

F. **Urine colors** (279–285). Normally, the urine color ranges from colorless to deep amber, depending on the concentration of urochrome, an endogenously produced pigment. The amount of urochrome excreted over 24 h is constant, and the concentration depends on the osmolality. Dilute urine is almost colorless, and concentrated is deep yellow to amber. Dyes from crayons may show up in the urine.

   1. **White or cloudy urine.** See crystalluria. **Cloudy urine may be associated with** bacteria, chyluria, crystals, lipuria (carbon monoxide intoxication, severe diabetes mellitus, nephrotic syndrome), phosphates, primidone intoxication, pyuria and urates. **Phosphates** clouds are very common (alkaline urine clouds disappear at pH of less than 7) and of no clinical importance. **Urate** are often exogenous from foods (liver, sweetbread), or endogenous from tissue nuclei destruction (leukemia, gout, normal newborns). The presence of urate does not mean excessive uric acid.

   2. **Red/pink urine.** Ampicillin, aminosalicylic acid (on contact with hypochlorite bleach on some toilet papers), aniline, anthocyanin (beets, some body powders (Soothe and Cool), blackberries, food coloring), deferoxamine, hematuria, ibuprofen, Kool-Aid, Jello, lead (chronic), lycopene (tomatoes and watermelon), mercury, myoglobinuria, naphthalene, phenacetin, phenolphthalein (purplish color to alkaline urine), phenazopyridine, phenytoin, porphyrins, pyridium, quinine, rifampin. *Serratia spp.* UTI gives a red urine.

TABLE 86-24. *Condition and possible substance causing hematuria*

Condition	Possible substances
Pseudohematuria	Phenytoin, ibuprofen, levodopa, nitrofurantoin, rifampin, quinine
Glomerulonephritis	Mercury and gold salts, penicillamine, heroin, probenecid, antivenin
Vasculitis	Allopurinol, colchicine, diphenhydramine, furosemide, hydantoins, isoniazid, penicillins
Loin-pain syndrome	Oral contraceptives
Thrombotic	Chemotherapeutic agents, cocaine microangiopathy
Acute interstitial nephritis	Penicillins, rifampin, ibuprofen, sulfonamides, phenidione, phenytoin
Chronic interstitial	
c. papillary necrosis	Analgesics, alcohol
s. papillary necrosis	Lithium
Intrarenal obstruction	Methotrexate, sulfonamide
Extrarenal obstruction	Methysergide
Nephrolithiasis	Triamterene, vitamin D, acetazolamide
Urinary tract carcinoma	Analgesic abuse
Interstitial cystitis	Cyclophosphamide, mitotane, penicillins, busulfan
Hematuria without urinary tract lesion	Anticoagulants
Hematuria site	Nonsteroidal antiinflammatory disease

3. **Red/orange urine.** Anthraquinone (alkaline) laxatives on standing. Anthocyanin (foods—beets [beta-cyanine beet pigment], blackberries), blood, candy dyes, cascara (alkaline), Azo-Gantrisin, bilirubin, canthanthines, congo red (alkaline urine), deferoxamine with iron intoxication, daunorubicin, dehydration, doxorubicin, fava beans, fluorescein, heavy metals, hematuria etiology, hemoglobinuria, indandiones, iron, lead, mercury, myoglobinuria, methyldopa, naphthalene, paprika, *p*-aminosalicylic acid on contact with hypochlorite bleach on toilet paper, phenytoin, phenazopyrine (acid urine), phenolphthalein (alkaline urine), phenothiazines, porphyrins, pyridium, quinacrine, riboflavin, red Kool Aid, rifampin, santonin, senna, sulfasalazine, urate (especially in newborns), vegetable dyes, vitamins (multivitamins, riboflavin, thiamine).

4. **Brown-black urine.** Aloe (seaweed), alcaptonuria (due to homogentisic acid turns brown on standing), bile or blood pigments (from old blood), benzene, cascara, bilirubin, chloroquine, creosol, dinitrophenol, furazolidone, hemoglobin pigments (acid hematin) from hemolysis, lead, L-dopa with hypochlorite in toilet, melanin, mercury, methemoglobinemia, methocarbamol, metronidazole, methyldopa with hypochlorite in toilet, methyldopa, metronidazole, naphthalene, nitrites, nitrofurantoin, phenacetin, phenazopyridium, phenols, phenothiazine, phenytoin, primaquine, porphyria, providine iodine, quinine, rhubarb, senna, sulfonamides, tyrosinosis.

5. **Blue/green urine.** Amitriptyline, anthraquinone, azuresin, biliverdin, boric acid, blue dyes, chlorophyll or Chlorets, indomethacin, iron, salts, methocarbamol, methylene blue, indigo blue, phenols, phenolphthalein (acid urine), Pseudomonas infection, resorcinol, triamterene.

6. **Diaper fluorescence.** Fluorescence of a porphyrin-soaked diaper under Wood's light occurs with congenital erythropoietic porphyria (Gunther disease) (284,285).

G. **Urinary odors** (286–294). See body and breath odors. The urine odors are as follows: ammonia odor is derived from the decomposition of urea after the urine is secreted; disagreeable mercaptan odor after asparagus has been eaten, fecal odor intestinal perforation, fruity odor of ketones, odor of violets after turpentine ingestion.

1. **Acetone.** Acetone, chloroform, isopropanol, metabolic ketoacidosis (methanol, salicylate, ethanol, ethylene glycol, isoniazid, iron) lacquer, phenol, salicylates.

2. **Ammonia.** Ammonia or uremia.

3. **Bleach (hypochlorite).** Hypochlorite.

4. **Carrots.** Cicutoxin of water hemlock.

5. **Disinfectants.** Creosote, phenol.

6. **Fish.** Zinc phosphide, tyrosinemia, trimethylaminuria (inborn errors of metabolism), hepatic failure, hypermethioninemia.

7. **Formaldehyde.** Formaldehyde, methanol.

8. **Foul or fetid.** Infection.

9. **Fruity.** Chloral hydrate, paraldehyde, acetone, and ketones.

10. **Garlic.** Arsine, arsenic, dimethylsulfoxide (DMSO), malathion, parathion, yellow phosphorous, phosphine, selenium, tellurium, thallium, zinc phosphide.

11. **Maple sugar.** Maple sugar urine disease.

12. **Mothballs.** Camphor, naphthalene, paradichlorobenzene.

13. **Musty.** Phenylketonuria.
14. **Pears.** Chloral hydrate, paraldehyde.
15. **Pine oil.** Pine oil.
16. **Rotten eggs.** Disulfiram, hydrogen sulfide, hepatic failure, mercaptans, *N*-acetyl-cysteine, sewer gas.
17. **"Sweaty feet."** Isovaleric aciduria
18. **Tobacco.** Nicotine (cotinine).
19. **Violets.** Turpentine.

H. **Crystalluria** (295). **Massive ingestion of the following drugs may cause crystalluria:** amoxicillin, cephalexin, methotrexate, primidone, and sulfonamides have been reported to produce crystalluria. Antihistamines, aspirin, phenacetin, sulfonamides can all produce subclinical crystalluria at therapeutic doses.

XV. **Genitourinary tract** (296,297)

A. **Urinary bladder.** The bladder mucosa is exposed to the local action of excreted toxins which may produce irritation, ulceration and hemorrhagic cystitis. **Neoplasms of the bladder** have been implicated from exposure to aniline, benzidine, beta-naphthylamine, cobalt, and paraffin.

   1. **Dysuria. Painful micturition** has been observed from anticholinergic agents, arsenic cantharidin (Spanish Fly), bubble bath detergents, chlorates, colchicine, chromates, cyclophosphamide (hemorrhagic cystitis), doxorubicin, mercuric chloride, methenamine, methylene blue, naphthalene, beta-naphthylamine, phenol, phenolphthalein, radiation, saponin, toluidine, and turpentine.

   2. **Urinary retention.** Urinary retention is defined as a volume of urine retained greater than expected bladder capacity (age in years + 2 = capacity in oz) in a patient who is unable to voluntarily empty the bladder. The bladder has the **capacity in an adult** of 350 to 450 mL. Micturition is carried out by activation of the parasympathetic system at sacral nerves S-2 to S-4, from which stimulatory impulses are sent to the detrusor muscle and inhibitory impulses to the sympathetic alpha-adrenergic neurons of the internal sphincter and trigone resulting in contraction of the bladder wall and relaxation of the sphincters. The external sphincter is under voluntary control through the pudendal nerve. **Parasympatholytic (sympathetic) drugs and ganglion blockade** can cause urinary retention. Urinary retention must be **differentiated from dehydration** by clinical evaluation, urine specific gravity and by a fluid challenge. **Comatose patients** from almost any cause may have urinary retention.

      a. The **medical and urologic causes of acute urinary retention** are divided into urinary tract obstructions (constipation, polyps, congenital, dysuria, neuromuscular disorders including neurogenic bladder and medications, trauma, postoperatively, hypermagnesemia, and psychogenic).

      b. The **following substances have been noted to cause urinary retention:** alpha-adrenergic simulators (amphetamines unopposed alpha stimulation at internal sphincter), antiasthma drugs (disrupt internal sphincter relaxation), anticholinergic agents (inhibit bladder contraction), antihistamines, antiparkinson agents, antispasmodic agents, beta-blockers (propranolol), calcium channel blockers (nifedipine decrease bladder contractility), disopyramide, ephedrine, guanethidine, isoniazid, L-dopa, lindane, magnesium excess, opioids, phenothiazines, TCA.

3. **Incontinence** (298). Incontinence may be due to abnormalities in bladder or urethral function, decreased compliance or increases in pressure, disturbances in reflex control, or overflow incontinence. The etiology of the potential causes can be remembered by the mnemonic of **DIAPERS: D**—delirium; **I**—urinary infection; **A**—atrophic urethritis; **P**—pharmaceuticals (sedative-hypnotics, loop diuretics, anticholinergics, adrenergic blockers and calcium channel blockers); **P**—psychologic; **E**—endocrine imbalances such as hypoglycemia or hypercalcemia; **R**—restricted mobility; **S**—stool impaction.

XVI. **Other toxicologic manifestations**

A. **Gynecomastia and galactorrhea** (299–302). Breast enlargement may be a physiologic phenomena in newborns, adolescent boys (30%), and elderly men.

1. The **mechanisms** may be an increase in free estrogens, decrease in endogenous free androgens, androgen receptor defects, and enhanced breast tissue sensitivity. It may be the result of estrogen-secreting tumors, or increased availability of estrogen precursors such in cirrhosis, relative changes in the estrogen/androgen ratios, testicular failure or drugs. The drugs may mimic estrogen action (digitalis), inhibit androgen action (cimetidine or spirolactone), or increase estrogen synthesis (chorionic gonadotropin).

2. **Gynecomastia has been reported to result** from street drugs (alcohol, i.e., ethanol*, androgens, marijuana, opioids); cancer chemotherapeutic agents; hormones and related drugs (androgens, bromocriptine, estrogens, oral hormonal contraceptives); and prescription drugs, including amiodarone, amphetamines, amitriptyline, bromocriptine*, cancer chemotherapeutic drugs* (alkylating agents, vincristine, busulfan), captopril, chlordiazepoxide, chlorpromazine, cimetidine*, clomiphene, cyproterone, diazepam, diethylpropion, digitalis, diltiazem, fluphenazine, gold, haloperidol, hormones* and related drugs (androgens and anabolic steroids, chorionic gonadotropin, estrogens and estrogen agonists, methyltestosterone, oral contraceptives), imipramine, isoniazid, itraconazole, ketoconazole, lovastatin, loxapine, marijuana, meprobamate, mesoridazine, methyldopa*, metoclopramide, metronidazole, molindone, nifedipine*, omeprazole, opioids (codeine, heroin, morphine), perphenazine, phenytoin, phenothiazines*, penicillamine, ranitidine*, reserpine, spirolactone, thioridazine, thiothixene, thioxanthenes, TCA, trifluoperazine

B. **Galactorrhea.** The cause of galactorrhea may include **prolactin secreting tumors** of the pituitary (prolactinoma, chromophobe adenoma, empty sellar syndrome) or ectopic bronchogenic carcinoma; **hypothalamic disorders** including inflammation (encephalitis), tumors (craniopharyngioma), infiltrative diseases (sarcoidosis), pituitary stalk trauma; **endocrinologic causes** such as hypothyroidism, "postpill" syndrome; **DA inhibition** by medications such as benzamides, butyrophenones, phenothiazines, reserpine and methyldopa; **PC; psychogenic; neurogenic** such as chest wall disease from herpes zoster, trauma, and lung tumors.

C. **Priapism** (303–307). Priapism is a painful, persistent, and abnormal penile erection, involving the corpus cavernosa but not corpus spongiosum or glans penis. It is due to the failure of the arteries and sinusoids to constrict and allow for detumescence. The erection is not accompanied by sexual desire or excitement.

1. **Priapism has been reported from** antidepressants (trazodone), antipsychotic drugs (chlorpromazine), antihypertensive (prazosin), anticoagulants (heparin), black widow spider bites, chlorpromazine, cocaine (304), corticosteroids, ethanol, doxazosin, fluphenazine, haloperidol, heparin, loxapine, metaclopramide, marijuana (low doses), neuroleptics, papaverine (307), phenytoin, prazosin, psychedelic "street" drugs, scorpion stings (305), sedative-hypnotics (methaqualone), sulfonylureas (tolbutamide), tamoxifen, terazosin, testosterone, thioridazine, trazodone.

2. Pharmacologic induction has been reported with papaverine, phentolamine, and yohimbine.

3. Medically, it is seen in males with sickle cell disease, with amyloidosis, and after dialysis.

D. **Impotence** (308). There are many medical causes of impotence, with diabetes mellitus a frequent cause. Alcohol* has been associated with 8% rate of impotence in young males, anticonvulsants (reduction in testosterone by enzyme induction), antidepressants, beta-adrenergic blockers. * cimetidine (antiandrogenic effect), clofibrate, *clonidine, cocaine (sometimes difficulty in erection), *digoxin (estrogen-like activity), diuretics (thiazides), guanethidine (24% impotence), marijuana (large doses only), methyldopa, MAOI, *opioids, nitrates and nitrites, *phenothiazines, *progesterone, *reserpine, *sedative-hypnotics, spirolactone.

E. **Splenomegaly** (309). The cause of enlarged spleen in an asymptomatic patient is usually hematopoietic, but the differential includes disorders of the portal system, infectious and inflammatory diseases. An enormous spleen suggests a myeloproliferative disorder or a tropical disease, a palpable spleen in a black patient suggests sickle cell variant such as thalassemia or sickle cell C disease. Ask about family members with anemia, jaundice and enlargement of the spleen (spherocytosis) and about foreign travel (malaria). **Laboratory tests** include a smear for spherocytes, tear shaped cells and hairy cells, leukemic cells, malaria, and giant platelets. Biochemical profile should include bilirubin, lactate, liver function, heterophile (Infectious mono), hemoglobin electrophoresis for hemoglobinopathies, immunologic analysis, Coomb's test, serum protein electrophoresis for IgM, tests for antinuclear antibodies and rheumatoid factor, bone marrow aspiration, technician imaging of the liver and spleen. **Hematologic disorders** include hereditary spherocytosis, acquired autoimmune hemolytic anemia, pyruvate kinase deficiency, hemoglobinopathies, myeloproliferative diseases, lymphoproliferative disorders (non-Hodgkin's lymphoma, chronic leukemia), and macroglobulinemia. **Portal system disorders** include hypersplenism associated with obstruction thrombosis, stenosis, atresia, congestive splenomegaly (Banti's syndrome portal hypertension associated with hepatic cirrhosis). **Infections** include infectious mononucleosis, bacterial endocarditis, malaria, schistosomiasis, leishmaniasis, brucellosis, and HIV. **Inflammatory disorders** include rheumatoid arthritis with pancytopenia (Felty's syndrome), systemic lupus erythematosus, sarcoidosis, and amyloidosis. **Miscellaneous disorders** include Gaucher's disease, cysts, and reticulendotheliosis.

References

1. Cone TE. Diagnosis and treatment: some diseases, syndromes and conditions associated with an unusual odor. *Pediatrics* 1968;41:993–995.
2. Mace JW, et al. The child with an unusual odor. *Clin Pediatr* 1976;15:57–62.
3. Shelley ED, et al. The fish odor syndrome. *JAMA* 1984;251:253–256.
4. Schiffman SS. Taste and smell. *N Engl J Med* 1983;308:1275–1279,1337–1342.
5. Goldfrank L, et al. Teaching the recognition of odors. *Ann Emerg Med* 1982;11:684–666.
6. Getchell TV, Bartoshuk LM, Doty L, Snow JB. *Smell and taste in health and disease*. New York: Raven Press, 1991.
7. Richman RA, Post EM, Sheehen PR, et al. Olfactory performance during childhood: development of an odorant identification test for children. *J Pediatr* 1992;121:911.
8. Woodward GA, Baldasso RN. Diphenhydramine toxicity in a five-year-old with varicella. *Pediatr Emerg Care* 1990;5:59–61.
9. Filloux F. Toxic encephalopathy caused by the topical application of diphenhydramine. *J Pediatr* 1986;25:163.
10. Davies JE, Dedbia H, Morgade C, et al. Lindane poisonings. *Arch Dermatol* 1983;119:142–144.
11. Rauch AF, Kowalsky SF, Lesar TS, et al. Lindane (Kwell)–induced aplastic anemia. *Arch Intern Med* 1990;150:2393–2395.
12. Garrettson LK. Acute poisoning from the use of isopropyl alcohol in tepid sponging. *JAMA* 1953;152:317.
13. Rubinstein AD, Musher DM. Epidemic boric acid poisoning simulating staphylococcal toxic epidermolysis in a newborn Ritter's disease. *J Pediatr* 1970;77:884.
14. Halling H. Suspected link between exposure to hexachlorophene and malformed infants. *Ann NY Acad Med* 1979;320:426–435.
15. Lockhart JD. How toxic is hexachlorophene. *Pediatrics* 1972;50:229–235.
16. Robson AM, Kissane JM, Elvick NH, et al. Pentachlorophenol poisoning in a nursery for newborn infants. I. Clinical features and treatment. *J Pediatr* 1969;75:309–316.
17. Armstrong RW, Eichner ER, Klein DE, et al. Pentochlorophenol poisoning in a nursery for newborn infants. II. Epidemiology and toxicologic studies. *J Pediatr* 1969;75:317–325.
18. Wysocki D, Flynt J, Golfield M, et al. Epidemic neonatal hyperbilirubinemia and the use of phenol disinfectant detergent. *Pediatrics* 1987;61:165–170.
19. Kearney T, et al. Chemically induced methemoglobinemia from aniline poisoning. *West J Med* 1984;140:282–286.
20. Gryboski J, Weinstein D, Ordway NK. Toxic encephalopathy apparently related to the use of an insect repellant. *N Engl J Med* 1961;264:289–291.
21. Zadikoff CM. Toxic encephalopathy associated with the use of insect repellant. *J Pediatr* 1979;95:140–142.
22. Hall AH, Hogan DJ. *Case studies in environmental exposures. Skin lesions and environmental exposures; rash decisions*. USDHSS, USPYHS, ATSDR. May 1993.
23. Adams RM. *Occupational skin disease*. 2nd ed. Philadelphia: WB Saunders, 1990.
24. Suskind RR. Environment and the skin. *Med Clin North Am* 1990;74:307–324.
25. AMA. The health effects of "Agent Orange" and polychlorinated dioxin contaminants: an update. Presented at the AMA Conference, Chicago, 1984.
26. Roujeaue JC, Stern RS. Severe adverse cutaneous reaction to drugs. *N Engl J Med* 1994;331:1272–1285.
27. Fine J-D. Management of acquired bullous skin diseases. *N Engl J Med* 1995;333:1475–1484.
28. Metzker A, Merlob P. Suction purpura. *Arch Dermatol* 1992;128:822–824.
29. Koechle MK, Hutton KP, Muller SA. Angiotensin converting enzyme inhibitor–induced pemphigus: three case reports and literature review. *Mayo Clin Proc* 1994;69:1166–1171.
30. Modly CE, et al. Evaluation of alopecia; a new algorithm. *Cutis* 1989;43:148–152.
31. Helk TN. Evaluation of alopecia. *JAMA* 1995;273:897–898.
32. Atton AV, Tunnessen WW. Alopecia in children: the most common causes. *Pediatr Rev* 1990;12:29.
33. Bergfeld WF, Helm ZTZN. Hair loss getting to the root of the problem. *Consultant* 1994;34:1390–1400.
34. Stratton MA. Drug-induced systemic lupus erythematosus *Clin Pharm* 1985;4:657–663.
35. Von Otteningen WF. *Poisoning*. Berlin: Germany: Paul V. Hoeber, 1952.
36. Dunn C, Held JL, Spitz J, et al. Coma blisters: a report and review. *Cutis* 1990;45:425–426.
37. Beveridge GW, Lawson AAH. Occurrence of bullous lesions in acute barbiturate intoxication. *BMJ* 1965;1:835–837.
38. Aldrich LB, Mottari AR, Vinik AJ. Distinguishing features of idiopathic flushing and the carcinoid syndrome. *Arch Intern Med* 1988;148:2614–2618.
39. Wallace MR, Mascola JR, Oldfield EC III. Red man syndrome incidence, etiology and prophylaxis. *J Infect Dis* 1991:164:1180–1185.
40. Sallit IE. Pseudo-red-man syndrome. *N Engl J Med* 1993;328:584–585.
41. Wilson EF. Estimation of the age of cutaneous contusions in child abuse. *Pediatrics* 1977;69:750–752.

42. Zanolli MD, McAlvany J, Krowchuk DP. Phenolphthalein-induced fixed drug eruption: a cutaneous complication of laxative use. *Pediatrics* 1993;91;119–1200.
43. Greaves MW. Chronic urticaria. *N Engl J Med* 1995;332:1767–1771.
44. Daniel CR, Sherr RK. Nail changes by systemic drugs or ingestants. *J Am Acad Dermatol* 1984;10:250.
45. Gaber CW, Lapkin RA. Metoprolol and alopecia. *Cutis* 1981:28:833–634.
46. Requena L. Chemotherapy-induced transverse ridging of the nails. *Cutis* 1991;68:129.
47. Kromann NP, Villhelmsen R, Stahl D. The dapsone syndrome. *Arch Dermatol* 1982;118:531–532.
48. Graber CW, Lapkin RA. Metoprolol and alopecia. *Cutis* 1981;28:633–634.
49. Ferguson MM, Simpson NB, Hammersley N. Severe nail dystrophy associated with retinoid therapy. *Lancet* 1983;2:974.
50. Daniel CR, Sherr RK. Nail changes caused by system drugs or ingestants. *J Am Acad Dermatol* 1984;10:250–258.
51. Kantor GR. Evaluation and treatment of generalized pruritus. *Cleve Clin J Med* 1990;6:52.
52. Kantor GR. Generalized pruritus: how do you manage it? *Emerg Med* 1993;25:19–26.
53. Clinical case solving: when you only live twice. *N Engl J Med* 1995;332:1221–1225.
54. Welens HJJ, Lemery RT, Smeets H, et al. Sudden arrhythmic death without overt heart disease. *Circulation* 1992;85:192–197.
55. Stratman HG, Kennedy HL. Torsades de pointes associated with drugs and toxins. Recognition and management. *Am Heart J* 1987;113:1470–1482.
56. Tzivoni D, et al. Magnesium therapy for Torsades de pointes. *Circulation* 1988;77:392.
57. Piccone A, et al. Magnesium infusion in treatment of Torsades de pointes. *Am Heart J* 1986;112:847.
58. Dec GW, Fuster V. Idiopathic dilated myocardiopathy. *N Engl J Med* 1994;1576:1564–1575.
59. Olsen KR, Pentel PR, Kelley MT. Physical assessment and differential diagnosis of the poisoned patient. *Med Toxicol* 1987;2:56–58,70–73.
60. Benowitz NL, Goldschalger N. Cardiac disturbances in the toxicologic patient. In: Haddad LM, Winchester FJ, eds. *Clinical management of poisoning and drug overdose*. Philadelphia: WB Saunders, 1983:65.
61. Levin RJ. Cardiac principles. In: Goldfrank LK, ed. *Emergency toxicology*. Norwalk, CT: Appleton-Century-Crofts, 1985:86.
62. Balazs T, Hanig JP, Herman EH. Toxic responses of the cardiovascular system. In: *Toxicology: the basic science of poison*. New York: Macmillan, 1985:367.
63. Mofenson HC, Carricco TR, Shauben J. Poisoning by antidysrhythmic drugs. *Pediatr Clin North Am* 1986;33:723.
64. von Oettingen WF. *Poisoning*. Germany: Paul B. Hoeber, 1952.
65. Rubin RB, Neugarten J. Cocaine-induced rhabdomyolysis masquerading as myocardial ischemia. *Am J Med* 1989;86:551–553.
66. Schnieder SM. Non-myocardial infarction chest pain: differential diagnosis, clinical clues and initial emergency management. *Emerg Med Rep* 1995:16:246–254.
67. Hollander JE, Hoffman RS. Cocaine-induced myocardial infarction: an analysis and review of the literature. *J Emerg Med* 1992;10:169–177.
68. Hollander JE, et al. Predictors of coronary artery disease in patients with cocaine associated myocardial infarction [Abstract 122]. *Clin Toxicol* 1995;33:532.
69. Hollander JE, et al. Cocaine-associated myocardial infarction: mortality and complications. *Arch Intern Med* 1995;155:1081–1086.
70. Eisler T, Hall RP, Kalavar KA, et al. Erythromelalgia-like eruption in parkinsonism patients treated with bromocriptine. *Neurology* 1981;31:1368–1370.
71. Olsen KR, Pentel P, Kelly MT. Physical assessment and differential diagnosis of the poisoned patient. *Med Toxicol* 1987;2:52.
72. Bernstein IL. Occupational asthma: coming of age. *Ann Intern Med* 1982;97:125–127.
73. Occupational disease surveillance: occupational asthma. *MMWR* 1990;39:116–123.
74. Glauser FL, Smith WR, Caldwell A, et al. Ethchlorvynol (Placidyl)–induced pulmonary edema. *Ann Intern Med* 1976;84:46–48.
75. Heffner JE, Sahn SA. Salicylate-induced pulmonary edema. *Ann Intern Med* 1981;95:405–409.
76. Rubsbenstein JL, Kaufman DM. A clinical study of an epidemic of heroin intoxication and heroin-induced pulmonary edema. *Am J Med* 1971;51:704–714.
77. Ashbaugh DG, Bielow DB, Petty TL. Acute respiratory distress in adults. *Lancet* 1967;2:319–323.
78. Horbar JD, Soll R, Sutherland JM, et al. A multicenter randomized placebo-controlled trial of surfactant in the development and treatment of adult respiratory distress syndrome. *N Engl J Med* 1989;320:959–965.
79. Menzel DB, McCellan RO. Response of the respiratory system. In: Doull J, et al., eds. *Toxicology: the basic science of poisons*. New York: Macmillan, 1987, pp. 1–200.
80. Da Silva AMT. Principle of respiratory therapy. In: Haddad LM, Winchester JF, eds. *Clinical management of poisoning and drug overdoses*. Philadelphia: WB Saunders, 138, 1996.

81. Olsen KR, Pantel PR, Kelley MT. Physical assessment and differential diagnosis of the poisoned patient. *Med Toxicol* 1987;2:52–81.

82. Garay SM. Pulmonary principles. In: Goldfrank LK, ed. *Toxicologic emergencies.* Norwalk, CT: Appleton-Century-Crofts, 1985:80.

83. von Oettingen WF. *Poisoning.* Germany: Paul B. Hoeber, 1952.

84. Done AK. Signs, symptoms and sources. *Emerg Med* 1982;Jan:42–77.

85. Arena JM, Drew RH. *Poisoning: toxicology, symptoms and treatment.* Springfield, IL: Charles C. Thomas Publisher, 1986.

86. Urizar RE, Goldrick MD, Cerda J. Pulmonary-renal syndrome. *NYS J Med* 1991;91:212–221.

87. Cooper JAD, ed. Drug-induced pulmonary disease. *Clin Chest Med* 1990;11:1–194.

88. Witorsch P. Drug-induced bronchopulmonary disorders. *Drug Ther* 1991;16:27–38.

89. Tomarken JL, Britt BA. Malignant hyperthermia. *Ann Emerg Med* 1987;16:1253.

90. Lorin MI. *The febrile child—clinical management of fever and other types of pyrexia.* New York: John Wiley and Sons, 1982.

91. Guze BH, Baxter LR. Neuroleptic malignant syndrome. *N Engl J Med* 1985;313:163.

92. Vassallo SC, Delaney KA. Pharmacologic effects of thermoregulation mechanisms of drug-related hyperthermia. *Clin Toxicol* 1990;27:199–224.

93. Rosenberg MR. Neuroleptic malignant syndrome: review of therapy. *Arch Intern Med* 1989;149:1927–1931.

94. Stine RT. Accidental hypothermia. *JACEP* 1977;59:364.

95. Martin TG. Near drowning and cold water immersion. *Ann Emerg Med* 1984;13:263.

96. Danzl DF, Pozos RS. Multicenter hypothermia survey. *Ann Intern Med* 1987;16:1042–1055.

97. Greenblatt DL. Fatal hyperthermia following haloperidol therapy for sedative-hypnotic withdrawal. *J Clin Psychiatry* 1978;39:673–675.

98. Dinubile MJ. Antibiotics: the antipyretic of choice. *Am J Med* 1990;89:787–788.

99. Schumock GT, Frazier JL. Drug-induced alterations in body temperature. *Clin Pharmacol Ther* 1991;16:264–277.

100. Callaway CW, Clark R. Hyperthermia in psychostimulant overdose. *Ann Emerg Med* 1994;24:68–74.

101. Stone RJ. Heat illness. *JACEP* 1979;8:154.

102. Tek DT, Olshaker JS. Heat illness. *Emerg Clin North Am* 1992;109:299–309.

103. Jolly T, Ghezzi KT. Accidental hypothermia. *Emerg Clin North Am* 1992;10:311.

104. Anom. Hypothermia-related deaths—North Carolina, November 1993 to March 1994. *MMWR* 1994;43:849–856.

105. Treatment of hypothermia. *Med Lett* 1994;36:116–118.

106. Danzi DF, Polzos RS. Accidental hypothermia. *N Engl J Med* 1994;331:1756–1760.

107. Bauer J, Roberts MB, Reisdorff EJ. Evaluation of behavioral and cognitive changes: the mental state. *Pediatr Clin North Am* 1991;9:1–111

108. Gastrointestinal mobility and neurologic diseases. *Mayo Clin Proc* 1990;65:844–845.

109. Anonymous. Drugs that cause psychiatric symptoms. *Med Lett* 1993;35:65–70.

110. Agnew JR, Stopard W. Mercury intoxication among dental personnel. *JAMA* 1983;250:822.

111. Johnson BL, Anger WK. Behavioral toxicology. In: Rom WN, ed. *Environmental and occupational medicine.* Boston: Little, Brown and Company, 1983.

112. Gianni AJ Nageotte C, Loiselle RH. Comparison of chlorpromazine, haloperidol, and primozide in the treatment of phencyclidine psychosis: DA-2 receptor specificity. *Clin Toxicol* 1985;22:573.

113. Ayd FJ. Haloperidol: twenty years clinical experience. *J Clin Psychiatr* 1978;39:807.

114. Sellars EM. Simplifying treatment of alcohol withdrawal: diazepam loading. *Clin Pharmacol Ther* 1982;31:268.

115. Wilson LM. Intensive care delirium. *Arch Intern Med* 1972;130:225.

116. Jacobs JW, et al. Screening for organic mental syndromes in the medically ill. *Ann Intern Med* 1977;86:40–46.

117. Bauer J, Roberts MB, Reisdorff EJ. Evaluation of behavioral and cognitive changes: the mental state. *Pediatr Clin North Am* 1991;9:1–11.

118. Lipowski ZJ. Delirium in the elderly patient. *N Engl J Med* 1989;320:578–582.

119. Lipowski ZJ. Delirium (acute confusional states). *JAMA* 1987;256:1789–1782.

120. Roca RP. Bedside cognitive examination: usefulness in detecting delirium. *Psychosomatics* 1987;28:71–76.

121. Brenner RP. The electroencephalogram in altered states of consciousness. *Neurol Clin* 1985;3:615–631.

122. Mahler ME, Cummings JL, Benson DF. Treatable dementias. *West J Med* 1987;146:705–712.

123. Council on Scientific Affairs, AMA. Dementia. *JAMA* 1986;256:2234–2238.

124. Meulam MM. Dementia: its definition, differential diagnosis and subtypes. *JAMA* 1985;253:2559–2561.

125. Consensus Conference. Differential diagnosis of dementing diseases. *JAMA* 1987;258:3411–3416.

126. Dubin WR, Weiss KJ, Zeccardi JA. Organic brain syndrome: the psychiatric imposter. *JAMA* 1983;249:60–62.

127. APA. *Diagnostic and statistical manual of mental disorders.* 3rd ed. Washington, DC: American Psychiatric Association, 1987.

128. Cummings JL. Dementia: the failing brain. *Lancet* 1995;345:1481–1484.
129. Fleming KC, Adams AC, Petersen RC. Dementia: diagnosis and evaluation. *Mayo Clin Proc* 1995/6:70:1093–1107.
130. Fleming K, Evans JM. Pharmacologic therapies for dementia. *Mayo Clin Proc* 1995;70:1116–1123.
131. Tomaszewski CA, Thom SR. Use of hyperbaric oxygen in toxicology. *Emerg Clin North Am* 1994;12:437–459.
132. Hampson NB, Dunford RG, Kramer CG, et al. Selection criteria utilized for hyperbaric oxygen treatment of carbon monoxide poisoning. *J Emerg Med* 1995;13:227–233.
133. *Hyperbaric oxygen therapy: a committee report.* Bethesda, MD: Undersea and Hyperbaric Medical Society, 1992.
134. Plum F, Posner J. *Diagnosis of stupor and coma.* Philadelphia: FA Davis Co, 1980.
135. Henry GL. Neurologic emergencies. 2. Altered mental status. *Emerg Med* 1988; March:24–57.
136. Sabin TD. The differential diagnosis of coma. *N Engl J Med* 1974;290:1062.
137. Zun L, et al. A survey of the form of mental status examination administered by emergency physicians. *Ann Emerg Med* 1986;15:916–922.
138. Jennett B, et al. Assessment of outcome after severe brain damage. A practical scale. *Lancet* 1975;1:480–484.
139. Teasdale G, Jennett B. Assessment of coma and impaired consciousness: a practical scale. *Lancet* 1974;2:81–84.
140. Levy DE, et al. Predicting the outcome from hypoxic-ischemic coma. *JAMA* 1985;253:1420–1427.
141. Strickbine-Van Reet P, et al. A preliminary prospective neurophysiological study of coma in children. *Am J Dis Child* 1984;138:492–495.
142. Singer J. Altered consciousness as an early manifestation of intussusception. *Pediatrics* 1979;64:93–94.
143. Sebire G, Devictor D, Huault G, et al. Coma associated with intense bursts of abnormal movements and long-lasting cognitive disturbances: an acute encephalopathy of obscure origin. *J Pediatr* 1993;121:845–851.
144. Levin M, Kay JDS, Gould JD, et al. Hemorrhagic shock and encephalopathy: a new clinical syndrome with a high mortality in young children. *Lancet* 1983;2:64–67.
145. Seizures: guidelines for record review, AAP. *Pediatr Rev* 1992;1.
146. Middleton DB. After a child's first seizure. *Emerg Med* 1993;181.
147. Scheuer ML, Pedley TL. The evaluation and treatment of seizures. *N Engl J Med* 1990;323:1468–1473.
148. Cascino GD. Epilepsy: contemporary perspectives on evaluation and treatment. *Mayo Clin Proc* 1994;69:1199–1211.
149. Zaccara G, Muscas GC, Messori A. Clinical features, pathogenesis and management of drug-induced seizures. *Drug Safety* 1990;5:109–151.
150. Delgardo-Escueta AV, Bajorek JG. Status epilepticus mechanisms of brain damage and rational management. *Epilepsia* 1982;23:29–41.
151. Shorvon SD. Epidemology, classification, natural history and genetics of epilepsy. *Lancet* 1990;336:93–96.
152. Young WF, Maddox DE. Spells: in search of a cause. *Mayo Clin Proc* 1995;70:757–765.
153. Day SC, et al. Evaluation and outcome of emergency room patients with transient loss of consciousness. *Am J Med* 1982;73:15–23.
154. Kapoor WN, et al. Diagnostic evaluation of syncope. *Am J Med* 1991;90:91.
155. Schwartz RH, et al. Seizures and syncope in adolescent cocaine abusers. *Am J Med* 1988;85:462.
156. Webb CL, et al. Quinidine syncope in children. *Am Coll Cardiol* 1987;9:1031.
157. Grubb BP, et al. Utility of upright tilt table testing in the evaluation and management of syncope of unknown origin. *Am J Med* 1991;90:6.
158. Cinbis B, Aysun G. Alice in Wonderland syndrome as an initial manifestation of Epstein Barr virus infection. *Br J Ophthalmol* 1992;76:316.
159. Plum F, Posner JB. *The diagnosis of stupor and coma.* Philadelphia: FA Davis Co, 1980.
160. Lessel S. Pediatric pseudotumor cerebri (idiopathic intracranial hypertension). *Surv Ophthalmol* 1992;37:155–166.
161. Quincke H. Unber meningitis serosa und verwandte Zustande. *Dtsch Z Nervenheilk* 1897;9:149–168.
162. Plum F, Posner JB. *The diagnosis of stupor and coma.* Philadelphia: FA Davis Co, 1980.
163. Malozowaski S, Tanner LA, Wysowski D, et al. Growth hormone, insulin-like growth factor 1, and benign intracranial hypertension. *N Engl J Med* 1993;329:665–666.
164. Radhakrishnan K, Ahlskog, Garrity JA. Idiopathic intracranial hypertension. *Mayo Clin Proc* 1994;69:169–180.
165. Carasiti ME. Drug-induced aseptic meningitis. *Resident Staff Physician* 1988;34:11–17.
166. Widener HL, Littman BH. Ibuprofen-induced aseptic meningitis in a patient with systemic lupus. *JAMA* 1978;238:1062.
167. Zaccara G, Muscas GC, Messori A. Clinical features, pathogenesis and management of drug-induced convulsions. *Drug Safety* 1990;5:109–151.
168. Dyck PJ. The causes classification and treatment of peripheral neuropathy. *N Engl J Med* 1982;307:283–286.
169. Lotti M, et al. Occupational peripheral neuropathy. *West J Med* 1982;137:493–498.
170. Schaumburg H, et al. Sensory neuropathy from pyridoxine abuse: a new megavitamin syndrome. *N Engl J Med* 1983;309:445–448.
171. McHardy KC. Weakness. *BMJ* 1984;288:1591–1594.
172. Rodenberg H, Gratton M, Rosenberg J. Left upper-extremity weakness in an 18-year-old man. *Ann Emerg Med* 1991;20:672–679.
173. Patterson MC, Gomez MR. Muscle disease in children: a practical approach. *Pediatr Rev* 1990;12:73–83.

174. Poltz PH. Not myositis. *JAMA* 1992;268:2074–2077.
175. Wijdicks EFM. *Neurology of critical illness*. Philadelphia: FA Davis Co, 1995.
176. Stumpf D. Acute ataxia. *Pediatr Rev* 1987;8:303.
177. Connlly AM, Dodson WE, Prensky AL, et al. Course and outcome of acute cerebellar ataxia. *Ann Neurol* 1994;35:673–679.
178. Engle EC. Case records of the Massachusetts General Hospital. *N Engl J Med* 1995;333:579–585.
179. Lanston JW. Chronic parkinsonism in human due to by product of meperidine analog synthesis. *Science* 1983;219:976.
180. Stevenson G, Humprey G, Sturman S. Monoamine oxidase B in parkinsonism. *Lancet* 1990;1:80.
181. Lang AE, Weiner WJ. *Drug-induced movement disorders*. New York: Futura Publishing, 1991.
182. Klawans HL, Brandaburg MM. Chorea in childhood. *Pediatr Ann* 1993;22:41–50.
183. Feldman V. Serious reactions to phenothiazines. *J Pediatr* 1976;89:163–164.
184. Corre KA, et al. Extended therapy for acute dystonic reactions. *Ann Emerg Med* 1984;13:194–197.
185. Granto J, Stern JR, Ringel A, et al. Neuroleptic malignant syndrome: successful treatment with dantrolene and bromocriptine. *Ann Neurol* 1983;14:89–90.
186. Kaplan HI, Sodock BJ. *Comprehensive textbook of psychiatry*. Baltimore: Williams & Wilkins, 1986:1315–1329.
187. Larson EW. Organic causes of mania. *Mayo Clin Proc* 1988;63:906–912.
188. Pane CA, Winiarski AM, Salness KA. Aggression directed toward emergency department staff at a university teaching hospital. *Ann Emerg Med* 1991;20:283–286.
189. Dubin WR, Weiss KJ. *Handbook of emergency psychiatric emergencies*. Springhouse, PA: Springhouse Corp, 1991.
190. Dubin WR, Feld JA. Rapid tranquilization of the violent patient. *Am J Emerg Med* 1989;7:313–320.
191. Dublin WR. Overcoming danger with violent patients: guidelines for safe and effective management. *Emerg Med Rep* 1992;13:112.
192. Drachman DA, Hart CW. An approach to the dizzy patient. *Neurology* 1972;22:323.
193. Brown RD, Wood CD. Vestibular pharmacology. *Trends Pharmacol Sci* 1980;150–153.
194. Jacobson GP, Newman CW. Dizziness inventory. *Arch Otolaryngol* 1990;116:424.
195. Samuels MA. Does dizziness = vertigo? *Emerg Med* 1991;Sept:59.
196. Froehling DA, Silverstein MDS, Mohr DN, et al. Does this dizzy patient have a serious form of vertigo. *JAMA* 1994;271:385–388.
197. Martyn LI, DiGeorge A. Selected eye defects of special importance in pediatrics. *Pediatr Clin North Am* 1987;34:1517.
198. Liu GT. Abnormalities of the pupil. When should you worry? *Contemp Pediatr* 1995;12:83–98.
199. Ellenberg DJ, Spector LD, Lee A. Flea collar pupil. *Ann Emerg Med* 1992;21:1170.
200. Brown DG, Hammill LF. Glutethimide poisoning: unilateral pupillary abnormalities. *N Engl J Med* 1971;285:806.
201. Froehling DA, Silverstein MDS, Mohr DN, et al. Does this dizzy patient have a serious form of vertigo. *JAMA* 1994;271:385–388.
202. Spyker DA, Gallianosa AG, Surati PM. Health effects of acute carbon disulfide exposure. *J Toxicol Clin Toxicol* 1982;19:87–93.
203. MacMahon B, Monson RR. Mortality in the U.S. rayon industry. *J Occup Med* 1988;30:698–705.
204. Smilkstein MJ, et al. Acute toxic blindness: unrecognized quinine poisoning. *Ann Emerg Med* 1987;16:98–101.
205. Kohn BA. The differential diagnosis of cataracts in infancy and childhood. *Am J Dis Child* 1976;130:184–192.
206. Ellenberg DJ. The flea collar pupil. *Ann Emerg Med* 1992;21:1170.
207. Friedenwald JS, et al. Acid burns of the eye. *Arch Ophthalmol* 1946;35:98.
208. Shingleton BJ. Eye injuries. *N Engl J Med* 1991;325:408–413.
209. Hughes WF, et al. Alkali burns of the eye. Clinical and pathologic course. *Arch Ophthalmol* 1946;36:189.
210. Davidson SI, Rennie IG. Ocular toxicity from systemic drug therapy: an overview of clinically important adverse reactions. *Med Toxicol* 1986:1:217–224.
211. Smith MS. Amitriptyline ophthalmoplegia. *Ann Intern Med* 1979;91:793.
212. Troutman WG. Drug-induced diseases. In: Knoben JE, Anderson PO, eds. *Handbook of clinical drug data*. 7th ed. Hamilton, IL: Drug Intelligence Publications, 1993.
213. Nadol JB. Hearing loss. *N Engl J Med* 1993;329:1092–1095.
214. von Oettingen WF. *Poisoning*. Berlin: Germany: Paul B. Hoeber, 1952.
215. Done AK. Signs, symptoms and sources. *Emerg Med* 1982;Jan:42–77.
216. Arena JM, Drew RH. *Poisoning: toxicology, symptoms and treatment*. Springfield, IL: Charles C. Thomas Publisher, 1986.
217. Goldfrank L, et al. *Toxicologic emergencies*. 3rd ed. Norwalk, CT: Appleton-Century-Crofts, 1986.
218. Busis SN. Questions and answers. Treatment of tinnitus. *JAMA* 1992;268:1467.
219. Bott S, MaCallum R. Medication-induced esophageal injury: survey of literature. *Med Toxicol* 1986;1:449–457.
220. Biller JA, Flores A, Bule T, et al. Tetracycline-induced esophagitis. *J Pediatr* 1992;120:144–145.
221. Romero Y, Evans JM, Fleming KC. Constipation and fecal incontinence in the elderly population. *Mayo Clin Proc* 1996;71:61–92.
222. Savitt DL, Hawkins HH, Roberts JR. The radiopacity of ingested medications. *Ann Emerg Med* 1987;16:331–339.

223. Handy CA. Radiopacity of oral nonliquid medications. *Radiology* 1971;98:525–533.
224. Greensher J, Mofenson HC, Gavin WJ. Usefulness of abdominal x-rays in diagnosis of poisoning. *Vet Hum Toxicol* 1979;211:45–46.
225. McCarron MM, Wood JD. The cocaine "body packer" syndrome—diagnosis and treatment. *JAMA* 1983;250:1417–1420.
226. Schabel SI, Rogers CI. Opaque artifacts in a health food fadist simulating ovarian neoplasm. *Am J Roentgenol* 1978;130:789–790.
227. Spitzer A, Caruthers SB, Stables DP. Radiopaque suppositories. *Radiology* 1976;121:71–73.
228. Woolf AD, Saperstein A, Zawin J, et al. Radiopaqicity of household air refresheners and moth repellents. *Clin Toxicol* 1993;31:415–428.
229. Langman MJS. Epidemiologic evidence and the association between peptic ulceration and non-steroidal anti-inflammatory drug use. *Gastroenterology* 1989;96:640–646S.
230. Cicale M. Stress ulcer bleeding: prophylaxis in the ICU. *Hosp Formum* 1992;27:584–587.
231. Tryba M. Stress bleeding prophylaxis. *Am J Med* 1989;86:85–93.
232. Tryba M, Zevounou F, Torok M, et al. Prevention of acute stress bleeding with sucralfate, antacids or cimetidine. A controlled study with pirezenpine as a basic medication. *Am J Med* 1985;79:55–61.
233. Tryba M. Risk of acute stress bleeding and nosocomial pneumonia in ventilated intensive care patients: sucralfate versus antacids. *Am J Med* 1987;83:117–124.
234. Lopez-Herce J, Dorao P, Elola P, et al. Frequency and prophylaxis of upper gastrointestinal hemorrhage in critically ill children: a prospective study comparing the efficacy of almagate, ranitidine and sucrafate. *Crit Care Med* 1992;20: 1082–1090.
235. Cook DJ, Reeve BK, Guyatt GH, et al. Stress ulcer prophylaxis in critically ill patients: resolving discordant meta-analysis. *JAMA* 1996;275:308–313.
236. Ochner RK. Drug-induced liver disease. In: *Hepatology: a textbook of liver disease*. Philadelphia: WB Saunders, 1982: 691–727.
237. Rakela J, et al. Fulminant hepatitis; Mayo Clinical experience with 34 cases. *Mayo Clin Proc* 1985;60:289.
238. Zimmerman HJ. Chemical hepatic injury. In: Haddad LM, Winchester JF, eds. *Clinical management of poisoning and drug overdose*. Philadelphia: WB Saunders, 1983:220–249.
239. Carson JL, Strom BI, Duff A, et al. Acute liver disease associated with erythromycin, sulfonamides and tetracycline. *Ann Intern Med* 1993;11:576–583.
240. Castielle A, Arenas JI. Fluoxetine hepatotoxicity. *Am J Gastroenterol* 1994;89:458–459.
241. Lee W. Acute liver failure. *N Engl J Med* 1993:329:1662–1872.
242. Caraceni P, Van Thiel D. Acute liver failure. *Lancet* 1995;345:163–169.
243. Vale JA, Proudfoot AT. Paracetamol (acetaminophen) poisoning. *Lancet* 1995;346:547–552.
244. Osterloh J, et al. Biochemical relationships between Reye's and Reye's-like metabolic and toxicologic syndromes. *Med Toxicol* 1989;7:272–294.
245. Jones J, Schafer T. Chapter 29. In: Boyers T, Zakin, eds. *Hepatology: a textbook of liver disease*. Philadelphia: WB Saunders, 1982:691–727.
246. Rakela J, et al. Fulminant hepatitis; Mayo Clinical experience with 34 cases. *Mayo Clin Proc* 1985;60:289.
247. Zimmerman HJ. Chemical hepatic injury. In: Haddad LM, Winchester JF, eds. *Clinical management of poisoning and drug overdose*. Philadelphia: WB Saunders, 1983:220–249.
248. Carson JL, Strom BI, Duff A, et al. Acute liver disease associated with erythromycin, sulfonamides and tetracycline. *Ann Intern Med* 1993;11:576–583.
249. Castielle A, Arenas JI. Fluoxetine hepatotoxicity. *Am J Gastroenterol* 1994;89:458–459.
250. Malloy A, Klein F Jr. Drug-induced pancreatitis: a critical review. *Gastroenterology* 1980;78:813.
251. Steinberg W. Acute drug- and toxin-induced pancreatitis. *Hosp Pract* 1985;20:95–102.
252. Berger TM, Cook WJ, O'Marcraigh AS. Acute pancreatitis in a 12-year-old girl after erythromycin overdose. *Pediatrics* 1992;90:624–626.
253. Cumaste VV. Erythromycin-induced pancreatitis. *Am J Med* 1989;298:190.
254. Hawksworth CRE. Acute pancreatitis associated with infusion of erythromycin lactbionate. *BMJ* 1989;298:190.
255. Mofenson HC, Caraccio TR, Naraz H, Steckler G. Acetaminophen-induced pancreatitis. *J Toxicol Clin Toxicol* 1991; 29:223–230.
256. Gilmore IT, Tourvas E. Paracetamol-induced acute pancreatitis. *BMJ* 1977;1:753–754.
257. Caldarola V, Hasset JM, Hall AH, et al. Hemorrhagic pancreatitis associated with acetaminophen overdose. *Am J Gastroenterol* 1986;91:579–582.
258. Steinberg W, Tenner S. Acute pancreatitis. *N Engl J Med* 1994;330:1198–1207.
259. Ranson JHC, Rifkind KM, Turner JW. Prognostic signs and nonoperative lavage in acute pancreatitis. *Surg Gynecol Obstet* 1976;145:209–219.
260. Imrie CW, Buist LJ, Shearer MG. Importance of cause and outcome of pancreatic pseudocysts. *Am J Surg* 1988;156: 159–162.

261. Feld LG, et al. Acute renal failure. 1. Pathophysiology and diagnosis. *J Pediatr* 1986;109:401–407.
262. Hook JB. Toxic responses of the kidney. In: Doull J, et al., eds. *Toxicology: the basic science of poisons*. New York: Macmillan, 1985.
263. Maher JF. Acute renal failure complicating intoxication. In: Haddad LM, Winchester JF, eds. *Poisoning and drug overdose*. Philadelphia: WB Saunders, 1983:170–184.
264. Matthews OP. Acute renal failure in children. *Pediatrics* 1980;65:57
265. Schrier RW. Acute renal failure: pathogenesis, diagnosis and management. *Hosp Pract* 1981;93–112.
266. Wrenn KD, et al. Sorting through the rhabdomyolysis: an enigma made manageable. *Emerg Med Rep* 1987;8:163.
267. Clinical conference: rhabdomyolysis. *NYS J Med* 1988;88:582–588.
268. Curry SC, et al. Drug- and toxin-induced rhabdomyolysis. *Ann Emerg Med* 1989;18:1064–1084.
269. Marks EA, Arsura EL. Cocaine-induced rhabdomyolysis. *Emerg Med* 1990;Aug:79–82.
270. Koppel C. Clinical features, pathogenesis, and management of drug-induced rhabdomyolysis. *Med Toxicol Adverse Drug Exp* 1989;4:108–126.
271. Qwen CA, Mubanak SJ, Hargens AF, et al. Intramuscular pressures with limb compression: clarification of pathogenesis of the drug-induced muscle compartment syndrome. *N Engl J Med* 1979;300:1169–1172.
272. Sinert R, Kohl L, Rainone T, Scalea T. Exercise-induced rhabdomyolysis. *Ann Emerg Med* 1994;23:1301–1304.
273. Patel R, et al. Myoglobinuric renal failure in phencyclidine overdose. Report of 8 cases. *Ann Emerg Med* 1980;9:549–553.
274. Wallach J. *Interpretation of diagnostic tests*. 5th ed. Boston: Little, Brown and Company, 1992.
275. Bergstein JM. Hematuria, proteinuria and urinary tract infections. *Pediatr Clin North Am* 1982;29:55.
276. Brewer ED, Benson GS. Algorithms for diagnosis: hematuria in a child. *JAMA* 1981;246:993–995.
277. Hymes LC, Warshaw BL. Thiazides in children with idiopathic hypercalcemia and hematuria. *J Urol* 1987;138:1217.
278. Norman ME. An office approach to hematuria and proteinuria. *Pediatr Clin North Am* 1987;34:595.
279. Cone TE. Some syndromes, diseases and conditions associated with abnormal coloration of the urine or diaper. *Pediatrics* 1968;41:654–658.
280. Said R. Contamination of the urine with povidone iodine. A cause of false-positive test for occult blood in urine. *JAMA* 1979;242:748–750.
281. Bakler MD, Baldassano RN. Povidone iodine as a cause of factitious hematuria and abnormal urine coloration in the pediatric emergency department. *Pediatr Emerg Care* 1989;5:240–241.
282. Shirked HC, ed. *Pediatric therapy*. 5th ed. St Louis: Mosby, 1975.
283. Raymond JR, Yager WE. Abnormal urine color. Differential diagnosis. *South Med J* 1988:837.
284. Pollack SS, Rosenthal MS. Diaper diagnosis of porphyria. *N Engl J Med* 1994;330:114.
285. Pierach CA, Ippen H. A porphyrin-soaker diaper. *N Engl J Med* 1994;330;1690.
286. Cone TE. Diagnosis and treatment: some diseases, syndromes and conditions associated with an unusual odor. *Pediatrics* 1968;41:993–995.
287. Mace JW, et al. The child with an unusual odor. *Clin Pediatr* 1976;15:57–62.
288. Shelley ED, et al. The fish odor syndrome. *JAMA* 1984;251:253–256.
289. Schiffman SS. Taste and smell. *N Engl J Med* 1983;308:1275–1279,1337–1342.
290. Goldfrank L, et al. Teaching the recognition of odors. *Ann Emerg Med* 1982;11:664–666.
291. Arena JM, Drew RH. *Poisoning: toxicology, symptoms, treatments*. Springfield, IL: Charles C. Thomas Publisher, 1986.
292. von Oettingen WF. *Poisoning*. Berlin: Germany: Paul B. Hoeber, 1952.
293. Henkin RJ. Hypersomia and depression following exposure to toxic vapors. *JAMA* 1990;264:2803.
294. Deems D. Smell and taste disorders: a study of 750 patients. *Arch Otolaryngol Head Neck Surg* 1991;117:519–521.
295. Clark RF. Crystalluria following cephalexin overdose. *Pediatrics* 1992;89:672–673.
296. York JJ. What to do about acute urinary retention. *Emerg Med* 1991;23:88–96.
297. Peter JR, Steinhart GF. Acute urinary retention in children. *Emerg Pediatr Care* 1993:4:205–207.
298. Cotton P. Physicians hear about incontinence. *JAMA* 1990;264:2361.
299. Carlson HE. Gynecomastia. *N Engl J Med* 1980;303:795–799.
300. Barnett G, et al. Effects of marijuana on testosterone in male subjects. *J Theor Biol* 1983;104:685–692.
301. Wilson JD. Gynecomastia. *N Engl J Med* 1991;324:334–335.
302. Braunstein GD. Gynecomastia. *N Engl J Med* 1993;328:490.
303. O'Brien W, et al. Priapism: current concepts. *Ann Emerg Med* 1989;18:980–983.
304. Forelli RL, et al. Priapism and other manifestations of cocaine abuse. *J Urol* 1990;143:584–585.
305. Amitai Y, Mines Y, Aker M, et al. Scorpion sting in children. A review of 51 cases. *Clin Pediatr* 1985;24:136–140.
306. Styles AD. Priapism following black widow spider bite. *Clin Pediatr* 1982;21:174–175.
307. Virag R. About pharmacologically induced prolonged erection. *Lancet* 1985;2:519.
308. Troutman WG. Sexual dysfunction. In: Knoben JE, Anderson PO, eds. *Handbook clinical drug data*. 7th ed. Hamilton, IL: Drug Intelligence Publications, 1993:71–77.
309. Eichner ER, et al. Splenomegly: an algorithic approach to the diagnosis. *JAMA* 1981;246:2858.

Selected Readings

Adler SN, Lam M, Connors A. *manual of differential diagnosis*. Boston: Little, Brown and Company, 1982.

Doull J, et al. *Toxicology: the basic science of poisons*. New York: Macmillan, 1987.

Haddad LM, Windchester FJ. *Management of poisoning and drug overdose*. Philadelphia: WB Saunders, 1983.

Noji EK, Kelen GD. *Manual of toxicologic emergencies*. Chicago: Year Book, 1989.

Subject Index

Page numbers in *italics* indicate figures. Page numbers followed by "t" indicate tables.